The Royal Marsden Hospital Manual of Clinical Nursing Procedures

The Royal Marsden Hospital Manual of Clinical Nursing Procedures

Seventh Edition

Edited by

Lisa Dougherty
OBE, RN, MSc
Nurse Consultant Intravenous Therapy
The Royal Marsden Hospital NHS Foundation Trust

and

Sara Lister
RN, PGDAE, BSc (Hons), MSc
Assistant Chief Nurse/Head of School
The Royal Marsden School of
Cancer Nursing & Rehabilitation
The Royal Marsden Hospital NHS Foundation Trust

THE ROYAL
MARSDEN

The Royal Marsden **NHS**
NHS Foundation Trust

WILEY-BLACKWELL
A John Wiley & Sons, Ltd., Publication

This edition first published 2008
© 1992, 1996, 2000, 2004, 2008 by The Royal Marsden Hospital

Blackwell Publishing was acquired by John Wiley & Sons in February 2007. Blackwell's publishing programme has been merged with Wiley's global Scientific, Technical, and Medical business to form Wiley-Blackwell.

Registered office
John Wiley & Sons Ltd, The Atrium, Southern Gate, Chichester, West Sussex, PO19 8SQ, United Kingdom

Editorial office
9600 Garsington Road, Oxford, OX4 2DQ, United Kingdom

For details of our global editorial offices, for customer services and for information about how to apply for permission to reuse the copyright material in this book please see our website at www.wiley.com/wiley-blackwell.

Library of Congress Cataloging-in-Publication Data

The Royal Marsden Hospital manual of clinical nursing procedures. – 7th ed. / edited by Lisa Dougherty and Sara E. Lister.
    p. ; cm.
  Includes bibliographical references and index.
  ISBN-13: 978-1-4051-6999-8 (pbk. : alk. paper)
  ISBN-10: 1-4051-6999-0 (pbk. : alk. paper)   1. Nursing–Technique–Handbooks, manuals, etc.   I. Dougherty, Lisa.   II. Lister, Sara E.   III. Royal Marsden NHS Trust.   IV. Title: Manual of clinical nursing procedures.
  [DNLM: 1. Nursing Care–methods.   2. Nursing Process.   3. Nursing Theory.   4. Patient Care Planning. WY 100 R8887 2008]

RT42.R68 2008
610.73–dc22   2007022389

A catalogue record for this book is available from the British Library.

Set in 9.5/11.5pt Sabon by Aptara Inc., New Delhi, India

Printed in Singapore by Fabulous Printers Pte Ltd

1   2008

Foreword to the seventh edition

As the new Chief Nurse of the Royal Marsden Hospital, but a contributor and clinical user for many years, it is a special pleasure and honour to be asked to introduce the seventh edition of *The Royal Marsden Hospital Manual of Clinical Nursing Procedures*. The Manual is internationally renowned and used by nurses across the world to help with their clinical practice. When a text is dedicated to clinical practice it is essential that it is regularly updated so that it reflects the most current evidence.

More than ever nurses need to be able to assure the public, patients and their families that care is based on the best available evidence. As nurses seeking to improve our care it is essential that we are able to critically analyse our judgements in the light of current knowledge about an area of practice. For all of us working with patients and their families there is an imperative to question and review our practice using the many sources of knowledge available to us. In the busy day-to-day clinical world it can be challenging to find time to search for the evidence and this is where *The Royal Marsden Hospital Manual of Clinical Nursing Procedures* can be a real practical help.

For the first time in this seventh edition reviewing the evidence or sources of knowledge has been made more explicit with each level of evidence graded. This grading provides the reader with an understanding of whether the reference comes from a randomized controlled trial, national or international guidance or from expert opinion. At its best, clinical nursing care is an amalgam of a sensitive therapeutic relationship coupled with effective care based on the best evidence that exists. Some areas of clinical practice have attracted international research so the evidence upon which to base care is more obvious. However there are many other areas of practice where very little rigorous or robust research has taken place so it is more of a challenge to ensure evidence based care. Perhaps this manual will stimulate us to reflect on the gaps in research and knowledge as well as provide the impetus to start further research in these areas.

As you look at the list of contributors to the manual you will see that this edition has continued to ask clinically active nurses to share their practice in their chapters. This has the added advantage of ensuring that this manual reflects the reality of practice but also ensures that nurses at the Royal Marsden NHS Foundation Trust are frequently reviewing the evidence and reflecting upon their care.

As I commend this seventh edition of *The Royal Marsden Hospital Manual of Clinical Nursing Procedures* to you I am aware that it will be used in many different countries and settings. Having had the privilege of visiting and meeting nurses across the world I know that there are more commonalities than differences between us. The common theme is of course that as nurses we strive to provide the best care that is individually and sensitively planned. I hope that this manual will continue to be a valuable resource as you seek to achieve this.

Finally, I would like to pay a warm tribute to the amazing amount of work undertaken by the two editors, Lisa Dougherty and Sara Lister, and to all the nurses and allied health professionals at the Royal Marsden Hospital who have worked so hard on this seventh edition.

Shelley Dolan
Chief Nurse
The Royal Marsden Hospital
2008

Introduction and guidelines for use

Core to nursing, wherever it takes place, is the commitment to care for individuals and to keep them safe. The first edition of *The Royal Marsden Hospital Manual of Clinical Nursing Procedures* was produced in the early 1980s as a core procedure manual for safe practice within The Royal Marsden Hospital, the first cancer hospital in the world. Twenty-five years and seven editions later the staff of the hospital are still working together to update it, ensuring that only current evidence-based practice is recommended. The Manual is informed by the day-to-day practice in the hospital and in reverse is the corporate policy and procedure document of the organization. It therefore does not cover all aspects of acute nursing practice or those relating to children's or community nursing. However, it does contain the procedures and changes in practice that reflect modern acute nursing practice.

In this edition, for the first time, the type of evidence that underpins procedures has been made explicit. The system used to categorize the evidence is broader than that generally used. It has been developed from the types of evidence described by Rycroft-Malone *et al.* (2004) in an attempt to acknowledge that 'in reality practitioners draw on multiple sources of knowledge in the course of their practice and interaction with patients' (Rycroft-Malone *et al.* 2004, p. 88). The framework still needs to be tested but has been useful in highlighting how little empirical research underpins nursing practice.

The sources of evidence, along with examples, are identified as follows:

1   *Clinical experience (E):*
- Encompasses expert practical know-how, gained through working with others and reflecting on best practice.
- If there is no written evidence to support clinical experience as a justification for undertaking a procedure the text will be referenced as an E but will not be preceded by an author's name.
- Example: (Dougherty 2008: E). This is drawn from the following article that gives expert clinical opinion: Dougherty, L. (2008) Obtaining peripheral vascular access. In: *Intravenous Therapy in Nursing Practice* (eds L. Dougherty & J. Lamb), 2nd edn. Blackwell Publishing, Oxford.

2   *Patient (P):*
- Gained through expert patient feedback and extensive experience of working with patients.
- Example: (Diamond 1999: P). This has been gained from a personal account of care written by a patient, Diamond, J. (1999) *C Because Cowards Get Cancer Too.* Vermillon, London.

3   *Context (C):*
- Can include Audit and Performance data, Social and Professional Networks, Local and National Policy, guidelines from Professional Bodies (e.g. Royal College of Nursing [RCN]) and manufacturer's recommendations.
- Example: (Department of Health 2001: C). This document gives guidelines for good practice: Department of Health (2001c) *Reference Guide to Consent for Examination or Treatment.* Department of Health, London.

4   *Research (R):*
- Evidence gained through research.
- Example: (Fellowes *et al.* 2004: R 1a). This has been drawn from the following evidence: Fellowes, D., Wilkinson, S. & Moore, P. (2004) Communication skills training for healthcare professionals working with cancer patients, their families and/or carers. *Cochrane Database Syst Rev*, 2, CD003751. DOI: 10.10002/14651858.CD003571.pub2.

The levels that have been chosen are adapted from Sackett, Strauss and Richardson (2000) as follows:

1 (a)   Systematic reviews of randomized controlled trials (RCTs).
(b)   Individual RCTs with narrow confidence limits.
2 (a)   Systematic reviews of cohort studies.
(b)   Individual cohort studies and low quality RCTs.
3 (a)   Systematic reviews of case-controlled studies.
(b)   Case-controlled studies.

4   Case series and poor quality cohort and case-controlled studies.
5   Expert opinion.

The rationale for the system and further explanation is outlined further in Chapter 1. This chapter also sets out the context of current nursing practice.

As well as making the evidence base for procedures explicit, all chapters have been reviewed and some expanded to encompass new material including the legislative changes that have impacted on nursing roles. Chapter 11, *Drug administration: general principles*, includes a section about non-medical prescribing and Chapter 47, *Violence: prevention and management*, incorporates the National Institute for Health and Clinical Excellence (NICE) guidance (NICE 2005) on the management of violent patients. The recent *National Evidence Based Guidelines for Preventing Healthcare Associated Infection in NHS Hospitals in England* (Pratt *et al.* 2007) are reflected in the updated Chapter 5, *Aseptic technique*, Chapter 18, *Elimination: urinary*, and Chapter 45, *Vascular access devices: insertion and management*. In response to an increasing essential emphasis on infection control, a number of additional procedures have been added including 'Putting on and removing a disposable plastic apron' and 'Use of non-sterile gloves' in Chapter 5, *Aseptic technique*. 'Anti-embolic management' in Chapter 30, *Perioperative care*, has been updated to include NICE (2007) Venous thromboembolism: reducing the risk of venous thromboembolism (deep vein thrombosis and pulmonary embolism) in inpatients undergoing surgery.

Communication and Assessment, the second chapter of the last edition, is now two distinct chapters. In this edition, Chapter 2, *Assessment and the process of care*, discusses the importance of assessing a patient's care needs in any situation and explores some of the different approaches to undertaking this; Chapter 3, *Communication*, is a more practical guide about issues to consider when talking to patients. Chapter 23, *Moving and handling*, has been replaced with Chapter 34, *Positioning*, a chapter specifically about how to position patients, giving details of procedures such as how to help a patient sit in bed, to stand and lie comfortably.

The format follows that of previous editions with the addition of colour photographs, figures and chapter coding. This, we hope, will make some of the steps in a procedure easier to follow.

Structure of chapters

The structure of each chapter is consistent throughout the book, as outlined below. An explanation of this structure can be found in Chapter 1.

- *Definition*: Each chapter begins with an explanation of the aspect of care, with any technical or difficult concepts explained.
- *Reference material:* This provides background and presents the research and expert opinion in this area.

Where appropriate the related anatomy and physiology is explained. Any specific psychological issues that the procedure may raise for the patient have also been included, so the nurse can carry out the procedure with the knowledge and the right attitude.

- *Procedure*: Each chapter includes the current procedures that are used in the acute hospital setting. They have been drawn from the daily nursing practice at The Royal Marsden NHS Foundation Trust. Only procedures where the authors have the knowledge and expertise have been included.
- Each procedure gives detailed step-by-step actions; these are supported by rationale. For the first time where available the known evidence underpinning this rationale has been indicated.
- *Illustrations*: For the first time colour illustrations of the steps of some procedures are included. This will enable the nurse carrying out the procedures to see in more detail such things as the correct position of hands or the angle of a needle.
- *Reference and reading list*: The chapter finishes with a combined reference and reading list. Only recent texts from the last 10 years have been included unless they are seminal texts.

This book is intended as a reference and a resource, not as a replacement for practice-based education. None of the procedures in this book should be undertaken without prior instruction and subsequent supervision from an appropriately qualified and experienced professional. We hope that *The Royal Marsden Hospital Manual of Clinical Nursing Procedures* will continue to be a resource and a contribution to 'continually improving the overall standard of clinical care' (NHSE 1999, p. 3).

References

NHSE (1999) *Clinical Governance: Quality in the New NHS.* Department of Health, London.

NICE (2005) *Violence. The Short-Term Management of Disturbed/Violent Behaviour in Psychiatric In-Patient Settings and Emergency Departments*. National Institute for Health and Clinical Excellence, London.

NICE (2007) *Venous thromboembolism: reducing the risk of venous thromboembolism (deep vein thrombosis and pulmonary embolism) in in-patients undergoing surgery*. National Collaborating Centre for Acute Care. Royal College of Surgeons for England, London. www.guidance-nice.org.uk/CG/published/CG46. Accessed 30/4/07.

Rycroft–Malone, J. *et al.* (2004) What counts as evidence in evidence based practice? *J Adv Nurs*, **47**(1), 81–90.

Pratt, R.J. *et al.* (2007) Epic 2: National evidence-based guidelines for preventing health-care associated infections in NHS hospitals in England. *J Hosp Infect*, **65**(1)(Suppl), S1–S12.

Lisa Dougherty
Sara Lister
Editors

Contents

Foreword to the seventh edition	*v*	
Introduction and guidelines for use	*vii*	
Quick reference to the guidelines	*xvii*	
Acknowledgements	*xxi*	
List of contributors to the seventh edition	*xxiii*	
List of abbreviations	*xxvii*	

PART ONE

1 The context of nursing ... 3
   Introduction ... 4
   What is nursing practice today? ... 4
   Patients' perspective ... 4
   What do organizations want from nurses? ... 8
   Conclusion ... 12
   References and further reading ... 12

2 Assessment and the process of care ... 15
   Introduction ... 16
   Principles of assessment ... 16
   Structure of assessment ... 17
   Methods of assessment ... 18
   Decision making and nursing diagnosis ... 20
   Planning and implementing care ... 22
   Evaluating care ... 23
   Summary of recommendations and guidance
      for practice ... 24
   Documenting and communicating care ... 25
   References ... 25

3 Communication ... 28
   Reference material ... 29
   Procedure guidelines: Provision of information ... 30
   Conclusion ... 39
   References ... 39

PART TWO

4 Abdominal paracentesis ... 43
   Reference material ... 44
   Procedure guidelines: Abdominal paracentesis ... 46
   Procedure guidelines: Intraperitoneal drain
      removal ... 47

Problem solving: Abdominal paracentesis ... 48
References and further reading ... 49

5 Aseptic technique ... 50
   Reference material ... 51
   Procedure guidelines: Apron: putting on and
      removing a disposable plastic apron ... 57
   Procedure guidelines: Aseptic technique ... 59
   Procedure guidelines: Hand washing ... 61
   Procedure guidelines: Non-sterile gloves use ... 64
   References and further reading ... 67

6 Barrier nursing: nursing the infectious or
   immunosuppressed patient ... 70
   Barrier nursing ... 71
   Reference material ... 71
   Source isolation ... 74
   Reference material ... 74
   Procedure guidelines: Isolation of source
      of infection ... 79
   Protective isolation ... 83
   Reference material ... 85
   Procedure guidelines: Neutropenic patient care ... 88
   Acquired immune deficiency syndrome ... 90
   Reference material ... 90
   Human immunodeficiency virus 2 ... 93
   Reference material ... 93
   Procedure guidelines: Acquired immune
      deficiency syndrome (AIDS): patient care in
      a general ward ... 93
   Antimicrobial-resistant organisms ... 100
   Reference material ... 100
   Aspergillosis ... 104
   Reference material ... 104
   Clostridium difficile ... 105
   Reference material ... 106
   Cryptosporidiosis ... 107
   Reference material ... 107
   Hepatitis ... 108
   Hepatitis A ... 108
   Reference material ... 108
   Procedure guidelines: Hepatitis A: patient care ... 110
   Hepatitis B ... 111

Reference material   111
Procedure guidelines: Hepatitis B: patient care   113
Non-A non-B hepatitis   116
Reference material   116
Procedure guidelines: Non-A non-B hepatitis:
    patient care   117
Hepatitis C   117
Reference material   117
Hepatitis D   118
Reference material   118
Hepatitis E   118
Reference material   118
Hepatitis B genotype F   119
Reference material   119
Hepatitis G (HBV/G)   119
Reference material   119
The herpesviruses   119
Cytomegalovirus   119
Reference material   119
Epstein–Barr virus   120
Reference material   120
Herpes simplex virus   121
Reference material   121
Varicella zoster virus   122
Reference material   122
Legionnaires' disease   123
Reference material   123
Listeriosis   124
Reference material   124
Pneumocystosis   125
Reference material   125
Tuberculosis   126
Reference material   126
Transmissible spongiform encephalopathies   128
Reference material   129
References and further reading   130

7   Breast aspiration and seroma drainage   146
Breast aspiration   147
Reference material   149
Procedure guidelines: Breast aspiration   149
Seroma drainage   151
Procedure guidelines: Seroma drainage   153
References and further reading   154

8   Cardiopulmonary resuscitation   155
Reference material   156
Procedure guidelines: Cardiopulmonary
    resuscitation (CPR)   163
References and further reading   167

9   Compression therapy in the management of
    lymphoedema   169
Reference material   170
Assessment of the patient with lymphoedema   171
Measurement of limb volume   171
Reference material   172

Procedure guidelines: Compression therapy:
    limb volume calculation   173
Phases of treatment   174
Maintenance phase of treatment   174
Intensive phase of treatment   175
Procedure guidelines: Compression garments
    (elastic): application of   178
Procedure guidelines: Compression bandaging
    (standard multilayer)   179
References and further reading   185

10 Discharge planning   187
Reference material   188
Procedure guidelines: Discharge planning   196
References and further reading   200

11 Drug administration: general principles   202
Reference material   203
Injections and infusions   212
Summary   219
Procedure guidelines: Self-administration of drugs   220
Procedure guidelines: Oral drug administration   221
Procedure guidelines: Injections: administration   224
Procedure guidelines: Rectal medication
    administration   231
Procedure guidelines: Vaginal medication
    administration   231
Procedure guidelines: Topical applications of
    medication   232
Procedure guidelines: Administration of
    medication in other forms   233
Procedure guidelines: Continuous infusion of
    intravenous drugs   235
Procedure guidelines: Intermittent infusion of
    intravenous drugs   238
Procedure guidelines: Injection (bolus or push)
    of intravenous drugs   241
Problem solving: Injection and infusion of
    intravenous fluids and drugs   244
References and further reading   251

12 Drug administration: cytotoxic drugs   254
Reference material   255
Procedure guidelines: Cytotoxic drugs:
    environmental precautions   257
Procedure guidelines: Cytotoxic drugs:
    accidental exposure   261
Routes of administration   262
Intravenous administration   262
Reference material   262
Procedure guidelines: Cytotoxic drugs:
    intravenous administration   264
Extravasation of vesicant drugs   266
Reference material   266
Procedure guidelines: Extravasation
    management: peripheral cannula   272
Oral administration   274

Reference material   274
Intramuscular and subcutaneous injection   275
Reference material   275
Topical application   275
Reference material   275
Intrathecal administration   276
Reference material   277
Intrapleural instillation   278
Reference material   278
Procedure guidelines: Cytotoxic drugs:
    intrapleural administration   279
Problem solving: Intrapleural cytotoxic drug
    administration   280
Intravesical instillation   280
Reference material   280
Procedure guidelines: Cytotoxic drugs:
    intravesical instillation   281
Problem solving: Intravesicular instillation of
    cytotoxic drugs   282
Intraperitoneal administration   283
Reference material   283
Procedure guidelines: Cytotoxic drugs:
    intraperitoneal instillation   284
Problem solving: Intraperitoneal instillation of
    cytotoxic drugs   285
Intra-arterial administration   285
Reference material   285
Problem solving: Intra-arterial administration
    of cytotoxic drugs   287
References and further reading   288

13 Drug administration: delivery (infusion devices) 290
Reference material   291
Infusion devices   296
Gravity infusion devices   296
Infusion pumps   298
Summary   301
Procedure guidelines: Subcutaneous
    administration of drugs using a syringe
    driver (e.g. Sims (Graseby) Medical MS26)   302
Procedure guidelines: Syringe driver:
    preparation of the syringe and priming the
    infusion set for 24-hour drug administration
    using the Sims (Graseby) Medical MS26   303
Procedure guidelines: Syringe driver: inserting
    the winged infusion set or cannula and
    connecting syringe   304
Problem solving: Syringe drivers   307
References and further reading   309

14 Elimination: bladder lavage and irrigation   310
Reference material   311
Procedure guidelines: Bladder lavage   314
Procedure guidelines: Urinary catheter:
    maintenance solution administration   316
Procedure guidelines: Continuous bladder
    irrigation   318

Bladder irrigation recording chart   319
Problem solving   321
References and further reading   321

15 Elimination: bowel care   324
Reference material   325
Procedure guidelines: Bedpan use: assisting
    a patient   325
Procedure guidelines: Commode use: assisting
    a patient   326
Enemas   335
Reference material   335
Procedure guidelines: Enema administration   336
Problem solving: Enema administration   338
Suppositories   338
Reference material   338
Procedure guidelines: Suppository administration 339
Digital rectal examination   340
Procedure guidelines: Digital rectal examination 341
Manual evacuation   342
Procedure guidelines: Manual evacuation of faeces 343
Rectal irrigation   344
Reference material   345
References and further reading   345

16 Elimination: continent urinary diversions   348
Reference material   349
Teaching intermittent self-catheterization of a
    continent urinary diversion stoma   355
Reference material   355
Procedure guidelines: Continent urinary
    diversion stoma: self-catheterization   355
Procedure guidelines: Continent urinary
    diversion stoma drainage tubes: flushing   357
Problem solving: Continent urinary diversion
    stoma   358
Useful addresses   359
References and further reading   359

17 Elimination: stoma care   361
Reference material   362
Procedure guidelines: Stoma care   370
Procedure guidelines: Urine specimen
    collection (ileal conduit or urostomy)   372
Procedure guidelines: Stoma bridge or rod
    removal   373
Problem solving: Stoma care   374
Useful addresses   375
References and further reading   375

18 Elimination: urinary   377
Reference material   378
Procedure guidelines: Urinary catheterization   384
Procedure guidelines: Urinary catheterization:
    intermittent self-catheterization   388
Procedure guidelines: Urine specimen
    collection: catheter (CSU)   390

Procedure guidelines: Urinary catheter bag:
        emptying   392
Procedure guidelines: Urinary catheter removal   392
Problem solving: Urinary catheter   393
Penile sheaths   395
Reference material   395
Procedure guidelines: Penile sheath application 396
References and further reading   397

19 Gene therapy for the management of cancer   400
Reference material   401
Procedure guidelines: Gene therapy: patient care 405
Further advice   410
References and further reading   410

20 Haematological procedures   412
Reference material   413
Bone marrow procedures   414
Apheresis procedures (donor or therapeutic)   417
Procedure guidelines: Bone marrow aspiration
        and trephine biopsy   419
Procedure guidelines: Bone marrow harvest   422
Problem solving: Bone marrow harvest   425
References and further reading   426

21 Intrapleural drainage   428
Reference material   429
Procedure guidelines: Intrapleural drain insertion 434
Procedure guidelines: Intrapleural drain:
        changing the drain bottle   438
Procedure guidelines: Intrapleural drain removal 439
Problem solving: Intrapleural drainage   441
References and further reading   442

22 Last offices   444
Reference material   445
Procedure guidelines: Last offices   446
Issues specific to critical care   449
Procedure guidelines: Last offices: additional
        considerations in critical care   450
Problem solving: Last offices   451
Procedure guidelines: Last offices:
        requirements for people of different religious
        faiths   452
References   456
Further reading on religious faiths   457

23 Lumbar puncture   459
Reference material   460
Procedure guidelines: Lumbar puncture   463
Problem solving: Lumbar puncture   465
References and further reading   466

24 Nutritional support   467
Reference material   468
Procedure guidelines: Weighing the patient   479
Procedure guidelines: Feeding an adult   481

Procedure guidelines: Nasogastric intubation
        with tubes using an introducer   482
Procedure guidelines: Nasogastric intubation
        with tubes without using an introducer, e.g.
        a Ryle's tube   484
Procedure guidelines: Percutaneous
        endoscopically placed gastrostomy (PEG)
        tube care   486
Procedure guidelines: Radiologically inserted
        gastrostomy (RIG) tube care   488
Procedure guidelines: Jejunostomy feeding tube
        care   488
Procedure guidelines: Enteral feeding tubes:
        administration of medication   489
Procedure guidelines: Enteral feeding tube:
        unblocking   490
Problem solving: Swallowing difficulties   491
References and further reading   494

25 Observations   496
Pulse   497
Reference material   497
Procedure guidelines: Pulse measurement   501
Twelve-lead electrocardiogram (ECG)   502
Procedure guidelines: Electrocardiogram (ECG)   502
Blood pressure   504
Reference material   504
Procedure guidelines: Blood pressure (manual)   510
Respiration   512
Reference material   513
Procedure guidelines: Pulse oximetry   520
Peak flow   521
Reference material   521
Procedure guidelines: Peak flow reading using
        manual peak flow meter   522
Temperature   522
Reference material   524
Urinalysis   528
Procedure guidelines: Temperature measurement   529
Reference material   530
Characteristics of urine   530
Procedure guidelines: Urinalysis   532
Blood glucose   533
Reference material   533
Procedure guidelines: Blood glucose monitoring   536
Central venous pressure   538
Reference material   538
Procedure guidelines: Central venous pressure
        measurement   539
Problem solving: Central venous pressure (CVP)   540
References   541

26 Observations: neurological   545
Reference material   546
Procedure guidelines: Neurological
        observations and assessment   553
References and further reading   556

27 Pain management and assessment 557
    Reference material 558
    Procedure guidelines: Pain control: assessment
        and education of patient prior to surgery 572
    Procedure guidelines: Pain assessment chart:
        chronic 573
    References and further reading 573

28 Pain management: Entonox administration 577
    Reference material 579
    Procedure guidelines: Entonox administration 581
    Problem solving: Entonox administration 582
    References and further reading 583

29 Pain management: epidural and intrathecal
    analgesia 585
    Reference material 586
    Epidural/intrathecal analgesia for patients with
        intractable chronic and cancer pain 591
    Procedure guidelines: Epidural/intrathecal
        catheter for chronic pain: preinsertion
        management 592
    Procedure guidelines: Epidural/intrathecal
        catheter insertion 593
    Procedure guidelines: Epidural/intrathecal
        infusion: setting up utilizing an ambulatory
        pump 594
    Procedure guidelines: Epidural/intrathecal
        catheter for chronic pain management:
        post-insertion management 595
    Procedure guidelines: Epidural/intrathecal exit
        site dressing change 596
    Procedure guidelines: Epidural/intrathecal
        analgesia top up (bolus) 597
    Procedure guidelines: Discharge planning for
        patients with epidural/intrathecal catheter
        in situ 597
    Procedure guidelines: Epidural/intrathecal
        catheter removal 599
    Problem solving: Epidural/intrathecal infusions
        of local anaesthetic agents and opioids:
        management of side-effects 599
    Problem solving: Epidural/intrathecal
        insertion: complications 601
    Problem solving: Epidural/intrathecal catheter:
        issues with pump and site 602
    References and further reading 603

30 Perioperative care 605
    Preoperative care 606
    Reference material 606
    Procedure guidelines: Antiembolic stockings:
        fitting and wearing 608
    Procedure guidelines: Preoperative care 611
    Intraoperative care 613
    Reference material 613
    Procedure guidelines: Intraoperative care 616

    Postanaesthetic recovery 617
    Reference material 617
    Procedure guidelines: Postanaesthetic recovery 620
    Problem solving: Postanaesthetic recovery 623
    Procedure guidelines: Postoperative recovery 625
    References and further reading 627

31 Personal hygiene: eye care 629
    Reference material 630
    Procedure guidelines: Eye swabbing 637
    Procedure guidelines: Artificial eye care 638
    Procedure guidelines: Contact lens care 639
    Procedure guidelines: Eye drop instillation 641
    Procedure guidelines: Eye ointment instillation 642
    Procedure guidelines: Eye irrigation 643
    Procedure guidelines: Eyelid closure for
        comatose patients 645
    References and further reading 646

32 Personal hygiene: mouth care 647
    Reference material 648
    Procedure guidelines: Mouth care 654
    Problem solving: Mouth care 656
    References and further reading 657

33 Personal hygiene: skin care 660
    Reference material 661
    Procedure guidelines: Bed bathing a patient 664
    References and further reading 666

34 Positioning 668
    Reference material 669
    Principles of positioning 669
    Medical considerations 669
    Positioning in bed 670
    Procedure guidelines: Positioning the patient
        supine 670
    Procedure guidelines: Positioning the patient
        sitting in bed 671
    Procedure guidelines: Positioning the patient
        side lying 672
    Guidance for assisting patients to move 673
    Procedure guidelines: Moving from lying to
        sitting: assisting the patient 674
    Procedure guidelines: Positioning the patient in
        a chair 675
    Procedure guidelines: Moving from sitting to
        standing: assisting the patient 675
    Procedure guidelines: Walking: assisting the
        patient 681
    Procedure guidelines: Positioning to minimize
        the work of breathing 682
    Procedure guidelines: Positioning to maximize
        ventilation/perfusion (V/Q) matching and
        oxygenation 683
    Positioning of patients with cardiorespiratory
        compromise 684

Positioning to maximize the drainage of
  respiratory secretions   684
Positioning the patient with neurological
  impairment   684
Procedure guidelines: Positioning the
  neurological patient with tonal problems   686
Procedure guidelines: Positioning the
  preoperative and postoperative amputee patient 688
Positioning and amputee management   688
References and further reading   689

35 Radioactive source therapy: sealed sources   691
Sealed radioactive source therapy   692
Reference material   692
Remote afterloading   698
Reference material   698
Procedure guidelines: Sealed radioactive
  sources insertion: patient care   702
Procedure guidelines: Intraoral sealed
  radioactive sources: patient care   704
Procedure guidelines: Iridium and caesium
  gynaecological sources (manual and
  afterloaded): patient care   705
Procedure guidelines: Gynaecological caesium
  and iridium wires removal   706
Problem solving: Gynaecological caesium and
  iridium wires   708
Procedure guidelines: Selectron treatment:
  patient care   708
Procedure guidelines: Selectron applicator
  removal   709
Problem solving: Selectron treatment   710
Procedure guidelines: Radioactive seeds (e.g.
  iodine-125): patient care   711
Procedure guidelines: Breast sealed radioactive
  sources: patient care   712
Procedure guidelines: Interstitial perineal
  template (Hammersmith hedgehog)   712
Useful websites   714
References and further reading   714

36 Radioactive source therapy and diagnostic
  procedures: unsealed sources   716
Reference material   717
Procedure guidelines: Iodine-131:
  pre-administration care   726
Procedure guidelines: Iodine-131 thyroid
  treatment: patient care   726
Procedure guidelines: Iodine-131 mIBG
  treatment: patient care   727
Procedure guidelines: Unsealed source therapy:
  patient care post-administration   727
Procedure guidelines: Unsealed radioactive
  sources for diagnostic investigations:
  patient care   730
Procedure guidelines: Unsealed radioactive
  sources: emergency procedures   731

Regulations   733
Web resources   733
References and further reading   733

37 Renal replacement therapy: peritoneal dialysis
  and continuous venovenous haemodiafiltration   735
Reference material   736
Peritoneal dialysis   736
Reference material   736
Continuous renal replacement therapy   739
Reference material   739
Procedure guidelines: Peritoneal dialysis   740
Problem solving: Peritoneal dialysis   742
Procedure guidelines: CVVHDF: utilizing a
  CVVHDF device   744
References and further reading   747

38 Respiratory therapy   749
Reference material   750
Continuous positive airway pressure   756
Reference material   756
Hazards of oxygen therapy   758
Procedure guidelines: Pre-continuous positive
  airway pressure (pre-CPAP)   760
Procedure guidelines: Continuous positive
  airway pressure (CPAP): setting up   761
Procedure guidelines: Humidification for
  respiratory therapy   761
Problem solving: Oxygen therapy by nasal
  cannulae or oxygen mask   762
Problem solving: Continuous positive airway
  pressure (CPAP)   763
References and further reading   765

39 Scalp cooling   766
Reference material   767
Procedure guidelines: Scalp cooling   770
Problem solving: Scalp cooling   772
References and further reading   772

40 Specimen collection for microbiological analysis   774
Reference material   775
Procedure guidelines: Specimen collection:
  section swabs   781
Procedure guidelines: Specimen collection:
  body fluid   784
Procedure guidelines: Cervical uterine smear or
  Pap smear   789
References and further reading   793

41 Spinal cord compression management   795
Reference material   796
Procedure guidelines: Moving and handling
  a person with suspected spinal cord
  compression   800
Procedure guidelines: Spinal cord compression
  (suspected): assessment   801

Procedure guidelines: Spinal cord compression
    (suspected): treatment   803
Procedure guidelines: Spinal cord compression
    (suspected): rehabilitation   804
Problem solving: Spinal cord compression
    (suspected)   806
References   807

42 Tracheostomy care and laryngectomy care
    (including voice rehabilitation)   809
Tracheostomy and laryngectomy care   810
Reference material   810
Laryngectomy voice rehabilitation   819
Reference material   820
Procedure guidelines: Tracheostomy dressing
    change   822
Procedure guidelines: Tracheostomy suction   823
Humidification   824
Procedure guidelines: Humidification of
    patient with tracheostomy   825
Procedure guidelines: Tracheostomy tube change   825
Problem solving: Tracheostomy   827
Procedure guidelines: Changing a Blom–Singer
    type non-indwelling voice prosthesis   828
References and further reading   829

43 Transfusion of blood and blood products   831
Reference material   832
Procedure guidelines: Blood product request   843
Problem solving: Requesting a blood product   843
Procedure guidelines: Blood sampling:
    pre-transfusion   844
Problem solving: Blood sampling:
    pre-transfusion   844
Procedure guidelines: Transfusion of blood
    components   845
Problem solving: Transfusion of blood
    components   847
References and further reading   847

44 The unconscious patient   849
Reference material   850
Procedure guidelines: Unconscious patient care   852
References and further reading   853

45 Vascular access devices: insertion and
    management   855
Reference material   856
Peripheral cannulae   860
Reference material   860
Midline catheters   865
Reference material   865
Central venous access devices   866
Peripherally inserted central catheters   866
Reference material   866
Short-term percutaneous central venous
    catheters (non-tunnelled)   869

Reference material   869
Skin-tunnelled catheters   872
Reference material   872
Implantable ports   874
Reference material   874
Discharging patients home with a VAD in situ   876
Quality-of-life issues: living with a VAD   877
Procedure guidelines: Peripheral cannula
    insertion   878
Procedure guidelines: Midline catheter insertion   882
Procedure guidelines: Peripherally inserted
    central catheter (PICC) insertion and removal   884
Procedure guidelines: Central venous catheter
    insertion site dressing change   887
Procedure guidelines: Central venous access
    device: maintaining patency   888
Procedure guidelines: Central venous access
    device: taking blood samples   889
Procedure guidelines: Central venous access
    device: unblocking an occlusion   891
Procedure guidelines: Implanted ports:
    insertion and removal of non-coring needles   894
Procedure guidelines: Central venous catheter
    (non-cuffed/tunnelled): removal   896
Procedure guidelines: Central venous catheter
    (skin-tunnelled): surgical removal   897
Problem solving: Central venous access devices   899
Arterial cannulae   902
Reference material   902
Procedure guidelines: Arterial puncture: radial
    artery   904
Procedure guidelines: Arterial cannula
    insertion: preparation and setting up of
    monitoring set   907
Procedure guidelines: Arterial cannula: taking
    a blood sample   909
Procedure guidelines: Arterial cannula: removal   911
Problem solving: Arterial cannulation   912
References and further reading   913

46 Venepuncture   919
Reference material   920
Procedure guidelines: Venepuncture   924
Problem solving: Venepuncture   928
References and further reading   931

47 Violence: prevention and management   932
Reference material   933
Procedure guidelines: Violence: prevention and
    management   938
References and further reading   940

48 Wound management   942
Wound healing and management   943
Reference material   943
Pressure ulcers or decubitus ulcers   955
Reference material   955

Fungating wounds   960
Reference material   960
Radiotherapy skin damage   964
Reference material   965
Plastic surgery wounds   965
Reference material   966
Scarring   968
Reference material   968
Methods of wound closure   969
Procedure guidelines: Wound dressings change
  for acute and surgical wounds   970
Procedure guidelines: Suturing a simple
  wound   971
Procedure guidelines: Sutures, clips or staples
  removal   974
Procedure guidelines: Wound drain dressing
  (Redivac: closed drainage systems)   975

Procedure guidelines: Change of vacuum
  drainage system   976
Procedure guidelines: Wound drain removal
  (Yeates vacuum drainage system)   977
Procedure guidelines: Wound drain shortening
  (Penrose: open drainage systems)   978
Procedure guidelines: Topical negative pressure
  (TNP) therapy   978
References and further reading   980

Appendices
  Appendix 1: The Code: Standards of conduct,
   performance and ethics for nurses and
   midwives   985
  Appendix 2: Contributors to previous editions   993

Index   996

Quick reference to the guidelines

Abdominal paracentesis	46
Acquired immune deficiency syndrome (AIDS): patient care in a general ward	93
Administration of medication in other forms	233
Antiembolic stockings: fitting and wearing	608
Apron: putting on and removing a disposable plastic apron	57
Arterial cannula insertion: preparation and setting up of monitoring set	907
Arterial cannula: removal	911
Arterial cannula: taking a blood sample	909
Arterial puncture: radial artery	904
Artificial eye care	638
Aseptic technique	59
Bed bathing a patient	664
Bedpan use: assisting a patient	325
Bladder lavage	314
Blood glucose monitoring	536
Blood pressure (manual)	510
Blood product request	843
Blood sampling: pre-transfusion	844
Bone marrow aspiration and trephine biopsy	419
Bone marrow harvest	422
Breast aspiration	149
Breast sealed radioactive sources: patient care	712
Cardiopulmonary resuscitation (CPR)	163
Central venous catheter (non-cuffed/tunnelled): removal	896
Central venous access device: maintaining patency	888
Central venous access device: taking blood samples	889
Central venous access device: unblocking an occlusion	891
Central venous catheter (skin-tunnelled): surgical removal	897
Central venous catheter insertion site dressing change	887
Central venous pressure measurement	539
Cervical uterine smear or Pap smear	789
Change of vacuum drainage system	976
Changing a Blom–Singer type non-indwelling voice prosthesis	828
Commode use: assisting a patient	326
Compression bandaging (standard multilayer)	179
Compression garments (elastic): application of	178
Compression therapy: limb volume calculation	173
Contact lens care	639
Continent diversion stoma: self-catheterization	355
Continent urinary diversion stoma drainage tubes: flushing	357
Continuous bladder irrigation	318
Continuous infusion of intravenous drugs	235
Continuous positive airway pressure (CPAP): setting up	761
CVVHDF: utilizing a CVVHDF device	744
Cytotoxic drugs: accidental exposure	261
Cytotoxic drugs: environmental precautions	257
Cytotoxic drugs: Intraperitoneal instillation	284
Cytotoxic drugs: intrapleural administration	279
Cytotoxic drugs: intravenous administration	264
Cytotoxic drugs: intravesical instillation	281
Digital rectal examination	341
Discharge planning	196
Discharge planning for patients with epidural/intrathecal catheter in situ	597
Electrocardiogram (ECG)	502
Enema administration	336
Enteral feeding tube: unblocking	490
Enteral feeding tubes: administration of medication	489
Entonox administration	581
Epidural/intrathecal catheter for chronic pain management: post-insertion management	595
Epidural/intrathecal catheter removal	599
Epidural/intrathecal catheter for chronic pain: preinsertion management	592
Epidural/intrathecal catheter insertion	593
Epidural/intrathecal analgesia top up (bolus)	597
Epidural/intrathecal exit site dressing change	596
Epidural/intrathecal infusion: setting up utilizing an ambulatory pump	594
Extravasation management: peripheral cannula	272
Eye drop instillation	641
Eye irrigation	643
Eye ointment instillation	642
Eye swabbing	637
Eyelid closure for comatose patients	645
Feeding an adult	481
Gene therapy: patient care	405

Gynaecological caesium and iridium wires removal   706
Hand washing   61
Hepatitis A: patient care   110
Hepatitis B: patient care   113
Humidification for respiratory therapy   761
Humidification of patient with tracheostomy   825
Implanted ports: insertion and removal of
    non-coring needles   894
Injection (bolus or push) of intravenous drugs   241
Injections: administration   224
Intermittent infusion of intravenous drugs   238
Interstitial perineal template (Hammersmith
    hedgehog)   712
Intraoperative care   616
Intraoral sealed radioactive sources: patient care   704
Intraperitoneal drain removal   47
Intrapleural drain insertion   434
Intrapleural drain removal   439
Intrapleural: changing the drain bottle   438
Iodine-131 mIBG treatment: patient care   727
Iodine-131 thyroid treatment: patient care   726
Iodine-131: pre-administration care   726
Iridium and caesium gynaecological sources
    (manual and afterloaded): patient care   705
Isolation of source of infection   79
Jejunostomy feeding tube care   488
Last offices   446
Last offices: additional considerations in critical care   450
Last offices: requirements for people of different
    religious faiths   452
Lumbar puncture   463
Manual evacuation of faeces   343
Midline catheter insertion   882
Mouth care   654
Moving and handling a person with suspected
    spinal cord compression   800
Moving from lying to sitting: assisting the patient   674
Moving from sitting to standing: assisting a patient   675
Nasogastric intubation with tubes using an
    introducer   482
Nasogastric intubation with tubes without using
    an introducer, e.g. a Ryle's tube   484
Neurological observations and assessment   553
Neutropenic patient care   88
Non-A non-B hepatitis: patient care   117
Non-sterile gloves use   64
Oral drug administration   221
Pain assessment chart: chronic   573
Pain control: assessment and education of patient
    prior to surgery   572
Peak flow reading using manual peak flow meter   522
Penile sheath application   396
Percutaneous endoscopically placed gastrostomy
    (PEG) tube care   486
Peripheral cannula insertion   878
Peripherally inserted central catheter (PICC)
    insertion and removal   884

Peritoneal dialysis   740
Positioning the neurological patient with tonal
    problems   686
Positioning the patient in a chair   675
Positioning the patient side lying   672
Positioning the patient sitting in bed   671
Positioning the patient supine   670
Positioning the preoperative and postoperative
    amputee patient   687
Positioning to maximize ventilation/perfusion
    (V/Q) matching and oxygenation   683
Positioning to minimize the work of breathing   682
Postanaesthetic recovery   620
Postoperative recovery   625
Pre-continuous positive airway pressure (pre-CPAP)   760
Preoperative care   611
Provision of information   30
Pulse measurement   501
Pulse oximetry   520
Radioactive seeds (e.g. iodine-125): patient care   711
Radiologically inserted gastrostomy (RIG) tube care   488
Rectal medication administration   231
Scalp cooling   770
Sealed radioactive sources insertion: patient care   702
Selectron applicator removal   709
Selectron treatment: patient care   708
Self-administration of drugs   220
Seroma drainage   153
Specimen collection: body fluid   784
Specimen collection: section swabs   781
Spinal cord compression (suspected): assessment   801
Spinal cord compression (suspected): rehabilitation   804
Spinal cord compression (suspected): treatment   803
Stoma bridge or rod removal   373
Stoma care   370
Subcutaneous administration of drugs using a
    syringe driver (e.g. Sims (Graseby) Medical MS26)   302
Suppository administration   339
Sutures, clips or staples removal   974
Suturing a simple wound   971
Syringe driver: inserting the winged infusion set or
    cannula and connecting syringe   304
Syringe driver: preparation of the syringe and
    priming the infusion set for 24-hour drug
    administration using the Sims (Graseby)
    Medical MS26   303
Temperature measurement   529
Topical applications of medication   232
Topical negative pressure (TNP) therapy   978
Tracheostomy dressing change   822
Tracheostomy suction   823
Tracheostomy tube change   825
Transfusion of blood components   845
Unconscious patient care   852
Unsealed radioactive sources for diagnostic
    investigations: patient care   730
Unsealed radioactive sources: emergency procedures   731

Unsealed source therapy: patient care
 post-administration 727
Urinalysis 532
Urinary catheter bag: emptying 392
Urinary catheter removal 392
Urinary catheter: maintenance solution administration 316
Urinary catheterization 384
Urinary catheterization: intermittent
 self-catheterization 388
Urine specimen collection (ileal conduit or urostomy) 372
Urine specimen collection: catheter (CSU) 390
Vaginal medication administration 231

Venepuncture 924
Violence: prevention and management 938
Walking: assisting the patient 681
Weighing the patient 479
Wound drain dressing (Redivac: closed drainage
 systems) 975
Wound drain removal (Yeates vacuum drainage
 system) 977
Wound drain shortening (Penrose: open drainage
 systems) 978
Wound dressings change for acute and surgical
 wounds 970

Acknowledgements

Since the first edition was conceived by Robert Tiffany, and then published in 1984, *The Royal Marsden Hospital Manual of Clinical Nursing Procedures* has been supported by innovative and enthusiastic editors (including Phylip Pritchard, Jennifer Hunt, Jill David, Valerie Anne Walker, Chris Bailey and Jane Mallett) as well as many previous members of staff. We are continuing their legacy of providing a manual that underpins good nursing practice.

Yet again we have encouraged nursing and allied health professionals at all levels to be involved in contributing to the various chapters, some of whom are contributing for the first time. It has been more challenging for all the authors due to the change in the procedure section and the provision of evidence for each rationale and so the time and effort of all chapter authors should be especially acknowledged in this edition.

We would also like to extend our thanks to some key people who helped in various ways: Sylvie Hampton, Tissue Viability Consultant, for her help in reviewing the wound management chapter; Jo Rycroft Malone whose work on evidence-based nursing has been invaluable in providing a pragmatic and comprehensive system for grading the source of evidence underpinning the procedures in this manual; Dale Russell and Erika Suchanova of the David Adams Library, The Royal Marsden School of Cancer Nursing and Rehabilitation for their help and support in finding and providing the references required by the authors.

Finally, our thanks go to Beth Knight and Katherine Unwin at Blackwell Publishing for their advice and continual support in all aspects of the publishing process.

Lisa Dougherty
Sara Lister
Editors

List of contributors to the seventh edition

Karen Allan RN, BSc (Hons)
Senior Staff Nurse, Smithers Ward
(Chapter 33: Personal hygiene: skin care)

Michael Bailey RN, MSc, BSc (Hons), Dip Theo, Dip HE
Senior Staff Nurse, Wilson
(Chapter 25: Observations)

Amanda Baxter RN, RMN, ONC, BSc (Hons), PG Dip
Clinical Nurse Specialist, Pelvic Care
(Chapter 16: Elimination: continent urinary diversions;
   Chapter 17: Elimination: stoma care)

Jo Bull RN, BN (Hons) Dip ONC
Senior Staff Nurse, Burdet Coutts Ward
(Chapter 14: Elimination: bladder lavage and irrigation)

Louise Causer RN, ONC, MBA
Clinical Nurse Specialist, Nuclear Medicine
(Chapter 36: Radioactive source therapy and
   diagnostic sources: unsealed sources)

Suzanne Chapman BSc, MSc
Clinical Nurse Specialist, Pain Management
(Chapter 27: Pain: management and assessment;
   Chapter 28: Pain: Entonox administration;
   Chapter 29: Pain: epidural and intrathecal analgesia)

Jill Cooper Dip COT, DMS
Head Occupational Therapist
(Chapter 41: Spinal cord compression management)

Maria Crisford RN, BSc (Hons), Dip Nursing,
   Slice 1 & 2
Colorectal Specialist Sister
(Chapter 15: Elimination: bowel care)

Sharyn Crossen RN, BN, Dip Cancer Nursing
Sister, Wilson Ward
(Chapter 25: Observations)

Andrew J. Dimech RN, BN, Dip Oncology,
   PG Dip Intensive Care
Lecturer Practitioner, Cancer Critical Care
(Chapter 37: Renal replacement therapy: peritoneal dialysis
   and continuous venovenous haemodiafiltration)

Nigel Dodds RN, MSc, BSc (Hons), Dip HE,
   RHV, PG Cert Education
Lead Nurse Hospital and Home Programme
(Chapter 22: Last offices)

Shelley Dolan RN, MSc, BA (Hons)
Chief Nurse
(Chapter 8: Cardiopulmonary resuscitation; Chapter 38:
   Respiratory therapy)

Lisa Dougherty OBE, RN, MSc
Nurse Consultant Intravenous Therapy
(Chapter 11: Drug administration: general principles;
   Chapter 12: Drug administration: cytotoxic drugs;
   Chapter 39: Scalp cooling; Chapter 45: Vascular access
   devices: insertion and management)

Ann Duncan RN, ONC
Ward Sister, Smithers Ward
(Chapter 41: Spinal cord compression management)

Ann Farley RN, BA (Hons)
Specialist Sister, Palliative Care
(Chapter 11: Drug administration: general principles)

Jagdesh K. Grewal RN, BA (Hons), PG Dip
   Nurse Education, DMS
Senior Sister, Theatres
(Chapter 30: Perioperative care)

Diz Hackman Dip Physiotherapy, MCSP, PG Dip Advanced
   Practice, MSc
Clinical Specialist Physiotherapist in Neurology/Oncology,
   Physiotherapy Department
(Chapter 34: Positioning)

James Neale Hanvey RMN, RN, Dip HE, MSc
Divisional Nurse Director, Rare Cancers Division
(Chapter 43: Transfusion of blood and blood products)

Sarah Hart RN, BSc (Hons), MSc
Clinical Nurse Specialist Infection Control Radiation
    Protection
(Chapter 5: Aseptic technique; Chapter 6: Barrier nursing:
nursing the infectious or immunosuppressed patient;
Chapter 19: Gene therapy for the management of cancer;
Chapter 35: Radioactive source therapy: sealed sources;
Chapter 36: Radioactive source therapy and diagnostic
procedures: unsealed sources)

Beverley Henderson RN, PG Dip Counselling &
    Psychotherapy, BSc (Hons)
Clinical Nurse Specialist, Psychological Care
(Chapter 47: Violence: prevention and management)

Justine Hofland RN, BA (Hons), Dip HE, MSc
Lecturer Practitioner
(Chapter 25: Observations)

Hilary Hollis RN, BSc (Hons), MSc, PG Dip, RNT
Formerly Programme Leader
(Chapter 1: The context of nursing)

Victoria Hollis RN, BN (Hons)
Specialist Sister, Transitional Care Unit
(Chapter 25: Observations)

Lynne Hopwood RN, BSc (Hons)
Assistant Chief Nurse (Operations)
(Chapter 11: Drug administration, general principles)

Sonja Hoy RN, PG Dip, PG Cert, BSc (Hons), Dip Nursing
Lecturer Practitioner
(Chapter 40: Specimen collection for microbiological
    analysis)

Patricia Hunt RN, MSc, PG Dip
Lecturer Practitioner
(Chapter 44: The unconscious patient)

Lorraine Hyde RN, ONC, BSc (Hons)
Senior Sister, Day Care Services
(Chapter 12: Drug administration: cytotoxic drugs)

Kate Jones Dip Physiotherapy, MSc, MCSP
Clinical Specialist Physiotherapist Musculoskeletal/
    Oncology, Physiotherapy Department
(Chapter 34: Positioning)

Audrey Kelly RN, Dip HE
Specialist Sister, Breast Care
(Chapter 7: Breast aspiration and seroma drainage)

Jennifer Kelynack RN, BN, Certificate in Intensive
    Care
Nursing Sister, Critical Care Unit
(Chapter 44: The unconscious patient)

Maria Law RN, ONC Cert
Ward Sister, Kennaway Ward
(Chapter 4: Abdominal paracentesis)

Sally Legge RN, MSc
Clinical Nurse Specialist, Gastrointestinal Unit
(Chapter 4: Abdominal paracentesis)

Sara Lister RN, BSc (Hons), PGDAE, MSc
Assistant Chief Nurse/Head of School
(Chapter 1: The context of nursing)

Anne McLoughlin RN, BSc (Hons) Nursing
Specialist Sister, Breast Care
(Chapter 7: Breast aspiration and seroma drainage)

Chris McNamara RN, BSc (Hons), MSc
Lecturer Practitioner
(Chapter 40: Specimen collection for microbiological
    analysis)

Neve Mann RN, BSc (Hons), ONC
Formerly Practice Development Facilitator
(Chapter 30: Perioperative care)

David Mathers RN, Dip HE, BSc (Hons)
Deputy Charge Nurse, University Hospitals of Leicester
    NHS Trust
(Chapter 27: Pain management and assessment)

Jennifer Miller BSc (Hons), MSc, State Registered
    Occupational Therapist
Senior Occupational Therapist, Occupational
    Therapy Department
(Chapter 41: Spinal cord compression management)

Carolyn Moore MCSP
Superintendent Physiotherapist, Physiotherapy Department
(Chapter 34: Positioning)

Gillian M. Parker RN, BSc, ONC
Senior Staff Nurse, Burdett Coutts Ward
(Chapter 18: Elimination: urinary)

Sinéad Parry RN, BSc (Hons)
Project Lead, End of Life Care, Learning Disabilities, Trinity
    Hospice formerly Complex Discharge Co-ordinator,
    Royal Marsden Hospital
(Chapter 10: Discharge planning)

Natalie Pattison BSc (Hons), MSc, N92 Dip Cancer Nursing
Nurse Researcher, Critical Care Nursing
(Chapter 22: Last offices)

Barry Quinn RN, BACC Phil, BD, MSc, PG Cert Teaching
Lecturer Practitioner Haemato-oncology
(Chapter 23: Lumbar puncture; Chapter 32: Personal
    hygiene: mouth care)

Louise-Ann Ritchie RN, BN, MSc
Nurse Practitioner, Haematology
(Chapter 20: Haematological procedures)

Lara Roskelly RN, Dip General, Psychiatric, Community nursing and midwifery, Dip Critical Care Nursing, Cardiothoracics and Trauma
Critical Care Outreach Sister
(Chapter 21: Intrapleural drainage)

Kevin Russell RN, BSc Dip HE, Dip Cancer Nursing, BSc (Hons)
Charge Nurse, Critical Care Unit
(Chapter 26: Observations: neurological; Chapter 31: Personal hygiene: eye care)

Mave Salter RN, NDN (Cert), ONC, Cert Ed, Dip Couns, BSc (Hons), MSc
Complex Discharge Co-ordinator
(Chapter 10: Discharge planning)

Catherine Sandsund Dip Physiotherapy, Advanced Cert Cardiorespiratory Physiotherapy, MSc
Senior Physiotherapist, Physiotherapy Department
(Chapter 34: Positioning)

Neelam Sarpal RN, BSc, PG Dip Teaching and Learning
Teaching Sister
(Chapter 11: Drug administration: general principles; Chapter 13: Drug administration: infusion devices)

Steve Scholtes RN, BSc, MSc
Charge Nurse, Burdett Coutts Ward
(Chapter 14: Elimination: bladder lavage and irrigation; Chapter 18: Elimination: urinary)

Clare Shaw RD (Registered Dietitian), BSc (Hons), PhD
Consultant Dietitian
(Chapter 24: Nutritional support)

Caroline Soady RN, BSc (Hons), MSc
Clinical Nurse Specialist Head and Neck
(Chapter 42: Tracheostomy care and laryngectomy care (including voice rehabilitation))

Catherine South RN, Dip Nursing Studies, BA (Hons)
Specialist Sister, Head and Neck
(Chapter 48: Wound management)

Anna-Marie Stevens RN, RM, ONC, BSc (Hons), MSc
Clinical Nurse Specialist Palliative Care
(Chapter 27: Pain management and assessment; Chapter 44: Unconscious patient)

Mary Anne Tanay RN, BSc (Hons), Dip Oncology
Research Nurse, Head and Neck
(Chapter 48: Wound management)

Nicola Tinne RN, BSc, Dip Health Studies
Specialist Sister Head, Neck and Thyroid Cancer and Chair Wound Management Group
(Chapter 48: Wound management)

Richard Towers RN, Dip Oncology, BSc (Hons), MSc
Lecturer Practitioner Psychological Care
(Chapter 3: Communication)

Jen Watson RN, BSc
Senior Sister, Critical Care Unit
(Chapter 45: Vascular access devices: insertion and management)

Caro Watts RN, BSc (Hons), MSc, Dip Oncology, Cert Mgt
Nurse Consultant Transitional Care (Cancer)
(Chapter 2: Assessment)

Alexandra Westbrook RN, BSc (Hons), MSc, PG Dip Teaching and Learning
Programmer Leader
(Chapter 2: Assessment and the process of care; Chapter 15: Elimination: bowel care)

Barbara Witt RN
Nurse Phlebotomist
(Chapter 46: Venepuncture)

Miriam Wood RN, ONC, BSc (Hons)
Senior Practice Development Facilitator
(Supporting role)

Mary Woods RN, BSc (Hons), MSc, ONC
Clinical Nurse Specialist/Head of Lymphoedema Services
(Chapter 9: Compression therapy in the management of lymphoedema)

List of abbreviations

5-FU	5-fluorouracil
A&E	Accident and Emergency
AAMI	Association for the Advancement of Medical Instrumentation
ABG	arterial blood gas
ACoP	Approved Codes of Practice
ADH	antidiuretic hormone
ADL	activities of daily living
AED	automated external defibrillator
AFO	ankle foot orthosis
AHA	American Heart Association
AIDS	acquired immune deficiency syndrome
ALARP	as low as reasonably practicable
ALS	advanced life support
ANH	acute normovolaemic haemodilution
AORN	Association of Perioperative Registered Nurses
AP	alternating pressure
APTR	activated partial thromboplastin ratio
ARDS	acute respiratory distress syndrome/adult respiratory distress syndrome
ARF	acute renal failure
ARSAC	Administration of Radioactive Substances Advisory Committee
ATC	around the clock
AV	atrioventricular
BAL	bronchoscopy with bronchoalveolar lavage
BCC	basal cell carcinoma
BCG	bacille Calmette-Guérin
BCSH	British Committee for Standards in Haematology
BIA	bioelectrical impedance analysis
BLS	basic life support
BMA	British Medical Association
BME	biomedical engineering
BMI	body mass index
BMT	bone marrow transplantation
BOC	British Oxygen Company
BPI	Brief Pain Inventory
Bq	becquerel
BSE	bovine spongiform encephalopathy
BSO	Biological Safety Officer
BUN	blood urea nitrogen
C&R	control and restraint
CAPD	continuous ambulatory peritoneal dialysis
CARES	Cancer Rehabilitation Evaluation System
CAVD	central venous access device
CAVH	continuous arteriovenous haemofiltration
CBE	charting by exception
CCU	coronary care unit
CDC	Centers for Disease Control
CDs	controlled drugs
CE	*Conformité Europèene*
cfu	colony-forming units
cGy	centigray
CJD	Creutzfeldt-Jakob disease
CLP	continuous low pressure
CMF	cyclophosphamide, methotrexate and fluorouracil
CMV	cytomegalovirus
CNS	central nervous system
CO	carbon monoxide or cardiac output
CO_2	carbon dioxide
COPD	chronic obstructive pulmonary disease
COSHH	Control of Substances Hazardous to Health
CPAP	continuous positive airway pressure
CPR	cardiopulmonary resuscitation
Cr	creatinine
CRP	C-reactive protein
CRRT	continuous renal replacement therapy
C-SAS	Chemotherapy Symptom Assessment Scale
CSF	cerebrospinal fluid
CSS	Central Sterile Services
CT	computed tomography
CVAD	central venous access device
CVC	central venous catheter
CVP	central venous pressure
CVVHDF	continuous venovenous haemodiafiltration
DBP	diastolic blood pressure
DEFRA	Department of the Environment Food Rural Affairs
DH	Department of Health
DIC	disseminated intravascular coagulation
DMSO	dimethyl sulfoxide
DNA	deoxyribonucleic acid
DNAR	do not attempt resuscitation

DRE	digital rectal examination	HIV 1	human immunodeficiency virus 1
DVLA	Driver and Vehicle Licensing Agency	HIV 2	human immunodeficiency virus 2
DVT	deep vein thrombosis	HIV	human immunodeficiency virus
EAPC	European Association of Palliative Care	HLA	human leucocyte antigen
EBV	Epstein–Barr virus	HME	heat and moisture exchange(r)
ECG	electrocardiogram	HNIg	human normal immunoglobulin
EDTA	ethylenediaminetetra-acetic acid	HPA	Health Protection Agency
EGF	epidermal growth factor	HSC	Health Service Circular
ELISA	enzyme-linked immunosorbent assay	HSE	Health and Safety Executive
EMEA	European Medicines Evaluation Agency	HSV	herpes simplex virus
EMRSA	epidemic strains of MRSA	HTLV	human T-leukaemia/lymphoma virus
ENT	ears, nose and throat	HTLV-1	human T-leukaemia/lymphoma virus type 1
EPO	erythropoietin	I-131	Iodine-131
EPP	exposure-prone procedures	IASP	International Association for the Study of Pain
ERV	expiratory reserve volume		
ESRD	end-stage renal disease	IBCT	Incorrect Blood Component Transfused
ESRF	end-stage renal failure	IC	inspiratory capacity
EUPAP	European Pressure Ulcer Advisory Panel	ICD	implantable cardioverter defibrillator
FEC	fluorouracil, epirubicin and cyclophosphamide	ICP	intracranial pressure
FFI	fatal familial insomnia	ICS	intra-operative cell salvage
FFP	fresh frozen plasma	ICU	intensive care unit
FGF	fibroblast growth factor	IDDM	insulin-dependent diabetes mellitus
FNA	fine needle aspirate/fine needle aspiration	IGF-1	insulin-like growth factor 1
FRC	functional residual capacity	IgG	immunoglobulin G
FTSG	full-thickness skin graft	IgM	immunoglobulin M
FWB	fully weight bearing	IHD	intermittent haemodialysis
G	giga	ILCOR	International Liaison Committee on Resuscitation
GCS	Glasgow Coma Scale		
G-CSF	granulocyte-colony stimulating factor	IMV	intermittent mandatory ventilation
GFR	glomerular filtration rate	INR	international normalized ratio
GI	gastrointestinal	IRMER	Ionising Radiation (Medical Exposure) Regulations
GINA	Global Initiative for Asthma		
GISA	glycopeptide intermediate *Staphylococcus aureus*	IRR	infrared radiation
GM-CSF	granulocyte macrophage-colony stimulating factor	IRR99	Ionising Radiations Regulations 1999
GMM	genetically modified micro-organisms	IRV	inspiratory reserve volume
GP	general practitioner	ISC	intermittent self-catheterization
GRE	glycopeptides-resistant enterococci	IV	intravenous
GSL	general sales list	JAPAC	Joint UKBTS/NIBSC Professional Advisory Committee
GTAC	Gene Therapy Advisory Committee		
GVHD	graft-versus-host disease	k	kilo
Gy	gray	KGF	keratinocyte growth factor
HAAg	hepatitis A antigen	KVO	keep the vein open
HAART	highly active antiretroviral therapy	LANSS	Leeds Assessment of Neuropathic Symptoms and Signs
HACCP	Hazard Analysis Critical Control Points		
HCAI	health care-acquired infection	LBC	liquid-based cytology
HAV	hepatitis A virus	LCT	long-chain triglycerides
HBcAg	hepatitis B core antigen	LDR	low dose rate
HBIg	hepatitis B immunoglobulin	M	mega
HBsAg	hepatitis B surface antigen	MAC	*Mycobacterium avium intracellulare*
HBV	hepatitis B virus	MAP	mean arterial pressure
HCV	hepatitis C virus	MBP	mean blood pressure
HDN	haemolytic disease of the newborn	MBq	megabecquerel
HDR	high dose rate	mc	millicuries
HDV	hepatitis D virus	MCT	medium-chain triglycerides
HEPA	high-efficiency particulate air	MDA	Medical Devices Agency
HEV	hepatitis E virus	MDR-TB	multi-drug resistant TB
HGV	hepatitis G virus	MeV	megaelectron volts

MHRA	Medicines and Healthcare Products Regulatory Agency		PEFR	peak expiratory flow rate
MHSWR	Management of Health and Safety at Work Regulations		PEG	percutaneous endoscopically placed gastrostomy
MI	myocardial infarction		PGD	patient group direction
mIBG	meta-iodobenzylguanidine		PHCT	primary health care team
MPQ	McGill Pain Questionnaire		PHN	postherpetic neuralgia
MRI	magnetic resonance imaging		PICC	peripherally inserted central catheter
MRSA	methicillin-resistant *Staphylococcus aureus*		PN	parenteral nutrition
MSAS	Memorial Symptom Assessment Scale		PNS	peripheral nervous system
MSSA	methicillin-sensitive *Staphylococcus aureus*		POCT	point-of-care testing
mSv	millisieverts		POM	prescription only medicine
MV	minute ventilation		PPE	personal protective equipment
N_2O	nitrous oxide		PSAR	Pain and Assessment Records
NANB	non-A, non-B (hepatitis)		psi	pounds per square inch
NANDA	North American Nursing Diagnosis Association		PTFE	polytetrafluoroethylene
			PVC	polyvinylchloride
NANDA-I	North American Nursing Diagnosis Association – International		PWB	partially weight bearing
			PWO	partial withdrawal occlusion
NCI-CTC	National Cancer Institute Common Toxicity Criteria		RAS	reticular activating system
			RCN	Royal College of Nursing
NGF	nerve growth factor		RCS	Royal College of Surgeons for England
NHS	National Health Service		RCT	Randomized controlled trial
NHSE	National Health Service Executive		RCUK	Resuscitation Council UK
NICE	National Institute for Health and Clinical Excellence		Re186 HEDP	rhenium-186 hydroxyethylidene diphosphonate
NIDDM	non-insulin-dependent diabetes mellitus		Rh	rhesus
NINSS	Nosocomial Infection National Surveillance Service		RIDDOR	Reporting of Incidents, Diseases and Dangerous Occurrences Regulations 1995
NMC	Nursing and Midwifery Council		RIG	radiologically inserted gastrostomy
NMDA	N-methyl-D-aspartate		RNI	reference nutrient intake
NONPF	National Organization of Nurse Practitioner Faculties		RNIB	Royal National Institute of the Blind
			RNID	Royal National Institute of the Deaf
NPSA	National Patient Safety Agency		RTO	Resuscitation Training Officer
NRPB	National Radiological Protection Board		RV	residual volume
NRS	Numerical Rating Scales		SA	sinoatrial
NSAID	non-steroidal anti-inflammatory drug		SABRE	Serious Adverse Blood Reactions and Events
NVQ	National Vocational Qualification		SARS	severe acute respiratory syndrome
NWB	non-weight bearing		SBP	systolic blood pressure
O_2	oxygen		SCC	spinal cord compression
OAG	Oral Assessment Guide		SCNS	Supportive Care Needs Survey
OMI	Oral Mucositis Index		SGA	subjective global assessment
P	pharmacy medicines		SHOHTS	Safe Handling of Hazardous Therapeutic Substances
$PaCO_2$	partial pressure of carbon dioxide		SHOT	Serious Hazards of Transfusion
PAD	preoperative autologous donation		SI	Système International
PASV	pressure-activated safety valve		SIMV	simulated intermittent mandatory ventilation
PBSCs	peripheral blood stem cells		SIRS	systemic inflammatory response syndrome
PC	*Pneumocystis carinii*			
PCA	patient-controlled analgesia		SLE	systemic lupus erythematosus
PCEA	patient-controlled epidural analgesia		SLT	speech and language therapist
PCP	*Pneumocystis carinii* pneumonia		SNBTS	Scottish National Blood Transfusion Service
PCR	polymerase chain reaction		SPI	Social Problems Inventory
PD	peritoneal dialysis		SRHH	Self Report Health History
PDGF	platelet derived growth factor		SSD	sterile supplies department
PE	pulmonary embolism/pulmonary embolus		SSG	split-thickness or split skin graft
PEA	pulseless electrical activity		SSRI	selective serotonin reuptake inhibitor
PEEP	positive end expiratory pressure		SVC	superior vena cava

swg	standard wire gauge		*V/Q*	ventilation/perfusion
T$_3$	triiodothyronine		VAC	vacuum-assisted closure
T$_4$	tetraiodothyronine		VAD	vascular access device
TACO	transfusion-associated circulatory overload		VC	vital capacity
TA-GVHD	transfusion-associated graft-versus-host disease		vCJD	variant Creutzfeldt–Jakob disease
TB	tuberculosis		VDRL	venereal disease research laboratory
TCI	target controlled infusion		VDS	Verbal Descriptor Scales
TEDS	thromboembolic deterrent stockings		VEGF	vascular endothelial growth factor
TENS	transcutaneous electrical nerve stimulation		VF	ventricular fibrillation
TGF	transforming growth factor		VGF	vascular endothelial growth factor
TIME	tissue, infection, moisture and edge advancement		VISA	vancomycin intermediate *Staphylococcus aureus*
TIVA	total intravenous anaesthesia		VRI	vancomycin-resistant enterococci
TLC	total lung capacity		VRSA	vancomycin-resistant *Staphylococcus aureus*
TLD	thermoluminescent		VT	ventricular tachycardia
TNP	topical negative pressure therapy		VTE	venous thromboembolism
TPI	*Treponema pallidum* immobilization		VTM	viral transport medium
TRALI	transfusion-related acute lung injury		VZIg	varicella zoster immunoglobulin
TRSC	Therapy Related Symptom Checklist		VZV	varicella zoster virus
TSEs	transmissible spongiform encephalopathies		WBP	wound bed preparation
TTO	to take out		WHO	World Health Organization
TV	tidal volume		WR	Wasserman test

Part one

Chapter 1

The context of nursing

Introduction 4
What is nursing practice today? 4
Patients' perspective 4
What do organizations want from nurses? 8
Conclusion 12
References and further reading 12

Introduction

Nursing encompasses autonomous and collaborative care of individuals of all ages, families, groups and communities, sick or well and in all settings. Nursing includes the promotion of health, prevention of illness, and the care of ill, disabled and dying people. Advocacy, promotion of a safe environment, research, participation in shaping health policy and in patient and health systems management, and education are also key nursing roles.

(International Council of Nursing 2007)

Modern nursing practice is explored from two perspectives in this chapter, reminding the reader of the professional context within which any nursing procedure should be undertaken, as well as explaining how the manual can be used by nurses whether at the beginning of their career or in advanced practice roles.

What is nursing practice today?

By nature this book is very procedurally focused, but just carrying out those procedures as tasks without recognizing the humanity of the patient you are caring for is not nursing. If nurses in the UK were asked to describe their job today phrases such as: 'Too much to do too little time . . . too much paper work.' would be heard. With increasing pressure on time nursing can become about performing tasks, but the essence of nursing is not doing but being open in whatever arises in the interaction with the client. It is about being fully present in the moment with unconditional acceptance of the client's experience; with compassion and respect for their choice. Nursing involves the interaction of individuals and is a socially compassionate as well as a scientific profession (Coventry 2006).

Patients' perspective

One of the drivers for nursing practice today is expectations of patients: 'They are more knowledgeable and expect to be treated as partners and equals, and to have choices and options available to them' (DH 2006, p. 6). We know that patients want more than just a person who can carry out a series of procedures and interventions dictated by their medical condition. Recent research has explored what patients want from their nurse (Milburn et al. 1995; Williams & Iruita 2004). In these two studies the interpersonal aspect of the nurse's role was emphasized as being high on the priority list for patients. From one perspective the time to listen and talk, i.e. performing a social function, helps patients to feel respected and valued as human beings. The social interaction while intimate or difficult procedures are being carried out also provides a valuable distraction. As a patient recently commented, 'Having my chemo was so much better when it was given by a friendly chatty nurse, we talked and gossiped about all sorts'.

Specific therapeutic communication is also highly valued by patients:

. . . I want them to listen to me when I need them. When I get bad news (about this cancer) I need somebody to sit and listen and to know they don't leave you when you get bad news. They take their time . . . when you are low, they are there.

(Milburn et al. 1995, p. 1096)

Frequently even this therapeutic conversation takes place while the nurse is involved in another procedure or care activity with the patient.

Patients also talk about the importance of the nurse in the 'little things'. Reflecting on an episode of hospital care for the treatment of cancer, K.B. Schwartz wrote in *The Boston Globe* that: 'It is quiet acts of humanity that have felt more healing than the high dose radiation and chemotherapy' (Schwartz 1995). These 'little things' such as changing soiled linen or cleaning up the leaking stoma bag have been described by Darbyshire (1999) as having profound meaning for recovery and, indeed, for cure. He describes this as the essence of nursing, a caring praxis that includes the ability to be with another, sensitively minimizing embarrassing and humiliating experiences.

Practices such as these little yet very complex ones are what helps a patient towards recovery. Giving baths and getting patients to the bathroom are often considered to be the basics of nursing, so are often taken for granted and their complexity and importance are often overlooked. It is when they are carried out by an experienced nurse purposefully and with a patient-centred approach that they make a difference to patients because of the nursing knowledge and skill that is drawn upon (Macleod 1994). The depth of knowledge of the patient and possibilities for recovery influences the timing, pacing and sustainability of action (Benner 1991). Knowledge of the patient is a key component of excellent nursing practice and must be drawn upon when any care activity or procedure is carried out.

Research by Williams and Irurita (2004) found that attention to these interpersonal therapeutic aspects of care provides emotional comfort for patients, which in turn helped patients to feel in control over what was happening to them.

Dignity

When Milburn (Milburn et al. 1995, p. 1094) asked patients, 'What care they would like from a nurse?' one of the responses was, 'Being acknowledged and treated as an individual'. They described this as being treated with respect, which meant kind, prompt care and regular contact from the nurses. Patients felt care was dignified not only when they were appropriately dressed or covered but also when there was adequate allocation of time, acknowledgement of their views and feelings and the demonstration of discretion and consideration of their feelings (Walsh & Kowanko 2002).

One of the principles of the revised Nursing and Midwifery Council (NMC) Code is: 'Make the care of people your first concern, treating them as individuals and respecting their dignity' (NMC 2008). There has been much philosophical debate about the concept of dignity, particularly in the provision of care to a diverse population and the challenges of respecting the values, beliefs and practices of different cultures (Willis 1999), age groups and individuals (Coventry 2006). What does this mean in day-to-day nursing practice?

> The most powerful tool a nurse possesses to maintain and promote dignity is herself, to work with feelings, use them constructively to understand patients and to treat them as valid worthy and important at a time when they are vulnerable. In order to promote the dignity of another, feelings need to be clarified and understood, to ensure interactions and interventions are patient focused.   (Haddock 1996, p. 931)

When involved with a physical procedure for a patient, nurses can respect the dignity of the patient by discussing with the patient:

- If they would like the procedure to take place?
- When is the best time for the procedure to take place?
- Where would they like it to take place?
- Who would they like to be there?
- If they need any medication before it begins?
- If they have any questions?
- How much information they would like about the procedure?

(Adapted from Price 2004.)

Patients need to feel that they have an equal and influential role in health care. Communication not only conveys respect but it is also often the only way of assuring patients that we are interested in their experiences, perceptions and needs. Chapter 3 discusses in more depth the skills of communicating effectively with patients.

Consent

Dignity exists when an individual is capable of exerting control over his or her behaviour, surroundings and the way in which he or she is treated by others. He or she should be capable of understanding information and making decisions. He or she should feel comfortable with his or her physical and psychological status quo (Mairis 1994). Formally and legally this involves ensuring that an individual can give full and appropriate consent for the care and treatment they receive. It would be expected that a nurse would gain a patient's consent for any procedure included in this manual. The NMC (2008) states four over-riding professional responsibilities with regard to obtaining consent:

1 You must ensure that you gain informed consent before you begin any treatment or care.
2 You must be able to demonstrate that you have acted in someone's best interests if you have provided care in an emergency.

3 You must respect and support people's rights to accept or decline treatment and care.
4 You must uphold people's rights to be fully involved in decisions about their care.

'Consent' is a patient's agreement for a nurse and other health professionals to provide care (DH 2001c). The consent process is a partnership between the patient and the nurse involved. It is a two-way process that is dependent upon competence (of the provider and requester of consent) and information. Consent is a core clinical activity and is fundamental to patient care, best practice and clinical governance. Patients may indicate consent non-verbally (for example, by presenting their arm for their pulse to be taken), verbally or in writing (DH 2001c). The Department of Health (DH) guidelines, *Reference Guide to Consent for Examination or Treatment* (DH 2001c), give more details about implementing and having a robust process of consent.

Patients have a fundamental legal and ethical right to determine what happens to their own bodies. Valid consent to treatment is therefore absolutely central in all forms of health care, from providing personal care to undertaking major surgery. Seeking consent is also a matter of common courtesy between health professionals and patients.

While there is no English statute setting out the general principles of consent, case law ('common law') has established that touching a patient without valid consent may constitute the civil or criminal offence of battery. Further, if as a nurse you fail to obtain proper consent and the patient subsequently suffers harm as a result of a procedure or treatment, this may be a factor in a claim of negligence against the health professional involved. Poor handling of the consent process may also result in complaints from patients through the National Health Service (NHS) complaints procedure or to professional bodies (DH 2001c).

English common law identifies three components of a valid consent:

1 Competency.
2 Information.
3 Voluntariness.

This means the nurse has a duty to ensure the person is 'competent' to consent, has adequate information about what is going to take place and is agreeing to it voluntarily (DH 2001c). Adhering to these principles is as important whether you are seeking consent to catheterize a patient or insert a peripheral cannula. If an examination, procedure or treatment is carried out without these requirements being fulfilled then a civil action may be brought in the tort of battery, which protects a person from unwanted touching, or in the tort of negligence, where harm results directly from the procedure.

Documentation

For significant procedures, it is essential for nurses to document clearly both a patient's agreement to the intervention and the discussions that led up to that agreement.

6

Table 1.1 Examples of patient procedures that may be carried out by a nurse and the type of consent suggested.

Procedures requiring informed written consent by completion of standard consent form	Procedures requiring informed verbal consent and documentation in patient record	Implied consent (procedure discussed with patient but no formal record required)
Therapeutic ■ Chemotherapy (including instillation of chemotherapy via pleural or peritoneal aspiration; oral chemotherapy, e.g. 6 MP, methotrexate, hydroxyurea, and intrathecal chemotherapy) ■ Pleural/abdominal aspiration, drainage ■ IV/sedation for any procedure requiring it ■ Insertion of any indwelling central venous access device ■ Plasma exchange ■ Peripheral blood stem cell harvest (patient or donor) ■ Leucopheresis (therapeutic) ■ Bone marrow harvest (patient or donor) ■ Blood product transfusions *Diagnostic* ■ Breast diagnosis ■ Percutaneous biopsy, e.g. liver, breast, stereotactic wire localization ■ CT-guided biopsies *Other* ■ HIV testing and counselling ■ Photography ■ Genetic testing	■ Female patients undergoing pelvic simulation requiring insertion of vaginal tampon ■ Physio procedures (specific procedures) ■ Complementary therapies	■ Students'/visitors' attendance during treatment procedure ■ Diagnostic tests: – Plain X-ray ■ Clinical examination ■ Breast, rectal, genital examination ■ Urinary catheterization ■ Nasogastric tube insertion ■ Fine-needle aspiration ■ Bone marrow aspiration ■ Bone marrow trephine ■ Skin biopsy ■ Use of patient information ■ Venepuncture

Table 1.1 gives examples of procedures that should have written consent and those where informal consent is adequate. This may be done either through the use of a consent form (with further detail recorded in the patient's notes if necessary) or through documenting in the patient's notes that they have given oral consent.

A standard consent form should provide space for a nurse to identify what information they have provided to the patient and to sign confirming that they have done so. The nurse who provides this information must be competent to do so.

Consent is often wrongly equated with a patient's signature on a consent form. A signature on a form is *evidence* that the patient has given consent but is not *proof* of valid consent (DH 2001c). Patients who are rushed into signing a form or are given too little information or too little time may not have given valid consent, despite the signature. Similarly, if a patient has given valid verbal consent, the fact that they are physically unable to sign the form is no bar to treatment (DH 2001c). Patients are entitled to withdraw consent any time after signing a consent form; their signature acts only as evidence of the process of consent giving, it is not a binding contract.

It is rarely a legal requirement to seek written consent, but it is good practice to do so if any of the following circumstances apply:

■ The treatment or investigative procedure is complex or involves significant risks (the term 'risk' is used throughout to refer to any adverse outcome, including those which some health professionals would describe as 'side-effects' or 'complications') (DH 2001c), e.g. breast aspiration.

■ The procedure involves a local or general anaesthetic or sedation, e.g. lumbar puncture.

■ The clinical care being provided is not the primary purpose of the procedure, e.g. photography (DH 2001c).

■ There may be significant consequences for the patient's employment, social or personal life (DH 2001c), e.g. human immunodeficiency virus (HIV) testing.

■ For each course of anticancer medical therapy (cytotoxic, radiotherapy, hormonal, biological or other). NB. Course = planned treatments, e.g. one treatment, six treatments or maintenance therapy.

■ The treatment is part of a project or programme of research approved by a research ethics committee.

Consent for one procedure or course of treatment does not give any automatic right to undertake any further treatment or procedure.

Once signed, completed consent forms should be filed in the patient's medical notes. If any changes are made to a form after the patient has signed it, these should be initialed and dated by both the patient and health professional. Patients should be given a copy of the consent form that they have signed.

It is generally not necessary to document a patient's consent to routine and low-risk procedures, such as providing personal care or taking a routine blood sample. However, if the nurse has any reason to believe that the consent may be disputed later or if the procedure is of particular concern to the patient (for example, if they have declined, or become very distressed about, similar care in the past), it would be appropriate to do so (DH 2001c). The record should be put in the patient's medical notes and should specify the actual information given to the patient. The health professional carrying out the procedure is ultimately responsible for ensuring that the patient has given valid consent for what is to be done, it is they who will be held responsible in law if this is challenged later (DH 2001c).

Competent staff

Milburn (Milburn *et al.* 1995) probably not unsurprisingly found that patients considered: A good nurse is one who knows what she is doing.

The NMC Code states:

Keep your skills and knowledge up to date.
- You must have the knowledge and skills for safe and effective practice without direct supervision.
- You must keep your knowledge and skills up to date throughout your working life.
- You must recognize and work within the limits of your competence.

(NMC 2008)

As a qualified nurse there is an expectation that you will have the competence on qualifying to carry out fundamental procedures. Competence is defined in the dictionary as having, 'The ability to do something successfully or efficiently' (Pearsall 1998, p. 374). There is considerable debate as to what is needed to achieve this, whether it is just technical ability to perform a skill or whether associated knowledge and the appropriate attitude is also important (Ray 1987; Darbyshire 1999; Arthur *et al.* 2001; Musk 2004). However the NMC states that a registered nurse 'must have the knowledge and skills for safe and effective practice when working without direct supervision'. The manual has been structured to reflect this approach to professional education recognising that competence is not just about knowing how to do something but also about understanding the rationale for doing it and the impact it may have on the patient (see Table 1.2).

Competence develops over time. Benner's (1984) model of skill acquisition offers a framework to define the development from novice through to clinical expert. Based on the Dreyfus model (1982), which distinguishes between the level of skilled performance that can be achieved through principles and theory based in the classroom and context-

Table 1.2 Structure of chapters.

Definition	Each chapter begins with an explanation of the aspect of care, with any technical or difficult concepts explained
Reference material	This provides background and presents the research and expert opinion in this area. Where appropriate, the related anatomy and physiology is explained. Any specific psychological issues that the procedure may raise for the patient have also been included, so the nurse can carry out the procedure with the knowledge and the right attitude
Procedure	Each chapter includes the current procedures that are used in the acute hospital setting. They have been drawn from the daily nursing practice at The Royal Marsden NHS Foundation Trust. Only procedures where the authors have the knowledge and expertise have been included Each procedure gives detailed step-by-step actions; these are supported by rationale. For the first time, where available, the known evidence underpinning this rationale has been indicated
Illustrations	For the first time colour illustrations of the steps of some procedures are included. This will enable the nurse carrying out the procedures to see in more detail such things as the correct position of hands or the angle of a needle
Reference and reading list	The chapter finishes with a combined reference and reading list. Only recent texts from the last 10 years have been included unless they are seminal texts

dependant judgements and skill that can only be acquired in real situations (Dreyfus 1982), the manual is relevant to competence development at all levels.

Stage 1: Novice As a novice the reference material will give 'objective attributes' (Benner 1984), knowledge of features of the task that can be gained away from the situation, e.g. understanding of venous anatomy of the arm. The procedures will give 'context free rules' (Benner 1984) to guide actions that are not determined by the patient as an individual. This is the first step to technical competence (Ray 1987).

Stage 2: Advanced beginner The advanced beginner who has got some clinical experience and can use the reference material to understand what they have seen in practice and the procedures as a reminder of the steps to follow to undertake a procedure. Chapters such as Assessment (Chapter 2) and Communication (Chapter 3) will also be important at this stage to introduce the nurse to professional aspects of care that are essential in carrying out any procedure holistically as they progress to becoming a competent practitioner.

Stage 3: Competent At this stage the nurse should be familiar with carrying out core procedures, but they may need to develop problem-solving skills in respect of specific procedures. The problem-solving sections will help them to develop these techniques.

Stage 4: Proficient   Proficient nurses perceive situations as wholes. They will have integrated the knowledge skills and attitudes (Benner 1984). The manual will provide a useful reference to alert them to changes in practice and heighten awareness of the evidence underpinning practice.

Stage 5: Expert   The manual will be useful to the expert to highlight areas where further research needs to be done to establish the evidence underpinning practice. It will also be a useful reference to guide them as they learn those procedures that are new to their role.

What do organizations want from nurses?

The expert nurse is frequently being asked to take on new roles and perform procedures to meet the demands of the changing health service. The following factors in the UK are identified as driving the changes needed in nursing (DH 2006, p. 6).

- Society in the UK today is more complex, giving rise to greater social, cultural, racial and geographical diversity.
- There are more people in the older age range so long-term conditions are more prevalent. As a consequence demand for health and social care will continue to rise.
- Major causes of morbidity and mortality such as heart disease and some cancers can respond well to preventative measures, but these frequently require life style changes that can be hard to achieve.
- Health is not distributed equally and inequalities continue to be a major challenge.
- The working population is smaller so fewer people are available to enter the nursing profession.
- Rapid advances in technology mean more effective treatments as well as the ability to provide care in different settings.
- The cost of new treatments, information and communication technology means a greater focus on value for money.

Health care organizations are therefore redefining what they want from their nursing workforce.

Advanced practice

In response to the increasing complexity of health care and the diverse environments in which care takes place, advanced practice nursing roles have developed.

Initially *The New Deal* for doctors (NHSME 1991) began the debate about the areas of medical practice that could be taken over by nurses, with bold statements being made about the potential cost savings (Richardson & Maynard 1995).

With the publication of *The Scope of Professional Practice* (UKCC 1992) procedures previously carried out by doctors became the responsibility of nurses and new advanced practice roles evolved. 'Advanced practice' is an umbrella term relating to the skills, knowledge, expertise and attitude that are firmly grounded in clinical practice, and encompasses aspects of education, research, consultation and case management (Hawkins & Holcombe 1995; NMC 1999; Royal Marsden NHS Trust 2003). The new advanced practice senior clinical roles such as clinical nurse specialists, nurse consultants and nurse practitioners ensure experienced and highly skilled nurses stay close to patient care (DH 2006). The Chief Nursing Officer's '10 key roles' for Nurses in England (DH 2000) provided the legitimacy and authority needed to assume new responsibilities, like the freedom to admit and discharge patients, or order diagnostic investigations. In practice this means that nurses are undertaking procedures that are more numerous, invasive and complex than 20 years ago when the first edition of this manual was published; for example, seroma drainage, the insertion of a peripherally inserted central catheter and removal of a skin-tunnelled catheter. One of the challenges has been assessing competence at this higher level of practice (Lillyman 1998). Benner's (1984) model of skill acquisition offers a framework to define the development from novice through to clinical expert. This and her subsequent work (Benner *et al.* 1996) have been used extensively to articulate the qualities that distinguish an expert nurse and to define expert nursing care. This framework has been used to develop role development profiles, tools that:

> Support competence acquisition in relation to role developments, enabling individuals to take responsibility for planning, managing and evaluating learning and to provide the opportunity for the individual to maintain a record of their own developing competence.

(Royal Marsden Hospital 2004)

Those activities that have not previously fallen within the scope of nursing practice and for which the nurse has not received education and training may be considered to be role developments. Procedure guidelines are integral to role development and are part of the process of ensuring clinical effectiveness in 'doing the right thing the right way'. Within the UK there are constant challenges for employers to define and manage these roles because currently there is no national legislative statement of what constitutes an advanced practitioner. This also has implications for the general public as any nurse can call themselves an advanced practitioner. The NMC initiated national consultation on this aspect of nursing practice in 2005 with the view of establishing a specific part of the register for nurses who were functioning as advanced practitioners. The competencies required to undertake this role are one aspect of the consultation. These competencies have no legal standing at present but are currently being considered by the Privy Council. For further information see www.nmc.org.uk. These competences are based on those used by Royal College of Nursing Advanced Nursing Practice Programme, that were adapted for use in 2002 from the established work of the National Organization of Nurse Practitioner Faculties (NONPF) in the USA.

Cost effectiveness and patient safety

Developing new roles has obvious risks attached to it and although every individual nurse is accountable for their own actions, every health care organization has to take vicarious liability for the care, treatment and procedures that take place. An organization will have expectations of all its nurses in respect of keeping patients, themselves and the environment safe, for example having knowledge of and complying with the recent publication from the NPSA regarding the standardization of wrist bands in order to improve patient safety, which sets out the details that should be provided and the processes that should be followed on the checking and applying of wrist bands (NPSA 2007). There are the obvious ethical and moral reasons for this: 'Nurses have a moral obligation to protect those we serve and to provide the best care we have available' (Wilson 2005, p. 118).

With increasing emphasis on cost effectiveness the necessity of a registered nurse to carry out all procedures is constantly questioned. A study entitled *Improving the Effectiveness of the Nursing Workforce* (Centre for Health Economics 2003) has highlighted the shift in roles at the other end of the novice-to-expert continuum, with health care assistants taking responsibility for an increasing number of procedures that historically have been the professional domain of nursing (O'Dowd 2003). Although on a day-to-day basis this may look more cost effective, it has been demonstrated that the higher the ratio of registered nurses to patients the lower the mortality rates (Lancaster 1998; Aiken *et al.* 2002). Aiken described nurses as 'the surveillance system' (Lancaster 1998). It is not just the action of taking the vital signs, dressing the wound or starting the intravenous drip. It is the watchfulness that is always part of the nurse's thinking process while activities such as these are completed (Meyer & Lavin 2005). This has been described as vigilance. Vigilance is the search for signals. Signals are events that the individual determines to be indicators of something significant. Vigilance is not seen, it is only an action that occurs as the result of watching out and responding to the signals that others will infer that vigilance has been happening. Meyer and Lavin (2005) propose that vigilance has five components. The manual can help the nurse develop competence in vigilance:

1 Attaching meaning to what is: This is described as the ability to differentiate 'adverse signals' that indicate that there are dangers from the ordinary noise, the normal signs and symptoms. Developing theoretical and professional knowledge is an important part of learning to identify these signals. The reference material in the introductory chapters is essential to developing an understanding of the underlying physiological function or psychological response of the individual so the nurse understands what is normal.

2 Anticipating what might be: Observe, as the normal procedures and responses are described so the abnormal becomes more apparent.

3 Calculating risks: Understanding that there is an inherent risk in every situation. Problem-solving sections help to increase risk awareness and knowledge of the implications of untoward situations associated with procedures.

4 Readiness to act: Developed from a knowledge base, this allows the nurse to know what things might be required in a situation and to make sure interventions can be carried out quickly when necessary. The manual has been written by experts who are sharing years of experience of carrying out the procedures. Therefore they know what equipment is needed, have knowledge of the potential problems that might occur and, over time, they have built up solutions to address them.

5 Monitoring the results of interventions: Experts writing chapters have made explicit the source of rationale for steps in intervention process, i.e. professional knowledge.

If qualified nurses deliver care there is also an increased opportunity for patients to benefit from therapeutic nursing. Evidence demonstrates that this does contribute positively to the patient's experience of care (Spilsbury & Meyer 2001). As well as this often hidden aspect of nursing being essential to organizations, it is also essential for patients as they want to feel secure with the nurses caring for them (Williams & Irurita 2004). They want to be assured that the nurses have the ability to assess their needs as individuals as well as recognize their personal limitations and potential risks.

Clinical governance means that health care providers have a statutory duty for quality improvement to:

Continually improve the overall standard of clinical care, whilst reducing variations in outcomes of, and access to, services as well as ensuring that clinical decisions are based on the most up-to-date evidence of what is known to be effective.

(NHSE 1999a, p. 3)

With this has come an increasing focus on risk management. Risk can be defined as the possibility of incurring misfortune or loss resulting in:

- Harm to patients.
- Resources being diverted to provide extra treatment to correct the initial injury.
- Resources being diverted to the investigation of complaints, adverse incidents and medical negligence.
- Harm to the reputation of the provider because of poor performance.
- Reduction in confidence of the public.

(Adapted from Swage 2000.)

Risk management is a means of reducing the risks of adverse events occurring in organizations by systematically assessing, reviewing and then seeking ways to prevent their occurrence (NHSE 1999b).

Having robust evidence-based procedures is a necessary part of the infrastructure of effective risk management and the evidence bases for this edition of the manual will now be considered.

Evidence-based practice

Historically, nursing and specifically clinical procedures have been based upon rituals rather than research (Walsh & Ford 1989; Ford & Walsh 1994). Despite the 1972 Committee on Nursing Report chaired by Briggs identifying that nursing should become a research-based profession (Committee on Nursing 1972), this was slow to happen. Walsh and Ford in 1989 were still challenging some of the rituals that continued in nursing; for example, salt in bath water, nil by mouth from midnight (Walsh & Ford 1989). However, since this time the concept of evidence-based practice or evidence-based nursing has been introduced into health care by the DH through government policy (DH 1997).

Today, evidence-based practice is becoming an integral part of practice, education management and health care strategy and policy, with infrastructures established by the government such as the National Institute for Health and Clinical Excellence (NICE), the Centre for Evidence Based Nursing and the NHS Centre for Reviews and Dissemination at York University. These will increase the likelihood of the care that is delivered to patients being based upon evidence of what works (Rycroft-Malone *et al.* 2004a). With its roots in medicine, questions have been raised as to whether the concept of evidence-based medicine can be transferred to other disciplines within health care including nursing (Freshwater 2004). It is necessary to explore the term evidence-based practice and establish what evidence is used to base practice upon.

What is evidence-based practice?

David Sackett, a leader in the field of evidence-based medicine, defines this as:

> ... the conscientious, explicit and judicious use of current best evidence in making decisions about the care of the individual patients. The practice of evidence-based medicine means integrating individual clinical expertise with the best available external clinical evidence from systematic research. (Sackett 1996, p. 72)

Consequently it can be seen that from its inception in medicine, with the emphasis on the use of research evidence to underpin evidence-based practice, there is today an increasing emphasis on the limitations of using this alone as a basis for decisions. Rather the ability to use research evidence and clinical expertise together with the preferences and circumstances of the patient to arrive at the best possible decision for that patient is recognized (Guyatt *et al.* 2004). This then opens up challenges as to what can be regarded as evidence to facilitate clinical decision making.

When making clinical decisions clinicians use evidence that relates to the four principal interests of:

1 Feasibility: practical and possible.
2 Appropriateness: fits or is apt for a situation.
3 Meaningfulness: personal experience, opinions, values of the patient.
4 Effectiveness: achieves the intended outcome. (Pearson *et al.* 2007.)

The leaders of evidence-based practice in the past have focused more upon the evidence of effectiveness through research; however, this is beginning to change. Thus the evidence required today to support all of these principles needs to come from a range of sources, as proposed by Higgs and Jones who consider that evidence should be: 'Knowledge derived from a variety of sources that has been subjected to testing and has found to be credible' (Higgs & Jones 2000, p. 311). Knowledge can be gained that is both propositional, that is from research and generalizable, and non-propositional, that is implicit knowledge derived from practice (Rycroft-Malone *et al.* 2004b). Likewise evidence-bases can be drawn from a number of different sources, and this pluralistic approach needs to be set in the context of the complex clinical environment in which nurses work in today's NHS (Rycroft-Malone *et al.* 2004b; Pearson *et al.* 2007). The evidence-bases that can be drawn upon fall under four main areas:

1 Research.
2 Clinical experience/expertise/tradition.
3 Patient, clients and carers.
4 The local context and environment. (Rycroft-Malone *et al.* 2004b; Pearson *et al.* 2007.)

In the clinical environment, practitioners will draw upon and integrate these forms of evidence in order to deliver person-centred care.

Of the sources of evidence available, research has been regarded as the best form. However, in some areas of nursing practice there is a lack of evidence available to use to support decisions made in practice (Pearson *et al.* 2007). In addition there is also debate about the types of evidence available to support practice. Within nursing qualitative research is the prevalent design used, whilst within the field of evidence-based practice there is the perception that evidence that is quantitative in nature is superior to that which is qualitative (Rolfe & Gardner 2006). Whilst there are different opinions on the value of qualitative research to evidence-based practice it is important to consider as Mulhall suggests: 'No single design has precedence over another, rather the design chosen must fit the particular research question' (Mulhall 1998, p. 5). In practice this can be a challenge and currently there will continue to be debate and discussion on the relative merits of different research designs to evidence-based practice. This will be discussed further when considering the grading of evidence.

Clinical experience and expertise play a fundamental role in terms of evidence-based practice. However, there remains some contention in relation to the terminology, role and status within the literature (Rolfe & Gardner 2006; Pearson *et al.* 2007). A clear distinction is apparent between experience as a source of knowledge or evidence and expertise, which is the application of evidence to practice, but these terms are often used interchangeably. So a nurse may have many years of experience, been qualified for 20 years, but may not have developed knowledge as a result of this and thus is not able to apply this to develop expertise when making decisions related to her clinical practice. On the other hand a nurse may have both experience and expertise but these are difficult to capture, make explicit and ensure they are verified for a wider audience (Rycroft-Malone *et al.* 2004b). Expert opinion does have a role within evidence-based practice both within hierarchies of evidence and within the definitions of evidence-based practice, although it is often regarded as poorer evidence compared to research (Rolfe & Gardner 2006). What is perhaps most important is the blending of this knowledge with research and the sharing of this with others to contribute to the evidence-based decision making in practice (Rycroft-Malone *et al.* 2004b).

The involvement of patients in decision making about their own care and wider consultation in relation to the development of services within the NHS is a principle that has been developed and supported by the DH in relation to health care generally and cancer care more specifically (DH 1995; DH 2000). Whilst individual's experiences and preferences should be central to the practice of evidence-based health care, a study by Evans *et al.* (2003) with cancer patients found that the concept of user involvement was an alien one to a significant proportion of cancer service users. The inclusion of patient's values, experiences and preferences into evidence-based practice is complicated and difficult to achieve (Rycroft-Malone *et al.* 2004b). For example, a patient may request a new treatment but the research evidence may not be there to support it, or the patient may decline a treatment for which there is research evidence because from their experience it has unwelcome side-effects. This should not stop us from working towards the patient and carer having a greater role in the decision and care they receive. We must also be mindful that without patient participation the research we use as evidence to underpin our practice would not be possible.

The context within which health care is delivered, whilst not traditionally recognized as a base for evidence, has been suggested to contain sources of evidence that would impact upon evidence-based patient care (Rycroft-Malone *et al.* 2004b). Practitioners will draw upon both local and national sources to underpin their practice and these would include, for example, policies, patient stories, cultural context and professional networks. For some it may include the use of some of the procedures that are contained in this edition. Moreover, in today's NHS in cancer and other specialties it is evident that NICE guidance, the NHS Cancer Plan,

published patient stories, patient satisfaction surveys and other sources will influence and impact upon the delivery of patient care. What we have yet to determine is how to appraise and integrate this systematically into the evidence-based agenda in which we work.

Systems and challenges of grading evidence

Within the arena of evidence-based practice today there is requirement for the quality of the evidence to be assessed before it is used to inform practice. To do this hierarchies of evidence have been developed by a range of individuals and organizations in an attempt to identify the 'best' evidence to inform a particular decision that is required to be made in relation to a particular treatment, procedure or area of practice (Sackett 2000; Joanna Briggs Institute, NHS Centre for Reviews and Dissemination). A key underlying assumption of using such a system is that not all evidence is equivalent (Rycroft-Malone 2006) and the quality of the evidence base therefore needs to be judged in some way. Making such judgements about evidence is complex and difficult to achieve. However, the use of an explicit approach as you will find in this edition may help to facilitate critical appraisal of these judgements, provide confidence when applying evidence in practice and improve communication of this information (Grade Working Group 2004).

One of the challenges for nursing is that many of the hierarchies of evidence do not consider some of the evidence-bases discussed in this chapter and put a lower value on research evidence that is not a randomized controlled trial (RCT). To address this problem, some writers such as Rolfe and Gardner (2006) have sought to challenge this and move from an 'exclusive' hierarchy to an 'inclusive' hierarchy that does not only consider evidence from research programmes but considers all sources of evidence together. How this is achieved is under discussion in the literature, so in the interim we have established after much debate a process to grade the procedures in this edition which capture all the evidence-bases not only the research.

Grading evidence in The Royal Marsden Manual of Clinical Nursing Procedures

The evidence underpinning all the procedures has been reviewed and updated. To reflect the current trends in evidence-based practice, the evidence presented to support the procedures within the current edition of *The Royal Marsden Manual of Clinical Practice Procedures* have been graded, with this grading made explicit to the reader. The rationale for the system adopted in this edition will now be outlined.

As we have seen there are many sources of evidence and ways of grading evidence, and this has led us to a decision to consider both of these factors when referencing the

Table 1.3   Levels of evidence. Adapted from Sackett *et al*. (2000).

1a	Systematic reviews of RCTs
1b	Individual RCTs with narrow confidence limits
2a	Systematic reviews of cohort studies
2b	Individual cohort studies and low quality RCTs
3a	Systematic reviews of case-controlled studies
3b	Case-controlled studies
4	Case series and poor quality cohort and case-controlled studies
5	Expert opinion

RCTs, randomized controlled trials.

procedures. You will therefore see that references will identify if the source of the evidence was from:

- Clinical experience (Dougherty 2003: E)
- Patient (Diamond 1999: P)
- Context (DH 2000: C)
- Research (Fellowes *et al*. 2004: R)

If there is no written evidence to support a clinical experience as a justification for undertaking a procedure the text will be referenced as an 'E' but will not be preceded by an author's name.

For the evidence that comes from research this referencing system will be taken one step further and the research will be graded using a hierarchy of evidence. The levels that have been chosen are adapted from Sackett *et al*. (2000) and can be found in Table 1.3.

Taking the example above of Fellowes *et al*. (2004) 'Communication skills training for healthcare professionals working with cancer patients, their families or carer', this is a systematic review of RCTs from the Cochrane Centre and so would be identified in the references as: Fellowes *et al*. (2004: R 1a).

Through this process we hope that you the reader will be able to more clearly identify the nature of the evidence upon which the care of patients is based and that this will assist you when using these procedures in practice. You may also like to consider the evidence-base for other procedures and policies in use in your own organization and consider the evidence-base that underpins these.

Implementing evidence in practice

The implementation of evidence in practice in an organization, be that at a local level in a ward, throughout a hospital or in the community, can be demanding and requires planning, determination and time and the participation of individuals, teams and organization to effect this change. It is beyond the scope of this chapter to consider the process in detail but some key factors to consider in the successful implementation of evidence-based practice are the evidence which has been explored in detail in this chapter, the context and facilitation (Rycroft-Malone *et al*. 2002). Implementa-

tion of evidence in practice is most likely to occur when evidence is robust and inclusive, the context is receptive to change and the process is facilitated by someone who has the skills to effect change. Practice development teams in organizations may be best placed to assist with the implementation of evidence in practice.

Conclusion

This chapter has discussed the current context of health care, identifying the issues that influence the use and development of nursing procedures in the delivery of patient-centred care. The procedures in this book affect the whole person. They range from those that are observational and physically non-invasive to those involving intrusion into both the physical body and the psychological persona. The intent also varies; some are diagnostic, others therapeutic, and some are supportive with the aim of increasing well-being. This chapter seeks to remind you of the importance of seeing procedures not just as tasks but as part of the whole for the patient.

It is important to remember that even if a procedure is very familiar to us and we are very confident in carrying it out, it may be new to the patient, so time must be taken to explain it and gain consent, even if this is only verbal consent. The diverse range of technical procedures that patients may be subjected to should act as a reminder not to lose sight of the unique person undergoing such procedures and the importance of individualized patient assessment in achieving this:

> When a nurse
> Encounters another
> What occurs is never a neutral event
> A pulse taken
> Words exchanged
> A touch
> A healing moment
> Two persons
> Are never the same
>
> (Anon)
> (Dosey Keegan & Guzzetta 2005)

Nurses have a central role to play in helping patients to manage the demands of the procedures described in this manual. It must not be forgotten that for the patient the clinical procedure is part of a larger picture, which encompasses an appreciation of the unique experience of illness. Alongside this we need to be mindful of the evidence upon which we are basing the care we deliver. We hope that through increasing the clarity with which the evidence for the procedures in this edition are presented you will be better able to underpin the care you deliver to your patients in your day-to-day practice.

References and further reading

Aiken, L. *et al*. (2002) Hospital nurse staffing and patient mortality, nurse burnout and job satisfaction. *JAMA*, **288**, 1987–93.

Arthur, D., Pang, S. & Wong, T. (2001) The effect of technology on the caring attributes of an international sample of nurses. *Int J Nurs Stud*, **38**, 37–43.

Benner, P. (1984) *From Novice to Expert*. Addison Wesley, California.

Benner, P. (1991) The role of experience, narrative and community in skilled ethical comportment. *Adv Nurs Sci*, **14**(2), 1–21.

Benner, P., Tanner, C.A. & Chesla, C.A. (1996) *Expertise in Nursing Practice*. Springer, New York.

BMA (1995) *Advance Statements About Medical Treatment*. BMJ Publishing, London.

Briggs, A. (1972) *Report of the Committee on Nursing*. Cmnd 5115. HMSO, London.

Centre for Health Economics (2003) *Improving the Effectiveness of the Nursing Workforce*. University of York, York.

Committee on Nursing (1972) *Report of the Committee on Nursing*. HMSO, London.

Coventry, M. (2006) Care with dignity: a concept analysis. *J Gerontol Nurs*, **32**(5), 42–8.

Cox, C.L. & Reyes-Hughes, A. (2002) Clinical effectiveness, nursing diagnosis and the role of the clinical nurse specialist and nurse practitioner. In: *Clinical Effectiveness in Practice* (eds C.L. Cox & A. Reyes-Hughes). Palgrave, Basingstoke, pp. 1–17.

Darbyshire, P. (1999) Nursing, art and science: revisiting the two cultures. *Int J Nurs Pract*, **5**(3), 123–31.

DH (1995) *Improving the Quality of Cancer Services–A Report by the Expert Advisory Group on Cancer to the Chief Medical Officers of England and Wales*. HMSO, London.

DH (1997) *The New NHS. Modern, Dependable*. HMSO, London.

DH (1998) *A First Class Service*. Department of Health, London.

DH (2000) *The NHS Cancer Plan*. Department of Health, London.

DH (2001a) *National Service Framework for Older People*. Department of Health, London.

DH (2001b) *Essence of Care Benchmarks*. Department of Health, London.

DH (2001c) *Reference Guide to Consent for Examination or Treatment*. Department of Health, London.

DH (2002a) *Chief Nurses. Ten Key Roles*. Department of Health, London.

DH (2002b) *Discharge from Hospital: Pathway, Process and Practice*. Department of Health, London.

DH (2006) *Modernising Nursing Careers*. Department of Health, London.

Dosey, B., Keegan, L. & Guzzetta, C. (2005) *Holistic Nursing Practice*, 4th edn. Jones and Bartlett, Sudbury, MA.

Dreyfus, S.E. (1982) Formal models vs. human situational understanding: inherent limitations on modeling of business expertise. *Office: Technology and People*, **1**, 133–55, cited in Benner, P. (1984) *From Novice to Expert*. Addison Wesley, CA.

Evans, S. *et al.* (2003) User involvement in UK cancer services: bridging the policy gap. *Eur J Cancer Care*, **12**, 331–8.

Fellowes, D., Wilkinson, S. & Moore, P. (2004) Communication skills training for healthcare professionals working with cancer patients, their families and/or carers. *Cochrane Database of Syst Rev*, **2**, CD003751.

Ford, P. & Walsh, M. (1994) *New Rituals for Old*. Butterworth Heinemann, Oxford.

Fowell, A. *et al.* (2002) An integrated care pathway for the last two days of life: Wales-wide bench-marking in palliative care. *Int J Palliat Nurs*, **8**(12), 566–73.

Freshwater, D. (2004) Aesthetics and evidence based practice in nursing: an oxymoron. *Int J Human Caring*, **8**(2), 8–12.

GMC (1998) *Seeking Patients' Consent. The Ethical Considerations*. General Medical Council, London.

Goding, L. & Edwards, K. (2002) Evidence-based practice. *Nurse Res*, **9**(4), 45–57.

Grade Working Group (2004) Grading quality of evidence and strength of recommendations. *BMJ*, **328**, 1490–8.

Guyatt, G., Cook, D. & Haynes, B. (2004) Evidence based medicine has come a long way, Editorial. *BMJ*, **29**, 990–1.

Haddock, J. (1996) Towards clarification of the concept 'dignity'. *J Adv Nurs*, **24**(5), 924–31.

Hawkins, J.W. & Holcombe, J.K. (1995) Titling for advanced practice nurses. *Oncol Nurs Forum*, **22**(8), 5–9.

Higgs, J. & Jones, M. (2000) *Clinical Reasoning in the Health Professionals*, 2nd edn. Butterworth Heinemann, Oxford.

International Council of Nursing (2007) www.ICN.ch/definition. Accessed 30/3/07.

Kelson, M. (2001) Patient involvement in clinical governance. In: *Advancing Clinical Governance* (eds M. Lugon & J. Secker-Walker). Royal Society of Medicine Press, London, pp. 5–18.

Kibbe, D.C., Kaluzny, A.D. & McLaughlin, C.P. (1994) Integrating guidelines with continuous quality improvement: doing the right thing the right way to achieve the right goals. *J Quality Improvement*, **20**(4), 181–91..

Kitson, A., Harvey, G. & McCormack, B. (1998) Enabling the implementation of evidence based practice: a conceptual framework. *Qual Health Care*, **7**(3), 149–58.

Lancaster, R. (1998) Powerful nurses protecting patients. *Nurs Stand*, **13**(7), 30–1.

Lillyman, S. (1998) Assessing competence. In: *Advanced and Specialist Nursing Practice* (eds G. Castledine & P. McGee). Blackwell Science, Oxford, pp. 119–129.

Ling, J. (1997) Clinical trials, palliative care and the research nurse. *Int J Palliat Nurs*, **3**(4), 192–6.

Macleod, M. (1994) It's the little things that count: the hidden complexity of every day clinical nursing practice. *J Clin Nurs*, **3**, 361–8.

Mairis, E.D. (1994) Concept clarification in professional practice–dignity. *J Adv Nurs*, **19**, 947–53.

Mann, T. (1996) *Clinical Audit in the NHS*. NHSE, Leeds.

Meyer, G. & Lavin, M.A. (2005) Vigilance: the essence of nursing. www.nursing world.org/ojin/topic22/tpc22_6.htm. Accessed 20/4/07.

Milburn, M. *et al.* (1995) Nursing care that patients value. *Br J Nurs*, **4**(18), 1094–8.

Mulhall, A. (1998) Nursing, research, and the evidence. *Evid Based Nurs*, **1**(1), 4–6.

Musk, A. (2004) Proficiency with technology and the expression of caring: can we reconcile these polarized views? *Int J Human Caring*, **8**(2), 13–20.

NHSE (1996) *Achieving Effective Practice: A Clinical Effectiveness and Research Information Pack for Nurses, Midwives and Health Visitors*. Department of Health, Leeds.

NHSE (1997) *The New NHS: Modern, Dependable*. Department of Health, London.

NHSE (1999a) *Clinical Governance: Quality in the New NHS*. Department of Health, London.

NHSE (1999b) *Clinical Governance in London Region, Draft Template of Audit Risk Management Report for a Trust Board*. NHSE London Region, London (www.doh.gov.uk/ntro/risktemp.htm).

NHSE (2000) *The NHS Plan. A Plan for Investment, a Plan for Reform*. Department of Health, London.

NHSME (1991) *Junior Doctors: The New Deal*. NHS Management Executive, London.

NICE (2001) *Pressure Ulcer Risk Assessment and Prevention*. National Institute for Health and Clinical Excellence, London.

NICE/NHS Modernization Agency (2003) *Protocol-Based Care*. Department of Health, London (www.modern.nhs.uk/protocolbasedcare/default.htm).

NMC (1999) *A Higher Level of Practice*. Nursing and Midwifery Council, London.

NMC (2006) A–Z advice sheet: consent. www.nmc-uk.org.

NMC (2008) *The Code: Standards of Conduct, Performance and Ethics for Nurses and Midwives*. Nursing and Midwifery Council, London.

NONPF www.nonpf.org. Accessed 6/8/07.

NPSA (2007) *Standardizing wrist bands improves patient safety*. Safer Practice Notice, 3 July no. 24, National Patient Safety Agency, London.

O'Dowd, A. (2003) Who should perform the caring role? *Nurs Times*, 99(10), 10–11.

Pearsall, J. (1998) *The New Oxford Dictionary of English*. Oxford University Press, Oxford.

Pearson, A., Field, J. & Jordan, Z. (2007) *Evidence-based Clinical Practice in Nursing and Health Care*. Blackwell Publishing, Oxford.

Price, B. (2004) Demonstrating respect for patient dignity. *Nurs Stan*, 19(12), 45–51.

Ray, M.A. (1987) Techological caring: a new model in critical care. *Dimens Crit Care Nurs*, 6(3), 166–73.

Rees, E. (2001) The ethics and practicalities of consent in palliative care research: an overview. *Int J Palliat Nurs*, 7(10), 489–92.

Resuscitation Council (UK) (2000) *Resuscitation Council Guidelines*. Resuscitation Council (UK), London.

Richardson, G. & Maynard, A. (1995) *Fewer Doctors? More Nurses? A Review of the Knowledge Base of Doctor–Nurse Substitution*. Centre for Health Economics, University of Leeds, Leeds.

Rolfe, G. (2001) *Closing the Theory Practice Gap: A New Paradigm for Nursing*. Butterworth Heinemann, Oxford.

Rolfe, G. & Gardner, L. (2006) Towards a geology of evidence based practice–a discussion paper. *Int J Nurs Stud*, 43, 903–13.

Royal Marsden Hospital (2004) *Developing your role: a guide for nurses*. Royal Marsden NHS Foundation Trust, London (unpublished).

Royal Marsden Hospital Quality Assurance Department (2001) *The Relationship Between Clinical Audit and Clinical Effectiveness*. Royal Marsden NHS Trust, London.

Royal Marsden NHS Trust (2003) *Advanced Nursing Practice at The Royal Marsden NHS Trust 1999–2002*. Royal Marsden NHS Trust, London.

Rycroft-Malone, J. *et al.* (2002) Getting evidence into practice: ingredients for change. *Nurs Stan*, 16(37), 38–43.

Rycroft-Malone, J. *et al.* (2004a) An exploration of the factors that influence the implementation of evidence into practice. *J Clin Nurs*, 13, 913–24.

Rycroft-Malone, J. *et al.* (2004b) What counts as evidence in evidence-based practice? *J Adv Nurs*, 47(1), 81–90.

Rycroft-Malone, J. (2006) The politics of the evidence-based practice movements: legacies and current challenges. *J Res Nurs*, 11 (2), 95–108.

Sackett, D.L. (1996) Evidence based medicine; what it is and what it isn't. *BMJ*, 312, 71–2.

Sackett, D.L. *et al.* (2000) *Evidence-based Medicine: How to Practice and Teach EBM*, 2nd edn. Churchill Livingstone, New York.

Schwartz, K.B. (1995) 'A patient's story, 16th July'. *The Boston Globe Magazine*. www.thescwartzcentre.org/story/index.html. Accessed 2/4/07.

Smith, R. (1998) Informed consent: edging forwards (and backwards). Informed consent is an unavoidably complicated issue. *BMJ*, 316(7136), 949–51.

Spilsbury, K. & Meyer, J. (2001) Defining the nursing contribution to patient outcome: lessons from a review of the literature examining nursing outcomes, skill mix and changing roles. *J Clin Nurs*, 10(1), 3–14.

Swage, T. (2000) *Clinical Governance in Health Care Practice*. Butterworth Heinemann, Oxford.

UKCC (1992) *Scope of Professional Practice*. UKCC, London.

Walsh, K. & Kowanko, I. (2002) Nurses and patients perceptions of dignity. *Int J Nurs Pract*, 8(3), 143–51.

Walsh, M. & Ford, P. (1989) *Nursing Rituals, Research and Rational Actions*. Heinemann Nursing, Oxford.

Williams, A. & Irurita, V.F. (2004) Therapeutic and non-therapeutic interpersonal interactions: the patients' perspective. *J Clin Nurs*, 13, 806–15.

Willis, W.O. (1999) Culturally competent nursing care during the perinatal period. *J Perinat Neonatal Nurs*, 13(3), 45–59.

Wilson, C. (2005) Said another way: my definition of nursing. *Nurs Forum*, 40(3), 116–18.

Wilson, J.H. (1999) Risk reviews and using a risk management strategy. In: *Clinical Risk Modification, a Route to Clinical Governance?* (eds J. Wilson & J. Tingle). Butterworth Heinemann, Oxford, pp. 39–65.

World Health Alliance (2002) *Factsheet*. www.whpa.org/factptsafety.htm. Accessed 20/8/07.

World Medical Association (2002) *Declaration of Helsinki: Ethical Principles for Medical Research Involving Human Subjects*. World Medical Association General Assembly, Washington, DC.

Chapter 2

Assessment and the process of care

Introduction **16**
Principles of assessment **16**
Structure of assessment **17**
Methods of assessment **18**
Decision making and nursing diagnosis **20**
Planning and implementing care **22**
Evaluating care **23**
Summary of recommendations and guidance for practice **24**
Documenting and communicating care **25**
References **25**

Introduction

For many years, nurses have been expected to demonstrate their contribution to the process of patient care in a structured and comprehensive manner (RCN 2003; NMC 2005; NMC 2008). To achieve this, there is a growing body of evidence underpinning the development of common nursing languages, to enable clearer and more consistent communication and delivery of such care (Muller-Staub *et al.* 2006). In addition to this, there has been an increasing amount of emphasis placed on the importance of critical thinking skills, through thorough assessment, to form accurate clinical judgements and make evidence-based decisions, in order to provide appropriate and individualized care to patients/clients (Daly 1998; Di Vito-Thomas 2000; Seymour *et al.* 2003). Furthermore, as nursing becomes a more autonomous profession in itself, and with continuous developments of new roles and responsibilities it is of utmost importance that we are able to identify what it is that nurses are providing for patients (interventions), for what reason (nursing diagnosis) and with what results (outcomes) (Clark 1999).

Critical thinking is therefore a pivotal skill that underpins clinical judgement and decision making, and culminates in the application of knowledge and experience to clinical practice. However, many authors highlight the lack of a consensus definition around this fundamental, yet complex cognitive process (Daly 1998; Clarke & Holt 2001; Alfaro-Lefevre 2004). Based on some concept analysis work done at The Royal Marsden Hospital in 2004, the following is a definition that integrates many of the key components of critical thinking offered within the nursing literature.

> Critical thinking is a purposeful, reflective and thorough process of reasoning, using cognitive skills including synthesising, interpreting, analysing and evaluating inferences, that enables a clinical issue to be explored from all angles, before arriving at a sound judgement or decision to enhance patient care.
>
> (The Royal Marsden Hospital 2004, unpublished)

The critical thinking approach to nursing care is more than seeking a solution to a problem; it is about challenging assumptions and exploring alternatives in order to most effectively achieve a desired outcome. Critical thinking has arguably the most significant role to play in delivering a consistently high standard of nursing care with demonstrated benefits including improved documentation and enhanced clinical outcomes (Keller *et al.* 2001).

This chapter will consider the role that assessment plays, as an ongoing and central component of everyday care, which nurses achieve by using skills of observation, critical thinking, clinical judgement and communication, and by applying relevant theoretical knowledge (Crow *et al.* 1995; O'Neill & Dluhy 1997; Kennedy 1999; Alfaro-Lefevre 2002). It will then go on to explore the process of identifying nursing diagnoses, as a focus for evidence-based nursing care and identification of measurable and realistic patient outcomes. Some consideration will then be given to how such processes of care can be most effectively communicated and recorded.

Principles of assessment

Assessment is a systematic, deliberate and interactive process that underpins every aspect of nursing care (Heaven & Maguire 1996). It is the process by which the nurse and patient together identify needs and concerns and is seen as the cornerstone of individualized care. It is the only way that the uniqueness of each patient can be recognized and considered in the care process (Holt 1995). Assessment forms an integral part of patient care and should be viewed as a continuous process (Cancer Action Team 2007).

The process of assessment requires nurses to make accurate and relevant observations, to gather, validate and organize data and to make judgements to determine care and treatment needs. A nursing assessment should have physical, psychological, emotional, spiritual, social and cultural dimensions, and it is vital that these are explored with the person being assessed. The patient's perspective of their level of daily activity functioning (Horton 2002) and their educational needs are essential to help maximize their understanding and self-care abilities (Alfaro-Lefevre 2002). It is only after making observations of the person and involving them in the process that the nurse can validate his or her perceptions and make appropriate clinical judgements.

Effective patient assessment is integral to the safety, continuity and quality of patient care and fulfils nurses' legal and professional obligations in practice. The main principles of assessment are outlined below:

1 Patient assessment is patient-focused, being governed by the notion of an individual's actual, potential and perceived needs.
2 It provides baseline information on which to plan the interventions and outcomes of care to be achieved.
3 It facilitates evaluation of the care given and is a dimension of care that influences a patient's outcome and potential survival.
4 It is a dynamic process that starts when problems or symptoms develop, which continues throughout the care process, accommodating continual changes in the patient's condition and circumstances.
5 It is essentially an interactive process in which the patient actively participates.
6 Optimal functioning, quality of life and the promotion of independence should be primary concerns.
7 The process includes observation, data collection, clinical judgement and validation of perceptions.
8 Data used for the assessment process is collected from several sources by a variety of methods, depending on the health care setting.
9 To be effective the process must be structured and clearly documented.
  (Teytelman 2000; Alfaro-Lefevre 2002; White 2003; NMC 2008.)

Structure of assessment

Structuring patient assessment is vital to monitor the success of care and to detect the emergence of new problems. Different conceptual or nursing models, such as Roper *et al.* (2000), provide frameworks for a systematic approach to assessment (such as Roper's Activities of Daily Living) implying that there is a perceived value in the coexistence of a variety of perspectives. There remains, however, much debate about the effectiveness of such models for assessment in practice, some arguing that individualized care can be compromised by fitting patients into a rigid or complex structure (Tierney 1998; Kearney 2001). Nurses therefore need to take a pragmatic approach and utilize assessment frameworks that are useful and appropriate to their particular area of practice. This is particularly relevant in today's rapidly changing health care climate where nurses are taking on increasingly advanced roles, working across boundaries and setting up new services to meet patients' needs (DH 2006).

Nursing models represent a set of concepts and statements integrated into a meaningful conceptual framework (Kozier *et al.* 2003) representing different theoretical approaches to nursing care.

Nursing models can serve as a guide to the overall approach to care within a given health care environment and therefore provide a focus for the clinical judgements and decision-making processes that result from the process of assessment. It has been argued that whilst nursing models have not been widely implemented in clinical practice, nurses do use them as a way to consider the process of nursing (Wimpenny 2001). During any patient assessment, nurses engage in a collection of cognitive, behavioural and practical steps but do not always recognize them as discrete decision-making entities (Ford & McCormack 1999). Nursing models give novice practitioners a structure with which to identify these processes and to reflect on their practice in order to develop analytical, problem-solving and judgement skills needed to provide an effective patient assessment.

Nursing models have been developed according to different ways of perceiving the main focus of nursing. These include adaptation models (e.g. Roy 1984), self-care models (e.g. Orem *et al.* 2001) and activities of daily living models (e.g. Roper *et al.* 2000). Each model represents a different view of the relationship between four key elements of nursing: namely health, person, environment and nursing. It is therefore important that the appropriate model is used to ensure the focus of assessment data collected is effective for particular areas of practice (Murphy *et al.* 2000; Alfaro-Lefevre 2002). Nurses must also be aware of the rationale for implementing a particular model since the choice will determine the nature of patient assessment in their day-to-day work. The approach should be sensitive enough to discriminate between different clinical needs and flexible enough to be updated on a regular basis (Smith & Richardson 1996; Allen 1998).

In the context of cancer care, the Cancer Action Team (2007) have published guidance for an holistic common assessment for assessing the supportive and palliative care needs of adults with cancer. The content of the assessment is divided into five domains including background information and assessment preferences, physical needs, social and occupational needs, psychological well-being and spiritual well-being. The guidance recommends that a structured assessment should be undertaken at key points throughout the person's cancer illness trajectory, recognizing the importance of assessment as an ongoing process (Cancer Action Team 2007).

Incorporating these key dimensions, the framework of choice at The Royal Marsden Hospital is based on Gordon's Functional Health Patterns (Gordon 1994; Box 2.1). The framework facilitates an assessment that focuses on patients' and families' problems and functional status and applies clinical cues to interpret deviations from the patient's usual patterns (Johnson 2000). The model is applicable to all levels of care and allows all problem areas to be identified, and the information derived from the patient's initial functional health patterns is crucial for interpreting both the patient's and their family's pattern of response to the disease and treatment. It is therefore considered particularly applicable for the cancer and palliative care settings where patient's needs and responses vary enormously along their illness trajectory.

Box 2.1   Gordon's Functional Health Patterns (Gordon 1994)

- Health perception–health management
- Nutrition–metabolic
- Elimination
- Activity–exercise
- Sleep–rest
- Cognitive–perceptual
- Self-perception–self-concept
- Coping–stress tolerance
- Role–relationship
- Sexuality–reproductivity
- Value–belief

The structure of a patient assessment depends not only on the speciality and care setting but also on the purpose of the assessment. A different type of assessment will be required for an acutely ill patient where early recognition of potential or actual deterioration is essential (Ahern & Philpot 2002), from the type of assessment used for a patient with rehabilitation needs. The appropriate type of assessment depends then on the priorities of care and this varies at specific times along the patient's pathway (see Box 2.2 for a summary of the types of assessment). The single assessment process outlined in *The National Service Framework for Older People* (DH 2001) acknowledges the importance of this and highlights that assessment is a unified process where different professionals are involved in a number of stages. The process utilizes a variety of assessment levels to explore the health and social needs of a particular patient group and facilitates

Types of patient assessment (Ahern & Philpot 2002; Holmes 2003; White 2003)

Mini assessment

A snapshot view of the patient based on a quick visual and physical assessment. Consider patient's ABC (airway, breathing and circulation), then assess mental status, overall appearance, level of consciousness and vital signs before focusing on the patient's main problem.

Comprehensive assessment

An in-depth assessment of the patient's health status, physical examination, risk factors, psychological and social aspects of the patient's health that usually takes place on admission or transfer to a hospital or health care agency. It will take into account the patient's previous health status prior to admission.

Focused assessment

An assessment of a specific condition, problem, identified risks or assessment of care; for example, continence assessment, nutritional assessment, neurological assessment following a head injury, assessment for day care, outpatient consultation for a specific condition.

Ongoing assessment

Continuous assessment of the patient's health status accompanied by monitoring and observation of specific problems identified in a mini, comprehensive or focused assessment.

a collaborative, systematic and comprehensive profile of the patient's needs.

Methods of assessment

Assessment information is collected in many different formats and consists of both objective and subjective data. Nurses working in different settings rely on different observational and physical data that may include assessment of vital signs, physical systems, symptoms and laboratory results. Subjective data is based on what the patient perceives and experiences and may include descriptions of their concerns, support network, their awareness and knowledge of their abilities/disabilities, their understanding of their illness and their attitude to and readiness for learning (Coyne et al. 2002; White 2003). A variety of methods have been developed to facilitate nurses in eliciting both objective and subjective assessment data on the assumption that if assessment is not accurate, all other nursing activity will also be inaccurate.

Studies of patient assessment by nurses are few but they indicate that discrepancies between nurses' perceptions and those of their patients are common (Lauri et al. 1997; McDonald et al. 1999; Parsaie et al. 2000; Brown et al. 2001). Communication is therefore key for as Suhonen et al. (2000) suggest, 'there are two actors in individual care, the patient and the nurse' (Suhonen et al. 2000, p. 1254). Gaining

insight into patients' preferences and individualized needs is facilitated by meaningful interaction and depends both on patients' willingness and capability in participating in the process and in nurses' interviewing skills. The initial assessment interview not only allows the nurse to obtain baseline information about the patient, but also facilitates the establishment of a therapeutic relationship (Crumbie 2006). Patients may find it difficult to disclose some problems and these may only be identified once the nurse–patient relationship develops and the patient trusts that the nurse's assessment reflects concern for his or her well-being.

Assessment interviews

An assessment interview needs structure to progress logically in order to facilitate the nurse's thinking (an example of such a structure can be found in Box 2.3) and to make the patient feel comfortable in telling their story. It can be perceived as being in three phases: the introductory, working and end phases (Crumbie 2006). It is important at the beginning to emphasize the confidential nature of the discussion and to take steps to reduce anxiety and ensure privacy since patients may modify their words and behaviour depending on the environment (Neighbour 1987). In the middle working phase, various techniques can be employed to assist with the flow of information. Open questions are useful to identify broad information that can then be explored more specifically with focused questions to determine the nature and extent of the problem. Other helpful techniques include restating what has been said to clarify certain issues, verbalizing the implied meaning, using silence and summarizing (Morton 1993). It is important to recognize that there may be times when it is not possible to obtain vital information directly from the patient; they may be too distressed, unconscious or unable to speak clearly, if at all. In such situations appropriate details should be taken from relatives or friends and recorded as such. Effort should equally be made to overcome language or cultural barriers by the use of interpreters.

The end phase involves a further summary of the important points and an explanation of any referrals made. In order to gain the patient's perspective on the priorities of care and to emphasize the continuing interest in their needs, a final question asking about their concerns can be used (Alfaro-Lefevre 2002). Examples include: 'Tell me the most important things I can help you with.', 'Is there anything else you would like to tell me?', 'Is there anything that we haven't covered that still concerns you?', or 'If there are any changes or you have any questions do let me know'.

Assessment tools

The use of assessment tools enables a standardized approach to be used to obtain specific patient data. This can facilitate the documentation of change over time and the evaluation of clinical interventions and nursing care (Conner & Eggert 1994). Perhaps more importantly, assessment tools encourage patients to engage in their care and provide a vehicle for communication to allow nurses to follow patients'

Box 2.3   Carrying out a patient assessment using Functional Health Patterns (adapted from Gordon 1994)

Pattern	Assessment and data collection is focused on
Health perception–management	■ The person's perceived level of health and well-being, and on practices for maintaining health. ■ Habits that may be detrimental to health are also evaluated. ■ Actual or potential problems related to safety and health management may be identified as well as needs for modifications in the home or needs for continued care in the home.
Nutrition and metabolism	■ The pattern of food and fluid consumption relative to metabolic need. ■ Actual or potential problems related to fluid balance, tissue integrity. ■ Problems with the gastrointestinal system.
Elimination	■ Excretory patterns (bowel, bladder, skin). ■ Excretory problems such as incontinence, constipation, diarrhoea and urinary retention may be identified.
Activity and exercise	■ The activities of daily living requiring energy expenditure, including self-care activities, exercise and leisure activities. ■ The status of major body systems involved with activity and exercise is evaluated, including the respiratory, cardiovascular and musculoskeletal systems.
Sleep and rest	■ The person's sleep, rest and relaxation practices. ■ Dysfunctional sleep patterns, fatigue, and responses to sleep deprivation may be identified.
Cognitive and perceptual ability	■ The ability to comprehend and use information. ■ The sensory functions, neurologic functions.
Perception/concept of self	■ The person's attitudes toward self, including identity, body image and sense of self-worth. ■ The person's level of self-esteem and response to threats to his or her self-concept may be identified.
Stress and coping	■ The person's perception of stress and on his or her coping strategies. ■ Support systems are evaluated, and symptoms of stress are noted. ■ The effectiveness of a person's coping strategies in terms of stress tolerance may be further evaluated.
Roles and relationships	■ The person's roles in the world and relationships with others. ■ Satisfaction with roles, role strain or dysfunctional relationships may be further evaluated.
Sexuality and reproduction	■ The person's satisfaction or dissatisfaction with sexuality patterns and reproductive functions. ■ Concerns with sexuality may be identified.
Values and belief	■ The person's values, beliefs (including spiritual beliefs) and goals that guide his or her choices or decisions.

experiences more effectively. An example of this comes from the European-wide cancer nursing WISECARE project (Kearney 2001). Nurses developed systematic measurements for four chemotherapy treatment-related symptoms and this enhanced care by directly linking nursing interventions to patients' reports of their experience. Improvements in outcomes were demonstrated and patients perceived their feelings and experience had been better considered in their treatment plan (Kearney 2001).

Assessment tools in clinical practice can be used to assess patients' general needs, e.g. the supportive care needs survey (Bonevski et al. 2000) or to assess a specific problem, e.g. the oral assessment guide (Eilers et al. 1988). The choice of tool depends on the clinical setting although in general the

aim of using an assessment tool is to link the assessment of clinical variables with measurement of clinical interventions (Frank-Stromborg & Olsen 1997). To be useful in clinical practice, an assessment tool must be simple, acceptable to patients, have a clear and interpretable scoring system and demonstrate reliability and validity (Brown et al. 2001).

Nurse researchers and clinicians have developed a broad spectrum of tools to assess the problems frequently encountered by people with cancer (Box 2.4). More tools are used in practice to assess treatment-related symptoms than other aspects of care, possibly because these symptoms are predictable and of a physical nature and are therefore easier to measure. The most visible symptoms are not always those that cause most distress however (Holmes & Eburn 1989),

---

Box 2.4   Examples of assessment tools used in cancer care

Generic assessment tools

Cancer Rehabilitation Evaluation System (CARES) (Ganz *et al*. 1992)
Problems checklist (Osse *et al*. 2004)
Supportive Care Needs Survey (SCNS) (Bonevski *et al*. 2000)

Specific assessment tools

Piper Fatigue Scale (Piper 1997)
Oral assessment (Eilers *et al*. 1988)
Chemotherapy Symptom Assessment Scale (C-SAS) (Brown *et al*. 2001)
Pain and Assessment Records (PSAR) (Bouvette *et al*. 2002)

---

and acknowledgement of the patient's subjective experience is therefore an important element in the development of assessment tools (McClement *et al*. 1997; Rhodes *et al*. 2000).

The use of patient self-assessment tools appears to facilitate the process of assessment in a number of ways. It enables patients to indicate their subjective experience more easily, give patients an increased sense of participation (Kearney *et al*. 2000) and prevent patients from being distanced from the process by nurses rating their symptoms and concerns (Brown *et al*. 2001). Many authors have demonstrated the advantages of increasing patient participation in assessment by the use of patient-self-assessment questionnaires (Rhodes *et al*. 2000). A number of patient self-report tools have been developed for cancer patients as a result, and whilst many have been established for research purposes, an increasing number are being used very effectively in everyday clinical practice (Box 2.5).

The methods used to facilitate patient assessment are important adjuncts to assessing patients in clinical practice. There is a danger that too much focus can be placed on the framework, system or tool that prevents nurses thinking about the significance of the information that they are gathering from the patient (Harris *et al*. 1998). Rather than

following assessment structures and prompts rigidly, it is essential that nurses utilize their critical thinking and clinical judgement throughout the process in order to continually develop their skills in eliciting information about patients' concerns and using this to inform care planning (Edwards & Miller 2001).

Decision making and nursing diagnosis

The purpose of collecting information through the process of assessment is to enable the nurse to make a series of clinical judgements, otherwise known as nursing diagnoses, and subsequently decisions about the nursing care each individual needs. The decision-making process is based upon the cues observed, analysed and interpreted and it has been suggested that expert nurses assess the situation as a whole and make judgements and decisions intuitively (King & Clark 2002; Peden-McAlpine & Clark 2002; Hedburg & Larsson 2003), reflecting Benner's (1984) renowned novice-to-expert theory. However, others argue that all nurses use a logical process of clinical reasoning in order to identify patients' needs for nursing care and that, while this becomes more automated with experience, and perhaps more subconscious, it should always be possible for a nurse to explain how he or she arrives at a decision about an individual within their care (Putzier & Padrick 1984; Gordon 1994; Rolfe 1999). A further notion is that of a continuum, where our ability to make clinical judgements about our patients lies on a spectrum, with intuition at one end and linear, logical decisions (based on clinical trials, for example) at the other (Thompson 1999; Cader *et al*. 2005). Factors that may influence the process of decision making include time, complexity of the judgement or decision to be made, as well as the knowledge, experience and attitude of the individual nurse.

Nursing diagnosis is a term to describe both a clinical judgement that is made about an individual's response to health or illness, and the process of decision making that leads to that judgement (Box 2.6 illustrates the process of making a nursing diagnosis). The importance of thorough assessment within this process cannot be underestimated. The gathering of comprehensive and appropriate

---

Box 2.5   Examples of specific patient self-assessment tools used in cancer care

- Self Report Health History (SRHH) (Skinn & Stacey 1994)
- Memorial Symptom Assessment Scale (MSAS) (Portenoy *et al*. 1994)
- Concerns Checklist in Oncology Outpatient Setting (Dennison & Shute 2000)
- Therapy Related Symptom Checklist (TRSC) (Williams *et al*. 2001)
- Social Problems Inventory (SPI) (Wright *et al*. 2001)
- Symptoms and Concerns Checklist (Lidstone *et al*. 2003)

Box 2.6   The process of nursing diagnosis (Tanner *et al*. 1987; Gordon 1994)

- Collect information using an appropriate assessment framework.
- Identify clusters of information and consider possible nursing judgements (nursing diagnoses).
- Collect further information to verify these judgements.
- Arrive at an accurate nursing judgement (nursing diagnosis).

data from patients, including the meanings attributed to events by the patient, is associated with greater diagnostic accuracy and thus more timely and effective intervention (Gordon 1994; Hunter 1998; Alfaro-Lefevre 2002).

The concept of 'nursing diagnosis' has historically generated much debate within British literature, and it is therefore important to clarify the difference between a nursing diagnosis and a patient problem or care need. 'Patient problems' or 'needs' are common terms used within nursing to facilitate communication about nursing care (Hogston 1997). As patient problems/needs may involve solutions or treatments from disciplines other than nursing, the concept of 'patient problem' is similar to but broader than nursing diagnosis. Nursing diagnoses describe problems that may be dealt with by nursing expertise (Leih & Salentijn 1994) (Box 2.7).

Box 2.7 Characteristics of conditions labelled as nursing diagnoses (Gordon 1994)

1 Nurses can identify the condition through a process of diagnostic reasoning (assessment, problem identification).
2 The condition can be resolved primarily by nursing interventions.
3 Nurses assume accountability for patient/outcomes.
4 Nurses assume responsibility for research on the condition and its treatment.

The term nursing diagnosis also refers to a standardized nursing language, to describe patients' needs for nursing care, that originated in America over 30 years ago and has now been developed, adapted and translated for use in numerous other countries. The language of nursing diagnosis provides a classification of over 200 terms (NANDA-I 2007) representing judgements that are commonly made with patients/clients about phenomena of concern to nurses, enabling more consistent communication and documentation of nursing care (see Box 2.8 for an example of a nursing diagnosis). There are different types of nursing diagnoses within the North American Nursing Diagnosis Association–International (NANDA-I) classification system (2007), including actual nursing diagnoses (e.g. acute pain), risk nursing diagnoses (e.g. risk for falls) and wellness diagnoses (e.g. readiness for enhanced nutrition). The different types of diagnoses and the number that already exist have begun to demonstrate the diversity and complexity of nursing practice; however, it should be noted that this language is still under development and is by no means an exhaustive classification of nursing practice. Similar common languages have also been developed for nursing interventions and outcomes, as well as specific languages that have been developed for community nurses and health visitors. Whilst there are claimed to be some disadvantages to using such a standardized system to express nursing care, these are far outweighed by the advantages of having a structured and consistent system to articulate the care that is provided by nurses.

Most significantly, the use of common language enables nurses to clearly and consistently express what they do for patients and why; making the contribution of different nursing roles clearly visible within the multidisciplinary care pathway (Grobe 1996; Moen *et al.* 1999; Payne 2000; Delaney 2001; Elfrink *et al.* 2001). Secondly, an increasingly important reason for trying to structure nursing terms in a systematic way has been the need to create and analyse nursing information in a meaningful way for electronic care records (Clark 1999; Westbrook 2000). The term 'nursing diagnosis' is not commonly used within the UK as no

---

Box 2.8 An example of a nursing diagnosis (adapted from NANDA-I 2007)

Label	Acute pain
Definition Provides clear meaning of the diagnosis.	An unpleasant sensory and emotional experience associated with actual or potential tissue damage or described in terms of such damage (International Association for the Study of Pain, 2007). Sudden or slow onset of any intensity from mild to severe with an anticipated or predictable end and a duration of < 3 months.
Defining characteristics Cues to determine if the condition or response described by the diagnosis is present for the patient/client.	For example: ■ The patient states they have pain. ■ Pain assessment: numerical rating scale (0–10) pain score > 2. ■ Evidence of noxious stimuli, e.g surgery, trauma. ■ Guarding of injury. ■ Reduction on patient's normal mobility. Refer to NANDA-I (2007) for a complete list of defining characteristics.
Related factors Factors that contribute to the diagnosis being present. Individualized to each patient or client.	Injury agents (biological, chemical, physical, psychological).

definitive classifications, or common languages, are in general use; however, for the aforementioned reasons, the adaptation and implemention of standard nursing languages within clinical practice in the UK is currently being explored (Chambers 1998; Westbrook 2000; Lyte & Jones 2001).

Planning and implementing care

Nursing diagnoses provide a focus for planning and implementing effective and evidence-based care. This process consists of identifying nursing-sensitive patient outcomes and identifying appropriate interventions that will enable the individual to reach their desired outcome. However, while nurses may gather valuable information through the assessment process, it is often the case that very little of this is translated into the documentation (Ford & Walsh 1994), resulting in the standard of care bearing little relationship to the written documentation (Ford & Walsh 1994; Ballard 2006). Therefore, when planning care it is vital:

- To determine the immediate priorities and recognize whether patient problems require nursing care or whether a referral should be made to someone else.
- To identify the anticipated outcome for the patient, noting what the patient will be able to do and in what time frame. The use of 'measurable' verbs that describe patient behaviour or what the patient says facilitates the evaluation of patient outcomes (Box 2.9).
- To determine the nursing interventions, i.e. what nursing actions will prevent or manage the patient's problems so that the patient's outcomes may be achieved.
- To record the care plan for the patient which may be written or individualized from a standardized/core care plan or a computerized care plan.
  (Shaw 1998; Alfaro-Lefevre 2002; White 2003.)

Outcomes should be patient focused and realistic, stating how the outcomes or goals are to be achieved and when

---

Box 2.9 Examples of measurable and non-measurable verbs for use in outcome statements (Alfaro-Lefevre 2002, pp. 134–5)

Measurable verbs (use these to be specific)

- State; verbalize; communicate; list; describe; identify
- Demonstrate; perform
- Will lose; will gain; has an absence of
- Walk; stand; sit

Non-measurable verbs (do not use)

- Know
- Understand
- Think
- Feel

---

the outcomes should be evaluated. Patient-focused outcomes centre on the desired results of nursing care, i.e. the impact of care on the patient, rather than on what the nurse does. Outcomes may be short, intermediate or long term, enabling the nurse to identify the patient's health status and progress (stability, improvement or deterioration) over time. Setting realistic outcomes and interventions requires the nurse to distinguish between nursing diagnoses that are life threatening or are an immediate risk to the patient's safety and those that may be dealt with at a later stage. Identifying which nursing diagnoses/problems contribute to other problems (for example, difficulty breathing will contribute to the patient's ability to mobilize) will make the problem a higher priority. By dealing with the breathing difficulties, the patient's ability to mobilize will be improved.

The nature of the patient outcomes will differ according to the specific patient group or focus of the patient's nursing diagnoses. For example, patient outcomes related to safety, physiological and behavioural responses are defined in the peri-operative patient-focused model (Kleinbeck & McKennett 2000). However, in the community setting, patient and family outcomes relate to the knowledge, behaviour and signs and symptoms as described in the Omaha nursing classification system (Martin & Scheet 1992). Health visitors in the UK are now using this framework to demonstrate the effectiveness of care and to facilitate the assessment process and identify clients' progress (Clark et al. 2001). Nursing has been shown to influence patient outcomes in the hospital setting according to Lee (1999) in a review of the literature, but more research is necessary to evaluate further the interrelationship. No benefit has been identified from any studies between written care planning, record keeping and patient outcomes (Moloney & Maggs 1999; Currell et al. 2003).

The formulation of nursing interventions is dependent on adequate information collection and accurate clinical judgement during patient assessment. As a result specific patient outcomes may be derived and appropriate nursing interventions undertaken to assist the patient to achieve those outcomes (Hardwick 1998). Nursing interventions should be specific to help the patient achieve the outcome and should be evidence based. When determining what interventions may be appropriate in relation to a patient's problem, it may be helpful to clarify the potential benefit to the patient after an intervention has been performed, as this will help to ensure its appropriateness.

It is important to continue to assess the patient on an ongoing basis whilst implementing the care planned. Assessing the patient's current status prior to implementing care will enable the nurse to check whether the patient has developed any new problems that require immediate action. During and after providing any nursing action, the nurse should assess and reassess the patient's response to care. The nurse will then be able to determine whether changes to the patient's care plan should be made immediately or at a later stage. If there are any patient care needs that need immediate action, for example consultation or referral to a doctor, recording the actions taken is essential. Involving the patient and their family or friends will promote the patient's well-being and self-care abilities. The use of clinical documentation in nurse handover will help to ensure that the care plans are up to date and relevant (Alfaro-Lefevre 2002; White 2003).

Evaluating care

Effective evaluation of care requires the nurse to critically analyse the patient's health status to determine whether the patient's condition is stable, has deteriorated or improved. Seeking the patient's and family's views in the evaluation process will facilitate decision making. By evaluating the patient's outcomes the nurse is able to decide whether changes need to be made to the care planned. Evaluation of care should take place in a structured manner and on a regular basis by a registered nurse. The frequency of evaluation depends on the clinical environment within which the indi-

vidual is being cared for as well as the nature of the nursing diagnosis (problem) to which the care relates. Questions such as:

- What are the patient's self-care abilities?
- Is the patient able to do what you expected?
- If not, why not?
- Has something changed?
- Are you missing something?
- Are there new care priorities?

will help to clarify the patient's progress (Alfaro-Lefevre 2002, p. 5; White 2003). It is helpful to consider what is observed and measurable to indicate that the patient has achieved the outcome. There are a variety of different approaches to evaluating care. At The Royal Marsden Hospital a strategy known as 'charting by exception' (CBE) has been implemented, in which only exceptions to the documented care are recorded. This method is reliant on an up-to-date and individualized care plan being maintained

---

Box 2.10 Guidelines for nursing documentation (Royal Marsden NHS Trust 2005)

General principles

1 Records should be written legibly in black ink in such a way that they cannot be erased and are readable when photocopied.
2 Entries should be factual, consistent, accurate and not contain jargon, abbreviations or meaningless phrases (e.g. observations fine).
3 Each entry must include the date and the time (using the 24-hour clock).
4 Each entry must be followed by a signature and the name printed as well as:
 - the job role (e.g. Staff Nurse or Clinical Nurse Specialist);
 - if a nurse is a temporary employee (i.e. an agency nurse) the name of the agency must be included under the signature.
5 If an error is made this should be scored out with a single line and the correction written alongside with date, time and initials. Correction fluid should not be used at any time.
6 All assessment and entries made by student nurses must be countersigned by a registered nurse.
7 Health care assistants:
 - can write on fluid balance and food intake charts;
 - who have demonstrated achievement of the learning outcomes for observing and monitoring the patient's condition as defined in *The Royal Marsden Hospital Health Care Assistant Role Assessment and Development Profile* (2001) can write on observation charts;
 - must not write on prescription charts, assessment sheets, care plans or progress notes.

Assessment and care planning

1 The first written assessment and the identification of the patient's immediate needs must begin within 4 hours of admission. This must include any allergies or infection risks of the patient and the contact details of the next of kin.
2 The following must be completed within 24 hours of admission and updated as appropriate:
 - completion of nutritional, oral, pressure sore and manual handling risk assessments;
 - other relevant assessment tools, e.g. pain and wound assessment.
3 All sections of the Nursing Admission Assessment must be completed at some point during the patient's hospital stay with the identification of the patient's care needs. If it is not relevant or if it is inappropriate to assess certain Functional Health Patterns, e.g. *the patient is unconscious*, then indicate the reasons accordingly.
 The ongoing nursing assessment should identify whether the patient's condition is stable, has deteriorated or improved.
4 Care plans should be written wherever possible with the involvement of the patient, in terms that they can understand, and include:
 - patient focused, measurable, realistic and achievable goals;
 - nursing interventions reflecting best practice;
 - relevant core care plans that are individualized, signed, dated and timed.
5 Update the care plan with altered or additional interventions as appropriate.
6 The nursing documentation must be referred to at shift handover so it needs to be kept up to date.

Summary of recommendations and guidance for practice

Principles of assessment

- Assessment should be a systematic, deliberate and interactive process that underpins every aspect of nursing care (Heaven & Maguire 1996: R 5).
- Assessment should be seen as a continuous process (Cancer Action Team 2007: C).

Structure of assessment

- The structure of a patient assessment should take into consideration the speciality and care setting and also the purpose of the assessment (E).
- When caring for individuals with cancer, assessment should be carried out at key points during the cancer pathway and dimensions of assessment should include background information and assessment preferences, physical needs, social and occupational needs, psychological well-being and spiritual well-being (Cancer Action Team 2007: C).
- Functional Health Patterns provide a comprehensive framework for assessment, which can be adapted for use within a variety of clinical specialities and care settings (Gordon 1994: R 5).

Methods of assessment

- Methods of assessment should elicit both subjective and objective assessment data (E).
- An assessment interview must be well structured to progress logically in order to facilitate the nurse's thinking and to make the patient feel comfortable in telling their story (E).
- Specific assessment tools should be used, where appropriate, to enable nurses to monitor particular aspects of care, such as symptom management (e.g. pain, fatigue), over time. This will help to evaluate the effectiveness of nursing interventions whilst often providing an opportunity for patients to become more involved in their care (Conner & Eggert 1994: R 5).

Decision making and nursing diagnosis

- Nurses should be encouraged to provide rationale for their clinical judgements and decision making within their clinical practice (NMC 2005: C; E).
- The language of nursing diagnosis is a tool that can be used to make clinical judgements more explicit and enable more consistent communication and documentation of nursing care (Clark 1999; Westbrook 2000: R 5).

Planning and implementing care

- When planning care it is vital that nurses recognize whether patient problems require nursing care or whether a referral should be made to someone else (E).
- When a nursing diagnosis has been made, the anticipated outcome for the patient must be identified in a manner which is specific, achievable and measurable (NMC 2005: C; E).
- Nursing interventions should be determined in order to address the nursing diagnosis and achieve the desired outcomes (Gordon 1994: R 5).

Evaluating care

- Nursing care should be evaluated using measurable outcomes on a regular basis and interventions adjusted accordingly (The Royal Marsden Hospital; Box 2.10: C).
- Progress towards achieving outcomes should be recorded in a concise and precise manner. Using a method such as charting by exception can facilitate this (Murphy 2003: R 5).

Documenting and communicating care

- The content and quality of record keeping are a measure of standards of practice relating to the skills and judgement of the nurse (NMC 2005: C).
- In addition to the written record of care, the important role that the nursing shift report, or 'handover', plays in the communication and continuation of patient care should be considered, particularly when considering the role of electronic records (Ballard 2006: R 5).

and is based on the assumption that, through observation and assessment, the nurse makes a judgement that the care has been provided according to the care plan. If for any reason this is not the case, i.e. if particular interventions have not been provided or if they are now deemed inappropriate, then this would be documented as an exception to the care planned (Murphy 2003).

Documenting and communicating care

Nurses have a professional responsibility to ensure that health care records provide an accurate account of treatment, care planning and delivery, and are viewed as a tool of communication within the team. There should be 'clear evidence of the care planned, the decisions made, the care delivered and the information shared' (NMC 2005, p. 8). The content and quality of record keeping are a measure of standards of practice relating to the skills and judgement of the nurse (NMC 2005). Thus communication and assessment skills are integral to providing quality care.

The ability to develop good practice in record keeping is considered to be an area for improvement by nurses (Frank-Stromborg & Christensen 2001a, b; Rodden & Bell 2002; Wood 2003). Record keeping is an integral part of nursing care (NMC 2005), and the purpose of health records is to ensure that those coming after you can see what has been done, or not done, why and by whom (NHSE 1999). This will ensure not only that patient care is not compromised but also that any decisions made can be justified or reconsidered at a later date (NHSE 1999). Box 2.10 provides some key guidance for documentation.

In addition to the written record of care, it is also important to consider the significant role that the nursing shift report, or 'handover', plays in the communication and continuation of patient care, particularly when considering the role of electronic records in enhancing such systems of communication (Ballard 2006). Inter-shift reports can be classified into four different styles, namely the recorded, bedside, written and the verbal (Miller 1998) and each has its benefits and disadvantages. Whilst often seen as a ritual, it is suggested that handover is a ritual that is necessary for team building and continuity of care (Strange 1996; Williams 1998; Lally 1999); however, the question often arises as to what extent such a variety of approaches to handover actually reflect documented care, and vice versa. Rather than referring to the care plan during handover, it has been found that elements such as vital signs, comfort measures and medications are most often referred to (Lally 1999). However if a care plan-orientated style was to be used, it is suggested this can result in improved documentation and the realization that nursing diagnoses (care needs), rather than medical diagnoses, are the primary focus when delivering nursing care (Wallum 1995; Webster 1999). As nursing moves towards electronic methods of documentation, the issue of how such electronic records of nursing care are integrated into shift reports warrants greater attention.

References

Ahern, J. & Philpot, P. (2002) Assessing acutely ill patients on general wards. *Nurs Stand*, 16(47), 47–52.

Alfaro-Lefevre, R. (2002) *Applying Nursing Process: Promoting Collaborative Care*. Lippincott, Williams & Wilkins, Philadelphia.

Alfaro-Lefevre, R. (2004) *Critical Thinking and Clinical Judgement: a Practical Approach*, 3rd edn. Saunders, MO.

Allen, D. (1998) Record-keeping and routine practice: the view from the wards. *J Adv Nurs*, 27(6), 1223–30.

Ballard, E. (2006) Improving information management in ward nurses practice. *Nurs Stand*, 20(50), 43–8.

Benner, P. (1984) *From Novice to Expert: Excellence and Power in Clinical Nursing Practice*. Addison Wesley, Menlo-Park, CA.

Bonevski, B. *et al.* (2000) Evaluation of an instrument to assess the needs of patients with cancer. *Cancer*, 88, 215–17.

Bouvette, M., Fothergill-Bourbonnais, F. & Perreault, A. (2002) Implementation of the Pain and Symptom Assessment Record (PSAR). *J Adv Nurs*, 40(6), 685–700.

Brown, V. *et al.* (2001) The development of the Chemotherapy Symptom Assessment Scale (C-SAS): a scale for the routine clinical assessment of the symptom experiences of patients receiving cytotoxic chemotherapy. *Int J Nurs Stud*, 38(5), 497–510.

Cader, R., Campbell, S. & Watson, D. (2005) Cognitive continuum theory in nursing decision-making. *J Adv Nurs*, 49(4), 397–405.

Cancer Action Team (2007) *Holistic Common Assessment of Supportive and Palliative Care Needs for Adults with Cancer: Assessment Guidance*. Cancer Action Team, London.

Chambers, S. (1998) Nursing diagnosis in learning disabilities nursing. *Br J Nurs*, 7(19), 1177–81.

Clark, J. (1999) A language for nursing. *Nurs Stand*, 13(31), 42–7.

Clark, J. *et al.* (2001) Professional briefing. New methods of documenting health visiting practice. *Community Pract*, 74(3), 108–12.

Clarke, D.J. & Holt, J. (2001) Philosophy: a key to open the door to critical thinking. *Nurse Educ Today*, 21, 71–8.

Conner, F.W. & Eggert, L.L. (1994) Psychosocial assessment for treatment planning and evaluation. *J Psychosoc Nurs Ment Health Serv*, 32(5), 31–42.

Coyne, P.J., Lyne, M.E. & Watson, A.C. (2002) Symptom management in people with AIDS. *Am J Nurs*, 102(9), 48–57.

Crow, R.A., Chase, J. & Lamond, D. (1995) The cognitive component of nursing assessment: an analysis. *J Adv Nurs*, 22, 206–12.

Crumbie, A. (2006) Taking a history. In: *Nurse Practitioners Clinical Skills and Professional Issues* (ed. M. Walsh). Butterworth Heinemann, Edinburgh, pp. 14–26.

Currell, R., Wainwright, P. & Urquhart, C. (2003) Nursing record systems: effects on nursing practice and health care outcomes. *Cochrane Database of Systematic Reviews*, Issue 3.

Daly, W.M. (1998) Critical thinking as an outcome of nursing education. What is it? Why is it important to nursing practice? *J Adv Nurs*, 28(2), 323–31.

Delaney, C. (2001) Health informatics and oncology nursing. *Semin Oncol Nurs*, 17(1), 2–6.

Dennison, S. & Shute, T. (2000) Identifying patient concerns: improving the quality of patient visits to the oncology outpatient department–a pilot audit. *Eur J Oncol Nurs*, 4(2), 91–8.

DH (2001) *The National Service Framework for Older People*. Department of Health, London.

DH (2006) *Modernising Nursing Careers: Setting the Direction*. Department of Health, London.

Di Vito-Thomas, P. (2000) Identifying critical thinking behaviours in clinical judgements. *J Nurses Staff Dev*, 16(4), 174–80.

Edwards, M. & Miller, C. (2001) Improving psychosocial assessment in oncology. *Prof Nurse*, 16(7), 1223–6.

Eilers, J., Berger, A.M. & Peterson, M.C. (1988) Development, testing and application of the oral assessment guide. *Oncol Nurs Forum*, 15(3), 325–30.

Elfrink, V. et al. (2001) Standardised nursing vocabularies: a foundation for quality care. *Semin Oncol Nurs*, 17(1), 18–23.

Ford, P. & McCormack, B. (1999) Determining older people's need for registered nursing in continuing health care: the contribution of The Royal College of Nursing's Older People's Assessment Tool. *J Clin Nurs*, 8(6), 731–42.

Ford, P. & Walsh, M. (1994) *New Rituals for Old. Nursing Through the Looking Glass*. Butterworth Heinemann, Oxford.

Frank-Stromborg, M. & Christensen, A. (2001a) Nurse documentation: not done or worse, done the wrong way–part I. *Oncol Nurs Forum*, 28(4), 697–702.

Frank-Stromborg, M. & Christensen, A. (2001b) Nurse documentation: not done or worse, done the wrong way–part II. *Oncol Nurs Forum*, 28(5), 841–6.

Frank-Stromborg, M. & Olsen, S.J. (1997) *Instruments for Clinical Healthcare–Research*, 2nd edn. Jones & Bartlett, London.

Ganz, P.A. et al. (1992) The CARES: a generic measure of health-related quality of life for patients with cancer. *Quality of Life Research*, 1, 19–29.

Gordon, M. (1994) *Nursing Diagnosis, Process and Application*. Mosby, St. Louis.

Grobe, S.J. (1996) The nursing intervention lexicon and taxonomy. Implications for representing nursing care in automated patient records. *Holist Nurs Pract*, 11(1), 48–63.

Hardwick, S. (1998) Clarification of nursing diagnosis from a British perspective. *Assignment*, 4(2), 3–9.

Harris, R. et al. (1998) Patient assessment: validation of a nursing instrument. *Int J Nurs Stud*, 35, 303–13.

Heaven, C.M. & Maguire, P. (1996) Training hospice nurses to elicit patient concerns. *J Adv Nurs*, 23, 280–6.

Hedburg, B. & Larsson, U.S. (2003) Observations, confirmations and strategies–useful tools in decision-making process for nurses in practice. *J Clin Nurs*, 12(2), 215–22.

Hogston, R. (1997) Nursing diagnosis and classification systems: a position paper. *J Adv Nurs*, 26, 496–500.

Holmes, H.N. (ed.) (2003) *Three-minute Assessment*. Lippincott, Williams & Wilkins, Philadelphia, pp. 1–32.

Holmes, S. & Eburn, E. (1989) Patients' and nurses' perceptions of symptom distress in cancer. *J Adv Nurs*, 14(7), 575–81.

Holt, P. (1995) Role of questioning in patient assessment. *Br J Nurs*, 4, 1145–6.

Horton, R. (2002) Differences in assessment of symptoms and quality of life between patients with advanced cancer and their specialist palliative care nurses in a home care setting. *Palliat Med*, 16(6), 488–94.

Hunter, M. (1998) Rehabilitation in cancer care: a patient focused approach. *Eur J Cancer Care*, 7, 85–7.

Johnson, T. (2000) Functional health pattern assessment on-line: lessons learned. *Comput Nurs*, 18(5), 248–54.

Kearney, N. (2001) Classifying nursing care to improve patient outcomes; the example of WISECARE. *NT Research*, 6(4), 747–56.

Kearney, N. et al. (2000) Collaboration in cancer nursing practice. *J Clin Nurs*, 9, 429–35.

Keller, C.A., Carolin, K. & Fedoronko, K. (2001) Bone marrow transplant teaching rounds: promoting excellence in nursing care. *Oncol Nurs Forum*, 28(3), 457–8.

Kennedy, C. (1999) Decision making in palliative nursing practice. *Int J Palliat Nurs*, 5(3), 142–6.

King, L. & Clark, J.M. (2002) Intuition and the development of expertise in surgical ward and intensive care nurses. *J Adv Nurs*, 37(4), 322–9.

Kleinbeck, S. & McKennett, M. (2000) Challenges of measuring intraoperative patient outcomes. *AORN J*, 72(5), 845–50, 853.

Kozier, B. et al. (2003) *Fundamentals of Nursing: Concepts, Process and Practice*, 7th edn. Addison Wesley, Menlo Park CA.

Lally, S. (1999) An investigation into the functions of nurses' communication at the inter-shift handover. *J Nurs Manag*, 7(1), 29–36.

Lauri, S., Lepisto, M. & Kappeli, S. (1997) Patients' needs in hospital: nurses' and patients' views. *J Adv Nurs*, 25, 339–46.

Lee, J. (1999) Does what nurses do affect clinical outcomes for hospitalized patients? A review of the literature. *Health Serv Res*, 34(5), 1011–32.

Leih, P. & Salentijn, C. (1994) Nursing diagnosis: a Dutch perspective. *J Clin Nurs*, 3, 313–20.

Lidstone, V. et al. (2003) Symptoms and concerns amongst cancer outpatients: identifying the need for specialist palliative care. *Palliat Med*, 17, 588–95.

Lyte, G. & Jones, K. (2001) Developing a unified language for children's nurses, children and their families in the United Kingdom. *J Clin Nurs*, 10, 79–85.

Martin, K. & Scheet, N. (1992) *The Omaha System: a Pocket Guide for Community Health Nursing*. W.B. Saunders, Philadelphia, pp. 37–41.

McClement, S.E., Woodgate, R.L. & Degner, L. (1997) Symptom distress in adults with cancer. *Cancer Nurs*, 20(4), 236–43.

McDonald, M.V. et al. (1999) Nurses' recognition of depression in their patients with cancer. *Oncol Nurs Forum*, 26(3), 593–9.

Miller, C. (1998) Ensuring continuing care: styles and efficiency of the handover process. *Aust J Adv Nurs*, 16(1), 23–7.

Moen, A. et al. (1999) Representing nursing judgements in the electronic record. *J Adv Nurs*, 30(4), 990–7.

Moloney, R. & Maggs, C. (1999) A systematic review of the relationships between written manual nursing care planning, record keeping and patient outcomes. *J Adv Nurs*, 30(1), 51–7.

Morton, P.G. (1993) *Health Assessment in Nursing*, 2nd edn. Springhouse, Philadelphia.

Muller-Staub, M., Lavin, M. & Needham, I. (2006) Nursing diagnoses, interventions and outcomes: application and impact on nursing practice: systematic review. *J Adv Nurs*, 56(5), 514–31.

Murphy, E.K. (2003) Charting by exception. *AORN J*, 78(5), 821–3.

Murphy, K. et al. (2000) The Roper, Logan and Tierney (1996) model: perceptions and operationalization of the model in psychiatric nursing within a Health Board in Ireland. *J Adv Nurs*, 31(6), 1333–41.

NANDA-I (2007) *Nursing Diagnoses: Definitions and Classification 2007–2008*. North American Nursing Diagnosis Association – International, Philadelphia.

Neighbour, R. (1987) *The Inner Consultation*. MTP Press, Lancaster.

NHSE (1999) *For the Records: Managing Records in NHS Trusts and Health Authorities (HSC 199/53 1999)*. NHSE, London.

NMC (2008) *The Code: Standards of Conduct, Performance and Ethics for Nurses and Midwives*. Nursing and Midwifery Council, London.

NMC (2005) *Guidelines for Records and Record Keeping*. Nursing and Midwifery Council, London.

O'Neill, E.S. & Dluhy, N.M. (1997) A longitudinal framework for fostering critical thinking and diagnostic reasoning. *J Adv Nurs*, 26, 825–32.

Orem, D.E., Taylor, S.G. & Renpenning, K. (2001) *Nursing: Concepts of Practice*, 6th edn. Mosby, St. Louis.

Osse, B.H. *et al.* (2004) Towards a new clinical tool for needs assessment in the palliative care of cancer patients: the PNPC Instrument. *J Pain Symptom Manage*, 28(4), 329–41.

Parsaie, F.A., Golchin, M. & Asvadi, I. (2000) A comparison of nurse and patient perceptions of chemotherapy treatment stressors. *Cancer Nurs*, 23(5), 371–4.

Payne, J. (2000) The nursing interventions classification: a language to define nursing. *Oncol Nurs Forum*, 27(1), 99–103.

Peden-McAlpine, C. & Clark, N. (2002) Early recognition of client status changes: the importance of time. *Dimens Crit Care Nurs*, 21(4), 144–50.

Piper, B.F. (2004) Measuring fatigue. In: *Instruments for Clinical Health Care Research* (eds M. Frank-Stromborg & S.J. Olsen), 3rd edn. Jones & Bartlett, MA, pp. 538–569.

Portenoy, R.K. *et al.* (1994) The Memorial Symptom Assessment Scale: an instrument for the evaluation of symptom prevalence, characteristics and distress. *Eur J Cancer*, 30(a), 1326–36.

Price, C.I.M., Han, S.W. & Rutherford, I.A. (2000) Advanced nursing practice; an introduction to physical assessment. *Br J Nurs*, 12(4), 22–5.

Putzier, D.J. & Padrick, K.P. (1984) Nursing diagnosis: a component of nursing process and decision-making. *Top Clin Nurs*, 5(1), 21–9.

RCN (2003) *Defining Nursing*. Royal College of Nursing: London.

Rhodes, V.A. *et al.* (2000) An instrument to measure symptom experience: symptom occurrence and symptom distress. *Cancer Nurs*, 23(1), 49–54.

Rodden, C. & Bell, M. (2002) Record keeping: developing good practice. *Nurs Stand*, 17(1), 40–2.

Rolfe, G. (1999) Insufficient evidence: the problems of evidence-based nursing. *Nurse Educ Today*, 19(6), 433–42.

Roper, N., Logan, W. & Tierney, A.J. (2000) *The Roper Logan Tierney Model of Nursing: Based on Activities of Living*. Churchill Livingstone, Edinburgh.

Roy, C. (1984) *Introduction to Nursing: an Adaptation Model*, 2nd edn. Prentice Hall, New Jersey.

Royal Marsden NHS Trust (2001) The Royal Marsden Hospital Health Care Assistant Role Assessment and Development profile. Unpublished.

Royal Marsden NHS Trust (2005) Guidelines for Nursing Documentation. Unpublished.

Seymour, B., Kinn, S. & Sunderland, N. (2003) Valuing both critical and creative thinking in clinical practice: narrowing the research–practice gap. *J Adv Nurs*, 42(3), 288–96.

Shaw, M. (1998) *Charting Made Incredibly Easy!* Springhouse Corporation, Springhouse PA.

Skinn, B. & Stacey, D. (1994) Establishing an integrated framework for documentation: use of a self-reporting health history and outpatient oncology record. *Oncol Nurs Forum*, 21(9), 1557–66.

Smith, G. & Richardson, A. (1996) Development of nursing documentation for use in the outpatient oncology setting. *Eur J Cancer Care*, 5, 225–32.

Strange, F. (1996) Handover: an ethnographic study of ritual in nursing practice. *Intensive Crit Care Nurs*, 12(2), 106–12.

Suhonen, R., Valimaki, M. & Katajisto, J. (2000) Developing and testing an instrument for the measurement of individual care. *J Adv Nurs*, 32(5), 1253–63.

Tanner, C.A. *et al.* (1987) Diagnostic reasoning strategies of nurses and nursing students. *Nurs Res*, 36(6), 358–62.

Teytelman, Y. (2000) Effective nursing documentation and communication. *Semin Oncol Nurs*, 18(2), 121–7.

Thompson, C. (1999) A conceptual treadmill: the need for 'middle ground' in clinical decision making theory in nursing. *J Adv Nurs*, 30(5), 1222–9.

Tierney, A.J. (1998) Nursing models; extant or extinct? *J Adv Nurs*, 28(1), 77–85.

Wallum, R. (1995) Using care plans to replace the handover. *Nurs Stand*, 9(32), 24–6.

Webster, J. (1999) Practitioner-centred research: an evaluation of the implementation of the bedside hand-over. *J Adv Nurs*, 30(6), 1375–82.

Wenzel, G. (2002) Creating an interactive interdisciplinary electronic assessment. *Comput Inform Nurs*, 20(6), 251–60.

Westbrook, A. (2000) Learning curve. Nursing language. *Nurs Times*, 96(14), 41.

White, L. (2003) *Documentation and the Nursing Process*. Delmar Learning, Clifton Park, NY.

Williams, J. (1998) Managing change in the nursing handover. *Nurs Stand*, 12(18), 39–42.

Williams, P.D. *et al.* (2001) Treatment type and treatment severity among oncology patients by self-report. *Int J Nurs Stud*, 38, 359–67.

Wimpenny, P. (2001) The meaning of models of nursing to practising nurses. *J Adv Nurs*, 40(3), 346–54.

Wood, C. (2003) The importance of good record-keeping for nurses. *Nurs Times*, 99(2), 26–7.

Wright, E.P. *et al.* (2001) Feasibility and compliance of automated measurement of quality of life in oncology practice. *J Clin Oncol*, 21(2), 374–82.

27

Chapter 3

Communication

29 Reference material
30 *Procedure guidelines*: Provision of information
39 Conclusion
39 References

Definition

Communication is a reciprocal process that involves the exchange of both verbal and non verbal messages to convey feelings, information, ideas and knowledge (Wilkinson 1999; Wallace 2001).

Reference material

High quality communication is crucial for the delivery of nursing care and connects the psychological, social and physical domains of patient care.

Good communication involves careful consideration of the patient's perspective. Listening to and supplying patients with the information to understand their illness, treatment and care will support those patients to get what they want from health care services. This will contribute to the efficacy of treatment and result in better care delivery, the promotion of more successful psychological support and consequent patient satisfaction.

It might never be possible to capture a pure and all encompassing description of communication to follow as a procedure; however, it is possible to isolate and define the ingredients of 'communication' and the strategies required to interact well and therefore learn the skills of good communication (Hargie & Dickson 2004; Back *et al.* 2005).

Specific consideration is given to communication in cancer care, although it can be argued that good communication follows similar patterns across a range of situations and disciplines.

Where 'patient' is described this can be extended to include conversations with family members and significant acquired relationships. Extending communication and support to family members (with the consent of the patient) is a crucial way of including personal and social aspects of life, promoting self help, informal support and a genuine understanding of the patient.

People with potentially life-limiting illnesses such as cancer want, among other things:

- Open communication (Heyland *et al.* 2006).
- Clear, honest information (Baile *et al.* 2000; Jenkins *et al.* 2001; Smith *et al.* 2005).
- Emotional support (Smith *et al.* 2005).

Relevant issues in communication

'Psychological distress is common among people affected by cancer' (NICE 2004, p. 9) and effective communication is widely regarded to be a key determinant of patient satisfaction, compliance and recovery (Chant *et al.* 2002), yet poor communication is one of the commonest causes of complaints in health care (Cambell 2006).

It is therefore necessary to have appropriate communication skills and be confident enough to utilize them in our clinical practice.

Numerous issues have been highlighted by the National Institute for Health and Clinical Excellence (NICE) that res-

onate powerfully when considering how nurses communicate with patients and relatives in cancer care.

Our responsibility lies in ensuring that, 'All patients undergo systematic psychological assessment at key points and have access to appropriate psychological support' (NICE 2004, p. 9).

This means more than referring psychological issues on to appropriate services, it means:

- Recognizing psychological needs on a par with physical needs.
- Being able to maintain a compassionate dialogue.
- Addressing psychological needs with exploratory communication skills.
- Providing emotional support via the skills illustrated in this chapter.
- Understanding the concerns of patients and relatives.

Issues in service provision

Health professionals and nurses especially are considered to be caring. The human suffering generated by illnesses such as cancer might be expected to stimulate an instinctive ability for human connection and empathy.

It might also be sensibly assumed that experience in the field of oncology nursing would have developed communication skills to a level where emotional and psychological support is consistently and skilfully provided to patients and relatives.

The evidence however can contradict these assumptions: 'Research suggests communication skills do not reliably improve with experience' (Cantwell & Ramirez 1997).

Psychological support needs improvement (Maguire *et al.* 1996) and this is highlighted when considering why patients' needs are not always met: 'Professionals are not eliciting the patients' problems or concerns' (NICE 2004, p. 16). 'Patients and carers frequently report the communication skills of health practitioners to be poor' (NICE 2004, p. 8).

Data from the Department of Health (DH) in the UK for the period 2003–04 illustrated that complaints relating to the attitude of staff and communication (written and oral) accounted for nearly 20 000 out of 90 000 complaints (22%) (DH 2005).

The close relationship between good communication and emotional support (NICE 2004, p. 56) should compel our profession to pay greater attention to communication skill development and use.

Reasons for communication problems

A bias towards physical and task related functions in nurse education and problems in the style of communication training may be partly responsible for the evidence seen (Chant *et al.* 2002).

It is still not uncommon to hear qualified nurses outlining the limitations of their education in relation to communication with patients. In practice, confidence is frequently reported to be low in managing commonly occurring emotive situations, e.g. patient's emotional distress.

Evidence also suggests that internal and institutional social barriers can exist within health services that make patient-centred communication difficult and less valued than technical ability (Chant *et al*. 2002; McCabe 2004).

Ward sisters/charge nurses can have a major impact on the style and quality of communication in the workplace (Wilkinson 1991) and therefore have some responsibility for role modelling good communication.

Working in high mortality areas is not without its burdens, and issues like 'death anxiety' are hypothesized to have an impact on our 'comfort level' when talking about serious illness and issues relating to death (Deffner & Bell 2005). End-of-life discussions and high degrees of emotional disclosure are areas that we find difficulty engaging with (Booth *et al*. 1996; Edwards 2005).

Good practice in end-of-life care is, however, not out of reach and is demonstrated by psycho-socially mature staff with well-developed communication skills.

Institutional anxiety about communication and psychological distress/crises is likely to have a negative impact upon the successful management of such issues.

The potential to feel unskilled and inadequately trained to deal with emotional distress and end-of-life issues can be addressed via focused and proven learning of fundamental communication skills. Once applied in the clinical environment these skills are potentially sufficient to provide the necessary emotional support to most patients. These skills are tools by which we can connect more effectively with people, but will only remain effective when coupled with a genuine sense of caring and compassion.

Guidelines for providing information to patients and discussing procedures to be carried out

With any procedure explained within this manual, it is essential that the patient (assuming consciousness and ability to make rational decisions) is psychologically prepared and consented. This requires careful explanation and discussion before a procedure is carried out.

It is easy perhaps for us to become so familiar with procedures that we expect them to be considered 'routine' by our patients. This can prevent us from providing thorough and necessary information and gaining acceptance and co-operation from our patients.

We therefore need to avoid assuming that repetitive or frequent procedures do not require consent, explanation and potential discussion, e.g. taking a temperature.

Procedure guidelines **Provision of information**

Procedure

Action	Rationale
1 Review the changing context of the patient's situation.	
2 Prepare for discussion.	
3 Consider whether the procedure is necessary.	
4 Make use of appropriate patient leaflets.	
5 If possible discuss the procedure some time before it is to be carried out.	Give patients the opportunity to digest information in their own time (Lowry 1995: E). In certain groups it can be demonstrated to improve clinical outcomes; satisfaction; chances of meeting the targeted discharge date; and return to prior functional status sooner (Lookinland & Pool 1998: R 2b).
6 Introduce yourself.	Ensure patient understands who you are and your role and specific aim. Promote patient satisfaction (Delvaux *et al*. 2004: R 1b).
7 Maintain a warm and approachable demeanour. Do not rush.	Promote patient satisfaction (Delvaux *et al*. 2004: R 1b).
8 Explain that you have a procedure to carry out, considering privacy in giving information.	Promote dignity/preserve confidentiality (NMC 2008: C).
9 Name the procedure. Elicit, clarify and check the information gathered by the patient.	Promote understanding and patient satisfaction.

10	Explain the procedure avoiding the use of medical jargon. Be prepared to repeat information or rephrase until understanding at the patient's desired level is reached. (If understanding is not achieved, consent has not been achieved.)	Establish mutual understanding. Gain compliance with procedure: minimize risk (NMC 2008: C). Improve outcome and reduce nurses' stress (Fellowes *et al.* 2004: R 1a). Help patients manage side effects and adhere to care and treatment (Chelf *et al.* 2001: R 3a).
11	Confirm consent: ensure that the patient is happy for you to proceed. Allow the patient an opportunity to ask further questions or say no to the procedure. (Full understanding may reveal that the patient is not ready to proceed.)	Respecting the rights of the individual (NMC 2008). Obtaining consent correctly (DH 2001: C; NMC 2006: C).
12	Start the procedure, reiterating the main issues as you go along and keeping the patient updated by progress.	To maintain open dialogue and address issues and questions, as they arise.
13	Make it clear when the procedure has finished and what has been achieved. Offer opportunity for discussion of implications and situation, disclosing information at a level the patient wishes.	So that the patient is aware and has the information they need and want (Jenkins *et al.* 2001: R 2b).

It is important to consider giving information in small amounts and check whether the patient understands what has been said after each part has been explained. Keep language simple and clarify common and complex medical terms, e.g. 'cannula', 'catheter'.

Check frequently whether the patient wishes you to continue to provide them with the same level of information. If confusion is arising, consider whether you are providing too much detail, or using too many medical terms. Be aware whether the patient is paying attention or appears anxious (e.g. fidgety/non-attentive behaviour). Do not ignore these cues: name them. For example: 'I notice you seem a little anxious while I am describing this…' or, 'You seem concerned about the procedure, what can I do to help'? This recognition of behaviour will help to fully explore and support the patient's concerns.

Prior to starting, establish how the patient can communicate with you during the procedure, e.g. confirm they can ask questions, request more analgesia or ask for the procedure to stop (if this is realistic).

Information must be presented accurately and calmly and without 'false reassurance', e.g. do not say something 'will not hurt' or it 'will not go wrong', when it might. It is better to explain the risk and likely outcome. Explain that working with the nurse and co-operating with instructions is likely to improve the outcome and that every effort will be made to reduce risk and manage any problems efficiently.

Respect any refusal unconditionally; however, you may wish to explore the reasons for refusal and explain the potential (realistic) consequences. Document carefully and discuss with the multidisciplinary team. If a patient has had a procedure before do not assume they are fully aware of the potential experience or risk involved, which may well have changed.

Attention to good communication, honesty, confidence and calmness will help to reassure the patient, thus gaining their compliance and improving the potential outcome (Maguire & Pitceathly 2002).

Giving the right amount of information is important; for example, it has been shown that getting the level of information wrong (too much or too little) at diagnosis can significantly impact upon the subsequent level of coping (Fallowfield *et al.* 2002). Getting the level right can be achieved by simply asking how much people want to know and frequent checking if the level of information is satisfactory for the individual.

Recognizing our own agenda

When meeting and caring for patients we do so with our role and purpose clearly identified. Information needs to be gathered in order to provide safe and efficient care. This occurs in a time-pressured environment with practical and technical issues requiring dedicated and simultaneous attention for several patients. In summary, nurses are required to manage a lot and therefore there may be a tendency to impose a structure of control upon the working environment to facilitate organization and safety. Although this is clearly necessary to get the job done, it controls the environment to an extent where it may be difficult to hand control over to the patient to lead their own care, or initiate a discussion involving psychological and emotional needs. In addition, factors like the wearing of uniform and the physical environment are likely to influence the type of dialogue that occurs (Hargie & Dickson 2004; Edwards 2005).

Patients may expect that the principal reason for communication is the physical problem: this is frequently confirmed by the questioning and communication bias that nurses can use.

Combine this with a tendency for patients to withhold or delay the disclosure of psycho-social concerns until later in a conversation (Silverman *et al.* 2005) and we can partly understand why a patient's psycho-social needs may not be being met.

Resolving demands upon time and meeting psychological support needs

Part of the answer lies in a change of emphasis and a shift in the culture of health care (Smith *et al.* 2005). Psychological care issues need to be considered on a par with physical and technical care. Psychological support can be integrated with everyday nursing activity and may take a lot less time than anticipated. Investing time in listening and managing psychological care issues (like anxiety) early in a patient's journey might significantly reduce the overall demands made upon the nursing team over a longer period (Carlson & Bultz 2004): consider how much an anxious patient seeks frequent attention, often disrupting the flow of work. Early recognition and appropriate management of psychological issues will promote understanding and compliance, demanding less nursing time and crucially improve the patient's experience.

Investing time in psychological care is essential for the patient's experience to improve and this time will develop empathy and promote a less technological and more human bias to delivering care with nurses getting more reward from their working environment.

If we can adopt a position where the patient is allowed to take the lead in dialogue, all the required information can still be gathered but the patient's priorities will have been acknowledged and we can contextualize this information within a broader bio-psycho-social framework. This offers a better understanding of the patient's experience and will enable us to care for patients more holistically.

Communication skills

Listening

Listening is a skill often assumed to be natural. Rarely would we consider we were physically unable to listen and perhaps this makes us pay little attention to this crucial skill area.

How to let someone know you are listening to them

- Non-verbal encouragement
- Verbal characteristics
- Questioning
- Paraphrasing
- Clarifying
- Summarizing
- Empathy

The physical act of hearing is distinct from that of 'listening'.

Hearing can be seen to be passive, but listening requires active processing and the attachment of meaning.

It might be difficult for us to answer the question 'How do we listen?' and perhaps a procedure of 'How to listen' wouldn't do justice to the sophistication and success of good listeners. However there are ways of describing the constituent parts of listening which, if followed, would make the person speaking appreciate that they were being listened to.

Problems can emerge as two people may interpret the meaning of the same dialogue differently. For example if you have asked the question, 'How are you?' and the patient replies 'Getting by', do you assume they are doing well and coping or do you assume that this means they are struggling and 'Putting on a brave face'?

Hopefully we will be attending to numerous non-verbal cues to decipher what the patient actually means. If there is a suggestion of 'incongruence' where the patient says, 'Getting by' with a low and sad sounding voice, coupled with a simultaneous lowering of the head, we might consider the latter assumption. Alternatively if the patient sounds upbeat and looks you in the face with a smile you might be reassured they mean the former (for further information see the Non-verbal communication section below).

One thing is certain: an amount of concentration is required to make sure we are getting the right message. In a difficult working environment for intimate and in-depth discussion (Edwards 2005) we need to make the best use of available space, minimize potential distractions, setting time aside by confidently letting your colleagues know you are going to 'talk'. Challenge any indication that this isn't a legitimate use of nursing time.

There are strategies to promote successful listening, e.g. 'summarizing' and 'clarifying' (at suitable moments) what the patient is saying (see sections below). Listening remains the fundamental skill in communication and is the way that we are most likely to show care and provide support.

Verbal responses

The way things are said makes a big difference, so attention needs to be paid to the tone, rate and depth of speech. This means sounding alert, interested and caring, but not patronizing. Speech should be delivered at an even rate: not too fast or too slow (unless presenting difficult or complex information).

Non-verbal characteristics of speech should naturally correspond with the verbal message.

Non-verbal responses

Non-verbal communication generally indicates information transmitted without speaking. Included in this would be the way you sit or stand, facial expression, gestures and posture, whether you nod or smile, the clothes worn: all will have an impact on the total communication taking place (Hargie & Dickson 2004).

Egan (2002) usefully describes the acronym SOLER to summarize the constituent elements of non-verbal communication. The acronym indicates: facing the patient **Squarely**; maintaining an **Open** posture; **Leaning** slightly towards the patient to convey interest; having appropriate **Eye** contact, not staring, nor avoiding (a cultural dimension needs to be considered); and being **Relaxed**. By learning an awareness of these factors and making this behaviour part of your normal demeanour, patients will be encouraged to talk more openly, facilitating emotional disclosure.

Saying nothing says something, so there is always communication however reluctant you or the patient are.

It can be argued that non-verbal information is more powerful than verbal information, e.g. in the case of 'incongruence' where the verbal message indicates one thing and the non-verbal suggests another (see above). There is a tendency to believe the non-verbal message over the verbal in these instances.

This highlights the need to communicate with genuine compassion. Without this, communication can be severely reduced in its effectiveness.

Non-verbal communication becomes even more important in the case of people whose verbal communication is impaired, e.g. by stroke, trauma or surgery. Patients need to be supported, ensuring, for example, they have constant access to pen and paper; the use of communication boards can be used to good effect and it is worth considering the use of information technology and communication software, if available. The experience of losing the ability to speak can be very isolating and frustrating and preparation of the patient and practice with communication aids is important to maximize the success of communication. It is essential that people with a speech deficit are given more time to communicate their needs, and we must be patient and persist with interaction until a satisfactory level of understanding is gained.

We can use non-verbal behaviour to encourage patients to talk by nodding/making affirming noises, e.g. 'Hmmm'. This 'affirming' is mostly done naturally, e.g. at points of eye contact, as specific points are made and during slight pauses in dialogue. It can be especially important to affirm when the patient is talking about psychological or emotional issues as they will need you to validate that this is an acceptable topic of conversation.

Paying attention to and tailoring the environment facilitates good communication, e.g. promoting privacy, removing distractions and sitting at the same level as the patient to talk are the minimum necessary considerations.

Questioning

One skill that needs to be used in close collaboration with listening is that of questioning. When specific information is required, e.g. in a crisis, closed questions are indicated. Closed questions narrow the potential answer (Silverman *et al.* 2005) and allow the gathering of specific information for a purpose. Closed questions therefore are ones which are likely to generate a short yes or no answer, e.g. 'Are you alright'?

In cancer care however a broader assessment of the patient's perspective is required and there is a need to show compassion and support psycho-social issues. Open questions and listening are therefore required. Open questions do the opposite of closed questions; they broaden the potential answer (Silverman *et al.* 2005) and hand the initiative

and agenda over to the patient. So instead of asking, 'Are you alright?' ask, 'How are you today?' or, 'What has your experience of treatment been like'?

It is good to include a psychological focus to make it clear that this is part of what you are interested in; for example, 'How did that make you feel?' or, 'What are your main concerns'?

Open questions cannot be used in isolation as the opportunity for open discussion can easily be blocked by failing to ensure that the rest of the fundamental communication elements are in place. Attention therefore must be paid to providing sufficient time, verbal space (not interrupting) and encouragement (in the form of non-verbal cues, paraphrasing, clarifying and summarizing), so that the patient and/or relative can express their feelings and concerns.

Open questions may not be appropriate with people who have a communication problem: perhaps following head and neck surgery, or where complex communication is going to be difficult, as with a difficulty talking in the English language.

Try to use one question at a time: it is easy to ask more than one question in a sentence and this can make it unclear where your focus is and lead the patient to answer only one part of your question.

Reflecting back

You can repeat the same words back to the patient: this signals that their focus is a legitimate topic for discussion (Perry & Burgess 2002), but if this technique is overused it can sound unnatural (Silverman *et al.* 2005).

When it is used it needs to be done with thought and include, 'Something of you in your response' (Egan 2002, p. 97), meaning that you remain alert and caring.

Paraphrasing

This technique involves telling the patient what they have told you but using different words that retain the same meaning; for example:

Patient: I need to talk to them but whenever they start to talk to me about the future, I just start to get wound up and shut down.
Nurse: So when your family try to talk, you get tense and you stop talking . . . .

Clarifying

The aim of this technique is to reduce ambiguity and help the patient define and explore the central or pivotal aspect of issues raised. Many of us may be reluctant to explore emotional or psychological issues too much; just in case issues are raised that are emotional and hard to deal with (Perry & Burgess 2002). However, if the principles of good communication are applied and a focus on the patient's agenda is maintained, distressing and difficult situations can be moved forward positively.

34

Once open questions have opened dialogue, it is likely that certain issues will be raised that would benefit from further exploration. Clarification encourages the expression of detail and context to situations and may help to draw out pertinent matters, perhaps not previously considered by either patient or health professional. A mixture of open or closed questions can be used in clarification; for example:

- 'Are you feeling like that now'?
- 'You say that you've not had enough information: can you tell what you do know'?
- 'You mention that you are struggling: what kinds of things do you struggle with'?
- 'You say it's been hard getting this far: what has been the hardest thing to cope with'?
- 'You seem to be down today, am I right'?
- 'Can you describe how the experience made you feel'?

It might be necessary for you to clarify your own position too: perhaps acknowledge that you don't know something and cannot answer certain questions, e.g. 'Will the treatment work'?

Sometimes not knowing can be a valuable position, enabling you to seek out the patient's experience and not just imagine it. Our imagination and experience might be relevant but each patient and relative will require the opportunity to tell it in their words and need to feel 'heard'.

Summarizing

This intervention can usefully be used as a way of opening or closing dialogue. An opening can be facilitated by recapping over a previous discussion or outlining your understanding of the patient's position. Summarizing can be used to punctuate a longer conversation and highlight specific issues raised.

This serves several purposes:

- It informs your patient that you have listened and understood their position.
- It allows the patient to correct any mistakes or misconceptions generated.
- It brings the conversation from the specific to the general (which can help in recontextualizing issues within a bigger picture).
- It gives an opportunity for agreement to be made about what may need to happen.

An example of summarizing:

It sounds like you are tired and are struggling to manage the treatment schedule: it also sounds like you don't have enough information and we could support you more with that . . . .

Summarizing can be a useful opportunity to plan and agree what actions are necessary. Avoid getting caught up with planning though: the important issue is that you have listened and understood. In our nursing role we are familiar with 'doing' and correcting problematic situations, and although interventions can be helpful in psycho-social issues, sometimes it is necessary not to act and to just 'be' with the patient, accepting their experience as it is, however emotionally painful.

Recognizing when to act and when to sit with distress can be difficult but it is important for us to develop this awareness and accept that sometimes there are no solutions to difficult situations and the temptation to always correct problems might only serve to negate the patient's experience.

Empathy

Sharing time and physical space with other people demands the development of a relationship. In nursing, the relationship with patients is defined by many factors, e.g. physical and medical care. In clinical roles it might be possible to be emotionally detached and to exist behind a 'professional mask' (Taylor 1998, p. 74), but to work in a supportive role a shared experience and bond is generated, inclusive of feelings.

Recognizing our own feelings is important to allow us to understand and to 'tolerate another person's pain' (McKenzie 2002, p. 34).

As nurses we demonstrate empathy when there is a 'desire to understand the client (patient) as fully as possible and to communicate this understanding' (Egan 2002, p. 97).

This means attempting to understand what the patient might be going through, taking into consideration their physical, social and psychological environment. This inferred information can be used to 'connect' with the patient, all the time checking that our interpretation of their experience is accurate (we can be wrong even if we have experienced similar things).

As the patient's environment can change considerably in short spaces of time it is essential to remain alert to the consequent change and interdependency of bio-psycho-social elements.

Rogers seminally described the skill of empathy as: 'The ability to experience another person's world as if it were one's own, without losing the "as if" quality' (Rogers 1975, p. 2). That means allowing ourselves to get into the patient's shoes and experience some of what they might be experiencing, without allowing ourselves to enter the experience wholly (it isn't our experience to own). Empathy allows for an opportunity to 'taste' and therefore to attempt to understand the patient's perspective. Understanding emotions and behaviours in this way encourages an acceptance and positive negotiation of them. Maintaining the 'as if' quality protects us from adopting too great an emotional load. Having too much of a sense of loss or sorrow may prevent us from offering effective support, as we are drawn to focus on our own feelings more than is necessary or helpful (for ourselves or the patient).

Empathy may not always come easily, especially if a patient is angry. What can be very useful in the development and use of empathy is the ability to step back from the situation and reflect upon what it is that you, as the nurse feel and how this relates to what is happening for the patient.

Supporting ourselves

Sharing a patient's distress is difficult and we can help ourselves by sharing and reflecting upon these experiences.

If you communicate well and allow patients to talk, you will be exposed to weighty emotional experiences, e.g. fear, loss and profound sadness. This emotional experience is part of working as a nurse in oncology and arguably health services in general.

Sitting with emotional pain is not without its consequence or burden (Dunne 2003) and it is therefore essential that our own needs are recognized and nurses learn ways of processing this burden.

Historically the nursing culture is more synonymous with 'getting on with it' than with the idea of self care. However 'getting on with it' means disowning the feelings that emotive situations generate within us (Johns & Freshwater 1998). If we do this then we are failing to empathize and may deprive patients and relatives of supportive and good quality care. To facilitate empathy and the subsequent management of psycho-social issues there needs to be an equivalent commitment to 'self care'.

The first challenge is to recognize this need and develop the emotional maturity to accept that a person cannot support without being 'supported' themselves.

Secondarily it will require institutions and the senior staff within them to place psychological care on a par with physical care and to do more than pay lip service to a holistic concept of care. This also means making a commitment to communication training that follows a proven approach (for examples of these see Razavi *et al.* 2000a, b; Wilkinson *et al.* 2002, 2003; Delvaux *et al.* 2004; Boyd 2005).

Thirdly there must be action on the part of the institution and individual to take on the responsibility for safe and effective clinical supervision to allow people to reflect on issues in a non-threatening environment (Dunne 2003).

The more developed our communication skills are, the more effectively we can manage situations. This can provide greater job satisfaction and reduce stress (Fellowes *et al.* 2004).

Everyone needs to be able to reflect upon their skills of communication and everyone can develop their skills via appropriate training (Jenkins & Fallowfield 2002; Wilkinson *et al.* 2002; Delvaux *et al.* 2004; Fellowes *et al.* 2004).

Specific issues

Blocking

Blocking means avoiding addressing the patient's agenda by:

- Failing to pick up on cues (ignoring).
  e.g. Not responding to a patient's disclosure of concern.
- Selectively focusing on the physical aspects of care.
  e.g. Making it clear that your priority is physical care.
- Premature or false reassurance.
  e.g. Where someone is worried, telling them it will be okay.

- Inappropriate encouragement or trivializing.
  e.g. Telling someone they look fine when they have expressed altered body image.
- Passing the buck.
  e.g. Suggesting it is another professional's responsibility to answer questions or sort out the problem.
- Changing the subject.
- Jollying along.
  e.g. 'Don't worry, the sun is still shining (!)'
- Using closed questions.

(Faulkner & Maguire 1994.)

The greater the emotional disclosure, the more nurses use blocking behaviours (Booth *et al.* 1996) and the highest blocking behaviour by health professionals occurs with patients with recurrent cancer (Wilkinson 1991). Interestingly nurses who felt supported practically and emotionally by supervisors decreased their blocking behaviours (Booth *et al.* 1996).

For further discussion about blocking and how nurses and health professionals lack (or perceive a lack of) necessary skills to communicate and support people effectively, readers are directed to Wilkinson 1991; Booth *et al.* 1996; Wilkinson *et al.* 1998 and Fallowfield 2002.

Recognizing blocking tactics and honestly considering how much this occurs in our own practice can help us to reduce this behaviour and support our patients better.

Language and cultural issues

Illness and medical environments are not culturally neutral (Moore & Spiegel 2004, p. 17). We work with and need to care for people from different cultures who may have a primary language other than English. Beliefs and values may be very different from our own and lead to misunderstanding. Consideration must be given to patients speaking a different language and, 'Suitably trained and skilled interpreters and advocates should be available for patients' (NICE 2004, p. 57).

It is not possible to list all the cultural considerations required when communicating with people from different cultural backgrounds; however, it is vital that we remain aware that our assumptions about good communication may not span all cultures. Offence can easily be caused by inappropriate eye contact or touch and an open attitude, and sensitivity to these issues will serve us well in practice.

Including a cultural dimension to nursing care involves addressing these issues by observing acceptable interaction between family members and simply asking patients from different cultural backgrounds about specific considerations, preferences and things to avoid.

Depression and anxiety

Depression in cancer patients is a frequently occurring phenomenon, with the type of cancer and stage of progression influencing the prevalence (Fallowfield *et al.* 2002; Massie 2004). In our daily work with cancer patients we need to be able to assess low mood and the level of coping amongst patients in our care. At diagnosis a good proportion of patients and families are understandably in a state of shock and have anxiety and low mood as part of a stress reaction. Importantly, 'A substantial minority go on to develop persistent psychological disorders' (Moorey & Greer 2002, p. 5).

Where persistent and unrealistic negative predictions and expressions of hopelessness are apparent we need to recognize them and act. Concern about a patient's behaviour, e.g. significant lethargy that isn't accounted for by treatment side effects, should be sensitively explored and further support offered.

Frequently depression can present with anxiety. Anxiety occurs frequently and to some extent can be seen as 'normal' given the threats and stresses inherent in treatment and potentially life-threatening disease (Stark *et al.* 2002).

It is important to avoid labelling and pathologizing normal anxiety reactions to stressful experiences. When patients are anxious they require support and realistic reassurance, not a psychological diagnosis.

Significant and prolonged anxiety can lead to 'panic attacks' which require calm management. Various symptoms can be experienced by the person, e.g. abdominal discomfort, dizziness, tingling in fingers and toes, mostly caused by changes in breathing. This is a very distressing state for the patient, who may attribute the sensations to more serious causes.

Anxiety can be avoided by making time for patients to talk things through, eliciting and addressing concerns realistically and giving accurate information. Where fears are realistic, work with the patient to explore and focus upon their strengths and what will help them get through difficult situations. 'Ignorance is the parent of fear' (Melville 1994, p. 40).

Supporting patients with severe anxiety/suffering panic attacks

- Stay with the patient, remain calm. Ensure the patient is suffering anxiety and not something more serious.
- Reassure the patient that they will feel better shortly if they follow your advice. Gain eye contact, speak confidently and calmly. Offer to hold their hand but be aware that some people may not want this.
- Encourage the person to breathe deeply and slow their breathing down (it might help to demonstrate). Get them to breathe with you: count slowly one, two, three to breathe in, pause, and one, two, three to breathe out.
- As their breathing slows, encourage them with positive affirmation that they are controlling the situation.
- Once the crisis has passed it is important to reflect upon what prompted the anxiety in that situation, how it builds up, and for the person to raise their awareness of their breathing. The patient needs to recognize how shallow or rapid breathing can cause many of the symptoms they have experienced and are afraid of, e.g.

light-headedness, tingling in fingers and toes, abdominal discomfort.
- Refer for further exploration and psychological support if occurring frequently or there is a history of anxiety.
- Use of prescribed benzodiazepines may help if the above strategy is not immediately helpful.

Denial and collusion

Denial is a coping mechanism to enable people to deal with shocking, painful or distressing information (Goldbeck 1997) and for this reason many patients with cancer use it functionally. Denial frequently generates discomfort and uncertainty for the health professional. There is a potential risk of using the term to explain away certain patient behaviours, or to avoid tackling difficult issues with people. Careful management of denial is required, but is within the scope of someone with good communication skills.

Denial and collusion: key points

- Denial is a coping mechanism.
- We need to consider carefully when to respect it and when to challenge it, sharing this with colleagues.
- Collusion needs to be understood and recognized in staff and or in families. It is best addressed and worked through as early as possible to avoid the situation becoming too complicated.

The degree of denial varies considerably and has different implications for the health professional.

It is often inappropriate to challenge functional denial; however, this can become complex when trying to ensure whether someone has understood his or her diagnosis and the implications of treatment.

If the process of information giving and the delivery of bad news is handled professionally and the process is clearly documented it can be easier to assess whether denial or ignorance is represented by certain behaviours.

Once the duty to disclose information has been met, the degree to which the patient accepts the information is variable and needs to be respected.

It can generally be assumed that where denial does not affect the treatment regime or damage family relationships then it need not be confronted.

Breaking denial down and forcing someone to confront their reality can be particularly harmful. An individual's ability to cope with further information can change, so it can be useful to 'test' denial from time to time; for example: 'How do you feel things are going for you?' or, 'Do you require any further information or clarification of information'?

Exploring what and how much a patient wants to know can indicate whether they want to retain their denial as a coping mechanism or are ready to confront their situation further. Remember that 'most patients want as much information as possible about treatment and illness' (Jenkins *et al.* 2001, p. 49).

Working in oncology we may feel pressured to provide and maintain hope for patients (Houldin 2000). The maintenance of hope is very valuable for patients when they are confronting and going through tough physical and psychological times. Maintaining inappropriate hope however is similar to providing premature or inappropriate encouragement (see Blocking section above), and may say more about our own difficulty in tackling difficult emotional issues than the patient's ability to deal with the consequences of reality.

At the point where hopes for a cure or significantly prolonged life become unrealistic, we need to recognize the issue and make it explicit, i.e. share information with the patient and their family (with consent) as well as other professional colleagues involved in care. If this doesn't occur then collusive relationships may develop and health professionals might attempt to conceal reality from the patient.

Poor professional communication can lead to the patient receiving mixed messages about their situation, which is potentially far more distressing than confronting reality.

Collusion can leave health professionals feeling confused, deceitful and disturbed. There can be a feeling that nurses should not challenge the information giving of medical staff and it certainly offers no advantage to be contradicting one another in the health setting. In a nursing role however we should acknowledge our ability to recognize collusion where it occurs and face up to the situation with colleagues. With good planning, honest information can be given to the patient and family, to allow them to make decisions about their care, treatment and future, however short that time may be.

Collusion within families can also occur with family members expressing a desire to protect the patient from bad news, or alternatively the patient wishes to do the same for their family. The motive in these situations is frequently one of protection and arises from love.

Managing collusion with professionals and patients and their families requires an exploration of the consequences of maintaining the silence. If delicately managed, this exploration will often lead to some acceptance that the truth is less harmful, e.g. by the realization that people will not be able to say things they wish to say, or organize things they wish to happen. If agreement cannot be gained, then it must be pointed out that there is a duty to be truthful if the party lacking information 'wants to know'. A statement can be made that if the patient or relative states clearly that they do not wish to know bad news then this wish will be respected.

Breaking bad news

Bad news is: 'Any information that produces a negative alteration to the person's expectations about their present and future' (Buckman 1992, p. 15). Being involved with breaking bad news is an unavoidable part of oncology nursing. Bad news is often formally given by doctors; however, nurses often clarify and confirm the information given either immediately or in the following hours and days.

The use of a breaking bad news model is indispensable, e.g. SPIKES (a six-step approach). Models provide a valuable framework to ensure that we meet the individual information needs of our patients. The SPIKES model involves:

- **S**etting up the interview.
- Assessing the patient's **P**erception (of their current situation).
- Obtaining the patient's **I**nvitation (to disclose information).
- Giving **K**nowledge and information.
- Addressing the **E**motions with **E**mpathy.
- **S**trategy and **S**ummary (making a plan for the future/ avoiding abandoning the patient). (Baile *et al.* 2000.)

A poorly planned and insensitive approach to breaking bad news has been shown to increase patient distress with a possible lasting impact on coping ability, potentially even influencing psychological pathology, e.g. anxiety and depression (Maguire 1998; Fallowfield & Jenkins 2004).

Communicating with the blind or partially sighted

Sight loss can be very variable, ranging from mild to complete. Any sight disturbance is a significant issue in caring for patients. It might simply mean ensuring glasses are kept safely, within reach and clean, or providing large print documents, braille or audio information.

Blind people will rely more heavily on other senses, especially their hearing and it might therefore be necessary to read things carefully for them. Be open about the visual impairment: ask what helps and what doesn't.

Good communication practice becomes more important, e.g. introducing yourself even when the person may have met you on numerous occasions (as your voice may not always be distinguishable). A lack of non-verbal information can compromise verbal meaning. Consider describing something complex on the phone: it takes a lot more verbal information. Careful explanation and repetitive checking of understanding is a key technique. To some extent you may be the eyes of the patient and you need to relay information that they will not be aware of, e.g. the patient's relative has arrived on the ward but is waiting.

There will be an increased demand for empathic skills.

Make it clear when you are leaving to avoid confusion (visual cues are not always available to the blind or partially sighted).

In situations where confusion may occur as to whom is being spoken to, use the patient's name or a light touch when addressing them.

- Blind and partially sighted people have the same information needs as everyone else and need accessible information in a suitable format.
- Access to information facilitates informed decisions and promotes independence.

- No single method will suit all. Even the same person might use different methods at different times and under different circumstances. It is important to identify the preferred method(s) for each person.
- It is also important to remember the blind or partially sighted person does not necessarily have a hearing loss.

There is now a legal duty to meet the information needs of blind and partially sighted people (Disability Discrimination Act 1999).

Ethnic minorities

There is very little material available in large print, Braille or on tape in ethnic languages.

Resources

Royal National Institute of the Blind (RNIB): See It Right, 105 Judd Street, London, WC1H 9NE. Tel. 020 7391 2397. Email: www.seeitright@rnib.org. Helpful website of the RNIB: www.rnib.org.uk.

Communicating with the deaf or hard of hearing

As with blindness, the extent of the impairment varies significantly. Mild hearing loss might simply require more care with clarity of speech and ensuring the patient is able to see your face clearly. If a hearing aid is used, make sure it is in use and working. Reduce noise in the environment: hearing aids amplify everything, even background noise. More severe hearing problems will not benefit from a hearing aid and these patients reply more on lip reading and/or signing.

Lip reading is a difficult skill and requires a lot of concentration. Not all sounds/words produce a shape on the lips and so the lip-reader has to piece together meaning from what they do distinguish. What information you do convey via your facial expression and lip movement needs to be accentuated, hence pay attention to the direction of light (not behind you) and ensure the patient is ready to begin. Contextualize your discussion by giving the topic for conversation first. Try to relax and allow your body language and gesture to flow normally. Speak normally: not too fast or too slow (although slightly slower speech may be beneficial).

Keep your hands away from your face, avoid using complex words and be prepared to repeat yourself as many times as it takes. If you cannot make yourself understood, write things down. Use sentences not single word answers: this again helps to contextualize information.

Suggestions when communicating with someone who is deaf or hard of hearing

- Find a suitable place to talk, with good lighting and no noise or distractions.
- Be patient and allow extra time for the consultation/conversation.

- If the person is wearing a hearing aid, do not assume they can hear you. Ask if it is on and if they still need to lip read.
- If an interpreter is required always remember to talk directly to the person you are communicating with, not the interpreter.
- Make sure you have the listener's attention before you start to speak.
- Talk clearly, but not too slowly, and do not exaggerate your lip movements.
- Use natural facial expressions and gestures.
- Use plain language; avoid waffling, jargon and unfamiliar abbreviations.
- Check the person understands you.
- Depending on the purpose of the consultation, writing down a summary of the key points made might be helpful.

Resources

Royal National Institute of the Deaf (RNID): 19–23 Featherstone Street, London, EC1Y 8SL. Tel. 0207296 8264. Textphone 020 7296 8246. Fax 020 7196 8199. Email: supporterservices@rnid.org.uk. Website: www.rnid.org.uk.

Communicating with a person with aphasia (complex disorder of language processing)

- Make an early referral to a speech and language therapist (SLT).
- Be aware of where the aphasic patient is within their disease trajectory.
- Be aware if the patient has impaired attention, concentration and/or memory.
- Minimize distractions, both visual and auditory.
- Allow enough time, with a calm, friendly, encouraging approach.
- Make sure the aphasic patient understands the purpose of the conversation.
- Talk directly to the aphasic patient and ask them what is/isn't helpful.
- Have a pen and paper for both people to use: writing or drawing can support what is being said.
- Speech should be clear, slightly slower and of normal volume.
- Use straightforward language and avoid jargon (medical terminology).
- Say one thing at a time and pause between 'chunks' of information.
- Structure questions carefully and check the patient understands.
- Make it clear when there is a change of topic.
- Support the spoken language with appropriate non-verbal communication.
- Abilities may fluctuate, so what helps one moment might not work another.
- Be prepared for their and your frustration. You might have to come back to a topic at another time.

■ Confusion or miscommunication can be avoided by using a notebook to record salient/key information, especially when the information is new and/or complex, anxiety is present or memory function is impaired.

Conclusion

As nurses we have a profound responsibility to include good communication and psychological support as part of our role. These skills need to be incorporated as a priority, alongside technological advances and extended roles. We cannot afford to forget that people have emotions and psychological needs that require as much, if not more, attention than the physical and technical care delivered. Without this consideration the processes of successful treatment and recovery can be seriously impaired and undermined. Everyone can develop and improve their communication skills, and by paying attention to this crucial aspect of the nursing role, may be pleased to discover how rewarding and valuable this investment is for both nurse and patient.

References

Back, A.L. *et al.* (2005) Approaching difficult communication tasks in oncology. *CA Cancer J Clin*, **55**, 164–77.

Baile, W.F. *et al.* (2000) SPIKES – a six-step protocol for delivering bad news: application to the patient with cancer. *Oncologist*, 5(4), 302–11.

Booth, K. *et al.* (1996) Perceived professional support and the use of blocking behaviours by hospice nurses. *J Adv Nurs*, **24**, 522–7.

Booth, K., Maguire, P. & Hillier, V.F. (1999) Measurement of communication skills in cancer care: myth or reality? *J Adv Nurs*, **30**(5), 1073–97.

Boyd, K. J. (2005) *Enhancing clinical communication: developing an education programme for consultants in SE Scotland*. MMedSci Clinical Education Thesis, University of Nottingham (unpublished).

Buckman, R. *Breaking Bad News: A Guide for Health Care Professionals*. Baltimore: Johns Hopkins University Press, 1992, p. 15.

Cambell, S. (2006) A project to promote better communication with patients. *Nurs Times*, **102**(19), 28–30.

Cantwell, B.M. & Ramirez, A.J. (1997) Doctor–patient communication: a study of junior house officers. *Med Educ*, **31**(1), 17–21. In: Fellowes, D., Wilkinson, S. & Moore, P. (2004) Communication skills for health care professionals working with cancer patients, their families and/or carers. *Cochrane Database Syst Rev*, 2, CD003751.

Carlson, L.E. & Bultz, B.D. (2004) Efficacy and medical cost offset of psychosocial interventions in cancer care: making the case for economic analyses. *Psychooncology*, 13, 837–49.

Chant, S. *et al.* (2002) Communication skills: some problems in nurse education and practice. *J Clin Nurs*, **11**, 12–21.

Chelf, J.H. *et al.* (2001) Cancer-related patient education: an overview of the last decade of evaluation and research. *Oncol Nurs Forum*, **28**(7), 1139–47.

Cooley, C.M. (2005) Communication skills in palliative care. In: *Handbook of Palliative Care* (eds C. Faull, Y. Carter & L. Daniels), 2nd edn. Blackwell Publishing, Oxford, pp. 86–97.

Deffner, J.M. & Bell, S.K. (2005) Nurses' death anxiety, comfort level during communication with patients and families regarding death, and exposure to communication education : a quantitative study. *J Nurses Staff Dev*, **21**(1), 19–23.

Delvaux, N. *et al.* (2004) Effects of a 105 hours psychological training program on attitudes, communication skills and occupational stress in oncology: a randomised study. *Br J Cancer*, **90**, 106–14.

DH (2005) www.performance.doh.gov.uk/hospitalactivity/data_requests/download/nhs_complaints/complaint_04_summary.xls. Accessed 11/5/05.

DH (2001) *Consent: What You Have a Right to Expect (A Guide for Adults)*. Department of Health, London.

DH (2000) *The NHS Cancer Plan*. Department of Health, London.

Disability Discrimination Act Section 21 (1999) www.opsi.gov.uk/acts/acts2005/200513.htm, DDA 2005. Accessed 10/05.

Drew, A. & Fawcett, T.N. (2002) Responding to the information needs of patients with cancer. *Prof Nurse*, **17**(7), 443–6.

Dunne, K. (2003) The personal cost of caring. Guest editorial. *Int J Palliat Nurs*, **9**(6), 232.

Edwards, P. (2005) An overview of the end-of-life discussion. *Int J Palliat Nurs*, **11**(1), 21–27.

Egan, G. (2002) *The Skilled Helper. A Problem–Management and Opportunity–Development Approach to Helping*, 7th edn. Brooks/Cole, Pacific Grove, CA.

Fallowfield, L. & Jenkins, V. (2004) Communicating sad, bad, and difficult news in medicine. *Lancet*, **363**, 312–19.

Fallowfield, L., Jenkins, V.A. & Beveridge, H.A. (2002) Truth may hurt but deceit hurts more: communication in palliative care. *Palliat Med*, **16**, 297–303.

Faulkner, A. & Maguire, P. (1994) *Talking to Cancer Patients and their Relatives*. Oxford University Press, Oxford.

Fellowes, D., Wilkinson, S. & Moore, P. (2004) Communication skills for health care professionals working with cancer patients, their families and/or carers. *Cochrane Database Syst Rev*, **2**, CD003751.

Goldbeck, R. (1997) Denial in physical illness. *J Psychosom Res*, **43**(6), 575–93.

Hargie, O. (2006) *The Handbook of Communication Skills*, 3rd edn. Routledge, London.

Hargie, O. & Dickson, D. (2004) *Skilled Interpersonal Communication: Research Theory and Practice*, 4th edn. Routledge, London.

Heyland, D.K. *et al.* (2006) What matters most in end-of-life care: perceptions of seriously ill patients and their family members. *CMAJ*, **174**(5), 627–33.

Houldin, A.D. (2000) *Patients with Cancer: Understanding the Psychological Pain*. Lippincott, Philadelphia.

Jenkins, V.A. & Fallowfield, L.J. (2002) Can communication skills training alter physicians' beliefs and behaviour in clinics? *J Clin Oncol*, **20**, 765–9.

Jenkins, V.A., Fallowfield, L.J. & Saul, J. (2001) Information needs of patients with cancer: results from a large study in UK cancer centres. *Br J Cancer*, **84**(1), 48–51.

Johns, C. & Freshwater, D. (1998) *Transforming Nursing through Reflective Practice*. Blackwell Science, London.

Lookinland, S. & Pool, M. (1998) Study on effect of methods of pre-operative education in women. *AORN J*, **67**(1), 203–13.

Lowry, M. (1995) Knowledge that reduces anxiety: creating patient information leaflets. *Prof Nurse*, **10**(5), 318–20.

McCabe, C. (2004) Nurse–patient communication: an exploration of patients' experiences. *J Clin Nurs*, **13**, 41–9.

McKenzie, R. (2002) The importance of philosophical congruence for therapeutic use of self in practice. In: *Therapeutic*

Nursing. *Improving Patient Care through Self-awareness and Reflection* (ed. D. Freshwater). Sage Publications, London, pp. 22–38.

Maguire, P., Faulkner, A., Booth, K., Elliott, C. & Hillier, V. (1996) Helping cancer patients disclose their concerns. *Eur J Cancer*, **32 A**, No. 1 78–81.

Maguire, P. (1998) Breaking bad news. *Eur J Surg Oncol*, 24(3), 188–91.

Maguire, P. & Pitceathly, C. (2002) Key communication skills and how to acquire them. *Br Med J*, 325, 697–700.

Massie, M.J. (2004) Prevalence of depression in patients with cancer. *J Natl Cancer Inst*, 32, 57–71.

Melville, H. (1994) *Moby Dick*. Penguin Classics, London.

Moore, R.J. & Spiegel, D. (2004) *Cancer, Culture and Communication*. Kluwer Academic/Plenum Publishers, New York.

Moorey, S. & Greer, S. (2002) *Cognitive Behaviour Therapy for People with Cancer*. Oxford University Press, Oxford.

NICE (2004) *Improving Supportive and Palliative Care for Adults with Cancer*. National Institute for Health and Clinical Excellence, London.

NMC (2006) *A–Z Advice Sheet Consent*. www.nmc.org.

NMC (2008) *The Code: Standards of Conduct, Performance and Ethics for Nurses and Midwives*. Nursing and Midwifery Council, London.

Perry, K.N. & Burgess, M. (2002) *Communication in Cancer Care*. Blackwell Publishing, Oxford.

Razavi, D. *et al.* (2000a) Testing health care professionals' communication skills: the usefulness of highly emotional standardized role-playing sessions with simulators. *Psychooncology*, 9(4), 293–302.

Razavi D. *et al.* (2000b) Does training increase the use of more emotionally laden words by nurses when talking with cancer patients? A randomized study. *Br J Cancer*, 87, 1–7.

Rogers, C.R. (1975) Empathic: An Unappreciated Way of Being. *Counselling Psychologist*, 5, 2–10.

Scott, T. (2004) *Integrative Psychotherapy in Healthcare. A Humanistic Approach*. Palgrave, Basingstoke.

Silverman, J., Kurtz, S. & Draper, J. (2005) *Skills for Communicating with Patients*, 2nd edn. Radcliffe Publishing, Abingdon.

Smith, C., Dickens, C. & Edwards, S. (2005) Provision of information for cancer patients: an appraisal and review. *Eur J Cancer Care*, 14, 282–8.

Stark, D. *et al.* (2002) Anxiety disorders in cancer patients: their nature, associations and relation to quality of life. *J Clin Oncol*, 20(14), 3137–48.

Street, R. (2003) Interpersonal communication skills in health care contexts. In: *Handbook of Communication and Social Interaction Skills* (eds J. Greene & B. Burleson). Lawrence Erlbaum Associates, Mahwah, NJ, pp. 909–35.

Taylor, B. (1998) Ordinariness in nursing as therapy. In: *Nursing as Therapy* (eds R. McMahon & A. Pearson). Stanley Thornes, Cheltenham, pp. 64–75.

Van de Molen, B. (1999) Relating information needs to the cancer experience, part 1: information as a key coping strategy. *Eur J Cancer Care*, 8(4), 238–44.

Wallace, P.R. (2001) Improving palliative care through effective communication. *Int J Palliat Nurs*, 7(2), 86–90.

Wilkinson, S. (1999) Communication: it makes a difference. *Cancer Nurs*, 22(1), 17–20.

Wilkinson, S., Roberts, A. & Aldridge, A. (1998) Nurse–patient communication in palliative care: an evaluation of a communication skills programme. *Palliat Med*, 12(1), 13–22.

Wilkinson, S.M. (1991) Factors which influence how nurses communicate with cancer patients. *J Adv Nurs*, 16, 677–88.

Wilkinson, S.M., Gambles, M. & Roberts, A. (2002) The essence of cancer care: the impact of training on nurses' ability to communicate effectively. *J Adv Nurs*, 40(6), 731–8.

Wilkinson, S.M. *et al.* (2003) Can intensive 3-day programmes improve nurses' communication skills in cancer care? *Psychooncology*, 12(8), 747–59.

Part two

Chapter 4

Abdominal paracentesis

Reference material **44**
Procedure guidelines: Abdominal paracentesis **46**
Procedure guidelines: Intraperitoneal drain removal **47**
Problem solving: Abdominal paracentesis **48**
References and further reading **49**

Definition

Abdominal paracentesis is a technique used to drain an abnormal collection of ascitic fluid from the abdomen (Campbell 2001). This is achieved by inserting a fenestrated catheter through the abdominal muscles into the peritoneal cavity (Kouraklis 2002). This procedure is usually performed in the patient with cancer for the relief of symptoms caused by ascites.

Indications

Abdominal paracentesis is indicated under the following circumstances:

- To obtain a specimen of fluid for analysis for diagnostic purposes.
- To relieve the symptoms associated with ascites, both physical and psychological.
- To administer substances such as cytotoxic drugs (e.g. bleomycin, cisplatin) or other agents into the peritoneal cavity, to achieve regression of serosae deposits responsible for fluid formation.

(Hosttetter *et al*. 2005.)

Reference material

Anatomy and physiology

The peritoneum is a semi-permeable serous membrane consisting of two separate layers.

- Parietal layer: this covers the abdominal and pelvic walls and the undersurface of the diaphragm.
- Visceral layer: this lines and supports the abdominal organs and the parietal peritoneum (Figure 4.1).
- Peritoneal cavity: the space between the parietal and visceral layers (Thibodeau & Patton 2007).
- Fluid is produced from the capillaries lining the peritoneal cavity and is drained by lymphatic vessels under the diaphragm. The fluid is collected by the right lymphatic duct which drains into the vena cava. The peritoneum forms the largest serous membrane in the body (Tortora & Grabowski 2003). However, in patients with malignant ascites, this balance of production and drainage is disrupted and ascitic fluid collects in the peritoneal cavity.

Functions of the peritoneum

- The peritoneum is a serous membrane that enables the abdominal contents to glide over each other without friction.
- It forms partial or complete cover for the abdominal organs.
- It forms ligaments and mesenteries which help to keep the organs in position.

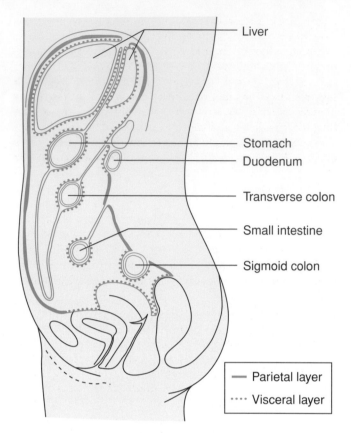

Figure 4.1 Peritoneum of female in lateral view.

- The mesenteries contain fat and act as a store for the body.
- The mesenteries can move to engulf areas of inflammation and this prevents the spread of infection.
- It has the power to absorb fluids and exchange electrolytes. (Tortora & Grabowski 2003; Thibodeau & Patton 2007.)

Malignant ascites

Malignant ascites can be caused by non-malignant conditions such as cirrhosis of the liver, advanced congestive heart failure and chronic pericarditis or by malignant conditions such as metastatic cancer of the ovary, stomach, colon or breast. Cirrhosis of the liver is the most common cause of ascites. In non-malignant causes of ascites, other interventions are usually considered before performing abdominal paracentesis (Hewish 2006). It should be noted that in about one-third of patients with cancer, ascites has a non-malignant cause (Hosttetter *et al*. 2005). The incidence of ascites in patients with cancer is not well recorded; however, it is known to occur in many different cancer types (Cope 2005). Malignant ascites accounts for about 10% of ascites of which 34–54% are from ovarian cancers (Winkelman 2004).

Ascites is often accompanied by debilitating symptoms as large amounts of fluid collect in the peritoneal cavity causing an increase in intra-abdominal pressure and resulting in pressure on internal structures. Symptoms initially include vague abdominal discomfort, which can go on to affect the respiratory and gastrointestinal systems. Gastric pressure may cause anorexia, indigestion or hiatus hernia. Intestinal pressure may result in constipation, bowel obstruction or decreased bladder capacity. Pressure on the diaphragm decreases the intrathoracic space and causes shortness of breath. Patients also become increasingly fatigued finding simple daily tasks difficult (Winkelman 2004). Even minimal distension of the abdomen can cause the patient distress with concerns relating to body image.

Malignant ascites accumulates owing to a number of causes and is different in pathogenesis than benign ascites (Hosttetter *et al.* 2005). Venous obstruction or liver metastases may also lead to ascites. Other co-morbid conditions, such as cardiac or renal impairment, can also increase the risk of developing malignant ascites (Winkelman 2004).

In patients with advanced cancer, malignant ascites is the most likely diagnosis of an abdominal fluid collection and often reflects end-stage disease. However, in some cases such as ovarian cancer and lymphoma, ascites can be an early presentation and efforts to obtain tumour shrinkage and prolongation of survival should be undertaken (Marincola & Schwartzentruber 2001). If a definitive diagnosis is needed to establish cause to aid staging and possible surgical intervention then a peritoneal tap and analysis of fluid will be useful (Marincola & Schwartzentruber 2001). Fentiman (2002) states that cytological confirmation of malignant cells is difficult with only a 50% chance of success. Interventions used to treat ascites range from an aggressive approach to a purely palliative approach. There have been few definitive studies that have evaluated the different approaches in the treatment of malignant ascites (Hosttetter *et al.* 2005).

Treatment for ascites may include:

- Paracentesis: the most common way of managing ascites as it has an immediate effect in 90% of cases (Campbell 2001; Marincola & Schwartzentruber 2001).
- Diuretics: useful mainly in cirrhotic-type ascites. This may be used for malignant ascites together with a restriction of salt and fluid intake, and has been found to be effective in about one-third of patients (Hosttetter *et al.* 2005).
- Peritoneovenous shunt: generally used in patients with long-term prognosis.
- Instillation of intraperitoneal agents: cytotoxics, sclerosants and biological substances have been tried in an attempt to control the recurrence of ascites. As yet intraperitoneal agents have not been proven, unequivocally, to have a greater beneficial effect than the use of diuretics (Fentiman 2002).

This chapter describes only abdominal paracentesis, a procedure which is carried out because it is relatively easily performed and gives immediate effective relief of symptoms. However, it is not undertaken lightly because of the poten-

tial risks of inducing hypovolaemia, hypokalaemia, hyponatraemia and visceral injury (Hosttetter *et al.* 2005). Ascites tends to recur and requires repeated drainage and this may lead to protein depletion because ascitic fluid contains proteins. Further ascitic fluid may become loculated in the peritoneal cavity making it difficult to drain the fluid away. A mark is often placed on the skin at the time of an ultrasound to find the area of maximum fluid collection and to guide the physician as to where to place the catheter or the catheter may be placed directly under ultrasound guidance; this reduces the occurrence of bowel perforation. The introduction of infection during insertion of the ascitic drain is a risk which can be reduced by following an aseptic technique (Lee *et al.* 2000). Other complications include haemorrhage into the peritoneal cavity, pulmonary emboli and peritonitis (Campbell 2001).

Nursing care

Nursing and medical care of patients with malignant abdominal ascites should be aimed at improving quality of life by relieving suffering caused by the symptoms (Cope 2005). Each patient should be carefully assessed with consideration of their individual circumstances, maintaining respect for their wish to have or not have interventional treatment (Campbell 2001). It is an invasive procedure performed at present by a doctor assisted by a nurse at the patient's bedside.

There is much debate about whether it is safe to drain large volumes of fluid rapidly from the abdomen. One concern is that profound hypotension may follow because of the sudden release of intra-abdominal pressure and consequent possible vasodilatation (Lee *et al.* 2000). However, Stephenson and Gilbert (2002), following a local study and literature search, suggest that up to 5 litres of fluid may be safely drained over a few hours. They also state that it is not necessary to drain the abdomen until dry. McNamara (2000) supports this by pointing out that the maximum relief of symptoms may be achieved after the initial few litres are drained. This is further supported by Moorsom (2001) who suggests that several litres can be drained on free flow over 1 hour. It is generally not necessary to have intravenous fluid or albumin replacement. However, patients with ascites who have large tumours, cirrhosis of the liver or renal impairment may require slower drainage of fluid and possible fluid replacement depending on their clinical condition. Abdominal and peritoneal tumours can cause ascites to develop independently of the circulatory system and therefore hypotension is not usually seen as the ascites is drained (Klee 2004). Further, it is known that prolonged drainage times can lead to catheter infection and peritonitis (Stephenson & Gilbert 2002).

In all cases regular observations must be carried out to detect early signs of shock, cardiovascular compromise and infection so that the doctor can be informed and action can be taken promptly. Drainage of the fluid must be monitored regularly, volumes recorded and blockages detected and managed. Patients may require assistance to move and position themselves, and may experience pain requiring careful repositioning or appropriate analgesia. The drain should be taken out when the desired amount of fluid has been removed. The patient's renal function should be checked following this procedure. This is to ensure that any signs of dehydration or pre-renal failure are treated as early as possible. Clinical practice at The Royal Marsden Hospital reflects a drainage pattern that is dependent on the individual assessment of the patient and their medical condition.

Nursing interventions for patients undergoing abdominal paracentesis include education about the nature of the procedure, about what results can realistically be expected, and the risks and benefits. Information should also be given about post-procedure care of the puncture site and about the importance of diet and fluid intake to replace proteins and fluid lost in the ascitic fluid. It is essential that the patient, family and carer are involved in the discussion so that an informed and joint decision may be made in order to achieve the best possible outcome.

Preparatory investigations

The patient's clinical condition and purpose of the procedure must be taken into account when deciding what investigations are necessary but most pre-procedure investigations include a blood screen and ultrasound examination. To keep intrusion to a minimum for palliative patients, fewer investigations may be performed. Blood is usually checked for: full blood picture; urea and electrolytes, creatinine; liver function test, plasma proteins and coagulation screen (Hewish 2006).

Procedure guidelines   Abdominal paracentesis

Equipment

1 Sterile abdominal paracentesis set containing forceps, scalpel blade and blade holder, swabs, towels, suturing equipment, trocar and cannula (or other approved catheter and introducer), connector to attach to the cannula and guide fluid into the container.
2 Sterile dressing pack.
3 Sterile receiver.
4 Sterile specimen pots.
5 Local anaesthetic.

6 Needles and syringes.
7 Chlorhexidine 0.5% in 70% alcohol.
8 Adhesive dressing.
9 Large sterile drainage bag or container (with connector if appropriate to attach to cannula).
10 Gate clamps.
11 Sterile gloves.
12 Weighing scales if appropriate.
13 Tape measure if appropriate.

Procedure

Action	Rationale
1 Explain and discuss the procedure with the patient.	To ensure that the patient is involved in the decision and understands the procedure, the agreed aim, the risks and benefits. Informed consent may then be obtained (Campbell 2001: R 5; DH 2001: C; Cope 2005: R 5; NMC 2006: C).
2 Ask the patient to empty his/her bladder.	If the bladder is full there is a chance of it being punctured when the trocar is introduced (E).
3 Weigh patient before and after procedure and record.	To assess weight changes and the fluid loss (E; RMH Guidelines: C).
4 Ensure privacy.	To maintain dignity (P; E; DH 2006: C).
5 Measure patient's girth around umbilicus before and after procedure and record.	This provides an indication of fluid shift and how much fluid has reaccumulated (E).
6 The patient should lie supine in bed with the head raised 45–50 cm with a back rest.	Normally the pressure in the peritoneal cavity is no greater than atmospheric pressure, but, when fluid is present, pressure becomes greater than atmospheric pressure. This position will then aid gravity in the removal of fluid and the fluid will drain of its own accord until the pressure is equalized (E).

7   The procedure is performed by a doctor assisted by a
    nurse throughout:

(a)	The abdomen is prepared aseptically and draped with sterile towels. Local anaesthetic is administered.	To reduce the risk of local and/or systemic infection. The peritoneal cavity is normally sterile (E; Lee *et al*. 2000: R 5; DH 2005: C).
(b)	Once the anaesthetic has taken effect the doctor makes an incision.	To minimize pain during the procedure and thus maximize patient comfort and facilitate co-operation (E).
(c)	The trocar and cannula are inserted via the incision.	
(d)	The trocar is removed.	

8	Ascitic fluid is collected (20–100 ml as instructed by the doctor) and sent for cytology.	If necessary, in order to diagnose the cause of ascites (E; Fentiman 2002; Hosttetter *et al*. 2005: R 5).
9	If the cannula is to remain in position, sutures may be inserted.	To ensure cannula remains *in situ*. To reduce risk of trauma to the patient (E).
10	A closed drainage system is now attached to the cannula using a connector if appropriate. A secure dry dressing should be applied to ensure the drain site is protected and taped firmly in position.	A sterile container with a non-return valve is necessary to maintain sterility. To reduce local and/or systemic infection (E).
11	Monitor the patient's blood pressure, pulse and respirations and observe the rate and nature of the drainage. A clamp should be available on the tubing to reduce the flow of fluid if necessary.	To observe for signs of shock and/or infection and to ensure unobstructed drainage (P; E).
12	Monitor the patient's fluid balance. Encourage a high-protein and high-calorie diet.	After removal of large amounts of peritoneal fluid, fluid moves from the vascular space and reaccumulates in the peritoneal cavity. Ascitic fluid contains protein in addition to sodium and potassium. Problems of dehydration and electrolyte imbalance may be present (E).
13	Drainage of fluid may be free flowing up to 5 litres unless adverse symptoms present. Alternatively, drainage may be controlled at 2 litres every 4 hours.	If patient shows adverse signs then clamp drain, inform medical team and reopen after medical intervention and advice (Stephenson & Gilbert 2002: R 3b).

Procedure guidelines   Intraperitoneal drain removal

Equipment

1   Sterile dressing pack.
2   Sterile gloves.
3   Stitch cutter (if drain has a suture holding it in place).
4   Adhesive tape.

5   Transparent dressing.
6   Gauze (low linting).
7   Bactericidal alcohol handrub (if appropriate).

Procedure

This procedure is usually carried out by a member of the nursing team who has been instructed in the removal of intraperitoneal drains. Removal of the drain should be done in consultation with the medical team.

Action	Rationale
1 Explain and discuss the procedure with the patient.	To ensure the patient understands the procedure and is ready to proceed (E; DH 2001: C).

Procedure guidelines *(cont.)*

2	Establish that the patient is comfortable, and is not in pain or allergic to the tape to be used.	To reduce unnecessary discomfort and to ensure the patient will not have a local reaction to the tape (P; E).
3	Wash hands with bactericidal soap and water or bactericidal alcohol handrub.	To reduce the risk of infection (DH 2005: C).
4	Prepare equipment using aseptic technique. Apply gloves from dressing pack.	To minimize the risk of contamination (DH 2005: C).
5	Remove the old dressing.	To allow access to the relevant area (E).
6	Cut the knot from the purse-string suture (if present).	To allow mobility of the suture (E).
7	Cut the suture holding the drain in place if present and remove the suture.	To free the drain and prevent it falling out (E).
8	Instruct patient to breathe normally, explain that you are about to take the drain out and steadily pull the drain out.	To ensure that the patient is fully aware of what is about to happen so as not to cause unnecessary distress (P; E).
9	Place gauze over the site and secure it firmly. A transparent dressing may also be used to provide a seal.	To prevent leakage of fluids (P; E).
10	Explain to the patient that the procedure is complete and that there may be some temporary leakage. In the event of this occurring, the dressing will be changed or a stoma bag may be placed over the site for a short period of time.	To reduce the risk of leakage and prevent the patient becoming distressed if there is leakage and to reduce risk of contamination to clothes (P; E).
11	Ensure the patient is comfortable and clear the equipment away.	To reduce the risk of cross-infection (DH 2005: C).
12	Wash hands with bactericidal soap and water.	To reduce the risk of cross-infection (DH 2005: C).
13	Measure fluid drained and record in appropriate document.	To provide an accurate record (NMC 2005: C).
14	Record vital signs and document procedure done.	To ascertain that the patient is stable and to promote continuity of care and for future reference (E).
15	Check renal function on the following day.	To check for signs of dehydration or pre-renal failure (E).

Problem solving: Abdominal paracentesis

Problem	Cause	Suggested action
Patient exhibits shock.	Major circulatory shift of fluid or sudden release of intra-abdominal pressure, vasodilatation and subsequent lowering of blood pressure.	Clamp the drainage tube with a gate clamp to prevent further fluid loss. Record the patient's vital signs. Refer to the medical staff for immediate intervention.
Cessation of drainage of ascitic fluid.	Abdomen is empty of ascitic fluid.	Check with the total output of ascitic fluid given on the patient's fluid balance chart. Measure the patient's girth; compare this measurement with the pre-abdominal paracentesis measurement. Suggest to medical staff that the cannula should be removed. Discontinue the drainage system.

Problem	Cause	Suggested action
	Patient's position is inhibiting drainage.	Change the patient's position, i.e. move the patient upright or onto his or her side to encourage flow by gravity. Encourage patient to mobilize.
	The ascitic fluid has clotted in the drainage system.	'Milk' the tubing. If this is unsuccessful, change the drainage system aseptically.
Signs of local or systemic infection.	Bacterial invasion at site of abdominal paracentesis cannula.	Obtain a swab from the site of the cannula for culture review. Apply a dry dressing. Antibiotics may be necessary and instructions to check site and clean wound until resolved. Refer to the medical staff.
Cannula becomes dislodged.	Ineffective sutures or trauma at the puncture site.	Apply a secure dry dressing. Reassure patient. Inform the medical staff.
Pain.	Pressure of ascites or position of drain.	Identify cause. Anchor drain securely to avoid pulling at insertion site or movement within abdomen. Assist patient with repositioning. Administer appropriate prescribed analgesic, monitor the patient's response and inform medical staff.

References and further reading

Campbell, C. (2001) Controlling malignant ascites. *Eur J Palliat Care*, **8**(5), 187–90.

Cope, D. (2005) Malignant effusions and edema. In: *Cancer Nursing Principles and Practice* (eds C. Yarbro, M. Frogge & M. Goodman), 6th edn. Jones & Bartlet, Sudbury, MA, pp. 826–40.

DH (2001) *Good practice in consent: achieving the NHS Plan commitment to patient-centred consent practice*. HSC 2001/023. Department of Health, London.

DH (2005) Saving lives. A delivery programme to reduce healthcare infection including MRSA. www.dh.gov.uk/publications. Accessed 20/8/06.

DH (2006) About dignity in care. www.dh.gov.uk/PolicyAndGuidance/HealthAndSocialCareTopics/SocialCare/DignityInCare/DignityInCare-Article. Accessed 25/2/06.

Fentiman, I. (2002) *Oxford Text Book of Oncology*, 2nd edn. Oxford University Press, Oxford.

Hewish, P. (2006) Ascites tapping. www.patient.co.uk/showdoc/40002410/. Accessed 20/8/06.

Hosttetter, R., Marincola, F. & Schwartzentruber, D. (2005). Malignant ascites. In: *Cancer Principles and Practice of Oncology* (eds V. Devita, S. Hellman & S. Rosenberg), 7th edn. Lippincott Williams & Wilkins, Philadelphia, pp. 2392–8.

Klee, M. (2004) Symptom control info. www.symptomcontrol.com/88.0.html. Accessed 20/8/06.

Kouraklis, G. (2002) Post-operative drainage in patients with malignant ascites: a safe method. *J Surg Oncol*, **79**, 124–5.

Lee, A., Lau, T.N. & Yeong, K.Y. (2000) Indwelling catheters for the management of malignant ascites. *Support Care Cancer*, **8**(6), 493–9.

Marincola, F.M. & Schwartzentruber, D.J. (2001) *Cancer Principles and Practice of Oncology*, 6th edn. Lippincott, Williams & Wilkins, Philadelphia, pp. 2745–52.

McNamara, P. (2000) Paracentesis – an effective method of symptom control in the palliative care setting? *Palliat Med*, **14**, 62–4.

Moorsom, D. (2001) Paracentesis in a home care setting. *Palliat Med*, **15**, 169–70.

NMC (2005) *Guidelines for Records and Record Keeping*. Nursing and Midwifery Council, London.

NMC (2006) *A–Z Advice Sheet Consent*. www.nmc.org.

Stephenson, J. & Gilbert, J. (2002) The development of clinical guidelines on paracentesis for ascites related to malignancy. *Palliat Med*, **16**, 213–18.

Thibodeau, G. & Patton, K. (2007) Anatomy of the digestive system. In: *Anatomy and Physiology* (eds G. Thibodeau & K. Patton), 6th edn. Mosby, St. Louis, pp. 925–60.

Tortora, G. & Grabowski, S. (2003) The digestive system. In: *Principles of Anatomy and Physiology* (ed B. Roesch), 10th edn. John Wiley & Sons, Inc., New York, pp. 825–905.

Winkelman, L.M. (2004) Malignant ascites. In: *Cancer Symptom Management* (eds C. Yarbo, M. Frogge & M. Goodman), 3rd edn. Jones & Barlett, London, pp. 401–19.

Chapter 5

Aseptic technique

51 Reference material

57 *Procedure guidelines:* Apron: putting on and removing a disposable plastic apron

59 *Procedure guidelines:* Aseptic technique

61 *Procedure guidelines:* Hand washing

64 *Procedure guidelines:* Non-sterile gloves use

67 References and further reading

Definition

Aseptic means 'without micro-organisms'. Aseptic technique refers to the practice used to prevent the risk of infection. There are two aims of an aseptic technique: first, to protect the patient from contamination by pathogenic organisms during medical and nursing procedures; secondly, to protect the health care worker during nursing and medical procedures from being exposed to potentially infectious blood and body fluids. This can be achieved by ensuring that only sterile equipment and fluids are used during invasive medical and nursing procedures. The aseptic technique procedure has continually developed and is a skill-based procedure evolved from ritualistic and evidence-based practice (Preston 2005).

Ayliffe *et al.* (2000) suggest that there are two types of asepsis: medical and surgical asepsis. Medical or clean asepsis reduces the number of organisms and prevents their spread; surgical or sterile asepsis includes procedures to eliminate micro-organisms from an area and is practised by nurses in operating theatres and treatment areas.

A randomized prospective study has been undertaken to evaluate whether some procedures should be included in the medical or surgical category. Using a medical aseptic non-touch technique compared to a surgical technique when changing central venous devices, fluids or lines caused no difference in infection rates, indicating that it was safe to use the simpler non-touch medical aseptic technique (Larwood *et al.* 2000). However, limiting entry to sterile sites by adopting a closed system for intravascular devices (Rosenthal & Maki 2004) and urinary catheterization (Stephan *et al.* 2006) reduces the incidence of intravenous (IV) and urinary catheter-associated infection.

Indications

Patients have a right to be protected from preventable infection and nurses have a duty to safeguard the well-being of their patients, as health care-acquired infection is recognized as a major and increasing problem for our patients (Chalmers & Straub 2006). An aseptic technique should be implemented during any invasive procedure that bypasses the body's natural defences, e.g. the skin and mucous membranes, or when handling equipment such as IV cannulae and urinary catheters that have been used during these procedures.

Whilst it is difficult to maintain sterility, it is important to prevent contamination of sterile equipment. Poor aseptic techniques can lead to contamination. A 22% syringe contamination rate was observed for syringes prepared by intensive care unit nurses, compared to a 1% rate for the syringes prepared by pharmaceutical technicians (Van Grafhorst *et al.* 2002).

A study to establish nurses' actions whilst carrying out aseptic techniques suggested that not all nurses followed the same actions and that the rationale for the practice of aseptic techniques is not always research based (Preston 2005). Similar discrepancies were found amongst medical staff (Stein *et al.* 2003). Nurses can feel uncertain about how to undertake an aseptic technique (Hallett 2000). Unfortunately some infection control practices routinely used cannot be rigorously studied for ethical or logistical reasons; for example, wearing versus not wearing gloves (Mangram *et al.* 1999). Other problems relate to nurses not always understanding that research is an important part of a nurse's role (Kuuppelomaki & Tuomi 2005).

Chalmers and Straub (2006) suggest that incorporating risk management strategies during health care can help to prevent and control health care-associated infection. By predicting and planning for potential problems asepsis can be maintained.

Reference material

Health care-acquired infection (HCAI) (also called nosocomial infection) is defined as infection occurring in patients after admission to any health care facility that was neither present nor incubating at the time of admission. Infections acquired in hospital but not manifest until after the patient is discharged are included in the definition (Ayliffe *et al.* 2000). Crowe and Cooke (1998) reviewed the case definition for nosocomial infections, finding areas of consensus and variation which made comparisons of infection rates difficult.

No single factor explains why patients acquire an infection, but it is estimated that one in 10 National Health Service (NHS) hospital patients will acquire a HCAI, which is costing at least £1 billion a year. The commonest sites of infection are:

Table 5.1 Surgical site infections can be further divided by surgical category.

Surgical category	Infection risk
Clean (non-traumatic wound where respiratory, alimentary and genitourinary tracts were not entered)	1.5–4.2%
Clean/contaminated (non-traumatic wound in which respiratory, alimentary and genitourinary tracts were entered without significant spillage)	<10%
Contaminated (fresh traumatic wound from a relatively clean source or an operative wound with gross spillage from the gastrointestinal tract or entrance into genitourinary or biliary tract in the presence of infected urine or bile)	10–20%
Dirty or infected (traumatic wound from a dirty source or delayed treatment, faecal contamination, foreign bodies, a devitalized viscus or pus)	20–30%

- urinary (23%) (80% of urinary tract infections are associated with indwelling urinary catheters);
- lung (22%);
- wound (9%);
- blood (6%) (the UK has one of the highest rates of meticillin-resistant *Staphylococcus aureus* blood isolates in Europe. Sixty per cent of blood infections are associated with intravascular devices).

(DH 2003.)

Immunocompromised patients have an increased risk of HCAI. Risk factors include underlying disease, invasive procedures, medical devices and length of hospital stay. Prevention of infection for those immunocompromised patients with multiple risk factors cannot always be achieved (DH 2003). Infections acquired by neutropenic patients differ from those of general hospitalized patients. Bloodstream infections are the most common infections for neutropenic patients with haematological malignancies (Glauser & Calandra 2000) and recovery from these is often poor (Garrouste-Orgeas *et al.* 2000).

Risk factors associated with HCAI include invasive procedures, indwelling devices, malignancy, a stay in intensive care or surgical department and length of hospital stay (DH 2003).

The cost of infection is high, to both the patient and the hospital. HCAI increases mortality and morbidity (DH 2003) and causes an increase in pain and suffering, slower recovery, longer hospital stay, loss of earnings and disability experienced by the patients (Chalmers & Straub 2006). The hospital will have increased waiting lists and increased hospital costs. Breaks in aseptic techniques have been implicated in post-operative wound infections (Michalopoulos & Sparos 2003). It is essential when aseptic techniques are used as a method of preventing infection that these procedures are sound in theory and are carried out correctly.

Hospitals recognize the significance of nosocomial infections and employ infection control teams to:

- Reduce the likelihood of patients being exposed to infectious micro-organisms while in hospital.
- Provide adequate care for patients with communicable infections.
- Minimize the likelihood of employees, visitors and communicable contacts being exposed to infectious micro-organisms.
- Develop policies for appropriate management of patients with communicable infections.
- Provide surveillance systems which give adequate feedback to appropriate staff.
- Provide education in techniques to prevent the emergence and spread of infection.

Prevention of HCAI requires specific expertise (Gordts 2005). Analysis has demonstrated that infection control programmes are not only clinically effective but also cost effective (Scheckler *et al.* 1998).

Factors that influence compliance with infection control procedures included lack of knowledge, lack of time, shortage of staff, lack of facilities such as hand wash basins, lack of isolation rooms (Wilcox 2005) and bed occupancy and turnover intervals (Cunningham *et al.* 2005) as relevant indicators. It was suggested that greater emphasis and knowledge may motivate staff to make time for correct compliance with infection-control procedures.

All staff involved in patient care must receive education and training in the prevention of HCAI (DH 2001a). Creativity is required when facilitating learning related to infection control (Ford & Koehler 2001). Feedback of infection rates can achieve changes in practice (Reilly 2002).

When cross-infection does occur, the cost of investigating and controlling even a small outbreak is high. It has been estimated that an infection increases the costs of health care by more than 300% (Whitehouse *et al.* 2002), emphasizing how important it is to prevent infection. The Infection Control Standards Working Party has prepared standards for practice to make prevention, detection and control of infection in hospitals as effective as possible (Infection Control Standards Working Party 1993). Surgical wound infections are the third most common nosocomial infection in England and Wales (DH 2003) (see Table 5.1). Between October 1997 and June 2001, 140 English hospitals participated in the Nosocomial Infection National Surveillance Service (NINSS) of surgical site infection. One of the findings found that mortality rates were significantly higher following hip prostheses if the patient developed a wound infection (Coello *et al.* 2005). This data emphasizes the need for flawless aseptic technique principles in the operating theatre and the wards.

The diagnosis of infection relies on classic signs of inflammation such as local redness, swelling and pain, although decreased numbers of neutrophils produce minimal or atypical clinical signs of infection (van der Meer & Kuijpers 2000). These local signs and symptoms can precede a further sequence of events, which can be lymphangitis, lymphadenitis, bacteraemia and septicaemia, which, if not promptly recognized and treated, can result in death.

Some patients die each year as a result of HCAI. Whilst many of these fatalities occur in patients already dying from other causes and/or in patients whose infections were not preventable, a proportion of these deaths are avoidable (DH 1995; Taylor *et al.* 2001). The risk of death increases with the severity of the patient's underlying disease.

A survey completed by nurses working on wards assessed adherence to aspects of aseptic technique, and revealed an enormous level of variability, with 3% not washing their hands when delivering medication via a peripherally inserted central line (Galway *et al.* 2003). Nurses' heavy workload has been reported as a contributing factor in poor compliance with hygiene measures (Cunningham *et al.* 2005), which suggests that unnecessary time-consuming aspects of an aseptic technique should be avoided. This view is supported by Bree-Williams and Waterman's (1996) study, which highlighted that the practice of aseptic technique has become ritualistic and complex, and simpler practices are easier, cheaper and not detrimental to the patients.

Continuous education in basic infection control procedures and policies is essential, followed by audits to measure improvements (Michalopoulos & Sparos 2003). Reviews of the literature suggest that the majority of nurses have an incomplete knowledge on how to prevent cross-infection. This should be provided during pre-registration as well as in-service training (Roberts 2000). Bissett (2006) suggests that it is impossible to completely remove the risk of infection. But the National Audit Office estimates that if infection control guidelines were adhered to, HCAI could be reduced by 15% (Taylor *et al.* 2001). One multiple education approach targeted at central venous catheters was found to reduce infection rates and improve compliance to catheter care policies (Lobo *et al.* 2005). A different educational approach using local incidents of non-compliance to standard precautions may also enhance training (Ferguson *et al.* 2004) as a creative approach to training is often needed when undertaking in-service training for a large number of staff (Ford & Koehler 2001).

Principles of asepsis

Infection is caused by organisms which invade the host's immunological defence mechanisms, although susceptibility to infection may vary from person to person (Chalmers & Straub 2006). The risk of infection is increased if the patient is immunocompromised by:

- Age. Neonates and the elderly are more at risk because their immune systems are less efficient.
- Underlying disease. For example, those patients with severe debilitating or malignant disease.
- Prior drug therapy, such as the use of immunosuppressive drugs or the use of broad-spectrum antimicrobials.
- Patients undergoing surgery.

(Calandra 2000.)

The following factors must be considered when nursing immunocompromised patients:

- Classic signs and symptoms of infection are often absent.
- Untreated infection may disseminate rapidly.
- Infections may be caused by unusual organisms or organisms which, in most circumstances, are non-pathogenic.
- Some antibiotics are less effective in immunocompromised patients.
- Repeated infections may be caused by the same organism.
- Superinfections, where a patient acquires a more pathogenic organism (of the same or different species) than the one already causing infection (Laurence & May 2003), require nursing care of the highest standard, including strict adherence to aseptic technique to prevent such infections.

Chalmers and Straub (2006) suggest that a basic principle of infection control for all patients is to assess the risk of the transmission of infection from one patient to another and to plan nursing care accordingly before action is taken. Ryan *et al.* (2006) discusses how an awareness of risk amongst anaesthetists contributes to compliance to infection control guidelines. A prospective study investigating whether a risk asessment programme was effective, found that infections could be prevented which increased patients' safety (Segers *et al.* 2005). This suggests that if each patient is evaluated individually it is possible to focus more closely on those patients who are most susceptible to infection. The most usual means for spread of infection include:

- Hands of the staff involved.
- Inanimate objects, e.g. instruments and clothes.
- Dust particles or droplet nuclei suspended in the atmosphere.

Hand washing

Hand washing is well researched and uncontroversial, having been found to be the single most important procedure for preventing nosocomial infection as hands have been shown to be an important route of transmission of infection (DH 2001a). The type and amount of micro-organisms colonizing health care workers and patients' intact skin can vary from 102 to 106/cm² (Akyol *et al.* 2006). Contamination of hands can easily occur: one study evaluating contamination of gloves during a surgical aseptic technique found that contamination occurred in 55% of gloved hands (Kocent *et al.* 2002). Unfortunately, recent studies (McArdle *et al.* 2006) support those done earlier showing that hand washing is rarely carried out in a satisfactory manner. Studies have shown that up to 89% of staff miss some part of the hand surface during hand washing (Taylor 1978) (Figure 5.1), with the most important factor inhibiting hand washing being busyness (Blatnik & Lesnicar 2005) or inaccessible

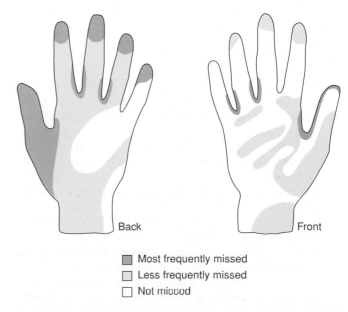

■ Most frequently missed
□ Less frequently missed
□ Not missed

Figure 5.1 Areas most commonly missed following hand washing. (Reproduced by kind permission of *Nursing Times*, where this article first appeared in 1978.)

sinks (Harris *et al.* 2000), with compliance improving when hand washing facilities were installed close to each patient's bed (Cam 2004). Compliance can improve and be sustained when new products are introduced accompanied by an associated behavioral modification programme (Whitby *et al.* 2006).

Hands must be cleaned before and after every patient contact (DH 2001a). Hand washing can be achieved by three methods:

- Soap and water are effective in removing physical dirt or soiling and transient micro-organisms (Grinbaums *et al.* 1995). Bars of soap can become slimy and be heavily contaminated during use and should not be used in patient areas. Therefore liquid soap in closed containers that do not come into contact with the user's hands should be used (Subbannayya *et al.* 2006).
- Antimicrobial detergent is effective in removing physical dirt and soiling and more effective in removing resident micro-organisms than soap and water.
- Alcohol-based handrub, whilst not effective in removing physical dirt or soiling, is more effective in destroying transient bacteria than more time-consuming hand wash methods. Therefore, hands that are visibly soiled or potentially contaminated with dirt or organic matter must be washed first with liquid soap and running water before using alcohol-based handrub (DH 2001a).

Hand washing must include the following:

1 Roll up sleeves, remove rings and wristwatches.
2 Use continuously running water.
3 Use soap.
4 Position hands to avoid contaminating arms.
5 Avoid splashing clothing or floor.
6 Rub hands together vigorously.
7 Use friction on all surfaces.
8 Rinse hands thoroughly with hand held down to rinse.
9 Dry hands thoroughly.

Hand washing should be undertaken after patient contact and before an aseptic technique is performed (DH 2001a). The use of 'glow and tell' hand washing inspection cabinets to assess the effectiveness of hand washing has been seen to improve hand washing technique (Bissett & Craig 2005).

A dispenser of alcoholic handrub should be placed on the lower shelf of all trolleys used for aseptic techniques to allow hands to be cleaned during the aseptic procedure. A nurse with 'socially clean' hands will not need to wash them during the aseptic procedure, but should use a bactericidal alcoholic handrub whenever disinfection is required, e.g. after opening the outer wrappers of dressings. The use of a handrub will also remove the need for the nurse to leave the patient during the procedure to wash the hands at the nearest basin, during which time contamination may occur.

Compliance with hand washing can be improved through multifaceted approach to training (Aragon *et al.* 2005). Ward-based infection-control link nurses can increase infection-control awareness and motivate staff to improve practice (Dawson 2003). It has been suggested that successful campaigns to improve hand washing will reduce infection rates but hospital management support is required (Pittet 2003). The wearing of rings increases the number of bacteria under the ring compared to adjacent skin or the opposite hand (Kelsall *et al.* 2006). Effective hand washing is difficult to achieve if watches and rings are not removed; rings can also cause micro-tears around the base of the finger which could expose patients to bacterial contamination (Kelsall *et al.* 2006). Artificial nails harbour microbes and cannot be cleaned as effectively as short, natural nails and must not be worn by those undertaking aseptic techniques (Porteous 2002).

Washed, wet and poorly dried hands can more easily transfer micro-organisms to other surfaces than dry hands (Gould 2000): the damper the hands, the greater the number of micro-organisms (Taylor *et al.* 2000). Thorough drying of hands after hand washing is essential but lapses in hand drying do occur (Chandra & Milind 2001). Electric air drying or disposable paper towels are the usual method of hand drying; the choice depends on the area where the hand washing is being undertaken and on issues such as noise and heat generation, waste disposal and the availability of a regular supply of paper towels. Research indicates that bacteria counts on palms and hands can increase after being dried using warm air, whilst paper towels were the most useful for removing bacteria from fingertips (Yamamoto *et al.* 2005). This suggests that the preferred method is the drying of hands with a good-quality paper towel (DH 2001a). Towel holder type and position must be considered, to ensure they are in the correct position for ease of use and that a paper towel can be removed without contaminating the remaining towels and the holder does not jam or allow the towels to fall out (Harrison *et al.* 2003). Care must be taken not to contaminate the hand wash area. Taps and the paper towel dispenser exit are the most likely areas to be contaminated, which can lead to contamination of the hands of the next user of the hand wash area (Griffith *et al.* 2003).

Non-touch technique

A non-touch technique is essential to ensure that hands, even though they have been washed, do not contaminate the sterile equipment or the patient. This can be achieved by the use of either forceps or sterile gloves (DH 2001a). However, it must be remembered that forceps may damage tissue (David 1991) and gloves can become damaged during use (Kelsall *et al.* 2006). There is no direct evidence that gloves that leak result in transmission of infection (DH 2001a). However, gloves can become contaminated during use with firm touching of the skin rather than light touching, leading to increased contamination (Kocent *et al.* 2002). Gloves must be removed carefully to prevent hands becoming contaminated during removal. Hands must be washed following removal of gloves (DH 2001a). Gloves are single-use items and must not be washed during use (Chalmers & Straub 2006).

Inanimate objects

All instruments, fluids and materials that come into contact with the wound must be sterile if the risk of contamination is to be reduced. Crow (1994) suggests four principles of asepsis, which are: (i) know what is sterile; (ii) know what is not sterile; (iii) keep these two types of items separate; and (iv) replace contaminated items immediately. There will be times when wounds will be in contact with tap water, maybe to remove dressings or during routine showering/bathing (Heal *et al.* 2006). A small double-blind randomized controlled trial comparing tap water and normal saline found no difference in healing or infection rates (Griffiths *et al.* 2001). Once the exposure to tap water is finished, the wound should be redressed using aseptic technique.

The sterile supplies department should normally provide all sterile instruments. The Department of Health (DH) (NHSE 2000) requires that all surgical instruments are traceable to the process that washed, packed and autoclaved the pack, and on whom the pack has been used. A traceability system means that the cleaning, packing and sterilization process can be checked. This ensures that the correct procedure had been undertaken at all stages of the process. If a problem occurs either with the pack or with the patient on whom the pack has been used, the instruments can be traced. These systems involve the instrument pack being labelled to prove it has gone through a sterile process. Prior to the pack being released from the autoclave, a trained person inspects the autoclave cycle responsible for the sterilization of the pack, to ensure the autoclave cycle was completed satisfactorily (NHSE 2000). When using the pack it must be checked for conformance; this includes whether the steam indicator has changed colour, the product is in date and it is undamaged. Once the pack has been used, the label has to be removed from the pack and put in the patient's notes.

All medical devices must carry the *Conformité Européene* (CE) marking which allows patients, clinicians and other users to be confident that the medical device will perform as the manufacturer intends and is safe when used as instructed (MHRA 2006). Any faults or incidents with medical devices must be reported (MHRA 2005).

The manufacturer's recommendations for all clinical supplies must be followed at all times. The reuse of single-use items must not occur and could result in legal, economic and ethical consequences (Medical Devices Agency 2000).

Forceps can be used to arrange the dressing pack, and then to remove the used dressing before being discarded. Alternatively the washed hands can be inserted into the polythene waste bag to arrange the pack before removing the used dressing. The bag which contains the used dressing is then inverted, before the bag is attached to the dressing trolley. Any equipment that becomes contaminated during a procedure must be discarded. On *no* account should it be returned to the sterile field. Care must also be taken to ensure that equipment and lotions are sterile and that packaging is undamaged before use (Ayliffe *et al.* 2000).

While following aseptic technique, it is important to evaluate the whole procedure to ensure that the principles are followed throughout the whole process. Potential problems such as reusing left-over dressings or taking tape from a contaminated roll (Oldman 1991) will therefore be avoided.

The dressing trolley

Most disinfectants are not sporicidal, have a limited antimicrobial spectrum and must be used only on clean surfaces or equipment, e.g. instruments, as they may fail to penetrate blood or pus (Ayliffe *et al.* 2000). Therefore it is essential that equipment such as a trolley is cleaned daily and, when it becomes contaminated, with a detergent solution and dried carefully with paper towels. This will remove a high proportion of micro-organisms, including bacterial spores (Ayliffe *et al.* 2000). Prior to use for aseptic technique, trolleys should be wiped over with chlorhexidine in 70% ethanol alcohol using a clean paper towel (Ayliffe *et al.* 2000). Trolleys used for aseptic procedures must not be used for any other purpose.

Personal protective equipment

Personal protective equipment (PPE) means all equipment that is intended to be worn to protect a person against risks to their health and that which may compromise their safety. The *Personal Protective Equipment at Work Regulations* (HSE 1992) requires employers to carry out a formal assessment of the PPE needs of their employees. The aim of the assessment is to identify any foreseeable risks that cannot be controlled by other means and the suitable PPE available to reduce risk (Masterson & Teare 2001). All PPE must have an appropriate British Standard kitemark or European Community CE mark. Staff required to wear PPE must be provided with information, instruction and training on the hazards from which the PPE does or does not protect the wearer, and the purpose, correct use, limitations, maintenance and storage information related to the PPE (HSE 1992). If an individual is carrying out any task that involves blood or body fluids they require PPE for the following reasons:

- To prevent the user's clothing becoming contaminated with pathogenic micro-organisms, which may subsequently be transferred to other patients in their care.
- To prevent the user's clothing becoming soiled, wet or stained during the course of their duties.
- To prevent transfer of potentially pathogenic micro-organisms from user to patient.
- To prevent the user acquiring infection from the patient (DH 2001a).

Uniform and other protective clothing should not be taken home for laundering. Changing facilities should be provided for staff to encourage them to change out of their uniform in the workplace (NHSE 2002). Nurses' uniforms can become contaminated with pathogenic micro-organisms (Perry *et al.* 2001). It is therefore recommended that a disposable plastic apron, which is impermeable to bacteria, is worn during aseptic procedures. Plastic aprons are single-use items and are worn for one procedure or episode of patient care and then removed (DH 2001a). Gowns must be worn when undertaking invasive surgical procedures; for example, when inserting central venous catheters (DH 2001b). Surgical masks are an integral part of theatre clothing. However, it has never been shown that wearing a surgical mask decreases post-operative wound infections (Lipp & Edwards 2005). Masks must be worn as part of routine universal precautions when there is a risk of airborne aerosol of blood or body fluids, administration of toxic drugs or contact with patients who are smear positive with drug-resistant tuberculosis (DH 2001a; NICE 2006). These masks must comply with the Control of Substances Hazardous to Health (COSHH) (DH 2002) regulations. For surgical procedures undertaken on the wards, masks are generally not required. There is no evidence that wearing a face mask is important in preventing catheter-related infection during central catheter insertion (DH 2001b).

Gloves

Disposable gloves are available in latex and synthetic materials, in sterile and non-sterile form, with and without powder. Gloves must conform to European Community (CE) standards, must not be powdered nor made from polythene. Alternatives to latex gloves must be available because of the increase in sensitivity to latex amongst patients and health care workers (DH 2001a).

Latex allergy guidelines pertaining to the safety of patients and staff must be available. All health care workers must be knowledgeable about latex allergy and its related issues (Wright *et al.* 2001). Problems related to latex allergies must be reported to the Occupational Health Department immediately for early diagnosis and treatment (Medical Devices Agency 1996). Incidences of latex sensitivity are reportable to the Health and Safety Executive under the Reporting of Injuries, Diseases and Dangerous Occurrences Regulations (1985) (RIDDOR) (HSE 1995; NHSE 1999).

Boxed, clean, non-sterile, powder-free gloves made from materials other than latex are safe for routine use (Rossoff *et al.* 1993), in particular to protect hands from contamination with organic matter and micro-organisms (DH 2001a). However, boxed, clean, non-sterile gloves should not be used for aseptic techniques as there is insufficient evidence to justify a practice change to non-sterile gloves for aseptic techniques (St. Clair & Larrabee 2002). Efforts must be made when wearing gloves to avoid glove contamination (Kocent *et al.* 2002) and glove damage (Cork *et al.* 1995).

Failure to change gloves after each patient contact does occur particularly when handling food (Blenkharn 2006). Generally compliance with correct glove use is poor (Girou *et al.* 2004).

Protective footwear

Micro-organisms can be found on the bottom of footwear (Haigh 1993). However, the risk of acquiring infection from floors (Ayliffe *et al.* 2000) and the bottom of health care workers' footwear is low (Haigh 1993). Whilst washable shoes must be kept for those entering the operating theatre (Ayliffe *et al.* 2000), footwear worn elsewhere in the hospital is chosen to comply with risk management rather than infection control.

Environmental cleanliness

The NHS requires that patients are nursed in a clean, comfortable and safe environment (DH 2003). The NHS Performance Assessment Framework (NHSE 2001) includes a cleanliness standard. The standard can be used to monitor and improve cleaning services. The standard has five key objectives: (i) take cleaning seriously; (ii) listen to patients; (iii) infection control; (iv) education; (v) development and monitoring. Included in the standard are lists of elements and their cleaning requirements. These include odour control and a tidy, uncluttered, well-maintained environment (NHSE 2001).

Good hospital hygiene is an integral and important component for preventing HCAI. Unfortunately extensive contamination of the hospital environment is known to occur (Oie *et al.* 2002). Cleaning and disinfecting programmes and protocols for patient care areas must be clearly defined and carefully monitored to ensure high standards of cleanliness are achieved (DH 2003), to ensure that the patient area must be visibly clean, free of dust and soilage before an aseptic technique is commenced. Therefore thorough cleaning, clean laundry, safe collection of waste and food hygiene and pest control are essential (DH 2001a).

Routine cleaning of the environment is the responsibility of the hospital domestic staff. Cleaning must be suspended during aseptic techniques (Ayliffe *et al.* 2000).

Patient hygiene

The majority of infections in susceptible patients are caused by the patient's own endogenous flora (Glauser & Calandra 2000). Preoperative bathing or showering is a well-accepted procedure for reducing skin micro-organisms (Webster & Osborne 2006). Bathing and showering using an antiseptic detergent to eliminate meticillin-resistant *Staphylococcus aureus* (MRSA) colonization of skin is well documented (Rohr *et al.* 2003), although a study comparing routine skin cleaning with soap and water to chlorhexidine solution found no difference in wound infections (Kalantar-Hormozi & Davami 2005). The general population's showering habits vary considerably (Wilkes *et al.* 2005). It is well documented that illness affects patients' well-being which may influence their energy levels (Munch *et al.* 2005); therefore, nurses must be prepared to assist patients with their daily bath or shower.

Studies have established that it is not detrimental for stitches of surgical wounds to get wet (Heal *et al.* 2006). After showering any non-waterproof dressing should be changed immediately. The use of a transparent film dressing allows continuous inspection and more secure anchorage as well as being comfortable and protecting against wetting during showering (Cosker *et al.* 2005).

Airborne contamination

The spread of airborne infection is most likely to occur following procedures such as bed making (Shiomori *et al.* 2002) and cleaning, which can disperse organisms into the air. Airborne contamination of sterile goods can occur (Dietze *et al.* 2001). Ideally such activities should cease 30 minutes before a dressing is to be undertaken. To reduce further the risk of airborne contamination of open wounds, the wound should be exposed for as short a time as possible (Ayliffe *et al.* 2000). Dirty dressings should be placed carefully in a yellow clinical waste bag, which is sealed before disposal (DH 2006a). Clean wounds should be dressed before contaminated wounds. Colostomies and infected wounds should be dressed last of all to minimize environmental contamination and cross-infection.

Air movement should be kept to a minimum during the dressing. This means that adjacent windows should be closed and the movement of personnel within the area discouraged.

Procedure guidelines   Apron: putting on and removing a disposable plastic apron

Action	Rationale
1 Adequate supply of disposable aprons in a dispenser made for this purpose to be available.	Staff are more likely to put on an apron if they are readily available (E).
2 Dispenser to be positioned away from any source of contamination, but near enough to the point of use to be readily available. For example outside a barrier nursing room.	Plastic aprons generally are in rolls or packs of 100 or 200. Micro-organisms such as MRSA and VRE will survive on contaminated equipment (Dietze *et al.* 2001: R 1b).
3 Colour-coded aprons to be in areas of high risk, for example in Critical Care Units, where each bed has a different colour apron designated for that bed space.	By colour coding aprons it is possible to see if the correct colour apron is being used for the correct task or environment (E).
4 Plastic aprons are single-use items and must be only worn for one procedure or episode of patient care.	Single patient-use items only and cannot be cleaned and reused for another patient (MHRA 2002: E).
5 Used aprons must be discarded and disposed of in a yellow clinical waste bag.	All waste contaminated with blood, body fluids, excretions, secretions and micro-organisms disposed as clinical waste. Yellow is the recognized colour for clinical waste (DH 2005: C; DH 2006a: C).
6 Plastic aprons must be worn during close contact with a patient, patient equipment or the environment when contamination with pathogenic micro-organisms or blood and body fluids is expected. Perspiration is an exception (Pratt *et al.* 2007).	To protect the clothing that is covered by the plastic apron from contamination (Pratt *et al.* 2007: R 1a).
7 Remove a plastic apron from the dispenser making sure no other aprons are dislodged at the same time. If this does occur the dislodged unwanted apron should be disposed of as domestic waste in a black polythene bag.	Dislodged aprons can become contaminated; as this apron has not been used and therefore is not contaminated it can be disposed of as domestic waste (DH 2005: C; DH 2006a: C).
8 Pull the apron over your head, avoid touching your hair and uniform (see Action figure 8).	Hands may become contaminated when touching hair and skin as hair and skin can be colonized with micro-organisms such as *Staphylococcus aureus* and *epidemidis*, which can cause infections (Mims *et al.* 2004: R 1a).
9 Tie the apron loosely at the back.	Tightly tied aprons can cause the wearer to become hot and uncomfortable, as well as make the apron more difficult to remove (E).

Procedure guidelines *(cont.)*

10 Cleanse hands, using an alcoholic handrub.	Hands must be cleansed before and after every contact with patients and their equipment. As hands would have been cleansed after the previous patient's contact, hands would have been clean before putting on the apron (Pratt *et al.* 2007: R 1a).
11 If required put on single-use disposable gloves. Gloves should be put on after the apron is put on and removed before the apron is removed.	Sterile gloves to be worn for invasive procedures, contact with sterile sites, non-intact skin or mucous membranes. Clean gloves to be worn when exposure to blood, body fluids, secretions and excretions is likely to occur (Pratt *et al.* 2007: R 1a).
12 Undertake procedure. On completion of the procedure remove the apron. This is achieved by pulling on the apron to break the loop around the neck and the ties behind the back. This is achieved by pulling on the part of the apron that is clean for example the neck and sides (see Action figures 12a–c).	Hands may become contaminated during the procedure by removing the apron, unhooking the neck loop or untying the apron's ties, which could contaminate the wearer's neck, hair and the back of their clothing (E).
13 Clean hands using a liquid soap and warm running water and carefully dry with a paper towel.	Alcoholic handrub is only suitable for clean hands, whilst liquid soap and water removes contamination (Pratt *et al.* 2007: R 1a).
14 If extensive splashing of blood, body fluids, secretions and excretions are expected a full body fluid-repellent gown must be worn as a single-use item.	A gown offers more protection than a plastic apron which only covers the front of the wearer's uniform (Pratt *et al.* 2007: R 1a).

Action 8   Pull the apron over your head, avoiding touching your hair and uniform.

Action 12a   To remove apron, pull apron to break loop around neck and ties behind the back.

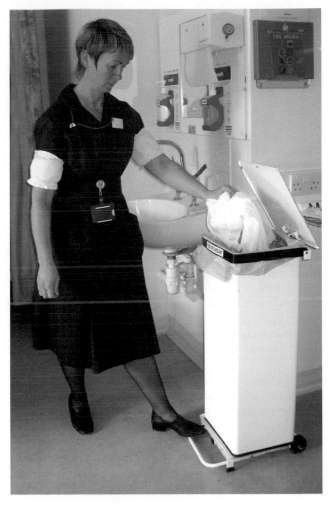

Action 12b   Avoid touching uniform whilst removing apron.

Action 12c   Dispose of used plastic apron as clinical waste.

Procedure guidelines   Aseptic technique

Equipment

1 Sterile dressing pack* containing gallipots or an indented plastic tray, low-linting swabs and/or medical foam, disposable forceps, gloves, sterile field, disposable bag.
2 Fluids for cleaning and/or irrigation.
3 Hypo-allergenic tape.
4 Appropriate dressing (see Chapter 48).
5 Appropriate hand hygiene preparation.
6 Any other material will be determined by the nature of the dressing: special features of a dressing should be referred to in the patient's nursing care plan.

7 Any extra equipment that may be needed during procedure, e.g. sterile scissors.
8 Chlorhexidine in 70% spirit and paper towels for cleaning trolley.
9 Total traceability system for surgical instruments and patient record form.

Procedure guidelines (cont.)

Procedure

Action	Rationale
1 Explain and discuss the procedure with the patient.	To ensure that the patient understands the procedure and gives his or her valid consent (NMC 2006: C; Wilson 2006: E).
2 Clean hands with bactericidal alcohol rub.	Hands must be cleaned before and after every patient contact and before commencing the preparations for aseptic technique, to prevent cross-infection (DH 2005: C).
3 Clean trolley with chlorhexidine in 70% spirit with a paper towel.	To provide a clean working surface (Ayliffe et al. 2000: C).
4 Place all the equipment required for the procedure on the bottom shelf of the clean dressing trolley.	To maintain the top shelf as a clean working surface (E).
5 Take the patient to the treatment room or screen the bed. Position the patient comfortably so that the area to be dealt with is easily accessible without exposing the patient unduly.	To allow any airborne organisms to settle before the sterile field (and in the case of a dressing, the wound) is exposed (Ayliffe et al. 2000 C). Maintain the patient's dignity and comfort (E).
6 If the procedure is a dressing and the wound is infected or producing copious amounts of exudate, put on a disposable plastic apron.	To reduce the risk of cross-infection (DH 2005: C).
7 Take the trolley to the treatment room or patient's bedside, disturbing the screens as little as possible.	To minimize airborne contamination (Ayliffe et al. 2000: C).
8 Loosen the dressing tape.	To make it easier to remove the dressing (E).
9 Clean hands with a bactericidal alcohol handrub.	To reduce the risk of wound infection (DH 2005: C).
10 Check the pack is sterile (i.e. the pack is undamaged, intact and dry. If autoclave tape is present, check that it has changed colour from beige to beige and brown lines), open the outer cover of the sterile pack and slide the contents onto the top shelf of the trolley.	To ensure that only sterile products are used (MHRA 2005: E).
11 Open the sterile field using only the corners of the paper.	So that areas of potential contamination are kept to a minimum (E).
12 Check any other packs for sterility and open, tipping their contents gently onto the centre of the sterile field.	To prepare the equipment and, in the case of a wound dressing, reduce the amount of time that the wound is uncovered. This reduces the risk of infection and a drop in temperature of the wound which will delay wound healing (Naylor et al. 2001: R 1a).
13 Clean hands with a bactericidal alcohol rub.	Hands may become contaminated by handling outer packets, etc. (DH 2005: C).
14 Place hand in disposable bag, arrange contents of dressing pack.	To maintain sterility of pack (E).

15	Remove used dressing with hand covered with the disposable bag, invert bag and stick to trolley.	To minimize risk of contamination, by containing dressing in bag (E).
16	Where appropriate, swab along the 'tear area' of lotion sachet with chlorhexidine in 70% spirit/swab saturated with 70% isopropyl alcohol. Tear open sachet and pour lotion into gallipots or on indented plastic tray.	To minimize risk of contamination of lotion (E).
17	Put on sterile gloves, touching only the inside wrist end.	To reduce the risk of infection. Gloves provide greater sensitivity than forceps and are less likely to cause trauma to the patient (David 1991: E).

Carry out procedure

18	Make sure the patient is comfortable.	
19	Dispose of waste in yellow plastic clinical waste bags. Remove gloves.	To prevent environmental contamination. Yellow is the recognized colour for clinical waste (DH 2006a: C).
20	If necessary, draw back curtains or, if appropriate, help the patient back to the bed area and ensure the patient is comfortable.	
21	Check that the trolley remains dry and physically clean. If necessary, wash with liquid detergent and water and dry throughly with a paper towel.	To reduce the risk of spreading infection (Ayliffe *et al.* 2000: C).
22	Clean hands with bactericidal alcohol handrub.	To reduce the risk of spreading infection (DH 2005: C).
23	Place sterility label from the outside of any surgical instrument packs used during the procedure on the patient record form which is to be placed in the patient's notes.	Provides a record, as the sterility label proves the pack has gone through a sterile process and that prior to release has been inspected by a trained person in the Sterile Services Department (NHSE 2000).

NB. Please note that for some procedures it may be more appropriate to use different types of sterile packs (e.g. IV packs). Since usage of these will vary locally reference is generally made to 'sterile dressing pack'.

Procedure guidelines   Hand washing

Hands must be cleaned before and after each patient contact, and after any task that may have resulted in the hands becoming contaminated. There is substantial evidence to indicate that hand washing is the single most important action to reduce the incident of hospital-acquired infection (DH 2001a).

Equipment and facilities

Wrist/knee/elbow or automatic taps should be used in all clinical areas in order to prevent dirty hands contaminating the taps, which could lead to cross-contamination of the next person who uses the taps. Hand basins should be located conveniently near to where they are required. They must be maintained in good working order and always kept stocked with a plentiful supply of paper towels and liquid soap in disposable containers. This ensures the soap containers are not topped up from a larger container. Soap containers can become contaminated (Ayliffe *et al.* 2000) and by renewing them on a regular basis, a potential source of infection is removed. It is important that the design of the paper towel dispenser allows for easy removal of the paper towel without contaminating the remaining towels. Contaminated paper towels could lead to cross-infection.

Procedure guidelines *(cont.)*

Procedure

Action	Rationale
1 Remove rings, bracelets and wristwatch.	Jewellery inhibits good hand washing. Dirt and bacteria can remain beneath jewellery after hand washing (DH 2001a: C).
2 Roll up sleeves.	Long sleeves prevent washing of wrists (E).
3 Cover cuts and abrasions on hands with waterproof dressing.	Cuts and abrasions can become contaminated with bacteria and cannot be easily cleaned. Repeated hand washing can increase the injury (DH 2001a: C).
4 Remove nail varnish and artificial nails. Nails must also be short and clean.	Long nails and false nails may be a source of infection by harbouring dirt and bacteria. Nail varnish can become cracked, which could lead to contamination if the nail polish fell into a patient's wound. Nail polish can also inhibit effective hand washing by potentially harbouring bacteria in microscopic imperfections of nail varnish (DH 2001a: C).
5 Hands that are visibly or potentially soiled or contaminated with dirt or organic material should be washed with liquid soap from a dispenser and running hand-hot water.	Liquid soap is very effective in removing dirt, organic material and any loosely adherent transient flora, but has little antimicrobial activity. Liquid soap must be used, as tablets of soap can become contaminated (DH 2001a: C).
(a) Turn on the taps using wrist/elbow or foot and direct the water flow away from the plughole. Run the water at a flow rate that prevents splashing.	Plugholes are often contaminated with micro-organisms that could be transferred to the environment or the user if splashing occurs (NHSE 2002: C).
(b) Run the water until hand hot.	Hand-hot water to be used to ensure that the skin of hands is not damaged by cold water. Water that is too hot could cause scalding. Soap is more effective in breaking down dirt and organic matter when used with hand-hot water (DH 2001a: C).
(c) Wet the surface of hands and wrists.	Soap applied directly onto dry hands may damage the skin. The water will also quickly mix with the soap to speed up hand washing (DH 2001a: C).
(d) Apply liquid soap and water to all surfaces of the hands.	To ensure all surfaces of the hands are cleaned (DH 2001a: C).
(e) Rub hands together for a minimum of 10–15 seconds, with particular attention to between the fingers and the tips of fingers and thumbs.	To ensure all surfaces of the hands are cleaned. Areas that are missed can be a source of cross-infection (DH 2001a: C).
(f) Nail brushes should not be used.	Nail brushes may damage the skin and result in increased shedding of bacteria from the hands (Winnefeld *et al.* 2000: C).

(g) Rinse soap thoroughly off hands.

A residue of soap can lead to irritation and damage to the skin. Damaged skin does not provide a barrier to infection for the health care worker and can become colonized with potentially pathogenic bacteria, leading to cross-infection (DH 2001a: C).

(h) Care must be taken not to contaminate the taps, sink or nozzle of the soap dispenser with dirt or organic material that is washed off hands.

Contamination of the nozzle of the soap dispenser can result in contamination of the liquid soap, leading to cross-infection (E).

(i) Dry hands thoroughly with a good-quality disposable paper towel from a towel dispenser.

Damp hands encourage the multiplication of bacteria and can potentially become sore (DH 2001a: C).

(j) Dispose of used paper towels in a black bag on a foot-operated stand.

Black is the colour coding for paper waste. Using a foot-operated waste bag stand prevents contamination of the hands (E).

6 Hands that are visibly clean and not soiled or contaminated with dirt, organic material or toxic substances can be cleaned using an alcoholic handrub.

The antimicrobial activity of alcohol is due to its ability to denature proteins. Alcoholic handrub solutions are a quick convenient method of cleansing clean hands of Gram-negative, Gram-positive vegetative bacteria, tuberculosis and a variety of fungi, but have poor activity against bacterial spores and cannot remove dirt, organic material or toxic substances such as drugs or radioactivity. Alcoholic handrub comes in a variety of solutions, gels and foams with an emollient (which reduces the drying effect of the alcohol) (DH 2001a: C).

(a) Follow the manufacturer's instructions for the amount of handrub to be used.

The instructions must be followed so that the correct amount of handrub is used to ensure effective hand cleaning. Too much will cause delays and leave hands sticky, too little will not clean hands adequately (E).

(b) Rub an alcoholic handrub into **all** areas of the hands, until the hands are dry.

To ensure all areas of the hands are cleaned. Alcohol is a rapid-acting disinfectant, with the added advantage that it evaporates, leaving the hands dry. This prevents contamination of equipment, whilst facilitating the application of unpowdered gloves (DH 2001a: C).

7 Hand washing using a bacterial detergent for surgical procedures to be undertaken outside the operating theatre:

Rapid multiplication of bacteria occurs under surgical gloves if hands are washed with a non-bactericidal soap. The use of bactericidal soap reduces the resident skin flora. Bactericidal detergents have a persistent activity, which means that following use the bacteria appear to reproduce slowly on hands.

(a) Turn on the taps using wrist/elbow or foot and direct the water flow away from the plughole. Run the water at a flow rate that prevents splashing.

Plugholes are often contaminated with micro-organisms that could be transferred to the environment or the user if splashing occurs (DH 2001a: C).

(b) Run the water until hand hot.

Hand-hot water to be used to ensure that the skin of hands is not damaged by cold water. Water that is too hot could cause scalding. Soap is more effective in breaking down dirt and organic matter when used with hand-hot water (DH 2001a: C).

Procedure guidelines *(cont.)*

64

(c) Wet hands with hand-hot water.

Applying bactericidal detergent directly onto dry hands increases the risk of skin damage/irritation (E).

(d) Apply the amount of bactericidal detergent advised by the manufacturer.

The correct amount of detergent must be used to ensure effective hand cleaning (E).

(e) The following washing/rubbing actions should be undertaken five times:

All surfaces of hands must be thoroughly washed for effective hand washing to have taken place (DH 2001a: C).

- Rotational rubbing of wrists.
- Palm to palm.
- Right palm to back of left hand.
- Left palm to back of right hand.
- Palm to palm, fingers interlaced.
- Back of fingers of one hand to palm of other hand with fingers interlaced.
- Rotational rubbing of right thumb in left palm and left thumb in right palm.
- Rotational rubbing of fingers in clasped palm of opposite hand.

(f) Holding hands upright, rinse them and wrists under hand-hot running water to remove soap.

Soap residue can cause skin damage. Hands must be held upright to ensure water splashes from unwashed areas of arm do not run down onto clean hands (E).

(g) Dry hands carefully using a good-quality paper towel.

Wet hands can encourage the growth of bacteria and may lead to sore hands (Gould & Chamberlain 1994: R 1a).

Hand washing for surgical procedures in theatre

8 The routine is the same as above but the forearms are included. The hand washing is extended to 2 minutes during which time repeated applications of the bactericidal detergent are required. Hands are dried using a sterile disposable paper towel.

The optimal length of the hand washing is unknown. The important factor is that all areas have been effectively cleaned and rinsed (E).

   To prevent contamination from unsterile paper towels (E).

Procedure guidelines   Non-sterile gloves use

Equipment

Gloves are single-use items. Single-use items cannot be cleaned and reused for the same or another patient (MHRA 2002: E). Clean boxed gloves are suitable for non-touch aseptic techniques and when there is a risk of exposure to blood, body fluids, excretions, secretions and micro-organisms. Gloves provide a barrier to the hands from contamination from blood, body fluids, excretions, secretions and micro-organisms (Pratt *et al.* 2007: C). Gloves that are CE marked must be available in all clinical areas. CE marking denotes the standard and suitability of the product (Pratt *et al.* 2007: C). Gloves should be stored safely to ensure they are protected from contamination. Powdered and polythene gloves should not be used. Alternatives to natural rubber latex gloves must be available for all staff who have a history of latex sensitivity. Emphasis should be placed on providing alternatives to latex for all staff.

   A full range of small, medium and large gloves must be accessible to ensure a correctly fitting glove is available for all staff. Incorrectly fitting gloves decreases dexterity of the wearer and could lead to accidents or poor care (E).

65

Action	Rationale
1 Hands to be cleaned prior to putting on gloves.	Hands must be cleansed before and after every patient contact or contact with patient's equipment (Pratt *et al.* 2007: C).
2 Gloves should be removed from the box singly, to prevent contamination of the lower down gloves.	To prevent cross-infection (E).
3 Holding the cuff of the gloves, pull the glove into position taking care not to contaminate the glove from the wearer's skin. This is particularly important when the second glove is being put on, as the gloved hand of the first glove can touch the skin of the ungloved second hand if care is not taken.	To prevent cross-infection (E).
4 During the procedure or when undertaking two procedures with the same patient, it may be necessary to change gloves. Gloves are single-use items and must not be cleansed and reused.	Gloves are single patient-use items only and cannot be cleaned and reused for the same or another patient (MHRA 2002: C).
5 Similarly if gloves become damaged during use they must be replaced.	Damaged gloves do not provide protection (E).
6 When the procedure is completed and the gloves are to be removed, care must be taken to ensure contamination of the wearer does not occur.	The outside of the glove may be contaminated (E).
7 The first glove can be removed by firmly holding the glove wrist and pulling off the glove in such a way as to turn it inside out.	Whilst removing the first glove the second gloved hand continues to be protected. By turning the glove inside out during removal the contamination is contained inside the glove (E).
8 The second glove is removed by slipping the fingers of the other ungloved hand inside the wrist of the glove and pulling it off whilst at the same time turning it inside out.	By putting the fingers inside the glove, the fingers will not be in contact with the potentially contaminated outer surface of the glove (E).
9 Used gloves are to be disposed of in the yellow clinical waste bag.	All waste contaminated with blood, body fluids, excretions, secretions and micro-organisms should be disposed of as clinical waste. Yellow is the recognized colour for clinical waste (DH 2005: C; DH 2006a: C).
10 Hands to be cleansed after taking off gloves, ideally by washing with liquid soap and running water.	Hands may have become contaminated. Alcoholic handrub is only suitable for clean hands whilst liquid soap and water removes contamination (Pratt *et al.* 2007 C).
11 If an apron is being worn at the same time as the gloves, the gloves are to be removed first followed by the apron and then the hands should be washed.	The gloves are more likely to be contaminated than the apron and therefore should be removed first to prevent cross-infection (E).

Procedure guidelines *(cont.)*

Action 2   Carefully remove gloves to prevent contamination of remaining gloves.

Action 3   Holding the cuff of the glove, pull the glove into position.

Action 7   Holding the cuff, remove the first glove, turning it inside out.

Action 8   Remove second glove by inserting fingers inside the wrist of the glove; pull it off whilst turning it inside out.

References and further reading

Akyol, A., Ulusoy, H. & Ozen, I. (2006) Handwashing: a simple, economical and effective method for preventing nosocomial infections in intensive care units. *J Hosp Infect*, **62**(4), 395–405.

Aragon, D., Sole, M.L. & Brown, S. (2005) Outcomes of an infection prevention project focusing on hand hygiene and isolation practices. *AACN Clin Issues*, **16**(2), 121–32.

Ayliffe, G.A.J. *et al.* (2000) *Control of Hospital Infection. A Practical Handbook*, 4th edn. Arnold, London.

Bissett, L. (2006) Reducing the risk of acquiring antimicrobial-resistant bacteria. *Br J Nurs*, **15**(2), 68–71.

Bissett, L. & Craig, K. (2005) Hand inspection cabinets as an aid to washing technique. *Nurs Times*, **1001**(31), 38–40.

Blatnik, J. & Lesnicar, G. (2005) Propagation of Methicillin-resistant *Staphylococcus aureus* due to the overloading of medical nurses in intensive care units. *J Hosp Infect*, **63**(2), 162–6.

Blenkharn, J.I. (2006) Glove use by ancillary and support staff: a paradox of prevention? *J Hosp Infect*, **62**(4), 519–20.

Bree-Williams, E.J. & Waterman, H. (1996) An examination of nurses' practices when performing aseptic technique for wound dressing. *J Adv Nurs*, **23**, 48–54.

Calandra, T. (2000) Practical guide to host mechanisms and the predominant infections encountered in immunocompromised patients. In: *Management of Infections in Immunocompromised Patients*, Part I (Section 1) (eds M.P. Glauser & P.A. Pizzo). W.B. Saunders, London, pp. 3–17.

Cam, J. (2004) What does it take to ensure effective hand decontamination by nurses? *Prof Nurse*, **19**(12), 26–8.

Chalmers, C. & Straub, M. (2006) Standard principles for preventing and controlling infection. *Nurs Stand*, **20**(23), 57–65.

Chandra, P.N. & Milind, K. (2001) Lapses in measures recommended for preventing hospital-acquired infection. *J Hosp Infect*, **47**(3), 218–22.

Coello, R. *et al.* (2005) Adverse impact of surgical site infections in English hospitals. *J Hosp Infect*, **60**(2), 93–103.

Cork, R.C. *et al.* (1995) Leak rate of latex gloves after tearing adhesive tape. *Am J Anesthesiol*, **22**(3), 133–7.

Cosker, T. *et al.* (2005) Choice of dressing has a major impact on blistering and healing outcomes in orthopaedic patients. *Wound Care*, **14**(1), 27–9.

Crow, S. (1994) Asepsis: a prophylactic technique. *Semin Perioper Nurs*, **3**(2), 93–100.

Crowe, M.J. & Cooke, E.M. (1998) Review of case definition for nosocomial infection – towards a consensus. Presentation by nosocomial infection surveillance unit to hospital infection liaison group, subcommittee of Federation of Infection Societies. *J Hosp Infect*, **39**(1), 3–11.

Cunningham, J.B., Kernohan, W.G. & Sowney, R. (2005) Bed occupancy and turnover interval as determinant factors in MRSA infections in acute settings in Northern Ireland: 1 April 2001 to 31 March 2003. *J Hosp Infect*, **61**(3), 189–93.

David, J. (1991) Letters. *Wound Manage*, **1**(2), 15.

Dawson, S.J. (2003) The role of the infection control link nurse. *J Hosp Infect*, **54**(4), 251–7.

DH (1995) *Hospital Infection Control: Guidance on the Control of Infection in Hospitals*. Department of Health, London.

DH (1998) *Prevention and Control of Tuberculosis in the United Kingdom* (HSC 1998/196). Department of Health, London.

DH (2001a) Standard principles for preventing hospital-acquired infection. *J Hosp Infect*, **47**(Suppl), S21–37.

DH (2001b) Guidelines for preventing infections associated with the insertion and maintenance of central venous catheters. *J Hosp Infect*, **47**(Suppl), S49–67.

DH (2002) *Control of Substances Hazardous to Health Regulations*. COSSH, Department of Health, London.

DH (2003) *Winning Ways*. Department of Health, London.

DH (2005) *Hazardous Waste (England) Regulations*. Department of Health, London.

DH (2006a) *Health Technical Memorandum 07-01: Safe management of healthcare waste*. Department of Health, London.

DH (2006b) *Saving Lives: A Delivery Programme to Reduce Healthcare Associated Infection including MRSA*. Department of Health, London.

Dietze, B. *et al.* (2001) Survival of MRSA on sterile goods packaging. *J Hosp Infect*, **49**(4), 255–61.

Ferguson, K.J. *et al.* (2004) Critical incidents of nonadherence with standard precautions guidelines among community hospital-based health care workers. *J Gen Intern Med*, **19**(7), 808–9.

Ford, D.A. & Koehler, S.H. (2001) A creative process for reinforcing aseptic technique practices. *AORN J*, **73**(2), 446–50.

Galway, R. *et al.* (2003) Central venous access and handwashing: variability in policies and practice. *Paediatr Nurs*, **15**(10), 14–18.

Garrouste-Orgeas, M. *et al.* (2000) A one-year prospective study of nosocomial bacteraemia in ICU and non-ICU patients and its impact on patients' outcome. *J Hosp Infect*, **44**(3), 206–13.

Girou, E., Chai, S.H. & Oppein, F. (2004) Misuse of gloves: the foundation for poor compliance with hand hygiene and potential for microbial transmission. *J Hosp Infect*, **57**(2), 162–9.

Glauser, M.P. & Calandra, T. (2000) Infections in patients with hematologic malignancies. In: *Management of Infections in Immunocompromised Patients*, Part II (Section 4) (eds M.P. Glauser & P.A. Pizzo). W.B. Saunders, London, pp. 141–88.

Gordts, B. (2005) Models for the organisation of hospital infection control and prevention programmes. *Clin Microbiol Infect*, Suppl **1**, 19–23.

Gould, D. (2000) Innovations in hand hygiene: manual from SSL International. *Br J Nurs*, **9**(20), 2175–80.

Gould, D. & Chamberlain, A. (1994) Gram-negative bacteria. The challenge of preventing cross-infection in hospital wards: a review of the literature. *J Clin Nurs*, **3**(6), 339–45.

Griffith, C.J. *et al.* (2003) Environmental surface cleanliness and the potential for contamination during handwashing. *Am J Infect Control*, **31**(2), 93–6.

Griffiths, R.D., Fernandez R.S. & Ussia, C.A. (2001) Is tap water a safe alternative to normal saline for wound irrigation in the community setting. *J Wound Care*, **10**(10), 407–11.

Grinbaums, R.S., de Mendonca, J.S. & Cardo, D.M. (1995) An outbreak of handscrubbing-related surgical site infections in vascular surgical procedures. *Infect Control Hosp Epidemiol*, **16**(4), 198–202.

Haigh, C. (1993) A study of micro-organism levels on nurses' footwear. *Br J Nurs*, **2**(22), 1109–12.

Haley, R.W. *et al.* (1985a) The efficiency of infection surveillance and control programmes in preventing nosocomial infections in US hospitals. *Am J Epidemiol*, **121**, 182–205.

Hallett, C.E. (2000) Infection control in wound care: a study of fatalism in community nursing. *J Clin Nurs*, **9**(1), 103–9.

Hambraeus, A. (1973) Transfer of *Staphylococcus aureus* via nurses' uniform. *J Hyg*, **71**, 799–814.

Hampton, S. (2002) The appropriate use of gloves to reduce allergies and infection. *Br J Nur*, **11**(17), 1120–4.

Harris, A.D. *et al.* (2000) A survey on handwashing practices and opinions of health care workers. *J Hosp Infect*, **45**(4), 318–21.

Harrison, W.A. *et al.* (2003) Techniques to determine contamination exposure routes and the economic efficiency of folded paper-towel dispensing. *Am J Infect Control*, **31**(2), 104–8.

Heal, C. *et al.* (2006) Can sutures get wet? Prospective randomised controlled trial of wound management in general practice. *BMJ*, **332**(7549), 1053–4.

HSE (1992) *Personal Protective Equipment at Work Regulations*. Department of Health, London.

HSE (1995) *Reporting of Injuries, Diseases and Dangerous Occurrences Regulations (RIDDOR)*. Department of Health, London.

Infection Control Standards Working Party (1993) *Standards in Infection Control in Hospitals*. HMSO, London.

Kalantar-Hormozi, A.J. & Davami, B. (2005) No need for preoperative antiseptics in elective outpatients plastic surgical operations: a prospective study. *Plast Reconstr Surg*, **116**(2), 529–31.

Kelsall, N.K.R. *et al.* (2006) Should finger rings be removed prior to scrubbing for theatre? *J Hosp Infect*, **62**(4), 450–2.

Kocent, H. *et al.* (2002) Washing of gloved hands in antiseptic solution prior to central line insertion reduces contamination. *Anaesth Intensive Care*, **30** (3), 338–40.

Kuuppelomaki, M. & Tuomi, J. (2005) Finnish nurses' attitudes towards nursing research and related factors. *Int J Nurs Stud*, **42**(2), 187–96.

Larwood, K.A., Anstey, C.M. & Dunn, S.V. (2000) Managing central venous catheters: a prospective randomised trial of two methods. *Aust Crit Care*, **13**(2), 44–50.

Lawrence J. & May D. (2003) *Infection Control in the Community*. Churchill Livingstone, Edinburgh.

Lipp, A. & Edwards, P. (2005) Disposable surgical face masks: a systematic review. *Can Oper Room Nurs J*, **23**(3), 20–1.

Lobo, R.D. *et al.* (2005) Impact of an educational program and policy changes on decreasing catheter-associated bloodstream infections in a medical intensive care unit in Brazil. *Am J Infect Control*, **33**(2), 83–7.

Mangram, A.J. *et al.* (1999) Guideline for prevention of surgical site infection, 1999. Centers for Disease Control and Prevention [CDC] Hospital Infection Practices Advisory Committee. *Am J Infect Control*, **27**(2), 97–132.

Masterson, R.G. & Teare, E.L. (2001) Clinical governance and infection control in the United Kingdom. *J Hosp Infect*, **47**(1), 25–31.

McArdle, F.I. *et al.* (2006) How much time is needed for hand hygiene in intensive care? A prospective trained observer study of rates of contact between healthcare workers and intensive care patients. *J Hosp Infect*, **62**(3), 304–10.

Medical Devices Agency (1996) *Latex Sensitivities in Health Care Setting (Use of Latex Gloves)*. MDA DB 9601. Medical Devices Agency, London.

Medical Devices Agency (2000) *Equipped to Care. The Safe Use of Medical Devices in the 21st Century*. Medical Devices Agency, London.

MHRA (2005) *Safeguarding Public Health. Guidance for Manufacturers on Clinical Investigations to be Carried out in the UK*. Medicines and Healthcare Products Regulatory Agency. Department of Health, London.

MHRA (2006) *The CE Mark*. Bulletin No 2. Medicines and Healthcare Products Regulatory Agency. Department of Health, London.

MHRA (2002) Devices labeled single use only. *One Liners*, **19**. Department of Health, London.

Michalopoulos, A. & Sparos, L. (2003) Post-operative wound infections. *Nurs Stand*, **17**(44), 53–6, 58, 60.

Mims, C. *et al.* (2004) Infection of the skin, soft tissue, muscle and associated systems. In: *Medical Microbiology Updated*, Vol. 4(26), 3rd edn, pp. 350–77. Mosby, Edinburgh.

Munch, T.N. *et al.* (2005). The association between anaemia and fatigue in patients with advanced cancer receiving palliative care. *J Palliat Med*, **8**(6), 1144–9.

Naylor, W. *et al.* (2001) *The Royal Marsden Hospital Handbook of Wound Management in Cancer Care*. Blackwell Science, Oxford.

NHSE (1999) *Latex Medical Gloves and Powdered Latex Medical Gloves*. Department of Health, London.

NHSE (2000) *Decontamination of Medical Devices*. Department of Health, London.

NHSE (2001) *National Standards of Cleanliness for the NHS*. Department of Health, London.

NHSE (2002) *Infection Control in the Built Environment*. Department of Health, London.

NICE (2006) *Tuberculosis*. National Institute for Health and Clinical Excellence, London.

NMC (2006) *A–Z Advice Sheet Consent*. www.nmc.org.

North Thames Audit and Clinical Effectiveness in Occupational Health (2000) *Report on Latex Gloves Policies and Procedures*. Royal Free Hampstead Centre, London.

Oie, S., Hosokawa, I. & Kamiya, A. (2002) Contamination of room handles by Methicillin-sensitive/Methicillin-resistant *Staphylococcus aureus*. *J Hosp Infect*, **51**(2), 140–3.

Oldman, P. (1991) A sticky situation – microbiological study of adhesive tape used to secure IV cannulae. *Prof Nurse*, **6**(5), 265–9.

Pereira, L.J., Lee, G.M. & Wade, K.J. (1997) An evaluation of five protocols for surgical handwashing in relation to skin condition and microbial counts. *J Hosp Infect*, **36**, 49–65.

Perry, C., Marshall, R. & Jones, E. (2001) Bacterial contamination of uniforms. *J Hosp Infect*, **48**(3), 238–41.

Pittet, M.W. (2003) Hand hygiene: improve standards and practice for hospital care. *Curr Opinion Infect Dis*, **16**(4), 327–35.

Porteous, J. (2002) Artificial nails: very real risk. *Can Oper Room Nurs*, **20**(3), 16–17, 20–1.

Pratt, R.J. *et al.* (2007) Epic 2 national evidence-based guidelines for preventing healthcare-associated infection in NHS hospitals in England. *J Hosp Infect*, **65**(Suppl 1), S2–12.

Preston, R.M. (2005) Aseptic technique: evidence-based approach for patients' safety. *Br J Nurs*, **14**(10), 540–2, 544–6.

Reilly, J. (2002) Changing surgical practice through feedback of performance data. *J Adv Nurs*, **38**(6), 607–14.

Roberts, C. (2000) Universal precautions: improving knowledge of trained nurses. *Br J Nurs*, **9**(1), 43–7.

Rohr, U. *et al.* (2003) Methicillin-resistant *Staphylococcus aureus* whole body decolonization among hospitalized patients with variable site colonization by using mupirocin in combination with octenidine dihydrochloride. *J Hosp Infect*, **54**(4), 305–9.

Rosenthal, V.D. & Maki, D.G. (2004) Prospective study of the impact of open and closed infusion stems on rates of central venous catheter-associated bacteraemia. *Am J Infect Control*, **32**(3), 135–41.

Rossoff, L.J. *et al.* (1993) Is the use of boxed gloves in an intensive care unit safe? *Am J Med*, **94**(6), 602–7.

Ryan, A.J. *et al.* (2006) A national survey of infection control practices by New Zealand anaesthetists. *Anaesth Intensive Care*, **34**(1), 68–74.

Scheckler, W.E. *et al.* (1998) Requirements for infrastructure and essential activities of infection control and epidemiology in hospitals: a consensus panel report. Society for Healthcare Epidemiology of America. *Infect Control Hosp Epidemiol*, **19**(2), 114–24.

Segers, P. *et al.* (2005) Risk control of surgical site infection after cardiothoracic surgery. *J Hosp Infect*, **62**(4), 437–45.

Shiomori, T. *et al.* (2002) Evaluation of bed making-related airborne and surface Methicillin resistant *Staphylococcus aureus* contamination. *J Hosp Infect*, **50**(1), 30–5.

St. Clair, K. & Larrabee, J.H. (2002) Clean versus sterile gloves; which to use for postoperative dressing changes? *Outcomes Manag*, **6**(1), 17–21.

68

Stein, A.D., Makarawo, T.P. & Ahmad, M.F.R. (2003) A survey of doctors' and nurses' knowledge, attitude and compliance with infection control guidelines in Birmingham teaching hospitals. *J Hosp Infect*, **54**(1), 68–73.

Stephan, F. *et al.* (2006) Reduction of urinary tract infection and antibiotic use after surgery: a controlled, prospective, before–after intervention study. *Clin Infect Dis*, **42**(11), 1544–51.

Subbannayya, K. *et al.* (2006) Can soap act as fomites in hospitals? *J Hosp Infect*, **62**(2), 244–5.

Taylor, J.H. *et al.* (2000) A microbiological evaluation of warm air hand driers with respect to hand hygiene and the washroom environment. *J Appl Microbiol*, **89**(6), 910–19.

Taylor, K., Plowman, R. & Roberts, J.A. (2001) *The Challenge of Hospital Acquired Infection*. National Audit Office, London.

Taylor, L. (1978) An evaluation of handwashing techniques 1. *Nurs Times*, **74**(2), 54–5.

van der Meer, J.W.M. & Kuijpers, T.W. (2000) Infections in patients with primary (congenital) immunodeficiences. In: *Management of Infections in Immunocompromised Patients*, Part II (Section 1) (eds M.P. Glauser & P.A. Pizzo). W.B. Saunders, London, pp. 47–78.

Van Grafhorst, J.P. *et al.* (2002) Unexpected high risk of contamination with Staphylococci species attributable to standard preparation of syringes for continuous intravenous drug administration in a simulation model in intensive care units. *Crit Care Med*, **30**(4), 833–6.

Ward, V. *et al.* (1997) *Preventing hospital acquired infection. Clinical guidelines*. Public Health Laboratory Service, London.

Webster, J. & Osborne, S. (2006) Preoperative bathing or showering with skin antiseptics to prevent surgical site infection. *Cochrane Database Syst Rev*, **19**(2), CD004985.

Whitby, M., McLaws, M.L. & Ross, M. (2006) Why healthcare workers don't wash their hands: a behavioral explanation. *Infect Control Hosp Epidemiol*, **27**(5), 484–92.

Whitehouse, J.D. *et al.* (2002) The impact of surgical-site infections following orthopaedic surgery at a community hospital and a university hospital: adverse quality of life, excess length of stay and extra cost. *Infect Control Hosp Epidemiol*, **23**(4), 183–9.

Wilcox, A. (2005) Preventing healthcare-associated infection in primary care. *Primary Health Care*, **15**(8), 43–50.

Wilkes, C.R., Mason, A.D. & Hern, S.C. (2005) Probability distribution for showering and bathing water-use behavior for various US subpopulations. *Risk Anal*, **25**(2), 317–37.

Wilson, J. (2006) *Infection Control in Clinical Practice*, 3rd edn. Bailliere Tindall, London.

Winnefeld, M. *et al.* (2000) Skin tolerance and effectiveness of two hand decontamination procedures in everyday hospital use. *Br J Dermatol*, **1**(393), 546–50.

Wright, L., Spickett, G. & Stoker, S. (2001) Latex allergy awareness among hospital staff. *Nurs Times*, **97**(38), 49–52.

Yamamoto, Y., Ugai, K. & Takahashi, Y. (2005) Efficiency of hand drying for removing bacteria from washed hands: comparison of paper towel drying with warm air drying. *Infect Control Hosp Epidemiol*, **26**(3), 316–20.

Chapter 6

Barrier nursing: nursing the infectious or immunosuppressed patient

71   **Barrier nursing**
71   Reference material
74   **Source isolation**
74   Reference material
79   *Procedure guidelines:*
      Isolation of source of infection
83   **Protective isolation**
85   Reference material
88   *Procedure guidelines:* Neutropenic
      patient care
90   **Acquired immune deficiency syndrome**
90   Reference material
93   **Human immunodeficiency virus 2**
93   Reference material
93   *Procedure guidelines:* Acquired
      immune deficiency syndrome
      (AIDS): patient care in a general
      ward
100 **Antimicrobial-resistant organisms**
100 Reference material
104 **Aspergillosis**
104 Reference material
105 *Clostridium difficile*
106 Reference material
107 **Cryptosporidiosis**
107 Reference material
108 **Hepatitis**
108 **Hepatitis A**
108 Reference material
110 *Procedure guidelines:* Hepatitis A:
      patient care
111 **Hepatitis B**
111 Reference material
113 *Procedure guidelines:* Hepatitis B:
      patient care

116 **Non-A non-B hepatitis**
116 Reference material
117 *Procedure guidelines:* Non-A non-B
      hepatitis: patient care
117 **Hepatitis C**
117 Reference material
118 **Hepatitis D**
118 Reference material
118 **Hepatitis E**
118 Reference material
119 **Hepatitis B genotype F**
119 Reference material
119 **Hepatitis G (HBV/G)**
119 Reference material
119 **The herpesviruses**
119 **Cytomegalovirus**
119 Reference material
120 **Epstein–Barr virus**
120 Reference material
121 **Herpes simplex virus**
121 Reference material
122 **Varicella zoster virus**
122 Reference material
123 **Legionnaires' disease**
123 Reference material
124 **Listeriosis**
124 Reference material
125 **Pneumocystosis**
125 Reference material
126 **Tuberculosis**
126 Reference material
128 **Transmissible spongiform
      encephalopathies**
129 Reference material
130 References and further reading

Barrier nursing

Definition

Barrier nursing is the use of infection control practices aimed at controlling the spread of, and eradicating, pathogenic organisms (Garner 1996a, b). These practices may require the setting up of mechanical barriers to contain pathogenic organisms within a specified area.

Indications

Barrier nursing includes:

- Source isolation to segregate infected patients in single rooms to prevent the spread of infection.
- Cohort source isolation to segregate a number of patients with the same infection in one ward when there are inadequate number of single rooms, to prevent the spread of infection (NHS Estates 2002).
- Protective isolation (reverse barrier nursing) to segregate immunosuppressed patients (individuals with impaired immunity due to disease or treatment) to protect them from acquiring an exogenous infection.
- Strict source isolation to segregate patients infected with a serious contagious disease, e.g. viral haemorrhagic fever, in isolation units to prevent the spread of infection (DH 1998a).

Reference material

It is estimated that health care-associated infection (HCAI) affects one in 10 NHS patients each year, and costs the National Health Service (NHS) one billion pounds annually (DH 2003a). This means there are at least 100 000 infections a year, which results in about 5000 deaths where infection is the primary cause of death and a further 15 000 where infection is a substantial contributory factor in the death (DH 2002a). The indiscriminate and inappropriate use of antibiotics to treat infection promotes the emergence of antibiotic resistant micro-organisms (DH 2003a). Infection with a resistant micro-organism increases the risk of death from infection (Coia et al. 2006).

The main sites of infection are:

- Urinary (23%) (80% of these are related to urinary catheterization).
- Lung (22%) (with pneumonia occurring most frequently among patients who had been ventilated).
- Wound (9%).
- Blood (6%) (60% of blood infections were related to intravenous feeding devices, urinary catheters or similar devices (DH 2003a). In one matched cohort study of adult patients being cared for in intensive care units, it was found that blood stream infections increased the risk of death (42% with blood stream infection dying compared with 26% who did not; Laupland et al. 2006).

Those patients with a more serious illness, such as cancer, are particularly vulnerable and susceptible to infection (DH 2003a). Neutropenic patients with haematological malignancies are at increased risk of infectious morbidity and mortality. One USA study found a 6.8% inpatient mortality rate for neutropenia hospitalization (Caggiano et al. 2005), whilst another more recent study put the rate at 9.5% (Kuderer et al. 2006). A further prospective surveillance study of hematology–oncology patients found that the incidence of HCAI in neutropenic patients is significantly higher (up to 25.3%) than in immune-competent patients, with length of neutropenia a marker for risk of infection (Engelhart et al. 2002). The incidence of infection is directly related to the neutrophil count, with the probability that 25% of patients with a neutrophil count less than $100/mm^3$ for 1 week will develop an infection. Bloodstream infections are the most common type of infection (Glauser & Calandra 2000).

The risk of infection also depends on the patient's ability to respond to infection, rather than the number of neutrophils in the peripheral blood (Dale & Liles 1998). A careful patient medical history and physical examination provides an initial risk assessment of the patient's susceptibility to infection.

Risk assessment includes establishing the known or suspected risk, establishing what preventative measures are already in place and then producing an action plan, which should include specific precautions for the patient (HSE 2003a). Using this approach, inappropriate and unnecessary precautions are not adopted (Garner 1996a, b). An oncology centre in the USA has developed a risk assessment complication tool using risk factors from published studies and national guidelines. A retrospective survey of records found that the tool was effective in helping to determine which patients were at high risk of developing an infection (Donohue 2006).

Most precautions against transferring infection demand more effort, take more time and cost more when neutropenic patients are cared for, than the comparable procedures in normal circumstances. However, the cost of an outbreak of infection can be far more (Wilcox & Dane 2000).

For the infected patient the consequences can be considerable and may include:

- Delayed or prevented recovery.
- Increased pain, discomfort and anxiety.
- Extended hospitalization, which has implications for the patient, the family and the hospital:
  - If isolated the patient may receive less care (Evans et al. 2003).
  - Psychological stress as a result of loneliness and boredom from periods spent in isolation (Maunder et al. 2003). A study of the psychological and occupational impact of a severe acute respiratory syndrome (SARS) outbreak, found that isolated patients reported fear, loneliness, boredom, anger and worries about the risk to family and friends. Staff, however, were affected by fear of contagion and of infecting their family, friends and work colleagues (Maunder et al. 2003).

Sources of infection

Self-infection (endogenous infection)

Self-infection results when tissues become infected from other sites in the patient's body. The normal microbial flora of the human body consists largely of the organisms in the alimentary tract, upper respiratory tract, female genital tract and on the skin. This flora may include versatile pathogens (e.g. *Staphylococcus aureus*) that may cause disease in almost any tissue, as well as others (e.g. *Micrococcus* species and diphtheroids), which are usually of very low pathogenicity and rarely cause infection. Many organisms exist with capabilities between these extremes. Many infections acquired by immunosuppressed patients are caused by the patient's own microbial flora (Glauser & Calandra 2000). For example, septicaemia in neutropenic patients is often due to translocation of micro-organisms from the gut (Paulus *et al.* 2005).

Cross-infection (exogenous infection)

Cross-infection may be caused by infection from patients, hospital staff or visitors who are suffering from the relevant disease (cases) or who are symptomless carriers. Food and the environment may also be factors in cross-infection (Ayliffe *et al.* 2000). For example, blood stream infections in neutropenic patients can be due to contamination of a central venous catheter by micro-organisms not carried by the patient but acquired exogenously from the environment, other patients or staff (Paulus *et al.* 2005).

Transmission of infection is directly related to the environment and management, with insufficient working space, overcrowding of patients and understaffing predisposing to cross-infection (NHS Estates 2002).

Routes and reservoirs of infection

A reservoir of infection is anywhere where organisms can survive and multiply. For infection to occur there has to be a route of transmission between the reservoir and the susceptible host (Ayliffe *et al.* 2000).

The health care environment is a secondary reservoir for organisms with the potential for infecting patients. It is essential that all plans for new or renovated health care buildings are designed to ensure that HAI is reduced (NHS Estates 2002). Routes of spread include the following.

Direct contact

Organisms can be transmitted directly to susceptible people by the hands of health care workers and by contaminated equipment. Therefore it is essential that all equipment is cleaned following each and every episode of use (MDA 2002). Hand washing has been shown to reduce the spread of infection, so hands must be washed before and after every patient contact and contact with contaminated equipment (DH 2001a). However, studies of hand washing by nurses and others have shown that this procedure is generally not carried out efficiently (Creedon 2005), although

compliance does seem to improve during dirty high-risk situations (Kuzu *et al.* 2005). Teaching interventions, belief in the benefits of the activity, peer pressure of senior physicians, administrators' role modelling (Whitby *et al.* 2006) and feedback on performance (Kuzu *et al.* 2005) may all improve compliance with hand-washing requirements. Patient education programmes that enable the patient to ask the health care workers providing direct care to them, 'Did you wash your hands?' have also been seen to increase compliance with hand washing (McGuckin *et al.* 2004).

Hand washing with soap removes transient micro-organisms, whilst the use of bactericidal soap removes both transient and resident skin micro-organisms (DH 2001a). In clinical areas washing in running water is essential. Basins should be deep enough to contain any splashing water and should be plugless. Taps should not be operated by hand but by remote control, elbow, knee or foot, as appropriate (Chapter 5).

A quick, convenient and effective disinfectant for clean hands, without the use of soap and water, is an alcoholic handrub, which can remove organisms and reduce nosocomial infections (Johnson *et al.* 2005). This handrub is less drying to hands (Creedon 2005) and well liked if introduced following educational initiatives. Alcoholic handrubs are not effective on hands that are visibly soiled or potentially contaminated with dirt or organic matter. In such circumstances washing with soap and running water, followed by careful drying with a good-quality paper towel, is required (DH 2001a).

Any item or equipment used near or in a patient area may be a reservoir of micro-organisms. This can range from obvious items such as stethoscopes (Hill *et al.* 2006), commodes (Vardhan *et al.* 2000), children's toys (Fleming & Randle 2006), cot mattresses (Jenkins & Sherburn 2005), fabrics (Neely & Maley 2000) and blood pressure cuffs (Walker *et al.* 2006) to patients' files (Panhotra *et al.* 2005), computer keyboards (Wilson *et al.* 2006) and doctors' ties (Ditchburn 2006). This research emphasizes the importance of cleaning items after patient use.

Airborne

Organisms can be transmitted in dust or skin scales carried by air. This is likely to occur during procedures such as bed making (Sexton *et al.* 2006), when particles may land directly on open wounds or puncture sites. Doors of isolation rooms must be kept closed to minimize airborne spread of micro-organisms (Sexton *et al.* 2006). The hospital ward environment must be visibly clean, free from dust and soilage and acceptable to patients, their visitors and staff. The Secretary for State has stated that: 'Patients rightly expect hospitals to be clean.' The message it gives spreads far beyond infection to say to patients, 'You are in safe hands' (DH 2004a, p. 1). Sites most likely to fail a ward cleaning inspection are the toilets and kitchen (Griffith *et al.* 2000).

Airborne infection may also occur through droplets. Water from nebulizers or humidifiers may be contaminated by *Pseudomonas* species (Ayliffe *et al.* 2000). Fine droplet spray from ventilation cooling towers or showers contaminated with *Legionella pneumophila* correlates with the incidence of nosocomial Legionnaires' disease (Declerck *et al.* 2006).

Positive pressure air conditioning protects immunosuppressed patients by reducing the entry of outside air into the room. Negative pressure air conditioning reduces the amount of air leaving the room therefore keeping pathogenic micro-organisms within the barrier nursing room. When negative pressure air conditioning is being used, for example with a patient with tuberculosis, the air changes should be 12 per hour with the pressure regularly monitored (CDC 2003).

Food borne

Food poisoning occurs when contaminated foods are ingested, with *Campylobacter* species being one of the most common causes (Gillespie *et al.* 2006). *Salmonella* species continues to be a problem and is particularly associated with contaminated eggs (Gillespie *et al.* 2005) and chicken (Meldrum *et al.* 2005), and contamination was linked to cross-contamination and inadequate heat treatment (Gillespie *et al.* 2005). Prevention includes good infection control practices (Maguire *et al.* 2001). New food hygiene legislation (Food Standards Agency 2006) applies to all food businesses in the UK. An internationally recognized and recommended system for food hygiene, called Hazard Analysis Critical Control Points (HACCP), focuses on identifying the critical points in the entire food chain where problems could occur and then putting in steps to prevent the problems occurring (Food Standards Agency 2006). Hand washing, thorough cooking, storage, segregation of cooked and uncooked food, clean environment and equipment are essential. Hot food must be kept hot and cold food must be kept chilled. As some organisms such as *Listeria* can survive in low temperatures (Flessa *et al.* 2005), ideally ward refrigerators should be kept below 5°C. Food products must also be obtained from reputable suppliers (Ejidokun *et al.* 2000) (Table 6.1).

Blood borne

Blood, or bloodstained material, is potentially hazardous, transmitting infection through inoculation accidents, existing breaks in the skin, gross contamination of mucous membranes, sexual activity or, prenatally, from mother to baby (UK Health Department 2002a).

Vector borne (an insect or animal carrier/transmitter of disease)

International movement of people and products is associated with the emergence of infectious diseases (Mangili & Gendreau 2005) by introducing infectious agents into areas in which they had previously been absent (Gezairy 2003). Research on vaccines, environmentally safe insecticides, vector control and training programmes for health care workers can assist in disease control (Gezairy 2003). Although disease transmitted by biting insects is not a major problem in the UK, insects such as cockroaches can carry pathogenic organisms on their bodies and in their digestive tracts. This may infect the hospital environment, which includes food and sterile supplies (Lemos *et al.* 2006). Storage of supplies in dry, clean, well-ventilated areas is therefore essential. Statutory requirements related to pest control must also be met (DH 2001a).

Types of barrier nursing

1 Source isolation also termed 'transmission based precautions' (Garner 1996a, b).
2 Protective isolation.

Source isolation is designed to prevent the spread of pathogenic micro-organisms from an infected patient to other patients, hospital personnel and visitors. The need for isolation is determined by the ease with which the disease can be transmitted in hospital and, if it is transmittable, by its severity. As infectious diseases are transmitted by different routes, isolation procedures must, in order to be effective, provide appropriate barriers to the route of transmission.

Table 6.1 Temperature required to prevent food infections.

Refrigeration	A food temperature of 8°C or below is effective in controlling the multiplication of most micro-organisms. It is recommended that the temperature of refrigerators holding perishable food, i.e. milk, is at 5°C or below. Ward refrigerators must have their temperature checked and recorded regularly through the day. Any problems in maintaining the low temperature must be reported and repaired immediately. Food in refrigerators at a temperature above 8°C should not be used
Freezers	Freezing food at temperatures below −18°C will prevent micro-organisms multiplying
Cooking	Temperatures of 75°C or above are effective in destroying most bacteria
Hot food holding	Food should be delivered to the patient as soon as it is cooked and served. Temperatures above 63°C will control the multiplication of bacteria in correctly prepared and cooked food
Cooling	Cooked food that is served cold must be cooled as quickly as possible and then refrigerated
Reheating of cooked food	This must only be undertaken by staff with catering/food hygiene qualifications (Food Standards Agency 2006)

In addition, the procedures imposing these barriers must be adhered to universally by all hospital staff entering the isolation unit. Risk assessment of the patient to evaluate the risk of cross-infection to other patients must be undertaken, to ensure the most appropriate restrictions are implemented (HSE 2003a).

Protective isolation protects the patient from the hospital environment. Protective isolation techniques have also been referred to as reverse barrier nursing and reverse isolation, and include the use of high-efficiency particulate air (HEPA) filters (Cacciari *et al.* 2004; Wilson 2006) (see Protective isolation section, below).

Source isolation

Definition

Source isolation or transmission based precautions is a process of care whereby an infectious patient and any material that has been in contact with them or eliminated by them are isolated from others to prevent the spread of infection. This is achieved by achieving standard precautions for all patients, and adding airborne, droplet or contact precautions depending on the patient's causative organism (Garner 1996a, b).

Indications

The decision to isolate a patient will be influenced by the availability of facilities as well as by the physical condition of the area where the isolation is to take place. In determining the most suitable area, a number of criteria need to be met. Among these are the relative cleanliness of the ward, the standard of domestic services support, the infected patient's causative pathogen, the immune status of the other patients and the anticipated length of the isolation. A review of the effectiveness of different isolation polices and practices in the UK, suggests that a concerted effort that includes isolation of meticillin-resistant *Staphylococcus aureus* (MRSA) -positive patients, can reduce the incidence of MRSA, even when MRSA is endemic (Cooper *et al.* 2003).

Unfortunately facilities for the isolation of infected patients are not always available. The NHS Estates highlights that the NHS rarely provides more than 20% of single rooms in NHS hospitals (NHS Estates 2005). A 12-month prospective observational study of the demand and availability of single rooms carried out in a large UK teaching hospital found that there were 845 patients requiring isolation facilities, of whom 185 (22%) did not have this need met (Wigglesworth & Wilcox 2006).

The NHS Estates suggests that with the increase in antibiotic-resistant bacteria and immunocompromised inpatients, there is an increasing need for en-suite single rooms and negative as well as positive pressure isolation rooms (NHS Estates 2002).

Reference material

Source isolation may be achieved by:

1   Purpose-built infectious disease wards.
    Advantages:
    (a) decreased risk of cross-infection;
    (b) less disruption to general wards;
    (c) nurses often more informed and motivated;
    (d) improved, supervised cleaning;
    (e) improves decolonization of patients with MRSA (Fitzpatrick *et al.* 2000).
    Disadvantages:
    (a) increased costs;
    (b) when full, similar patients have to remain on general wards;
    (c) when there are no infectious patients requiring admission, beds are closed to the admission of patients without a contagious infection;
    (d) inadvisable to admit immunosuppressed patients who would be at significant risk of morbidity and mortality if cross-infection were to occur with virulent infections such as drug-resistant tuberculosis, although this can be prevented by ventilation systems. These are capable of being switched to negative pressure for infected patients and positive pressure for immunosuppressed patients (Cacciari *et al.* 2004);
    (e) problem of staff recruitment;
    (f) staff may not be conversant with patients' underlying clinical conditions (Chattopadhyay 2001);
    (g) isolation on general wards can result in isolated patients being seen less often than non-isolated patients (Evans *et al.* 2003).
2   Negative pressure plastic isolator used for dealing with patients who have highly contagious infections such as Ebola virus infection (Bruce & Brysiewicz 2002).
    Advantages:
    (a) provides a high degree of protection to those in contact with patient;
    (b) said to be comfortable and acceptable to patients (Trexler *et al.* 1977).
    Disadvantages:
    (a) not freely available;
    (b) expensive to obtain and maintain;
    (c) limited experienced health care workers to provide required care.
3   Single rooms on general wards.
    Advantages:
    (a) allows patients to remain on ward, which provides continuity of care;
    (b) will reduce cross-infection (Eveillard *et al.* 2001);
    (c) en-suite single rooms provide greater privacy and are preferred by many patients (NHS Estates 2002);
    (d) some patients suggest barrier nursing in a single room allows greater freedom for visitors and from routine (Newton *et al.* 2001).

74

Disadvantages:
(a) some patients report a negative experience of barrier nursing, with feelings of being 'a leper' (Newton *et al.* 2001);
(b) shortage of suitable single rooms, resulting in patients with known infections being cared for in open wards. Hospitals with 10% of their beds as single rooms often find these inadequate to cope with every infected patient (NHS Estates 2002).
4 Cohort barrier nursing: when a group of patients have the same infection, it may be necessary to cohort barrier nurse these patients in a small bay.
Advantage:
(a) undertaken correctly can successfully control and contain infection (Zafar *et al.* 1998).
Disadvantage:
(a) restrictions on admissions to these beds.

One small case-controlled study found that nursing catheterized patients in single rooms reduced the transmission rate of micro-organisms compared to those catheterized patients in shared rooms, as standard precautions were more likely to be adopted in single rooms (Fryklund *et al.* 1997). This supports the use of single rooms for infected patients as the bed around infected patients can often be contaminated with the infecting organism (Widdowson *et al.* 2002).

Effective source barrier nursing practice is achieved most easily by isolating the patient in a single room with the following:

- An anteroom area for protective clothing.
- Hand-washing facilities.
- Toilet facilities.

However, with good technique, an area in the ward away from especially vulnerable patients can be used. In some instances where cross-infection has occurred it may be more appropriate to cohort nurse these patients together in a small ward with designated staff, so containing the infection to one area, rather than using side rooms on different wards (NHS Estates 2002). Uninfected patients must not be admitted into this area until all the infected patients have been discharged and the area has been thoroughly cleaned.

General principles of source isolation

The main emphasis for successful source isolation nursing procedures is on hand washing and protection of clothes; both have been seen to reduce cross-infection (Lucet *et al.* 2005). Several general principles need to be adhered to if effective barrier nursing is to occur. Every effort must be made to ensure that instructions are kept simple and realistic. Regular assessment and evaluation of the situation must take place to ascertain whether barrier nursing continues to remain the most appropriate form of care.

Box 6.1   Standard barrier nursing precautions

Standard precautions include:
- Hospital environment clean, free from dust and soilage.
- Hands must be decontaminated immediately before and after every patient contact.
- Personal protective equipment worn when exposed to blood or body fluids, These include gloves, masks, eye protection, face shield, aprons and gowns.
- Safe use and disposal of waste in particular sharps (DH 2001a).
- Safe handling of used, foul or infected linen.
- All reusable shared equipment cleaned, disinfected or sterilized after each patient use.
- Health care workers fit and free from infection.

Standard precautions should be adopted for all patients (Box 6.1). When a patient has been found to have an infection that required source isolation, besides using standard precautions, additional precautions should be adopted based on transmission-based precautions. These included: droplet, airborne and contact precautions (Garner 1996a, b) (Box 6.2).

Box 6.2   Routes of transmission of infection and extra precautions used with standard precautions to prevent cross-infection

Airborne transmission

Passage of micro-organisms from a source person through aerosols spread.

Airborne precautions

Designed to reduce the transmission of micro-organisms in droplets and evaporated droplets that remain suspended in the air or dust particles containing infectious agents. Examples: tuberculosis and varicella.

Droplet transmission

Passage of airborne residue of a potentially infectious micro-organism aerosol from which most of the liquid has evaporated.

Droplet precautions

Designed to reduce the risk of transmission of infectious micro-organisms by air. This achieved by the use of masks, aprons and gloves. Examples: influenza, meningococcal meningitis.

Contact transmission

Passage of micro-organisms by direct or indirect contact.

Contact precautions

Designed to reduce the risk of transmission of micro-organisms by direct or indirect contact. This is achieved by wearing gloves and apron. Examples: MRSA, *Clostridium difficile.*

75

Protective clothing

Uniforms

Microbiological sampling of nurses' uniforms detected *Staphylococcus aureus*, *Clostridium difficile* and vancomycin-resistant enterococci (VRE) on uniforms both before and after wear (Perry *et al.* 2001). This study was supported by a laboratory study that tested the survival of micro-organisms on various hospital fabrics and plastics and found that *Staphylococcus aureus* survived on polyester material for up to 56 days (Neely & Maley 2000). These studies reiterate the need for uniforms to be changed daily and when soiled (Perry *et al.* 2001). Changing and laundry facilities must be provided to all staff (NHS Estates 2002). If health care workers take their uniforms home to wash, the uniforms must be washed, tumbled dry and ironed to ensure the effectiveness of home laundering (Patel 2005).

Plastic apron

The wearing of a plastic apron is an accepted part of barrier-nursing technique. Uniforms can become contaminated during close contact with infected patients (DH 2001a). The wearing of an apron can protect the uniform and prevent the spread of micro-organisms from one patient to the next (Callaghan 1998). Disposable plastic aprons are cheap, impermeable to bacteria and water, are easy to put on, protect the probable area of maximum contamination and are preferable to cotton gowns, which provide increased cover but are readily penetrated by moisture and bacteria (Belkin 2002).

Gowns

When there is a risk of extensive splashing of blood and body fluids, secretions and excretions, a full body, fluid-repellent gown should be worn to protect the wearer (DH 2001a), as well as patients, as wearing a gown and gloves has been shown to reduce the transmission of micro-organisms such as VRE (Srinivasan *et al.* 2002). However, another study found that wearing gowns and overshoes routinely did not prevent infection in patients undergoing bone marrow transplantation (BMT), and by eliminating the unnecessary use of gowns and overshoes saved nursing time and hospital resources (Duquette-Petersen *et al.* 1999). Belkin (2002) suggests that staff and visitors should select a gown that is appropriate for the task and degree of exposure anticipated, to prevent contamination of blood and body fluids to the wearer of the gown.

Doctors' white coats

Doctors should also be encouraged to change their white coats regularly as it has been shown that a white coat can easily be contaminated and that the design should be modified in order to facilitate hand washing (Loh *et al.* 2000).

Caps

Although the wearing of disposable head covering while nursing infected patients is still practised, hair that is clean and tidy has not been implicated in cross-infection. Therefore, unless heavy contamination or splashing is present or expected, the wearing of caps is not justified. However, head covering continues to be required in the operating theatre, as its use has been shown to reduce wound infections (Friberg *et al.* 2001).

Masks

Masks are worn to protect the wearer from infection, for example from severe respiratory infection (SARS), which requires a FFP 3 mask (Chia *et al.* 2005), or aerosol-generating procedures, when a PPF 2 mask is generally worn (Aisien & Ujah 2006). Masks are also worn by a person undertaking an aseptic technique to reduce the risk of airborne contamination during the surgical procedure (Friberg *et al.* 2001). A small randomized controlled trial showed a trend towards masks being associated with fewer infections, whilst a larger study found no difference in infection rates between masked and unmasked persons undertaking clean surgery (Lipp & Edwards 2002). Masks suitable to be worn as personal protective equipment (PPE) must meet the European standard EN 149 (2001) that is approved for use in the UK. Masks are graded depending on total inward leakage. FF 1 is the lowest level of protection and FFP 3 is the highest level of protection. If a mask needs to be worn it must be a filter type and fit the face closely (Ayliffe *et al.* 2000). Masks are single-use items and manufacturer's instructions must always be followed (Lipp & Edwards 2005).

Eye protection

Eye protection must be worn to prevent contamination by micro-organisms, blood and body fluids (DH 2001a), for example in the operating theatre (Keogh *et al.* 2001), when barrier nursing (Parker & Goldman 2006) or when a patient is bleeding (Ho *et al.* 2005).

Overshoes

The floors of hospital wards become easily contaminated by large numbers of bacteria (Ayliffe *et al.* 2000). Shoe coverings should be used when contamination of the environment occurs, as part of the Control of Substances Hazardous to Health (COSHH) requirements for PPE (HSE 2002). However, there is no evidence that shoe coverings reduce contamination of clean floors (Santos *et al.* 2005).

Gloves

Gloves reduce hand contamination by transient pathogens (Kac *et al.* 2005). Gloves must conform to *Conformité Européene* (CE) standards, be of acceptable quality and available in all clinical areas (DH 2001a). Gloves should be unpowdered (MDA 1998) and not made of latex (MDA 1996; NHS Executive 1999a), as latex allergies have serious implications for patients and health care workers (Wright *et al.* 2001). A 1-year longitudinal study of operating room personnel reported a significant decrease in natural rubber latex sensitivity after changing to powder-free low-protein gloves (Korniewicz *et al.* 2005).

Boxed, clean non-sterile gloves (termed examination gloves: DH 2005a) are adequate for routine non-invasive nursing care (Rossoff *et al.* 1993). Clean gloves must be worn when handling blood or body fluids, or cleaning (DH 2001a). Gloves must be changed between patients, and hands must be washed with bactericidal soap and water or bactericidal alcohol handrub after removing gloves.

The practice of double gloving is an option that can be adopted during surgical procedures when gloves may become damaged. It is suggested that double gloving can cause loss of tactile sensitivity and increased costs. However, it is a necessary and sensible practice when there is a risk of gloves being damaged during use (Twomey 2003).

Incorrect use of gloves has been found to be common, poor practice exposing patients to the risk of cross-infection (Girou *et al.* 2004). Examination gloves must be worn if there is a risk of exposure to body fluids. Sterile gloves must be worn for surgical aseptic techniques, for example for the insertion of medical devices (DH 2005a). Gloves are single-use items and must not be cleaned and reused for the same or another patient (NICE 2003).

Cleaning

Some bacteria can survive in the environment for long periods of time, for example *Enterococcus faecium* can survive for 60 days (Gastmeier *et al.* 2006). Thorough cleaning of the environment is essential, as dust from floors and surfaces contain organisms that, if transferred to patients, can cause infection (Dancer *et al.* 2006). All furniture must be damp dusted to remove organisms dispersed into the air from bed making. The floor must be vacuum cleaned with a machine fitted with a filter followed by damp mopping with hot, soapy water (the mop head must be laundered daily) and then the washed area must be dried carefully (De Lorenzi *et al.* 2006). Dry dusting or the use of a broom should be forbidden as studies have shown this method of cleaning simply redisperses the organisms into the air (Ayliffe *et al.* 2000). Cleaning equipment must be washed and dried after each use.

Ensuring a clean patient environment is every health care worker's responsibility; included in this objective is ensuring that maintenance of the environment is achieved. The Department of Health's (DH) Matron Charter, an action plan for cleaner hospitals (DH 2004b), has placed the responsibility for ensuring the patient environment is clean and well maintained within the remit of the Moden Matron (Gamble 2005).

Antibacterial surfaces and materials have been developed that will inhibit colonization and growth of micro-organisms. These surfaces may be designed to gradually diffuse agents into the surrounding area that prevent contamination of micro-organisms, or the surface is bonded with the agent that destroys micro-organisms on contact. Silver, for example, has been shown to have disinfectant activity against *Staphylococcus aureus* and *Pseudomonas* (Brady *et al.* 2003). However, the use of these products does not provide a substitute for careful cleaning of the environment and equipment.

Patient hygiene

Essence of care is a patient-focused benchmark for clinical governance. Included in the 10 bench marks is a benchmark for patients' personal and oral hygiene. All patients must be individually assessed to identify advice or care required to maintain and promote personal hygiene. Patients must be provided with hygiene information, education and assistance when required, as well as toiletries for their own personal use (DH 2003a). Maintaining patient hygiene is a fundamental part of nursing care and should not be delegated to unqualified staff (Whiting 1999). It is essential patients wash their hands and they should be encouraged to use alcoholic handrub to improve their compliance with hand washing (Banfield & Kerr 2005).

Patients should be encouraged, and when necessary helped, to shower or bath daily and more frequently, for example, if incontinent. Analysis of showering and bathing showed that age and level of education significantly influenced showering/bathing frequency. This information can be used to establish patient current hygiene practices, to establish where changes need to be made (Wilkes *et al.* 2005). As cancer is known to cause fatigue it is essential that nurses play a key role in identifying and managing unwillingness to maintain personal hygiene for what ever reason (Mock & Olsen 2003).

A study evaluating:

(a) daily soap and water baths;
(b) cleansing with cloths saturated with 2% chlorhexidine gluconate;
(c) cloths without chlorhexidine;

found that the incidence of VRE acquisition was reduced with all three methods but cleansing with chlorhexidine-saturated cloths was a simple and statistically effective strategy to reduce VRE contamination of patients' skin. It has led to a reduction of VRE in the environment and on health care workers' skin (Vernon *et al.* 2006).

It is essential that baths are cleaned and dried between patients with a non-abrasive cleaning agent, ideally incorporating a hypochlorite, as viable organisms can survive in bath scum (Ayliffe *et al.* 2000). If bed bathing is unavoidable, the patient should be supplied with their own bowl, which is washed and dried after use and stored at the bedside to prevent cross-infection.

Waste

Collection, transportation and disposal of hazardous and non-hazardous waste is regulated by the following: Environment Protection Act 1990; The Safe Management of Healthcare Waste 2006 (DH 2006a); The Carriage of Dangerous Goods (Classification, Packaging and Labelling) and Use of Transportable Pressure Receptacles Regulations

2004 (DH 2004d); and The Control of Substances Hazardous to Health Regulations (COSHH) (HSE 2002).

Domestic waste, which includes all waste not contaminated with blood, body fluids and toxic chemicals is disposed of in black polythene bags. From July 2005, Hazardous Waste (England and Wales) Regulations 2005 replaced The Special Waste Regulations 1996. Under the new regulations hazardous and non-hazardous waste must be separated.

Within a source barrier nursing room all waste other than sharps or unused drugs must be put into the appropriate waste bag, sealed securely in the room, labelled with ward, hospital and date and sent for incineration.

Sharps and unused drugs must be placed in disposal boxes (that conform to UN3291 and BS7320) at the point of use. These boxes must not be overfilled. When full, the container must be shut, labelled with ward, hospital and date and sent for incineration. Containers must not be left on the floor in public areas (DH 2001a).

Linen

Infected linen must be placed in a red alginate polythene bag. The bag is tied shut and then placed in a red linen bag to be sent in a safe manner to the laundry for barrier washing. This entails placing the full alginate bag in the washing machine where it dissolves, allowing the hot water to wash and disinfect the linen. In this way staff and the environment are protected from contamination (DH 1995a).

Cutlery and crockery

Crockery and cutlery can become contaminated with pathogenic organisms. Hands must be washed after handling utensils used by patients (NHS Executive 1995).

All crockery should have excess food removed (Stahl Wernersson et al. 2004) and must be machine washed in a dishwasher with a final rinse of 80°C for 1 minute to disinfect it (Ayliffe et al. 2000). Disposable crockery and cutlery are needed only when gross contamination has occurred or if a dishwasher is not available (Redpath & Farrington 1997).

Urine, faeces and vomit

These must be disposed of immediately and carefully to prevent contamination of the environment. This may be by using a bedpan washer or macerator. Gloves must be worn when handling and disposing of urine, faeces and vomit. Hands must be washed following removal of the gloves (DH 2001a).

Notification of infection

If a patient develops signs and symptoms of infection, or if bacteriological analysis identifies an organism that necessitates barrier nursing, swift communication and action are needed to instigate this. Any problems may be discussed with the infection control team.

Informing the patient and visitors

Giving careful explanation to the patient is essential so that they can co-operate fully with the restrictions (Ayliffe et al. 2000). This will include the provison of written information (Ward 2000). The nurse should have a full understanding of the epidemiology and transmission of the micro-organism that has necessitated the patient being barrier nursed (Stirling et al. 2004) and be sensitive to the psychological implications of being labelled 'infectious' and of being confined in isolation (Gammon 1999). It is important that nurses are aware of strategies for dealing with and preventing the effects of isolation (Madeo 2003).

The emergence of resistant micro-organisms has led to an increase in barrier nursing. A US study (Catalano et al. 2003) compared two groups of seriously ill patients, one of which required isolation because of resistant micro-organism infections. This study, using the Hamilton Depression Anxiety Rating Scale, found that the isolated group had significantly higher scores on both anxiety and depression at the time of follow up. A cross-sectional matched controlled UK study found that hospitalized patients with MRSA had higher levels of depression and anxiety symptoms than the MRSA negative group of patients (Tarzi et al. 2001). Tarzi and colleagues recommend that further studies are needed to examine the best ways of managing the detrimental effects of barrier nursing (Tarzi et al. 2001). Fortunately, many patients in fact preferred a single room, and adapted well to any subsequent loneliness and boredom. A review of the literature of nurses' perceptions of single rooms compared with shared rooms, found that nurses believed that a single room impacts positively on the patient's hospital experience, by increasing privacy, improving the interaction with staff and the patients' families and by reducing noise and anxiety (Chaudhury et al. 2006). The patient's visitors must also be told why the barrier nursing restrictions are necessary. Visitors will generally be allowed into the room at the discretion of the infection control team. They must be taught to observe the correct procedures for entering and leaving the room. As children are more susceptible to infection than adults, any visit by a child should be discussed with the infection control team.

Domestic staff

The domestic manager must be informed as soon as barrier nursing is commenced. He or she will then provide the ward domestic with written instructions.

The ward domestic staff must understand clearly why barrier nursing is required and should be instructed on the correct procedure. The nursing staff must check that the ward domestics understand and are following their instructions correctly. If the patient is in a single room, a mop (laundered daily), bucket (washed and dried after use), cleaning fluid and disposable cloths should be used solely for this patient's use. If the patient is in a general ward, special care must be taken with the cleaning so that potentially infectious material is not transferred from the area around the infected patient to other patient areas. The infected patient's area must be cleaned last and separately.

Staff allocation

A minimum number of staff should be involved in caring for an infected patient. The nurse concerned with the infected patient should not also attend to other susceptible patients. If barrier nursing is for an infectious disease such as chickenpox, it is important that only personnel who have already had the disease should attend this patient.

The protection of staff against the risk of infection is one of the main functions of the occupational health department. This department offers an immunization and counselling service.

Procedure guidelines   Isolation of source of infection

Equipment

1 Isolation suite if possible. A single room with en-suite facilities will prevent cross-infection (NHS Estates 2002).
2 All items required to meet the patient's nursing needs during the period of isolation, e.g. instruments to assess vital signs.

3 Protective clothing.
4 Alcoholic handrub.

Procedure

Isolation room preparation

Action	Rationale
1 Place a barrier nursing sign outside the door.	To inform anyone intending to enter the room of the situation (Dhaliwal & McGeer 2005: R 1b).
2 List requirements for personnel before entering and after leaving the isolation area.	To decrease entries to and exits from the room (E).
3 Remove all non-essential furniture. The remaining furniture should be easy to clean and should not conceal or retain dirt or moisture either within or around it.	To minimize the risk of furniture harbouring microbial spores or growth colonies (NHS Estates 2002: C).
4 Stock the hand basin with a suitable bactericidal soap preparation and paper towels for staff use.	Facilities for hand washing within the infected area are essential for effective barrier nursing (NHS Estates 2002: C).
5 Place yellow clinical waste bag in the room on a foot operated stand. The bag must be sealed before it is removed from the room.	For containing contaminated rubbish within the room. Yellow is the recognized colour for clinical waste (DH 2006a: C).
6 Place a container for sharps in the room.	To contain contaminated sharps within the infected area (DH 1996a: C).
7 When the sharps container is two-thirds full it must be firmly shut and sent for incineration.	To minimize the risk of leakage from the sharps container (DH 2006a: C).
8 Keep the patient's personal property to a minimum. Advise him/her to wear hospital clothing. All belongings taken into the room should be washable, cleanable or disposable.	The patient's belongings may become contaminated and cannot be taken home unless they are washable or cleanable (E).
9 Provide the patient with his/her own thermometer and sphygmomanometer, and all items necessary for attending to personal hygiene.	Equipment used regularly by the patient should be kept within the infected area to prevent the spread of infection (Walker et al. 2006: R 1b).

Procedure guidelines *(cont.)*

10 Keep dressing solutions, creams and lotions, etc., to a minimum and store them within the room.	All partially used materials must be discarded when barrier nursing ends (sterilization is not possible), therefore unnecessary waste should be avoided (Dietze *et al.* 2001: R 1b).
11 Set up a trolley outside the door to hold plastic aprons and bactericidal alcoholic handrub (this is contraindicated if the trolley causes an obstruction or is a hazard to staff and others).	Staff are more likely to use the equipment if it is readily available (E).

Entering the isolation room

Action	Rationale
1 Collect all equipment needed.	To avoid entering and leaving the infected area unnecessarily.
2 Roll up long sleeves to the elbow.	To allow hand washing to take place (E).
3 Put on a disposable plastic apron.	A plastic apron is inexpensive, quick to put on and protects the front of the uniform, which is the most likely area to come in contact with the patient (DH 2005a: R 1a).
4 Put on a disposable, impermeable gown when heavy contamination is anticipated.	To fully protect clothing from contamination to shoulders, arms and back, as permeable cotton gowns are an ineffective barrier against bacteria, particularly when wet (DH 2005a: R 1a).
5 Put on a disposable well-fitting mask if there is a risk of airborne contamination, i.e.: (a) Meningococcus meningitis. (b) Blood and body fluids. (c) Tuberculosis.	To reduce the risk of inhaling organisms and to comply with safe techniques and practices (DH 2005a: R 1a).
6 Safety glasses, visors and goggles should be put on when it is likely that aerosolized droplets of blood or body fluids are present in the air.	To give protection to the conjunctiva from blood and body fluid splashes (DH 2005a: R 1a).
7 Rinse hands with bactericidal alcoholic handrub.	Hands must be cleaned before and after patient contact to reduce the risk of cross-infection (DH 2005a: R 1a).
8 Put on disposable gloves only if you are intending to deal with blood, excreta or contaminated material.	To reduce the risk of hand contamination (DH 2005a: R 1a).
9 Enter the room, shutting the door behind you.	To reduce the risk of airborne organisms leaving the room (Kao & Yang 2006: R 1b).

Attending to the patient in isolation

Action	Rationale
1 *Meals*. Meals only need to be served on disposable crockery and eaten with disposable cutlery if deemed necessary by the infection control team. Disposables and uneaten food should be discarded in the appropriate bag.	Contaminated crockery is a potential disease vector (Ayliffe *et al.* 2000: E).
2 *Non-disposable crockery and cutlery* must be washed in a dishwasher with a hot disinfecting cycle.	Water at 80°C for 1 minute in a dishwasher will disinfect crockery and cutlery (Ayliffe *et al.* 2000: E).

3 *Excreta*. A toilet should be kept solely for the patient's use. If neither this nor disposable items are available, a separate bedpan or urinal and commode should be left in the patient's room. Gloves must be worn by staff when dealing with excreta. Bedpans and urinals should be bagged in the isolation room, emptied and then washed in a bedpan washer.	To minimize the risk of infection being spread from excreta, e.g. via a toilet seat or a bedpan (Hota 2004: R 1a).
4 *Accidental spills*. Any suspected contaminated fluids must be mopped up immediately and the area cleaned with disinfectant.	Surfaces must be left as dry as possible after cleaning (Ayliffe *et al.* 2000: E) as damp areas encourage microbial growth and increase the risk of spread of infection.
5 *Bathing*. If an en-suite bathroom is not available, an infected patient must be bathed last on the ward. Clean and dry the bath after the previous patient and after the infected patient.	Surfaces must be left as dry as possible after cleaning (Ayliffe *et al*. 2000: E). Leaving the bath dry after disinfection reduces the risk of microbes surviving and infecting others. Bacteria will not easily grow on clean, dry surfaces.
6 *Dressings*. Aseptic technique must be used for changing all dressings. Waste materials and dirty dressings should be discarded in the appropriate yellow clinical waste bag. Used lotions, creams, etc., must be kept in the room and not used for other patients. Sterile packs must be stored safely to protect them from contamination and damage.	Aseptic procedure minimizes the risk of cross-infection. Lotions and creams can become easily contaminated. Micro-organisms can survive on unopened sterile packs (Dietze *et al.* 2001: R 1a).
7 *Linen*. Place infected linen in a red alginate polythene bag, which must be secured tightly before it leaves the room. Just outside the room, place this bag into a red linen bag which must be secured tightly and not used for other patients. These bags should await the laundry collection in a safe area.	Placing infected linen in a red alginate polythene bag confines the organisms and allows staff handling the linen to recognize the potential hazard (DH 1995a: C).
8 *Waste*. Yellow clinical waste bags should be kept in the room for disposal of all the patient's rubbish. The top of the bag should be sealed and labelled with the name of the ward or department before it is removed from the room.	Yellow is the international colour for clinical waste (DH 2006 a: C).

Leaving the isolation room

Action	Rationale
1 If wearing gloves, remove and discard them in the yellow clinical waste bag. Clean hands with bactericidal alcoholic handrub.	To remove pathogenic organisms acquired during contact with patient before removing gown, so preventing contamination of uniform (DH 2005a: R 1a).
2 Remove apron and discard it in the appropriate bag. Clean hands with bactericidal alcoholic handrub.	Hands may be contaminated by a used plastic apron (DH 2005a: R 1a).
3 Reusable gowns must be worn once and then sent to the laundry.	To reduce the risk of cross-infection by contaminated uniforms, as staff find it hard to distinguish the inside/outside of a gown. If the gown is worn inside out, uniforms can be contaminated (E).
4 Leave the room, shutting the door behind you.	To reduce the risk of airborne spread of infection (Kao & Yang 2006: R 1a).
5 Rub hands with a bactericidal alcoholic handrub.	To remove pathogenic organisms acquired from such items as the door handle (Oie *et al.* 2002: R 1a).

Procedure guidelines *(cont.)*

Cleaning the isolation room

Action	Rationale
1 Domestic staff must be educated and trained to understand why barrier nursing is required to prevent a health care-acquired infection and should be instructed on the correct procedure when cleaning an isolation room.	To reduce the risk of mistakes and to ensure that barrier nursing is maintained (DH 2001a: R 1b).
2 The area where barrier nursing is being carried out must be cleaned last.	To reduce the risk of the transmission of organisms (Gould 2005: E).
3 Separate cleaning equipment must be kept for this area.	Cleaning equipment can easily become infected. Cross-infection may result from shared cleaning equipment (Wilson 2006: E).
4 Members of the domestic services staff must wear gloves and plastic aprons.	To reduce the risk of cross-infection (DH 2005a: R 1b).
5 Floor (hard surface). This must be washed daily with a disinfectant as appropriate. All excess water must be removed.	Daily cleaning will keep bacterial count reduced. Organisms, especially Gram-negative bacteria, multiply quickly in the presence of moisture and on equipment (Wilson 2006: E).
6 Cleaning solutions must be freshly diluted and the spray container emptied, cleaned and dried daily.	Cleaning fluid can easily become contaminated (Dharan *et al.* 1999: R 1b).
7 After use, the bucket must be cleaned and dried.	Bacteria will not easily survive on clean, dry surfaces (Ayliffe *et al.* 2000: E).
8 Mop heads should be laundered in a hot wash daily.	Mop heads become contaminated easily (Wilson 2006 E).
9 Floor (carpet). The use of carpets in clinical areas must be avoided (DH 2002b). If an infected patient has been admitted into a room with a carpet, a vacuum cleaner should be used which is fitted with an efficient filter. After use the dust bag must be changed and the brush head washed and dried.	Vacuum cleaning reduces the dust, thus reducing organisms (Trakumas *et al.* 2001: R 1b).
10 On discharge, the carpet must be carefully cleaned.	Micro-organisms can easily survive in carpet fibres (Malik *et al.* 2006: R 1b).
11 Furniture and fittings should be damp dusted using a disposable cloth and a detergent solution or a disinfectant if appropriate.	To remove any organisms (Wilson 2006: E).
12 The toilet, shower and bathroom area must be cleaned at least once a day using a non-abrasive hypochlorite powder or cream. A disinfectant will only be required if soiling of the area has occurred.	Non-abrasive powders or creams preserve the integrity of the surfaces. These areas recontaminate rapidly after cleaning and routine chemical disinfection is of little value and should be saved for terminal cleaning following discharge of the patient (Ayliffe *et al.* 2000: E).

Transporting infected patients outside the source isolation area

Action	Rationale
1 Inform the department concerned about the diagnosis.	To allow other departments time to make their own arrangements (E).
2 Arrange for the patient to have the last appointment of the day.	The department concerned, the hospital corridors, lifts, etc., will be less busy and will allow more time for special cleaning and disinfecting (E).
3 Any porters involved must be instructed carefully. The trolley or chair should be cleaned after use.	Protection and reassurance of porters are necessary to allay fear and to minimize the risk of the infection being spread to them (Ayliffe *et al.* 2000: E).
4 It may be necessary for the nurse to escort the patient.	To ensure the necessary precautions are maintained (E).
5 In some circumstances, for example meningococcus meningitis and tuberculosis, the patient should wear a mask when leaving the room.	To prevent airborne cross-infection (E).

Discharging the patient from isolation

Action	Rationale
1 Inform the infection control team when the patient is due for discharge.	The infection control team may need to provide advice on any special precautions (E).
2 The room should be stripped. All textiles must be changed and curtains sent to the laundry.	Curtains readily become colonized with bacteria (Patel 2005: E).
3 Impervious surfaces, e.g. lockers, stools and blinds, should be washed with soap and water.	Wiping of surfaces is the most effective way of removing contaminants. Relatively inaccessible places, e.g. ceilings, may be omitted; these are not generally relevant to any infection risk (Wilson 2006: E).
4 The floor must be washed and dried thoroughly.	To remove any organisms present (Ayliffe *et al.* 2000: E).
5 The room can be reused as soon as it has been correctly and thoroughly cleaned.	Most organisms will survive in the environment for long periods of time. Effective cleaning will remove these organisms. Once cleaning has been completed correctly, the room is ready to admit another patient (Samuelsson *et al.* 2003: R 1a).

Protective isolation

Definition

Protective isolation is a process of care which provides a safe environment for patients who are susceptible to infection by isolating them as far as possible from the risk of infection from all exogenous sources.

Indications

Protective isolation can be an appropriate form of care for many patients, e.g. patients with burns, neutropenia, receiving BMT, or children with immunodeficiency disease. The aim of protective isolation is to prevent and treat infection until the period of immunosuppression has passed.

Immunosuppression is a generalized depression of the immune system (Mims *et al.* 2004), which increases the risk of acquiring an infection. This necessitates protecting immunosuppressed patients from micro-organisms carried in the environment, on health care workers providing care, on visitors and on other patients.

Present-day treatments have increased the number of immunosuppressed patients, owing to their underlying disease and intensive treatment regimens. This is particularly noticeable with oncology and transplant patients. Increasingly aggressive treatment for haematologic malignancies has increased the challenge to prevent immunosuppressed patients developing a hospital acquired infection (Bodey 2005). At the same time the debate related to the need for protective isolation, which is costly and has been associated with psychological problems for the patient, continues (Mank *et al.* 2003).

At the same time changes have occurred in the organisms associated with infection (Dykewicz 2001), particularly the emergence of antimicrobial-resistant micro-organisms (Coia *et al.* 2006). Concurrently difficulties related to factors such as recruitment and retention of health care workers (Newman *et al.* 2002), as well as achieving high standards of cleanliness, decontamination and sterilization have occurred (Taylor *et al.* 2001).

Immunosuppressed patients can become infected with pathogens that can infect people with normal immune responses, as well as with opportunistic micro-organisms that do not usually cause disease in healthy persons (Gerberding 1998). Traditionally protective isolation has been used to eliminate sources of infection to protect the immunosuppressed patient during their hospital stay, so increasing their chances of recovery (Hayes-Lattin *et al.* 2005). Immunosuppression can be caused by many factors including:

- Primary disease such as leukaemia, lymphoma, acquired immune deficiency syndrome (AIDS) and severe combined immunodeficiency disease (SCID).
- Secondary disease, such as diabetes, which may complicate primary disease.
- Drugs, in particular cytotoxic drugs and corticosteroids.
- Antimicrobial therapy causing changes in the patient's microbial flora.
- Irradiation therapy: the degree of immunosuppression is related directly to the area being treated.
- Trauma and burns.
- Age: extremes of age due to developing immunity in the young and waning immunity in the elderly.

On admission a detailed clinical history of the patient's past and current health status must be obtained. This initial assessment, along with ongoing physical examination, is essential to assess for any complications that may affect the patient's recovery. Prior to commencing high-dose chemotherapy, a risk assessment to evaluate the patient's immune status must be undertaken to assess their risk of acquiring an infection. These risks include: underlying cause of immune defect, expected extent and duration of planned immunosuppression treatment, presence of invasive devices, damage to skin and mucous membranes, such as mucositis, and presence of underlying disease, such as diabetes mellitus (CDC 2003). This assessment will also ensure that practical measures can be adopted to reduce the risk of infection (Farrington & Pascoe 2001; Masterton & Teare 2001).

The risk of infection will be increased by breaches in the body's natural defence mechanisms, for example:

- Skin by, for example, indwelling catheters, repeated venepuncture, pressure ulcers.
- Mucous membranes, from oral ulceration.
- Body cavities by urinary catheters or endotracheal tubes (Calandra 2000).

Immunosuppressed patients are at increased risk of HCAI and for those most at risk HCAI cannot always be prevented (Taylor *et al.* 2001). The likelihood of developing an infection is related to the neutrophil count (Marrs 2006). This risk is greatest:

- The lower the count.
- With a rapidly falling count.
- If the length of neutropenia is extended (Glauser & Calandra 2000).

The recovery from HCAI by immunosuppressed patients is often poor (Garrouste-Orgeas *et al.* 2000), making infection the leading cause of death amongst allogeneic bone marrow transplant immunosuppressed patients (Working Group 2000). A study to analyse infectious complication during hematopoietic stem cell transplantation found that infection was still the main complication of transplantation (Park *et al.* 2006) (Table 6.2).

Immunosuppressed patients are at risk of infections that affect immunocompetent patients, as well as from opportunistic micro-organisms. Antibiotic-resistant infections are of particular concern. Prompt diagnosis of infection is essential (Wilson 2006). All signs and symptoms of infection or deteriorating health must be considered significant and swiftly investigated. Once microbiological samples have been obtained, antibiotics should be commenced as soon as possible. Delay in the initation of effective therapy significantly increases mortality rates (Anderson *et al.* 2006). These will generally be broad-spectrum antibiotics (Klastersky 2004), administered via the intravenous route to ensure speed of delivery since recovery is improved with early treatment (Greub *et al.* 2000).

Some patients have an increased risk of infection due to a combination of immunosuppressive factors. For example, a patient with leukaemia who is undergoing BMT and

Table 6.2 Overall morbidity and infection related morbidity rates following hematopoietic stem cell transplantation (SCT).

Stages of transplantation	Overall mortality rate during hematopoietic SCT (%)	Infection related mortality rates during hematopoietic SCT (%)
Pre-engraftment period	3.16	1.8
During mid-recovery period	7.9	4.1
Late recovery period	26.9	15.9

who develops graft-versus-host disease (GVHD) may require treatment with increased doses of immunosuppressive drugs (Marr *et al.* 2002). A study of adults and children with neutropenia following stem cell transplantation found the incidence of infection was 38.9 per 1000 days (Laws *et al.* 2006). The extrinsic risk factor reported for neutropenic patients is central venous catheterization (Urrea *et al.* 2004).

In the 1970s and 1980s trials to evaluate the effectiveness of protective isolation were undertaken. For example a study by Yates *et al.* (1973) found no difference in infection rates in the first 21 days following admission. However, after this time patients experienced fewer infections if they were being cared for in protective isolation rooms. Others have demonstrated that protective isolation with topical and non-absorbable antibiotics and low microbial diet significantly reduced the number of infections, but did not affect long-term survival (Levine *et al.* 1973; Ribas-Mundom *et al.* 1981). It has also been suggested that protective isolation reduces the incidence of GVHD in patients with aplastic anaemia (Storb *et al.* 1983), although in contrast a study by Petersen *et al.* (1987) suggested that the incidence of GVHD was not affected. Nevertheless, the results of Petersen's project indicated that infection rates were significantly reduced in patients in protective isolation compared to those patients in conventional hospital rooms. The Centers for Disease Control (CDC) in the USA (Garner & Simmons 1983) highlight that expensive isolation precautions do not prevent endogenous infections and therefore do not appear to be warranted for most compromised patients. This view is supported by Russell *et al.* (2000), who point out that the majority of infections will be endogenous and will have very little to do with the environment. However, Johnson *et al.* (2000) suggest that the incidence of systemic fungal infections in immunosuppressed patients is increasing and some preventive measures such as air filtration, cleanliness of the environment and hand washing before and after every patient contact helps to reduce the risk of fungal infection.

There are suggested links between flower and plant water becoming contaminated, the risk of *Aspergillus* on the dust found on flowers and plants and an infection risk to the immunocompromised patient. There is also the extra work for nursing staff in looking after plants/flowers. Therefore the sensible approach is to restrict flowers and plants from protective isolation facilities (Humphreys 2005).

A survey of 91 BMT units in the USA found that while all units used some type of protective environment practice, these varied between units. The researchers recommended that national standards for protective isolation need to be compiled, which could be used to rationalize nursing care (Poe *et al.* 1994). A later study in Italy found that more than 60% of bone marrow transplant centres used complex and multiple measures to prevent infection (Errico *et al.* 1999). Additional studies are required to evaluate the role of protective isolation in the care of hospitalized neutropenic patients (Larson & Nirenberg 2004).

Immunosuppressed patients require skilled nursing care (Radwin 2000). To prevent infection, all staff must receive infection control education, training and supervision (DH 2001a).

The British Committee for Standards in Haematology (BCSH) (1995) defines four levels of care required for the management of adult patients with haematological malignancies and bone marrow failure as:

1 Level 1 for patients with transient severe neutropenia. This involves rooms designated for neutropenic patients, which have skilled staff over the 24-hour period. Expert advice and support are available from a nurse specialist.
2 Level 2 for patients requiring induction chemotherapy for leukaemia.
3 Level 3 for patients undergoing autologous transplantation. Levels 2 and 3 management require single rooms with en-suite facilities. Level 2 requires experienced nurses with recognized certificates in haematology. The view of the BCSH (1995) is supported by the Croner's Health Service Risk Management and Practice Special Report (Croner 1998), which suggests that immunosuppressed patients require cubicle facilities and en-suite toilet facilities.
4 Level 4 for patients undergoing related allogeneic and autologous transplantation. Care at level 4 requires single rooms, en-suite facilities, laminar airflow or positive filtered air conditioning and a designated kitchen area. Levels 3 and 4 require nurses who are experienced, with at least 25% of nurses having certificates in haematology or oncology. The BCSH (1995) highlights the stresses experienced by nurses caring for BMT patients and recommends the provision of staff support.

Reference material

Protective isolation may be achieved by:

- Purpose-built units.
- Plastic isolators.
- Single rooms on a general ward.
- Shared rooms within a controlled environment on a general ward.
- Bioclean room, which is a new technology where a dust-free aseptic environment is created by circulating air containing ultra-fine water droplets with negative air ions, which collect and facilitate the removal of airborne organisms (Shinjo *et al.* 2002).

Purpose-built units

A purpose-built unit will include:

- Positive pressure filtered air supply, which is required for immunosuppressed patients in protective isolation (NHS Estates 2002). This involves at least 12 air changes per hour (Humphreys 2004). This will ensure airborne

85

micro-organisms outside the protective isolation ward do not enter the room.

- Single rooms with integral toilet, shower, a hatch system for the aseptic transfer of equipment into the room, and an entry area for visitors and staff where protective clothing can be donned and hands washed.
- Facilities to provide pathogen-free food.
- Gastrointestinal decontamination.

These units are expensive to build, maintain and staff.

Plastic isolators

An isolator consists of a framework erected around a bed from which a plastic tent is suspended (Trexler 1975). The tent has an air supply attached, which keeps the whole apparatus inflated. A positive air pressure is usually maintained within the isolator. In some cases, for example when nursing patients with Lassa fever, the pressure within the isolator is slightly below atmospheric pressure, which prevents the escape of any infected particles. Although patients may feel a strong sense of containment within the isolator, this system does have the advantage of achieving high standards of bacteriological control, and it can be assembled and dismantled rapidly.

Single rooms and shared rooms in general wards

Immunosuppressed patients are at risk of acquiring an infection from environmental micro-organisms (Kusne & Krystofiak 2001). Therefore the decision to isolate a patient will be influenced by the availability of facilities coupled to the general condition of the ward area where the isolation is to take place. In determining the most suitable area, a number of criteria need to be met. Among these are the relative cleanliness of the ward, the standard of domestic services support, the microbiological status of the other patients and the anticipated length of the isolation. This less vigorous method of protective isolation is unlikely to greatly reduce the acquisition of potential pathogens, as only person-to-person transfer of infection is prevented, since facilities such as clean air and pathogen-free food are not usually available on general wards. A survey by the European Group for Bone and Marrow Transplantation of 180 transplant units in Germany found that generally both autologous and allogeneic transplant pateints were isolated (Kruger *et al.* 2001). However, a review in Western Australia during a time when there were insufficient purpose-built protective isolation rooms for immunosuppressed patients, suggested that autologous transplants did not require the same level of protective isolation as allogeneic transplants (Dadd *et al.* 2003). Kruger and colleagues (Kruger *et al.* 2001) suggested that differences in opinion were due to the lack of clinical trials related to the need and effectiveness of protective isolation. These researchers suggested that for cost effectiveness and convenience it is necessary to abolish senseless measures (Kruger *et al.* 2001). Mank *et al.* (2003) undertook a systematic literature review and conducted a medical/nursing guidelines

study. Their findings suggested if improved hygienic measures were adopted for patients with severe neutropenia, protective isolation would be unnecessary.

When shared facilities are used, it is essential that all patients are carefully screened to ensure that those with infections are excluded.

Protective isolation environment

The prevention of exogenous transmission of infection is important and can be achieved by careful monitoring of the environment to remove items that could predispose to infection, for example fabric-covered chairs (Malik *et al.* 2006), as well as choosing dust-free options such as hidden heat panels instead of radiators (NHS Estates 2002). Scrupulous cleaning with special attention to furniture and equipment within the room will also prevent transmission (Boden 1999). All surfaces must be cleanable, especially items such as electric fans, air cooling systems and chairs (Custovic *et al.* 1998), with excess equipment and the patient's personal property removed to make the cleaning process easier and more effective (Humphreys 2006). The patient's area must be well maintained (CDC 2003). This was highlighted by Loach (1997), who discussed how her experience of protective isolation was badly affected by a shower being broken.

Patient hygiene

Studies have highlighted the overwhelming fatigue experienced by patients with leukaemia and lymphoma. Fatigue hinders patients' ability to take care of themselves and demonstrates the importance of expert nursing, intervention and assessment (Danaher *et al.* 2006).

The limiting of endogenous transmission of infection, which is the major cause of infection in immunosuppressed patients (Glauser & Calandra 2000), is difficult, but good patient hygiene and restriction of invasive devices and procedures are beneficial.

Infection

In the early period of immunosuppression, respiratory, gastrointestinal, skin, mucosa bacterial and fungal flora may cause infection. These include: *Staphylococcus aureus* and *S. epidermidis*, streptococci, *Candida*, enterococci and Gram-negative bacteria such as *Escherichia coli* and *Pseudomonas*. Later reactivation of latent infections or new infections such as herpes simplex, zoster, cytomegalovirus, Epstein–Barr virus, *Pneumocystis carinii*, *Aspergillus* and toxoplasmosis may occur (Working Group 2000). Unfortunately, signs and symptoms of infection are often altered in immunosuppressed patients (Sepkowitz 2005). Progression of infection in the immunosuppressed patient may be rapid and widespread, and the earliest signs of infection must be looked for (see Chapter 25). When fever appears, diagnostic and therapeutic measures must be instigated immediately (Barber 2001). Patient survival depends upon prompt recognition of problems and instigation of medical and nursing intervention. The initiation of empirical antibiotics in febrile neutropenia has been the most important advance in the management of immunocompromised patients (Sharma & Lokeshwar 2005). Investigations to establish the cause of infection include chest X-ray, bacteriological and viral culture of blood, urine and sputum, and swabs obtained from any suspicious lesion. Bowden (2000) states that the best approach to diagnose infection is the use of aggressive diagnostic procedures early to establish the cause of the infection. (see Chapter 40).

Hand washing

Immunosuppressed patients are at increased risk of nosocomial infection, and bacteria that cause infection are particularly easily disseminated by health care workers' hands. Strict hand washing before and after patient contact can reduce rates of infection (Slota et al. 2001) (see Chapter 5). Hand washing can be said to be the most important means of infection control (DH 2001a). The use of an alcohol handrub to cleanse clean hands improves compliance with hand-cleaning policies (Johnson et al. 2005). Hands should be washed with liquid soap and hand-hot water and dried carefully with a good quality paper towel when coming on or going off duty, before breaks, beverages, meals and when hands become contaminated. Once clean, before and after contact with patients, their equipment or specimens, hands can be cleansed using alcoholic handgel. Hot air hand dryers should not be used in clinical areas as they can only be used by one person at a time and may therefore impede hand washing. Bars of soap should not be used as they can become contaminated and lead to cross-infection (Nguyen et al. 2005).

Diet

Food is a potential source of infection (Meier & Lopez 2001) and good food hygiene practice is essential (Food Standards Agency 2006).

Generally, if non-absorbable gut antibiotics are prescribed, a neutropenic diet must be provided (Patterson 1993). This includes thoroughly cooked foods, canned foods and foods known to be pathogen free such as cereal (Moody et al. 2006). Reheated food is not likely to be pathogen free and should not be used. If pathogen-free food is unavailable the diet should consist only of food that has been well cooked, with foods known to have high bacterial counts avoided. Foods known to have an increased risk of being contaminated, for example fresh cream, shellfish, raw or lightly cooked eggs (Ejidokun et al. 2000), soft cheeses (Gillespie et al. 2001), pâté, raw vegetables, salads and fruit, must be eliminated from the diet (Moody et al. 2006). A study to evaluate a neutropenic diet in the outpatient setting found that adhering to the diet was difficult and problems included nausea, vomiting, sore mouth and diarrhoea (DeMille et al. 2006). This study found no significant difference in infec-

tion rates between compliant and non-compliant patients and concluded that more research was required (DeMille et al. 2006).

Drinking water should be obtained from filtered mains drinking water (Vonberg et al. 2005a) not from bottles (Klont et al. 2006). Infection from ice can also occur from contamination within the ice maker or from staff, patients or visitors. Surveys of hospital ward ice machines demonstrated a wide range of potentially opportunistic pathogenic microorganisms (King 2001). Ice for immunosuppressed patients should be made by putting filtered drinking water into single-use ice makers, then into a conventional freezer (NHS Estates 2002). It should be noted that microwave cookers have been found to be an unreliable means of heating food (Anaya et al. 2006) and therefore should not be used in these circumstances.

Well-nourished people undergoing BMT have a better survival rate and shorter hospital stay than undernourished patients (Henry 1997). Food provided for patients must be prepared following recognized General Food Hygiene Regulations (Food Standards Agency 2006), including thorough hand washing. Food cooked and brought in from home must be avoided as this may not have been prepared according to good food hygiene practices (Glauser & Calandra 2000). Visitors should be encouraged to bring in prepackaged food such as biscuits and crisps or tinned items, which will have been manufactured to the necessary food hygiene standards. A review of practice related to clean diets found evidence of a move away from stringent sterile diets towards more relaxed regimens with rational, justifiable food hygiene guidelines, has not been connected to incidence of infection; however, the lack of scientific basis for food restrictions means that the debate will continue (Wilson 2002).

Psychological issues

Protective isolation can cause increased stress for patients (Heinonen et al. 2005) and they should be prepared before they enter isolation; nurses can reduce anxiety by assisting patients to learn about their situation and by demonstrating compassion and sensitivity while delivering care and information (Quinn 2005). Research has shown that the overriding concern of patients in isolation was a desire to receive information about their disease and reassurance regarding their treatment (Krasuska et al. 2002). It is important that health care workers are aware of the impact of protective isolation on patients (Quinn 2003). One study of 39 leukaemia patients in isolation found that 16 (41%) experienced adjustment disorders, anxiety and/or depression (Sasaki et al. 2000).

Nursing care

The value of nursing care has been emphasized in improving the care of patients undergoing BMT. A descriptive longitudinal study of stem cell transplant patients' perception of care, found that those patients with a good clinical outcome reported higher quality of life and greater satisfaction with care. This study provided increased insight into patients' experiences and highlighted the need for refined educational and supportive interventions (Schulmeister *et al.* 2005). Therefore orientation, education and training for new and existing staff are essential, to allow nurses to keep up with developments and to understand that the evidence is not always available to direct nursing care but that infection control in this group of patients is prudent and reasonable (Larson & Nirenberg 2004).

It is suggested that cancer nursing can result in burn out, producing symptoms such as fatigue, anxiety, depression and poor concentration (Schraub & Marx 2004). Burn out can be detrimental to nurses, their colleagues and the patients in their care. A postal survey to cancer centres in Canada and a focus group of personnel from six major cancer centres found that job satisfaction was related to patient care and contact. Major job stresses related to heavy workload that decreased the quality of patient care. The authors of this study suggested that system changes that help to alleviate workloads would reduce nurses' stress (Grunfeld *et al.* 2005). Bernardi and colleagues suggest that support groups assist in the coping mechanisms to avoid burn out (Bernardi *et al.* 2005). While Medland and colleagues suggest that programmes designed to improve coping skills may reduce stress

and burn out and improve cancer nurse retention (Medland *et al.* 2004).

The risk of infection is the most common cause of mortality and morbidity for neutropenic patients (Shelton 2003). Whilst major gaps exist in empirical evidence regarding nursing intervention to prevent infection (Larson & Nirenburg 2004), nurses must recognize and adopt the factors that are known to reduce infection (DH 2005a). A study investigating compliance with infection control policies found that non-compliance was widespread (Kim *et al.* 2003). To provide optimum nursing care, infection control must be incorporated into nursing care (Shelton 2003).

Discharge home

Discharge planning should start early (see Chapter 10). Risk assessment of the home should be undertaken to ensure the home is clean and well maintained (Bloomfield & Scott 2003a), with a well-equipped kitchen for food preparation, storage and cooking (Bloomfield 2003b).

Caution should be taken when in contact with domestic pets, which may be carriers of infection. For example, dogs can be infected with a wide range of infections including *Cryptosporidium*, which can cause serious infection in an immunosuppressed person (Lefebvre *et al.* 2006).

Procedure guidelines   Neutropenic patient care

Procedure

Preparation of the room for neutropenic patient care and maintenance of general cleanliness

Action	Rationale
1 A single room or a designated shared room should be used if possible.	To reduce airborne transfer of micro-organisms (NHS Estates 2002: R 1a).
2 A toilet to be kept for the sole use of the patient.	To reduce the risk of cross-infection (NHS Estates 2002: R 1a).
3 Area to be cleaned meticulously before the patient is admitted.	To reduce the risk of infection (DH 2003a: R 1a).
4 Equipment and supplies to be kept for the sole use of the patient.	To reduce the risk of cross-infection. Equipment can easily become colonized with micro-organisms, which may cause cross-infection (Dietze 2001: R 1b).
5 Surfaces and furniture to be damp dusted daily using disposable cleaning cloths and detergent solution.	Damp dusting and mopping remove micro-organisms without distributing them into the air (DH 2005a: R 1a).
6 Floor to be mopped daily using soap and water.	To reduce the risk of cross-infection (Wilson 2006: E).
7 Mop head to be laundered daily.	As above.
8 Bucket and mop handle to be cleaned and dried.	As above.

Nursing procedure

Entering room of neutropenic patient

Action	Rationale
1 A disposable plastic apron to be worn when in contact with the patient.	To protect staff clothing from becoming contaminated, which could transfer organisms to the other patients in their care (DH 2005a: R 1a).
2 Clean hands with bactericidal alcoholic handrub.	Hands are regarded as the principal source of transfer of micro-organisms (for further information see Chapter 5) (DH 2005a: R 1a).
3 Door of room to be kept closed. Ideally the air in the room should be under slightly positive pressure. The air flow should be from the room into the corridor.	To reduce the risk of airborne transmission of infection from other areas of the ward (Sexton *et al.* 2006: R 1b).

Visitors to neutropenic patient

Action	Rationale
1 The patient should be asked to nominate close relatives and friends who may then, after instruction, visit freely. The patient or his or her representative should inform casual acquaintances or non-essential visitors that they should avoid visiting during the period of neutropenia.	The incidence of infection increases in proportion to the number of people visiting. Large numbers of visitors are difficult to screen and educate. Unlimited visiting by close relatives and friends diminishes the sense of isolation that the patient may experience (E).
2 Any visitor with an infection or who has been in contact with infection should be excluded.	Neutropenic patients are susceptible to infection (Calandra 2000: E).
3 Children, unless very close relatives, should be discouraged.	Children are more likely to have been in contact with infectious diseases which can have serious consequences if transmitted to a neutropenic patient (E).

Diet for neutropenic patient

Action	Rationale
1 Educate the patient to choose only cooked food from the hospital menu and eliminate raw fruit, salads and uncooked vegetables from the diet.	Uncooked foods are often heavily colonized by micro-organisms, particularly Gram-negative bacteria (Moody *et al* 2006: R 1A).
2 Food brought into the hospital by visitors must be restricted and: (a) obtained from well-known, reliable firms; (b) in undamaged, sealed tins and packets; (c) within the expiry date.	Correctly processed and packaged foods are more likely to be of an acceptable food hygiene standard (E).
3 Filtered water to be used (Vonberg *et al.* 2005b).	Tap water is safe to drink but can become colonized by organisms, particularly Gram-negative organisms found in the plughole of sinks or overflow outlet when the water is being filled (Campana *et al.* 2004: R 2b).
4 Sealed packets of fruit juice (long shelf-life varieties, particularly those rich in vitamins) are suitable. Juice should be poured directly into a clean jug and drunk the same day.	These juices have been pasteurized and remain pathogen free until they are opened (E).

Procedure guidelines *(cont.)*

Discharging the neutropenic patient

Action	Rationale
1 Crowded areas, for example shops, cinemas, pubs and discos, should be avoided.	Although the patient's white cell count is usually high enough for discharge, the patient remains immunocompromised for some time (Calandra 2000: E).
2 Pets should not be allowed to lick the patient, and new pets should not be obtained.	Pets are known carriers of infection (Lefebvre *et al.* 2006: R 1b).
3 Certain foods, for example take-away meals, soft cheese and pâté, should continue to be avoided.	Take-away meals are subject to handling by a large number of individuals and are stored for longer periods, both of which increase the likelihood of contamination (Gillespie *et al.* 2001: R 1b).
4 Salads and fruit should be washed carefully, dried and, if possible, peeled.	To remove as many pathogens as possible (Moody *et al.* 2006: R 1b).
5 Any sign or symptoms of infection should be reported immediately to the patient's general practitioner or to the discharging hospital.	Any infection may continue to have serious consequences if left unlocated (Anderson *et al.* 2006: R 2b).

Acquired immune deficiency syndrome

Definition

Acquired immune deficiency syndrome (AIDS) is a state of immunosuppression caused by the human immunodeficiency viruses 1 (HIV 1) and 2 (HIV 2), which causes a chronic, progressive disruption of the immune system. As no overall description can be made for AIDS, an internationally agreed case definition has been made. This definition provides uniform, simple criteria for categorizing HIV conditions to facilitate evaluation of treatment and care of persons with HIV (CDC 1992).

HIV infection is divided into four groups:

- Primary HIV infection (often associated with a rash and fever).
- Asymptomatic phase.
- Persistent generalized lymphadenopathy.
- Symptomatic infection, which is further subdivided. Some patients' symptoms may be classified as AIDS-defining conditions.

AIDS-defining conditions include:

- Certain opportunistic infections.
- Certain cancers.
- Wasting syndrome.
- Encephalopathy.

AIDS-defining cancers include:

- Kaposi's sarcoma, which is decreasing in prevalence.
- Primary central nervous system lymphoma.

- Non-Hodgkin's lymphoma (Burkitt's or immunoblastic).
- Invasive cervical cancer.

Highly active antiretroviral therapy (HAART) has reduced the incidence and significantly improved the prognosis of HIV-related cancers (Diamond *et al.* 2006a). This improvement has been seen for persons with Kaposi's sarcoma and lymphoma but not with HIV-associated anal cancer (Bower *et al.* 2004).

Reference material

People still question whether HIV is pathogenic, and what causes AIDS. Such doubt can lead to denial and a lack of action in tackling the problem of HIV. Scientific evidence shows that HIV is the cause of significant mortality and morbidity due to AIDS world-wide (Marx *et al.* 2004).

It is reported that the AIDS epidemic is slowing but huge challenges remain (Kuehn 2006). The epidemiology of HIV and AIDS is changing and although HIV is still incurable the introduction of antiretroviral therapy has reduced the need for HIV-positive patients to be admitted to hospital (Diamond *et al.* 2006a). However, the incidence of new problems, for example the increased incidence of anal cancer amongst HIV-positive persons, may be directly related to the increased survival of HIV-positive patients (which in turn has increased the risk of long-term survivors developing cancer [Diamond *et al.* 2005]). Unfortunately the emergence of HIV-drug resistance in patients receiving antiretroviral therapy does occur and decreases treatment options (Chen & Lee 2006).

At the Chelsea and Westminster Hospital, London, an attempt has been made to predict mortality on the basis of clinical characteristics. For example, a person with Kaposi's sarcoma with another AIDS-defining illness has a reduced prognosis compared to a person with AIDS aged 50 years and over with a rising CD4 count (Stebbing *et al.* 2006).

Antibody and antigen serological tests are used to diagnose HIV infection and to monitor the disease process (Saville *et al.* 2001). A rapid test is now available in the USA where results can be obtained in 30 minutes (CDC 2006). However, an increase in the incidence of false negative tests have been found when using this rapid test method (Jindal *et al* 2005). Limitations of the antibody tests include the absence of antibody in the early stages of seroconversion and changing levels of the virus, which may be missed by the antigen tests (Saville *et al.* 2001). The DH (DH 1996a) recommended that patients should not be tested for HIV antibodies without their consent, and that information should be offered to the patient before and after the test. The DH offer guidelines on what information should be included in the pre-test appointment meeting. During this discussion the patient should be informed about how HIV is transmitted and the significance of a negative and positive test. This provides a framework for obtaining HIV antibody test consent as previously there was a lack of consistency in the content of pre-test information given to the patient (DH 1996a).

The major disadvantage of diagnosis based on serology is the window period before immunoglobulin G (IgG) antibodies are produced in response to the HIV infection. p24 antigen is present in serum samples prior to and following seroconversion, when the antibody screening test is negative or indeterminate. p24 antigen tests can be used for diagnosis and monitoring levels of HIV from the time of seroconversion until late stages of disease (Flandre *et al.* 2006). Viral load in peripheral blood can be measured and used for diagnostic, prognostic and monitoring of antiviral therapy purposes (Wood *et al.* 2006).

Early diagnosis of HIV infection is important as it improves patient outcomes through better monitoring and provision of early treatment and care. An additional benefit is that if a person knows that they are HIV antibody positive, they can take steps to reduce transmission of HIV to others (Health Protection Agency 2006).

Transmission

Newly diagnosed HIV-positive test results are reported in a confidential manner to the Health Protection Agency. From the 5560 reports received to date in 2005, the agency predicted that the number of people diagnosed with HIV in 2005, once late reports had been received, would be 7750 (Health Protection Agency 2006). This number continues to rise each year. HIV has been isolated in the blood, semen, tears and saliva, breast milk, genital secretions of women, cerebrospinal fluid and the brain. Of the new HIV diagnoses reported in 2005 where the route of transmission was known, 52% had acquired HIV through sex between men and women, with most cases acquired outside the UK; 31.5% through sex between men; 2% through injecting drug use; and 1% from other routes (Health Protection Agency 2006).

The overall picture remains one of increasing prevalence of HIV infection and a continual rise in the incidence of sexually transmitted diseases with world-wide geographical variations. In the UK there is a higher incidence of HIV in inner London, 117 in a million of the population, compared with 42 in a million of the population in outer London. Prevention involves the use of a condom with new and casual partners and considering the possible risk before acquiring a new sexual partner.

Since HIV surveillance began in the UK in 1982, 76 850 people have been diagnosed with HIV, and of those who have been diagnosed with AIDS, 61% have died. Currently over 58 000 people are living with HIV in the UK with an estimated further 19 700 who remain unaware of their diagnosis (Health Protection Agency 2006).

Whilst HIV is predominantly transmitted by sexual contact, it can be less commonly transmitted by intravenous drug misuse, mother to infant, blood products (rare), blood/tissue transfer (rare), plus some other undetermined routes (Communicable Disease Surveillance Centre 2002a).

Whilst transmission of HIV by blood and blood products is rare, HIV is known to have been transmitted in the UK when the donor was in the HIV window period (Morris *et al.* 2005). During an antigen test of blood donated in Scotland one HIV-positive donor was found (1 in 0.7 million) who would have been missed using the routine antibody test (Jarvis *et al.* 2006). It was estimated that between 1996 and 2003 the risk of HIV infectious donations entering the blood supply in the UK was 0.14 per million blood donations (Soldan *et al.* 2005). This suggests initiatives such as donor deferrals for at-risk behaviours and the introduction of more sensitive viral screening assays should reduce the risk of blood and blood product transmission of HIV even further.

World-wide there have been two reports of possible transmission of HIV from infected health care workers to patients during exposure-prone procedures (EPP). All health care workers have an ethical and legal responsibility to protect the health and safety of their patients. All health care workers who believe they may have been exposed to HIV have to seek and follow confidential professional advice. Those known to be HIV positive are not to undertake EPP. If it is thought that any EPP have been performed by an HIV-positive person, the Consultant in Communicable Diseases has to be informed. An appraisal of the EPP will be made and, if necessary, a decision about whether a patient notification of exposure to HIV needs to be taken (DH 2005b). All new health care workers need to have standard health clearance for serious communicable diseases prior to training (DH 2003c).

World-wide there are up to 300 reports (102 confirmed) of occupational transmission of HIV to health care workers (McCarthy *et al.* 2002). The risk of HIV transmission during a percutaneous exposure is estimated to be three per 1000 injuries, whilst following a mucocutaneous exposure it is a one in 1000 incidence. The use of antiretroviral drugs for post-exposure prophylaxis needs to be fully explained to all health care workers exposed to blood and body fluids to ensure they respond quickly and correctly following such exposure (DH 2000a).

HIV is not a notifiable disease, although partner notification is encouraged. One study in the USA approached, interviewed, counselled and tested men aged 15–29 years old; of the 10% who tested positive for HIV, 59% had thought they were at low risk for HIV infection (MacKellar *et al.* 2005).

Women and children

Studies on the transmission of HIV infection in Britain found that risk factors for HIV were:

1 Women heterosexually infected:
 ▪ resident in London;
 ▪ widowhood;
 ▪ being a young black woman.
2 Women who shared needles:
 ▪ resident in London or Scotland;
 ▪ large number of sexual partners;
 ▪ termination of pregnancy.

These differences need to be considered when prevention and control policies are being planned.

Most antenatal units offer HIV testing to all women, and most HIV units offer antiretroviral therapy in pregnancy. Some women decline HIV antenatal screening (Boxall & Smith 2004; Conaty *et al.* 2005) even though HIV-positive pregnant women can be told how to reduce the risk of transmission of HIV to their baby, including advice on breast feeding (DH 2004c).

Perinatal transmission of HIV from mother to foetus can occur during intrauterine, intrapartum and postpartum periods. During the postpartum period it is mainly through breast feeding, as HIV has been found in both colostrum and breast milk (Luzuriaga *et al.* 2006). The emphasis for the management and care of children with HIV is on prevention, early recognition and treatment, with advances in, and the use of, antiretroviral therapy being beneficial in slowing the progression of HIV disease (DH 2004c).

Clinical presentation

Following HIV infection a period occurs during which an HIV antibody test will be negative. Following seroconversion and the production of HIV antibodies, the test will be positive and the incubation period begins. The progression to AIDS disease will occur following an increase in plasma viral load and a fall in the CD4 count. These are factors which will determine when treatment should be started.

It is clear that an AIDS diagnosis significantly increases mortality. Prognostic factors can be used to predict survival times of people with advanced disease. Those patients with good performance status will have a longer survival rate, while in those patients with low body weight and neuro-

logical manifestations it will be reduced (May *et al.* 2006). Mortality has now decreased in developing countries where access to HAART has become possible (Braitstein *et al.* 2006).

Treatment

Combination HAARTs have considerably improved the survival and the quality of life of HIV-positive persons (Gona *et al.* 2006). HAART is also associated with improved survival of HIV-positive persons with cancer (Diamond *et al.* 2006b). This improvement has led to the patients having fewer opportunistic infections, fewer hospital admissions and a reduction in mother-to-baby transmission of HIV. There are a number of disadvantages, including short- and long-term side-effects, lifelong commitment to treatment, food and diet restrictions and pill burden, all of which are difficult to incorporate into the patient's lifestyle and are constant reminders of illness and confidentiality issues (Deeks 2006). Drug-resistant strains of HIV have now developed (Deeks 2006). The emergence of resistance is strongly associated with an increased risk of mortality (Hogg *et al.* 2006). HIV-related cancer remains a significant problem, in particular Kaposi's sarcoma, non-Hodgkin's lymphoma and cervical cancer (Bernstein *et al.* 2006).

Vaccine

Containment of HIV will require an effective vaccine (McMichael 2006). Such a vaccine will need to be preventive to protect HIV-negative people and therapeutic to reduce infectivity in those already found to be HIV positive. Considerable effort is now being focused on evaluating different approaches in developing a vaccine (Haynes & Montefiori 2006).

Confidentiality

HIV/AIDS raises many ethical issues. Confidentiality related to testing, treatment and care is essential. Persons with HIV have highlighted confidentiality as one of five main concerns and prefer to receive care at a genitourinary medicine clinic that provides a strict confidentiality service (Petchey *et al.* 2000). The stigma and discrimination related to HIV persists (DH 2005b).

Psychological support

Anxiety is a universal problem for people with AIDS. Health care workers can also experience anxiety when caring for HIV-positive persons. It is possible that nursing staff specially prepared could be the most effective way of minimizing stigma and discrimination against HIV-positive persons in the health care sector (Hodgson 2006).

Counselling should include: pre- and post-test counselling, importance of reduction in high risk behaviour, natural history of HIV disease, family and relationships, and bereavement discussions. Telephone hotlines, outreach contacts and crisis intervention should also be provided. Crisis intervention should include a structured support programme and support groups (Walch *et al.* 2006).

HIV palliative care offers disease-specific therapy and comfort with symptom-oriented treatment throughout the clinical course of the disease, not just at the end of life. Issues such as treatment choices and resuscitation need to be discussed early and whenever physical status changes (Robinson *et al.* 2006).

Infection control

There is a legal requirement for employers under the general duties of the Health and Safety at Work, etc. Act 1974, Management of Health and Safety at Work Regulations 1999 and the Control of Substances Hazardous to Health Regulations 2002 (HSE 2002) to safeguard employees and others against occupational risk. This includes risk posed by blood-borne infection. Strategies must be in place to reduce the incidence of exposure to HIV including the use of needleless devices that reduce the risk of needlestick injuries (Vaughn *et al.* 2004). It is important that standard principles for preventing HAI are applied by all health care workers in the care of all patients and, in the instance of HIV, at all stages of HIV-positive patients' care even in death. One study that highlights this requirement has indicated that HIV remains viable for a considerable time even in a cadaver (Ball *et al.* 1991). (See Chapter 22.)

The risk of HIV infection in health care workers can be reduced by strict adherence to universal precautions. Employees have a responsibility to adopt universal precautions for all patients. Factors such as fatigue, stress, levels of training, skill and experience affect safe practices.

Nursing care

Nursing problems associated with HIV include pain, confusion, depression, anxiety, fatigue, fever, dyspnoea, nausea and vomiting, diarrhoea, wasting and dehydration (Kemp & Stepp 1995). Nutrition is a significant issue; early detection and intervention can decrease problems (Highleyman 2006).

Good care is essential for persons with HIV/AIDS, although surveys have indicated that patients are not universally satisfied with the care they are receiving (Wolosin 2005) or the information provided related to treatment options (Gellaitry *et al.* 2005). Education, training, management support and experience in HIV care increases job satisfaction (Hall & Sutton 2002; Liljestrand 2004).

Nurses must keep up to date with improvements that have occurred related to HIV and AIDS, through the earlier diagnosis of HIV and AIDS and the availability of better treatments coupled with the increased use of prophylaxis. They must be ready to adapt to these changes and be prepared and able to provide good care.

Human immunodeficiency virus 2

Definition

Human immunodeficiency virus 2 (HIV 2) is closely related to HIV 1 but is antigenically distinct and demonstrates distinct replication and cytopathic characteristics (Albert *et al.* 1990).

Reference material

HIV 2 was first recognized in 1986 (Clavel *et al.* 1986), although evidence existed that HIV 2 infections were present in many West Africans as far back as 1966 (Kawamura *et al.* 1989). Serological evidence supporting the existence of a second HIV was published in 1985 (Barin *et al.* 1985). HIV 2 appears less virulent than HIV 1. Infection with HIV 2 does not protect against HIV 1 (Schim van der Loeff *et al.* 2001).

In the UK, screening of blood donors and people attending genitourinary medicine clinics shows that the occurrence of HIV 2 infection is rare.

Transmission, care and treatment of HIV 2 follows the same pattern as HIV 1.

Procedure guidelines **Acquired immune deficiency syndrome (AIDS): patient care in a general ward**

Procedure

Action	Rationale
1 All staff should be familiar with the risk of blood-borne viruses in the workplace, and their own hospital's codes of practice.	To ensure all staff are aware of, and take, the necessary precautions (HSE 2005a: C).
2 Hospital staff should cover any broken skin with a waterproof dressing.	To prevent the entry of infectious material (HSE 2005a: C).

93

Procedure guidelines *(cont.)*

3 Staff suffering from eczema should not nurse patients who are HIV antibody positive.

Any break in staff member's skin should be covered with a waterproof dressing to prevent entry of HIV. This would be difficult to accomplish with eczema lesions and would exacerbate the eczema (HSE 2005: C).

4 Accidental inoculations must be avoided at all cost.

Serious inoculation accidents have been seen to be a means of transmission of HIV (HSE 2005: C).

5 In the event of gross contamination of intact skin the affected area must be washed thoroughly with soap under warm water. A scrubbing brush must not be used.

Intact skin is a natural barrier against infection. By thorough washing the infectious material can be removed. Scrubbing brushes can cause skin damage which allows infection to enter (HSE 2005: C).

6 Puncture wounds or cuts must be made to bleed freely and washed under hot running water.

To flush out infectious material (HSE 2005: C).

7 A waterproof dressing must be applied and medical advice sought for large wounds.

To prevent further infection to the wound (HSE 2005: C).

8 An accident form must be completed immediately and taken to bacteriology, the occupational health physician or other medical advisor as appropriate.

It is important to have accurate records of all accidents and incidents in order to monitor events (HSE 2005: C).

9 HIV postexposure prophylaxis should be considered for all significant exposure to HIV.

HIV postexposure prophylaxis antiviral therapy has been shown to prevent seroconversion following significant exposure to HIV (DH 2000a: C).

HIV-positive individuals: low risk (i.e. patients who are not bleeding, incontinent, confused or infected with a contagious disease)

Nursing assessment of the risk of contamination of the environment with pathogenic organisms, blood or body fluids from a patient known to be HIV antibody positive allows care to be more accurately planned.

Action

1 If the patient is not bleeding, incontinent, confused or infected with a contagious disease, he/she is considered to be of low risk of transmitting infection to others and can be nursed on an open ward using all the patients' facilities as normal.

Rationale

HIV cannot be transmitted by social contact that occurs in hospital wards (HSE 2005a: C).

2 If a low-risk, HIV-positive individual develops an infection, is undergoing invasive procedures or becomes incontinent, nursing care will commence as for high-risk, HIV-positive persons.

Contamination with blood and body fluids has the potential risk of transmitting the HIV virus to others (HSE 2005a: C).

HIV-positive individuals: increased risk

Action

1 Known or strongly suspected HIV antibody-positive patients who are bleeding, incontinent, infected with a contagious disease or receiving invasive procedures should be nursed in a single room with its own toilet and hand-washing facilities.

Rationale

To minimize the risk of transmitting infection via blood and body fluid (HSE 2005a: C).

Entering the room of patient with AIDS

Action	Rationale
1 When the patient is not bleeding, coughing, incontinent or receiving procedures, protective clothing is not required.	Transmission of HIV is not possible from general contact in the absence of blood and bloodstained body fluids.
2 When the patient is incontinent, bleeding or undergoing invasive procedures, disposable well-fitting gloves and a plastic apron are needed.	Transmission of HIV is possible from body fluids (HSE 2005a: C).
3 If there is a possibility of airborne contamination, a correctly fitting mask and safety spectacles should be worn.	Transmission of HIV is possible if contaminated material is allowed to contaminate mucous membranes (HSE 2005a: C).

95

Liquid waste from patient with AIDS

Action	Rationale
1 All liquid waste from HIV-positive patients must be disposed of in a bedpan washer immediately, taking care to avoid splashing.	To prevent contamination of the environment (Ayliffe *et al.* 2000: E).
2 Areas without bedpan washers will need to use the slop hopper. Great care must be taken to pour waste slowly and carefully down the hopper to avoid splashing.	To prevent contamination of the environment (E).

Non-disposable equipment used for patient with AIDS

Action	Rationale
1 All sterile service and similar staff who have to process used non-disposable equipment should be familiar with the risk of blood-borne viruses in the workplace, and their own hospital's codes of practice.	To ensure all staff are aware of, and take, the necessary precautions to protect themselves from the risk of blood and body fluids (HSE 2005a: C).
2 Cleaning of non-disposable equipment needs to be performed thoroughly and in a safe manner.	Careless cleaning, immersion, drying, etc., can increase contamination of the environment (E).
3 Gloves/aprons must be worn, together with masks/eye protection if appropriate, when cleaning non-disposable equipment.	To prevent self-contamination (DH 2005a: 1a).
4 Before disinfection, equipment must be cleaned with soap and water, avoiding splashing.	Decontamination is a combination of processes including cleaning, as disinfectants cannot completely penetrate organic matter (Wilson 2006: E).
5 The equipment must then be dried carefully.	Wet objects would alter the disinfectant's strength and could inactivate the solution if soap and soiling were still present (E).
6 Autoclaving is the method of choice for sterilizing non-disposable equipment. If the equipment would be damaged by autoclaving, it may be disinfected in a properly maintained and tested washer disinfecting machine, using a disinfectant that will remove all bacteria, viruses and spores.	All non-disposable equipment must be properly and thoroughly cleaned and disinfected after use to prevent cross-infection (Wilson 2006: E).

Procedure guidelines *(cont.)*

7 If the equipment can be autoclaved it must be placed in a sterile supplies department (SSD) bag and taped shut. The bag must then be taken to SSD.	Autoclaving is the most effective sterilization method. Correct bagging and transportation of the equipment will prevent contamination of the environment (Ayliffe *et al.* 2000: E).
8 Expensive, delicate items, e.g. a ventilator, will require ethylene oxide disinfection.	Ethylene oxide disinfection is the second process of choice after autoclaving (Ayliffe *et al.* 2000: E).
9 Before the ethylene oxide disinfection process, these items must have all their disposable parts, filters, etc., removed and the whole item must be cleaned completely and thoroughly with hypochlorite 1% solution and dried carefully.	To prevent contamination of the environment (E).
10 The transportation and ethylene oxide process will take some time. Thought must be given beforehand to the use of this equipment for actively bleeding, incontinent patients.	Ethylene oxide disinfection involves lengthy airing of equipment after the process to ensure it is safe to reuse. During this time other patients may be deprived of the item (E).
11 All staff handling contaminated equipment and disinfectants must comply with The Control of Substances Hazardous to Health Regulations (COSHH) (HSE 2002).	These regulations are designed to protect people against risks to their health including hazardous substances such as disinfectants and micro-organisms (HSE 2002: C).

Specimen and appointment considerations for patients with AIDS

Action	Rationale
1 It is essential that all request cards for items such as specimens have the biohazard label attached.	To ensure all departments are informed that the sample is potentially dangerous (HSE 2003b: C).
2 All specimens must have the biohazard label attached and be double bagged in a specimen polythene biohazard bag with a biohazard label attached to the bag.	To ensure the laboratory is aware of potential risk and that the specimen is correctly contained to prevent cross-infection (for further information see Chapter 40, Specimen collection) (HSE 2003b: C).
3 The specimen should be taken to the laboratory in a washable, covered container.	To prevent contamination of the environment. If leakage does occur, it can be simply contained and cleaned up (HSE 2003b: C).
4 The patient will normally be given the last appointment of the day if invasive procedures are planned.	The department will be less crowded and busy, thus allowing time for appropriate precautions to be taken (E).

Domestic staff: responsibilities when working with a patient with AIDS

Action	Rationale
1 All cleaning staff should be familiar with the risk of blood-borne viruses in the workplace, and their own hospital's codes of practice. The room must be cleaned daily. (For further information see Procedure guidelines: Isolation of source of infection, above.)	To ensure all staff are aware of, and take, the necessary precautions. To minimize the risk of cross-infection (HSE 2005a: C).
2 A nurse must check the patient's room to establish that it is suitable for the domestic staff to clean.	To ensure the room is not contaminated with blood or body fluids (E).

3 If contamination of the environment with blood or body fluids occurs it must be treated with a hypochlorite solution or granules containing 10 000 ppm available chlorine.	To prevent cross-infection (Wilson 2006: E).

Terminal cleaning of the room used by patient with AIDS

Action	Rationale
1 The room must be cleared of all equipment in appropriate manner (see above) before it is cleaned.	It is impossible to clean thoroughly if potentially contaminated items are in the room (E).
2 The walls should only be cleaned if contamination is known to have occurred.	Micro-organisms do not survive on intact walls (E).
3 The curtains must be changed if contamination has occurred.	Discretion and assessment need to be used. If the room has only been used for a short time for a patient who has not contaminated the environment, curtains would not need changing (E).

Approach to the patient with AIDS

Action	Rationale
1 As soon as possible, the probable/known diagnosis must be discussed with the patient and the hospital policy explained.	It is essential that the patient understands fully and agrees the reason for these restrictions which, while protecting contacts, also protect the patient from further risks of infection (Aveyard 2002: E).
2 Psychological support is essential.	Psychological dysfunction is likely and should be recognized and treated early to alleviate and contain the mental distress which an AIDS patient may experience (Hodgson 2006: E).
3 It is necessary that all nurses caring for HIV antibody-positive patients are familiar with treatment and care procedures.	To ensure appropriate nursing care is delivered (Hodgson 2006: E).
4 Staff should adopt a non-judgemental approach in their dealings with HIV antibody-positive patients.	It is the responsibility of all health professionals to care for patients and not to pass moral judgements (Hodgson 2006: E).
5 It may be appropriate to recommend voluntary agencies to HIV antibody-positive patients.	Support groups have knowledge and experience which can help HIV antibody-positive individuals (Walch *et al.* 2006 E).

Visiting the patient with AIDS

Action	Rationale
1 Visitors should be encouraged.	To prevent isolation (E).
2 The diagnosis of AIDS is confidential and should not be disclosed.	To maintain confidentiality (E).

Discharging the patient with AIDS

Action	Rationale
1 Almost all patients with AIDS will require community services at some time during their illness.	AIDS patients will need to be admitted to hospital for the treatment of clinical illness, but will be encouraged to resume their normal activities when at home (E).

Procedure guidelines *(cont.)*

2 If an AIDS patient requires community services, the patient must have given consent for HIV antibody-positive diagnosis to be given to the general practitioner and community care personnel.

Confidentiality must not be breached without the patient's consent (NMC 2006: C). However, health care workers such as ambulance personnel and district nurses will need to take precautions if bleeding, incontinence or infections are present (E).

Disposal of waste from the patient with AIDS in the community

Action

1 Excreta and infected fluids can be discarded into the toilet in the normal manner.

2 Infected waste such as dressings, gloves and aprons, must be placed in yellow clinical waste bags and the local authority asked to collect them.

3 Sharps must be placed in a sharps box and stored in a safe place when full, and collected by the local health authority.

Rationale

To prevent contamination of the environment (E).

Yellow is the international colour for infected waste bags, and they are available on request from the local authority (DH 2006a: C).

To prevent inoculation accidents (DH 2006a: C).

Laundry from the patient with AIDS in the community

Action

1 Clothes and linen which are heavily soiled or bloodstained should be washed separately by washing machine using a hot wash cycle, over 70°C for 3 minutes. Wash as above if using a public launderette.

2 If the person is not fit enough, infected linen should be placed in red alginate polythene bags and the local authority asked to arrange collection and laundering.

Rationale

Heat inactivation combined with the considerable dilution factor found in a washing machine renders linen safe for reuse (DH 1995a: C).

Red alginate polythene bags are recognized internationally for infected linen (DH 1995a: C).

Crockery and cutlery from the patient with AIDS in the community

Action

1 Ideally, crockery and cutlery should be washed in a dishwasher with a final rinse temperature of at least 80°C.

2 There is no need to keep a separate store of crockery and cutlery if washed appropriately.

Rationale

Heat is effective in destroying micro-organisms (Ayliffe *et al.* 2000: E).

Crockery and cutlery present no risk of contamination if washed in a dishwasher with a final rinse temperature of at least 80°C (E).

Protective clothing for healthcare workers working with the patient with AIDS in the community

Action

1 Disposable apron and gloves need be worn only when blood or excreta are being handled.

2 Disinfectants are required only if blood or excreta spillage has occurred. A strong hypochlorite solution (1 part household bleach to 10 parts water) is recommended.

Rationale

There is no risk of acquiring infection from general social contact (HSE 2005: C).

Unnecessary use of disinfectants is expensive and may be potentially hazardous to staff and the environment (Wilson 2006: E).

Visitors to the patient with AIDS in the community

Action	Rationale
1 Visitors should be encouraged.	There is no risk of acquiring infection from social contact (HSE 2005: C).
2 The patient should be encouraged to resume social activities.	To minimize effects of boredom and loneliness (E).

Prevention of further infection in the patient with AIDS

Action	Rationale
1 The patient should be encouraged to stay away from individuals with infections.	AIDS patients are susceptible to infections (E).
2 If the patient develops any signs and symptoms of ill health, the general practitioner or hospital must be informed immediately. (For further details on discharge planning see Chapter 10.)	Early treatment of symptoms will enhance the chances of containing the disease (E).

Death of the patient with AIDS

Action	Rationale
1 The body should be laid out as described in the Procedure guidelines: Last offices (see Chapter 22). In addition, the nurse should wear gloves and a plastic apron.	To prevent contamination (HSE 2005: C).
2 All orifices must be packed.	The body continues to secrete fluids after death has occurred. Any leakage may contaminate the environment (E).
3 Any wounds, intravenous sites or skin breakages must be sealed with waterproof dressings.	To prevent leakage of contaminated fluids (E).
4 All documentation relating to this procedure must have a biohazard label attached.	To alert administration, portering and mortuary staff of the infection risks (HSE 2003b: C).
5 Once the body has been laid out and the room made presentable, family and friends may view the body.	To allow family and friends to spend time with the deceased person, allowing them to adjust to their loss and express their grief (E).
6 The body must be placed in a body bag.	The body bag will prevent leakage (E).
7 Porters must be given help and support.	There is no infection risk when the body is sealed in a body bag unless the bag becomes torn or damaged in transportation. Gloves and aprons will prevent contamination of the staff handling the body (HSE 2005: C).

Funeral arrangements of the patient with AIDS

Action	Rationale
1 Ideally, the hospital administration should have a list of funeral directors who will attend to an HIV-antibody positive patient.	It is important that the bereaved relatives are given every help and support to prevent unnecessary distress (E).

Antimicrobial-resistant organisms

Definition

The term *antimicrobial resistance* denotes a strain of organism not killed or inhibited by antimicrobial agents to which the species is generally sensitive, leading to an increase in length of hospital stay and severity of illness (DH 2000a).

Reference material

The increase in antimicrobial-resistant organisms is the inevitable consequence of the widespread use of antibiotics (Chen *et al.* 2004). The importance cannot be overemphasized. The increasing resistance of organisms to antibiotics brings the prospect of a return to the pre-antibiotic era (Bissett 2006). The DH (2000a) UK Antimicrobial Resistance Strategy and Action plan aims to minimize the morbidity and mortality due to antibiotic-resistant infections and to maintain the effectiveness of antimicrobials for the treatment and prevention of infection in humans and animals. Key interrelated elements of this strategy include surveillance, prudent antimicrobial use and infection control. The Standing Medical Advisory Committee (1998) points out that micro-organisms are getting ahead in the development of new antibiotics and therapeutic options are narrowing (DH 1998b).

Some new antimicrobial drugs have been developed that are effective against some antimicrobial-resistant micro-organisms (Leuthner *et al.* 2006). Unfortunately the introduction of new antimicrobial drugs into clinical practice eventually leads to the emergence of strains of bacteria resistant to the new drugs (Potoski *et al.* 2006).

Emphasis on antibiotic resistance has shifted from recognition to prevention (DH 2003a). In addition, research has been aimed at improving understanding of resistance and transmissibility of resistant organisms (Coia *et al.* 2006). The widespread and often indiscriminate use of antibiotics for prophylactic and veterinary purposes, as well as the inappropriate selection of these antibiotics, is believed to be an important factor in the development of resistant forms of bacteria (Lefebvre *et al.* 2006).

The transmission of genetic material between bacteria by conjugation has been well documented. Conjugation accounts in part for the rapid spread of resistance, with mutation, transformation and transduction also being involved (Corkill *et al.* 2005; Tenover 2006). The possibility of VRE transferring the vancomycin resistance gene to MRSA is a growing concern. It is also important that the relevant national surveillance network is notified (Health Protection Agency) to ensure that accurate information about the epidemiology and spread of these organisms is gathered (Coia *et al.* 2006).

Patient risk factors for developing an infection with an antimicrobial-resistant organism include: advanced age, underlying disease, severity of illness, interinstitutional transfer of patient, especially from a nursing home, prolonged hospitalization, surgery or transplantation, invasive devices and antibiotic therapy (Safdar & Maki 2002). The consequences of a patient being infected with a resistant form of bacteria are demanding in terms of increased length of stay in hospital, costs of care and treatment (Coia *et al.* 2006). Resistance to antiviral drugs has also been seen (Longerich *et al.* 2005; Jabs *et al.* 2006).

The DH (2003a) states that compliance with infection control measures and restrictive use of antibiotics are the key measures to prevent epidemics of multi-resistant bacterial infection. When an outbreak of infection does occur, the control of contamination of the environment can control the outbreak without requiring ward closure (Wilks *et al.* 2006). Infection control includes establishing best practice, education and training, establishing and monitoring standards and organizational support (DH 2000b).

Theoretically any organism can develop antimicrobial resistance. In practice, MRSA, *Staphylococcus epidermidis*, VRE and Gram-negative micro-organisms are of particular concern (Jones 2001).

Gram-negative bacteria

Gram-negative bacteria normally inhabit the gut, but can cause infections in the urinary tract, respiratory tract and wounds. Antimicrobial resistant strains have emerged, which have caused significant mortality and morbidity (Wu *et al.* 2006) and pose a significant risk due to limited treatment options (Navon-Venezia *et al.* 2005). This may be the consequence of excessive use of broad-spectrum antibiotics (Rolston 2005). Important resistant Gram-negative bacteria include *Klebsiella pneumoniae*, *Escherichia coli*, *Proteus mirabilis*, *Pseudomonas aeruginosa*, *Acinetobacter* and *Stenotrophomonas maltophilia* (Picazo 2005). *Pseudomonas* species, *E. coli* and *Klebsiella* (Babay *et al.* 2005) cause particular problems, being ubiquitous in the hospital environment (Vianelli *et al.* 2006). Resistant strains spread easily in hospitals and communities (Landman *et al.* 2002). Resistance in many Gram-negative bacteria is caused by the β-lactamase production enzyme, which can inactivate antibacterial agents (McGowan 2006). These organisms can multiply in warm, moist conditions and have been identified in eye drops, soap solutions, lotions, tubing used for ventilators and incubators, and the environment (Dancer *et al.* 2002). Risk factors for spread include overcrowded wards, lapses in hygiene and poor infection control practices. Spread is primarily by direct or indirect person-to-person contact (Casolari *et al.* 2005). However, contamination of equipment such as humidifiers and nebulizers has also been implicated in spread (Rae 1998).

Gram-negative bacteraemia is associated with septic shock (Candel *et al.* 2005), which occurs primarily in debilitated, hospitalized patients, who are the group that also develop the resistant form of Gram-negative bacteraemia (Lin *et al.* 2006). The major problem regarding Gram-negative-resistant organisms is that shock progresses before antibiotic sensitivities are known, producing increased clinical mani-festations of infection, which can result in death (Blot *et al.* 2005). Therefore, timely initiation of antibiotic therapy is crucial for severe infection.

Prevention of Gram-negative resistant micro-organisms relies on improved antibiotic usage and infection control (Paterson 2006), along with appropriate investigations to allow accurate and speedy diagnosis, so that effective treatment can be achieved (Anderson *et al.* 2006). One measure that has reduced the incidence of *Pseudomonas* infection is the use of filters on water outlets (Trautmann *et al.* 2005).

Gram-positive bacteria

Meticillin-resistant *Staphylococcus aureus* (MRSA) (coagulase-positive *Staphylococcus aureus*)

Staphylococcus aureus is part of the normal human flora, with large numbers of the organism being found on the skin and mucosa. Colonization or infection by MRSA is therefore more likely to occur in the nose, lesions and sites of abnormal skin, and in indwelling devices such as catheters and tracheostomies (Ayliffe *et al.* 2000). MRSA bacteraemia is associated with an increased risk of death compared with meticillin-sensitive *Staphylococcus aureus* (MSSA) (Gastmeier *et al.* 2005). Soon after the introduction of benzyl penicillin in the 1940s incidences of resistance were seen. With penicillin usage, the prevalence of resistant strains increased. In the 1960s meticillin was introduced and MRSA was soon reported (Jevons 1961). *Staphylococcus aureus* resistance to meticillin results from the expression of cell wall synthesizing enzyme, which has a low affinity for all β-lactams (Fuda *et al.* 2004). In 1981 the first epidemic strains of MRSA (EMRSA) were reported. Since this time MRSA has become endemic in some hospitals, with some senior nurses suggesting it is out of control (Lines 2006). There are increased rates of MRSA in the UK compared to most other European countries. It is difficult to establish reasons for this, but it has been suggested that facilities and resources provided, coupled with senior management support in controlling infection is important (Humphreys 2006). The media has labelled MRSA 'the super bug'. A study to measure MRSA awareness among health care workers, patients and their visitors, found increased levels of awareness amongst all patients, visitors and staff, and concerns about their own safety (Gill *et al.* 2006).

Resistance to other antibiotics have emerged: vancomycin intermediate *Staphylococcus aureus* (VISA); glycopeptide intermediate *Staphylococcus aureus* (GISA); and vancomycin-resistant *Staphylococcus aureus* (VRSA). Inappropriate or unnecessary use of antibiotics will further increase this resistance (Coia *et al.* 2006). New drugs have been developed that are effective against MRSA (Leuthner *et al.* 2006), but resistance (Potoski *et al.* 2006) and toxicity have already been seen (Bishop *et al.* 2006). The patient with increased resistance may become a reservoir for further dissemination

of difficult-to-treat resistant strains of MRSA (Gales *et al.* 2006).

The use of mupirocin nose cream and chlorhexidine baths or showers has been seen to irradicate colonization of MRSA and decrease the incidence of MRSA cross-infection (Sandri *et al.* 2006). However, resistance to mupirocin cream is also occurring (Fawley *et al.* 2006). Other products such as fusidic acid continue to be effective for irradication of MRSA colonization (Nishijima & Kurikawa 2002). Fortunately, disinfectant agents used for hand washing and cleaning remain equally effective against sensitive and resistant antibiotic strains of bacteria if manufacturers' recommendations are followed (Payne *et al.* 1998). Revised guidelines for the control of MRSA in hospitals have been compiled (Coia *et al.* 2006). The guidelines include recommendations that emphasize the need for active and timely interventions in reducing the numbers of patients colonized and infected with MRSA (Coia *et al.* 2006).

While rates of patients colonized with MRSA appear to be greater than those infected with MRSA, these infections are significant due to the difficulties in treating systemic infection and the ability of the organism to spread and colonize debilitated patients. Deaths from MRSA infection have increased (Crowcroft & Catchpole 2002).

Risk factors for MRSA include previous hospitalization, particularly in high-dependency units, presence of intravenous catheters, tracheotomies, wounds and pressure ulcers, underlying disease and recent antibiotics. Colonization with MRSA has been seen to be a risk factor for acquiring a hospital infection (Coia *et al.* 2006). Actively seeking and treating carriers has been seen to lead to a reduction in MRSA (McNeil *et al.* 2002). Screening specimens include nose, throat, axilla, groin and wounds. Delay in initiation of effective therapy has been shown to be a significant morbidity factor (Coia *et al.* 2006).

MRSA infection results in increased workload (Farrington *et al.* 2000) and increased length of stay in hospital with associated costs, in particular intravenous antibiotics. In addition, the detrimental effects on patients, their family and friends, such as pain, anxiety and depression, are a vital consideration. In one study, five patients being barrier nursed due to MRSA infection expressed feelings of loneliness, stigma, monotony and issues of control (Oldman 1998).

Screening

Until recently microbiological testing of specimens for MRSA took 2–3 days. However, rapid polymerase chain reaction (PCR) tests are now available where same day results can be achieved (Davidson *et al.* 2006). This is important as it enables the diagnosis of MRSA more rapidly, which in turn allows appropriate treatment to be started earlier and the risk of MRSA cross-infection reduced.

Active screening of patients for MRSA should be performed. The 2006 MRSA guidelines suggest that certain high-risk patients should be screened routinely. These groups should be determined locally, based on local experience.

Generally those included in screening would be frequent readmissions to any health care facility, direct interhospital transfers and persons known to have been infected or colonized with MRSA in the past (Coia *et al.* 2006).

Patients transferred from all hospitals where MRSA infection/colonization is common should be screened on admission, and treated as suspect until the results of screening specimens are known. These restrictions may be minimal, with nursing care involving good hand washing following patient contact. However, if the patient is obviously ill, for example with a discharging wound, then this would necessitate source isolation nursing (see Source isolation section, above). Any patients in contact with infected patients must be screened to detect cross-infection. This would include nose swabs and swabs from skin lesions and urinary and intravenous catheters. If cross-infection occurs, it may be necessary to close a ward to new admissions, particularly to surgical or intensive care patients.

Screening of health care workers is not recommended routinely, but if MRSA cross infection occurs in wards, screening of staff should be considered as health care workers have been seen to acquire and transmit MRSA to patients. MRSA eradication and treatment for health care workers should be the same as for a patient (Coia *et al.* 2006).

In patients known to be colonized with MRSA, signs of infection must be treated as significant, with MRSA considered to be the possible cause. Early investigations, appropriate specimen collection and treatment are essential (see Chapter 40). Relapses may occur, especially in debilitated patients and particularly in sites such as tracheotomies (MacKinnon & Allen 2000). This means that source isolation must be maintained even after three negative cultures have been obtained. The presence of MRSA should be documented in the patient's records in order to alert staff should readmission be necessary (Coia *et al.* 2006).

Transmission

MRSA is mainly spread by hands; therefore, hand hygiene is the most important factor in controlling an outbreak of MRSA (Coia *et al.* 2006). Environmental cleanliness is also important, as MRSA can survive for a long period in the environment. Microbiological sampling of MRSA-positive patients' rooms in a hospital in Ireland found that the mattress, linen and furniture were all positive for MRSA. Increased contamination was found in patients infected with MRSA compared to those colonized with MRSA (Sexton *et al.* 2006). This study emphasized the importance of cleaning and keeping the door of the room closed to prevent the airborne spread of MRSA. Similarly it has been found that there is a correlation between increased rates of MRSA and bed occupancy, particularly with the rapid turnover of patients in acute hospitals (Cunningham *et al.* 2005).

Once patients have been discharged, the ward must be cleaned thoroughly before new patients are admitted (Coia *et al.* 2006). A prospective microbiological study of MRSA contamination of isolation rooms following the discharge of a MRSA-positive patient, found that daily routine cleaning over a 4-week period did not remove MRSA contamination. Inadequate cleaning and therefore the removal of exogenous MRSA predisposes to cross-infection with MRSA (Sexton *et al.* 2006).

A 3-year prospective study monitoring MRSA infection and daily workload of nurses, found a correlation between nurses with a very high workload and MRSA cross-infection (Blatnik & Lesnicar 2006). A year-long intensive care study found that segregation of MRSA-positive patients did not prevent the spread of MRSA, but did produce a potential risk to the patient by being segregated (Cepeda *et al.* 2005). Other studies emphasize the importance of hand washing but continue to advocate segregation of MRSA colonized or infected patients (Henderson 2006).

Patients with large wounds, eczema or respiratory tract infection with a productive cough will be heavy dispersers of MRSA and are often responsible for spread. Faulty ventilation systems (Cotterill *et al.* 1996) and crowded conditions have also been implicated in the spread of MRSA (Kibbler *et al.* 1998). Source isolation in a single room with the door closed and limiting the movement of MRSA-positive patients will minimize spread (Coia *et al.* 2006). Studies comparing isolation strategies found that when using single rooms there was a decrease in the risk of cross-infection due to the correct use of PPE on entry, signage and encouraging/reminding of the importance of hand washing (Dhaliwal & McGeer 2005).

When there are large numbers of MRSA-infected/colonized patients, cohort nursing in one ward is an effective means of controlling outbreaks. Other measures include:

- Correctly performed hand washing before and after patient contact. A bactericidal alcoholic handrub can be used when hands are clean.
- High standard of ward cleaning, as inanimate surfaces near affected patients are commonly contaminated with MRSA.
- Careful containment and disposal of waste.
- Careful segregation, containment and laundering of used linen.
- Careful education of the patient and their visitors to ensure compliance to policy, as familial carriage and subsequent infection have been reported.
- Planned cleaning of the ward, including difficult-to-clean areas such as blinds.
- Appropriate investigation and treatment of health care workers. While MRSA rarely causes infection in healthy persons, health care workers can become colonized with MRSA and go on to transmit MRSA to their patients. Staff screening is indicated if transmission of MRSA continues in spite of control measures being undertaken. Investigation and treatment of health care workers is the responsibility of the occupational health department, with the help of the infection control team.
- Wearing of masks during some procedures, e.g. suctioning, can reduce the risk of health care workers acquiring MRSA (Coia *et al.* 2006).

In areas where MRSA is endemic a risk assessment may need to be undertaken. The 2006 MRSA guidelines suggest there are some patients at increased risk of MRSA. These include:

1 Frequent readmissions to any health care facility.
2 Direct interhospital transfers.
3 Recent inpatient at hospitals abroad or hospitals in the UK which are known or likely to have high prevalence of MRSA.
4 Residents of residential care facilities where there is known or likely high prevalence of MRSA carriage (Coia *et al.* 2006).

Some patients are at increased risk of serious MRSA infection. These include: HIV-positive persons; patients with eczema, dermatitis, psoriasis; patients in intensive care; neonatal, burns, transplantation, cardiothoracic, orthopaedic, trauma, vascular surgery and renal patients (Coia *et al.* 2006). Attempts to control MRSA require a comprehensive approach to reduce the associated morbidity and mortality (Fairclough 2006).

Community care

Interhospital movement should be restricted to the absolute minimum. If the patient must be transferred to another hospital the receiving hospital must be informed in plenty of time for the necessary arrangements to be made. The ambulance service should be notified if it is being used to transfer an MRSA patient, mainly to prevent another patient being placed in the same vehicle before it is cleaned. Hand washing by the ambulance service staff and cleaning of local areas of patient contact, i.e. chair or stretcher, are all that is required after transport of an affected patient.

People colonized with MRSA do not present a risk to healthy people in the community, and should live their lives without restrictions. However, in care of the elderly wards and residential homes where other residents may have postoperative wounds, strict attention to hand washing, environmental cleanliness and compliance with aseptic technique is important, which generally makes segregation unnecessary (Coia *et al.* 2006).

Staphylococcus epidermidis (coagulase-negative staphylococci)

Staphylococcus epidermidis is part of the body's normal commensal flora (Ziebuhr *et al.* 2006) and an important cause of infection as well as a significant cause of morbidity and mortality (Yang *et al.* 2006). This is particularly problematic in immunosuppressed patients (Falcone *et al.* 2004) or in those with invasive devices such as intravenous catheters, particularly for those patients with cancer who are hospitalized for several days (Knauer *et al.* 2004). Significant levels of resistance are seen, reflecting antibiotic usage (Trueba *et al.* 2006), and are associated with a poor prognosis (Rabaud & Mauuary 2001). Cross-infection may occur, which can become endemic in hospitals (Monsen *et al.* 2005).

Staphylococcus epidermidis can organize into a complex multi-layer of cells covered with polysaccharide, called a biofilm. This biofilm allows the organism to adhere to foreign objects such as catheters and become less susceptible to antibiotics (Rohde *et al.* 2005). Research and technology continue to produce devices such as tracheostomy tubes that will inhibit the formation of biofilms (Jarrett *et al.* 2002).

Streptococcus pneumoniae

There are over 30 species of *Streptococcus pneumoniae*, some of which can cause programme cell death or apoptosis during pneumococcal meningitis and pneumonia (Marriott & Dockrell 2006). Different species have differing pathogenicity (Aricha *et al.* 2004). *Streptococcus pneumoniae* is the major cause of community-acquired pneumonia (File 2006) and can also be the cause of bacteraemia, otitis media, meningitis, peritonitis and sinusitis. Most patients who develop this infection have other risk factors that predispose them to infection, for example malignancy, splenectomy, AIDS, malnutrition, age (very young and elderly) and, in particular, alcohol consumption (de Roux *et al.* 2006).

Streptococcus pneumoniae is carried asymptomatically in the nose and throat of healthy persons and can be easily transmitted by person-to-person spread (Serrano *et al.* 2006).

Resistant *S.pneumoniae* was recognized in the 1960s, but was not seen in the UK until 1976 in a patient with a history of foreign travel (Meers & Matthews 1978). Since this time, resistance to penicillin has been increasing with a marked ability to cause cross-infection (File 2006). The increased incidence of *S.pneumoniae* infection has led to the increased use of vaccine. These vaccines are based on the serotype antigen of the *pneumoniae*; therefore, the serotype of the organism needs to be known to ensure the appropriate vaccine is given. Currently there are multi-valent vaccines available that contain the antibiotic-resistant serotypes (Berg *et al.* 2006).

Vancomycin-resistant enterococci

Vancomycin-resistant enterococci (VRE) are also referred to as glycopeptide-resistant enterococci (GRE) (Cookson *et al.* 2006). Enterococcus species were once considered normal bacterial flora which occasionally acted as opportunistic pathogens. The genus *Enterococcus* includes 21 species with *Enterococcus faecalis* and *faecium* an important cause of nosocomial infection (Cookson *et al.* 2006). The origin of VRE may be due to selection of VRE by the use of vancomycin, or introduced into the hospital by patients already colonized with VRE due to acquisition from animals or via the food chain. VRE infections are associated with greater rates of clinical treatment failures and mortality compared to vancomycin-sensitive enterococci infections (Brown *et al.* 2006a).

VRE infection and colonization are associated with previous vancomycin use and/or broad-spectrum antibiotic therapy, severe underlying disease, immunosuppression, intra-abdominal surgery and prolonged hospitalization, with the risk of acquisition of VRE directly proportional to the length of stay in hospital (McEvoy *et al.* 2006). Most VRE infections are endogenous, with the colonization of the human bowel prolonged often for months, sometimes years (Brown *et al.* 2006a). Cross-infection does occur (Samuelsson *et al.* 2003); however, transmission from patient to patient or by direct contact, particularly by unwashed hands or contamination of equipment or the environment, frequently occurs (Cookson *et al.* 2006). The food chain, especially raw minced meat, is thought to be responsible for the increased incidence of VRE in humans, due to use of the glycopeptide avoparcin as a food additive. However, a large German study of raw minced meat and pork failed to demonstrate a connection between 8% of meat samples positive for VRE and patients' clinical isolates, which were of different resistance patterns (Klein *et al.* 1998). A great cause of concern is the appearance of transferable high-level glycopeptide resistance in enterococci, producing some strains that are now resistant to all available antibiotics. Enterococci readily colonize the bowel, spread rapidly among hospital patients and transfer their antibiotic resistance widely among themselves and other Gram-positive species (French 1998). Patients with diarrhoea or incontinence pose a significant risk of cross-infection to others and should be segregated in a single room with an en-suite toilet (Mayer *et al.* 2003).

Contamination of the environment readily occurs (Wendt *et al.* 1998). Reducing environmental contamination will control spread (Hayden *et al.* 2006). VRE can survive temperatures of 71°C for 10 minutes or 80°C for 3 minutes (Bradley & Fraise 1996); it can survive in 150 parts per million available chlorine for 5 minutes (Kearnes *et al.* 1995) and in the environment for longer than 11 days (Neely & Maley 2000). Inoculation studies found that VRE can survive on stethoscopes and telephones for 30 minutes and on fingertips for 60 minutes (Noskin *et al.* 1995). Thorough cleaning of the environment and equipment both during the patient admission and on discharge of the patients is important in preventing cross-infection of VRE (Martinez *et al.* 2003). Strict attention to hand washing before and after patient contact is essential. Patients must wash their hands after visiting the toilet and before meals. While universal precautions are generally adequate for caring for VRE-positive patients, when patients have diarrhoea or cannot comply with infection control policies barrier nursing is required, particularly if other patients in the area are immunocompromised (Mayer *et al.* 2003).

From September 2003 it became compulsory for all Trusts in England to monitor VRE bacteraemia as part of the Healthcare Associated Infection Development Strategy to combat infectious diseases (Brown *et al.* 2006a).

Aspergillosis

Definition

Aspergillosis is an infection caused by a fungus of the genus *Aspergillus*, causing inflammatory granulomatous lesions on, or in, any organ (Nosari *et al.* 2001), and is a major complication for neutropenic patients (Afessa & Peters 2006).

Reference material

Aspergillus species are common saprophytic moulds, easily recognized by their conidiophores, which are swollen ends of hyphae, from which radiate large numbers of sterigmata which end in short chains of spores. Each *Aspergillus* conidiospore releases thousands of spores, which remain suspended in the air for long periods and are viable for many months in dry locations. They are among the most buoyant of fungal spores and are ubiquitous in the environment and present in all unfiltered air (Ronning *et al.* 2005). Over 200 species of *Aspergillus* have been characterized, but fewer than 20 are reported as being pathogenic to humans, the most common species causing allergic and invasive disease being *A. fumigatus* and *A. flavus*, which have emerged as important pathogens, particularly in invasive disease of immunosuppressed patients (Vonberg & Gastmeier 2006).

Aspergillus spores are commonly found in soil and vegetation (Lugauskas *et al.* 2005) as well as inside buildings, for example in carpets (Ali *et al.* 2006). One study found greater levels of *Aspergillus* indoors when compared with out of doors (Tormom Molina *et al.* 2002). Cases of allergic and invasive disease have been reported among individuals working in close contact with such substances and who inhale large numbers of *Aspergillus* spores. Examples include fungus inhalation during building work, continual prolonged exposure, such as farmers and gardeners (Monso 2004) and some factory workers (for example working in a herb factory) (Golec *et al.* 2004).

Generally, aspergillosis has been associated with building renovation, when large numbers of spores are often liberated into the environment (Gibb *et al.* 2006), which can lead to outbreaks of infection (Vonberg & Gastmeier 2006). These spores are then inhaled and deposited in the lungs. Ear, cutaneous, sinus and dental infections have also been known to occur. Other reported modes of transmission include airborne spread, which is associated with indwelling catheters (Manian 2003), and food-borne spread. *Aspergillus flavus* can generate a carcinogenic substance called aflatoxin in foodstuffs (Yu *et al.* 2005). Normal healthy people rarely develop invasive disease. Although incidence of infection in healthy people has been seen (see above), aspergillosis is primarily an infection of severely immunocompromised patients (Humphreys 2004). Diseases range from allergic bronchopulmonary aspergillosis in patients with asthma, aspergilloma in patients with lung cavities, chronic necrotizing aspergillosis in the mildly immunocompromised or those with chronic lung disease to invasive aspergillosis in immunocompromised patients, which is severe and can be fatal (Vonberg & Gastmeier 2006).

Incidence of invasive aspergillosis continues, possibly as a consequence of the widespread use of aggressive chemotherapy, increased transplantation and AIDS (Vonberg & Gastmeier 2006). The organism is capable of invasion across all natural barriers, including cartilage and bone, and has a propensity for invading blood vessels, causing thrombosis and infection. The major concern is the potential for severe haemorrhage, which may cause death and which occurs in about 10% of patients. Generally, infection is chronic, causing symptoms directly related to the site of infection. Infections requiring surgical treatment have been seen among transplantation patients (Ali *et al.* 2006).

Diagnosis

The early detection of infection to allow for the appropriate therapeutic approach to be commenced is essential (Ali *et al.* 2006). Diagnosis is difficult (Ali *et al.* 2006) as isolation of *Aspergillus* may be due to contamination of the specimen from environmental *Aspergillus*. Diagnosis relies on demonstration of *Aspergillus* by culture and microscopy along with consideration of the patient's clinical condition (Jayshree *et al.* 2006). Advances have been made in diagnoses using tests such as polymerase chain reaction (PCR) tests (Ali *et al.* 2006). Early chest X-ray and computed tomography (CT) scans are important diagnostic and management tools (Hauggaard *et al.* 2002).

Treatment

Despite improvements in early diagnosis and effective treatment, invasive pulmonary aspergillosis continues to cause significant morbidity and mortality (Ali *et al.* 2006). This may be due to poor penetration of antifungal agents into infected tissue (Paterson *et al.* 2003). Newer drugs for treatment and prophylaxis are now available which have fewer side-effects: Caspofungin (Pancham *et al.* 2005), Voriconazole (Sambatakou *et al.* 2006), AmBisome (Takemoto *et al.* 2006) and Itraconazole (Maertens & Boogaerts 2005). The outcome of aspergillosis is likely to depend on the extent of underlying pulmonary disease, delays in diagnosis, commencement of effective therapy. A study of cancer patients with invasive aspergillosis found that admission to the intensive care unit (ICU) was a prognostic factor for treatment failure (Lionakis *et al.* 2005). This study reflects the mortality and morbidity of *Aspergillus* infection associated with seriously ill patients who require ICU admission.

Prevention

Control measures are essential in preventing *Aspergillus* infection. Stringent environmental control in high-risk areas such as transplant units is required, as there is a strong correlation between fungal contamination and infection (Ali *et al.* 2006). Air conditioning systems must be functioning and well maintained, and the environment kept scrupulously clean, with emphasis placed on vacuuming, damp dusting and mopping. Instruments, dressings, equipment and linen must always be stored properly to prevent contamination by *Aspergillus*. This highlights the importance of removing wound dressings for the shortest period of time possible

before dressing changes to prevent contamination of open wounds.

The NHS Estates (2002) has produced a very comprehensive guidance document related to reducing the risk of infection during all the various stages of building projects and renovation work.

During constructive or renovation projects in hospital, infection control teams must identify the infection risks posed by each project and plan ways to minimize the risk. The use of barriers to prevent *Aspergillus* spores entering patient areas is essential (Cooper *et al.* 2003). Ideally, relocation of immune suppressed patients to unaffected areas is advisable, and thorough cleaning of work areas before the return of patients is imperative. Antifungal prophylaxis for patients with malignancy and profound prolonged neutropenia has been recommended (Glasmacher & Prentice 2005).

Person-to-person spread has not been demonstrated, and therefore barrier nursing is not required. However, sputum should be disposed of carefully and patients encouraged to cover the mouth and nose when coughing. It has been advised that practical measures to be followed by immunocompromised patients include regular hand washing and avoiding plants and flowers (Maertens *et al.* 2001). Prevention of air contamination in haematologic/oncology wards is essential (Hahn *et al.* 2002).

Clostridium difficile

Definition

Clostridium difficile is a slender, Gram-positive anaerobic rod which is spore forming, motile and widely distributed in soil and the intestinal tract of animals (DH 2003a). Approximately 3% of healthly adults are carriers of *C. difficile*. This increases to 7% in residents of long-term care facilities, 14% of hospitalized elderly on acute medical wards and 20% of elderly patients in chronic care wards (DH 2003b). *Clostridium difficile* is capable of surviving in the environment for prolonged periods (Cunha 1998). Bacteria of this type may be a normal component of gut flora and flourish when other gut organisms are eradicated by antibiotics (Mohan *et al.* 2006).

The typing system for *C. difficile* uses a test called ribatyping. Over 100 types have been identified. Type 027 has been identified as producing 16 times more toxin A and 23 times more toxin B and has been implicated in outbreaks associated with severe disease. Type 027, whilst rare in the UK, has been found in isolates obtained from the National Public Health Service for Wales that were tested as part of a research study with specimens from the USA and Canada (Warny *et al.* 2005). Recently multi-drug resistant strains with increased virulence have been found (Sebaihia *et al.* 2006), in particular the strain called Ribotype 1 (Hawkyard & Bignardi 2006) has caused outbreaks of infection in North America and Europe (McDonald *et al.* 2005; Warny *et al.* 2005). Typing of *C. difficile* isolates allows for investigation of outbreaks of infection (DH 2003b).

Reference material

Clostridium difficile causes gastrointestinal infection ranging from symptomless colonization to severe foul smelling diarrhoea, abdominal pain and fever, with toxin-producing strains causing pseudomembranous colitis (Mohan *et al.* 2006). It is now one of the most commonly detected enteric pathogens, an important cause of nosocomial infection in nursing homes and hospitals, and a common cause of mortality and morbidity in hospitalized patients. The incidence and severity has increased in the past several years (Oldfield 2006).

Diarrhoea can be caused by disruption of the normal flora of the gut by antibiotics which allow *C. difficile* to multiply. The colonic mucosa becomes covered with a characteristic fibrinous pseudomembrane. Signs and symptoms can be relatively mild, resolving when antibiotics are discontinued, or more severe, as in cases of pseudomembranous colitis, which may require surgical resection of parts of the colon and is associated with a significant mortality rate (Koss *et al.* 2006).

Since April 2003 NHS Trusts in England are required to report cases of *C. difficile* to their regional Communicable Disease Surveillance Centre as part of CoSurv (a systematic national alert organisms laboratory reporting system) (DH 2003b).

Diagnosis

Diagnosis is based on clinical findings, endoscopy and laboratory evaluation. Clinical findings range from profuse, watery, green, foul smelling or bloody diarrhoea, with cramping abdominal pains, tenderness and high fever, to hypovolaemic shock and overwhelming sepsis. Endoscopy may reveal effects similar to those seen in non-specific colitis, or may show the yellow–white raised plaques which go on to form a membrane on the inflamed intestinal mucosa (DH 2003b).

Laboratory diagnosis

All patients with diarrhoea should have a stool sample sent to microbiology. *Clostridium difficile* is difficult to isolate in ordinary culture because of overgrowth by other organisms. To overcome this, a selective culture medium is used. The presence of *C. difficile* in culture is not by itself an indication of infection, it simply marks the organism's presence. Infection or disease is indicated by the presence of toxins produced by the organism, which can be identified using screening tests such as commercially available neutralized cell cytotoxicity assay or an immunoassay that will detect both toxin A and toxin B (DH 2003b). Pathogenic strains of *C. difficile* produce two protein exotoxins, toxin A (enterotoxin) and toxin B (cytotoxin). *Clostridium difficile* toxin A induces detachment of human epithelial cells from the basement membrane and subsequent death by apoptosis. This process may be asymptomatic or cause mild diarrhoea or it can lead to pseudomembranous colitis (Voth & Ballard 2005). Recurrence is common (DH 2003b).

Treatment

Initial treatment involves discontinuing antibiotics and providing supportive care, which includes hydration to compensate for loss of electrolytes (Wiesen *et al.* 2006) and antidiarrhoeal oral medication (Aslam & Musher 2006). However, significant infection can be treated with antibiotics (DH 2003b). In extreme cases of pseudomembranous colitis, surgery will be required, which may include resectional or diversion procedures (Koss *et al.* 2006), but death can occur even when diagnosis is made early and appropriate therapy is given (Mohan *et al.* 2006).

Studies using probiotics, which are live organisms that improve the microbial balance of the host, are ongoing (Novak & Katz 2006), as well as intravenous immunoglobulin, which has been given for severe refractory or recurrent *C. difficile* diarrhoea after failed conventional treatment (McPherson *et al.* 2006).

Transmission

Pseudomembranous colitis develops from overgrowth of *C. difficile* already present in the gut, or from exogenous organisms acquired via person-to-person contact or the faecal–oral route following contamination of the environment or poor hand washing by patients, visitors or health care workers. *Clostridium difficile* leads to increased costs associated with increased length of hospital stay (DH 2003b), and outbreaks in hospital have resulted in deaths (Sunenshine & McDonald 2006). Bignardi (1998) identified nine risk factors that appear to influence the chance of acquiring *C. difficile*; these were increasing age, severity of underlying disease, non-surgical gastrointestinal procedures, presence of nasogastric tube, antiulcer medication, stay in Intensive Care Unit (ITU), duration of hospital stay, duration of antibiotic therapy and administration of multiple antibiotics.

Antibiotic use was shown to be statistically significantly associated with both diarrhoea and carriage of *C. difficile*. Risks include type of antibiotic, route of administration and dose (Dial *et al.* 2004). Accurate identification of risk factors allows for appropriate decisions to be made to reduce risk and thereby reduce incidence. High-risk patients can be monitored closely to facilitate early detection of infection, commencement of treatment and infection control precautions.

Prevention of spread and management of infection

Reservoirs of *C. difficile* have been found, which included carpets, blood pressure cuffs, thermometers, nurses' uniforms (DH 2003b), radiators, curtain rails, commodes, floors and toilets (Verity *et al.* 2001). *Clostridium difficile* spores are capable of being transferred during periods of air disturbances by, for example, air conditioning, open windows and floor buffing (Fawley *et al.* 2005).

Reducing the risk of cross-infection by *C. difficile* relies on the adoption of several factors, which include the restriction of the use of those antibiotics that encourage the growth of *C. difficile*, reducing the duration of antibiotic courses and the length of stay in hospital, careful hand washing, environmental decontamination and isolation of symptomatic patients (DH 2003b). Hands may become contaminated following contact with a patient with *C. difficile* who is incontinent or has diarrhoea, therefore they should be washed with detergent and water, dried carefully and have a final cleanse with alcoholic handrub (Boyce *et al.* 2006). Cross-infection has been seen to be reduced by thorough cleaning of the environment and the use of clean equipment for each patient. Cleaning with a hypochlorite has been seen to reduce the incidence of *C. difficile* (Wilcox *et al.* 2003).

Nursing care

Careful barrier nursing is required for all patients with toxin-producing *C. difficile* or unexplained diarrhoea. Segregation from other patients must continue until signs and symptoms of infection have ceased. Healthy staff and visitors who are not receiving antibiotics are not at risk (Sanderson 1999).

Cryptosporidiosis

Definition

Cryptosporidium is a protozoan coccidian parasite, first isolated in 1907. Human infection is usually caused by *Cryptosporidium parvum* (Caccio & Pozio 2006). *Cryptosporidium* has a complicated life cycle, both asexual and sexual. Infection occcurs by the ingesting of the oocyst stage of the life cycle, commonly found in faecally contaminated material (Mims *et al.* 2004).

Reference material

Cryptosporidium species are a major cause of diarrhoea infections in both immunocompetent and immunosuppressed persons and can cause life-threatening infections in the latter, resulting in deaths (El-Mahallawy *et al.* 2004). However, in otherwise healthy persons usually only a self-limiting illness occurs (Caccio & Pozio 2006).

Transmission

Cryptosporidium has a world-wide distribution (Caccio & Pozio 2006) and can infect livestock, particularly calves and lambs, whose faecal matter infects water supplies, which then can infect humans (Hunter & Thompson 2005). Based on epidemiological evidence, consumption of certain foods and water appears to be a risk factor (Smith, A *et al.* 2006). Infection can also occur following direct contact with animals (Kiang *et al.* 2006) by hand-to-mouth route, and is easily transmitted from one person to another (Caccio 2005). Only a small inoculum of organism such as that carried by flies is required to cause infection (Graczyk *et al.* 2004).

Cryptosporidiosis can occur by accidental ingestion of natural water during recreational activities (Coupe *et al.* 2006), and infection acquired by swimming in swimming baths has been reported (Smith, H.V *et al.* 2006).

Cryptosporidium is unaffected by chlorine in the concentrations that can be used in the treatment of drinking water, and is inactivated only by being frozen or heated to temperatures of 65–85°C for 5–10 minutes or by exposure to boiling water. Prevention relies on compliance with safe practices by water companies and health authorities in water treatment processes. Routine water disinfection by chlorination is ineffective in controlling the organism except in small numbers. Therefore, all domestic water supplies are filtered to remove harmful pathogens. As 30% of all public water supplies in England and Wales comes from ground water, contamination of the water supply generally occurs when heavy rains follow drought, which can lead to leakage of effluent or slurry into treated water. The public water supplies in the UK are generally of a very high standard (Casemore 1998), with outbreaks of cryptosporidiosis due to contamination of mains tap water in the UK being uncommon, although outbreaks can occur (Hunter & Syed 2002). Infection can also be acquired from ice cubes and contaminated drinking water, eating food that has been cleaned inadequately, cooked in contaminated water, and from milk (Dawson 2005).

Immunosuppressed patients and their families must be warned about the risk of *Cryptosporidium* and provided with advice, particularly about hand washing after contact with animals (Hemsworth & Pizer 2006) and food, to ensure that prevention of food-borne disease involves the whole food production chain 'from farm to table' (Schlundt *et al.* 2004) (see Protective isolation section above).

The time from ingestion of oocysts to the development of symptoms can vary: one investigation suggested a 2–13 day incubation period, whilst duration of symptoms was 4–10 days for healthy persons who had became infected after visiting a contaminated swimming pool (Insulander *et al.* 2005). Symptoms include watery stools, vomiting and weight loss, fever, nausea, vomiting and weakness. Recovery involves an intact humoral and cellular immune response. Excretion of oocysts can continue after symptoms have ceased (Ungar 1995). For severely immunocompromised patients, particularly those with AIDS and bone marrow transplant recipients, colonization is common (Baqai *et al.* 2005), infection is protracted, severe and sometimes life threatening (Caccio & Pozio 2006). Severity reflects the level of immunosuppression (Sunnotel *et al.* 2006). Symptoms include a debilitating cholera-like diarrhoea and vomiting which, when found in terminal AIDS patients, is particularly distressing. Remission and relapse of cryptosporidiosis probably reflects fluctuation in immune status (Caccio & Pozio 2006).

Respiratory tract involvement has been caused either through aspiration of oocysts during vomiting or through haematogenous spread. Coughing can result in aerosol transmission of oocysts to others. Rare presentations include cholecystitis, hepatitis, pancreatitis and reactive arthritis (Ungar 1995).

Prevention

Immunocompetent people who swim in or drink water may be regularly exposed to infection, and may have higher levels of immunity to infection. Proactive measures are required for hospitalized immunosuppressed patients, which include using filtered water for drinking and making ice cubes (NHS Estates 2002).

The Third Report of the Group of Experts on *Cryptosporidium* in Water Supplies (DH 1998c) states that there is a strong correlation between outbreaks of infection and inadequacy in the treatment of water supplies or where there is overloading of the treatment process. This group and others recommend that inpatients and outpatients who are immunocompromised should:

1   Boil or filter all tap and bottled water used for drinking.
2   Avoid contact with infected animals and people.
3   Avoid contaminated water during recreational activities.
4   Avoid uncooked food that may have been washed in contaminated water.
5   Avoid exposure to young farm animals and pets, and avoid acquiring new young pets, as young animals are particularly susceptible to crytosporidiosis.
6   Filter domestic water supplies. Currently water companies regularly monitor water supplies; if contamination occurs users are informed and told to boil all drinking water; supplies are not turned off as water is needed for flushing toilets and fighting fires, etc. Unfortunately, during outbreak situations when all drinking water has to be boiled, compliance is often poor (Willocks *et al.* 2000).
7   Refrain from swimming whilst immunosuppressed.

The Third Report from the Group of Experts on *Cryptosporidium* in Water Supplies (DH 1998c) highlighted how the reported cases of cryptosporidiosis in England and Wales have decreased (Smith, H.V *et al.* 2006) but prevention measures need to continue.

Diagnosis

Microbiological testing of stools, using conventional staining microscopy and molecular techniques, as well as newer commercially available immunoassays, provides a diagnosis as well as epidemiology data in outbreak situations (Weitzel *et al.* 2006).

Treatment

The host immune response prevents initial infection and facilitates clearance of infection; prolonged infection is seen in immunocompromised persons. There is no reliable curative treatment for cryptosporidiosis but patients have responded to drugs such as paromomycin and azithromycin (Trad *et al.* 2003).

Nursing care

Oocysts are shed in large numbers during infection and only a small number of oocysts are required to cause infection.

Strict barrier nursing is required while diarrhoea persists, with segregation from other patients continuing until clear specimens of stool cultures are obtained.

Special attention to hand washing is essential. Hands should be washed using detergent and running water, dried carefully, followed by application of alcoholic handrub.

Any sign of cross-infection must be pursued vigorously to prevent further spread. This will include close co-operation with health and local authorities and the appropriate water companies, and between the outbreak control team and the authority.

Hepatitis

Hepatitis may be caused by a variety of agents including viruses and certain chemicals, and it may be secondary to other illnesses. Nurses need to be aware of the epidemiology, modes of transmission and prevention of hepatitis (Table 6.3).

Hepatitis A

Definition

Hepatitis A virus (HAV) is an enterically transmitted positive strand RNA virus classified as a hepavirus, a member of the Picornaviridae family (Mims *et al.* 2004). It was first identified 35 years ago, and causes an acute, self-limiting infection of the liver (Martin & Lemon 2006). It can also cause significant infection in vulnerable people, for example pregnant women (Elinav *et al.* 2006).

Reference material

HAV is a small, symmetrical RNA virus (enterovirus type 72). The virus is unusually stable, resisting heat at 60°C for 1 hour, at 25°C for 3 months, indefinite cold storage (5°C), acidic conditions (pH 3) and non-ionic detergents. It can survive for several months in sewage and the environment (Brundage & Fitzpatrick 2006). One study found HAV in mussels following marinating in an acid marinade with a pH of 3.75 for 4 weeks (Hewitt & Greening 2004). However, HAV can be inactivated after 4 minutes at 70°C, after 5 seconds at 80°C and instantly at 85°C (Battegay *et al.* 1995).

HAV is spread predominantly by the faecal–oral route, which can lead to large outbreaks of infection (Perrett *et al.* 2003). Following infection, the virus enters the bloodstream from unknown sites in the gastrointestinal tract. It can then infect liver cells when passing via the biliary tract to the intestine and into the faeces. Viral replication probably occurs in the jejunum before transmission via the portal vein to the liver. HAV has been associated with the following:

■   Contaminated water, milk and food. Any uncooked food and drink could be responsible for infection. However, particular problems are due to contamination at the time

Table 6.3 Types and infection routes of hepatitis viruses.

Subtypes	A	B	C	D	E	F	G
Infection route	Oral–faecal, sexual	Sexual, contact with blood and body fluids	Contact with blood and body fluids; less commonly sexual	As hepatitis B	Oral–faecal	As hepatitis B	As hepatitis C
Vaccine	Yes	Yes	No	No/ indirect from hepatitis B vaccine	No	No	No
Natural history	Acute	Acute–chronic	Acute–chronic	Acute–chronic	Acute–chronic	Not clear	Not clear
Long-term prognosis	Recovery	Carrier, cirrhosis, cancer	Carrier, cirrhosis, cancer	Carrier, cirrhosis, cancer	Unknown	Unknown	Unknown

of harvesting and packaging of uncooked frozen foods, which are then thawed and used (Fiore 2004). Large outbreaks of hepatitis A can be due to contamination of uncooked or cooked food, by an infected food handler or infected food source (Koopmans & Duizer 2004).

- Poor general hygiene and low economic status, contact with children in day care centres and intensive care units. Outbreaks of HAV at school, as well as among health care workers, have been associated with lack of toilet paper, soap and hand towels, and poor hygiene in school toilets (Chodick et al. 2006).
- Foreign travel to countries where HAV is endemic (Wasley et al. 2006).
- Blood transfusions (Gowland et al. 2004).
- Contact with a case of hepatitis A in the home (Sonder et al. 2004), during social activities (Sundkvist et al. 2000) or in hospital due to breaches in infection control measures (Chodick et al. 2006).
- Sexual contact. HAV can be reduced among homosexual men by HAV vaccination (Franco et al. 2003).
- Perinatal transmission of hepatitis A is uncommon (Duff 1998).
- Intravenous drug misusers. Needle-sharing practices contribute to the spread of HAV (Wells et al. 2006).

Following ingestion of HAV, multiplication occurs as the virus moves through the stomach, small intestine and large intestine. The virus eventually reaches the liver after leaving the alimentary system via the blood. Further replication occurs in the liver before being released into bile (Cuthbert 2001).

Diagnosis of acute HAV infection is usually confirmed serologically, by detecting immunoglobulin M (IgM) antibodies to hepatitis A antigen (HAAg), which appear in serum 2–7 weeks after oral inoculation, and may persist for some time, occasionally for more than a year. Evidence of past infection, and therefore immunity which can persist for life, is obtained by detecting serologically the presence of IgG antibody to HAAg. HAV can be detected by a variety of immunological and molecular techniques (Mims et al. 2004).

HAV has an incubation period of 2–7 weeks. HAV usually causes a minor illness in children and young adults, with a few cases being symptomatic. The illness often presents as an upper respiratory infection with the following signs and symptoms: anorexia, malaise, weight loss, pyrexia, diarrhoea, vomiting and jaundice (Mims et al. 2004). Complications of HAV can occur, which can lead to fulminant hepatitis (Beyazit et al. 2006).

A population based seroprevalence study in England and Wales indicated a low incidence of hepatitis A infection (Morris-Cunnington et al. 2004). Control and prevention of HAV rely on provision of good sanitation facilities, clean drinking water and supervision of food handlers. Careful personal hygiene and the use of condoms will limit person-to-person spread (Leung et al. 2005). Passive immunization with intramuscular normal pooled immunoglobulin (human normal immunoglobulin [HNIg]) gives protection against clinical hepatitis for about 3 months in most people. Post-exposure prophylaxis is advisable for household contacts during outbreaks of HAV infection (DH 2006b).

Hepatitis A vaccine is available and immunization has been seen to be effective (Brundage & Fitzpatrick 2006). The vaccine should be administered to those travelling in developing countries (Dick 1998), in areas of moderate or high HAV endemicity, particularly where sanitation and food hygiene are poor, but it is not an alternative to preventive behaviours. The DH (2006b) has recommended that sewage workers, military personnel and foreign diplomats should be considered for vaccination. In institutions for the care of the mentally ill, and in children's centres where the children are not toilet trained, vaccination policy should be formulated according to local circumstances (DH 2006b).

A combined hepatitis A and B vaccine is also available, which increases convenience and compliance, and reduces costs whilst providing prolonged dual protection (Van der Wielen et al. 2006). HNIg offers short-term protection for up to 4 months and can be given to people who have been in close contact with infected cases and to those travelling to areas where the disease is endemic (DH 2006b; Fiore et al. 2006).

HAV infection does not generally require hospital treatment. If admitted, strict barrier nursing in a single room with en-suite toilet would be required. Outbreaks of HVA among health care workers have been attributed to inadequate hand washing and then eating on the ward (Chodick et al. 2006).

Procedure guidelines   Hepatitis A: patient care

Hepatitis A: outpatient care

Action	Rationale
1 It is not usually necessary to admit the individual to hospital.	Usually a self-limiting disease (Kyrlagkitsis *et al.* 2002: R 1b; Lewis & Martin 2006: R 1b).
2 Patient education is essential and must include advice on good personal hygiene and careful hand washing.	Limits the spread of the virus. Careful hand washing removes contamination from hands (Banfield & Kerr 2005: R 1b).
3 Separate soap, flannel and towel must be provided.	To minimize the risk of infection being spread via equipment used for hygiene purposes (E).
4 Meticulous cleaning of bath, wash basin and toilet with a cream cleaner and hot water.	To remove contamination (Ayliffe *et al.* 2000: 5).
5 Bath and wash basin must be allowed to dry after use.	Viruses will not live on clean dry surfaces (Weaving 2006: 5).
6 Soiled bed linen and underclothing should be washed.	To remove contamination (DH 1995a: C).
7 Patient should refrain from intimate kissing and sexual intercourse while symptoms are present.	To reduce risk of cross-infection (Sonder *et al.* 2004: 5).
8 People with hepatitis A should avoid contact with susceptible people, i.e. the very young or old or those with debilitating illness.	To reduce the likelihood of infection (Sonder *et al.* 2004: 5).
9 Crockery and cutlery must be washed and rinsed in hot water.	Heat destroys the virus (Ayliffe *et al.* 2000: C).
10 Close contacts of the infected person should seek medical advice from their general practitioner.	To enable the general practitioner to assess whether the contact person should receive human normal immunoglobulin (HNIg) prophylaxis (DH 2006b: C).

Hepatitis A: inpatient care

Action	Rationale
1 Whenever possible, the patient should have medical or surgical treatment postponed until he/she is symptom free.	Medical and surgical treatment will debilitate the patient further and recovery will be slower (E).
2 Ideally, the patient should be discharged.	Cross-infection is less likely to occur at home (E).
3 A single room with separate toilet should be made available for the patient.	To prevent cross-infection (Chodick *et al.* 2006: 5).
4 Blood, secretions and excreta (particularly faeces) must be disposed of immediately in a heat-disinfecting bedpan washer.	To prevent cross-infection (Ayliffe *et al.* 2000: 5).
5 Careful hand washing after patient contact.	To prevent cross-infection (Chodick *et al.* 2006: 5).

Hepatitis B

Definition

Hepatitis B is a serious infectious disease caused by the hepatitis B virus (HBV), which produces an inflammatory condition of the liver leading to acute and in some cases chronic infection (Mims *et al.* 2004).

Reference material

HBV is a 42 nm double-shelled particle, inside which is a 27 nm inner core particle that contains the viral nucleic acid and represents the intact infectious virion (Mims *et al.* 2004).

HBV infection is a serious global health problem with 2 billion people infected world-wide, with 350 million of these suffering from chronic HBV infection. HBV infection is the 10th leading cause of death world-wide, with 500 000 to 1.2 million deaths per year caused by chronic HBV infection, cirrhosis and hepatocellular carcinoma (Lavanchy 2004). The incidence of HBV in the UK is low. An analysis of routine laboratory surveillance data between 1995–2000 in England and Wales suggests the incidence is 7.4 per 100 000 of the population. Intravenous drug use was the most frequent route of transmission, with numbers due to heterosexual contact transmission remaining stable, and a reduction in the number of cases related to men having sex with men. Whilst transmission during childhood remains rare, it is more frequently reported among South Asians, where their risk factors were medical treatment overseas and heterosexual contact (Hahne *et al.* 2004).

Prevention of HBV includes vaccination, prophylaxis, improved infection control and safer sex practices (Aggarwal & Ranjan 2004).

Epidemiology

HBV may be found in virtually all body secretions and excreta of patients with acute hepatitis B and carriers of the virus. Blood, semen and vaginal fluids are mainly implicated in the transmission of infection, which occurs by:

- Sexual transmission, both vaginal and anal.
- Accidental inoculation of blood following, for example, a sharps injury, or by drug addicts sharing used needles and syringes.
- Contamination of mucous membranes, eye, nose or mouth.
- Contamination of non-intact skin.
- Perinatal route at or about the time of birth.
- Blood transfusion. The estimated frequency of HBV-positive blood donations entering the blood supply during 1996–2003 was 1.66 per million donations (Soldan *et al.* 2005).

HBV infection acquired during infancy and early childhood has a high likelihood of progressing to chronic infection, which can lead to chronic hepatitis, cirrhosis and primary hepatocellular carcinoma. Vaccination would reduce this risk (Hahne *et al.* 2003).

Clinical response

HBV infection is clinically extremely variable, with the incubation period varying from 4 weeks to as long as 6 months.

Symptoms of acute HBV infection include jaundice of skin and eyes, dark urine, fatigue, nausea, vomiting and abdominal pain. Recovery can take several months to a year. Chronic infection can predispose the infected person to develop cirrhosis or cancer of the liver. HBV reactivation can occur in patients following allogeneic BMT (Kempinska *et al.* 2005).

Infectivity

The progress of HBV can be monitored by serological testing. Hepatitis B surface antigen (HBsAg) is detected in the blood approximately 3–4 weeks after exposure, with antibodies to hepatitis B core antigen (HBcAg) developing about 2 weeks after HBsAg occurs. Anti-HBc will eventually be replaced by anti-HBs, the antibody to HBsAg, which marks the end of high infectivity and the development of immunity to subsequent HBV infection. The antigen HBeAg is an internal component of the core of HBs and is an indicator of high infectivity; it will be replaced eventually by anti-HBe, which correlates with loss of viral replication (Mims *et al.* 2004). HBV is capable of surviving outside the body (Thompson *et al.* 2003), but will not multiply in the environment (Weaving 2006).

Diagnosis

Diagnosis is confirmed by a virological blood test with regular monitoring of antigen and antibody status to evaluate progress (Burek 2005). The diagnosis of chronic HBV infection is made using a combination of serological, virological, biochemical and histological markers (Park & Keeffe 2004).

Screening policy for HBsAg

Screening of the entire hospital patient population would be an effective way to identify hepatitis B infection, but this would be costly and time consuming in terms of the benefits derived.

In general, the best compromise is to test those patients belonging to groups in which there is a high prevalence of hepatitis B. These include the following people:

- All new admissions who currently live or were born in countries where there is a high prevalence of hepatitis B.
- Drug addicts.
- Institutionalized people with learning difficulties.
- All patients acutely or recently jaundiced.

HBV is not transmitted by normal daily contact including coughing, sneezing, hugging, holding hands or sharing bathrooms and toilets, cups and crockery with an HBV-positive person (DH 2003c).

Transmission of HBV in the health care setting

Transmission of HBV to health care workers can be substantially reduced by vaccination and adoption of universal safe precautions (Talaat *et al.* 2003).

Following all accidents involving inoculation or exposure to mucous membranes or non-intact skin, the patient should be tested for HBV, with the incident fully evaluated by the Occupational Health Unit and appropriate care provided. Health care workers who are involved in an incident can experience considerable distress and anxiety. Transmission of HBV from infected health care workers to their patients has occurred (Puro *et al.* 2003). The DH (2003a) requires that HBeAg-positive staff are not to undertake EPP. Those staff who are HBeAg negative must have additional testing to establish viral load. Those persons with HBV DNA levels exceeding 10^3 genome equivalents per millilitre cannot undertake EPP. Those whose viral load is below this figure have to be retested yearly (DH 2003a).

Immunization and vaccination

Passive protection against hepatitis B

Specific hepatitis B immunoglobulin (HBIg), prepared from pooled plasma with a high titre of hepatitis B surface antibody, is available for passive protection and is usually used in combination with hepatitis B vaccine to confer passive/active immunity under certain defined conditions (DH 2006b), including:

- Persons who have an inoculation, ingestion or splashing accident with HBsAg-infected blood.
- Babies of mothers with hepatitis B. In these cases babies should receive HBIg no later than 48 hours after birth. All pregnant women should be offered HBV testing at the beginning of antenatal care (DH 2004c).
- Sexual partners and, in some cases, family contacts judged to be high risk, or individuals suffering from acute hepatitis B and who are seen within 1 week of onset of jaundice.

Active immunization

Active immunization is by hepatitis B vaccine. Hepatitis B vaccine is a genetically engineered vaccine. The basic regimen consists of three doses of vaccine over 6 months, with a booster dose every 5 years. An accelerated schedule of three doses over 3 months with a booster at 12 months and then every 5 years can be given when rapid acquisition of immunity is required.

Health care workers involved in EPP, including theatre nurses, are required to be immunized against HBV. This means theatre nurses will have to provide evidence of HBV vaccination prior to employment. Those who fail to respond to vaccine have to be tested for HBV every 6 months to prove their continuing non-carrier status (DH 2003c).

Indications for immunization include:

- Personnel including teaching, training and nursing staff directly involved over a period of time in patient care where there is a high prevalence of HBV or where blood and blood products are handled regularly.
- Laboratory workers.
- Dentists and dental personnel.
- Medical and surgical personnel.
- Health care personnel on secondment to work in areas of the world where there is a high prevalence of HBV.
- Patients on entry to residential institutions where there is a high prevalence of HBV.
- Patients treated by maintenance haemodialysis.
- Sexual contacts of patients with acute HBV or carriers of HBV.
- Infants born to mothers who are HBsAg positive.
- Health care workers who receive an inoculation accident from a needle used on a patient who is HBsAg positive, either used alone or in combination with HBIg.

In addition, HBV vaccine is offered to selected high-risk populations; this includes homosexual men attending genitourinary clinics, as studies indicate they are at the greatest risk of acquiring HBV (McMillan 2005). A combined HBV and HAV vaccine is now available, which has been seen to be safe and well tolerated (Van der Wielen *et al.* 2006).

Prevention of hepatitis B in health care workers

It is important that health care workers adopt safe techniques when in contact with blood and body fluids of all patients, regardless of their hepatitis status.

Avoiding inoculation accidents and contamination of mucous membranes and skin is an essential component of safe techniques (DH 2001a).

Death of patients with hepatitis B

When infected patients die, their bodies are no more hazardous than when they were alive, providing that appropriate precautions against contamination with blood and body fluids are maintained (Sa *et al.* 2006). Guidelines recommend that bodies of patients known to be infected with hepatitis should be placed in a body bag. Relatives and significant others should be permitted to view, touch and spend time with the deceased person. However, embalming should not be undertaken (Healing *et al.* 1995).

Patient education

The DH (2006b) recommends that individuals found to be HBsAg carriers should be educated about the ways in which hepatitis B may spread and the precautions that can be taken to reduce the risk to others. It is stressed that unnecessary restrictions and precautions may cause distress and should be avoided.

Antiviral therapy

Treatment is aimed at preventing the progression of infection to hepatocellular cancer and cirrhosis. Treatments to decrease viral replication and improve the immune response include interferon-α administered three times a week for 4–6 months, lamidivudine and adefovir dipivoxil, which blocks viral replication. Long-term therapy is required, which can lead to the development of resistance to treatment (Aggarwal & Ranjan 2004). Combinations of antiviral drugs have been tried in patients failing to respond to mono-therapy, which has been seen to reduce the levels of HBV in blood (Santos *et al.* 2006; Sokucu *et al.* 2006).

Excellent long-term results have been achieved following liver transplantation for chronic liver disease (Bruix *et al.* 2006). Prophylactic therapy is necessary following bone or stem cell transplantation to prevent reactivation of HBV (Kempinska *et al.* 2005).

Procedure guidelines   Hepatitis B: patient care

Procedure

Action	Rationale
1 The patient may be nursed on an open ward using all the patients' facilities as normal unless there is a high risk of blood contamination of the ward environment.	If adequate precautions can be adhered to on an open ward, there is no need to isolate the patient (HSE 2005: E).
2 The patient must be assessed daily to establish accurately any sites of bleeding. Changes in the patient's condition should be recorded in the care plan.	Sites of bleeding must be identified in order that the appropriate precautions can be taken (E).
3 Used sharps must be correctly disposed of in a sharps bin.	Contaminated sharps are a potential inoculation hazard to others, so particular caution must be taken in handling them. Overloaded sharps containers may cause needles to pierce the walls of the container or even protrude through the top (DH 2001a: C).
4 A yellow clinical waste bag should be kept on a regular holder with a lid for the patient's disposable waste. When full this should be securely closed, and sent for incineration.	To confine potentially contaminated material, e.g. bloodstained tissues. Yellow is the internationally recognized colour for clinical waste (DH 2006a: C).
5 The patient's personal hygiene equipment must be kept at the bedside.	To prevent accidental use of equipment by others (E).
6 Used linen that is not bloodstained is placed in the white linen bags in the usual way.	Linen free from blood stains is not contaminated and may be dealt with in the normal manner (DH 1995a: C).
7 During venepuncture or other procedures likely to cause bleeding, furniture, bedding and clothing in the adjacent area should be protected with polythene sheeting.	To prevent contamination of the environment with spilled blood (E).
8 All staff involved with the patient should cover any cuts or grazes on their hands with waterproof dressings.	Broken skin provides a portal of entry for the hepatitis virus in the event of contact with the patient's blood (E).
9 Routine daily cleaning procedures may be carried out as normal. As part of universal safe technique and practices, domestic staff will be aware of the potential hazard associated with any blood contamination.	Education is necessary so the domestic staff can understand the hazards involved (E).

Procedure guidelines *(cont.)*

Accidental inoculation or spillage of blood from patient with hepatitis B

Action	Rationale
1 Any accident involving skin penetration or heavy contamination of abraded skin or mucosal surfaces of staff should be recorded on an accident form and this taken to bacteriology immediately. Occupational health must be informed, who will make an assessment for the need of HBV vaccine or HBV IgG.	To protect personnel. To comply with legal and/or hospital requirements (HSE 2005: C).
2 Blood spillage onto unbroken skin should be washed off with soap and running water. A scrubbing brush should not be used as this could break the skin. Complete an accident form, as above, and inform occupational health.	To remove the source of potential contamination. To comply with legal and/or hospital requirements (HSE 2005: C).
3 Accidental inoculation sites should be cleaned under running water, encouraged to bleed freely and then covered with waterproof plaster. Complete an accident form, as above.	Bleeding helps to expel the inoculated virus from the site. To comply with legal and/or hospital requirements (HSE 2005: C).
4 Blood spilled on hard surfaces must be wiped up immediately with paper towels and the area washed well with a solution such as hypochlorite.	To prevent viral spread. Dried blood remains infectious for several days (Wilson 2006: E).
5 Linen stained with blood should be treated as infected linen and placed in a red alginate polythene bag before being placed in a red linen bag.	Bloodstained linen is highly infectious. All linen in red alginate polythene bags will be washed in a barrier wash at the laundry (DH 1995a: C).

Precautions if patient with hepatitis B is bleeding

Action	Rationale
1 If significant bleeding is present in the mouth: (a) Consider the use of disposable crockery and cutlery and, with any contaminated food, dispose of as clinical waste. (b) Keep a personal food tray and water jug at the bedside. (c) Disposable mouth-care equipment, sputum pot and tissues should be kept at the bedside.	Significant amounts of blood contamination on crockery and cutlery may contaminate the ward kitchen and lead to cross-infection (E). Significant blood can be removed from jug and tray before it leaves the room to be thoroughly cleaned in a dish washer, so preventing cross-contamination (E). The sputum may be contaminated with blood from the mouth, therefore precautions must include avoiding contact with the patient's sputum (E).
2 If haematuria or melaena is present: (a) Wear plastic gowns and gloves when handling excreta. (b) Keep a toilet and handbasin for the patient's sole use, if practicable.	Blood present in the urine or faeces makes the patient's excreta a potential source of hepatitis B contamination (HSE 2005: E). Blood present in the urine or faeces makes the patient's excreta a potential source of hepatitis B contamination (HSE 2005: E).

(c) If a toilet is not available for the patient's sole use, bedpans or urinals must be used. These should be washed in the usual manner in the bedpan washer. Disposable bedpans are dealt with in the routine manner.

Blood present in the urine or faeces makes the patient's excreta a potential source of hepatitis B contamination (HSE 2005: E).

3 If the patient has a wound or a break in the skin:
  (a) Cover the area adequately so that there is no seepage.

To prevent the spread of the virus from dried or fresh blood. Dried blood can remain infectious for several days (HSE 2005: C).

  (b) Used dressings should be sealed securely in a plastic bag before being disposed of as clinical waste.

To prevent the spread of the virus (HSE 2005: C).

  (c) All tapes, lotions and creams are kept solely for the patient's use.

To prevent contamination and therefore the spread of the virus (E).

  (d) The dressing trolley must be cleaned carefully before reuse.

To prevent contamination and therefore the spread of the virus (E).

  (e) Non-disposable equipment should be emptied and wiped clean, placed in a central sterile supplies department bag, securely stapled shut and sent to the sterile supplies department in a safe manner, to be resterilized.

To remove any contamination and therefore reduce the risk of cross-infection (E).

Invasive procedures, specimens and transport for patient with hepatitis B

Action

1 All departments and staff who will be undertaking invasive procedures to the patient must be made aware of the patient's hepatitis B diagnosis.

Rationale

To allow them to make their own precautionary arrangements (E).

2 All request cards to be labelled appropriately.

To alert the receiving department of the diagnosis (HSE 2003b: C).

3 All specimens to be labelled appropriately and correctly bagged. (For further information on specimen collection see Chapter 40.)

To alert the receiving department of the diagnosis and prevent contamination of the environment (HSE 2003b: C).

4 If a patient who is bleeding has to be transported elsewhere, a nurse must accompany the patient and the porter involved should be provided with the following:

To prevent the contamination of the porter or other patients (E).

  (a) Disposable gloves and aprons.

To prevent the contamination of the porter (E).

  (b) Cleaning equipment for the trolley or chair before use by the next patient.

To remove any contamination and therefore reduce the risk of cross-infection (E).

Discharging the patient with hepatitis B

Action

1 The majority of precautions can cease.

Rationale

Discharge normally implies that the risk of cross-infection is no longer present (E).

2 The patient should be advised not to share razors, toothbrushes or similar personal property likely to be contaminated by blood.

To reduce the risk of cross-infection (E).

Procedure guidelines *(cont.)*

3 If bleeding occurs, the patient clears up the blood himself/herself and disposes safely of such items as contaminated tissues by burning or flushing down the toilet. If regular persistent bloodstained waste is generated, the health authority must be requested to make special collections.	To reduce the risk of cross-infection (E).
4 If emergency treatment or dental care is required, the patient must inform the health care worker of the fact that he/she has a recent history of hepatitis B infection.	To allow the correct precautions to be taken (E).

Death of a patient with hepatitis B

Action	Rationale
1 There should be minimal handling of the body. However, routine last offices can be undertaken (see Chapter 22).	To reduce the risk of infecting the nursing staff (E).
2 Nurses should wear disposable plastic aprons and gloves when handling the body.	
3 The body should be totally enclosed in a body bag specifically designed for infected patients.	To reduce the risk of infecting the nursing staff (E).
4 The mortuary staff should be informed of the diagnosis.	To ensure that all staff are aware of the infection risk.
5 If the relatives want to view the body, they must be supervised. The body bag can be opened by a nurse to allow viewing.	To prevent contamination (E).

Non-A non-B hepatitis

Definition

Due to major advances in knowledge concerning hepatitis, hepatitis A, B, C, D, E, F, G and H have been identified. There remains the theoretical possibility of further hepatitis types being reported. Until this time, the hepatitis virus non-A, non-B (NANB) is the term given to all clinical hepatitis that does not fall into the above-mentioned categories. The aetiology of NANB hepatitis remains unclear (He *et al.* 2003).

Reference material

There are no accepted serological tests for NANB. Diagnosis is achieved by excluding infections associated with NANB. These include symptoms associated with hepatitis A, B and C, cytomegalovirus, Epstein–Barr virus, toxic and drug-induced liver injury (including alcoholic liver disease), circulatory abnormalities, shock, sepsis, biliary tract disease and metabolic liver disease (Hsu *et al.* 2002). As new hep-

atitis viruses are discovered, studies involving retesting patients previously diagnosed as NANB hepatitis continue to highlight patients who fall into none of the known hepatitis categories. A search for yet another hepatitis virus continues (He *et al.* 2003).

NANB hepatitis has been shown to occur in patients who have received:

- blood transfusions;
- clotting factors for coagulation disorders;
- haemodialysis;

as well as:

- outbreaks of epidemics in tropical areas;
- sporadic cases with no identifiable cause.

Transmission appears to be similar to that of hepatitis B, i.e. principally through blood and blood products. There is an increased incidence in drug addicts due to the sharing of contaminated needles and syringes. It is essential that safe techniques are used at all times when in contact with blood and body fluids. Human immunoglobulin should be given prophylactically following a previous history of needlestick injuries. Treatment and care is the same as for hepatitis B.

Procedure guidelines   Non-A non-B hepatitis: patient care

The procedure should be as for hepatitis B.

Hepatitis C

Definition

Hepatitis C is an acute infectious disease caused by the hepatitis C virus (HCV), which is a single-stranded RNA virus, and a member of the Flaviviridae. There are six genotypes based upon differences in molecular structure (Mims *et al.* 2004).

Reference material

HCV was discovered in 1989, and is a major health problem. with about 170 million chronic HCV carriers throughout the world. The prevalence of hepatitis C in the UK is uncertain but it is estimated that there are around 200 000 people clinically infected with HCV (DH 2002a). In England, HCV is mainly spread by injecting drug users sharing blood-contaminated equipment. Other less common routes include sexual intercourse, mother to baby, and skin piercing and tattooing when unsterile equipment is used. It is also possible for spread to occur from sharing bloodstained toothbrushes and razors (DH 2002a; Franco *et al.* 2003).

HCV can survive out of the body for several weeks (Thompson *et al.* 2003). Of 106 syringes collected from a South London park, HCV was detected in 4.7% (Nyiri *et al.* 2004).

Clinical response

The incubation period following infection varies with a mean of about 7 weeks (Mims *et al.* 2004). The clinical manifestations of hepatitis C infection are non-specific and in some cases symptomless, and include fatigue, malaise and nausea. The disease may be mild and go unnoticed by the infected person, with patients recovering spontaneously and completely. However, up to 80% of these patients develop chronic active hepatitis and some progress to cirrhosis and cancer of the liver (DH 2002a). Alcohol misuse presents an increased risk of hepatic complications associated with HCV (Wilson 2006). Reactivation of HCV occurs during periods of immunosuppression due to treatment for haematological tumours (Vento *et al.* 2002).

The DH (2002a) has compiled an HCV strategy for England. Included in the strategy are six action points:

1 Keeping people healthy.
2 Reducing health inequalities.
3 Shaping services around patients, their families and carers.

4 Working with others.
5 Providing a comprehensive service.
6 Responding to the needs of different populations and continuously improving services.

Transmission

A national HCV register related to HCV-infected people is maintained (Harris *et al.* 2000).

Transfusion services in the UK began to screen for antibodies to HCV in September 1991 (DH 1995b). The screening programme was estimated to have a considerable positive effect on the prevention of post-transfusion HCV infection. Since screening began, during 1996–2003, 0.8 per million blood donors have been found to be HCV positive (Soldan *et al.* 2005). Before screening commenced it was estimated that 1289 HCV-infected donors donated blood. These were separated to provide blood products to 64 424 different persons. Of these, 1350 blood recipients have been traced and 50% were found to be HCV positive (Editorial 2002). British patients infected with HCV through blood and blood products received up to £45 000 compensation: a lump sum of £20 000 with a further £25 000 if the person developed cirrhosis or liver damage (Dyer 2004).

Transmission of HCV has occurred in haemodialysis centres: a study prospectively investigating HCV transmission found that stringent isolation (Saxena *et al.* 2003) and improved nurse staffing levels reduced HCV transmission (Saxena & Panhotra 2004).

Unprotected sex, increased sexual partners and the use of sex toys increase the risk of HCV transmission (Turner *et al.* 2006). Other risk factors include vertical transmission from mother to child (DH 2002a).

Diagnosis

Diagnosis of acute hepatitis C infection is established by the presence of antibodies to hepatitis C (anti-HCV IgG) in the blood (Mims *et al.* 2004).

Treatment

Cases should be referred to a specialist team in liver disease for evaluation, close observation and care (Brant *et al.* 2005). This may involve liver biopsy and liver function tests. Treatment includes combination therapy with interferon-α and ribavirin (Parise *et al.* 2006). Relapses do occur and liver transplantation can improve survival (Takada *et al.* 2006). Risk factors such as obesity contribute to non-response to treatment (Tarantino *et al.* 2006).

Nursing care

Since there is no vaccine for HVC it is critical for health care workers to work safely to prevent exposure to blood and body fluids. One nurse who developed HCV following a needlestick injury, highlighted the gruelling treatment programme that she received (Wright 2005). Unfortunately despite education, knowledge and compliance to safe practice is poor (Trim *et al.* 2003). A survey of medical (Elliott *et al.* 2005) and nurses' knowledge of HCV found that their understanding of HCV was poor (Elliott *et al.* 2005).

The DH (2002a) has produced advice for HCV-infected health care workers undertaking or planning to undertake EPP, to ensure patients are not put at risk, and the action to be taken when a health care worker is occupationally exposed to HCV. Currently there is no post-exposure prophylaxis for HCV (Sarrazin *et al.* 2004), but early treatment may prevent chronic HCV developing.

Patients with HCV infection must receive education on how to prevent cross-infection. A national survey of people with haemophilia, found that this group knew little of the route of HCV transmission (Nazzaro *et al.* 2006).

Nursing care for the patient infected with hepatitis C is the same as for patients with hepatitis B (see Procedure guidelines: Hepatitis B: patient care).

Hepatitis D

Definition

Hepatitis D virus (HDV), also referred to as delta virus, is a very small RNA virus; genotype 1 and 2 have been described (Su, C.W *et al.* 2006). HDV is dependent on HBV for its life cycle and for its replication by sharing its envelope protein (Taylor 2006). Combined HBV/HDV infection causes both fulminant hepatitis and the accelerated progression of pre-existing HBV hepatitis (Gheorghe *et al.* 2005).

Reference material

Hepatitis D is uncommon in the UK and USA, but common in countries such as Mongolia (Takahashi *et al.* 2004) and Russia (Abe *et al.* 2004). HDV is transmitted in the same way as HBV and is usually associated with intravenous drug use, sexually transmitted infections (Li *et al.* 2006a) and from mother to child (Abe *et al.* 2004).

HDV has a relatively short incubation period of 3–6 weeks (Mims *et al.* 2004). Infection with HBV and HDV results in a more severe and symptomatic illness than infection with HBV alone (Tsatsralt-Od *et al.* 2005).

Diagnosis

Diagnosis relies on the detection of HDV antibody in serum, using a PCR assay (Jardi *et al.* 2001).

Prevention

Prevention is based on vaccination (Baker 1994) as HBV vaccine is also effective against HDV (Duff 1998). Transmission of HDV to a nurse via a needlestick injury has occurred (Knysz *et al.* 2005).

Treatment

Prognosis for combined HBV and HDV infection is poor (Gheorghe *et al.* 2005). It has been suggested that high-dose interferon-α may be beneficial in chronic HDV infection, although relapses can occur (Husa *et al.* 2005). Treatment involves interferon-α therapy with or without lamivudine for at least a year (Niro *et al.* 2005), or interferon and ribavirin (Gunsar *et al.* 2005). Liver transplantation for delta cirrhosis has proved to be a successful treatment for HDV cirrhosis, (Hadziyannis 1997).

Presenting symptoms and nursing care are the same as for hepatitis B.

Hepatitis E

Definition

Hepatitis E is caused by an acute icteric virus leading to self-limiting disease. Hepatitis E virus (HEV) is a member of the Calicivirus family (Mims *et al.* 2004). It is a common cause of hepatitis in developing countries where it is endemic (Preiss *et al.* 2006), while HEV infection is uncommon in developed countries (Peron *et al.* 2006), with only eight reported cases in the UK (Sadler *et al.* 2006).

Reference material

HEV is a faeco-orally transmitted hepatitis virus which has many features similar to HAV (Mims *et al.* 2004). Major outbreaks have occurred due to consumption of contaminated waste and food. HEV will survive internal temperatures of rare cooked meat (Emerson *et al.* 2005), although person-to-person transmission is rarely seen. Travelling to endemic areas carries a risk of HEV infection (Lin *et al.* 2000).

Experimental data suggest HEV may be a zoonosis as HEV is pathogenic for some domestic and wild animals (Lin *et al.* 2000). HEV is common in pregnancy (Oncu *et al.* 2006), with mother-to-child transmission resulting in significant perinatal morbidity and mortality (Kumar *et al.* 2001).

HEV has been transmitted via blood transfusions even in countries where HEV infection is rare (Boxall *et al.* 2006).

The incubation period ranges between 2 and 9 weeks, with an average of 6 weeks. The virus is eliminated from the body on recovery, which prevents carriage of the virus (Mims *et al.* 2004). HEV has been associated with other hepatotropic viruses and can induce fulminant hepatitis with or without the simultaneous presence of other viruses (Irshad

1997). In areas with endemic HEV, acute liver failure is found secondary to HEV infection (Hamid *et al.* 2002).

Diagnosis

Diagnosis is made by detecting HEV antibody in serum. Due to the evolving epidemiology of HEV in England and Wales, HEV infection should be considered with patients with acute or fulminant hepatitis (Lewis *et al.* 2006).

Vaccination

There is no vaccine for HEV prevention, but efforts are on-going to find a vaccine (Maloney *et al.* 2005).

Nursing care

Barrier nursing is necessary for patients with hepatitis E infection.

Hepatitis B genotype F

Definition

Hepatitis B genotype F is the name given to a recently discovered virus causing hepatitis. There are two distinct genotypes, F1 and F2. This virus is commonly referred to as HBV genotype F, as immunodiffusion experiments show that this virus is a serotype of HBV (Kato *et al.* 2005).

Reference material

HBV genotype F is regarded as indigenous to Central and South America. It appears to cause acute and chronic liver disease and is associated with serious disease, with outbreaks of HBV genotype F causing significant morbidity and mortality (Franca *et al.* 2004). PCR tests are now able to distinguish and identify hepatitis F virus (Kato *et al.* 2005), although much remains to be learned about the virus. Nursing care and treatment is as for hepatitis B.

Hepatitis G (HBV/G)

Definition

Hepatitis G virus (HGV) is a recently identified rare virus causing hepatitis (Gomes *et al.* 2004), and is a positive, single-stranded RNA virus, which is a co-infection with hepatitis B (Kato *et al.* 2002). HGV causes acute and chronic liver disease and fulminant hepatitis (Kato *et al.* 2001).

Reference material

HGV was first described in Egypt and Indonesia, but has also been found in the Americas, Europe and Australia.

HGV route of transmission is similar to hepatitis B and includes blood donation, sexual transmission (with transmission occurring more easily from male to female than vice versa), mother to child, blood-sucking insects and by needle-stick injury. Diagnosis is by PCR serology tests (Kato *et al.* 2001). HGV RNA levels are suppressed but not eradicated by interferon-α and are unaffected by ribavirin treatment. Much remains to be learned about HGV. Nursing care is as for hepatitis B.

The herpesviruses

There are four human herpesviruses that cause infection. These are detected more frequently in immunocompromised people than in immunologically intact individuals (Kedzierski 1991). The four types are:

- cytomegalovirus (CMV);
- Epstein–Barr virus (EBV);
- herpes simplex virus (HSV);
- varicella zoster virus (VZV).

Cytomegalovirus

Definition

Cytomegalovirus (CMV) is a member of the herpesvirus family.

Reference material

Primary CMV infection in an immunocompetent person causes a transient infectious mononucleosis-like illness, often in childhood (Mims *et al.* 2004), but it can occur throughout life in a non-immune person and often goes unnoticed (Manfredi *et al.* 2006). Following primary infection, CMV persists in a latent state in leucocytes where they can reactivate later in life, particularly when a person is immunosuppressed. Reactivation is generally controlled by the host's cell-mediated immune response (Sinclair & Sissons 2006). After a clinically silent infection in the upper respiratory tract, CMV spreads to the lymphoid tissue and then to the circulating lymphocytes and monocytes, involving lymph nodes and the spleen. Primary CMV causes significant infection in the immunosuppressed (e.g. immature neonates), in patients who are receiving a transplant and in HIV-positive patients (Afessa & Peters 2006).

CMV is distributed widely throughout the world. CMV can be transmitted by saliva, urine, blood, semen and cervical secretions (Mims *et al.* 2004) as well as via breast milk (Neuberger *et al.* 2006).

More children develop birth defects from congenital CMV infection than from any other more commonly known causes of congenital problems, such as Down's syndrome and spina bifida (Ross *et al.* 2006). Congenital CMV leads to psychomotor impairment and deafness (Lanari *et al.* 2006). A UK study reviewed the risk factors for congenital CMV infection and identified the following as increasing the risk of acquiring CMV infection: caring for preschool children; onset of sexual activity <2 years before delivery; sexually transmitted disease during pregnancy; household size >3 people; maternal age <25 years (Fowler & Pass 2006). Infection during pregnancy predisposes to more severe sequelae from CMV infection (Ornoy & Diav-Citrin 2006).

CMV is a common cause of mortality and morbidity in patients with malignancies, such as leukaemia, and stem cell transplant (Torres *et al.* 2006) and solid organ transplant recipients (Diaz-Pedroche *et al.* 2006). For example CMV disease during liver transplantation is strongly and independently associated with mortality (Limaye *et al.* 2006).

Infection in healthy adults is mild and the prognosis is good. However, infection in the immunosuppressed can be severe and can be a major cause of mortality and morbidity with interstitial pneumonitis, hepatitis, Guillain–Barré syndrome, meningoencephalitis, myocarditis, colitis, thrombocytopenia and haemolytic anaemia, plus retinitis in patients with AIDS (Jabs *et al.* 2006). It is also suggested that CMV infection increases the risk of graft rejection (Coaquette *et al.* 2004).

Patients with HIV infection have an increased risk of CMV infection, and is a cofactor in enhancing the progression of AIDS (Griffiths 2006).

Diagnosis

The diagnosis of CMV requires laboratory confirmation and cannot be made on clinical evidence alone. Laboratory tests include demonstration of the virus or serological antibody screening, using PCR assays (Ziyaeyan *et al.* 2006). CMV is readily found in urine, mouth swabs and the buffy coat of blood, bronchoalveolar lavage fluid, biopsy and autopsy specimens.

Treatment

Treatment relies on successful diagnosis and early commencement of therapy. Antiviral treatment with ganciclovir, foscarnet and cidofovir has been seen to reduce mortality from CMV infection. Antiviral drug resistance to CMV is an emerging problem. Newer antiviral drugs such as leflunomide continue to be evaluated and may be active against certain strains of virus-resistant CMV (Avery *et al.* 2004). Treatment options are further limited by the toxicity of antiviral drugs (Ehlert *et al.* 2006).

Despite the progress in diagnosis and treatment of CMV, infection remains a significant cause of morbidity and mortality among immunosuppressed patients.

Prevention

Prevention relies on decreasing the risk of virus acquisition and reactivation. Therefore, blood products used should either derive from CMV seronegative donors or be free from viable leucocytes, which can be achieved by the use of seronegative donors or by removing white blood cells from the donation (Vamvakas 2005), which will reduce the risk of CMV infection (Blajchman 2006).

Prophylactic ganciclovir has been seen to effectively prevent large numbers of CMV infection when given during treatments such as BMT (Boeckh *et al.* 2002).

Studies to establish the risks of CMV infection among health care workers have found that the prevalence of antibodies to CMV among the general population and health care workers does not differ (Sobaszek *et al.* 2000). This suggests that the risk of transmission is no greater for those health care workers in contact with CMV infections (De Schryver *et al.* 1999) and that pregnant health care workers are not at increased risk of acquiring CMV (Sobaszek *et al.* 2000). Routine blood and body fluid precautions are essential to avoid CMV transmission among health care workers (Boussemart *et al.* 1998).

Patients with CMV infection generally do not require barrier nursing as they feel ill and do not mix closely with other patients. Therefore, patient-to-patient transmission is unlikely.

Epstein–Barr virus

Definition

Epstein–Barr virus (EBV) is a herpesvirus which causes infectious mononucleosis. EBV is generally a self-limiting infection in young children which goes unnoticed; in older children and young adults it can cause fever, malaise, headache, anorexia, pharyngitis and adenopathy, which resolves spontaneously in 2–3 weeks. In older adults a more severe infection is seen (Tattevin *et al.* 2006), which can include hepatitis and aseptic meningitis, but generally complete recovery is normal (Mims *et al.* 2004). However, pathological changes may occur, which can cause complications that include lymphoid and epithelial malignancies (Tao *et al.* 2006).

EBV is also associated with being an aetiological agent for the development of Burkitt's lymphoma (Jarrett 2006).

Reference material

EBV is found in the saliva and on the cervix, and can be transmitted by kissing and sexual contact, but rarely by blood transfusion. Diagnosis relies on serological methods that detect the presence of IgG and IgM antibodies to EBV viral capsid antigen (Mims *et al.* 2004). Following transmission EBV replicates in B lymphocytes and also in the epithelial cells of the nasopharynx (Mims *et al.* 2004), leading to infection of B lymphocytes. The incubation period between exposure and clinical manifestation in normal people varies from 30 to 50 days. EBV infection in healthy people is generally self-limiting with spontaneous recovery. Management consists of basic supportive care, as the use of antiviral agents and corticosteroids in the treatment of EBV remains limited (Holmes & Sokol 2002; Codeluppi *et al.* 2005).

EBV can persist in the host and reactivate at a later time, particularly during immunosuppression (Fafi-Kremer *et al.* 2005a), commonly following transplantation (Nozzoli *et al.* 2006) or in people with cancer or leukaemia (Gottschalk *et al.* 2005). This is usually due to immunosuppression decreasing EBV-specific immune function (Fafi-Kremer *et al.* 2005b), which results in increased EBV load in peripheral blood and in the oropharynx (Haque *et al.* 1997).

Barrier nursing is not necessary for EBV infection, but the patient should avoid kissing and sexual contact while symptoms persist. The patient's personal hygiene articles must not be shared.

Herpes simplex virus

Definition

Herpes simplex virus (HSV) is a double-stranded DNA virus and causes a range of infections, from painful vesicular lesions (cold sores) to life-threatening illness in the immunocompromised patient (Mims *et al.* 2004). It has an affinity for the skin and nervous system.

Reference material

HSV is a common condition (Huber 2003) and presents in two ways:

1 HSV 1 infections (oral herpes or cold sores, which are tingling or painful spots) tend to occur on the face or lips. However, primary infection can occur in the conjunctiva, where it causes conjunctivitis and keratitis; in the fingers, where it causes herpetic whitlow; and in the mouth, where it causes herpes gingivomatitis. After infection the virus replicates in cells of the oral mucosa forming vesicles (Mims *et al.* 2004). The HSV 1 incubation period is 2–12 days.
2 HSV 2 infections (herpes genitalis or genital herpes, which are painful ulcers) are usually limited to the genital region. However, both types of herpes can be contracted either genitally or orally. The HSV 2 incubation period is 2–7 days. HSV 2 is a common infection affecting sexually active people and appears to be increasing (Snoeck & De Clercq 2002).

Herpes simplex infections are world-wide in distribution. HSV 1 usually infects children between the ages of 2 and 10 years. Latent infection is then life-long. Transmission is primarily by contact with oral secretions. HSV 1 is chiefly responsible for perioral, ocular and encephalitic infections in adults. HSV 2 is spread by genital contact and is one of the most common sexually transmitted diseases. HSV 2 is the major cause of penile vesicular lesions, cervicovaginitis and proctitis, as well as neonatal disseminated disease (Mims *et al.* 2004).

Recurrent infection occurs frequently, generally as a result of reactivation of the virus, since HSV 1 may become latent within the trigeminal sensory nerve ganglion, and HSV 2 within the corresponding sacral ganglion (Mims *et al.* 2004). Infection or reactivation in the normal host tends to be a mild, self-limiting disease. The reactivated disease tends to be less severe than the primary infection, except in immunocompromised persons when it is more severe (Mims *et al.* 2004). In most cases there are prodromal symptoms such as burning and tingling sensations before blisters appear. Reactivation tends to occur when the immune system is weakened, in situations of stress, during a common cold infection or on exposure to strong ultraviolet light (Mims *et al.* 2004).

Individuals who are immunocompromised are susceptible to more severe presentations of HSV infections, which include pneumonia, hepatitis and/or encephalitis, with HSV infection the most frequent cause of corneal blindness in the USA (Fillet 2002). Deaths can also occur (Pinna *et al.* 2002).

HSV transmission can occur both from asymptomatic and symptomatic excretors. One means of minimizing the risk of infection is to avoid contact with infected lesions. Gloves are essential for all health care staff in direct contact with lesions. The use of condoms is advisable to minimize the risk of transmission during sexual intercourse (Casper & Wald 2002).

Herpes simplex can be transmitted to the neonate (Brown *et al.* 2006b) causing serious morbidity and mortality and significant congenital deformities (Norgard *et al.* 2006). Vaginal delivery for symptomless women and caesarian section for women with symptoms is advised. The use of valaciclovir significantly reduces the risks of herpes simplex infections (Sheffield *et al.* 2006).

Diagnosis

Prompt diagnosis is essential in order to enable appropriate treatment to be given (Smith & Nathan 2002).

The oral presentation of blisters and inflammation of HSV 1 is easily recognizable. With HSV 2, inflammation at the site of infection, a general feeling of being unwell, and symptoms of burning when passing urine are common, followed by blisters or sores which are characteristic of infection. Reactivation is often accompanied by warning symptoms of itching, tingling or pain in the genital regions followed by blisters. Confirmation of diagnosis is obtained by isolation of the virus in cell culture, and by an increase in antibody levels using PCR or enzyme-linked immunosorbent assay (ELISA) (Galadari & Fowzan 2006).

Treatment

The majority of infections in normal hosts resolve spontaneously. For the immune compromised patient, prompt treatment with antiviral chemotherapy reduces morbidity and the risk of serious complications. Oral, intravenous and topical preparations are available (Arduino & Porter 2006). Therapy includes famciclovir (Whitley 2006), penciclovir,

121

ganciclovir and foscarnet (Abdel-Haq *et al.* 2006). Therapy for children will depend on the severity and time of acquisition (Kimberlin 2005). Resistance to therapy is being seen (Kriesel *et al.* 2005), which is often associated with prolonged antiviral therapy (Wyles *et al.* 2005). Newer drugs appear to be successful in reducing the severity and frequency of recurrence (Kleymann 2003). For immunocompromised patients, antiviral therapy during immunosuppression can prevent reactivation of HSV (Tan & Goh 2006a).

Nursing care

Barrier nursing is essential in cases of extensive infection with herpesvirus. Postherpetic neuralgia (PHN) is a common problem, which is reduced by antiviral therapy. However, adequate analgesia must also be administered (Fillet 2002).

Varicella zoster virus

Definition

Varicella (chickenpox) is an acute highly infectious disease caused by the varicella zoster virus (VZV). Initial infection with VZV causes varicella (chickenpox). Following clinical recovery, the virus persists in the latent form in the dorsal root ganglia of nerves; reactivation of the latent VZV causes zoster (shingles). Viral reactivation appears as cellular immunity wanes: 30% of immunosuppressed patients develop zoster (Boeckh *et al.* 2006).

Reference material

Varicella

Surveillance of VZV infection in England and Wales from 1991 to 2000 found varicella in 1291 per 100 000 of the population and zoster in 373 per 100 000 of the population (Brisson & Edmunds 2003). The varicella incubation period is 11–21 days. The illness usually starts with 1 or 2 days of fever and malaise, although this may be absent, particularly in young children (but can be severe the older the person) (Welsby 2006). Vesicles begin on the face and scalp, spreading to the trunk, abdomen and then limbs. After 3 or 4 days the vesicles begin to dry and develop into granular scabs, during this time further vesicles may continue to appear. The number of vesicles can vary from so few that they are missed, to numerous that can cover the whole body.

Varicella is transmitted during person-to-person contact with the skin lesions or by inhalation of droplets from respiratory secretions and saliva. The infectious period is generally 2 days before the rash and up to the time when all of the vesicles have dried up. This can be prolonged in immunocompromised persons. Outbreaks of chickenpox have occurred from infected patients to non-immune health care workers (Paul & Jacob 2006). Herpes zoster (shingles) is caused by the reactivation of the person's own varicella virus

that has been latent since the chickenpox illness. Virus from the zoster lesions can cause chickenpox if the person with herpes zoster is in close contact with those who have not had chickenpox. Shingles cannot develop in one person from contact with another person's shingle lesions. Zoster is more common in the elderly. Neuralgia often precedes the onset of herpes zoster (shingles), which is a localized, painful, vesicular rash involving one or adjacent dermatomes. Chronic pain may persist after the rash has healed and is referred to as PHN, which can often be severe and refractory to many forms of treatment. PHN is probably related to neuronal inflammation induced by the replicating VZV (Roxas 2006). In patients with HIV and those undergoing transplantation, recurrent zoster can occur (Tan & Goh 2006a).

Varicella infection is not always benign (Abdulmalik *et al.* 2006). Hospitalization may be required (Staat *et al.* 2006). Following local replication, the virus will be carried by the bloodstream to other sites. It is thought that infected lymphocytes persist in the circulation and can go on to carry virus to major organs, causing pneumonia, hepatitis or other life-threatening complications. Both chickenpox and shingles can lead to neurological infection and disease. The virus reaches the nervous system either through the bloodstream or by direct spread from sensory ganglia. The most frequent manifestations include cerebral ataxia, neuralgia, acute encephalitis, aseptic meningitis and myelitis. Recovery from varicella in a fit adult is usually spontaneous and without sequelae, but can result in serious life-threatening complications in healthy children. Surveillance of VZV infection in England and Wales from 1991 to 2000 found that number of inpatient days and case fatalities due to zoster was about four to six times greater than for varicella (Brisson & Edmunds 2003).

Immunocompromised patients with VZV infection are at greater risk for dissemination and development of complications than the immunocompetent person and can be associated with serious morbidity and significant mortality. Prognosis has improved since the use of aciclovir for treatment and prophylaxis (Boeckh *et al.* 2006). Emphasis must be placed on early diagnosis, prophylaxis and treatment of varicella infection in immunosuppressed persons, especially those patients on steroid therapy, to reduce morbidity and mortality associated with herpesvirus infections (Hill *et al.* 2005).

Pregnant women who contract varicella may develop complications for the mother and the child (Pinot de Moira *et al.* 2006). Varicella vaccine is now available and has reduced mortality due to chickenpox (Davis 2006).

Zoster

It is thought that zoster appears when cell-mediated immunity fails to curtail virus reactivation. This may happen as a result of age, the side-effects of drugs or disease. The virus reactivates randomly in the nerve ganglion and spreads down the peripheral nerve producing vesicular skin lesions at the site supplied by the affected neurons (Mims *et al.* 2004).

Diagnosis

The diagnosis of chickenpox can usually be made from the characteristic pattern of vesicles. Confirmation is possible by culture of vesicle fluid or by serological antibody tests. Neuralgia often proclaims the onset of zoster and can occur several days before skin signs occur. Erythematous patches are the first sign. They progress to macules then to papules and finally to vesicles. New outbreaks of vesicles continue in untreated persons for some time. Fever, headaches and malaise can accompany the rash (Mims *et al.* 2004). The vesicles generally correspond in distribution to one or more sensory nerves. To minimize the risk of infection, care must be taken not to break the vesicles. Daily hygiene must be meticulous. Dissemination of zoster in an immunosuppressed patient generally occurs 6–10 days after the onset of localized lesions, and is usually limited to cutaneous involvement. Occasional haemorrhagic complications and pneumonia can occur (Mims *et al.* 2004).

Treatment

Treatment of varicella is normally only necessary for immunosuppressed patients (Klassen *et al.* 2005), and involves the use of antiviral agents such as aciclovir (Klassen *et al.* 2005), which reduces the time of new lesion formation, fever and visceral complications. The sequential use of intravenous followed by oral aciclovir has been shown to be effective and results in reduction of intravenous therapy and hospitalization. Oral aciclovir administered to healthy people who have been exposed to varicella can effectively prevent or modify clinical varicella. Failure to respond to 7–10 days of aciclovir suggests drug resistance; in such cases foscarnet or ganciclovir would be the drug of choice (Andrei *et al.* 2005).

Prevention

Pregnant women who have not had chickenpox should be counselled to avoid contact with people with chickenpox, as infants born to women who acquire varicella during or shortly after pregnancy are at high risk of infection. Varicella of the newborn is a life-threatening illness (Tan & Koren 2006b).

Pregnant women and immunosuppressed patients without a history of varicella and, in some cases, patients with a history of varicella, but who are currently on high-dose chemotherapy, should receive varicella zoster immunoglobulin (VZIg) when exposed to varicella or zoster. To be effective, VZIg must be administered as soon after exposure as possible (DH 2006b), which will give protection for approximately 4 weeks. Second cases of chickenpox in healthy people are extremely rare. A varicella vaccine preparation containing live attenuated virus is available for those persons who have not had chickenpox. Two doses are required (DH 2006b). Studies evaluating the costs and benefits of vaccinating varicella-susceptible health care workers suggest there are cost benefits (O'Neill & Buttery 2003).

Nursing care

Nurses must identify those patients at increased risk of VZV infection, and plan and implement interventions to decrease this risk to prevent outbreaks of VZV among patients. Only staff who have had varicella should have contact with patients with varicella or zoster. Source isolation is essential (see Source isolation section, above). The door of the room must be kept closed to minimize airborne transmission of the virus (Kao & Yang 2006).

Legionnaires' disease

Definition

Legionnaires' disease is an acute bacterial pneumonia caused by infection with *Legionella pneumophila*. This is responsible for about 90% of infection caused by the *Legionella* family. *Legionella* is a Gram-negative, aerobic, non-sporeforming unencapsulated bacillus (Cunha 2006).

Reference material

In the summer of 1976 an outbreak of pneumonia occurred among about 5000 people who had attended an American Legion convention in Philadelphia. There were 182 cases and 29 deaths. The epidemic aroused enormous public interest. Epidemiological investigations showed that the focus was the lobby of a famous hotel, but the cause remained unidentified for months until a small Gram-negative organism was found, which subsequently became known as *Legionella pneumophila* (Fraser *et al.* 1977).

There are more than 40 species of the *Legionella* family, with more than 50 serotypes (Fields *et al.* 2002) which have been isolated from a range of environmental sites including lakes, rivers, soils and man-made water systems such as cooling towers (Lee *et al.* 2002) and spars (Su *et al.* 2006), where biofilm and the presence of warm water increases the *Legionella* count (van der Kooij *et al.* 2005). This ability to survive and multiply is responsible for the contamination of water systems and the difficulty in irradicating the disease (Borella *et al.* 2005). *Legionella pneumophila* is a thermophile which flourishes at temperatures from 25 to 42°C and can survive a range of temperatures from 5 to 60°C. However, it is unusual for this organism to proliferate in temperatures of below 20°C or above 60°C (DH 2006). The most critical temperature is 36°C (Patterson *et al.* 1997). The major route of *Legionella* infection is by aerosol dispersion and inhalation of the bacteria from, for example, shower heads or more commonly from air conditioning systems. Contaminated shower heads and tap water aerosolize low numbers of the organisms during use. The aerosols are small enough to penetrate the lower respiratory system and cause infection (Sabria & Yu 2002).

Numerous outbreaks of Legionnaires' disease have occurred (Sabria *et al.* 2006). Around 300–350 cases are currently reported each year in England (Health Protection Agency 2006). Advice on how to investigate cases of Legionnaires' disease are available (Lee *et al.* 2002). A cross-sectional multicentre survey of Italian hotels found 45.8% of water samples positive for *Legionella*, highlighting that hotels, particularly those located in old buildings, are a potential source of infection (Borella *et al.* 2005; Ozerol *et al.* 2006). Effective maintenance of water systems is essential to minimize the risk of *Legionella* infection (NHS Executive 1994). Every effort should be made to avoid stagnant water conditions and to store and supply water outside this critical temperature. The quality of cold water can be improved by a dedicated supply direct from the incoming mains, and circulating hot water should be kept at a temperature of 60°C (Patterson *et al.* 1997). Removal of 'dead legs' in plumbing systems where sludge has formed, which predisposes to proliferation of the organisms, plus regular flushing of water systems not in regular use, reduce *Legionella* to below detectable levels (HSE 2005b). Water systems incorporating cooling towers and evaporation condensers pose particular problems, as their mode of operation produces conditions for microbial growth, deliberately creating sprays and aerosols which can disperse the organisms over wide areas if not controlled properly. When water from this source evaporates, droplets containing *Legionella* may be drawn into the air intakes of the building or fall on people passing by (Crimi *et al.* 2006).

Virulence is coupled to a susceptible host. The disease tends to affect those who are already immunocompromised, for example cancer patients (Rolston 2001) and the elderly, who are all predisposed to infection. The incubation period is about 2–10 days following first exposure. The signs and symptoms include malaise, general aches and headache, diarrhoea and vomiting, followed by high temperature, cough, rigors and respiratory distress. Some patients do not develop pneumonia but progress to profound septicaemia with symptoms of diplopia and mental confusion. Pneumonia is the most common presentation of *Legionella* infection, but wound infections have followed immersion in contaminated water. Post-infection symptoms of ill health, in particular fatigue, can persist for as long as 1.5 years (Lettinga *et al.* 2002).

Diagnosis

Diagnosis relies on laboratory diagnosis by:

1 Isolation of the causative organism.
2 Demonstration of the presence of the organism, its antigen or its products in the patient's body fluids or tissues (Diederen & Peeters 2006).

The above are coupled with the clinical picture and chest X-ray findings.

Treatment

Historically, treatment has included the antibiotic erythromycin, although newer antibiotics are being used (Pedro-Botet & Yu 2006). Empirical antibiotics are often commenced from a clinical assessment of the patient's signs and symptoms of infection, with the antibacterial spectrum including the most likely pathogen to be the cause of the infection (Felmingham 2004). Supportive therapy is also required for complications as they arise, which may include pulmonary failure, shock and acute renal failure. Person-to-person spread has never been demonstrated and therefore barrier nursing is not required. However, careful disposal of sputum and encouraging patients to cover their mouth and nose when coughing are necessary precautions.

Prevention

The Approved Code of Practice (HSE 2000) provides a basic framework for preventing outbreaks of disease, as well as identifying and assessing risk. In the event of an outbreak of Legionnaires' disease, the outbreak committee is convened to protect public health and prevent further infections by identifying and controlling infection risks (HSE 2000; Ricketts & Joseph 2006).

Prevention relies on regular inspection and maintenance of the water system, including planning, installation and commissioning (Freije 2004). Discovery of a single case of hospital-acquired Legionnaires' disease is an important sign of additional undiscovered cases; therefore, each case must be investigated fully (Sabria & Yu 2002; O'Neill & Humphreys 2005). Point-of-use water filters are also available to filter out and prevent *Legionella* infections (Sheffer *et al.* 2005).

Listeriosis

Definition

Listeriosis is an infectious disease caused by *Listeria monocytogenes*, a Gram-negative bacterium, and is a serious life-threatening infection. There are 13 different serotypes of *L. monocytogenes* (Mims *et al.* 2004).

Reference material

Listeria has a widespread distribution in the environment, including in soil, dust and vegetation. It also inhabits the gastrointestinal tract of animals and humans who may remain symptomless (Mims *et al.* 2004). The genus *Listeria* includes many types that are non-pathogenic to humans. *Listeria monocytogenes* is recognized as being the cause of listeriosis in humans (Mims *et al.* 2004). *Listeria* has the ability to survive and multiply in low temperatures including 0°C (Taormina & Beuchat 2001). This means that it can survive in food stored in a refrigerator, and mild heating of food can facilitate the growth of *Listeria* species (Li *et al*. 2002). X-ray irradiation of food can destroy *Listeria* (Robertson *et al*. 2006).

High levels of *Listeria* can occur in raw foods, for example pork (Thevenot *et al*. 2006) and soft cheese (Gianfranceschi *et al*. 2006). A high-risk food has the following properties: has the potential for contamination; supports the growth of *Listeria*; ready to eat; requires refrigeration; and stored for extended periods (ILSI Research Foundation; Risk Science Institute 2005). Outbreaks of *Listeria* food infections frequently occur, including in hospitals (Dawson *et al*. 2006).

Infection in immunecompetent persons is mild, whilst infection in the immunocompromised adult varies from a mild, chill-like illness to bacteraemia, septicaemia and meningitis. In neonates it can cause meningitis and serious sepsis (Mims *et al*. 2004). Research also suggests that *Listeria* easily passes from maternal organs to the placenta. Once colonized the placenta becomes a reservoir of infection resulting in reseeding of maternal organs. This process is only interrupted by the expulsion of the infected placenta tissue (Bakardjiev *et al*. 2006). Infection can lead to abortion, premature delivery, neonatal septicemia, or pneumonia with abscesses or granulomas (Mims *et al*. 2004).

Diagnosis

Routine microbiology testing for culture and sensitivities can be undertaken on specimens such as blood cutures, cerebral spinal fluid or newborn skin lesions (Mims *et al*. 2004).

Treatment

Early diagnosis and prompt administration of appropriate antibiotics are essential; even so deaths will still occur. Ampicillin or penicillin is usually regarded as the drug of choice, often in combination with gentamicin (Mims *et al*. 2004).

Transmission

Contaminated food is the most important vehicle of spread (ILSI Research Foundation: Risk Science Institute 2005). There are increasing reports of *Listeria* found in raw meat, fruit and vegetables, which predispose to contamination of, for example, coleslaw.

Prevention

Prevention entails scrupulous preparation of cooked food for immunocompromised people and pregnant women, plus the avoidance of uncooked foods, in particular soft cheese, coleslaw and pate (Mims *et al*. 2004). New food hygiene legislation (Food Standards Agency 2006) applies to all food businesses in the UK. An internationally recognized and recommended system for food hygiene called Hazard Analysis Critical Control Points (HACCP) focuses on identifying the critical points in the entire food chain where problems could occur and putting in steps to prevent problems occurring (Food Standards Agency 2006).

Person-to-person transmission during normal contact is unlikely. However, careful disposal of blood and body fluids and thorough hand washing after contact with the patient are essential.

Pneumocystosis

Definition

Pneumocystosis is an infection caused by the organism *Pneumocystis carinii* (PC), also referred to as *Pneumocystis jiroveci* (Singhal *et al*. 2005), which is closely related to fungi (De Souza & Benchimol 2005). Infection is mainly the consequence of exaggerated inflammatory response to the organism (Carmona *et al*. 2006).

Reference material

PC was first discovered in 1909 and causes infection worldwide, with most individuals testing seropositive for pneumocystis early in childhood (Respaldiza *et al*. 2004). PC is associated with outbreaks of pneumonia (*Pneumocystis carinii* pneumonia [PCP]) in immunocompromised persons (Giglotti & Wright 2005), and is is a major cause of illness and death in immunocompromised patients (Sritangratanakul *et al*. 2004). Molecular epidemiological studies identified more than 50 strains of PC that are widely distributed in the environment, and most children demonstrate that they have been harmlessly exposed to PC at an early age.

Certain types of patients are at a greater risk:

1 Patients of all ages receiving immunosuppressive agents for the treatment of cancer and during organ transplantation, particularly if chronic graft-versus-host reaction is present. Deaths from PCP continue to occur (Gal *et al*. 2002).
2 Children and infants with primary immunodeficiency disorders, particularly SCID (Berrington *et al*. 2000), with severe malnutrition (Russian & Levine 2001) or malignancy (Neville *et al*. 2002).
3 Patients with HIV/AIDS (Gigliotti & Wright 2005).
4 Patients with diseases such as connective tissue disease (Li *et al*. 2006b).

PC infections in immune compromised children are reported to be slow and insidious in onset, with initial non-specific signs of restlessness, lethargy, poor feeding over a period of weeks, resulting in tachypnoea, severe dyspnoea, use of accessory muscles for breathing, marked cyanosis and exhausting non-productive cough. Children and adults with underlying disease such as neoplasm often experience an abrupt onset of illness, with high fever, tachypnoea and cough, which can progress to a fatal outcome even with treatment (Wazir & Ansari 2004).

Diagnosis

Bronchoscopy with bronchoalveolar lavage (BAL) is widely used to detect respiratory infections (Lehto *et al.* 2005). The specimen is then microbiologically tested with the use of PCR (Hohenthal *et al.* 2005). Survival is related directly to the aggressiveness with which the diagnosis is pursued in the early stages of disease and with the early institution of appropriate therapy.

Treatment

Advances in prevention and treatment of PCP have led to a decrease in the incidence and improved outcomes (Santamauro *et al.* 2002).

Co-trimoxazole (the combination of trimethoprim and sulphamethoxazole) is the treatment of choice for PCP (Sritangratanakul *et al.* 2004), but it can be toxic and it may fail, resulting in treatment changes. Alternative drugs may include alovaquone or dapsone (Goldie *et al.* 2002).

Aerosolized pentamidine prophylaxis has significantly improved the prognosis of immunocompromised patients at risk of PCP (Marras *et al.* 2002).

Nursing care

Hospitalized patients who develop PCP may well be cared for in areas where there are large concentrations of immuno-suppressed patients. Owing to reports of clustering of this disease and the difficulty of identifying whether this represents person-to-person spread, patients with a productive cough should be placed in a single room until the cough improves. Precautions other than careful hand washing following patient contact are unnecessary.

Tuberculosis

Definition

Tuberculosis (TB) is a destructive infectious disease caused by *Mycobacterium tuberculosis*, which is an acid-fast bacillus. Other species of *Mycobacterium* that cause infection are referred to as 'atypical' mycobacteria (Mims *et al.* 2004).

Reference material

Mycobacterium tuberculosis is defined as an acid-fast bacillus because of a waxy material in the cell wall, which resists simple laboratory staining techniques unless treated with hot carbol fuchsin, which allows impregnation by the dye. This is retained despite attempts to decolourize it with acid or alcohol. Mycobacteria are distributed widely throughout the world, but only a few species are pathogenic to humans. These include *M. tuberculosis*, whose main host is humans, and *M. bovis* (the bovine type of tubercle bacillus), which is pathogenic to humans as well as to cattle. *M. bovis* has been found in milk samples (Thoen *et al.* 2006).

There are also atypical mycobacteria associated with patients who are severely immunocompromised due to HIV infection (Miguez-Burbano *et al.* 2006). These are *M. avium intracellulare* (MAC), *M. malmoense*, *M. xenopi* and *M. kansasii* (Mims *et al.* 2004). A significant decrease in MAC infections has now been seen amongst HIV-positive patients receiving antiretroviral therapy (Gona *et al.* 2006). In the past, these types rarely caused disease in humans but now cause a disease which quickly disseminates to most organs in the body, and do not respond as readily to established tuberculosis drugs (Lam *et al.* 2006). Atypical mycobacteria are not highly adapted to humans like *M. tuberculosis* and are not transmitted from person to person, but can survive in the environment and pass to human hosts.

TB causes characteristically chronic granulamatous lesions, mainly in the lungs, but the glands, bones, joints, brain and meninges, and other internal organs may be affected (Mims *et al.* 2004). Infection in immunocompromised cancer patients varies and can often be initially misdiagnosed as cancer (Aisenberg *et al.* 2005).

Mycobacterium tuberculosis is a pathogenic organism because of its ability to reside in and restrict the ability of the host macrophages, as well as being able to adhere to, invade and multiply within respiratory epithelial cells (Mims *et al.* 2004).

Epidemiology

One-third of the world's population is currently infected with TB, with approximately 3 million deaths occurring each year. In the UK there are about 7000 cases of TB each year due to *M. tuberculosis* with only 17 to 50 new cases of *Mycobacterium bovis* infection (De la Rua-Domenech 2006).

Outbreaks of infection do occur: one outbreak occurred from contact in a south-west of England public house (Gaber *et al.* 2005); another among health care workers due to the delay in diagnosing the index case resulting in 28 health care workers becoming infected (De Vries *et al.* 2006).

Certain conditions predispose to the development of TB, including general physical debilitation and lowered resistance due to disease, immunosuppressive drugs and alcoholism. In a study, the significant risk factors identified included being born outside the UK or having contact with persons born outside the UK (Dale *et al.* 2005).

Transmission

The mode of spread for TB is occasionally by ingestion, for example by drinking infected milk, but principally by inhalation of small droplets produced by coughing, sneezing, shouting and singing (CDC 2005). These droplets are probably the most effective vehicle of spread since they dry rapidly in the air to yield droplet nuclei of less than 5 nm in diameter which, when inhaled, can reach the alveoli, where local infection may occur. This is followed by dissemination to draining

126

lymphatics and spread through the body via the blood, usually within 2–12 weeks after the initial infection (CDC 2005). The organism can survive in the environment and on inadequately cleaned instruments such as endoscopes, which can lead to cross-infection (Larson *et al.* 2003).

Diagnosis

TB should be suspected in all people with a cough with or without cause, which lasts more than 3 weeks, with or without weight loss, anorexia, fever, night sweats or haemoptysis (DH 1998d). Tuberculin skin tests are used to determine TB infection, and the size of the erythematous response is used to make a provisional diagnosis (Toivgoogin *et al.* 2005). Microbiology investigations to find the presence of acid-fast bacilli in, for example, sputum, tissue, urine or cerebrospinal fluid are required. This is termed 'smear positive'. Confirmation and species identification by culture may take longer and is termed 'culture positive'. Newer methods are now available that reduce the time required for identification (Mims *et al.* 2004).

Patients with smear-positive pulmonary disease are infectious, those with smear-negative or non-pulmonary disease are not. Once appropriate combination chemotherapy has commenced, smear-positive people are considered non-infectious after 2 weeks of treatment (NICE 2006).

Patients with a TB diagnosis tend to be worried, frustrated and disappointed by their diagnosis (Chang *et al.* 2004) experiencing social stigmatization, isolation, pill burden, sexual dysfunction, loss of income and fear of additional specific problems related to TB (Hansel *et al.* 2004). Attention to this issue experienced by people with TB may optimize adherence to treatment and therefore treatment success (Marra *et al.* 2004).

Treatment

Until the 1960s, treatment included bed rest and attention to diet, but chemotherapy is now the preferred treatment. It involves the use of combination drugs designed to reduce viable bacteria as rapidly as possible in order to minimize the risk of ineffective treatment in those patients infected by drug-resistant bacteria. A 6-month regimen with four standard drugs is recommended in the initial phase for all forms of TB excluding meningitis (which may need to be treated for a longer period).

The NICE (2006) guidelines recommend that:

- The patients should be supervised by physicians with full training and care provided by nurse specialists.
- A named key worker should be assigned to all persons with TB, to promote adherence to treatment.
- Patients must be involved in treatment decisions from the outset and the importance of compliance to treatment emphasized.
- Written patient information material in the appropriate language should be provided.

- If a patient defaults from treatment they must be sent reminder letters in the appropriate language, receive health education counselling, have home visits, interviews, asked to start a patient diary, given random urine tests and other monitoring such as pill counting.
- The patient should be provided with help and advice related to money, housing and social services as appropriate to each person.
- In a few cases it may be necessary to directly observe the taking of tablets.
- Once treatment is completed, follow up clinic appointments for patients with drug-sensitive TB are not required.
- Patients should be told to watch out for symptoms of relapse and how to contact the TB service if required.
- Patients with HIV or drug-resistant TB should be followed up even when treatment is completed, especially those persons with HIV (NICE 2006).

A risk assessment must be made to establish each new patient's risk of having drug-resistant TB. The risks include:

- History of prior TB treatment.
- Prior TB treatment failure.
- Contact with a person known to have drug-resistant TB.
- Born in country with a high incidence of drug-resistant TB, HIV infection.
- Resident in London.
- Age, higher in age group 25–44 years.
- Male gender (NICE 2006).

Response to all TB therapy must be monitored, if there is no clinical improvement or if cultures remain positive, drug resistance should be suspected (NICE 2006). Outbreaks of multi-drug resistant TB (MDR-TB) do occur (Heldal *et al.* 2003).

TB continues to be a notifiable disease (DH 1995c). It is the responsibility of the Medical Officer for Environmental Health to follow up all contacts of infected people. Once a person has been diagnosed with TB, the diagnosing physician must assess the need for contact tracing. Screening should be offered to all household contacts, plus other close contacts such as partners. Contact tracing involves identifying the index case plus those who may have become infected. As transmission requires prolonged close contact with a smear-positive case, contact tracing is generally limited to those from the same household or equivalent. Casual contacts such as work colleagues are normally considered casual contacts and are not normally followed up. All contacts should be informed and provided with advice (NICE 2006). If transmission is shown to have occurred among this close contact group, a wider contact tracing may be required, including family, friends and work colleagues (DH 1998d). The infection control doctor with the consultant in communicable disease will evaluate whether hospital contacts will be followed up; generally this will only involve immunocompromised patients and health care workers. Contact tracing is likely to start from the date 1 month before the patient became symptomatic. In cases without symptoms it may be necessary to look back over 3 months (DH 1998d). Advice on handling outbreaks of TB is available (DH 1998c).

The World Health Organization (WHO) recognizes that TB persists as a global health problem and has prepared guidance on TB control to reduce mortality, morbidity and transmission of the disease, whilst preventing drug resistance (WHO 2002).

Prevention

The priorities for TB control are early detection of cases, examination of contacts, barrier nursing if appropriate and immunization of people with a negative tuberculin skin test with bacille Calmette-Guérin (BCG) vaccine (NICE 2006).

Certain professions, for example those working in hospitals, veterinary and prison staff, should not start work until they have completed a TB screen and health check, or documentary evidence is provided of screening in the last year (NICE 2006).

Staff in contact with untreated, smear-positive patients for a week or more should be reported to the occupational health department and a chest X-ray arranged. However, if the employee develops suspicious symptoms such as an unexplained cough lasting longer than 3 weeks, persistent fever or weight loss, then a full examination must be undertaken. Staff in regular contact with TB patients or clinical material should receive annual reminders of TB symptoms (NICE 2006).

Patients infected with HIV are predisposed to develop TB. Preventive treatment against TB in adults infected with HIV has been seen to reduce the incidence of infection. Early diagnosis and effective treatment of TB among HIV-infected patients are critical for curing and minimizing the negative effects of TB on HIV progression, as TB increases the risk of death among HIV-positive persons (Amin 2006).

Nursing care

Patients with TB will only be admitted if they have clinical or socio-economic needs such as homelessness (NICE 2006). They should be admitted into a single room. Masks should be worn if MDR-TB is suspected or aerosol-generating procedures are being performed. If the patient needs to leave the room they should wear a mask until they have received 2 weeks of drug therapy. In general, segregation can be reduced following 2 weeks of treatment as long as MDR-TB is not suspected. The exception would be if there was an HIV-positive or immunosuppressed patient in the same ward area, which would require extended segregation of the infected person (NICE 2006). High awareness of the disease is essential, as most patients can be investigated and treated on an outpatient basis. As home contacts will have already been exposed and will be routinely contacted and investigated, no changes at home will be required unless poor hygienic practices are used. Segregation while undergoing tests or routine visits to the outpatient department is required to prevent

more people being exposed. Adequate resources and an appropriately skilled workforce, including specialist nurses and outreach workers, are necessary (NICE 2006).

Evaluation of infectivity will be necessary. Sputum smear-positive people are considered infectious and those whose results are not yet known are treated as potentially positive. People who have smear-negative culture-positive pulmonary disease, plus non-pulmonary disease, are considered not to be infectious (DH 1998d). Infectious and potentially infectious patients should be cared for in a single room with the door closed. Patients being cared for with immunocompromised persons must be placed in a negative pressure room that is continuously and automatically monitored. All patients with known or suspected MDR-TB must be placed in a negative pressure single room with the door closed. If the patient is HIV-antibody positive this room should be near but physically separated from the HIV ward (DH 1998d).

Patients require careful explanation to ensure both they and their visitors comply with the barrier nursing precautions. Initially visitors should be restricted to those who have already had contact. Visitors who themselves are immunocompromised should only visit after careful discussion with and agreement by their own physician. Paediatric facilities and restrictions should be the same as for adults.

Patients must be taught to cover their mouths when coughing to prevent droplet spread, and to wash their hands after coughing. Patients must expectorate into sputum pots with tight fitting lids, and the pots must be changed frequently. As compliance to therapy can be poor, patients must be encouraged and, if necessary, supervised to ensure compliance with the drug treatment. Unconscious patients will need to have their drugs administered via a nasogastric tube, intravenously or intramuscularly (Ormerod 1996).

Legislation

Patients with TB who are non-adherent to therapy or who have complicated medical and social problems may pose a threat to others. Sections 37 and 38 of the Public Health (Control of Disease Act) 1984 provide legal powers to control infected patients who refuse to comply with treatment and pose a threat to public health. The Control of Substances Hazardous to Health (COSHH) Regulations (HSE 2002) include issues such as TB and disinfectants. These guidelines require a risk assessment, and the provision of adequate information, instruction and training to be carried out where an employee is exposed to substances hazardous to health.

Transmissible spongiform encephalopathies

Definition

Transmissible spongiform encephalopathies (TSEs), also referred to as prion diseases, are fatal degenerative brain diseases which occur in humans and some animal species. A common feature of all TSEs is the appearance of microscopic holes in the grey matter of the brain, giving it a sponge-like appearance, from which the conditions derive their names. TSE is very rare, with about 1 per million people per year affected (DH 2003d).

Reference material

There are several TSEs. In humans these are:

- Creutzfeldt–Jakob disease (CJD), including sporadic (80%), familial (10 to 15%), iatrogenic and new variant Creutzfeldt–Jakob disease (vCJD) (small number of cases).
- Gerstmann–Straussler–Scheinker syndrome.
- Fatal familial insomnia.
- Kuru.

In animals these are:

- Scrapie, bovine spongiform encephalopathy (BSE) (which may be transmitted to humans by eating infected animal tissue).
- Transmissible mink encephalopathy.
- Chronic wasting disease.
- Feline spongiform encephalopathy in domestic cats and captured exotic felines and ungulates.
- CJD, including classic, sporadic, familial, iatrogenic and vCJD.
- There is a suggested link between vCJD and consuming BSE-infected beef. Advice has been provided for those involved in the management and care of patients with CJD on the handling of deceased patients to minimize the risk to other patients, visitors and staff (DH 2003d).

TSEs are caused by an infectious agent, thought to be an infectious protein called a prion. Prions are not uniformly spread in the tissues, but high levels are thought to be in neural tissue, less in spinal fluid and lymphoreticular tissue, with very little in blood and other body fluids and tissue. This means that the central nervous system tissue, including the retina, pose the highest risk; lymphoid tissue, cornea and dura mater are lower risk; and most body fluids and other tissue are of negligible risk as CJD has only been found to be transmitted by the reuse of experimental brain electrodes, neurosurgery, dura mater and corneal grafts, pituitary growth hormones and gonadotrophins (DH 2003d).

Of major concern is that TSEs exhibit a high resistance to conventional chemical and physical decontamination methods and are not affected by disinfectants, such as formalin and ethylene oxide, or autoclaving at conventional times and temperatures (134°C for 3 minutes) (DH 2003d).

TSEs have a preclinical phase that lasts for years, followed by a rapid progressive dementia, loss of memory and intellect, personality changes, progressive unsteadiness and clumsiness. In CJD involuntary muscular jerking is common. There is no known treatment or prophylaxis and all TSEs are invariably progressive and fatal once clinical signs appear (DH 2003d).

Risk assessment

The risk related to vCJD was raised when it was found in tonsillar tissue of people who had died of vCJD, indicating that CNS tissue is not the only risk. In 1999 the NHSE provided guidance on minimizing the risk of transmission of vCJD. Advice included:

- Single-use kits for all lumbar punctures.
- Using single-use instruments whenever possible.
- Properly cleaned and sterilized surgical instruments to be used at all times.
- Instruments and equipment used in the care of patients with confirmed TSEs should not be reused but disposed of by incineration.
- Instruments used on patients suspected of having CJD should be quarantined pending confirmation of diagnosis. Certain patients should be regarded as at particular risk, for example recipients of dura mater grafts (DH 2003d).

Concerns have been raised about the risk to workers from being exposed to the agent of CJD. Lists of workers with unintentional exposure to CJD have to be compiled and kept for 40 years after the last known exposure (NHSE 1999b). There is no confirmed occupationally acquired cases of transmission of TSE, but there has been a small number of reports of sporadic CJD in health care workers including a neurosurgeon, retired laboratory worker and a pathologist, but the link with their occupation is speculative (DH 2003d).

The DH (2003d) issued a risk assessment related to the transmission of vCJD via used surgical instruments. An effort was made to clarify the most important factors affecting this risk. The assessment suggests that the risk of surgical transmission of vCJD from instruments used on a patient with vCJD cannot be ruled out, even when the instruments have been decontaminated and sterilized following government guidelines. This poses a risk to public health (DH 2003d). In August 2002, a hospital patient was unexpectedly diagnosed with CJD following a brain biopsy. The instruments used for the brain biopsy had been used subsequently during other patients' operations. Twenty-four patients who had had surgery at this time had to be followed up. The enquiry that followed this case found 12 individual factors where practices could be improved; of particular concern was the leak of confidential information to the press (Kirkup 2002).

Blood transfusions

Concerns have been raised related to the potential risk of CJD being transmitted by blood transfusion. There is little evidence to support these fears. However, the importance of improving the safety of blood and maintaining a sufficient blood supply is becoming an increasing issue. The following precautionary measures have been put in place in the UK:

- All blood for transfusion to be leucodepleted.
- Plasma for blood products has to be sourced from outside the UK.
- Fresh frozen plasma for those patients born after 1 January 1996 is now sourced from the USA (DH 2003d) (see Chapter 43).

Nursing care

The nursing care for patients with known or suspected CJD infection is the same as for any patient with an infection carried by blood and body fluids.

Safe techniques and practices need to be maintained at all times, and care must be taken to avoid contamination or needlestick injuries. If an accident occurs, routine first aid care must be given and the occupational health department informed.

The patient must be carefully assessed. If there is no evidence or likelihood of blood or body fluid contamination no restrictions are necessary, although close observations will have to be undertaken for bleeding or incontinence, particularly if dementia is a problem.

All specimens must be labelled with a biohazard sticker, double bagged and taken to the laboratory in a safe manner. If the patient is being referred for an invasive procedure they should be told in advance of the restrictions.

Patients requiring an operation must be last on the theatre list to allow for thorough cleaning of the theatre at the end of the operation. Disposable instruments should be used whenever possible and non-disposable instruments sent for incineration.

When the patient is ready for discharge, discharge planning must be negotiated with the community staff, as standard infection control procedures should be continued to prevent transmission of infection in the community. General guidelines for the control of infection in residential and nursing homes are available (DH 2006d).

Legislation

Legislation, guidance, local safety policies, codes of practice, accident reporting and health surveillance must be used to reduce the risk of vCJD. These include:

- The Health and Safety at Work, etc. Act 1974.
- The Environment Protection Act 1990.
- Management of Health and Safety at Work Regulations 1999.
- Genetically Modified Organisms (Contained Use) Regulations 2000.
- Control of Substances Hazardous to Health Regulations 2002 (HSE 2002).
- Reporting of Incidents, Diseases and Dangerous Occurrences Regulations 1995 (RIDDOR).

- The Carriage of Dangerous Goods (Classification, Packaging and Labelling) Regulations 2004.
- Department of Health 2006 Environment and sustainability Health Technical Memorandum 07-01 Safe management of healthcare waste (DH 2006a).
- Health and Safety Executive (HSE). Safe working and the Prevention of Infection in Clinical Laboratories and Similar Facilities 2003.

Nursing care for patients infected or suspected of being infected with TSEs is the same as for those infected with HIV and hepatitis B. Advice should be sought from the infection control team.

References and further reading

Abdel-Haq, N. et al. (2006) New antiviral agents. Indian J Pediatr, 73(4), 313–21.

Abdulmalik, A. et al. (2006) Varicella-associated purpura fulminans: chickenpox is not always benign. Med Princ Pract, 15(3), 232–4.

Abe, K. et al. (2004) Molecular epidemiology of hepatitis B, C, D and E viruses among children in Moscow, Russia. J Clin Virol, 30(1), 57–61.

Afessa, B. & Peters, S.G. (2006) Major complications following hematopoietic stem cell transplantation. Semin Respir Crit Care Med, 27(3), 297–309.

Aggarwal, R. & Ranjan, P. (2004) Preventing and treating hepatitis B infection. BMJ, 329, 1080–6.

Aisenberg, G.M. et al. (2005) Extrapulmonary tuberculosis active infection misdiagnosed as cancer: Mycobacterium tuberculosis disease in patients at a Comprehensive Cancer Centre (2001–2005). Cancer, 104(12), 2882–7.

Aisien, A.O. & Ujah, I.A. (2006) Risk of blood splashes to masks and goggles during cesarean section. Med Sci Monit, 12(2), CR94–97.

Albert, J. et al. (1990) Replicative capacity of HIV-2 like HIV-1, correlates with severity of immunosuppression. AIDS, 4(4), 291–5.

Ali, R. et al. (2006) Invasive pulmonary aspergillosis: role of early diagnosis and surgical treatment in patients with acute leukemia. Ann Clin Microbiol Antimicrob, 5(1), 17–23.

Amin, Z. (2006) Clinical tuberculosis problems and management. Acta Med Indones, 38(2), 109–16.

Anaya, I. et al. (2006) Survivability of Salmonella cells in popcorn after microwave oven and conventional cooking. Microbiol Res, [Epub ahead of print].

Anderson, D.J. et al. (2006) Predictors of mortality in patients with blood stream infection due to ceftazidime-resistant Klebsiella pneumoniae. Antimicrob Agents Chemother, 50(5), 1715–20.

Andrei, G. et al. (2005) Susceptabilities of several clinical varicella-zoster virus (VZV) isolates and drug-resistant VZV strains to bicyclic furano pyrimidine nucleosides. Antimicrob Agents Chemother 49(3), 1081–6.

Arduino, P.G. & Porter, S.R. (2006) Oral and perioral herpes simplex type 1(HSV-1) infection: review of management. Oral Dis, 12(3), 254–70.

Aricha, B., Fishov, I. & Cohen, Z. (2004) Differences in membrane fluidity and fatty acid composition between phenotypic variants of Streptococcus pneumoniae. J Bacteriol, 186(14), 4638–44.

Aslam, S. & Musher, D.M. (2006) An update on diagnosis, treatment and prevention of Clostridium difficile-associated disease. Gastroenterol Clin North Am, 35(2), 315–35.

Avery, R.K. *et al.* (2004) Use of leflunomide in an allogeneic bone marrow transplant recipient with refractory cytomegalovirus infection. *Bone Marrow Transplant*, 34(12), 1071–5.

Aveyard, H. (2002) The requirement for informed consent prior to nursing care procedures. *J Adv Nurs*, 37(3), 243–9.

Ayliffe, G.A.J. *et al.* (2000) *Control of Hospital Infection. A Practical Handbook*, 4th edn. Arnold, London.

Babay, H.A. *et al.* (2005) Bloodstream infections in pediatric patients. *Saudi Med J*, 26(10), 1555–61.

Bakardjiev, A.I., Theriot, J.A. & Portnoy, D.A. (2006) *Listeria monocytogenes* traffics from maternal organs to the placenta and back. *PLoS Pathog*, 2(6), e66.

Baker, S.A. (1994) Hepatitis: protecting BMETs and CEs. *J Clin Eng*, 19(6), 446–51.

Ball, J. *et al.* (1991) Long lasting viability of HIV after patient's death. *Lancet*, 338(8758), 63.

Banfield, K.R. & Kerr, K.G. (2005) Could hospital patients' hands constitute a missing link? *J Hosp Infect*, 61(3), 183–8.

Baqai, R., Anwar, S. & Kazmi, S.U. (2005) Detection of *Cryptosporidium* in immunosuppressed patients. *J Ayub Med Coll Abbottabad*, 17(3), 38–40.

Barber, F.D. (2001) Management of fever in neutropenic patients with cancer. *Nurs Clin North Am*, 36(4), 631–44.

Barin, F. *et al.* (1985) Serological evidence for virus related to Simian T-lymphotropic retrovirus III in residents of West Africa. *Lancet*, ii, 1387–9.

Battegay, M., Gust, I.D. & Feinstone, S.M. (1995) Hepatitis A virus. In: *Principles and Practice of Infectious Diseases*, Vol. 2, 4th edn (eds G.L. Mandell, J.E. Bennett & R. Dolin). Churchill Livingstone, New York, pp. 1636–66.

BCSH (1995) Guidelines on the provision of facilities for the care of adult patients with haematological malignancies (including leukaemia and lymphoma and severe bone marrow failure). *Clin Lab Haematol*, 17, 3–10.

Belkin, N.L. (2002) A historical review of barrier materials. *AORN J*, 76(4), 648–53.

Berg, S. *et al.* (2006) Serotypes of *Streptococcus pneumoniae* isolated from blood and cerebrospinal fluid related to vaccine serotypes and to clinical characteristics. *Scand J Infect Dis*, 38(6), 427–32.

Bernardi, M., Catania, G. & Marceca, F. (2005) The world of nursing burn out. A literature review. *Prof Inferm*, 58(2), 75–9.

Bernstein, W.B. *et al.* (2006) Acquired immunodeficiency syndrome-related malignancies in the era of highly active antiretroviral therapy. *Int J Hematol*, 84(1), 3–11.

Berrington, J.E. *et al.* (2000) Unsuspected *Pneumocystis carinii* pneumonia at presentation of severe primary immunodeficiency. *Arch Dis Child*, 82(2), 144–7.

Beyazit, Y. *et al.* (2006) Acute pericarditis and renal failure complicating acute hepatitis A infection. *South Med J*, 99(1), 82–4.

Bignardi, G.E. (1998) Risk factors for *Clostridium difficile* infection. *J Hosp Infect*, 40, 1–15.

Bishop, E. *et al.* (2006) Good clinical outcomes but high rates of adverse reactions during linezolid therapy for serious infection: a proposed protocol for monitoring therapy in complex patients. *Antimicrob Agents Chemother*, 50(4), 1599–602.

Bissett, L. (2006) Reducing the risk of acquiring antimicrobial-resistant bacteria. *Br J Nurs*, 15(2), 68–71.

Blajchman, M.A. (2006) The clinical benefits of the leukoreduction of blood products. *J Trauma*, 60(6)(Suppl), S83–90.

Blatnik, J. & Lesnicar, G. (2006) Propagation of methicillin-resistant *Staphylococcus aureus* due to the overloading of medical nurses in intensive care units. *J Hosp Infect*, 63(2), 162–6.

Bloomfield, S.F. & Scott, E.A. (2003a) Developing an effective policy for home hygiene: a risk-based approach. *Int J Environ Health Res*, 13(Suppl 1), S57–66.

Bloomfield, S.F. (2003b) Home hygiene: a risk approach. *Int J Hyg Environ Health*, 206(1), 1–8.

Blot, S. *et al.* (2005) Colonization status and appropriate antibiotic therapy for nosocomial bacteria caused by antibiotic-resistant gram-negative bacteria in intensive care unit. *Infect Control Hosp Epidemiol*, 26(6), 575–9.

Boden, M. (1999) Contamination in moving and handling equipment. *Prof Nurse* 14(7), 484–7.

Bodey, G.P. (2005) Managing infections in the immunocompromised patient. *Clin Infect Dis*, 40(Suppl 4), S239.

Boeckh, M. *et al.* (2002) Late cytomegalovirus disease and mortality in allogeneic hematopoietic stem cell transplant recipients: importance of viral load and T-cell immunity. *Blood*, 101(2), 407–14.

Boeckh, M. *et al.* (2006) Long term acyclovir for prevention of varicella zoster virus disease after allogeneic hematopoietic cell transplantation – a randomized double-blind placebo-controlled study. *Blood*, 107(5), 1800–5.

Borella, P. *et al.* (2005) *Legionella* contamination in hot water of Italian hotels. *Appl Environ Microbiol*, 71(10), 5805–13.

Boussemart, T. *et al.* (1998) Cytomegalovirus, pregnancy and occupational risk. *Arch Pediatr*, 5(1), 24–6.

Bowden, R.A. (2000) Infection in blood and bone marrow transplant patients: allogeneic and autologous transplantation. In: *Management of Infections in Immunocompromised Patients*, Part II, Chapter 5 (eds M.P. Glauser & P.A. Pizzo). W.B. Saunders, London, pp. 189–218.

Bower, M. *et al.* (2004) HIV-associated anal cancer: has highly active antiretroviral therapy reduced the incidence or improved the outcome? *J Acquir Immune Defic Syndr*, 37(5), 1563–5.

Boxall, E.H. & Smith, N. (2004) Antenatal screening for HIV; are those who refuse testing at higher risk than those who accept testing? *J Public Health (Oxf)*, 26(3), 285–7.

Boxall, E. *et al.* (2006) Transfusion-transmitted hepatitis E in a 'nonhyperendemic' country. *Transfus Med*, 16(2), 79–83.

Boyce, J.M. *et al.* (2006) Lack of association between the increased incidence of *Clostridium difficile* associated disease and the increasing use of alcoholic-based handrub. *Infect Control Hosp Epidemiol*, 27(5), 479–83.

Bradley, C.R. & Fraise, A.P. (1996) Heat and chemical resistance of enterococci. *J Hosp Infect*, 34, 191–6.

Brady, M.J. *et al.* (2003) Persistent silver disinfectant for the environment control of pathogenic bacteria. *Am J Infect Control*, 31(4), 208–14.

Braitstein, P. *et al.* (2006) Mortality of HIV-1 infected patients in the first year of antiretroviral therapy: comparison between low-income and high-income countries. *Lancet*, 11(367; 9513), 817–24.

Brant, L. *et al.* (2005) Pathways of care and resource utilization in a national cohort of patients with transfusion-acquired hepatitis C. *J Viral Hepat*, 12(6), 618–26.

Brisson, M. & Edmunds, W.J. (2003) Epidemiology of varicella-zoster virus in England and Wales. *J Med Virol*, 70(Suppl 1), S9–14.

Brown, D.F.J. *et al.* (2006a) National glycopeptide-resistant enterococcal bacteraemia surveillance working group report to the Department of Health, August 2004. *J Hosp Infect*, 62(Suppl 1), 1–27.

Brown, E.L. *et al.* (2006b) Maternal herpes simplex virus antibody avidity and risk of neonatal herpes. *Am J Obstet Gynecol*, 195(1), 115–20.

Bruce, J. & Brysiewicz, P. (2002) Ebola fever: the African emergency. *Int J Trauma Nurs*, 8(2), 36–41.

Bruix, J. *et al.* (2006) New aspects of diagnosis and therapy of hepatocellular carcinoma. *Oncogene*, 25(27), 3848–56.

Brundage, S.C. & Fitzpatrick, A.N. (2006) Hepatitis A. *Am Fam Physician*, 73(12), 2162–8.

Burek, V. (2005) Laboratory diagnosis of viral hepatitis B and C. *Acta Med Croatica*, 59(5), 405–12.

Burnard, P. (1992) Nurse training needs in AIDS counselling. *Nurs Stand*, 6(34), 34–39.

Cacciari, P. *et al.* (2004) Consideration on isolation rooms and alternative pressure ventilation systems. *Ann Ig*, 16(6), 777–801.

Caccio, S.M. (2005) Molecular epidemiology of human cryptosporidiosis. *Parassitologia*, 47(2), 185–92.

Caccio, S.M. & Pozio, E. (2006) Advances in the epidemiology, diagnosis and treatment of cryptosporidiosis. *Expert Rev Anti Infect Ther*, 4(3), 429–43.

Caggiano, V. *et al.* (2005) Incidence, cost, and mortality of neutropenia hospitalization with chemotherapy. *Cancer*, 103(9), 1916–24.

Calandra, T. (2000) Practical guide to host defence mechanisms and the predominant infections encountered in immunocompromised patients. In: *Management of Infections in Immunocompromised Patients,* Part I, Chapter 1 (eds M.P. Glauser & P.A. Pizzo). W.B. Saunders, London, pp. 3–16.

Callaghan, I. (1998) Bacterial contamination of nurse's uniform: a study. *Nurs Stand*, 13(1), 37–42.

Campana, S. *et al.* (2004) Molecular epidemiology of *Pseudomonas aerginosa*, *Burkholderia cepacia* complex and methicillin-resistant *Staphylocccocus aureus* in a cystic fibrosis centre. *J Cyst Fibros*, 3(30), 159–63.

Candel, F.J. *et al.* (2005) Bacteremia and septic shock after solid-organ transplantation. *Transplant Proc*, 37(99), 4097–9.

Carmona, E.M. *et al.* (2006) Pneumocystis cell wall beta-glucans induce dentritic cell costimulatory molecule expression and inflammatory activation through a Fas-Fas ligand mechanism. *J Immunol*, 177(1), 459–67.

Casemore, D.P. (1998) *Cryptosporidium* and the safety of our water supplies. *Commun Dis Public Health*, 1(4), 218–19.

Casolari, C. *et al.* (2005) A simultaneous outbreak of *Serratia marcescens* and *Klebsiella pneumoniae* in a neonatal intensive care unit. *J Hosp Infect*, 61(4), 312–20.

Casper, C. & Wald, A. (2002) Condom use and the prevention of genital herpes acquisition. *Herpes*, 9(1), 10–14.

Castognola, E. *et al.* (2006) Fungal infections in children with cancer: a prospective, multicenter surveillance study. *Pediatr Infect Dis J*, 25(7), 634–9.

Catalano, G. *et al.* (2003) Anxiety and depression in hospitalized patients in resistant organism isolation. *South Med J*, 96(2), 141–5.

CDC (1992) Revised classification system for HIV infection and expanded surveillance case definition for AIDS among adolescents and adults. *MMWR Morb Mortal Wkly Rep*, 41, 1–19.

CDC (2003) Guidelines for environmental infection control healthcare facilities. *MMWR Morb Mortal Wkly Rep*, 52(RR10), 1–42.

CDC (2005) Guidelines for preventing the transmission of *Mycobacterium tuberculosis* in health care setting. *MMWR Morb Mortal Wkly Rep*, 54(RR17), 1–141.

CDC (2006) Rapid HIV test distribution – United States, 2003–2005. *MMWR Morb Mortal Wkly Rep*, 55(24), 673–6.

Cepeda, J.A. *et al.* (2005) Isolation of patients in single rooms or cohorts to reduce spread of MRSA in intensive-care units: prospective two-centre study. *Lancet*, 365(9456), 295–304.

Chang, B. *et al.* (2004) Quality of life in tuberculosis: a review of the English language literature. *Qual Life Res*, 10, 1633–42.

Chattopadhyay, B. (2001) Control of infection wards: are they worthwhile? *J Hosp Infect*, 47(2), 88–90.

Chaudhury, H., Mahmood, A. & Valente, M. (2006) Nurses perception of single-occupancy versus multioccupancy rooms in a city care environment: an exploratory comparative assessment. *Appl Nurs Res*, 19(3), 118–25.

Chen, C.Y. *et al.* (2004) Trends and antimicrobial resistance of pathogens causing bloodstream infection among febrile neutropenic adults with hematological malignancy. *J Formos Med Assoc*, 103(7), 526–632.

Chen, L. & Lee, C. (2006) Distinguishing HIV-1 drug resistance, accessory, and viral fitness mutations using conditional selection pressure analysis of treated versus untreated patients' samples. *Biol Direct*, 1(1), 14–30.

Chia, S.E. *et al.* (2005) Appropriate use of personal protective equipment among healthcare workers in public sector hospitals and primary healthcare polyclinics during the SARS outbreak in Singapore. *Occup Environ Med*, 62(7), 473–7.

Chodick, G., Ashkenazi, S. & Lerman, Y. (2006) The risk of hepatitis A infection among healthcare workers: a review of reported outbreaks and sero-epidemiologic studies. *J Hosp Infect*, 62(4), 414–20.

Clavel, F. *et al.* (1986) Isolation of a new human retrovirus from West African patients with AIDS. *Science*, 233, 343–6.

Coaquette, A. *et al.* (2004) Mixed cytomegalovirus glycoproteins B genotypes in immunocompromised patients. *Clin Infect Dis*, 39(2), 155–61.

Codeluppi, M. *et al.* (2005) Rituximab as treatment of posttransplant lymphoproliferative disorder in patients who underwent small bowel/multivisceral transplantation: report of three cases. *Transplant Proc*, 37(6), 2634–5.

Coia, J.E. *et al.* (2006) Guidelines for the control and prevention of methicillin-resistant *Staphylococcus aureus* (MRSA) in healthcare facilities by the joint BSAC/HIS/ICNA working party on MRSA. *J Hosp Infect*, 63(Suppl 1), S1–44.

Communicable Disease Surveillance Centre (2002a) *HIV and AIDS in the UK in 2001*. Public Health Laboratory Service, London.

Communicable Disease Report (CDR) (2002b) First report of the Department of Health's mandatory MRSA Bacteremia Surveillance Scheme in acute NHS Trusts in England April to September 2001. *CDC Weekly* Public Health Laboratory Service, London., 12(6), 1–15.

Conaty, S.J. *et al.* (2005) Women who decline antenatal screening for HIV infection in the era of universal testing: results of an audit of uptake in three London Hospitals. *J Public Health (Oxf)*, 27(1), 114–7.

Cookson, B.D. *et al.* (2006) Guidelines for the control of glycopeptide-resistant enterococci in hospital. *J Hosp Infect*, 62(1), 6–21.

Cooper, E.E. *et al.* (2003) Influence of building construction work on *Aspergillus* infection in a hospital setting. *Infect Control Hosp Epidemiol*, 24(7), 472–6.

Corkill, J.E., Anson, J.J. & Hart, C.A. (2005) High prevalence of the plasmid-mediated quinolone resistance determinant qnrA in multi-drug resistant Enterobacteriaceae from blood cultures in Liverpool, UK. *J Antimicrob Chemother*, 56(6), 1115–17.

Cotterill S. *et al.* (1996) An unusual source for the outbreak of methicillin resistant *Staphylococcus aureus* on an intensive therapy unit. *J Hosp Infect*, 329(3), 207–16.

Coupe, S. *et al.* (2006) Detection of *Cryptosporidium*, *Giardia* and *Enterocytozoon bieneusi* in surface water, including recreational areas: a 1-year prospective study. *FEMS Immunol Med Microbiol*, 47(3), 351–9.

Creedon, S.A. (2005) Healthcare workers hand decontamination practices: compliance with recommended guidelines. *J Adv Nurs*, **51**(3), 208–16.

Creeson, S.A. (2006) Health care workers hand decontamination practices: an Irish study. *Clin Nurs Res*, **15**(1), 6–26.

Crimi, P. *et al.* (2006) Correlation between *Legionella* contamination in water and surrounding air. *Infect Control Hosp Epidemiol*, **27**(7), 771–3.

Croner (1998) *Health Service Risk Management and Practice Special Report.* www.croner.co.uk

Crowcroft, N.S. & Catchpole, M. (2002) Mortality from methicillin resistant *Staphylococcus aureus* in England and Wales: analysis of death certificates. *Br Med J*, **325**(7377), 1390–1.

Cunha, B.A. (1998) Nosocomial diarrhoea. *Crit Care Clin*, **14**(2), 329–38.

Cunha, B.A. (2006) The atypical pneumonias: clinical diagnosis and importance. *Clin Microbiol Infect*, **12**(Suppl 3), 12–24.

Cunningham, J.B., Kernohan, W.G. & Rush, T. (2005) Bed occupancy, turnover intervals and MRSA rates in English hospitals. *Br J Nurs*, **15**(12), 656–60.

Custovic, A. *et al.* (1998) Domestic allergens in public places. *Clin Exp Allergy*, **28**(1), 53–9.

Cuthbert, J.A. (2001) Hepatitis A: old and new. *Clin Microbiol Rev*, **14**(1), 38–58.

Dadd, G., McMinn, P. & Monterosso, L. (2003) Protective isolation in hemopoietic stem cell transplants: a review of the literature and single institution experience. *J Pediatr Oncol Nurs*, **20**(6), 293–300.

Dale, D.C. & Liles, C. (1998) How many neutrophils are enough? *Lancet*, **351**(9118), 1752–3.

Dale, J.W. *et al.* (2005) Origins and properties of *Mycobacterium tuberculosis* isolates in London. *J Med Microbiol*, **54**, 575–82.

Danaher, E.H. *et al.* (2006) Fatigue and physical activity in patients undergoing hematopoietic stem cell transplant. *Oncol Nurs Forum*, **33**(3), 614–24.

Dancer, S., Raeside, J. & Boothman, M. (2002) Environmental organisms from different hospital wards. *Br J Infect Control*, **3**(94), 10–14.

Dancer, S.J. *et al.* (2006) Antibiotic use is associated with resistance of environmental organisms in a teaching hospital. *J Hosp Infect*, **62**(2),200–6.

Davidson, M.M., Evans, R. & Hay, A.J. (2006) Same day detection of methicillin-resistant *Staphylococcus aureus* from screening swabs by real time polymerase chain reaction. *J Hosp Infect*, **62** (4), 484–5.

Davis, M.M. (2006) Successes and remaining challenges after 10 years of varicella vaccination in the USA. *Expert Rev Vaccines*, **5**(2), 295–302.

Dawson, D. (2005) Foodborne protozoan parasites. *Int J Food Microbiol*, **103**(2), 207–27.

Dawson, S. *et al.* (2006) *Listeria* outbreak associated with sandwich consumption from a hospital retail shop, United Kingdom. *Euro Surveill*, **11**(6), 89–91.

De la Rua-Domenech, R. (2006) Human *Mycobacterium bovis* infection in the United Kingdom: incidence, risks, control measures and review of the zoonotic aspects of bovine tuberculosis. *Tuberculosis (Edinb)*, **86**(2):77–109.

De Lorenzi, S. *et al.* (2006) Comparison of floor sanitation methods. *J Hosp Infect*, **62**(3), 346–8.

De Schryver, A. *et al.* (1999) Risk of cytomegalovirus infection among educators and health care personnel serving mentally disabled children. *J Infect*, **38**(1), 36–40.

De Souza, W. & Benchimol, M. (2005) Basic biology of *Pneumocystis carinii*: a mini review. *Mem Inst Oswaldo Cruz*, **100**(8), 903–8.

De Vries, G., Sebek, M.M. & Lambregts-van Weezenbeek, C.S. (2006) Health care workers with tuberculosis infected during work in the Netherlands. *Eur Respir J*, **28**(6), 1216–21.

Declerck, P. *et al.* (2006) Detection and quantification of *Legionella pneumophila* in water samples using competitive PCR. *Can J Microbiol*, **52**(6), 584–90.

Deeks, S.G. (2006) Antiretroviral treatment of HIV infected adults *BMJ*, **332**, 1489.

DeMille, D. *et al.* (2006) The effect of the neutropenic diet in the outpatient setting: a pilot study. *Oncol Nurs Forum*, **33**(2), 337–43.

de Roux, A. *et al.* (2006) Impact of alcohol abuse in the etiology and severity of community-acquired pneumonia. *Chest*, **129**(5), 1219–25.

DH (1995a) *Hospital Laundry Arrangements for Used and Infected Linen.* Department of Health, London.

DH (1995b) *Hepatitis C and Blood Transfusion Look Back.* PL CMO (95)1. HMSO, London.

DH (1995c) *Hospital Infection Control, Guidance on the Control of Infection in Hospitals.* 2383 IP 25K. Health Publications Unit, Heywood, Lancashire.

DH (1996a) *Guidelines for Pre-Test Discussion on HIV Testing.* HMSO, London.

DH (1998a) *Management and Control of Viral Haemorrhagic Fevers. Summary of Guidance from the Advisory Committee on Dangerous Pathogens.* 12491 HP 14k 1P Mar 98 (MUL). HMSO, London.

DH (1998b) *Standing Medical Advisory Committee, Sub Group on Antimicrobial Resistance. The Path of Least Resistance.* HMSO, London.

DH (1998c) Third Report of the Group of Experts (1998) *Cryptosporidium in Water Supplies.* Department of the Environment, Transport and the Regions, and Department of Health, London.

DH (1998d) *The Prevention and Control of Tuberculosis in the United Kingdom.* HSC 1998/196. HMSO, London.

DH (2000a) *HIV Post Exposure Prophylaxis: Guidance from the UK Chief Medical Officer' Expert Advisory Group on AIDS.* Department of Health, London.

DH (2000b) *United Kingdom Antimicrobial Resistance Strategy and Action Plan.* Department of Health, London.

DH (2001a) Standard principles for preventing hospital-acquired infections. *J Hosp Infect*, **47**(Suppl), S21–37.

DH (2001b) *The Essence of Care: Patients Focused Benchmarking for Health Care Practitioners.* Department of Health, London.

DH (2002a) *Hepatitis C for England Strategy.* HMSO, London.

DH (2002b) *Getting Ahead of the Curve. A Strategy for Combating Infectious Diseases (Including Other Aspects of Health Promotion).* HMSO, London.

DH (2003a) *Winning Ways. Working Together to Reduce Healthcare Associated Infection in England.* Department of Health, London.

DH (2003b) *National Clostridium difficile Standards Group. Report to the Department of Health, February 2003.* Department of Health, London.

DH (2003c) *Health Clearance for Serious Communicable Diseases: New Health Care Workers.* Department of Health, London.

DH (2003d) *Transmissible Spongiform Encephalopathy Agents: Safe Working and Prevention of Infection.* Department of Health, London.

DH (2004a) *Towards Cleaner Hospitals and Lower Rates of Infection.* Department of Health, London.

DH (2004b) *Matrons Charter, an Action Plan for Cleaner Hospitals.* Department of Health, London.

DH (2004c) *Children in Need and Blood-borne Viruses: HIV and Hepatitis.* Department of Health, London.

134

DH (2004d) *The Carriage of Dangerous Goods (Classification, Packaging and Labelling) and Use of Transportable Pressure Receptacles Regulations*. SI 2004, No. 568. Department of Health, London.

DH (2005a) *Saving Lives: A Delivery Programme to Reduce Healthcare Associated Infection including MRSA*. Department of Health, London.

DH (2005b) *HIV-infected Healthcare Workers: Guidance on Management and Patient Notification*. Department of Health, London.

DH (2005c) *Hazardous waste (England) regulations*. Department of Health, London.

DH (2006a) *Environment and sustainability Health Technical Memorandum 07-01: Safe management of healthcare waste*. Department of Health, London.

DH (2006b) *Immunisation Against Infectious Disease*. HMSO, London.

DH (2006c) *Water systems Health technical memorandum 04-01: The control of legionella, hygiene, "safe" hot water, cold water and drinking water systems*. Department of Health, Leeds

DH (2006d) *Infection Control Guidance for Care Homes*. Department of Health, London.

Dhaliwal, J. & McGeer, A. (2005) *Does Isolation Prevent the Spread of Methicillin-resistant Staphylococcus aureus?* CMAJ, **172**(7), 875.

Dharan S. *et al.* (1999) Routine disinfection of patients' environmental surfaces. Myth or reality. *J Hosp Infect*, **42**(2), 113–7.

Dial, S. *et al.* (2004) Risk of *Clostridium difficile* diarrhea among hospital patients prescribed proton pump inhibitors: cohort and case-control studies. *CMAJ*, **171**(1), 3–38.

Diamond, C. *et al.* (2005) Increased incidence of squamous cell anal cancer among men with AIDS in the era of highly active antiretroviral therapy. *Sex Transm Dis*, **32**(5), 314–20.

Diamond, C. *et al.* (2006a) Changes in acquired immunodeficiency syndrome-related non-Hodgkin lymphoma in the era of highly active antiretroviral therapy: incidence, presentation, treatment and survival. *Cancer*, **106**(1), 128–35.

Diamond, C. *et al.* (2006b) Highly active antiretroviral therapy is associated with improved survival among patients with IDS-related primary central nervous system non-Hodgkin's lymphoma. *Curr HIV Res*, **4**(3), 375–8.

Diaz-Pedroche, C. *et al.* (2006) Valganciclovir preemptive therapy for the prevention of cytomegalovirus disease in high-risk seropositive solid-organ transplant recipients. *Transplantation*, **82**(1), 30–5.

Dick, L. (1998) Travel medicine: helping patients prepare for trips abroad. *Am Fam Physician*, **58**(2), 383–98.

Diederen, B.M. & Peeters, M.F. (2006) Evaluation of two new immunochromatographic assays (rapid U *Legionella* antigen test and SD Bioline *Legionella* antigen test) for detection of *Legionella pneumophila* serogroup 1 antigen in urine. *J Clin Microbiol*, **44**(8), 2991–3.

Dietze, B. *et al.* (2001) Survival of MRSA on sterile goods packaging. *J Hosp Infect*, **49**(4), 255–61.

Ditchburn, I. (2006) Should doctors wear ties? *J Hosp Infect*, **63**(2), 227–8.

Donohue, R. (2006) Development and implementation of a risk assessment tool for chemotherapy-induced neutropenia. *Oncol Nurs Forum*, **33**(2), 347–52.

Duff, P. (1998) Hepatitis in pregnancy. *Semin Perinatol*, **22**(4), 277–83.

Duquette-Petersen L. *et al.* (1999) The role of protective clothing in infection prevention in patients undergoing autologous bone marrow transplantation. *Oncol Nurs Forum*, **26**(8), 1319–24.

Dyer, C. (2004) Payments announced for patients infected with hepatitis C. *BMJ*, **328**, 246.

Dykewicz, C.A. (2001) Hospital infection control in hematopoietic stem cell transplant recipients. *Emerg Infect Dis*, **7**(2), 263–7.

Editorial (2002) Transfusion transmission of HCV infection before anti-HCV testing of blood donations in England: results of the national HCV Lookback program. *Transfusion*, **42**(9), 1146–53.

Ehlert, K. *et al.* (2006) Treatment of refractory CMV-infection following hematopoietic stem cell transplantation with the combination of foscarnet and leflunomide. *Klin Padiatr*, **218**(3), 180–4.

Ejidokun, O.O. *et al.* (2000) Four linked outbreaks of *Salmonella enteritidis* phage type 4 infection: the continuing egg threat. *Commun Dis Public Health*, **3**(2), 95–100.

Elinav, E. *et al.* (2006) Acute hepatitis A infection in pregnancy is associated with high rates of gestational complications and preterm labor. *Gastroenterology*, **130**(4), 1129–34.

Ellett, M.L. (1999) Hepatitis A, B, and D. *Gastroenterol Nurs*, **22**(6), 236–44.

Elliott, S.K., Keeton, A. & Holt, A. (2005) Medical students' knowledge of sharps injuries. *J Hosp Infect*, **60**(4), 374–7.

El-Mahallawy, H.A. *et al.* (2004) Epidemiologic profile of symptomatic gastroenteritis in pediatric oncology patients receiving chemotherapy. *Pediatr Blood Cancer*, **42**(4), 338–42.

Emerson, S.U., Arankalle, V.A. & Purcell, R.H. (2005) Thermal stability of hepatitis E virus. *J Infect Dis*, **1**(295), 930–3.

Engelhart, S. *et al.* (2002) Surveillance for nosocomial infections and fever of unknown origin among adult hematology–oncology patients. *Infect Control Hosp Epidemiol*, **23**(5), 244–8.

Errico, A. *et al.* (1999) Survey of measures for the prevention of infection in bone marrow transplantation centers. *Assist Inferm Ric*, **18**(2), 80–6.

European Standard EN 149 (2001) *Respiratory protective devices, filtering half masks to protect against particles. Requirements, testing, marking*. www.bsi-global.com/en/

Evans, B.G. *et al.* (1991) HIV 2 in the United Kingdom. A review. *Commun Dis Rep*, **1**(2), R19–32.

Evans, H.L. *et al.* (2003) Contact isolation in surgical patients: a barrier to care? *Surgery*, **134**(2), 180–8.

Evans, H.S. *et al.* (1998) General outbreaks of infectious intestinal disease in England and Wales, 1995–1996. *Commun Dis Public Health*, **1**(3), 165–71.

Eveillard, M. *et al.* (2001) Evaluation of the contribution of isolation precautions in prevention and control of multi-resistant bacteria in a teaching hospital. *J Hosp Infect*, **47**(2), 116–24.

Eveillard, M. *et al.* (2002) Prevalence of methicillin resistant *Staphylococcus aureus* carriage at the time of admission in two acute geriatric wards. *J Hosp Infect*, **50**(2), 122–6.

Fafi-Kremer, S. *et al.* (2005a) A prospective follow-up of Epstein–Barr virus LMP1 genotypes in saliva and blood during infectious mononucleosis. *J Infect Dis*, **192**(12), 2108–11.

Fafi-Kremer, S. *et al.* (2005b) Long-term shedding of infectious Epstein–Barr virus after infectious mononucleosis. *J Infect Dis*, **191**(6), 985–9.

Fairclough, S.J. (2006) Why tackling MRSA needs a comprehensive approach. *Br J Nurs*, **15**(2), 72–5.

Falcone, M. *et al.* (2004) Methicillin-resistant *Staphylococcus* bacteremia in patients with hematologic malignancies: clinical and microbiological retrospective comparative analysis of *S. haemolyticus*, *S epidermidis* and *S Aureus*. *J Chemother*, **16**(6), 540–8.

Farrington M. & Pascoe G. (2001) Risk management and infection control-time to get our priorities right in the United Kingdom. *J Hosp Infect*, **47**(1), 19–24.

Farrington M. *et al.* (2000) Effects on nursing workload of different methicillin-resistant *Staphylococcus aureus* (MRSA) control measures. *J Hosp Infect*, **46**(2), 118–22.

Fawley, W.N. *et al.* (2005) Molecular epidemiology of endemic *Clostridium difficile* significance of subtypes of the United Kingdom Epidemic (Ribotype 1). *J Clin Microbiol*, 43(6), 2685–96.

Fawley, W.N. *et al.* (2006) Surveillance for mupirocin resistance following introduction of routine peri-operative prophylaxis with nasal mupirocin. *J Hosp Infect*, 62(3), 327–32.

Felmingham, D. (2004) Comparative antimicrobial susceptibility of respiratory tract. *Chemotherapy*, 50(Suppl 1), 3–10.

Fields, B.S., Benson, R.F. & Besser, R.E. (2002) *Legionella* and Legionnaires' disease: 25 years of investigation. *Clin Microbiol Rev*, 15(3), 506–26.

File, T.M. (2006) Clinical implications and treatment of multiresistant *Streptococcus pneumoniae* pneumonia. *Clin Microbiol Infect*, 12(Suppl 3), 31–41.

Fillet, A.M. (2002) Prophylaxis of herpesvirus infections in immunocompetent and immunocompromised older patients. *Drugs Aging*, 19(5), 343–54.

Fiore, A.E. (2004) Hepatitis A transmitted by food. *Clin Infect Dis*, 1(38; 5), 705–15.

Fiore, A.E., Wasley, A. & Bell, B.P. (2006) Prevention of hepatitis A through active or passive immunization: recommendations of the advisory committee on immunization practices (ACIP). *MMWR Recomm Rep*, 55, RR-701–23.

Fitzpatrick, F. *et al.* (2000) A purpose built MRSA cohort unit. *J Hosp Infect*, 46(4), 271–9.

Flandre, P. *et al.* (2006) Analyzing plasma HIV-1 RNA measurements as multiple recurrent events in clinical trials. *HIV Clin Trials*, 7(3), 116–24.

Fleming, K. & Randle, J. (2006) Toys – friend or foe? A study of infection risk in a paediatric intensive care unit. *Paediatr Nurs*, 18(4), 14–18.

Flessa, S., Lusk, D.M. & Harris, L.J. (2005) Survival of *Listeria monocytogenes* on fresh and frozen strawberries. *Int J Food Microbiol*, 101(3), 255–62.

Food Standards Agency (2006) *Food Hygiene Legislation*. www.foodstandards.gov.uk

Forns, X. & Bukh, J. (1998) Methods for determining the hepatitis C virus genotype. *Viral Hep Rev*, 4(1), 1–19.

Fowler, K.B. & Pass, R.F. (2006) Risk factors for congenital cytomegalovirus infection in the offspring of young women: exposure to young children and recent onset of sexual activity. *Pediatrics*, 118(2), 286–92.

Franca, P.H. *et al.* (2004) Strong association between Genotype F and hepatitis B antigen-negative variants among HBV-infected Argentinians. *J Clin Microbiol*, 42(11), 5015–21.

Franco, E. *et al.* (2003) Risk groups for hepatitis A virus infection. *Vaccine*, 21(19–20), 2224–33.

Fraser, D.W. *et al.* (1977) Legionnaires' disease: description of an epidemic of pneumonia. *N Engl J Med*, 297, 1189–97.

Freije, M.R. (2004) The word of water: new CDC guidelines recommend a proactive approach to *Legionella*. *Health Facil Manage*, 17(10), 33–4.

French, G.L. (1998) Enterococci and vancomycin resistance. *Clin Infect Dis*, 27(Suppl 1), S75–83.

Friberg, B. *et al.* (2001) Surgical area contamination comparable bacterial counts using disposable head and mask and helmet aspirator system, but dramatic increase upon omission of head-gear: an experimental study in horizontal laminar air-flow. *J Hosp Infect*, 47(2), 110–15.

Fryklund, B. *et al.* (1997) Transmission of urinary bacterial strains between patients with indwelling catheters nursing in the same room and in separate rooms compared. *J Hosp Infect*, 36, 147–53.

Fuda, C. *et al.* (2004) The basis for resistance to beta-lactam antibiotics by penicillin-binding protein 2 a of methicillin-resistant *Staphylococcus aureus*. *J Biol Chem*, 279(39), 40802–6.

Gaber, K.A. *et al.* (2005) An outbreak of tuberculosis in the South West of England related to a public house. *Prim Care Respir J*, 14(1), 51–5.

Gal, A.A. *et al.* (2002) Granulomatous *Pneumocystis carnii* pneumonia complicating hematopoietic cell transplantation. *Pathol Res Pract*, 198(8), 553–8.

Galadari, I. & Fowzan, A.W. (2006) A comparative study between viral isolates and indirect immunofluorescence in diagnosis of herpes simplex virus. *Allerg Immunol*, 38(2), 62–4.

Gales, C. *et al.* (2006) Emergence of linezolid-resistant *Staphylococcus aureus* during treatment of pulmonary infection in a patient with cystic fibrosis. *Int J Antimicrob Agents*, 27(4), 300–2.

Gamble, M.J. (2005) Using the modern charter to improve hospital cleaning. *Nurs Times*, 101(15), 26–7.

Gammon, J. (1999) The psychological consequences of source isolation: a review of the literature. *J Clin Nurs*, 8(1), 13–21.

Garner, J.S. (1996a) Guidelines for isolation precautions in hospitals. Part 1: evaluation of isolation practices. Hospital Infection Control Practices Advisory Committee. *Am J Infect Control*, 24(1), 24–31.

Garner, J.S. (1996b) Guidelines for isolation precautions in hospitals. Hospital Infection Control Practices Advisory Committee. *Am J Infect Control*, 17(1), 53–80.

Garner, J.S. & Simmons, B.P. (1983) CDC guidelines for isolation precautions in hospital. *Infect Control*, 4(4), 245–325.

Garrouste-Orgeas, M. *et al.* (2000) A 1 year prospective study of nosocomial bacteraemia in ICU and non ICU patients and its impact on patient outcome. *J Hosp Infect*, 44(3), 206–13.

Gastmeier, P. *et al.* (2005) Mortality risk factors with nosocomial *Staphylococcus aureus* infections in intensive care units: results from the German Nosocomial Infection Surveillance System (KISS). *Infection*, 33(2), 50–5.

Gastmeier, P. *et al.* (2006) Correlation between genetic diversity of nosocomial pathogens and their survival time in intensive care units. *J Hosp Infect*, 62(2), 181–6.

Gellaitry, G. *et al.* (2005) Patients' perception of information about HAART: impact on treatment decisions. *AIDS Care*, 17(3), 367–76.

Gerberding, J.L. (1998) Nosocomial transmission of opportunistic infections. *Infect Control Hosp Epidemiol*, 19(8), 574–7.

Gezairy, H.A. (2003) Travel epidemiology: WHO perspective. *Int J Antimicrob Agents*, 21(2), 86–8.

Gheorghe, L. *et al.* (2005) Natural history of compensated viral B and D cirrhosis. *Rom J Gastroenterol*, 14(4), 329–35.

Gianfranceschi, M. *et al.* (2006) Listeriosis associated with gorgonzola (Italian blue-veined cheese). *Foodborne Pathog Dis*, 3(2), 105–9.

Gibb, A.P., Fleck, B.W. & Kepton-Smith, L. (2006) A cluster of deep bacterial infections following eye surgery associated with construction dust. *J Hosp Infect*, 63(2), 197–200.

Gigliotti, F. & Wright, T.W. (2005) Immunopathogenesis of *Pneumocystis carinii* pneumonia. *Exper Rev Mol Med*, 7(26), 1–16.

Gill, J. *et al.* (2006) Methicillin resistant *Staphylococcus aureus*: awareness and perceptions. *J Hosp Infect*, 62(3), 333–7.

Gillespie, I.A. *et al.* (2001) General outbreak of infectious intestinal disease associated with fish and shell fish, England and Wales, 1992–1999. *Commun Dis Public Health*, 4(2), 117–23.

Gillespie, I.A. *et al.* (2005) Foodborne general outbreaks of *Salmonella enteritidis* phage type 4 infection, England and Wales, 1992–2002: where are the risks? *Epidemiol Infect*, 133(5), 795–801.

Gillespie, I.A. *et al.* (2006) Investigating vomiting and/or bloody diarrhoea in *Campylobacter jejuni* infection. *J Med Microbiol*, 55(6), 741–6.

Girou, E. *et al.* (2004) Misuse of gloves: the foundation for poor compliance with hand hygiene and potential for microbial transmission. *J Hosp Infect*, **57**(2), 162–9.

Glasmacher, A. & Prentice, A.G. (2005) Evidence-based review of antifungal prophylaxis in neutropenic patients with haematological malignancies. *J Antimicrob Chemother*, **56**(Suppl 1), 123–32.

Glauser, M.P. & Calandra, T. (2000) Infections on patients with hematologic malignancies. In: *Management of Infections in Immunocompromised Patients*, Part II, Chapter 4 (eds M.P. Glauser & P.A. Pizzo). W.B. Saunders, London, pp. 141–88.

Goldie, S.J. *et al.* (2002) Prophylaxis for human immunodeficiency virus-related Pneumocystis cariniii pneumonia: using simulation modelling to inform clinical guidelines. *Arch Intern Med*, **162**(8), 921–8.

Golec, M. *et al.* (2004) Immunologic reactivity to work-related airborne allergens in people occupationally exposed to dust from herbs. *Ann Agric Environ Med*, **11**(1), 121–7.

Gomes, S.A. *et al.* (2004) Uncommon mutation pattern of a hepatitis B virus isolate from genotype F infection a patient with AIDS. *J Infect*, **48**(1), 102–8.

Gona, P. *et al.* (2006) Incidence of opportunistic and other infections in HIV-infected children in the HAART era. *JAMA*, **296**(3), 292–300.

Gottschalk, S., Roomey, C.M. & Heslop, H.E. (2005) Post-transplant lymphoproliferative disorders. *Annu Rev Med*, **56**, 29–44.

Gould, D. (2005) Infection control: the environment and service organisation. *Nurs Stand*, **20**(5), 57–65.

Gowland, P. *et al.* (2004) Molecular and serologic tracing of a transfusion-transmitted hepatitis A virus. *Transfusion*, **44**(11), 1555–61.

Graczyk, T.K. *et al.* (2004) Mechanical transmission of *Cryptosporidium parvum* oocysts by flies. *Wiad Parazytol*, **50**(2), 243–7.

Greub, G., Koh, A. & Calandra, T. (2000) Practical guide to antimicrobial agents commonly used in the immunocompromised patients. In: *Management of Infections in Immunocompromised Patients*, Vol. 2(3), (eds M.P. Glauser & P.A. Pizzo). W.B. Saunders, London, pp. 33–42.

Griffith, C.J. *et al.* (2000) An evaluation of hospital cleaning regimes and standards. *J Hosp Infect*, **45**(1), 19–28.

Griffiths, P.D. (2006) CMV as a cofactor enhancing progression of AIDS. *J Clin Virol*, **35**(4), 489–92.

Grunfeld, E. *et al.* (2005) Job stress and job satisfaction of cancer care workers. *Psychooncology*, **14**(1), 61–9.

Gunsar, F. *et al.* (2005) Two-year interferon therapy with or without ribavirin in chronic delta hepatitis. *Antivir Ther*, **10**(6), 721–6.

Hadziyannis, S.J. (1997) Review: hepatitis delta. *J Gastroenterol Hepatol*, **12**(4), 289–98.

Hahn, T. *et al.* (2002) Efficacy of high-efficiency particulate air filtration in preventing aspergillosis in immunocompromised patients with hematologic malignancies. *Infection Control Hosp Epidemiol*, **23**(9), 525–31.

Hahne, S. *et al.* (2003) Hepatitis B incidence among South Asian children in England and Wales: implications for immunisation policy. *Arch Dis Child*, **88**, 1082–3.

Hahne, S. *et al.* (2004) Incidence and routes of transmission of hepatitis B virus in England and Wales, 1995–2000: implications for immunisation policy. *J Clin Virol*, **29**(4), 211–20.

Hall, J. & Sutton, A. (2002) Non-HIV nurses knowledge of HIV therapy. *Nurs Stand*, **16**(43), 33–6.

Hamid, S.S. *et al.* (2002) Heptitis E virus super infection in patients with chronic liver disease. *Hepatology*, **36**(2), 474–8.

Hansel, N.N. *et al.* (2004) Quality of life in tuberculosis: patient and provider perspectives. *Qual Life Res*, **13**(3), 639–52.

Haque, T. *et al.* (1997) A prospective study in heart and lung transplant recipients correlating persistent Epstein–Barr virus infection with clinical events. *Transplantation*, **64**(7), 1028–34.

Harris, H.E. *et al.* (2000) The HCV national register: towards informing the natural history of hepatitis C infection in the UK. *J Viral Hepat*, **7**(6), 420–7.

Hauggaard, A., Ellis, M. & Ekelund, L. (2002) Early chest radiography and CT in the diagnosis management and outcome of invasive pulmonary aspergillosis. *Acta Radiol*, **43**(3), 292–8.

Hawkyard, C. & Bignardi, G.E. (2006) Has the severity of *Clostridium difficile* infection increased? *J Hosp Infect*, **63**(1), 111–12.

Hayden, M.K. *et al.* (2006) Reduction in acquisition of vancomycin-resistant enterococcus after enforcement of routine environmental cleaning measures. *Clin Infect Dis*, **42**(11), 1552–60.

Hayes-Lattin, B., Leis, J.F. & Maziarz, R.T. (2005) Isolation in the allogeneic transplant environment: how protective is it? *Bone Marrow Transplant*, **36**(5), 373–81.

Haynes, B.F. & Montefiori, D.C. (2006) Aiming to induce broadly reactive neutralizing antibody responses with HIV-1 vaccine candidates. *Expert Rev Vaccines*, **5**(3), 347–63.

He, Z. *et al.* (2003) Retrospective analysis of non-A–E hepatitis: possible role of hepatitis B and C virus infection. *J Med Virol*, **69**(1), 59–65.

Healing, T.D. *et al.* (1995) The infection hazards of human cadavers. *Commun Dis Rep*, **5**, R61–9.

Health Protection Agency (2006) www.hpa.org.uk. Accessed 26/11/06.

Heinonen, H. *et al.* (2005) Stress among allogeneic bone marrow transplantation patients. *Patient Educ Couns*, **56**(1), 62–71.

Heldal, E. *et al.* (2003) Risk factors for recent transmission of *Mycobacterium tuberculosis*. *Eur Respir J*, **22**(4), 637–42.

Hemsworth, S. & Pizer, B. (2006) Pet ownership in immunocompromised children – a review of the literature and survey of existing guidelines. *Eur J Oncol Nurs*, **10**(2), 117–27.

Henderson, D.K. (2006) Managing methicillin-resistant staphylococci: a paradigm for preventing nosocomial transmission of resistant organisms. *Am J Infect Control*, **34**(5 Suppl), S46–54.

Henry, L. (1997) Immunocompromised patients and nutrition. *Prof Nurse*, **12**(9), 655–9.

Hewitt, J. & Greening, G.E. (2004) Survival and persistence of norovirus, hepatitis A virus, and feline calicivirus in marinated mussels. *J Food Prot*, **67**(8), 1743–50.

Highleyman, L. (2006) Nutrition and HIV. *BETA*, **18**(2), 18–32.

Hill, C., King, T. & Day, R. (2006) A strategy to reduce MRSA colonization of stethoscopes. *J Hosp Infect*, **62**(1), 122–3.

Hill, G. *et al.* (2005) Recent steroid therapy increases severity of varicella infections in children with acute lymphoblastic leukemia. *Pediatrics*, **116**(4), 525–9.

Ho, E.C., Patriar, S. & Corbridge, R. (2005) How we do it: blood contamination during management of epistaxis-awareness, utilization and availability of barrier protection. *Clin Otolaryngol*, **30**(1), 71–2.

Hodgson, I. (2006) Empathy, inclusion and enclaves: the culture of care of people with HIV/AIDS and nursing implications. *J Adv Nurs*, **55**(3), 283–90.

Hogg, R.S. *et al.* (2006) Emergence of drug resistance is associated with an increase risk of death among patients first starting HAART. *PLoS Med*, **3**(19), 1–18.

Hohenthal, U. *et al.* (2005) Bronchoalveolar lavage in immunocompromised patients with haematological malignancy-value of new microbiological methods. *Eur J Haematol*, **74**(3), 203–11.

Holmes, R.D. & Sokol, R.J. (2002) Epstein–Barr virus and post-transplant lymphoproliferative disease. *Pediatr Transplant*, **6**(6), 456–64.

Horng, Y.T. *et al.* (2006) Development of an improved PCR–ICT hybrid assay for direct detection of *Legionellae* and *Legionella pneumophila* from cooling tower water specimens. *Water Res*, 40(11), 2219–21.

Hota, B. (2004) Contamination, disinfection and cross-colonization: are hospital surfaces reservoirs for nosocomial infection. *Clin Infect Dis*, 39(8), 1182–9.

HSE (2000) *Legionnaires' Disease*. Health and Safety Executive, London.

HSE (2002) *Control of Substances Hazardous to Health (COSHH) Approved Code of Practice*. Health and Safety Executive, London.

HSE (2003a) *Five Steps to Risk Assessment*. Health and Safety Executive, London.

HSE (2003b) *Safe Working and the Prevention of Infection in Clinical laboratories and Similar Facilities*. Health and Safety Executive, London.

HSE (2005a) *Blood-borne Viruses in the Workplace. Guidance for Employers and Employees*. Health and Safety Executive, London.

HSE (2005b) *European Working Party for Legionella Infection*. Health and Safety Executive, London.

Hsu, Y.S. *et al.* (2002) Long term outcome after spontaneous HbeAg seroconversion in patients with chronic hepatitis B. *Hepatology*, 35(6), 1522–57.

Huber, M.A. (2003) Herpes simplex type-1 virus infection. *Quintessence Int*, 34(6), 453–67.

Humphreys, H. (2004) Positive-pressure isolation and the prevention of invasive aspergillosis. What is the evidence? *J Hosp Infect*, 56(2), 93–100.

Humphreys, H. (2005) On the wrong scent: banning fresh flowers from hospitals. *J Hosp Infect*, 62(94), 527–8.

Humphreys, H. (2006) Implementing guidelines for the control of methicillin-resistant *Staphylococcus aureus* and vancomycin-resistant enterococci: how valid are international comparisons of success? *J Hosp Infect*, 62(2), 133–5.

Hunter, P.R. & Syed, Q. (2002) A community survey of self-reported gastroenteritis undertaken during an outbreak of cryptosporidiosis strongly associated with drinking water after much press interest. *Epidemiol Infect*, 128(3), 433–8.

Hunter, P.R. & Thompson, R.C. (2005) The zoonotic transmission of *Giardia* and *Cryptosporidium*. *Int J Parasitol*, 35(11–12), 1181–90.

Husa, P. *et al.* (2005) Hepatitis D. *Acta Viron*, 49(4), 219–25.

ILSI Research Foundation; Risk Science Institute (2005) Achieving continuous improvement in reductions in foodborne listeriosis – a risk-based approach. *J Food Prot*, 68(9), 1032–94.

Insulander, M. *et al.* (2005) An outbreak of cryptosporidiosis associated with exposure to swimming pool water. *Scand J Infect Dis*, 37(5), 354–60.

Irshad, M. (1997) Hepatitis E virus: a global view of its seroepidemiology and transmission pattern. *Trop Gastroenterol*, 18(2), 45–9.

Irshad, M. *et al.* (2006) Transfusion-transmitted virus in associated with hepatitis A–E viral infections in various forms of liver diseases in India. *World J Gastroenterol*, 12(15), 2432–6.

Jabs, D.A. *et al.* (2006) Detection of ganciclovir resistance in patients with AIDS and cytomegalovirus retinitis: correlation of genotypic methods and viral phenotypes and clinical outcome. *J Infect Dis*, 193(12), 1728–37.

Jardi, R. *et al.* (2001) Quantitative detection of hepatitis B virus DNA in serum by a new rapid real-time fluorescence PCR assay. *J Viral Hepat*, 8(6), 465–71.

Jarrett, R.F. (2006) Viruses and lymphoma/leukaemia. *J Pathol*, 208(2), 176–86.

Jarrett, W.A., Ribes, J. & Manaligot, J.M. (2002) Biofilm formation on tracheostomy tubes. *Ear Nose Throat J*, 81(9), 659–61.

Jarvis, L.M. *et al.* (2006) Detection of HCV and HIV-1 antibody negative infections in Scottish and Northern Ireland blood donations by nucleic acid amplification testing. *Vox Sang*, 89(3), 128–34.

Jayshree, R.S. *et al.* (2006) Microscopic, cultural and molecular evidence of disseminated invasive aspergillosis involving the lungs and the gastrointestinal tract. *J Med Microbiol*, 55(Pt 7), 961–4.

Jenkins, R.O. & Sherburn, R.E. (2005) Growth and survival of bacteria implemented in sudden infant death syndrome on cot mattress material. *J Appl Microbiol*, 99(3), 573–9.

Jevons, M.P. (1961) Celberin resistant staphylococci. *Br Med J*, 1, 124–5.

Jindal, N. *et al.* (2005) HIV-1 infection in early seroconversion stage missed by rapid or ELISA tests – two case reports. *Indian J Pathol Microbiol*, 48(3), 395–6.

Johnson, E. *et al.* (2000) Preventing fungal infections in immuno-compromised patients. *Br J Nurs*, 9(17), 1154–64.

Johnson, P.D. *et al.* (2005) Efficacy of an alcoholic/chlorhexidine hand hygiene program in a hospital with high rates of nosocomial methicillin resistant *Staphylococcus aureus* (MRSA) infection. *Med J Aust*, 183(10), 509–14.

Jones, R.N. (2001) Resistance patterns among nosocomial pathogens: trends over the past few years. *Chest*, 119(2 Suppl), S397–404.

Kac, G. *et al.* (2005) Microbiological evaluation of two hand hygiene procedures achieved by healthcare workers during routine patients care: a randomized study. *J Hosp Infect*, 60(1), 32–9.

Kao, P.H. & Yang, R.J. (2006) Virus diffusion in isolation rooms. *H Hosp Infect*, 62(3), 338–45.

Kawamura, M. *et al.* (1989) HIV 2 in West Africa in 1966. *Lancet*, i, (8634), 385.

Kato, H. *et al.* (2001) Determination of hepatitis B virus genotype G by polymerase chain reaction with hemi-nested primers. *J Virol Methods*, 98(2), 153–9.

Kato, H. *et al.* (2002) Hepatitis B e antigen in sera from individuals infected with hepatitis B virus of genotype G. *Hepatology*, 35(4), 922–9.

Kato, H. *et al.* (2005) Classifying genotype F of hepataitis B virus into F1 and F2 subtypes. *World J Gastroenterol*, 11(40), 6295–304.

Kearnes, A.M., Freeman, R. & Lightfoot, N.F. (1995) Nosocomial enterococci; resistance to heat and sodium hypochlorite. *J Hosp Infect*, 30, 193–9.

Kedzierski, M. (1991) Understanding virology. *Prof Nurse*, 7(2), 99–102.

Kemp, C. & Stepp, L. (1995) Palliative care for patients with acquired immunodeficiency syndrome. *Am J Hosp Palliat Care*, 12(6), 14, 17–27.

Kempinska, A.M., Kwak, E.J. & Angel, J.B. (2005) Reactivation of hepatitis B infection following allogeneic bone marrow transplantation in a hepatitis B-immune patient: case report and review of the literature. *Clin Infect Dis*, 41(9), 1277–82.

Keogh, I.J. *et al.* (2001) Blood splash and tonsillectomy: an underestimated hazard to the otolaryngologist. *J Laryngol Otol*, 115(6), 455–6.

Kiang, K.M. *et al.* (2006) Recurrent outbreaks of cryptosporidiosis associated with calves among students at an educational farm programme in Minnesota. *Epidemiol Infect*, 134 (4), 878–86.

Kibbler, C.C., Quick, A. & O'Neil, A.M. (1998) The effect of increased bed numbers on MRSA transmission in acute medical wards. *J Hosp Infect*, 39, 213–19.

137

Kim, P.W. *et al.* (2003) Rates of hand disinfection associated with glove use, patient isolation and changes between exposure to various body sites. *Am J Infect Control*, 31(2), 97–103.

Kimberlin, D.W. (2005) Herpes simplex virus infections in neonates and early childhood. *Semin Pediatr Infect Dis*, 16(4), 271–81.

King, D. (2001) Ice machines – an audit of their use in clinical practice. *Commun Dis Public Health*, 4(1), 49–52.

Kirkup, B. (2002) Incident arising in October 2002 from a patient with Creutzfeldt–Jakob disease in Middlesbrough. Report of incident review. www.dh.gov.uk. Accessed 25/11/06.

Klassen, T.P. *et al.* (2005) Acyclovir for treating varicella in otherwise healthy children and adolescents. *Cochrane Database Syst Rev*, 4, CD002980.

Klein, G., Pack, A. & Reuter, G. (1998) Antibiotic resistance patterns of enterococci and occurrence of vancomycin-resistant enterococci in raw minced beef and pork in Germany. *Appl Environ Microbiol*, 64(5), 1825–30.

Klastersky, J. (2004) Management of fever in neutropenic patients with different risks of complications. *Clin Infect Dis*, 39(Suppl 1), S32–7.

Kleymann, G. (2003) Novel agents and strategies to treat herpes simplex virus infections. *Expert Opin Investig Drugs*, 12(2), 165–83.

Klont, R.R. *et al.* (2006) *Legionella pneumophilia* in commercial bottles water. *FEMS Immunol Med Microbiol*, 47(1), 42–4.

Knauer, A. *et al.* (2004) Effect of hospitalization and antimicrobial therapy on antimicrobial resistance of colonizing *Staphylococcus epidermidis*. *Wien Klin Wochenschr*, 116(14), 489–94.

Knysz, B. *et al.* (2005) Hepatitis D virus superinfection – a rare cause of occupational disease. *Med Pr*, 56(4), 317–18.

Koopmans, M. & Duizer, E. (2004) Food borne viruses: an emerging problem. *Int J Food Microbiol*, 90(1), 23–41.

Korniewicz, D.M. *et al.* (2005) Impact of converting to powder-free gloves. Decreasing the symptoms of latex exposure in operating room personnel. *AAOHN J*, 53(3), 111–16.

Koss, K. *et al.* (2006) The outcome of surgery in fulminant *Clostridium difficile* colitis. *Colorectal Dis*, 8(2), 149–54.

Krasuska, M.E. & Stanislawek, A. (2003) Communication with patients and their families, who undergo bone marrow transplantation. *Ann Univ Mariae Curie Sklodowska*, 58(2), 168–73.

Krasuska, M.E. *et al.* (2002) Information needs of the patients undergoing bone marrow transplantation. *Ann Univ Mariae Curie Sklodowska*, 57(2), 178–85.

Kriesel J.D. *et al.* (2005) Recurrent antiviral-resistant genital herpes in an immunocompetent patient. *J Infect Dis*, 192(1), 156–61.

Kruger, W.H. *et al.* (2001) Practices of infectious disease prevention and management during hematopoietic stem cell transplantation: a survey from the European group for blood and marrow transplantation. *J Hematother Stem Cell Res*, 10(60), 895–903.

Kuderer, N.M. *et al.* (2006) Mortality, morbidity, and cost associated with febrile neutropenia in adult cancer patients. *Cancer*, 106(10), 2258–66.

Kuehn, B.M. (2006) UNAIDS report. AIDS epidemic slowing but huge challenges remain. *JAMA*, 296(1), 29–30.

Kumar, R.M. *et al.* 2001. Sero-prevalence and mother-to-infant transmission of hepatitis E virus among pregnant women in the United Arab Emirates. *Eur J Obstet Gynecol Reprod Biol*, 100(1), 9–15.

Kusne, S. & Krystofiak, S. (2001) Infection control issues after bone marrow transplantation. *Curr Opin Infect Dis*, 14(4), 427–31.

Kuzu, N. *et al.* (2005) Compliance with hand hygiene and glove use in university-affiliated hospital. *Infect Control Hosp Epidemiol*, 26(3), 312–15.

Kyrlagkitsis, I. *et al.* (2002) Acute hepatitis A virus infection: a review of prognostic factors from 25 years experience in a tertiary referral center. *Hepatogastroenterology*, 49(44), 524–8.

Lam, P.K. *et al.* (2006) Factors related to response to intermittent treatment of *Mycobacterium avium* complex lung disease. *Am J Respir Crit Care Med*, 173(11), 1283–9.

Lanari, M. *et al.* (2006) Neonatal cytomegalovirus blood load and risk of sequelae in symptomatic and asymptomatic congenitally infected newborns. *Pediatrics*, 117(1), 76–83.

Landman, Q. *et al.* (2002) City-wide clonal outbreak of multiresistant *Acinetobacter baumannii* and *Pseudomonas aerginosa* in Brooklyn NY. *Arch Intern Med*, 162(13), 1515–20.

Larson, E. & Nirenberg, A. (2004) Evidence-based nursing practice to prevent infection in hospitalized neutropenic patients with cancer. *Oncol Nurs Forum*, 31(4), 717–24.

Larson, J.L. *et al.* (2003) Potential nosocomial exposure to *Mycobacterium tuberculosis* from a bronchoscope. *Infect Control Hosp Epidemiol*, 24(11), 825–30.

Laupland, K.B. *et al.* (2006) Cost of intensive care unit-acquired bloodstream infections. *J Hosp Infect*, 63(2), 124–32.

Lavanchy, D. (2004) Hepatitis B virus epidemiology, disease burden, treatment, and current and emerging prevention and control measures. *J Viral Hepat*, 11(2), 97–107.

Laws, H.J. *et al.* (2006) Surveillance of nosocomial infections in paediatric recipients of bone marrow or peripheral blood stem cell transplantation during neutropenia, compared with adult recipients. *J Hosp Infect*, 62(1), 80–8.

Lee, J.V. *et al.* (2002) Guidelines for investigating single cases of Legionnaires' disease. *Commun Dis Public Health*, 5(2), 157–62.

Lefebvre, B. *et al.* (2006) Growth performance and shedding of some pathogenic bacteria in feedlot cattle treated with different growth-promoting agents. *J Food Prot*, 69(6), 1256–64.

Lefebvre, S.L. *et al.* (2006) Prevalence of zoonotic agents in dogs visiting hospitalized people in Ontario: implications for infection control. *J Hosp Infect*, 62(3), 458–66.

Lehto, J.T. *et al.* (2005) Bronchoscopy in the diagnosis and surveillance of respiratory infections in lung and heart–lung transplant recipients. *Transpl Int*, 18(5), 562–71.

Lemos, A.A. *et al.* (2006) Cockroaches as carriers of fungi of medical importance. *Mycoses*, 49(1), 23–5.

Lettinga, K.D. *et al.* (2002) Legionnaires disease at a Dutch flower show: prognostic factors and impact of therapy. *Emerg Infect Dis*, 8(12), 1448–54.

Leung, A.K., Kellner, J.D. & Davies, H.D. (2005) Hepatitis A: a preventable threat. *Adv Ther*, 22(6), 578–86.

Leuthner, K.D., Cheung, C.M. & Rybak, M.J. (2006) Comparative activity of the new lipoglycopeptide telavancin in the presence and absence of serum against 50 glycopeptide non-susceptible staphylococci and three vancomycin-resistant *Staphylococcus aureus*. *J Antimicrob Chemother*, 58(2), 338–43.

Levine, A.S., Siegal, S.E. & Schrieber, A.D. (1973) Protected environment and prophylactic antibiotics. A perspective controlled study of their utility in the therapy of acute leukaemia. *N Engl J Med*, 288, 477–83.

Lewis, A.M. & Martin, R.C. (2006) The treatment of hepatic metastases in colorectal carcinoma. *Am Surg*, 72(6), 466–73.

Lewis, H. *et al.* (2006) Indigenous hepatitis E virus infection in England and Wales. *BMJ*, 332, 1509–10.

Li, J. *et al.* (2006a) Epidemiology of hepatitis B, C, D and G viruses and cytokine levels among intravenous drug users. *J Huazhong Univ Sci Technolog Med Sci*, 26(2), 221–4.

Li, J. *et al.* (2006b) *Pneumocystis carinii* pneumonia in patients with connective tissue disease. *Clin Rheumatol*, 12(3), 114–17.

Li, Y. *et al.* (2002) Mild heat treatment of lettuce enhances growth of *Listeria monocytogenes* during subsequent storage at 5°C or 15°C. *J Appl Microbiol*, **92**(2), 269–75.

Liljestrand, P. (2004) HIV care: continuing medical education and consultation needs of nurses, physicians and pharmacists. *J Assoc Nurses AIDS Care*, **15**(2), 38–50.

Limaye, A.P. *et al.* (2006) Impact of cytomegalovirus in organ transplant recipients in the era of antiviral prophylaxis. *Transplantation*, **81**(12), 1645–52.

Lin, C.C. *et al.* (2000) Diagnostic value of immunoglobulin G (IgG) and IgM anti-hepatitis E virus (HEV) tests based on HEV RNA in an area where hepatitis E is not endemic. *J Clin Microbiol*, **38**(11), 3915–18.

Lin, Y.C. *et al.* (2006) Clinical characteristics and risk factors for attributable mortality in *Enterobacter cloacae* bacteremia. *J Microbiol Immunol Infect*, **39**(1), 67–72.

Lines, L. (2006) A study of senior nurses perception about MRSA. *Nurs Times*, **102**(15), 32–5.

Lionakis, M.S. *et al.* (2005) *Aspergillus* susceptibility testing in patients with cancer and invasive aspergillosis: difficulties in establishing correlation between *in vitro* susceptibility data and the outcome of initial amphotericin B therapy. *Pharmacotherapy*, **25**(9), 1174–80.

Lipp, A. & Edwards, P. (2002) Disposable surgical face masks for preventing surgical wound infection in clean surgery. *Cochrane Database Syst Rev*, **1**, CD002929.

Lipp, A. & Edwards, P. (2005) Disposable surgical masks: a systematic review. *Can Oper Room Nurs J*, **23**(3), 20–1.

Loach, L. (1997) Blue days. *Nurs Times*, **93**(32), 31–2.

Loens, K. *et al.* (2006) Development of conventional and real-time NASBA® for the detection of *Legionella* species in respiratory specimens. *J Microbiol Methods*, **67**(3), 408–15.

Loh, W., Ng, V.V. & Holton, J. (2000) Bacterial flora on the white coats of medical students. *J Hosp Infect*, **45**(1), 65–8.

Longerich, T. *et al.* (2005) Recurrent herpes simplex virus hepatitis after liver retransplantation despite acyclovir therapy. *Liver Transpl*, **11**(10), 1289–94.

Lucet, J.C. *et al.* (2005) Successsful long term program for controlling methicillin-resistant *Staphylococcus aureus* in intensive care units. *Intensive Care Med*, **31**(8), 1051–7.

Lugauskas, A., Repeckiene, J. & Novosinskas, H. (2005) Micromycetes, producers of toxins, detected on stored vegetables. *Ann Agric Environ Med*, **12**(2), 253–60.

Luzuriaga, K. *et al.* (2006) Vaccines to prevent transmission of HIV-1 via breast milk: scientific and logistical priorities. *Lancet*, **368**(9534), 511–21.

MacKellar, D.A. *et al.* (2005) Unrecognized HIV infection, risk behaviors, and perceptions of risk among young men who have sex with men: opportunities for advancing HIV prevention in the third decade of HIV/AIDS. *J Acquir Immune Defic Syndr*, **38**(5), 603–14.

MacKinnon, M.M. & Allen, K.D. (2000) Long-term MRSA carriage in hospital patients. *J Infect Control*, **46**(3), 216–21.

Madeo, M. (2003) The psychological impact of isolation. *Nurs Times*, **99**(7), 54–5.

Maertens, J. & Boogaerts, M. (2005) The place for itraconazole in treatment. *J Antimicrob Chemother*, **56**(Suppl 1), i33–8.

Maertens, J., Vrebos, M. & Boogaerts, M. (2001) Assessing risk factors for systemic fungal infections. *Eur J Cancer Care (Engl)*, **10**(1), 56–62.

Maguire, H. *et al.* (2001) Hospital outbreak of *Salmonella virchow* possibly associated with a food handler. *J Hosp Infect*, **44**(4), 261–6.

Mahan, S.S. *et al.* (2006) Lack of value of repeat stool testing for *Clostridium difficile* toxin. *Am J Med*, **119**(4), 356–8.

Malik, Y.S. *et al.* (2006) Disinfection of fabrics and carpets artificially contaminated with calicivirus: relevance in institutional and healthcare centres. *J Hosp Infect*, **63**(2), 205–10.

Maloney, B.J. *et al.* (2005) Challenges in creating a vaccine to prevent hepatitis E. *Vaccine*, **23**(15), 1870–4.

Manfredi, R., Calza, L. & Chiodo, F. (2006) Primary cytomegalovirius infection in otherwise healthy adults with fever of unknown origin: a 3-year prospective survey. *Infection*, **34**(2), 87–90.

Mangili, A. & Gendreau, M.A. (2005) Transmission of infectious diseases during commercial air travel. *Lancet*, **365**(9463), 989–96.

Manian, F.A. (2003) Vascular and cardiac infections in end-stage renal disease. *Am J Med Sci*, **325**(4), 243–50.

Mank, A. *et al.* (2003) Is there still an indication for nursing patients with prolonged neutropenia in protective isolation? An evidence based nursing and medical study of 4 years experience for nursing patients with neutropenia without isolation. *Eur J Oncol Nurs*, **7**(1), 17–23.

Marr, K.A. *et al.* (2002) Invasive aspergillosis in allogenic stem cell transplant recipients: change in epidemiology and risk factors. *Blood*, **100**(13), 4358–66.

Marra, C.A. *et al.* (2004) Factors influencing quality of life in patients with active tuberculosis. *Health Qual Life Outcomes*, **2**, 58.

Marras, T.K. *et al.* (2002) Aerosolized pentamidine prophylaxis for *Pneumocystis carinii* pneumonia after allogeneic marrow transplantation. *Transpl Infect Dis*, **4**(2), 66–74.

Marriott, H.M. & Dockrell, D.H. (2006) *Streptococcus pneumoniae*: the role of apoptosis in host defense and pathogenesis. *Int J Biochem Cell Biol*, **38**(11), 1848–54.

Marrs, J.A. (2006) Care of patients with neutropenia. *Clin J Oncol Nurs*, **10**(2), 164–6.

Martin, A. & Lemon, S.M. (2006) Hepatitis A virus: from discovery to vaccines. *Hepatology*, **43**(2 Suppl 1), S164–72.

Martinez, J.A. *et al.* (2003) Role of environmental contamination as a risk factor for acquisition of vancomycin-resistant enterococci in patients treated in a medical intensive care unit. *Arch Intern Med*, **163**(16), 1905–12.

Marx, P.A. *et al.* (2004) AIDS as a zoonosis? Confusion over the origin of the virus and the origin of the epidemics. *J Med Primatol*, **33**(5-6), 220–6.

Masterton, R.G. & Teare, E.L. (2001) Clinical governance and infection control in the United Kingdom. *J Hosp Infect*, **47**(1), 25–31.

Maunder, R. *et al.* (2003) The immediate psychological and occupational impact of the 2003 SARS outbreak in a teaching hospital. *CMAJ*, **168**(10), 1245–51.

May, M.T. *et al.* (2006) HIV treatment response and prognosis in Europe and North America in the first decade of highly active antiretroviral therapy: a collaborative analysis. *Lancet*, **368**(9534), 451–8.

Mayer, R.A. *et al.* (2003) Role of fecal incontinence in contamination of the environment with vancomycin-resistant enterococci. *Am J Infect Control*, **31**(4), 221–5.

McCarthy, G.M. *et al.* (2002) Transmission of HIV in the dental clinic and elsewhere. *Oral Dis*, **8**(Suppl 2), 126–35.

McDonald, L.C. *et al.* (2005) An epidemic toxic gene variant strain of *Clostridium difficile*. *N Eng J Med*, **353**(23), 2433–41.

McEvoy, S.P. *et al.* (2006) Risk factors for the acquisition of vancomycin-resistant enterococci during a single-strain outbreak at a major Australian teaching hospital. *J Hosp Infect*, **62**(2), 256–8.

McGowan, J.E. (2006) Resistance in nonfermenting gram-negative bacteria: multidrug resistance to the maximum. *Am J Infect Control*, **34**(5)(Suppl 1), S29–37.

McGuckin, M. *et al.* (2004) Evaluation of a patient education model for increasing hand hygiene compliance in an inpatient rehabilitation unit. *Am J Infect Control*, **32**(4)235–8.

McMichael, A.J. (2006) HIV vaccines. *Annu Rev Immunol*, **24**, 227–55.

McMillan, A. (2005) Hepatitis B vaccination of men who have sex with men: experience with an accelerated course of vaccination in a genitourinary medicine clinic. *Int J STD AIDS*, **16**(9), 633–5.

McNeil, S.A., Mody, L. & Bradley, S.F. (2002) Methicillin-resistant *Staphylococcus aureus*. Management of asymptomatic colonization and outbreaks of infection in long-term care. *Geriatrics*, **57**(6), 16–27.

McPherson, S. *et al.* (2006) Intravenous immunoglobulin for the treatment of severe refractory and recurrent *Clostridium difficile* diarrhea. *Dis Colon Rectum*, **49**(5), 640–5.

MDA (1996) *Latex Sensitisation in the Health Care Setting*. Department of Health, London.

MDA (1998) *Latex Medical Gloves*. Department of Health, London.

MDA (2002) *Sterilization, Disinfection and Cleaning of Medical Equipment*. Department of Health, London.

Medland, J., Howard-Ruben, J. & Whitaker, E. (2004) Fostering psychosocial wellness in oncology nurses. Addressing burnout and social support in the workplace. *Oncol Nurs Forum*, **31**(1), 47–54.

Meers, P.D. & Matthews, R.B. (1978) Multiple-resistant pneumococcus. *Lancet*, **2**(8082), 219.

Meier, J. & Lopez, L. (2001) Listeriosis: an emerging food-borne disease. *Clin Lab Sci*, **14**(3), 187–92.

Meldrum, R.J. *et al.* (2005) Survey of *Salmonella* and *Campylobacter* of whole raw poultry in sales in Wales in 2003. *J Food Prot*, **68**(7), 1447–9.

Meyer, I.D. (1986) Infection in bone marrow transplant recipients. *Am J Med*, **81**, 27–8.

Miguez-Burbano, M.J. *et al.* (2006) Non-tuberculous mycobacteria disease as a cause of hospitalization in HIV-infected subjects. *Int J Infect Dis*, **10**(1), 47–55.

Mims, C.A. *et al.* (2004) *Medical Microbiology*, 3rd edn. Mosby, London.

Miyakoshi, K. *et al.* (1998) Prenatal ultrasound diagnosis of small bowel torsion. *Obstet Gynecol*, **91**(5, Part 2), 802–3.

Mock, V. & Olsen, M. (2003) Current management of fatigue and anemia in patients with cancer. *Semin Oncol Nurs*, **19**(4 Suppl 2), 36–41.

Mohamed, M.K. *et al.* (2006) Transmission of hepatitis C virus between parents and children. *Am J Trop Med Hyg*, **75**(1), 16–20.

Mohan, S.S. *et al.* (2006) Lack of value of repeat stool testing for *Clostridium difficile*. *Am J Med*, **119**(4), 356–8.

Monsen, T., Karisson, C. & Wistrom, J. (2005) Spread of clones of multidrug-resistant coagulase negative staphylococcus within a university hospital. *Infect Control Hosp Epidemiol*, **26**(1), 76–80.

Monso, E. (2004) Occupational asthma in greenhouse workers. *Curr Opin Pulm Med*, **10**(2), 147–50.

Moody, K. *et al.* (2006) Feasibility and safety of a pilot randomized trial of infection rate: neutropenic diet versus standard food safety guidelines. *J Pediatr Hematol Oncol*, **28**(3), 126–33.

Morris, K. *et al.* (2005) First HIV 'window period' donation in a UK blood donor. *Transfus Med*, **15**(3), 249–50.

Morris-Cunnington, M.C. *et al.* (2004) A population-based seroprevalence study of hepatitis A virus using oral fluid in England and Wales. *Am J Epidemiol*, **159**(8), 786–94.

Navon-Venezia, S., Ben-Ami, R. & Carmeli, Y. (2005) Update on *Pseudomonas aerginosa* and *Acinetobacter baumannii* infection in the healthcare setting. *Curr Opin Infect Dis*, **18**(4), 306–13.

Nazzaro, A.M. *et al.* (2006) Knowledge, attitudes, and behaviours of youths in the US hemophilia population: results of a national survey. *Am J Public Health*, **96**(9), 1618–22.

Neely, A.N. & Maley, M.P. (2000) Survival of enterococci and staphylococci on hospital fabrics and plastic. *J Clin Microbiol*, **38**(1), 724–6.

Neuberger, P. *et al.* (2006) Case-control study of symptoms and neonatal outcome of human milk-transmitted cytomegalovirus infection in premature infants. *J Pediatr*, **148**(3), 326–31.

Neville, K., Renbarger, J. & Dreyer, Z. (2002) Pneumonia in the immunocompromised pediatric cancer patient. *Semin Respir Infect*, **17**(1), 21–32.

Newman, K., Maylor, U. & Chansarkar, B. (2002) The nurse satisfaction, service quality and nurse retention chain: implications for management of recruitment and retention. *J Manage Med*, **16**(4–5), 271–91.

Newton, J.T., Constable, D. & Senior, V. (2001) Patients perceptions of methicillin-resistant *Staphylococcus aureus* and source isolation: a qualitative analysis of source-isolated patients. *J Hosp Infect*, **48**(4), 275–80.

Nguyen, D.M., Mascola, L. & Brancoft, E. (2005) Recurring methicillin-resistant *Staphylococcus aureus* in a football team. *Emerg Infect Dis*, **11**(4), 526–32.

NHS Estates (2002) *Infection Control in the Built Environment. Design and Planning*. HMSO, Norwich.

NHS Estates (2005) *Ward Layouts with Single Rooms and Space for Flexibility*. National Health Service Estates, Leeds.

NHS Executive (NHSE) (1994) *The control of Legionellae in Health Care Premises*, Health Technical Memorandum 2040, Code of Practice NHS Estates. HMSO, London.

NHS Executive (NHSE) (1995) *Hospital Infection Control: Guidance on the Control of Infection in Hospitals*. HSG (95) 10 1995. HMSO, London.

NHS Executive (NHSE) (1999a) *Latex Medical Gloves and Powdered Latex Medical Gloves*. Department of Health, London.

NHS Executive (NHSE) (1999b) *Variant Creutzfeldt–Jakob Disease (vCJD). Minimising the Risk of Transmission*. Department of Health, London.

NICE (2003) *Infection control. Prevention of healthcare-associated infection in primary and community care*. National Institute for Health and Clinical Excellence, London.

NICE (2006) *Tuberculosis*. National Institute for Health and Clinical Excellence, London.

Niro, G.A. *et al.* (2005) Lamivudine therapy in chronic delta hepatitis: a multicentre randomized-controlled pilot study. *Aliment Pharmacol Ther*, **22**(3), 227–32.

Nishijima, S. & Kurikawa, I. (2002) Antimicrobial resistance of *Staphylococcus aureus* isolated from skin infections. *Int J Antimicrob Agents*, **19**(3), 241–3.

NMC (2005) *Guidelines for Records and Record Keeping*. Nursing and Midwifery Council, London.

NMC (2006) *A–Z Advice Sheet Consent*. www.nmc.org.

Norgard, B. *et al.* (2006) Maternal herpes labialis in pregnancy and neural tube defects. *Dev Med Child Neurol*, **48**(8), 674–6.

Nosari, A. *et al.* (2001) Invasive aspergillosis in haematological malignancies: clinical findings and management for intensive chemotherapy completion. *Am J Hematol*, **68**(4), 231–6.

Noskin, G.A. *et al.* (1995) Recovery of vancomycin-resistant enterococci on fingertips and environmental surfaces. *Infect Control Hosp Epidemiol*, **16**(10), 577–81.

Novak, J. & Katz, J.A. (2006) Probiotics and prebiotics for gastrointestinal infections. *Curr Infect Dis Rep*, **8**(2), 103–9.

Nozzoli, C. *et al.* (2006) Epstein–Barr virus-associated post-transplant lymphoproliferative disease with central nervous system involvement after unrelated allogeneic hematopoietic stem cell transplantation. *Leuk Lymphoma*, 47(1), 167–9.

Nyiri, P. *et al.* (2004) Sharps discarded in inner city parks and play grounds—risk of bloodborne virus exposure. *Commun Dis Public Health*, 7(4), 287–8.

Oie, S., Hosokawa, I. & Kamiya, A. (2002) Contamination of room door handles by methicillin resistant *Staphylococcus aureus*. *J Hosp Infect*, 51(2), 140–3.

Oldfield, E.C. (2006) *Clostridium difficile*-associated diarrhea: resurgence with a vengeance. *Rev Gastroenterol Disord*, 6(2), 79–96.

Oldman, T. (1998) Isolated cases. *Nurs Times*, 94(11), 67–71.

Oncu, S. *et al.* (2006) Prevalence and risk factors for HEV infection in pregnant women. *Med Sci Monit*, 12(1), CR36–9.

O'Neill, E. & Humphreys, H. (2005) Surveillance of hospital water and primary prevention of nosocomial legionellosis: what is the evidence? *J Hosp Infect*, 59(4), 273–9.

O'Neill, J. & Buttery, J. (2003) Varicella and paediatric staff: current practice and vaccine cost-effectiveness. *J Hosp Infect*, 53(2), 117–19.

Ormerod, L.D. *et al.* (1998) Rapidly progressive herpetic retinal necrosis: a blinding disease characteristic of advanced AIDS. *Clin Infect Dis*, 26(1), 34–45.

Ormerod, L.P. (1996) Tuberculosis and immigration. *Br J Hosp Med*, 56(5), 209–12.

Ornoy, A. & Diav-Citrin, O. (2006) Fetal effects of primary and secondary cytomegalovirus infection in pregnancy. *Reprod Toxicol*, 21(4), 399–409.

Ozerol, I.H. *et al.* (2006) Legionnaires' disease: a nosocomial outbreak in Turkey. *J Hosp Infect*, 62(1), 50–7.

Pancham, S. *et al.* (2005) Caspofungin for invasive fungal infections: combination treatment with liposomal amphotericin B in children undergoing hemopoietic stem cell transplantation. *Pediatr Transplant*, 9(2), 254–7.

Panhotra, B.R., Saxena, A.K. & Al-Mulhim, A.S. (2005) Contamination of patients' files in intensive care units: an indication of strict hand washing after entering case notes. *Am J Infect Control*, 33(7), 398–401.

Parise, E.R. *et al.* (2006) Response to treatment with interferon-α and ribavirin in patients with chronic hepatitis C virus genotypes 2 and 3 depends on the degree of hepatic fibrosis. *Braz J Infect Dis*, 10(2), 78–81.

Park, S.H. *et al.* (2006) Current trends of infectious complications following hematopoietic stem cell transplantation in a single center. *J Korean Med Sci*, 21(2), 199–207.

Park, W. & Keeffe, E.B. (2004) Diagnosis and treatment of hepatitis B. *Minerva Gastroenterol Dietol*, 50(4), 289–303.

Parker, M.J. & Goldman, R.D. (2006) Paediatric emergency department staff perceptions of infection control measures against server acute respiratory syndrome. *Emerg Med J*, 23(5), 349–53.

Patel, S. (2005) Minimising cross-infection risks associated with beds and mattresses. *Nurs Times*, 101(8), 52–3.

Patel, S.N., Murray-Leonard, J. & Wilson, A.P.R. (2006) Laundering of hospital staff uniforms at home. *J Hosp Infect*, 62(1), 89–93.

Paterson, D.L. (2006) Resistance in gram-negative bacteria: Enterobacteriaceae. *Am J Infect Control*, 34(5 Suppl 1), S20–8.

Paterson, P.J. *et al.* (2003) Treatment failure in invasive aspergillosis: susceptibility of deep tissue isolates following treatment with amphotericin B. *J Antimicrob Chemother*, 52(5), 873–6.

Patterson, A.J. (1993) Review of current practices in clean diets in the UK. *J Hum Nutr Diet*, 6, 3–11.

Patterson, W.J. *et al.* (1997) Colonization of transplant unit water supplies with *Legionella* and protozoa: precautions required to reduce the risk of legionellosis. *J Hosp Infect*, 37(1), 7–17.

Paul, N. & Jacob, M.E. (2006) An outbreak of cadaver-acquired chickenpox in a health care setting. *Clin Infect Dis*, 43(5), 599–601.

Paulus, S.C. *et al.* (2005) A prospective study of septicaemia on a paediatric oncology unit: a 3-year experience at the Royal Liverpool Children's Hospital, Alder Hey UK. *Eur J Cancer*, 41(14), 2132–40.

Payne, D.N., Gibson, S.A. & Lewis, R. (1998) Antiseptics: a forgotten weapon in the control of antibiotic resistant bacteria in hospital and community setting. *J R Soc Health*, 118(i), 18–22.

Pedro-Botet, L. & Yu, V.L. (2006) *Legionella*: macrolides or quinolones? *Clin Microbiol Infect*, 12(Suppl 3), 25–30.

Peron, J.M. *et al.* (2006) Hepatitis E is an autochthonous disease in industrialized countries. Analysis of 23 patients in South-West France over a 13-month period and comparison with hepatitis A. *Gastroenterol Clin Biol*, 30(5), 757–62.

Perrett, K. *et al.* (2003) Changing epidemiology of hepatitis A: should we be doing more to vaccinate injecting drug users? *Commun Dis Public Health*, 6(2), 97–100.

Perry, C., Marshall, R. & Jones, E. (2001) Bacterial contamination of uniforms. *J Hosp Infect*, 48(3), 238–41.

Petchey, R. *et al.* (2000) The last resort would be to go to the GP. Understanding the perceptions and use of general practitioner services among people with HIV/AIDS. *Soc Sci Med*, 50(2), 233–45.

Petchey, R., Farnsworth, W. & Heron, T. (2001) The maintenance of confidentiality in primary care: a survey of policies and procedures. *AIDS Care*, 13(2), 251–6.

Petersen, F.B. *et al.* (1987) Infectious complications in patients undergoing marrow transplantation: a prospective randomized study of the additional effects of contamination and laminar air flow isolation among patients receiving prophylactic systemic antibiotics. *Scand J Infect Dis*, 19(5), 559–67.

Picazo, J.J. (2005) Management of febrile neutropenic patients. *Int J Antimicrob Agents*, 2(Suppl), S12–22.

Pinna, A.D. *et al.* (2002) Five cases of fulminant hepatitis due to herpes simplex virus in adults. *Dig Dis Sci*, 47(4), 750–4.

Pinot de Moira, A., Edmunds, W.J. & Breuer, J. (2006) The cost-effectiveness of antenatal varicella screening with post-partum vaccination of susceptibles. *Vaccine*, 24(9), 1298–307.

Poe, S.S *et al.* (1994) A national survey of infection prevention practices on bone marrow transplant units. *Oncol Nurs Forum*, 21(10), 1687–93.

Potoski, B.A. *et al.* (2006) Epidemiology profile of linezolid-resistant coagulase-negative staphylococci. *Clin Infect Dis*, 43(2), 165–71.

Preiss, J.C. *et al.* (2006) Autochthonous hepatitis E virus infection in Germany with sequence similarities to other European isolates. *Infection*, 34(3), 173–5.

Puro, V., Scognamiglio, P. & Ippolito, G. (2003) HIV, HBV, or HDV transmission from infected health care workers to patients. *Med Lav*, 94(6), 556–68.

Quinn, B. (2003) Exploring nurses experiences of supporting a cancer patient in their search for meaning. *Eur J Oncol Nurs*, 7(3), 164–71.

Quinn, B. (2005) Cancer and the treatment: does it make sense to patients. *Hematology*, 10(Suppl 1), 325–8.

Rabaud, C. & Mauuary, G. (2001) Infection and/or colonization by methicillin-resistant *Staphylococcus epidermidis* (MRSE). *Pathol Biol (Paris)*, 49(10), 812–14.

Radwin, L. (2000) Oncology patients' perception of quality nursing care. *Res Nurs Health*, 23(3), 179–90.

141

Rae, G.G. (1998) Risk factors for the spread of antibiotic-resistant bacteria. *Drugs*, 55(3), 323–30.

Redpath, C. & Farrington, M. (1997) Dispose of disposables. *J Hosp Infect*, 35(4), 313–17.

Reglier-Poupet, H. *et al.* (2005) Evaluation of the quality of hospital food from the kitchen to the patients. *J Hosp Infect*, 59(2), 131–7.

Respaldiza, N. *et al.* (2004) High seroprevalence in *Pneumocystis* infection in Spanish children. *Clin Microbiol Infect*, 10(11), 1029–31.

Ribas-Mundom, M., Granena, A. & Rozman, C. (1981) Evaluation of a protective environment in the management of granulocytopenic patients. A comparative study. *Cancer*, 48, 419–24.

Ricketts, K.D. & Joseph, C.A. (2006) The impact of new guidelines in Europe for the control and prevention of travel-associated Legionnaires' disease. *Int J Hyg Environ Health*, 209(6), 547–52.

Robertson, C.B. *et al.* (2006) Effect of X-ray irradiation on reducing the risk of listeriosis in ready-to-eat vacuum-packaged smoked mullet. *J Food Prot*, 69(7), 1561–4.

Robinson, L. *et al.* (2006) Palliative home nursing interventions for people with HIV/AIDS: a pilot study. *J Assoc Nurses AIDS Care*. 17(3), 37–46.

Rohde, H. *et al.* (2005) Induction of *Staphylococcus epidermidis* biofilm formation via proteolytic processing of the accumulation associated protein by *Staphylococcus* and host proteases. *Mol Microbiol*, 55(6), 1883–995.

Rolston, K.V. (2001) The spectrum of pulmonary infections in cancer patients. *Curr Opin Oncol*, 13(4), 218–23.

Rolston, K.V. (2005) Challenges in the treatment of infections caused by gram-positive and gram-negative bacteria in patients with cancer and neutropenia. *Clin Infect Dis*, 40(Suppl 4), S246–52.

Ronning, C.M. *et al.* (2005) Genomics of *Aspergillus fumigatus*. *Rev Iberoam Micro*, 22(4), 223–8.

Ross, D.S. *et al.* (2006) The epidemiology and prevention of congenital cytomegalovirus infection and disease: activities of the Centers for Disease Control and Prevention Workgroup. *J Womens Health (Larchmt)*, 15(3), 224–9.

Rossoff, L.J. *et al.* (1993) Is the use of boxed gloves in an intensive care unit safe? *Am J Med*, 94, 602–7.

Roxas, M. (2006) Herpes zoster and postherpetic neuralgia: diagnosis and therapeutic considerations. *Altern Med Rev*, 11(2), 102–13.

Russell, J.A. *et al.* (2000) Early outcomes after allogeneic stem cell transplantation for leukaemia and myelodysplasia without protective isolation: a 10 year study. *Biol Blood Marrow Transplant*, 6(2), 109–14

Russian, D.A. & Levine, S.J. (2001) *Pneumocystis carinii* pneumonia in patients with HIV infection. *Am J Med Sci*, 321(1), 56–65.

Sa, D.H. *et al.* (2006) Practice of universal precautions among healthcare workers. *J Natl Med Assoc*, 98(5), 722–6.

Sabria, M. & Yu, V.L. (2002) Hospital acquired legionellosis: solutions for a preventable infection. *Lancet Infect Dis*, ii(6), 368–73.

Sabria, M. *et al.* (2006) A community outbreak of Legionnaires' disease: evidence of a cooling tower as the source. *Clin Microbiol Infect*, 12(7), 642–7.

Sadler, G.J. *et al.* (2006) UK acquired hepatitis E – an emerging problem?*J Med Virol*, 78(4), 473–5.

Safdar, N. & Maki, D.G. (2002) The commonality of risk factors for nosocomial colonization and infection with antimicrobial-resistant *Staphylococcus aureus*, enterococcus, Gram negative bacilli, *Clostridium difficile* and *Candida*. *Ann Intern Med*, 136(11), 834–44.

Sambatakou, H. *et al.* (2006) Voriconazole treatment for subacute invasive and chronic pulmonary aspergillosis. *Am J Med*, 119(6), 527.e17–24.

Samuelsson, A. *et al.* (2003) Clustering of enterococcal infections in a general intensive care unit. *J Hosp Infect*, 54(3), 188–95.

Sanderson, P.J. (1999) What should we do about patients with *Clostridium difficile*? *J Hosp Infect*, 43(4), 251–3.

Sandri, A.M. *et al.* (2006) Reduction in incidence of nosocomial methicillin-resistant *Staphylococcus aureus* (MRSA) infection in an intensive care unit: role of treatment with mupirocin ointment and chlorhexidine baths for nasal carriers of MRSA. *Infect Control Hosp Epidemiol*, 27(2), 185–7.

Santamauro, J.T., Aurora, R.N. & Stover, D.E. (2002) *Pneumocystis carinii* pneumonia in patients with and without HIV infection. *Compr Ther*, 28(2), 96–108.

Santos, A.M., Lacerda, R.A. & Graziano, K.U. (2005) Evidence of control and prevention of surgical site infection by shoe cover and private shoes: a systematic literature review. *Rev Lat Am Enfermagem*, 13(1), 86–92.

Santos, S.A. *et al.* (2006) Effect of switching to tenofovir with emtricitabine in patients with chronic hepatitis B failing to respond to an adefovir containing regimen. *Eur J Gastroenterol Hepatol*, 18(12), 1253–7.

Sarrazin, U. *et al.* (2004) Postexposure prophylaxis after occupational exposure to HBV, HCV and HIV. *Radiologe*, 44(2), 181–94.

Sasaki, T. *et al.* (2000) Mental disturbance during isolation in bone marrow transplant patients with leukemia. *Bone Marrow Transplant*, 25(3), 315–18.

Saville, R.D. *et al.* (2001) Fourth-generation enzyme linked immunosorbent detection of human immunodeficiency virus antigen and antibody. *J Clin Microbiol*, 39(7), 2518–24.

Saxena, A.K. & Panhotra, B.R. (2004) The impact of nurse understaffing on the transmission of hepatitis C virus in a hospital-based hemodialysis unit. *Med Princ Pract*, 13(3), 129–35.

Saxena, A.K. *et al.* (2003) Impact of dedicated space, dialysis equipment, and nursing staff on the transmission of hepatitis C virus in a hemodialysis unit of the middle east. *Am J Infect Control*, 31(1), 26–33.

Schim van der Loeff, M.F. *et al.* (2001) HIV-2 does not protect against HIV-1 infection in a rural community in Guinea-Bissau. *AIDS*, 15(17), 2303–10.

Schlundt, J. *et al.* (2004) Emerging food-borne zoonoses. *Rev Sci Tech*, 23(2), 513–33.

Schraub, S. & Marx, E. (2004) Burn out syndrome in oncology. *Bull Cancer*, 91(9), 673–6.

Schulmeister, L., Quiett, K. & Mayer, K. (2005) Quality of life, quality of care, and patient satisfaction: perception of patients undergoing outpatient autologous stem cell transplantation. *Oncol Nurs Forum*, 32(1), 57–67.

Sebaihia, M. *et al.* (2006) The multidrug-resistant human pathogen *Clostridium difficile* has a highly mobile, mosaic genome. *Nat Genet*, 38(7), 779–86.

Sepkowitz, K.A. (2005) Treatment of patients with hematologic neoplasm, fever and neutropenia. *Clin Infect Dis*, 40(Suppl 4), S253–6.

Serrano, I., Melo-Cristino, J. & Ramirez, M. (2006) Heterogeneity of pneumococcal phase variants in invasive human disease. *BMC Microbiol*, 6(1), 67.

Sexton, T., Clarke, P. & O'Neill, E. (2006) Environmental reservoirs of methicillin-resistant *Staphylococcus aureus* in isolation rooms: correlation with patient isolates and implications for hospital hygiene. *J Hosp Infect*, 62(2), 187–94.

Sharma, A. & Lokeshwar, N. (2005) Febrile neutropenia in haematological malignancies. *J Postgrad Med*, 51(Suppl 1), S42–8.

142

Sheffer, P.J. *et al.* (2005) Efficacy of new point-of-use water filter for preventing exposure to *Legionella* and waterborne bacteria. *Am J Infect Control*, **33**(5 Suppl 1), S20–5.

Sheffield, J.S. *et al.* (2006) Valacyclovir prophylaxis to prevent recurrent herpes at delivery: a randomized clinical trial. *Obstet Gynecol*, **108**(1), 141–7.

Shelton, B.K. (2003) Evidence-based care for the neutropenic patients with leukaemia. *Semin Oncol Nurs*, **19**(2), 133–41.

Shinjo, K. *et al.* (2002) Efficacy of the Shinki bioclean room for preventing infection in neutropenic patients. *J Adv Nurs*, **37**(3), 227–33.

Sinclair, J. & Sissons, P. (2006) Latency and reactivation of human cytomegalovirus. *J Gen Virol*, **87**(Pt 7), 1763–79.

Singhal, R., Mirdha, B.R. & Guieria, R. (2005) Human pneumocystosis. *Indian J Chest Dis Allied Sci*, **47**(4), 273–83.

Sixbey, J.W. *et al.* (1984) Epstein–Barr virus replication in oropharyneal epithelial cells. *N Engl J Med*, **310**(19), 1225–30.

Slota, M. *et al.* (2001) The role of gown and glove isolation and strict handwashing in the reduction of nosocomial infection in children with solid organ transplantation. *Crit Care Med*, **29**(2), 405–12.

Smith, A. *et al.* (2006) Outbreaks of waterborne infectious intestinal disease in England and Wales, 1992–2003. *Epidemiol Infect*, **134**(6), 1141–9.

Smith, H.V. *et al.* (2006) Tools for investigating the environmental transmission of *Cryptosporidium* and *Giardia* infections in humans. *Trends Parasitol*, **22**(4), 160–7.

Smith, T.L. & Nathan, B.R. (2002) Central nervous system infections in the immune-competent adult. *Curr Treat Options Neurol*, **4**(4), 323–32.

Snoeck, R. & De Clercq, E. (2002) Role of cidofovir in the treatment of DNA virus infections, other than CMV infections, in immunocompromised patients. *Curr Opin Investig Drugs*, **3**(11), 1561–6.

Sobaszek, A. *et al.* (2000) Prevalence of cytomegalovirus infection among health care workers in pediatric and immunosuppressed adult units. *J Occup Environ Med*, **42**(11), 1109–14.

Sokucu, S. *et al.* (2006) Comparison of interferon monotherapy with interferon-lamivudine combination treatment in children with chronic hepatitis B. *Indian J Gastroenterol*, **25**(3), 136–9.

Soldan, K., Davison, K. & Dow, B. (2005) Estimates of the frequency of HBV, HCV, and HIV infectious donations entering the blood supply in the United Kingdom, 1996 to 2003. *Euro Surveill*, **10**(2), 17–19.

Sonder, G.J. *et al.* (2004) Hepatitis A virus immunity and seroconversion among contacts of acute hepatitis A patients in Amsterdam, 1996–2000: an evaluation of current prevention policy. *Am J Public Health*, **94**(9), 1620–6.

Special Waste Regulations (1996) HMSO, London.

Srinivasan, A. *et al.* (2002) A prospective study to determine whether cover gowns in addition to gloves decrease nosocomial transmission of vancomycin-resistant enterococci in the intensive care unit. *Infect Control Hosp Epidemiol*, **23**(8), 424–8.

Sritangratanakul, S., Nuchprayoon, S. & Nuchprayoon, I. (2004) Pneumocystis pneumonia: an update. *J Med Assoc Thai*, **87**(2), S309–17.

Staat, M.A. *et al.* (2006) Varicella-related hospitalization and emergency department visit rates, before and after introduction of varicella vaccine, among white and black children in Hamilton County, Ohio. *Pediatrics* **117** (5), e833–9.

Stahl Wernersson, S., Johansson, E. & Hakanson, H. (2004) Cross contamination in dishwashers. *J Hosp Infect*, **56**(4), 312–17.

Stebbing, J. *et al.* (2006) A prognostic index for AIDS-associated Kaposi's sarcoma in the era of highly active antiretroviral therapy. *Lancet*, **367**(9521), 1495–502.

Stirling, B., Littlejohn, P. & Willbond, M.L. (2004) Nurses and the control of infectious disease. Understanding epidemiology and disease transmission is vital to nursing care. *Can Nurse*, **100**(9), 16–20.

Storb, R. *et al.* (1983) GVHD and survival in patients with aplastic anaemia treated by bone marrow grafts with HLA identifiable siblings. *N Engl J Med*, **308**, 302–7.

Su, C.W. *et al.* (2006a) Genotypes and viremia of hepatitis B and D viruses are associated with outcomes of chronic hepatitis D patients. *Gastroenterology*, **130**(6), 1625–35.

Su, H.P. *et al.* (2006b) A legionellosis case due to contaminated spa water and confirmed by genomic identification in Taiwan. *Microbiol Immunol*, **50**(5), 371–7.

Sundkvist, T. *et al.* (2000) Outbreak of hepatitis A spread by contaminated drinking glasses in a public house. *Commun Did Public Health*, **3**(1), 60–2.

Sunenshine, R.H. & McDonald, L.C. (2006) *Clostridium difficile*-associated disease: new challenges from an established pathogen. *Cleve Clin J Med*, **73**(2), 187–97.

Sunnotel, O. *et al.* (2006) *Cryptosporidium*. *Lett Appl Microbiol*, **43**(1), 7–16.

Takada, Y. *et al.* (2006) Clinical outcomes of living donor living transplantation for hepatitis C virus (HCV)-positive patients. *Transplantation*, **81**(3), 350–4.

Takahashi, M. *et al.* (2004) High prevalence of antibodies to hepatitis A and E viruses and viremia of hepatitis B, C and D viruses among apparently healthy populations in Mongolia. *Chin Diag Lab Immunol*, **11**(2), 392–98.

Takemoto, K. *et al.* (2006) Comparative study on the efficacy of AmBisome and Fungizone in a mouse model of pulmonary aspergillosis. *J Antimicrob Chemother*, **57**(4), 724–31.

Talaat, M. *et al.* (2003) Occupational exposure to needlestick injuries and hepatitis B vaccination coverage among health care workers in Egypt. *Am J Infect Control*, **31**(8), 469–74.

Tan, H.H. & Goh, C.L. (2006a) Viral infections affecting the skin in organ transplant recipients: epidemiology and current management strategies. *Am J Clin Dermatol*, **7**(1), 13–29.

Tan, M.P. & Koren, G. (2006b) Chickenpox in pregnancy: revisited. *Reprod Toxicol*, **21**(4), 410–20.

Tao, Q. *et al.* (2006) Epstein–Barr virus (EBV) and its associated human cancers – genetics, epigenetics, pathobiology and novel therapeutics. *Front Biosci*, **11**, 2672–713.

Taormina, P.J. & Beuchat, L.R. (2001) Survival and heat resistance of *Listeria monocytogenes* after exposure to alkali and chlorine. *Appl Environ Microbiol*, **67**(6), 2555–63.

Tarantino, G. *et al.* (2006) Metabolic factors involved in the therapeutic response of patients with hepatitis C virus-related chronic hepatitis. *Gastroenterol Hepatol*, **21**(8), 1266–8.

Tarzi, S. *et al.* (2001) Methicillin resistant *Staphylococcus aureus*: psychological impact of hospitalization and isolation in the older adult. *J Hosp Infect*, **49**(4), 250–4.

Tattevin, P. *et al.* (2006) Increasing incidence of severe Epstein–Barr virus-related infectious mononucleosis: surveillance study. *J Clin Microbiol*, **44**(5), 1873–4.

Taylor, J.M. (2006) Hepatitis delta virus. *Virology*, **344**(1), 71–6.

Taylor, K., Plowman, R. & Roberts, J.A. (2001) *The Challenge of Hospital Acquired Infection*. National Audit Office, London.

Tenover, F.C. (2006) Mechanisms of antimicrobial resistance in bacteria. *Am J Med*, **119**(6 Suppl 1), S3–10.

Thevenot, D., Dernburg, A.M. & Vernozy-Rozand, C. (2006) An updated review of *Listeria monocytogenes* in the pork meat industry and its products. *J Appl Microbiol*, **101**(1), 7–17.

Thoen, C., Lobue, P. & De Kantor, I. (2006) The importance of *Mycobacterium bovis* as a zoonosis. *Vet Microbiol*, **112**(2–4), 339–45.

Thompson, S.C., Boughton, C.R. & Dore, G.J. (2003) Blood-borne viruses and their survival in the environment: is public concern about community needlestick exposures justified? *Aust N Z J Public Health*, 27(6), 602–7.

Toivgoogin, A. *et al.* (2005) Validity of using tuberculin skin test erythema measurement for contact investigation during a tuberculosis outbreak in schoolchildren previously vaccinated with BCG. *J Epidemiol*, 15(2), 56–64.

Tormom Molina, R. *et al.* (2002) Pollen and spores in the air of a hospital out-patient ward. *Allergol Immunopathol (Madr)*, 30(4), 232–8.

Torres, H.A. *et al.* (2006) Cytomegalovirus infection in patients with lymphoma: an important cause of morbidity and mortality. *Clin Lymphoma Myeloma*, 6(5), 393–8.

Trad, O. *et al.* (2003) Eradication of *Cryptosporidium* in four children with acute lumphoblastic leukemia. *J Trop Pediatr*, 49(2), 128–30.

Trakumas, S. *et al.* (2001) Particle emission characteristics of filter-equipped vacuum cleaners. *Am Ind Hyg Assoc J*, 62(4), 482–93.

Trautmann, M., Lepper, P.M. & Haller, M. (2005) Ecology of *Pseudomonas aeruginosa* in the intensive care unit and the evolving role of water outlets as a reservoir of the organism. *Am J Infect Control*, 33(5 Suppl 1), S41–9.

Trexler, P.C. (1975) Microbial isolators for use in the hospital. *Biomed Eng*, 10(2), 63–7.

Trexler, P.C., Emond, R.T. & Evans, B. (1977) Negative pressure plastic isolator for patients with dangerous infections. *Br Med J*, ii(6086), 559–61.

Trim, J.C., Adams, D. & Elliott, T.S. (2003) Healthcare workers' knowledge of inoculation injuries and glove use. *Br J Nurs*, 12(4), 215–21.

Trueba, F. *et al.* (2006) High prevalence of teicoplanine resistance among *Staphylococcus epidermidis* strains in a 5 year study. *J Clin Microbiol*, 44(5), 1922–3.

Tsatsralt-Od, B. *et al.* (2005) High prevalence of dual or triple infection of hepatitis B, C and delta viruses among patients with chronic liver disease in Mongolia. *J Med Virol*, 77(4), 491–9.

Tsiodras, S. *et al.* (2000) Infection and immunity in chronic lymphocytic leukemia. *Mayo Clin Proc*, 75(10), 1039–54.

Turner, J.M. *et al.* (2006) Behavioural predictors of subsequent hepatitis C diagnosis in a UK clinic sample of HIV positive men who have sex with men. *Sex Transm Infect*, 82(4), 298–300.

Twomey, C.L. (2003) Double gloving: a risk reduction strategy. *Jt Comm J Qual Saf*, 29(7), 369–78.

UK Health Department (2002a) *AIDS/HIV Infected Health Care Workers: Guidance on the Management of Infected Health Care Workers and Patient Notification*. UK Health Department, Wetherby.

UK Health Department (2002b) *Guidance for Clinical Health Care Workers. Protection against Infection with Blood Borne Viruses*. UK Health Department, Wetherby.

Ungar, B.L.P. (1995) *Cryptosporidium*. In: *Principles and Practices of Infectious Disease*, 4th edn, Vol. 2 (eds G.L. Mandell, J.E. Bennett & R. Dolan). Churchill Livingstone, New York, pp. 2500–10.

Urrea, M. *et al.* (2004) Nosocomial infections among pediatric hematology/oncology patients: results of a prospective incidence study. *Am J Infect Control*, 32(4|), 205–8.

Vamvakas, E.C. (2005) Is white blood cell reduction equivalent to antibody screening in preventing transmission of cytomegalovirus by transfusion? A review of the literature and meta-analysis. *Transfus Med Rev*, 19(3), 181–99.

van der Kooij, D., Veenendaal, H.R. & Scheffer, W.J. (2005) Biofilm formation and multiplication of *Legionella* in a model warm water system with pipes of copper, stainless steel and cross-linked polyethylene. *Water Res*, 39(13), 2789–98.

van der Wielen, M. *et al.* (2006) Hepatitis A/B vaccination of adults over 40 years old: comparison of three vaccine regimens and effect of influencing factors. *Vaccine*, 24(26), 5509–15.

Vardhan, M.S., Allen, K.D. & DeRuiter, G. (2000) Commodes: a health hazard. *J Hosp Infect*, 44(4), 320–1.

Vaughn, T.E. *et al.* (2004) Factors promoting consistent adherence to safe needle precautions among hospital workers. *Infect Control Hosp Epidemiol*, 25(7), 548–55.

Vento, S., Cainelli, F. & Longhi, M.S. (2002) Reactivation of replication of hepatitis B and C viruses after immunosuppressive therapy: an unresolved issue. *Lancet Oncol*, 3(6), 333–40.

Verity, P. *et al.* (2001) Prospective evaluation of environmental contamination by *Clostridium difficile* in isolation side rooms. *J Hosp Infect*, 49(3), 204–9.

Vernon, M.O. *et al.* (2006) Chlorhexidine gluconate to cleanse patients in medical intensive care units: the effectiveness of source control to reduce the bioburden of vancomycin-resistant enterococci. *Arch Intern Med*, 166(3), 306–12.

Vianelli, N. *et al.* (2006) Resolution of a *Pseudomonas aerginosa* outbreak in a hematology unit with the use of disposable sterile water filters. *Haematologica*, 91(7), 983–5.

Vonberg, R.P. & Gastmeier, P. (2006) Nosocomial aspergillosis in outbreak settings. *J Hosp Infect*, 63(3), 246–54.

Vonberg, R.P. *et al.* (2005a) Reusable terminal tap water filters for nosocomial legionellosis prevention. *Ann Hematol*, 84(6), 403–5.

Vonberg, R.P. *et al.* (2005b) Use of terminal tap water filter systems for prevention of nosocomial legionellosis. *J Hosp Infect*, 60(2), 159–62.

Voth, D.E. & Ballard, J.D. (2005) *Clostridium difficile* toxins: mechanism of action and role in disease. *Clin Microbiol Rev*, 18(2), 247–63.

Walch, S.E., Roetzer, L.M. & Minnett, T.A. (2006) Suppport group participation among persons with HIV: demographic characteristics and perceived barriers. *AIDS Care*, 18(4), 284–9.

Walker, N., Gupta, R. & Cheesbrough, J. (2006) Blood pressure cuffs, friend or foe? *J Hosp Infect*, 63(2), 167–9.

Ward, D. (2000) Infection control: reducing the psychological effects of isolation. *Br J Nurs*, 9(3), 162–70.

Warny, M. *et al.* (2005) Toxin production by an emerging strain of *Clostridium difficile* associated with outbreaks of severe disease in North America and Europe. *Lancet*, 366(9491), 1079–84.

Wasley, A., Fiore, A. & Bell, B.P. (2006) Hepatitis A in the era of vaccination. *Epidemiol Rev*, 28(1), 101–11.

Wazir, J.F. & Ansari, N.A. (2004) *Pneumocystis carnii* infection. Update and review. *Arch Pathol Lab Med*, 128(9), 1023–7.

Weaving, P. (2006) Treatment strategies for bacteria and viruses. Why clinical management must be different. *Nurs Times*, 102(24), 42–3.

Weitzel, T. *et al.* (2006) Evaluation of seven commercial antigen detection tests for *Giardia* and *Cryptosporidium* in stool samples. *Clin Microbiol Infect*, 12(7), 656–9.

Wells, R. *et al.* (2006) Hepatitis A prevalence among injection drug users. *Clin Lab Sci*, 19(1), 12–17.

Welsby, P.D. (2006) Chickenpox, chickenpox vaccination, and shingles. *Postgrad Med J*, 82(967), 351–2.

Wendt, C. *et al.* (1998) Survival of vancomycin-resistant and vancomycin-susceptible enterococci on dry surfaces. *J Clin Microbiol*, 36(12), 3734–6.

Whitby, M., McLaws, M.L. & Ross, M.W. (2006) Why healthcare workers don't wash their hands: a behavioral explanation. *Infect Control Hosp Epidemiol*, 27(5), 484–92.

Whiting, L.S. (1999) Maintaining patients' personal hygiene. *Prof Nurse*, 14(5), 338–40.

Whitley, R. (2006) New approach to the therapy of HSV infections. *Herpes*, 13(2), 53–5.

Whitley, R.J. (2002) Herpes simplex virus in children. *Curr Treat Options Neurol*, **4**(3), 231–7.

Widdowson, M.A. *et al.* (2002) An outbreak of diarrhea in a neonatal medium care unit caused by a novel strain of rotavirus: investigation using both epidemiologic and microbiological methods. *Infect Control Hosp Epidemiol*, **23**(11), 665–70.

Wiesen, P., Van Gossum, A. & Preiser, J.C. (2006) Diarrhoea in the critically ill. *Curr Opin Crit Care*, **12**(2), 149–54.

Wigglesworth, N. & Wilcox, M.H. (2006) Prospective evaluation of hospital isolation room capacity. *J Hosp Infect*, **63**(2), 156–61.

Wilcox, M.H. & Dane, J. (2000) The cost of hospital-acquired infection and the value of infection control. *J Hosp Infect*, **45**(2), 81–4.

Wilcox, M.H. *et al.* (2003) Comparison of the effect of detergent versus hypochlorite cleaning an environmental contamination and incidence of *Clostridium difficile* infection. *J Hosp Infect*, **54**(2), 109–14.

Wilkes, C.R., Mason, A.D. & Hern, S.C. (2005) Probability distribution for showering and bathing water-use behavior for various US subpopulations. *Risk Anal*, **25**(2), 317–37.

Wilks, M. *et al.* (2006) Control of an outbreak of multidrug-resistant *Acinetobacter baumannii-calcoaceticus* colonization and infection in an intensive care unit without closing the ICU or placing patients in isolation. *Infect Control Hosp Epidemiol*, **27**(7), 654–8.

Willocks, L.J. *et al.* (2000) Compliance with advice to boil drinking water during an outbreak of cryptosporidiosis. *Commun Dis Public Health*, **3**(2), 137–8.

Wilson, A.P. *et al.* (2006) Computer keyboards and the spread of MRSA. *J Hosp Infect*, **62**(3), 390–2.

Wilson, B.J. (2002) Dietary recommendations for neutropenic patients. *Semin Oncol Nurs*, **81**(1), 44–9.

Wilson, J. (2006) *Infection Control in Clinical Practice*, 3rd edn. Bailliere Tindall, London.

Wilson, L.E. *et al.* (2006) Progression of liver fibrosis among injection drug users with chronic hepatitis C. *Hepatology*, **43**(4), 788–95.

Wolosin, R.J. (2005) HIV/AIDS patient satisfaction with hospitalization in the era of highly active antiretroviral therapy. *J Assoc Nurses AIDS Care*, **16**(5), 16–25.

Wood, E. *et al.* (2006) Impact of baseline viral load and adherence on survival of HIV-infected adults with baseline CD4 cell counts $\geq$200 cells/μL. *AIDS*, **20**(8), 1117–23.

Woodman, C.B. *et al.* (2005) Role of sexual behaviour in the acquisition of asymptomatic Epstein–Barr virus infection: a longitudinal study. *Pediatr Infect Dis J*, **24**(6), 498–502.

Working Group (2000) Guidelines for preventing opportunistic infections among hematopoietic stem cell transplant recipients. *Biol Blood Marrow Transplant*, **6**(6A), 7–83.

WHO (2002) *Framework for Effective Tuberculosis Control*. World Health Organization, Geneva.

Wright, D. (2005) Hepatitis C nightmare. Interview by Charlotte Alderman. *Nurs Stand*, **20**(5), 26–7.

Wright, L., Spickett, G. & Stoker, S. (2001) Latex allergy awareness among hospital staff. *Nursing Times Plus*, **97**(38), 4–8.

Wu, C.J. *et al.* (2006) Predominance of gram-negative bacilli and increasing antimicrobial resistance in nosocomial blood stream infections at a university hospital in southern Taiwan 1996–2003. *J Microbiol Immunol Infect*, **39**(2), 135–43.

Wyles, D.L. *et al.* (2005) Development of herpes simplex virus disease in patients who are receiving cidofovir. *Clin Infect Dis*, **41**(5), 676–80.

Yang, X.M. *et al.* (2006) Comparative proteomic analysis between invasive and commensal strains of *Staphylococcus epidermidis*. *FEMS Microbiol Lett*, **261**(1), 32–40.

Yates, J.W. *et al.* (1973) A controlled study of isolation and endogenous microbial suppression in acute myelocytic leukaemia patients. *Cancer*, **32**, 1490–8.

Yu, J. *et al.* (2005) *Aspergillus fiavus* genomics: gateway to human and animal health, food safety, and crop resistance to diseases. *Rev Iberoam Micol*, **22**(4), 194–202.

Zafar, A.B. *et al.* (1998) Effectiveness of infection control program in controlling nosocomial *Clostridium difficile*. *Am J Infect Control*, **26**(6), 588–93.

Ziebuhr, W. *et al.* (2006) Nosocomial infections by *Staphylococcus epidermidis*: how a commensal bacterium turns into a pathogen. *Int J Antimicrob Agents*, Suppl 1: S14-20.

Ziyaeyan, M. *et al.* (2006) Diagnosis and monitoring of human cytomegalovirus infection in bone marrow transplant recipients by quantitative competitive PCR. *Exp Clin Transplant*, **4**(1), 470–4.

Chapter 7

Breast aspiration and seroma drainage

147 **Breast aspiration**
149 Reference material
149 *Procedure guidelines:* Breast aspiration
151 **Seroma drainage**
153 *Procedure guidelines:* Seroma drainage
154 References and further reading

Breast aspiration

Definition

Both benign and malignant conditions can present as breast lumps (Blamey *et al.* 2000). Breast aspiration is a quick and easy diagnostic tool for obtaining a cell sample from a breast lump using a needle and syringe (Dixon 2006). A fine needle aspirate can be useful for differentiating between solid and cystic masses, and fine needle aspiration (FNA) is a useful diagnostic tool.

Reference material

Anatomy and physiology

The breast lies over the pectoral muscles of the chest wall between the 2nd and 6th ribs in the mid-clavicular line. It is composed of glandular, fatty and fibrous tissues and is connected to the chest wall by fibrous strands called Cooper's ligaments. Each breast is formed by 15–20 lobes surrounding the nipple, each of which contains multiple ducts and lobules (Figure 7.1). This is the functional unit of the breast. Milk formed in the breast lobules travels via the lactiferous ducts and empties into the nipple. Breasts begin to develop around the 6th week of foetal life and progress to the budding stage at the 12th week. They are formed from the ectodermal mammary ridge that runs from the axilla to the groin, often referred to as the nipple line. They are rudimentary in both sexes until the age of puberty, when, in response to ovarian hormones, they begin to develop visually (Grimsey 2004). Under the influence of the pituitary gland, follicle stimulating hormone and luteinizing hormone are produced. As the levels of these hormones rise the egg follicles within the ovary begin to produce oestrogen, which is responsible for the first stages of breast development. At around 10 years of age the mammary tissue behind the nipple enlarges, producing the characteristic swelling referred to as the breast bud. Oestrogen induces the connective tissue and vascular growth that is required to support the ductal system. The connective tissue in turn stimulates fat deposition. Once ovulation begins, the increased output of progesterone balances the oestrogen output and results in the maturation of glandular tissue (Hughes *et al.* 2000). During the menstrual cycle the breasts undergo cyclical changes due to the changing levels of the hormone prolactin, which controls the secretion of oestrogen and progesterone. These hormones cause the breast tissue and ducts to enlarge. As a result the breast may change in size and become tender and nodular in the luteal phase (the second half) of the menstrual cycle. This nodularity or lumpiness is more pronounced in some women more than others and may result in the formation of benign breast conditions such as cysts. Cyclical nodularity is so common that it can be regarded as physiological rather than pathological (Dixon 2006). Changes in the breast are also common during pregnancy. These changes are due first to oestrogen and progesterone and then to hormones produced by the placenta (Grimsey 2004). When ovarian activity ceases at the menopause, the levels of oestrogen and progesterone decrease and as a result the glandular tissue in the breast starts to involute and atrophy. The glandular tissue is then replaced by fat and the breasts feel softer and more pendulous. Most benign conditions and almost all breast cancers arise within the terminal duct lobular unit (Dixon 2006). Changes in the glandular tissue include the development of benign (non-cancerous) conditions such as fibroadenomas and cysts as well as breast cancer.

Breast cancer

Breast cancer is a disease that affects almost 42 000 women in the UK every year. This accounts for almost one in three of all cancer cases in women, and the lifetime risk for breast cancer in women is one in nine (Cancer Research UK 2006). Although breast cancer in men is rare, around 300 men are also diagnosed with breast cancer each year (Cancer Research UK 2006).

Invasive ductal carcinoma is the most common type of breast cancer accounting for over 70% of cases. Invasive lobular carcinoma forms the next biggest group, although only 9% are of this histological type. The remainder are made up of less common tumours such as Paget's disease, inflammatory carcinoma, mucinous carcinoma, medullary carcinoma, tubular carcinoma and very rare types such as lymphomas or sarcomas of the breast (Dixon & Sainsbury 1998; Brogi & Harris 1999; Diab *et al.* 1999; Pederson *et al.* 1999). Most breast cancers are invasive, i.e. the cells have spread through the linings of the ducts into surrounding tissues, but a few may be non-invasive or in situ. Some breast cancers may

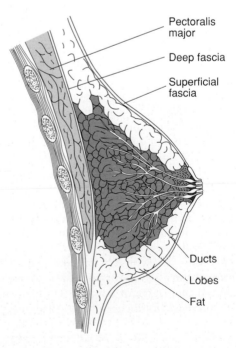

Figure 7.1 Anatomy of the breast.

(Labels: Pectoralis major; Deep fascia; Superficial fascia; Ducts; Lobes; Fat)

never become invasive and those that do may disseminate at different points in their development, dependent on their individual nature, varying from weeks in some, to years or never in others (Pointon & Day 1998).

Most lumps in the breast are found by patients themselves and these are far more likely to represent a benign condition such as a cyst or a fibroadenoma. Nine out of every ten breast lumps investigated in the hospital setting are benign (Cancer Research UK 2006). Consequently the majority of women are undergoing investigations to exclude malignancy. It is therefore important to find a simple, non-invasive test that can determine malignancy within given resources at minimal inconvenience to the patient.

Ideally less than 10% of all new patients with breast symptoms should be required to attend the hospital on more than two occasions for diagnostic purposes (BASO 2005).

Diagnostic methods

When a lump is found in the breast it is necessary to differentiate between benign and malignant disease in order to provide the appropriate treatment and care. Guidelines suggest the diagnostic process should be carried out in a designated breast clinic, which should provide an environment that allows effective multi-disciplinary clinical practice, whilst providing privacy for each individual patient (BASO 2005). Nowadays, diagnosis should be based on triple assessment, when an initial clinical assessment may be followed by appropriate imaging, FNA and/or core biopsy (BASO 2005). Not every patient will require each aspect of the triple assessment (Dixon 2006). However combining all three is recommended as the standard assessment approach and leads to a marked improvement in diagnostic accuracy (Wilson et al. 2001; BASO 2005) and enables a definitive diagnosis to be made in the vast majority of patients (Dixon & Sainsbury 1998). Consequently patients will know the diagnosis prior to any surgical intervention and can be prepared and informed beforehand. Health care professionals are also less reliant on surgery in the first instance, at a time when chemotherapy and hormone therapy are increasingly used as primary treatments for breast cancer. Triple assessment has a low, but definitive false negative rate (when the disease is present but not identified by the diagnostic test performed), which is higher in younger patients (BASO 2005).

An alternative method to FNA is core biopsy. An incision is made in the breast under local anaesthetic and a wide bore needle used to take a core of breast tissue. This method is helpful in differentiating between invasive and non-invasive disease. However, the procedure is more time consuming and, unlike FNA, the result cannot be made available immediately (Blamey et al. 2000).

Many other prognostic markers can now be measured from FNAs. In conjunction with immunocytochemistry, it is possible to measure oestrogen receptor, progesterone receptor and other markers such as the p53 enzyme and HER2/neu (McManus & Anderson 2001), although currently these are still more commonly performed on histological material.

Such markers indicate the likely growth mechanisms of the cancer and which medical treatments may be appropriate.

Fine-needle aspiration cytology
Accuracy

It is now possible to obtain very high accuracy rates in diagnosing breast cancer with FNA cytology. Both sensitivity (the number of cancers reported as cancer) and specificity (the number of benign lesions reported as benign) with this technique are reported as between 90 and 98% (Rocha et al. 1997; Arisio et al. 1998; Dixon 2006). Evidence suggests that most centres report false positive rates (i.e. mistaken diagnosis of cancer) of less than 0.5% (Dixon 2006) and false negative rates of about 5% (Dixon 2006). However, it is acceptable to plan treatment on the basis of malignant cytology supported by a diagnosis of malignancy on clinical examination and imaging. In symptomatic breast disease, FNA cytology used alongside clinical and radiological assessment allows a rapid, innexpensive and accurate diagnosis (Roskell & Buley 2004). False negative readings can occur when insufficient cells are obtained for analysis or when cancer cells are missed. Therefore accuracy is largely dependent on the expertise of the individuals performing the aspiration and interpreting the results (Shumate 1996; McKenzie & Dalrymple 1998). It is essential that professionals undertaking this procedure have expertise in this area (Roskell & Buley 2004) and practise several times a week to ensure consistent results (Ljung et al. 1994).

Application

Advantages of FNA, as mentioned previously, are that it is a quick, relatively non-invasive test and can be performed in the outpatient department. It also enables solid and cystic lesions to be differentiated. If the lump is a cyst then the fluid will drain out on aspiration and the lump will disappear. Therefore FNA has a therapeutic role in the symptomatic relief of a painful cyst, as well as a diagnostic role in the presence of a solid lesion. Clear fluid aspirated from breast cysts need not have cytological examination unless the lump has not disappeared. When blood is detected in the aspirate, it is recommended that the fluid is sent for cytology since often intracystic carcinomas yield bloodstained fluid (Querci Della Rovere et al. 2005).

A limitation with the application of FNA to breast diagnosis is that it may not be possible to reliably distinguish between in situ and invasive carcinoma, due to the lack of structural information derived from cells (McManus & Anderson 2001) when compared with that derived from tissues (histology). Internal consistency during FNA cytology is classified according to the degree of hardness (soft, rubbery or hard) and the presence or absence of a gritty texture during the procedure (Ousch et al. 2003). This description can give the operator some indication as to whether a lump is more likely to be benign or malignant.

Table 7.1 Classification of fine needle aspiration cytology.

C1	**Inadequate:** this is reported when scanty material has been obtained, which is insufficient for a diagnosis to be made (Dixon & Sainsbury 1998)
C2	**Benign**
C3	**Atypia:** atypical cells are seen but the majority of these will still be benign
C4	**Suspicious of malignancy:** 70–90% of these will eventually turn out to be malignant (McManus & Anderson 2001)
C5	**Malignancy confirmed**

Reporting

Reports have a numerical score (1–5) as well as a 'C score' (standing for cytology) and are categorized (Table 7.1).

The patient's experience

Many patients undergoing this procedure may be highly anxious due to concern over the possible diagnosis of cancer. Maguire (2006) acknowledges that a substantial proportion of women whose lumps prove to be benign remain distressed and as a result are at risk of anxiety and depression. Anxiety may increase the perceived pain of the procedure and if the patient is restless due to anxiety they may move when the needle is inserted. This may affect the accuracy of the procedure and increase the risk of complications. Burnett (Burnett & Purushotham 2001) identifies that it is hypothetically possible to pierce the lung and cause a pneumothorax when performing this procedure. Care should therefore be taken when performing aspiration in those areas of the breast where there is little breast tissue. Tumours are often vascular and there is also a risk of haematoma formation if care is not taken. This in turn can cause distortion of a mammogram and therefore difficulty in interpretation. For this reason mammogram investigations should be carried out prior to any needle biopsies being performed (BASO 2005). The process of aspiration can be uncomfortable or even painful when a 23 G needle is used routinely (Daltrey & Kissin 2000). However, a recent study provides evidence that a 27 G FNA cytology is suitable for obtaining cytology in palpable breast lumps (Querci della Rovere *et al.* 2005). Local anaesthetic is not normally used because it may distort the area to be needled and decrease the accuracy. However, a recent study showed that the use of local anaesthetic helped the tolerance of patients to the procedure and gave the operator a better chance of obtaining an adequate sample for diagnosis (Tutton 2001).

It is essential that patients receive explanations about each step of the procedure and are given a chance to discuss it or ask questions as required. Information delivered at a pace and in a language the patient can understand may result in decreased anxiety, decreased pain levels and improved compliance (Poroch 1995; Daltrey & Kissin 2000).

Summary

FNA of the breast is cost effective, rapid and accurate (McManus & Anderson 2001) and causes less discomfort and emotional distress than open biopsy (Layfield *et al.* 1993). With the proviso that experienced personnel undertake the procedure and examination of cells, for the majority of centres this is now the preferred method of diagnosis in breast cancer.

Procedure guidelines   Breast aspiration

Equipment

1 70% isopropyl alcohol swabs.
2 Sterile syringes (10 or 20 ml).
3 Sterile needles (21 or 23 G).
4 Microscope slides.
5 Universal container.
6 Slide tray.
7 Fixative (ethanol).
8 Low-linting gauze.
9 Plaster/surgical tape.
10 Sharps container.
11 Cytology request form.
12 Microscope slide holders.

Procedure

Action	Rationale
1 Place the patient lying down on a couch in a position that facilitates access to the site on the breast requiring aspiration. This may require them to roll slightly on their side or to lift their arm above the head.	To ensure the patient is comfortable and to ensure safety should the patient feel faint during the procedure (P).
2 Explain and discuss the procedure with the patient.	To ensure that the patient understands the procedure and gives his/her valid consent (E; NMC 2006: C).

Procedure guidelines *(cont.)*

3 Place slides on a tray.	In preparation for breast aspirate (E).
4 Prepare syringe by introducing 2 ml of air into the barrel.	To prevent aspirated material being sucked into the syringe (E).
5 Choose appropriate size needle and attach to the syringe.	Preferably 23 G, but for a large breast or deep lesion 21 G may be necessary (Walker 1998: R1; Daltrey & Kissin 2000: R1).
6 Clean area of patient's skin with single-use sterile swab saturated with 70% isopropyl alcohol.	To reduce the risk of infection (E).
7 Firmly fix breast lump or area of clinical interest between the fingers of one hand.	To stabilize the area before introducing the needle to ensure the correct area sampled (E).
8 Warn the patient that a needle is about to be inserted.	To reduce the risk of the patient moving (P).
9 Push the needle tip into the centre of the lump or area of clinical interest. Note consistency (see Action figure 9).	To obtain specimen from appropriate area. Consistency can be a diagnostic indicator, i.e. gritty (malignant) or rubbery (benign). This information is of use to the cytologist (E).
10 If the lump is thought to be cystic be careful not to move the needle whilst withdrawing fluid. Withdraw the needle when no further fluid appears in the syringe. If the fluid is discoloured send for cytological examination.	The needle must be kept in place in the cyst sack whilst withdrawing fluid to enable complete drainage of the cyst and reduce chances of it refilling. Clear fluid is indicative of a cyst only. Anything else should be sent to the laboratory to exclude malignancy (E).
11 Aspirate a solid lesion or area of clinical interest using the maximum amount of suction moving the tip of the needle back and forth and in different directions without withdrawing the needle through the skin.	To enable sampling of different areas and to obtain an adequate sample for transferring to the slide. There is no evidence that tumour cells can be disseminated along the needle tract (E).
12 After aspiration, allow the barrel of the syringe to return to 2 ml before withdrawing the needle to eliminate any negative pressure in the syringe.	To avoid the contents of the needle being sucked into the syringe (E).
13 After withdrawal of the needle from the breast, express the aspirate on to the slides. If the aspirate is thick then more slides will be required. Smear the cells evenly on the slides, with a second slide.	To prepare the cells for cytodiagnosis. A monolayer is required because if the smear is bloodstained or there is too much material on the slide, staining can be a problem and the cytologist cannot make a diagnosis (E).
14 Dry gauze should be placed over the puncture site and pressure applied for at least 1 minute or until bleeding has stopped.	To reduce the risk of haematoma formation (E).
15 Leave one slide to dry in the air and add fixative to the other as required by the cytologist. Label appropriately.	When such a small amount of material is available the cytologist will require different staining techniques for accurate diagnosis (E).

16 If the aspirate is lost into the barrel of the needle 5 ml of 0.9% sodium chloride should be drawn into the syringe through the same needle and the resultant suspension placed in a universal container.	So that the sample can be recovered by centrifugation and then stained as normal. A large percentage of the cells will still be lost (E).
17 Dispose of needle and syringe in sharps container.	To reduce risk of injury and infection to staff (E).
18 Label slides with name, number and which breast.	To ensure correct identification of specimen (E).
19 Apply a plaster or non-allergenic dressing to puncture site.	To protect clothing (P).
20 Complete cytology forms with full details.	To ensure correct identification and most accurate information for diagnosis (E).
21 Place slides in slide holder. Slide holder and cytology forms to be placed in plastic specimen bag.	To ensure safe transfer to laboratory (E).

151

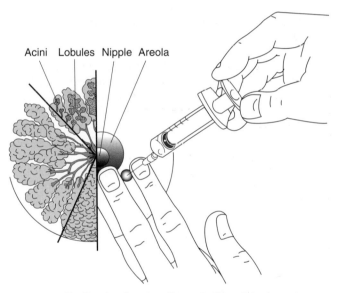

Acini   Lobules   Nipple   Areola

Action 9   Performing fine-needle aspiration of the breast.

Seroma drainage

Definition

A seroma is defined as a clinically identifiable collection of serous fluid within any *surgical* cavity (Woodworth *et al.* 2000). Seroma formation is a common complication of breast surgery. Dixon (2006) identified that seroma formation occurred in one-third to one-half of all patients following mastectomy and axillary surgery.

Possible causes of seroma formation after breast surgery

There are no proven causes of seroma formation. It is normal for haemo-serous fluid to collect postoperatively at the site of excision. Fluid collects where there is a space following tissue removal and it will continue to do so until the underlying tissues adhere (Harmer 2004). However, the likelihood of seroma formation appears to be dependent on the median yield of axillary lymph nodes excised and the surgical level of axillary dissection performed. There is no relationship between seroma formation and the patient's age, tumour size, grade or body mass index (Woodworth *et al.* 2000). Following breast surgery, drains are inserted and removed according to hospital policy, surgeon's preference and the volume drained over a 24-hour period. It is common for serous fluid to collect after removal of the drain. Depending on the amount that it has drained, a surgeon or specialist nurse may aspirate this as required.

Effects of seroma formation on the patient

Patients who develop seromas will commonly experience pain and discomfort, which may in turn prevent them from performing postoperative arm exercises which are recommended to restore mobility and minimize the risk of lymphoedema. A recurrent seroma if left untreated may increase the risk of infection. This can result in a delay in the initiation of adjuvant therapy. In more extreme circumstances the patient is at risk of skin flap necrosis if they have undergone breast reconstruction (Miller 1998).

Indications for seroma drainage

The following list indicates when it is appropriate for a nurse to undertake the procedure of seroma drainage:

- A seroma is visible to the naked eye, is located under the skin in the axilla, chest wall or back, has a 'water-bed' consistency when depressed and released, and the area is free from infection.
- A seroma is causing pain, discomfort or pressure/ tightness.
- A seroma is causing the patient restricted mobility, i.e. they are unable to maintain their exercise regime or daily activities.

- The patient has been adequately informed and is physically and psychologically prepared to undergo the procedure.
- The individual nurse has attained a level of proficiency and is competent to drain seromas independently.

Contraindications for seroma drainage

The following list indicates when it is inappropriate for a nurse to undertake the procedure of seroma drainage:

- An infection is clinically evident or suspected.
- The presence of a haematoma is suspected.
- The patient has a breast implant in situ (secondary to breast reconstruction), unless the seroma is located on the back as a result of autologous tissue transfer.
- The seroma is not causing discomfort or pain and is not affecting the patient's ability to continue their postoperative exercise regime or daily activities.
- The individual nurse has not attained a level of proficiency to be competent to drain seromas independently.

Potential complications arising during or following seroma drainage

Table 7.2 is a list of complications and subsequent actions required if they are suspected.

Summary

Seroma drainage is a relatively quick and atraumatic procedure that can relieve pain and discomfort and improve mobility and healing, with the proviso that it is conducted by proficient and appropriately trained nurses who ensure their competence is kept up to date by regularly incorporating it into their practice.

Table 7.2 Complications and actions required following seroma drainage.

Complication	Action required
Suspected pneumothorax on insertion of needle	Withdraw needle and call medical staff for assistance immediately
Suspected local infection (characterized by inflammation and erythema at wound site but with no exudate) (Miller 1998)	Continue with seroma drainage, referring to medical staff if the symptoms do not resolve after drainage as the patient may require antibiotic therapy
Suspected systemic infection (characterized by the patient feeling unwell and feverish with a pyrexia of 38°C or greater and inflammation and exudate present at the wound site) (Miller 1998)	Discontinue seroma drainage, referring to medical staff as the patient will require antibiotic therapy and may need further investigations
Drainage fails to resolve the seroma	Refer to medical staff for advice and assistance
Fluid aspirated is suspected to contain blood or pus in addition to or instead of serous fluid	Send fluid sample to microbiology for culture and sensitivity and inform the medical staff
The seroma is recurrent, filling again in excess of five times with the amount of fluid removed remaining static or increasing	Drain the seroma and refer to medical staff for advice on any further action required, such as insertion of a wound drain

Procedure guidelines Seroma drainage

Equipment

1 Sterile dressing pack containing indented plastic tray, dry gauze swabs, disposable gloves, sterile field and disposable bag.
2 Sterile syringes (30 and 50 ml).
3 Sterile needles (21 G).
4 Chlorhexidine in 70% alcohol solution (or equivalent).
5 Sterile dressing (non-adherent, 5–7 cm) or hypo-allergenic tape and gauze.
6 Sharps container.
7 Universal container.

Procedure

Action	Rationale
1 Place the patient lying down on a couch in a position that facilitates access to the seroma.	To ensure the patient is comfortable and the seroma is visible and accessible (E).
2 Explain and discuss the procedure with the patient.	To ensure that the patient understands the procedure and gives valid consent and co-operation (E; NMC 2006: C).
3 Open dressing pack on a clean trolley and lay out equipment, adhering to an aseptic technique as stated in Chapter 5.	To ensure no equipment is missing and to maintain asepsis (E).
4 Clean identified puncture site for drainage of seroma with chlorhexidine-soaked gauze and allow to dry.	To prevent infection and minimize 'stinging' when the needle is inserted (E).
5 Insert needle at a 45° angle towards seroma fluid.	To minimize discomfort and optimize the seroma drainage.
6 Gently draw back on the syringe. If the syringe becomes full, disconnect and discard in a yellow waste bag. Connect a new syringe and repeat.	To drain the fluid from the seroma and to ensure safe disposal of waste products (E; DH 2005: C).
7 When fluid ceases to flow, remove both the needle and the syringe together (do not disconnect them). Dispose both immediately in a sharps container.	To ensure the safe disposal of sharps and to minimize the risk of needlestick injury (E).
8 Apply pressure with gauze over the puncture site for at least 1 minute, after removal of the needle.	To reduce the risk of leakage and to allow the puncture site to close (E).
9 Apply a non-adherent dressing or non-allergenic tape and gauze over the puncture site. Instruct the patient to remove this 24 hours from the time of drainage.	To protect the patient's clothing and the puncture site, and to reduce the risk of infection (P).
10 Ensure the patient understands what to do in the event of reaccumulation of the seroma.	To maximize patient education and to ensure the safe discharge of the patient (P).
11 Complete the appropriate paperwork.	To ensure accurate record keeping and to promote continuity of patient care (P; NMC 2005: C).

References and further reading

Arisio, R. *et al.* (1998) Role of fine-needle aspiration biopsy in breast lesions: analysis of a series of 4110 cases. *Diagn Cytopathol*, 18(6), 462–7.

BASO (2005) The Association of Breast Surgery guidelines for the management of symptomatic breast disease. *Eur J Surg Oncol*, 31, S1–S21.

Berger, K. & Bostwick, J. (1998) Breast anatomy and physiology. In: *A Woman's Decision: Breast Care, Treatment and Reconstruction*, 3rd edn. Quality Medical Publishing, St. Louis, MO, pp. 7–12.

Blamey, R.W., Wilson, A.R.M. & Patnick, J. (2000) Screening for breast cancer. *BMJ*, 321(7262), 689–93.

British Association of Surgical Oncologists (2005) Guidelines for the management of symptomatic breast disease. *Eur J Surg Oncol*, 31, S1–21.

Brogi, E. & Harris, N. (1999) Lymphomas of the breast: pathology and clinical behaviour. *Semin Oncol*, 26(3), 357–64.

Burnett, K.L & Purushotham, A. (2001) *Holistic Breast Care*. Bailliere Tindall, Edinburgh.

Cancer Research UK (2006) www.canceresearchuk.org

Chaplin, B. (1996) Breast cancer: knowledge for practice. *Nurs Times*, 92(10), 1–4.

Daltrey, I.R. & Kissin, M.W. (2000) Randomised controlled trial of the effect of needle gauge and local anaesthetic on the pain of breast fine needle aspiration cytology. *Br J Surg*, 87, 777–9.

DH (2005) *Hazardous waste (England) regulations*. Department of Health, London.

Diab, S. *et al.* (1999) Tumour characteristics and clinical outcome of tubular and mucinous breast carcinomas. *J Clin Oncol*, 17(5), 1442–8.

Dixon, M. (2006) Symptoms, assessment and guidelines for referral. In: *ABC of Breast Diseases*, 3rd edn (ed. M. Dixon). BMJ Books, London.

Dixon, M. & Sainsbury, R. (1998) *Handbook of Diseases of the Breast*, 2nd edn. Churchill Livingstone, London.

Grimsey, E. (2004) An overview of breast cancer. In: *Breast Cancer Nursing Care and Management* (ed. V. Harmer). Whurr Publishers, London, pp. 1–17.

Harmer, V. (2004) Surgery as a treatment for breast cancer. In: *Breast Cancer Nursing Care and Management* (ed. V. Harmer). Whurr Publishers, London, pp. 82–95.

Hughes, L.E., Mansel, R.E. & Webster, T.J.G. (2000) *Benign Disorders and Diseases of the Breast: Concepts and Clinical Management*. W.B. Saunders, London.

Layfield, L. *et al.* (1993) The Palpable breast nodule: a cost effectiveness analysis of alternate diagnostic approaches. *Cancer*, 72(5), 1642–51.

Ljung, B.-M. *et al.* (1994) Fine needle aspiration techniques for the characterization of breast cancers. *Cancer*, 74, 1000–5.

Maguire, P. (2006) Psychological aspects. In: *ABC of Breast Diseases*, 3rd edn, pp. 85–89 (ed. M. Dixon). BMJ Publishing, London.

McKenzie, J.G. & Dalrymple, J. (1998) Fine needle aspiration. In: *Early Breast Cancer: From Screening to Multidisciplinary Management* (eds M. Morgan, R. Warren & G. Querci Della Rovere). Harwood Academic Publishers, Canada.

McManus, D.T. & Anderson, N.H. (2001) Fine needle aspiration cytology of the breast. *Curr Diagnost Pathol*, 7, 262–71.

Miller, M. (1998) How do I diagnose and treat wound infection? *Br J Nurs*, 7(6), 335–8.

National Cancer Institute (1997) The uniform approach to breast fine needle aspiration biopsy. *Am J Surg*, 174(4), 371–85.

NMC (2005) *Guidelines for Records and Record Keeping*. Nursing and Midwifery Council, London.

NMC (2006) *A–Z Advice Sheet Consent*. www.nmc.org

Online Management of Breast Diseases (1997) Anatomy of the breast and axilla: standard axillary lymphadenectomy. www.breastdiseases.com. Accessed on 15/07/06.

Osborne, M.P. (2000) Breast anatomy and development. In: *Diseases of the Breast*, 2nd edn (eds J.R. Harris *et al.*). Lippincott, Williams and Wilkins, London.

Ousch, J.R *et al.* (2003) Breast Aid: Clinical results from early development of a clinical decision rule for palpable solid breast masses. *Ann Surg*, 238(5), 728–37.

Pederson, L. *et al.* (1999) Prognostic comparison of three classifications for medullary carcinoma of the breast. *Histopathology*, 34(2), 175–8.

Pointon, L.J. & Day, N.E. (1998) The background of screening for breast cancer. In: *Early Breast Cancer: From Screening to Multidisciplinary Management* (eds M. Morgan, R. Warren & G. Querci Della Rovere). Harwood Academic Publishers, Canada.

Poroch, D. (1995) The effect of preparatory patient education on the anxiety and satisfaction of cancer patients receiving radiation therapy. *Cancer Nursing*, 18(3), 206–14.

Querci Della Rovere, G., Trott, P., Filshie, J., Ashley, S. & Hassanally, D. (2005) A prospective randomised study to evaluate the effectiveness of standard 23 gauge fine needle compared with a thinner 27 gauge needle for breast cytology. *The Breast*, 15(4), 567–9.

Rocha, P., Nadkarni, N. & Menezes, S. (1997) Fine needle aspiration biopsy of breast lesions and histopathological correlation. An analysis of 837 cases in 4 years. *Acta Cytol*, 41(3), 705–12.

Roskell, D.E. & Buley, I.D. (2004) Fine needle aspiration cytology in cancer diagnosis. *BMJ*, 329, 244–5.

Shumate, C. (1996) Surgical evaluation and treatment of breast cancer. In: *Diagnosis and Management of Breast Disease* (eds R. Blackwell & J. Grotting). Blackwell Science, Boston, MA.

Soo, M.S. & Williford, M.E. (1995) Seromas in the breast: imaging findings. *Crit Rev Diagnost Imag*, 36(5), 385–440.

Steering Committee on Clinical Practice Guidelines for the Care and Treatment of Breast Cancer (1998) Axillary dissection. *Can Assoc Radiat Oncol*, 158(3), 22–6.

Tutton, R. (2001) The effect of needle gauge and local anaesthetic on the diagnostic accuracy of breast fine needle aspiration cytology. *Eur J Surg Oncol*, 25, 42–5.

Walker, S. (1998) A randomized controlled trial comparing a 21G needle with a 23G needle for fine needle aspiration of breast lumps. *J R Coll Surg*, 43(5), 322–3.

Wilson, R. *et al.* (2001) *Clinical Guidelines for Breast Cancer Screening Assessment*. NHS Cancer Screening Programmes, Sheffield.

Woodworth, P.A. *et al.* (2000) Seroma formation after breast cancer surgery: incidence and predicting factors. *Am J Surg*, 66(5), 444–50.

154

Chapter 8

Cardiopulmonary resuscitation

Reference material **156**
Procedure guidelines: Cardiopulmonary resuscitation (CPR) **163**
References and further reading **167**

Definition

Sudden death as a result of cardiac arrest is responsible for 60% ischaemic heart disease deaths across Europe (RCUK 2005). Survival to hospital discharge is cited as 10.7% of all types of cardiac arrest with survival being higher (21.2%) in ventricular fibrillation arrests (RCUK 2005).

The term cardiac arrest implies a sudden interruption of cardiac output. It may be reversible with appropriate treatment (Handley 2004). The patient will collapse, lose consciousness, stop breathing and will be pulseless (Jevon 2001).

The four arrhythmias that cause cardiac arrest are:

- Asystole.
- Ventricular fibrillation (VF).
- Pulseless ventricular tachycardia (VT).
- Pulseless electrical activity (PEA).

For the purposes of resuscitation guidelines these rhythms are divided into two groups by their treatment.

- VF and pulseless VT, which require defibrillation
- Non-VF/VT, which do not require defibrillation (RCUK 2005).

Indications

The patient is unconscious, has absent or agonal (gasping) respirations and has no pulse (Perkins *et al.* 2005). Other clinical features such as pupil size, cyanosis and pallor are unreliable and so the practitioner should not waste time looking for them (Skinner & Vincent 1997).

Reference material

Principles

Failure of the circulation for 3–4 minutes will lead to irreversible cerebral damage (Docherty & Hall 2002). Basic life support (BLS) acts to slow down the deterioration of the brain and the heart until defibrillation and/or advanced life support (ALS) can be provided (RCUK 2005).

Resuscitation is the emergency treatment of any condition in which the brain fails to receive enough oxygen. The basic technique involves a rapid simple assessment of the patient followed by the BLS resuscitation. The first international consensus evidence based guidelines on resuscitation were published in 2000 (AHA/ILCOR 2000). These guidelines were reviewed in 2004/05 by the International Liaison Committee on Resuscitation and published in 2005 (International Liaison Committee on Resuscitation 2005). These internationally agreed guidelines based on research and audit now form the basis for the European Resuscitation Guidelines (European Resuscitation Council 2005) as well as the UK Resuscitation Guidelines (RCUK 2005).

Assessment

There are two stages of assessment.

1   An immediate assessment by the rescuer to ensure that cardiopulmonary resuscitation (CPR) may safely proceed

Figure 8.1   Initial verbal assessment.

(i.e. checking there is no immediate danger to the rescuer from any hazard, for example electrical power supply).

2   Assessment by the rescuer of the likelihood of injury sustained by the patient, particularly injury to the cervical spine. Although there may be no external evidence of injury, the immediate situation may provide the necessary evidence. For example, trauma to the cervical spine should be suspected in an accelerating/decelerating injury such as a road traffic accident with a motorbike travelling at speed. Once these two aspects have been assessed, the patient's level of consciousness should be checked by gently shaking his shoulders and asking loudly if he is alright (Figure 8.1). If there is no response the rescuer should commence the BLS assessment (Figure 8.2) immediately.

Note: if the arrest is witnessed or monitored, and a defibrillator is not immediately to hand, a single precordial thump should be administered. If delivered within 30 seconds after cardiac arrest, a sharp blow with a closed fist on the patient's sternum may convert VF back to a perfusing rhythm (RCUK 2005).

Basic life support

Basic life support (BLS) is sometimes known as the 'ABC'.

Airway

The rescuer should look in the mouth and remove any visible obstruction (leave well-fitting dentures in place). The most likely obstruction in an unconscious person is the tongue. The head tilt/chin lift manoeuvre (Figure 8.3), which removes the tongue from occluding the oropharynx, is an effective method of opening an airway and relieving obstruction in 80% of patients (Simmons 2002).

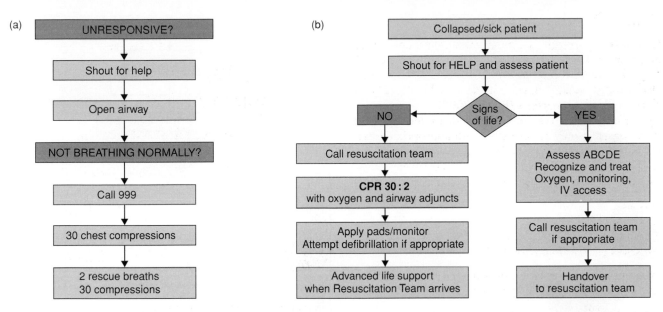

Figure 8.2 (a) Basic life support algorithm. (b) In-hospital resuscitation algorithm. CPR, cardiopulmonary resuscitation; IV, intravenous. Courtesy of RCUK (2005).

Note: if there is any suspicion of cervical spine injury (see above) try to avoid head tilt.

Breathing

Keeping the airway open, the rescuer should look, listen and feel for breathing (more than an occasional gasp or weak attempts at breathing) for up to 10 seconds. If the patient is breathing they should be turned into the recovery position (Figure 8.4). If the adult patient is not breathing and there is no suspicion of trauma or drowning, an immediate call for the cardiac arrest team should be made. It should be noted that in 40% of cases a person who has arrested still has agonal (gasping) respirations and these can be mistaken for normal breaths (Hauff *et al.* 2003). Artificial ventila-

tion must then be commenced and maintained. If there are no aids to ventilation available then direct mouth-to-mouth ventilation should be used (Figure 8.5). The recommended length for each breath is now 1 second (RCUK 2005). When cardiac arrest occurs in hospital, the RCUK (2005) recommend the use of adjuncts such as the pocket mask or the bag mask unit. They can be used to avoid direct person-to-person contact and some devices may reduce the risk of cross-infection between patient and rescuer (RCUK 2005). In 2005 in recognition of the concern in providing mouth-to-mouth resuscitation, the guidelines changed and the BLS

Figure 8.3 Head tilt/chin lift manoeuvre.

Figure 8.4 The recovery position.

158

Figure 8.5 If patient is not breathing, expired air resuscitation must be started immediately. Courtesy of Colqhoun *et al.* (1999).

Figure 8.6 The advanced life support algorithm for the management of cardiac arrest in adults. CPR, cardiopulmonary resuscitation; IV, intravenous; PEA, pulseless electrical activity; VF, ventricular fibrillation; VT, ventricular tachycardia. Courtesy of RCUK (2005).

algorithm now starts with chest compressions and then proceeds to two breaths (RCUK 2005).

One of the most easily learnt aids is the 'mouth-to-face mask' method. This is where a valved exhaled air ventilation mask with an oxygen attachment valve is used. The mask directs the patient's exhaled air and any fluid away from the rescuer and the oxygen port allows attachment of oxygen with enrichment up to 45%.

If the operator is skilled in airway management, an Ambu bag and mask may be used. When the bag is attached to oxygen, high levels, of up to 85%, can be obtained. However, it should be emphasized that to manipulate the head tilt, and hold on a face mask while squeezing a bag is a procedure that requires practice and is most safely achieved by two people, one holding the mask and one squeezing the bag (Hodgetts & Castle 1999).

The most effective method of airway management is to use an endotracheal tube, thus enabling the application of 100% oxygen (Bossaert *et al.* 1998). This method of airway management is included in the advanced life support algorithm (Figure 8.6).

Circulation

Circulation is assessed by looking for any signs of movement, including swallowing or breathing. If trained to do so, a check should also be made for the carotid pulse (Figure 8.7) for up to 10 seconds. If no circulation is detected it must be maintained by compressions. The correct place to compress is in the centre of the lower half of the sternum (Figure 8.8). The rescuer should position themselves vertically above the patient with arms straight and elbows locked. The sternum should be pressed down to depress it by 4–5 cm. This should be repeated at a rate of about 100 times a minute. After 30 compressions two rescue breaths are given, continuing compressions and rescue breaths in a ratio of 30:2 (RCUK 2005). There is evidence that chest compressions are often interrupted and that this is associated with a reduction in the chance of survival, it is therefore imperative that interruptions to chest compressions are minimized by effective coordination between rescuers (Eftestol *et al.* 2002; Van Alem *et al.* 2003).

Figure 8.7 If patient does not have a pulse in a major artery (carotid), or if there is a neck injury, the femoral artery may be felt. Circulation must then be established with compression. Courtesy of Colqhoun *et al.* (2004).

Figure 8.8 Establishing circulation with compression. Note fingers are clear of chest wall. Courtesy of Colqhoun *et al.* (1999).

Potentially reversible causes of a cardiopulmonary arrest

During cardiac arrest, potential causes or aggravating factors for which specific treatment exists should be considered. For ease of memory there are eight common causes of arrest, four of which begin with the letter H and four with the letter T:

- Hypoxia.
- Hypovolaemia.
- Hypothermia.
- Hypo/hyperkalaemia.
- Thromboembolism.
- Tension pneumothorax.
- Tamponade.
- Toxicity (metabolic or drug induced) (RCUK 2005).

Hypoxia

There are many reasons why a patient may become severely hypoxic (see Chapters 25 & 38), the most common being the following:

- Acute respiratory failure.
- Airway difficulties.
- Acute lung injury.
- Severe anaemia.
- Neuromuscular disorders.

For healthy cell metabolism the body requires a constant supply of oxygen. When this is interrupted for more than 3 minutes in most situations (except when there is severe hypothermia) cell death occurs, followed by lactic acidosis and very rapidly a cardiorespiratory arrest. The risk of hypoxia is minimized by ensuring that the patient's lungs are ventilated adequately with 100% oxygen (RCUK 2005).

Hypovolaemia

Hypovolaemia in adults that results in PEA is usually due to severe blood loss. While it is not the nurse's role to make a medical diagnosis, they may be aware of significant factors in the history of a patient that may have led to PEA.

The most common causes of severe blood loss are:

- Trauma.
- Surgical procedure.
- Gastrointestinal mucosa erosion.
- Oesophageal varices.
- Peripheral vessel erosion (by tumour usually).
- Clotting abnormality.

Note: blood loss, although usually overt, can be covert such as a gastrointestinal bleed which may only become apparent when the patient collapses.

The treatment for hypovolaemia is identifying and stopping the source of fluid or blood loss, and replacing the circulating volume with the appropriate fluid. Fluid resuscitation is normally started with a crystalloid, e.g. 0.9% sodium chloride, and/or colloid, e.g. Gelofusin (depending on local protocols). Blood is likely to be required rapidly if the blood loss exceeds 1500–2000 ml in an adult (RCUK 2005).

159

Hypothermia

Hypothermia should be suspected in any submersion or immersion injury. During a prolonged resuscitation attempt, a patient who was normothermic at the onset of cardiac arrest may become hypothermic (RCUK 2005). A low reading thermometer should be used if available. Resuscitation in the presence of hypothermia may be prolonged.

Hypo/hyperkalaemia and other metabolic disorders

Because potassium is so closely linked with muscle and nerve excitation, any imbalance will affect both the nervous conduction and the muscular working of the heart. Therefore a severe rise or fall in potassium can cause arrest arrhythmias. The causes of hypokalaemia are:

- Gastrointestinal fluid losses.
- Urinary fluid loss.
- Drugs that affect cellular potassium, e.g. antifungal agents such as amphotericin.

The immediate treatment for hypokalaemia that has resulted in an arrest is to give concentrated infusions of potassium while carefully monitoring the serial potassium measurements. Most intensive care unit (ICU)/Accident and Emergency (A&E) departments and coronary care units (CCUs) will have an arterial blood gas analyser that enables the potassium to be measured in 1 minute.

The patients who are most at risk of hyperkalaemia are those with renal failure or Addison's disease. The immediate treatment for hyperkalaemia is to give intravenous calcium. This has the effect of protecting the myocardium during the cardiac arrest. If the patient is successfully resuscitated it will be essential to monitor their serum potassium and if it remains high to commence therapy to lower or remove the potassium (RCUK 2006).

Thromboembolism

The commonest cause of thromboembolic or mechanical circulatory obstruction is a massive pulmonary embolus. Options for definitive treatment include thrombolysis or, if available, cardiopulmonary bypass and operative removal of the clot (RCUK 2005).

Tension pneumothorax

A tension pneumothorax is the sudden collapse of a lung, usually under pressure, which results in a severe change in intrathoracic pressure and cessation of the heart as a pump (Bersten & Soni 2003). The most common causes are:

- Trauma.
- Acute lung injury.
- Mechanical ventilation of the newborn.

The immediate treatment is the insertion of a large-bore cannula into the second intercostal space at the mid-

clavicular line of the affected side (RCUK 2005). Arrangements should be made for the insertion of a formal chest tube and underwater seal drain (see Chapter 21).

Tamponade

This is where there is an acute effusion of fluid in the pericardial space and as it enlarges, the heart is splinted and finally cannot beat. The fluid is usually blood but can be malignant or infected fluid (Dolan & Preston 2006). The most common cause for a sudden tamponade is trauma. The immediate treatment is the insertion of a catheter or surgical drainage of the fluid. After drainage, the cause of the tamponade should be sought and corrected where possible, for example with appropriate antibiotic therapy for a bacterial aetiology or surgical repair of a myocardial laceration (Shoemaker 2000).

Toxicity: poisoning and drug intoxication

Poisoning rarely leads to cardiac arrest but it is a leading cause of death in patients less than 40 years old. Self-poisoning with therapeutic or recreational drugs is the main reason for hospital admission (RCUK 2005). There are few specific therapeutic measures for poisons that are useful in the immediate situation. The emphasis must be on intensive supportive therapy, with correction of hypoxia, acid/base balance and electrolyte disorders. Specialist help can be obtained by telephoning one of the regional National Poisons Information Service Centres (RCUK 2005).

Drugs

Only a few drugs are indicated during the immediate management of a cardiac arrest and there is only limited scientific evidence supporting their use. Drugs should be considered only after a sequence of shocks has been delivered (if indicated) and chest compressions and ventilation started (RCUK 2005). Central venous access is optimum as it allows for drugs to be delivered rapidly. However, this is dependent on the skills available. If a peripheral intravenous cannula is already in place it should be used first (RCUK 2005). Selected drugs (epinephrine, atropine, naloxone and lidocaine) can be administered down the endotracheal tube but the dose of the drug should be increased to 2–3 times the intravenous dose (AHA/ILCOR 2000). It is also possible to administer drugs using the intraosseous route, which is used commonly in the resuscitation of children.

The drugs used in the treatment of cardiac arrest are:

1   Epinephrine (adrenaline) 1 mg (10 ml of a 1 : 10 000 solution) given intravenously. The main purpose of adrenaline is to utilize its inotropic effect to maintain coronary and cerebral perfusion during a prolonged resuscitation attempt. It is the first drug used in cardiac arrest of any aetiology. Epinephrine is included in the ALS universal algorithm (see Figure 8.6), 1 mg to be given every 3–5 minutes (RCUK 2005).

2 Atropine 3 mg given intravenously once only reduces cardiac vagal tone, increases the rate of discharge of the sinoatrial node and increases the speed of conduction through the atrioventricular node. Its use is advocated in asystolic cardiac arrest and bradycardic PEA of less than 60 beats per minute. Note: although there is no conclusive evidence that atropine is of value in asystole during a cardiac arrest, there are anecdotal accounts of success following its administration (RCUK 2005).

3 Amiodarone (300 mg in 20 ml) should be considered in VF or pulseless VT. It increases the duration of the action potential in the atrial and ventricular myocardium; thus the QT interval is prolonged. In refractory VT or VF following recovery from cardiac arrest a further 300 mg may be given followed by an infusion of 900 mg over 24 hours (RCUK 2005). Note: lidocaine can still be considered if amiodarone is not available (RCUK 2005).

4 Calcium chloride (10 ml of 10%) is only given during resuscitation when specifically indicated, i.e. for the treatment of PEA caused by hyperkalaemia, hypocalcaemia or overdose of calcium channel blocking drugs (RCUK 2005). Although it plays a vital role in the cellular mechanisms underlying myocardial contraction there are very few data supporting any beneficial action for calcium following most cases of cardiac arrest (RCUK 2005).

5 Sodium bicarbonate 8.4% is only used in prolonged cardiac arrest or according to serial blood gas analyses. Potential adverse effects of excessive sodium bicarbonate administration include hypokalaemia, exacerbation of respiratory acidosis and increased affinity of haemoglobin for oxygen. The high concentration of sodium can also exacerbate cerebral oedema. Other adverse effects are increased cardiac irritability and impaired myocardial performance. Sodium bicarbonate is usually given in 25–50 mmol aliquots and repeated as necessary. It can also be given in the special circumstances of tricyclic overdose or hyperkalaemia (Winser 2001).

6 Magnesium sulphate. Magnesium (4–8 mmol of 50%) should be given in cardiac arrest where there is a suspicion of hypomagnesaemia as this may precipitate refractory VF/VT (Winser 2001). The normal value for magnesium is 0.8–1.2 mmol/l (Wakeling & Mythen 2000).

Defibrillation

Defibrillation causes a simultaneous depolarization of the myocardium and aims to restore normal rhythm to the heart. This is the definitive treatment for VF/pulseless VT. It has been suggested that 80–90% of adults who collapse because of non-traumatic cardiac arrest are found to be in VF when first attached to a monitor (Varon *et al.* 1998). In hospital cardiac arrest is more likely to present as non-VF/VT. Early defibrillation is a vital link in the chain of survival and developments in public access defibrillation and first responder defibrillation by ward nurses in hospitals are focusing firmly on this link. Delay in defibrillation decreases

the chances of success by 7–10% each minute (Bossaert *et al.* 1998). Nurses are often first on the scene at a cardiac arrest, highlighting the obvious need for nurse-led defibrillation at ward level. While not all nurses are trained in defibrillation, they should understand why it is necessary and how it is done and be able to assist in an emergency (Austin & Snow 2000).

Safe defibrillation practice

Defibrillation in an environment where high flows of oxygen are present could represent a danger to patients and rescuers. It is essential therefore to ensure that oxygen tubing and equipment is moved away from the chest when defibrillation is performed. Using adhesive electrodes to deliver the shock as opposed to paddles may also minimize the danger (RCUK 2005).

Placement of paddles or self-adhesive electrodes

The right paddle or electrode should be placed to the right of the sternum below the clavicle and the left vertically in the mid-axillary line approximately level with the position V6 used in electrocardiogram (ECG) monitoring (see Figure 8.6 for the universal ALS algorithm for the management of cardiac arrest in adults).

Cardiopulmonary resuscitation standards and training

The Resuscitation Council UK (RCUK), formed in 1981, aims to promote the education of lay and professional personnel in the most effective methods of resuscitation appropriate to their needs. In its report *CPR Guidance for Clinical Practice and Training in Hospitals* (RCUK 2004), the Council made a number of recommendations relating to the provision of a resuscitation service in hospital:

- A resuscitation committee. This should comprise of medical and nursing staff who advise on the role and composition of the cardiac arrest team, resuscitation equipment and resuscitation training equipment.
- A Resuscitation Training Officer (RTO), who should be responsible for training in resuscitation, equipment maintenance and the auditing of resuscitation/clinical trials.
- Resuscitation training. Hospital staff should receive at least annual resuscitation training appropriate to their level and role. Medical and nursing staff should receive basic resuscitation training and should be encouraged to recognize patients who are at risk of having a cardiac arrest and call for appropriate help early. This is the most effective method of improving outcome (Jevon 2002). All medical staff should have advanced resuscitation training and senior nurses and doctors working in acute specialities (CCU, ITU, A&E) should hold a valid RCUK ALS certificate.
- A cardiac arrest team. Each hospital should have a team of about five people including a minimum of two

doctors (physician and anaesthetist), an ALS trained nurse, the RTO and a porter when possible. Clear procedures should be available for calling the cardiac arrest team. The Resuscitation Council has recommended the development of a medical emergency team who recognize patients who are at risk of having a cardiac arrest and initiate the most appropriate clinical intervention to prevent it (Jevon 2002).

- Resuscitation equipment. Ideally this should be standardized throughout the hospital (see Procedure guidelines: Cardiopulmonary resuscitation, below). Defibrillators should also be standardized. The widespread deployment of automated or shock advisory defibrillators is a realistic strategy to reduce mortality from cardiac arrests related to ischaemic heart disease (Jevon 2002). Bossaert (1997) believes that defibrillation should be a basic skills requirement of all nurses. With the advent of automated external defibrillators (AEDs) this may become a possibility in the near future.
- Audit and reporting of standards. All resuscitation attempts should be audited, ideally using a nationally recognized template such as Utstein template (recommended for use by the RCUK).
- Decisions relating to CPR. Every hospital should have a 'Do not attempt resuscitation' (DNAR) policy based on national guidelines (Jevon 2001; BMA, RCN, RCUK 2001).

If these recommendations are implemented, the standards in resuscitation and resuscitation training should improve (Jevon 2002).

Ethics

The increase in skills, knowledge, technology and pharmacological support has proved effective in prolonging quality of life for many patients. Many patients have good reason to be thankful for CPR and the numbers rise daily (RCUK 2005). Resuscitation attempts in the mortally ill, however, do not enhance the dignity that most people hope for in death. Ideally, resuscitation should only be attempted in patients who have a high chance of successful revival for a good quality of life (i.e. as deemed acceptable by the individual patient). There are many important factors that need to be considered when deciding whether or not to resuscitate a patient:

- The patient's own wishes.
- The views of relatives or close friends, who may be aware of the wishes of a patient who cannot communicate.
- The patient's disease and prognosis.
- The quality of life of the patient and expected quality should resuscitation be 'successful'.

Decision making: do not attempt resuscitation

In an attempt to reduce the number of futile resuscitation attempts many hospitals have introduced formal DNAR policies, which can be applied to individual patients in specific

circumstances. Health care professionals must be able to show that their decisions relating to CPR are compatible with the human rights set out in the Human Rights Act 1998 implemented on 2 October 2000 (e.g. the right to life, the right to be free from inhuman or degrading treatment and freedom of expression) (BMA 2000). The following guidelines are based on those provided in a joint statement by the British Medical Association (BMA), the Royal College of Nursing (RCN) and the RCUK (BMA, RCN, RCUK 2001). (Note: where no decision has been made and the express wishes of the patient are unknown, CPR should be performed without delay.)

- Sensitive advance discussion between experienced medical/nursing staff and patients regarding attempting CPR should be encouraged but not forced. Where patients lack competence to participate, people close to them can be helpful in reflecting their views. (Note: in England, Wales and Northern Ireland, no person is legally entitled to give consent to medical treatment on behalf of another adult.) Information about CPR needs to be realistic. Written information explaining CPR should be available for patients and those close to them to read. The BMA, in liaison with the RCUK, has published an information leaflet that may help patients and families discuss DNAR with medical and nursing staff (BMA 2002).
- Patients are entitled to refuse CPR even when there is a reasonable chance of success.
- Some patients may ask that no DNAR order be made. Patients cannot demand treatment which the health care team judges to be inappropriate, but all efforts should be made to accommodate their wishes and preferences.
- An advance DNAR order should only be made after consideration of the likely clinical outcome, the patient's wishes and the patient's human rights. It should be considered on an individual patient basis where:

1   Attempting CPR will not start the patient's heart and breathing.
2   There is no benefit in restarting the patient's heart and breathing.
3   The expected benefit is outweighed by the burdens (RCUK 2005).

- The overall responsibility for decisions about CPR and DNAR orders rests with the consultant in charge of the patient's care. Issues should, however, be discussed with other members of the health care team, the patient and people close to the patient where appropriate.
- There are exceptional cases where resuscitation discussions with a patient may be inappropriate, e.g. where senior members of the medical and nursing team consider that CPR would be futile and that such a discussion would cause the patient unnecessary distress and anguish. This could apply to patients in the terminal phase of their illness.
- The most senior members of the medical and nursing team available should clearly document any decisions

made about CPR in the patient's medical and nursing notes. The decision should be dated and the reasons for it given. This information must be communicated to all other relevant health care professionals. Unless it is against the wishes of the patient, their family should also be informed.

- The DNAR order should be reviewed on each admission or in light of changes in the patient's condition (BMA, RCN, RCUK 2001).

Finally, it should be noted that a DNAR order applies only to CPR and should not reduce the standard of medical or nursing care.

Procedure guidelines: Cardiopulmonary resuscitation (CPR)

Equipment

All hospital wards and appropriate departments, e.g. theatre, computed tomography (CT) scanning, should have a standardized cardiac arrest trolley or box. Resuscitation equipment should be checked on a daily basis (RCUK 2005) by the staff on the wards or clinical areas responsible for it, and a record of this check should be maintained. Below is a list of the minimum equipment recommended by the Resuscitation Council for the management of an adult cardiac arrest.

Airway management
- Pocket masks with oxygen port.
- Self-inflating resuscitation bag with oxygen reservoir and tubing.
- Clear face masks in sizes 4, 5 and 6.
- Oropharyngeal airways in sizes 2, 3 and 4.
- Yankauer suckers × 2.
- Endotracheal suction catheters × 10.
- Laryngeal mask airway (size 4) or Combitube (small).
- McGill forceps.
- Endotracheal tubes: oral, cuffed, sizes 6, 7 and 8.
- Gum elastic bougie.
- Lubricating jelly.
- Laryngoscopes × 2: normal and long blades.
- Spare laryngoscope bulbs and batteries.
- 1 inch ribbon gauze/tape.
- Scissors.
- Syringe: 20 ml.
- Clear oxygen mask with reservoir bag.
- Oxygen cylinders × 2 (if no wall oxygen).
- Cylinder key.

Circulation equipment
- Intravenous cannulae: 18 gauge × 3, 14 gauge × 3.
- Hypodermic needles: 21 gauge × 10.
- Syringes: 2 ml × 6, 5 ml × 6, 10 ml × 6, 20 ml × 6.
- Cannula fixing dressings and tapes × 4.
- Seldinger wire central venous catheter kits × 2.
- 12 gauge non-Seldinger central venous catheter × 2.
- Intravenous administration sets × 3.
- 0.9% sodium chloride: 1000 ml bags × 2.

Additional items
- ECG electrodes.
- Defibrillation gel pads/unless using fast patch electrodes.
- Clock.
- Gloves/goggles/aprons.
- A sliding sheet or similar device should be available for safe handling.

Drugs
Immediately available prefilled syringes of:
- Atropine: 3 mg × 1.
- Amiodarone: 300 mg × 1.
- Epinephrine/adrenaline: 1 mg (1 : 10 000) × 4.

Other readily available drugs
- Epinephrine (adrenaline): 1 mg (1 : 10 000) × 4.
- Sodium bicarbonate 8.4%: 50 ml × 1.
- Calcium chloride 10%: 10 ml × 2.
- Lidocaine/lignocaine: 100 mg × 2.
- Atropine: 1 mg × 2.
- 0.9% sodium chloride: 10 ml ampoules × 10.
- Naloxone: 400 g × 2.
- Epinephrine/adrenaline 1 : 1000 × 2.
- Amiodarone: 150 mg × 4.
- Magnesium sulphate 50% solution: 2 g (4 ml) × 1.
- Potassium chloride 40 mmol × 1.
- Adenosine: 6 mg × 10.
- Hydrocortisone: 200 mg × 1.
- Glucose 10%: 500 ml × 1.

Procedure

Action	Rationale
1 Note time of arrest, if witnessed.	Lack of cerebral perfusion for approximately 3–4 minutes can lead to irreversible brain damage (E).
2 Give patient precordial thump.	This may restore cardiac rhythm, which will give a cardiac output (E).

Procedure guidelines (cont.)

3 Summon help. If a second nurse is available, he/she can call for the cardiac arrest team, bring emergency equipment and screen off the area.

Maintain patient's privacy and dignity. CPR is more effective with two rescuers. One is responsible for inflating the lungs, and the other for chest compressions. Continue until medical help arrives (RCUK 2005: C).

4 Lie patient flat on a firm surface/bed. If on a chair, lower the patient to the floor, ensuring that the head is supported.

Effective external cardiac massage can be performed only on a hard surface (E; RCUK 2005: C).

5 If patient is in bed, remove bed head, and ensure adequate space between back of bed and wall.

To allow easy access to patient's head in order to facilitate intubation (E).

6 Ensure a clear airway. If cervical spine injury is excluded, extend, not hyperextend, the neck (thus lifting the tongue off the posterior wall of the pharynx). This is best achieved by lifting the chin forwards with the finger and thumb of one hand while pressing the forehead backwards with the heel of the other hand (see Figure 8.3). If this fails to establish an airway, there may be obstruction by a foreign body. Try to remove the obstruction if visible.

To establish and maintain airway, thus facilitating ventilation (RCUK 2005: C).

Do not remove well-fitted dentures.

They help to create a mouth to mask seal during ventilation (E).

7 Place the heel of one hand in the centre of the sternum and place the other on top, ensuring that the hands are located between the middle and the lower half of the sternum. Ensure that only the heel of the dominant hand is touching the sternum.

To ensure accuracy of external cardiac compression and reduced delay in commencing cardiac compressions (RCUK 2005: C).

Place the other hand on top, straighten the elbows and make sure shoulders are directly over the patient's chest.

The sternum should be depressed sharply by 4–5 cm. The cardiac compressions should be forceful, and sustained at a rate of 100 per minute.

This produces a cardiac output by applying direct downward force and compression (Smith 2000: R3).

8 Compress the Ambu bag in a rhythmical fashion: the bag should be attached to an oxygen source. In order to deliver 85% oxygen, a reservoir may be attached to the Ambu bag. If, however, oxygen is not immediately available, the Ambu bag will deliver ambient air.

Room air contains only 21% oxygen. In shock, a low cardiac output, together with ventilation–perfusion mismatch, results in severe hypoxaemia. The importance of providing a high oxygen gradient from mouth to vital cells cannot be exaggerated and so oxygen should be added during CPR as soon as it is available (80–100% is desirable) (Simmons 2002. R3).

9 Maintain cardiac compression and ventilation at a ratio of 30 : 2. This rate can be achieved effectively by counting out loud 'one and two', etc. There should be a slight pause to ensure that the delivered breath is sufficient to cause the patient's chest to rise. This must continue until cardiac output returns and the patient has a palpable blood pressure.

Counting aloud will ensure co-ordination of ventilation and compression ratio. To maintain circulation and oxygenation, thus reducing risk of damage to vital organs (E).

10 When the cardiac arrest team arrives, it will assume responsibility for the arrest in liaison with the ward staff.	To ensure an effective expert team co-ordinates the resuscitation (E; RCUK 2005: C).
11 Attach patient to ECG monitor using three electrodes or defibrillation patches/paddles.	To obtain adequate ECG signal. Accurate recording of cardiac rhythm will determine the appropriate treatment to be initiated (E).

Intubation in CPR

Action	Rationale
12 Continue to ventilate and oxygenate the patient before intubation.	The risks of cardiac arrhythmias due to hypoxia are decreased (RCUK 2005: C).
13 Equipment for intubation should be checked before handing to appropriate medical/nursing staff: (a) Suction equipment is operational. (b) The cuff of the endotracheal tube inflates and deflates. (c) The endotracheal tube is well lubricated. (d) That catheter mount with swivel connector is ready for use.	
14 During intubation, the anaesthetist may request cricoid pressure. This involves compressing the oesophagus between the cricoid ring and the sixth cervical vertebra.	To prevent the risk of regurgitation of gastric contents and the consequent risk of pulmonary aspiration (RCUK 2006: C).
15 Recommence ventilation and oxygenation once intubation is completed.	Intubation should interrupt resuscitation only for a maximum of 16 seconds to prevent the occurrence of cerebral anoxia (Handley et al. 1997: R 3).
16 Once the patient's trachea has been intubated, chest compressions, at a rate of 100 per minute, should continue uninterrupted (except for defibrillation and pulse check when indicated) and ventilation should continue at approximately 12 breaths per minute.	Uninterrupted compression results in a substantially higher mean coronary perfusion pressure. A pause in chest compressions allows the coronary perfusion pressure to fall. On resuming compressions, there is some delay before the original coronary perfusion pressure is restored (RCUK 2005: C).

Intravenous access in CPR

Action	Rationale
17 Venous access must be established through a large vein as soon as possible.	To administer emergency cardiac drugs and fluid replacement (RCUK 2005: C).
18 Asepsis should be maintained throughout.	To prevent local and/or systemic infection (DH 2005:C).
19 The correct rate of infusion is required.	To ensure maximum drug and/or solution effectiveness (E).
20 Accurate recording of the administration of solutions infused and drugs added is essential.	To maintain accurate records, provide a point of reference in the event of queries and prevent any duplication of treatment (NMC 2005: C).

Defibrillation
Used to terminate VF or VT.

Post-resuscitation care
After cardiac arrest, return of spontaneous circulation is just the first phase in a continuum of resuscitation. To return the patient to a state of normal cerebral function with no neurological deficit, a stable cardiac rhythm and normal haemodynamic function requires further resuscitation tailored to each patient's individual needs (RCUK 2005).

165

Procedure guidelines *(cont.)*

Action	Rationale
1 Check patient by assessing airway, breathing, circulation, blood pressure and urine output.	To ensure a clear airway, adequate oxygenation and ventilation and aim to maintain normal sinus rhythm and a cardiac output adequate for perfusion of vital organs. To ensure adequacy of ventilation and oxygenation (E).
2 Check arterial blood gases.	To ensure correction of acid/base balance (RCUK 2005: C).
3 Check full blood count, clotting and biochemistry.	To exclude anaemia as a contributor to myocardial ischaemia. A clotting disorder may have contributed to a major haemorrhage. Replacement stored blood for transfusion has less clotting factors and the patient may require replacement of clotting factors usually in the form of fresh frozen plasma (E). To assess renal function and electrolyte balance ($K+$, Mg^{2+} and Ca^{2+}). To ensure normoglycaemia. To commence serial cardiac enzyme assay (RCUK 2006: C).
4 Monitor patient's cardiac rhythm and record 12-lead ECG.	Normal sinus rhythm is required for optimum cardiac function (RCUK 2006: C). An assessment of whether cardiac arrest has been associated with a myocardial infarction should be made, as the patient may be suitable for coronary angioplasty or thrombolytic therapy.
5 A chest X-ray should be taken.	To establish correct siting of tracheal tube, gastric tube and central venous catheter. To exclude left ventricular failure, pulmonary aspiration and pneumothorax. To establish size and shape of heart (E).
6 Continue respiratory therapy.	Hypoxia and hypercarbia both increase the likelihood of a further cardiac arrest (RCUK 2006: C).
7 Assess patient's level of consciousness. This can be done by use of the Glasgow Coma Scale. Although this is intended primarily for head injury, it is clinically relevant. It contains five levels of consciousness: (a) Conscious and alert. (b) Drowsy but responsive to verbal commands. (c) Unconscious but responsive to minimal painful stimuli. (d) Unconscious and responsive to deep painful stimuli. (e) Unconscious and unresponsive. (See Chapter 26).	Once a heart has been resuscitated to a stable rhythm and cardiac output, the organ that influences an individual's survival most significantly is the brain (RCUK 2006: C). Initial assessment and regular monitoring will alert the nurse to any changes in function.
8 The patient should be made comfortable and nursed in the appropriate position, i.e. upright or in the recovery position. Avoid nursing supine as this physiologically hinders cardiac output and respiration. Careful explanation and reassurance is vital at all times, particularly if the patient is conscious and aware.	

9 Following stabilization of the patient's condition, consideration should be given to moving them to an appropriate critical care environment. All established monitoring should continue during transfer.

To facilitate a safe transfer of the patient between the site of resuscitation and an appropriate place of definitive care (E).

. . . .

A critical care outreach service, if available, may contribute to the care of the patient during stabilization and transfer.

To export the expertise of critical care to the patient and enhance the skills and understanding of ward staff in the delivery of critical care (Ridley 2002 :E; RCUK 2006:C).

. . . .

Please note: whether the resuscitation attempt was successful or not, the patient's relatives will require considerable support. Equally, the pastoral needs of all those associated with the arrest should not be forgotten (RCUK 2005:C).

References and further reading

AHA/ILCOR (2000) Guidelines 2000 for CPR and emergency care: an international consensus on science. *Resuscitation*, 46(1), 73–92, 109–14.

Austin, R. & Snow, A. (2000) Defibrillation. In: *Resuscitation: A Guide for Nurses* (ed. A. Cheller). Harcourt, London, pp. 141–57.

Baskett, P.J.F., Steen, P.A. & Bossaert, L. (2005) European Resuscitation Council Guidelines for Resuscitation 2005. Section 8: The ethics of resuscitation and end of life decisions. *Resuscitation*, 67(Suppl 1), S171–80.

Bersten, A.D. & Soni, N. (2003) *Oh's Intensive Care Manual*, 5th edn. Butterworth Heinemann, Edinburgh.

BMA (2000) *The Impact of the Human Rights Act on Medical Decision-Making*. British Medical Association, London.

BMA (2002) *Decisions Relating to Cardiopulmonary Resuscitation: Model Information Leaflet*. British Medical Association, London.

BMA, RCN, RCUK (2001) *Decisions Relating to Cardiopulmonary Resuscitation: A Joint Statement*. Resuscitation Council UK, London.

Bossaert, L. (1997) Fibrillation and defibrillation of the heart. *Br J Anaesth*, 79(2), 203–13.

Bossaert, L. et al. (1998) European Resuscitation Council Guidelines for adult advanced life support. *Resuscitation*, 37(1), 81–94.

Colqhoun, M., Handley, A.J. & Evans, T.R. (2004) *ABC of Resuscitation*, 5th edn. BMJ Publishing Group, London.

DH (2005) *Saving Lives: A Delivery Programme to Reduce Healthcare Associated Infection including MRSA*. Department of Health, London.

Docherty, B. & Hall, S. (2002) Basic life support and AED. *Prof Nurse*, 17(12), 705–6.

Dolan, S. & Preston, N.J. (2006) Malignant effusions. In: *Nursing Patients with Cancer* (eds N. Kearney & A. Richardson). Elsevier, Churchill Livingstone, Edinburgh, pp. 619–33.

Eftestol, T., Sunde, K. & Steen, P.A. (2002) Effects of interrupting precordial compressions on the calculated probability of defibrillation success during out-of-hospital cardiac arrest. *Circulation*, 105, 2270–3.

European Resuscitation Council (2005) *European Resuscitation Council Guidelines for Resuscitation*, 67(Suppl 1), S1–190.

Gabbott, D. et al. (2005) Cardiopulmonary resuscitation standards for clinical practice and training in the UK. *Resuscitation*, 64, 13–19.

Handley, A.J. (2004) Basic life support. In: *ABC of Resuscitation* (eds M. Colqhoun, A. Handley & T. Evans), 4th edn. BMJ Books, London, pp. 1–4.

Handley, A.J. et al. (1997) Single rescuer adult basic life support: an advisory statement by the Basic Life Support Working Group of the International Liaison Committee on Resuscitation. *Resuscitation*, 34, 101–7.

Hauff, S.R. et al. (2003) Factors impeding dispatcher-assisted telephone cardiopulmonary resuscitation. *Ann Emerg Med*, 42, 731–7.

Hodgetts, T. & Castle, N. (1999) *Resuscitation Rules*. BMJ Books, London.

International Liaison Committee on Resuscitation (2005) International consensus on cardiopulmonary resuscitation and emergency cardiovascular care science with treatment recommendations. *Resuscitation*, 67, 157–341.

Jevon, P. (2001) Cardiopulmonary resuscitation. Initial assessment. *Nurs Times*, 97(42), 41–2.

Jevon, P. (2002) Resuscitation in hospital: Resuscitation Council (UK) recommendations. *Nurs Stand*, 16(33), 41–4.

NMC (2005) *Guidelines for Records and Record Keeping*. Nursing and Midwifery Council, London.

Perbedy, M.A. et al. (2003) Cardiopulmonary resuscitation of adults in the hospital: a report of 14 720 cardiac arrests from the National Registry of Cardiopulmonary Resuscitation. *Resuscitation*, 58, 297–308.

Perkins, G.D. et al. (2005) Birmingham assessment of breathing study (BABS). *Resuscitation*, 53, 29–36.

RCUK (2001) *Decisions Relating to Cardiopulmonary Resuscitation: A Joint Statement from the British Medical Association, the Resuscitation Council (UK) and the Royal College of Nursing*. Resuscitation Council, UK, London.

RCUK (2004) *CPR Guidance for Clinical Practice and Training in Hospitals*. Resuscitation Council UK, London.

RCUK (2005) *Adult Basic Life Support: Resuscitation Guidelines*. Resuscitation Council UK, London.

RCUK (2006) *Advanced Life Support*, 5th edition. Resuscitation Council UK, London.

Ridley, S. (2002) Critical care – modality, metamorphosis and measurement. In: (ed S.A. Ridley) *Outcomes in Critical Care*. Butterworth Heinemann, Oxford, pp. 1–21.

Shoemaker, W.C. (2000) Pericardial tamponade. In: *Oxford Textbook of Critical Care* (eds A. Webb et al.). Oxford University Press, London, pp. 276–9.

Simmons, R. (2002) The airway at risk. In: *ABC of Resuscitation* (eds M. Colqhoun, A. Handley & T. Evans), 5th edn. BMJ Books, London, pp. 25–31.

Skinner, D. & Vincent, R. (1997) *Cardiopulmonary Resuscitation.* Oxford University Press, London.

Smith, D. (2000) Basic life support. In: *Resuscitation: A Guide for Nurses* (ed. A. Cheller). Harcourt, London, pp. 65–80.

Van Alem, A., Sanou, B. & Koster, R. (2003) Interruption of CPR with the use of the AED in out of hospital cardiac arrest. *Ann Emerg Med*, **42**, 449–57.

Varon, J., Marik, P.E. & Fromm, R.E. Jr (1998) Cardiopulmonary resuscitation: a review for clinicians. *Resuscitation* **36**(2), 133–45.

Wakeling, H.G. & Mythen, M.C. (2000) Hypomagnesemia. In: *Oxford Textbook of Critical Care* (eds A. Webb *et al.*). Oxford University Press, London pp. 561–4.

Winser, H. (2001) An evidence base for adult resuscitation. *Prof Nurse*, **16**(7), 1210–13.

Chapter 9

Compression therapy in the management of lymphoedema

Reference material **170**
Assessment of the patient with lymphoedema **171**
Measurement of limb volume **171**
Reference material **172**
Procedure guidelines: Compression therapy: limb volume calculation **173**
Phases of treatment **174**
Maintenance phase of treatment **174**
Intensive phase of treatment **175**
Procedure guidelines: Compression garments (elastic): application of **178**
Procedure guidelines: Compression bandaging (standard multilayer) **179**
References and further reading **185**

Definitions

Compression therapy in the management of lymphoedema involves the use of compression garments or low-stretch bandages (Asmussen & Strossenreuther 2003). Clinical and physical indications determined during a full assessment of the patient will facilitate the most appropriate choice of compression therapy for the individual patient.

The type of material from which the garments or bandages are made can determine the degree of pressure exerted on the tissues below, although the level of pressure achieved is dependent upon a complex combination of factors including the size and shape of the limb and the activity of the wearer (Clark 2003):

- Elastic compression garments apply an external force to the limb which pulls in to exert pressure on the tissues below (Eagle 2001). The pressure can be sustained over long periods of time both during activity and inactivity of the limb, providing a high working pressure whilst the muscle is active and a high resting pressure during inactivity of the muscle at rest (Todd 2000).
- Inelastic garments and low-stretch bandages provide a firm external encasement to the limb, and pressure arises from the body tissues and muscles as they push outwards against the firm encasement provided by the garment or bandage (Thomas & Nelson 1998). Inelastic garments and low-stretch bandages provide a relatively low resting pressure when the muscle is inactive during rest, which contrasts with a high working pressure during exercise of the muscle, as it contracts within the inelastic garment or bandage and produces a massaging effect on the tissues below to stimulate lymph drainage (Todd 2000).

The pressure exerted by the garment or bandage is also influenced by the circumference of the limb, with the highest pressure achieved where the limb is narrowest (Clark 2003). When a garment or bandage is applied to a limb of normal proportions therefore, the highest pressure will be achieved at the ankle or wrist, with graduated, reducing pressure along the length of the limb as the circumference increases (Todd 2000).

Indications

Compression therapy is the mainstay of conservative management for lymphoedema. It initiates physiological effects within the arterial, venous and lymphatic systems in order to:

- Ensure that lymphatic fluid in the limb travels towards the root of the limb.
- Limit the formation of fluid in the tissues.
- Contain the tissues of the swollen limb and help to maintain a normal shape to the limb.
- Maximize the effect of the muscle pump (Partsch 2003).

Elastic compression garments are usually used when the lymphoedema is mild and uncomplicated (Todd 2000) and to maintain the reduced size of a swollen limb after the use of low-stretch bandages.

Inelastic and low-stretch bandages are indicated when the lymphoedema is moderate to severe and the limb has swollen out of shape (Williams & Keller 2005). They are also effective when fibrosis of the subcutaneous tissues is present, due to the massaging effect on the tissues caused by the low resting pressures and high working pressures (Foldi et al. 2005).

Contraindications for compression therapy

- Arterial disease in the affected, swollen limb.
- Acute stages of deep vein thrombosis in the leg.
- Acute infections of the affected swollen limb, e.g. cellulitis.
- Cardiac oedema (Callam et al. 1997).

Reference material

There are many reasons why a limb may swell and the appearance of oedema represents an increase in extracellular fluid volume (Mortimer 2003a). Dependency or gravitational oedema is commonly seen in the immobile patient when the immobility results in a failure to activate the muscle pump causing an increase in capillary filtration and reduced lymph drainage in the dependent limb (Mortimer 2003a). Swelling can also occur in chronic venous disease of the lower limbs as a result of lymph drainage failure and increased capillary filtration (Mortimer 2003a).

Lymphoedema occurs because the lymphatics are reduced in number, obstructed, obliterated or simply fail to function (Stanton et al. 2000). Tissue swelling then appears due to the failure of lymph drainage (Stanton et al. 2000). Lymphoedema is most commonly seen in cancer patients as a result of damage to lymph nodes following surgery and/or radiotherapy, but it can also occur as a result of local tumour obstruction in lymph node areas. A survey of 1200 breast cancer patients reported the prevalence of chronic arm oedema as 28% (Mortimer et al. 1996). The prevalence increased with time following treatment in patients who had received postoperative radiotherapy (Mortimer et al. 1996). There is limited research to indicate the incidence of leg oedema following treatment for abdominal and pelvic tumours, soft tissue sarcomas and melanomas, although lymphoedema is known to occur following treatment for these tumours (Keeley 2000). In a study to determine the prevalence of lower limb lymphoedema in women receiving treatment for gynaecological cancers, Ryan et al. (2003) reported an overall incidence of lymphoedema in 18% of the study participants and suggested a prevalence of 47% for women with vulval cancer following surgery and radiotherapy to lymph node areas.

Lymphoedema can affect any part of the body including the face and head, but it most commonly affects a limb. The swelling can have physical, psychological and psychosocial implications for the patient and is associated with a number of complications arising from its development (Woods 2000a). Limb heaviness may lead to impaired function, reduced mobility and musculoskeletal problems (Tobin *et al*. 1993). Skin and tissue changes develop with increased lymph stasis in the oedematous limb and give rise to the characteristic deepened skin folds, distorted limb shape and hyperkeratosis associated with long-standing lymphoedema. There is an increased risk of local and systemic infection as a result of poor lymph drainage and recurrent acute inflammatory episodes are common (Mortimer 2003b).

The experience of living with lymphoedema as a long-term chronic condition is a unique experience for each patient and can have an impact on many areas of the individual's life. Studies of breast cancer patients with arm swelling have highlighted the degree of psychological and psychosocial distress that can be experienced when lymphoedema develops (Tobin *et al*. 1993; Woods 1993; Woods *et al*. 1995). The physical and psychological effects of lymphoedema are not short-lived and enormous motivation and perseverance coupled with adaptation are demanded in order to achieve control or reduction of the swelling (Mason 2000).

Assessment of the patient with lymphoedema

Assessment should include the following elements:

- *Details of the patient's medical history*: To determine whether external graduated pressure can be used safely. Arterial insufficiency of the lower limb must be excluded prior to the use of external graduated pressure and patients with a history of diabetes or cardiac failure should undergo a medical assessment prior to the commencement of treatment and follow close supervision during its progress (Eagle 2001).
- *Physical assessment*: To determine the cause of the swelling and any symptoms or complicating factors, i.e. the cause and extent of the oedema, assessment of skin condition and limb shape, disease status.
- *Psychological assessment*: To determine the effect of the swelling on the patient, i.e. effect on relationships, personal concerns and fears.
- *Psychosocial assessment*: To determine the influence of the swelling upon the patient's life, i.e. influence upon limb function and mobility, employment, hobbies, activities, personal roles.
- *Problem identification*: To determine actual and potential patient focused problem areas combined with patient strengths and preferences.

When the use of compression therapy is being considered, a full and careful assessment will highlight the patient's main problems and any co-existing complications. This information is then used to set realistic treatment goals and to determine the approach to treatment. A number of treatments are used in combination during the management of lymphoedema and their choice and usefulness can be determined by the therapist and patient at the time of assessment. Clarifying the influence of the lymphoedema on the patient's lifestyle, occupation and chosen social activities will help to identify patient-focused problem areas that may require adjustment. By gaining an understanding of the impact that the swelling may be having upon personal feelings and emotions, relevant supportive strategies can be identified (Woods 2000a).

Assessment should also include:

- *Planning*: To improve problems and utilize patient strengths. The health care professional should work in partnership with the patient to enable them to take appropriate action in order to manage their lymphoedema and work towards long-term control. Planning should focus on the patient's objectives so that immediate problems can be addressed and long- and short-term goals can then be identified.
- *Implementation*: To determine the appropriateness of interventions and modify where required. An individualized, holistic approach will incorporate education and support, particularly if personal changes are required to minimize the risk of complications developing. Success will be achieved when the patient possesses positive motivational factors and is an active participant in the management of their lymphoedema.
- *Evaluation*: To assess progress, modify and stop the intervention if necessary. In order to evaluate the outcome of a plan of treatment, suitable outcome indicators are required (Jenns 2000). No standardized method of evaluating the outcome of a plan of treatment has been adopted, but the measurement of limb volume using surface measurement is the most frequently used means of assessing response to treatment in lymphoedema management (Jenns 2000). The effect of treatment on the patient's psychological and psychosocial well-being should, however, also be monitored, and this is frequently achieved in a more subjective manner where the patient's views are sought (Woods 2002).

Measurement of limb volume

Definition

A frequently used method of assessing response to lymphoedema treatment is the measurement of limb size (Stanton *et al*. 2000). This can be established by recording and comparing measurements taken of both limbs with a tape measure positioned at fixed points on a limb; usually the wrist and 10 cm above and below the olecranon or 15 cm above and below the patella (Piller 1999). Although this method is easy and quick to complete, its use is primarily to track broad changes in limb circumference only and the method is prone to error if the tape measure is not positioned in the same place on each consecutive occasion.

A more accurate method of assessing response to treatment is the measurement of limb volume. Multiple circumferential measurements taken of both limbs at 4 cm intervals and applied to the formula for the volume of a cylinder provide a reliable method of determining the size of the limb and is the most widely used method of establishing limb volume (Moffatt *et al.* 2006a; Taylor *et al.* 2006). Reproducibility is accurate if care is taken with the procedure and a standard format for the recording of the measurements is used (Badger 1993; Woods 1994).

Indications

Circumferential measurements of the swollen and contralateral limb taken with a plastic-coated tape measure at 4 cm intervals and applied to the formula for the volume of a cylinder can provide a useful, objective means of determining response to treatment. Limb volume measurements can be calculated in order to:

- Determine the total excess volume of the swollen limb compared to the patient's contralateral normal limb.
- Establish the distribution of the swelling along the limb.
- Provide information to assist in the choice of compression therapy (Woods 2002).

Measurements can also be used to provide an objective method of determining response to treatment by indicating:

- Changes in the size and shape of the limb over time.
- Changes in the excess volume.
- The distribution of any volume loss or gain in the limb (Sitzia 1995).

Reference material

A variety of methods to measure limb volume have been used, including:

- Volume measured by water displacement (Kettle *et al.* 1958; Engler & Sweat 1962; Bernas *et al.* 1996).
- Volume measured using an optoelectronic device (Stanton *et al.* 1997).
- Volume calculated from circumferential measurements (Sitzia 1995).

Each of these methods has advantages and disadvantages. The calculation of limb volume from circumferential measurements, taken with a tape measure however, is uncomplicated and inexpensive.

The following points should be considered when using surface measurements in order to calculate limb volume (Badger 1993):

1 Ensure that the same position is used for the same patient each time the limb is measured. The position of the limb will affect the measurements taken because the degree to which muscles are flexed or relaxed will influence the shape and size of the limb.
2 The limb should be marked afresh on each measuring occasion with a washable ink, even when measuring on consecutive days. Any increase or decrease in limb volume will influence the position of the marks on the limb.
3 Tension should not be exerted on the tape measure during measuring. If tension is applied it will vary between measurers and recordings will not be consistent.
4 The tape measure should be positioned so that it is horizontal around the limb, taking care to ensure that it is not pulled tightly.
5 The same number of measurements should be taken on both limbs each time measurements are taken. The normal limb would not be expected to change significantly in volume except following vigorous exercise or where there has been weight loss or gain; therefore, the normal limb acts as a control in patients with unilateral swelling.
6 The starting point for the taking of measurements should be clearly identified by measuring and clearly recording the distance from the tip of the middle finger to the wrist. This starting point on the wrist should be used each time.
7 A standard format for the recording of measurements should be adopted to ensure that key points can be referred to.

Once measurement of the limb has been completed, a number of formulae may be used to calculate the limb volume (Badger 1993; Sitzia 1995). The formula for the volume of a cylinder (Box 9.1) considers the limb as a series of cylinders, each with a height of 4 cm, and limb volume is calculated by totalling the volume of each section.

Box 9.1 Procedure for calculating volume from circumferences

The formula for calculating the volume of a cylinder is $\frac{circumference^2}{\pi}$. The formula must be applied to each circumference measurement ($circ_1$, $circ_2$, ... $circ_n$) in order to calculate the volume of each segment; the volumes are totalled to give the total limb volume.

$$So\left(\frac{circ_1 \times circ_1}{3.1415}\right) + \left(\frac{circ_2 \times circ_2}{3.1415}\right) + \left(\frac{circ_3 \times circ_3}{3.1415}\right) + \cdots etc.$$

Use of a programmable calculator will speed up the process of calculation.

Procedure guidelines   Compression therapy: limb volume calculation

Equipment

1 Ruler, preferably 30 cm or longer.
2 Tape measure; avoid those made from fabric which tends to stretch.
3 Felt-tip pen for marking the limb.
4 Record chart and pen.

Measurement of lower limbs for compression therapy

Action	Rationale
1 Explain and discuss the proposed procedure with the patient.	To ensure that the patient understands the procedure and gives his/her valid consent (NMC 2006: C; NMC 2008: C).
2 Place the patient in a sitting position with the legs outstretched horizontally, preferably on a firm couch with adjustable height.	To ensure the lower limbs are relaxed and supported and the adjustable height means that the measurer can work without straining their back (E).
3 Standing on the outside of the leg, ask the patient to flex the foot to a right angle. Measure the distance from the base of the heel to the ankle, along the inside of the leg; mark the ankle, allowing at least 2 cm of leg to lie below the mark, and record the distance on the chart.	To establish and clearly record a reproducible fixed starting point for all subsequent measurements (Badger 1993: C). *Note*: the marks represent a point midway through each cylinder segment, they do not represent the base of the cylinder, therefore at least half the segment (i.e. 2 cm) must lie below the mark.
4 Ask the patient to relax the foot. From the starting point using a ruler mark the inside of the leg at 4 cm intervals along the length of the leg up to the groin.	To reduce the limb to 4 cm segments improves the accuracy of measurement since these segments resemble a cylinder more closely than does the whole limb. The formula used here assumes that the measurements are 4 cm apart (Sitzia 1995: R 5).
5 Place the tape measure around the limb and measure the circumference at each marked point, recording measurement on the chart. Make sure that the tape lies smoothly around the relaxed limb and that it does not lie at an angle. (Decide at the outset whether the tape is to be placed above, below or on the mark and keep to the same position every time.)	To ensure that there are no gaps between the limb and the tape and to ensure that the procedure is the same each each time reduces error (Aslem *et al.* 1996: R 3b).
6 Repeat the process on the other leg, whether or not it is swollen.	If only one limb is affected the normal limb acts as the patient's own control (Piller 1999: R 5).
7 If desired, a circumference measurement may be taken of the foot but this is *not* included in the calculation of volume.	The foot cannot be considered to be a cylinder and it is therefore inappropriate to include it in the calculation of volume (Taylor *et al.* 2006: R 5).
8 Ensure that the same number of measurements are made and clearly recorded on the record sheet for each leg.	Accurate documentation will ensure accuracy during limb volume calculation for each limb (Badger 1993: E).

Measurement of upper limbs for compression therapy

Action	Rationale
1 Explain and discuss the proposed procedure with the patient.	To ensure that the patient understands the procedure and gives his/her valid consent (NMC 2006: C; NMC 2008: C).

Procedure guidelines *(cont.)*

2 Sit the patient in a chair with the arms extended in front and resting on the back of a chair. The arms should be as close to an angle of 90° to the body as possible.	To ensure the arms are supported and accessible at a standard height. Changing the angle of the arms to the body will result in changes in the measurements (Boland & Adams 1998: R 5).
3 Measure the distance from the tip of the middle finger to the wrist. Mark the wrist, allowing at least 2 cm from where the hand joins the arm, and note down the distance.	To establish and clearly record a reproducible fixed starting point for all subsequent measurements (Badger 1993: E). *Note*: The marks represent a point midway through each cylinder segment, they do not represent the base of the cylinder, therefore at least half the segment (i.e. 2 cm) must lie below the mark.
4 From the starting point using a ruler mark along the inside length of the arm at 4 cm intervals up to the axilla.	Reducing the limb to 4 cm segments improves the accuracy of measurement since these segments resemble a cylinder more closely than does the whole limb (Sitzia 1995: R 5).
5 Place the tape measure around the limb and measure the circumference at each marked point, recording each measurement on the chart. Make sure that the tape lies smoothly around the relaxed limb and that it does not lie at an angle. Decide at the outset whether the tape is to be placed above, below or on the mark and keep to the same position every time.	To ensure that there are no gaps between the limb and the tape and to ensure that the procedure is the same each time reduces error (Aslem *et al*. 1996: R 3b).
6 Repeat the process on the other arm whether or not it is swollen.	If only one limb is affected the normal limb acts as the patient's own control (Piller 1999: R 5).
7 If desired, a circumference measurement may be taken of the hand but this is *not* included in the calculation of volume.	The hand cannot be considered to be a cylinder and it is therefore inappropriate to include it in the calculation (Taylor *et al*. 2006: R 5).
8 Ensure that the same number of measurements are made and clearly recorded on the record sheet for each leg.	Accurate documentation will ensure accuracy during limb volume calculation for each limb (Badger 1993: E).

174

Phases of treatment

Treatment of lymphoedema can be approached in two phases: the maintenance phase and the intensive phase (Jenns 2000).

During the maintenance phase, the concept of self-care is promoted to encourage the patient to become independent in the long-term management and control of their swelling. Elastic compression garments are used and the therapist evaluates progress at regular intervals to ensure that they remain appropriate and that any problems can be identified at an early stage (Doherty *et al.* 2006).

The intensive phase of treatment is a short, planned period of therapist-led treatment in which specific aims are identified, discussed and agreed between the patient and the therapist. Low-stretch bandages are applied daily to the swollen limb and left in place until they are reapplied the next day (Moffatt *et al.* 2006c).

Not all patients will follow both phases of treatment, and many may only need to follow the maintenance phase.

Maintenance phase of treatment

Indications

Elastic compression garments are used during the maintenance phase of lymphoedema management and are usually combined with other elements of treatment including:

- A skin-care regimen to minimize the risks of infection.
- Exercise to promote lymph drainage.
- Simple lymph drainage administered by the patient to stimulate lymph drainage (Jenns 2000).

Indications for this phase of treatment may include:

- Mild, uncomplicated swelling with a normal limb shape (Jenns 2000).
- The maintenance of limb shape and size following a course of intensive therapy (Moffatt *et al.* 2006b).
- A limb volume less than 20% of the opposite limb if the shape of the limb has been preserved (Badger *et al.* 2000).
- To control swelling and provide support in the palliative treatment of oedema (Woods 2000b).

Contraindications

Elastic compression garments should not be used where there is:

- Arterial disease; blood supply may be further compromised.
- Distortion of limb shape; the garment will not fit.
- Skin folds; the garment will cause ridges and a torniquet effect to the limb.
- Open wounds; the garment will become soiled and pose an infection risk.
- Fragile skin; application and removal of the garment may cause further damage to the skin.
- Lymphorrhoea; the garment will become wet and may cause skin excoriation.
- An acute infective episode (cellulitis); application and removal of the garment may be painful and cause damage to the friable skin (Moffatt *et al.* 2006b).

Choosing elastic compression garments

Choosing the correct garment for the patient can be a difficult decision and should always follow a detailed assessment of the patient (Eagle 2001) and should only be attempted by a health care professional with the knowledge and appropriate skills to ensure patient safety.

The use of compression garments:

- Provides support for inelastic tissues.
- Promotes lymph movement along superficial and deep lymphatics.
- Provides an external counterforce during activity which enhances muscle pump action (Todd 2000).

A wide range of garments are available which differ in construction, compression class and style, in addition to size and colour:

- *Construction*: Garments are manufactured as either round knit or flat knit. Round-knit garments are produced in one piece from synthetic fibres and are readily available in a variety of sizes 'off the shelf' to accommodate the needs of most patients. Flat-knit garments are manufactured from one piece of material sewn together with a seam. The shape can be adjusted during manufacture to suit patients' specific needs and the provision

of accurate measurements before manufacture ensures a good fit (Todd 2000).

- *Compression class*: The degree of pressure exerted by the garment on the surface of the skin it surrounds determines the classified compression of the garment (Asmussen & Strossenreuther 2003). The highest compression provided by a garment when fitted can be found at the wrist or the ankle. The compression is then graduated along the length of the limb to encourage movement of the fluid out of the limb. Elastic compression garments are made in a number of compression classes, and in lymphoedema management are usually provided in a compression class of an International Standard which provides greater compression than garments made to the British Standard (Todd 2000). These strong compression class garments are available through a hospital or specialist orthotic supplier and an increasing number can now be obtained on prescription (FP10).
- *Style*: All areas influenced by swelling must be contained within the compression garment or further swelling will develop. The patient should be instructed concerning the application, removal and care of the garment to ensure that maximum effectiveness is achieved through its use. Consideration of the patient's ability must be taken into account when choosing a garment as a high degree of dexterity and strength may be required during its application and removal and this may be impractical for the patient (Todd 2000).
- *Size*: The correct garment is one that fits well and is comfortable for the patient with no loose pockets of material where swelling can develop and no areas of constriction where a tourniquet effect can occur. The manufacturer's guidance for choosing the correct size is based on simple limb measurements and particular attention should be made to the fit at the ankle or wrist where high levels of compression can occur (Todd 2000).

Intensive phase of treatment

The intensive phase of treatment is usually carried out for a short specified period of 2–3 weeks, necessitating daily bandaging of the swollen limb with low-stretch bandages. This phase of treatment should always be carried out by a skilled therapist with the necessary skills and experience to apply bandages to the swollen limb, ensuring that pressure is graduated towards the root of the limb and evenly applied (Hampton 1998). Damage to the skin and tissues can occur if the bandages are incorrectly or inappropriately applied (Thomas & Nelson 1998).

During the intensive or reduction phase of treatment, low-stretch bandages are applied to the swollen limb daily as part of a multilayer system to provide a semi-rigid encasement to the limb. This aspect of treatment is usually combined with other elements of treatment including:

- A skin-care regimen to minimize the risks of infection.
- Specific exercises to promote lymph drainage.
- Manual lymphatic drainage administered by a specially trained therapist to stimulate lymph drainage (Jenns 2000).

Indications

Indications for this phase of treatment include:

- *Large limbs*: Containment hosiery used on large swollen limbs may be ineffective due to the difficulties of applying sufficient tension to compress the limb (Stillwell 1973; Badger *et al*. 2000).
- *Misshapen limbs*: Containment hosiery will promote the development of deep skin folds when the limb is awkwardly shaped (Todd 2000). Foam or soft padding under bandages will smooth out the folds and restore normal shape to the limb (see Figures 9.1 & 9.2 for examples of a misshapen limb before and after bandaging).
- *Severe lymphoedema*: Large limbs with long-standing oedema require high pressures to break down tissue fibrosis. Bandages provide a low resting and high active pressure which enables hardened tissues to soften (Moffatt *et al*. 2006c).

- *Lymphorrhoea*: The leakage of lymph fluid from the skin responds readily to external pressure provided by bandages (Jenns 2000).
- *Damaged or fragile skin*: Containment hosiery can cause damage to fragile skin. Bandages should be used until the skin condition improves (Jenns 2000).

Contraindications

Low-stretch bandages should not be used where there is:

- Arterial disease; tissue ischaemia can occur.
- Infection in the swollen limb; pain may occur.
- Uncontrolled cardiac failure; fluid overload can occur.
- Deep vein thrombosis; anticoagulation therapy should be commenced prior to the use of bandages.
- Physical or psychological unsuitability of the patient to comply with treatment (Todd 2000).

Palliative care

Bandaging can be versatile and extremely useful in the palliative care setting when volume reduction may be unrealistic

Figure 9.1 Example of a misshapen limb before bandaging.

Figure 9.2 Example of a misshapen limb after bandaging.

or not indicated. Support and comfort can be provided to a limb using a low level of pressure with a modified technique of bandaging designed around the patient's needs. The bandages can be left in place for 2–3 days and should not prevent the patient from maintaining full movement in their bandaged limb (Woods 2000b).

Preparation of the patient

The bandaging materials used on a swollen limb can be bulky and patients will therefore require appropriate information and advice concerning suitable loose fitting, easily applied clothing and, if the leg is being bandaged, appropriate wide opening footwear, which will accommodate the bulk of the bandages during the course of treatment. As the bandages are worn for 24 hours a day, advice will also be required concerning personal hygiene. The timing of appointments for the bandages to be replaced may need to consider opportunities to attend to personal hygiene, travel arrangements and accommodate family and work commitments. The therapist should also discuss and outline with the patient an appropriate exercise regimen to be followed during the course of treatment, to ensure that maximum effectiveness is gained from the course of bandaging. Verbal information given should be supported by written information and include details of what the patient should do if problems develop with the bandages and whom to contact (Williams & Keller 2005).

Principles to be followed in multilayer bandaging

Low-stretch, inelastic bandages should always be used. These provide a low resting pressure to the swollen limb when the muscle is inactive and a high working pressure during activity when the muscle is pumping against the resistance created by the bandage (Todd 2000).

For bandaging to be effective the following principles must be considered.

- *An even pressure should be provided around the circumference of the limb*. Where the limb shape is irregular or distorted by swelling, an even profile can be achieved with the use of padding or foam to add bulk to an area where shape requires correcting (Williams & Keller 2005).
- *The pressure from the bandages must be graduated along the length of the limb to ensure that the most pressure is achieved distally and the least proximally*. Graduated pressure will be achieved naturally in a regularly shaped limb where the circumference of the wrist or ankle is smaller than the circumference of the root of the limb. Graduated pressure can also be achieved by selecting the correct bandage width for the size of the limb and con-

trolling the amount of bandage tension and overlap used (Todd 2000). Moderate tension only should be used and the bandages should never be stretched to their maximum length.
- *The pressure applied to the limb should be adequate to counter the limb circumference*. Greater pressure is required when the circumference of the limb is large. This can be achieved by using more than one layer of bandages and selecting the correct width of bandage for the circumference of the limb (Todd 2000).

The bandages should be left in place day and night and removed once every 24 hours. This enables skin hygiene to be attended to and the condition of the skin to be checked. Reapplication of the bandages then ensures that effective compression is maintained on the changing limb shape (Todd 2000).

The bandages should be comfortable for the patient and removed at any time if they cause any pain, numbness or discoloration (blueness) in the fingers or toes. This may indicate a variety of causes including too great a compression on the limb. A satisfactory outcome of treatment should be achieved within 2–3 weeks. The patient may then begin the maintenance phase of treatment where containment hosiery is fitted.

Evaluation of the bandaging procedure

Evaluation of each stage of the bandaging procedure is essential to ensure that the bandage and padding have been used appropriately and correctly.

The process of evaluation must be thorough and should include:

1 Continuous attention to the colour of the digits. Too much pressure will result in compromised circulation.
2 Continuous attention to the sensations experienced in the bandaged limb. The bandages should not cause pain, numbness or tingling.
3 The shape of the limb. A cylindrical contour should be achieved with the use of soft foam and padding.
4 The overlap of the bandages. This should be even and consistent with no gaps in the bandages.
5 The pressure achieved. This should feel even to the patient and there should be no creases in the bandages. Layers should be used appropriately (Todd 2000).

Patient evaluation

The patient should feel comfortable and able to move their limb. Information should be given concerning when and how to remove the bandages if necessary.

Procedure guidelines   Compression garments (elastic): application of

The application of elastic garments can be greatly eased by the wearing of household rubber gloves during application, which facilitate control of the garment and prevent damage to the fabric of the garment. Application aids are also available commercially and may assist some patients who experience difficulties. Any moisturizing cream should be applied at night-time rather than in the morning before putting the garment on. A very fine layer of talcum powder applied to hot sticky skin can ease application. If this is the first time that the patient has worn elastic compression garments, the therapist should explain to the patient that the feeling of pressure may feel strange for the first few hours, but that it should not cause pain in the limb or numbness in the digits or toes.

Applying elastic compression garments to the leg

Action	Rationale
1 Explain and discuss the procedure with the patient.	To ensure that the patient understands the procedure and gives his/her valid consent (NMC 2006: C; NMC 2008: C).
2 If possible, position the patient seated upright on a bed or couch and raise the height to a comfortable level.	To ensure the comfort of both the patient and nurse (C).
3 Turn the stocking inside-out to the heel.	This makes it easier to ease the stocking up (E).
4 Pull the foot of the stocking over the patient's foot.	
5 Turn the rest of the stocking back over the foot and up the leg.	To prevent a torniquet effect developing at the ankle and enable the stocking to be eased up the leg (E).
6 Ask the patient to keep the leg straight and if possible to push against the nurse.	To ensure that a good grip can be gained on the stocking (E).
7 Starting at the foot, gradually ease the stocking into place over the heel and up the leg a bit at a time, until it is in its final position.	Since it is the material of the stocking that provides the pressure, it must be distributed evenly to ensure an even distribution of pressure (Juzo 2006: C).
8 Do not pull from the top.	This will cause the stocking top to become overstretched and will lead to an uneven distribution of the stocking material (Juzo 2006: C).
9 Once the stocking is in place, check that there are no creases or wrinkles, particularly around the joints.	Wrinkles cause chafing of the skin and constricting bands of pressure (E).
10 Check that the patient finds the stocking comfortable and ask that any feelings of pain, tingling or numbness be reported.	Pain, tingling or numbness indicates that the stocking has been either inappropriately applied or fitted (E).
11 To remove the stocking, peel the stocking off the limb from the top downwards. Do not roll it down.	Rolling the stocking can result in tight bands of material forming, which are difficult to move (E).
12 Document the manufacturer, style, and size of garment that the patient has been provided with.	To maintain accurate records (NMC 2005).

Applying elastic compression garments to the arm

Action	Rationale
1 Explain and discuss the procedure with the patient.	To ensure that the patient understands the procedure and gives his/her valid consent (NMC 2006: C; NMC 2008: C).

2 The patient may be seated or standing.	
3 Turn the sleeve inside-out to the wrist. Pull over the patient's hand. *Note*: if a glove or separate handpiece is worn, always put the sleeve on *after* the glove or handpiece.	To avoid increasing swelling in the hand (E).
4 Turn the rest of the sleeve back over the hand and up the arm.	To prevent a torniquet effect developing at the wrist and enable the sleeve to be eased up the arm (E).
5 Ask the patient to grip something stable, such as a towel rail or the back of a chair.	This steadies the arm and gives the patient something to pull against (E).
6 Working from the hand or wrist, gradually ease the sleeve up the arm.	Since it is the material that provides the pressure, it must be evenly distributed to ensure an even distribution of pressure (C).
7 Do not pull up from the top.	To prevent the top becoming overstretched which will result in an uneven distribution of pressure (C).
8 Once the sleeve is in place, check that there are no creases or wrinkles, particularly around the joints.	Wrinkles and creases cause chafing of the skin and constricting bands of pressure (E).
9 Check that the patient finds the sleeve comfortable and ask that any signs of pain, tingling or numbness be reported.	Pain, tingling or numbness indicate that the sleeve has been either inappropriately applied or fitted (E).
10 To remove the sleeve, peel the sleeve off the limb from the top. Do not roll it down.	Rolling the sleeve down can lead to tight bands of material forming which are difficult to move (E).
11 Document the manufacturer, style, and size of garment that the patient has been provided with.	To maintain accurate records (NMC 2005).

Procedure guidelines   Compression bandaging (standard multilayer)

This procedure should not be attempted by anyone who has not had specialist education in this area. The swollen limb should be clean and well moisturized with a bland cream (e.g. E45) before being bandaged. Pressure must be applied in a graduated profile, i.e. highest over the hand or foot, and gradually reducing as the limb is bandaged upwards, to ensure that fluid is encouraged to drain towards the root of the limb.

Thus, on a normally shaped limb, maintaining the same amount of bandage tension and the same amount of bandage overlap all the way up the limb will result in a natural graduation of pressure due to the gradual increase in the size of the limb from ankle to groin, or wrist to axilla. In cases where swelling has distorted the shape of the limb, additional padding is used to create a suitable profile on which to bandage, and adjustments may be needed in bandage tension and bandage overlap. Very large limbs may also require extra layers of bandage to be used in order to ensure that sufficient pressure is applied.

Equipment for bandaging an arm

1 Tubular stockinette.
2 Light retention bandages, 6 and 10 cm to bandage digits and to hold foam padding in place.
3 Padding, 6 cm roll.
4 Sheet of low-density foam.
5 Low-stretch bandages, 6 and 8 cm.
6 Tape.
7 Scissors.

Procedure guidelines *(cont.)*

Bandaging an arm and the fingers

Action	Rationale
1 Explain and discuss the procedure with the patient.	To ensure that the patient understands the procedure and gives his/her valid consent (NMC 2006: C; NMC 2008: C).
2 If possible, the patient should be seated in a chair. The nurse should be positioned in front of the patient.	To ensure the comfort of both the patient and nurse (C).
3 Cut a length of tubular stockinette long enough to fit the patient's arm. Cut a small hole for the thumb and slip over the patient's arm.	To protect the skin from chafing (Williams & Keller 2005: E).
4 The fingers must be bandaged (see Action figure 4a). Using a narrow light retention bandage anchor the bandage loosely at the wrist and bring across the back of the hand to the thumb. Bandage around the thumb from the tip downwards (start at the level of the nail bed). Do not pull the bandage tight but go gently and firmly. Take the bandage under the wrist and back over the back of the hand to the index finger (see Action figure 4b). Again, bandage from the nail bed down to the webs of the finger. Repeat the same procedure for all fingers. Finish by tucking in the end of the bandage (see Action figure 4c).	To reduce or prevent swelling (Williams & Keller 2005: E).
5 Check the colour and temperature of the tips of the fingers.	To ensure that the blood supply is not compromised (Partsch 2003: E).
6 Check that the patient can move the fingers and make a fist.	To check that the bandage is not too tight (Partsch 2003: E).
7 Using the roll of padding, cover the hand in a figure of eight, padding out the palm and back of the hand (see Action figure 7).	Padding out the hand ensures even pressure distribution and protects the bony areas of the hand (Williams & Keller 2005: E).
8 Using foam and padding, even out any exaggerated contours of the limb.	To create a smooth profile on which to apply the bandage (Williams & Keller 2005: E).
9 Cut foam to fit the length of the arm from the wrist to axilla. Ensure that the width is sufficient to encircle the arm with a small overlap.	To protect the elbow joint and provide a smooth, even profile on which to bandage (Williams & Keller 2005: E).
10 Wrap the foam around the arm, securing with a light retention bandage. Finish by tucking in the end of the bandage (see Action figure 10).	
11 Take a 6 cm compression bandage and start by anchoring it loosely at the wrist. Advise the patient to hold their fingers apart whilst the hand is bandaged and take the bandage across the dorsum of the hand to wrap it twice around the hand close to the base of the fingers. Continue bandaging the hand firmly in a figure of eight until all of the hand is covered (see Action figure 11). Continue the rest of the bandage up the forearm in a spiral, covering half of the bandage with each turn. Keep the bandage as smooth as possible.	The bandage width must relate to the circumference of the limb with the narrowest bandage used on the smallest circumference (Thomas 2003: R 5).

180

12 Take an 8 or 10 cm bandage and, starting at the wrist, bandage in a spiral, still covering half of the bandage with each turn, up to the top of the arm (see Action figure 12).

Two layers are used on the forearm to ensure that pressure is highest distally (Thomas 2003: R 5).

13 Secure the end of the bandage with tape.

14 Once again, check the colour and sensations of the finger tips and check that the patient can move all joints.

To check that the blood flow is not compromised (Partsch 2003: E).

15 Remind the patient to use the limb as normally as possible, to exercise as advised and to remove the bandages if any pain, tingling or numbness is experienced.

To ensure good lymph flow and to prevent complications developing (Partsch 2003: E).

16 Record the details of the procedure followed in the patient's relevant documentation.

To maintain accurate records and provide a point of reference for subsequent treatment (NMC 2005: C).

Action 4(a)   Bandaging swollen fingers.

Action 4(b)   Bandage is taken under wrist, back over hand, to index finger.

Action 4(c)   Finished bandage.

Action 7   Palm and back of hand are padded out.

Procedure guidelines *(cont.)*

Action 10   Foam is wrapped around arm, secured with a light retention bandage.

Action 11   Hand is bandaged firmly in a figure of eight using a 6 cm compression bandage.

Action 12   Starting at wrist, an 8 or 10 cm bandage is used to cover to top of arm, in a spiral fashion.

Equipment for bandaging a leg

1 Tubular stockinette.
2 Light retention bandages, 6 and 10 or 12 cm.
3 Padding, 10 and 20 cm.
4 Sheet of low-density foam.

5 Low-stretch compression bandages, 8, 10 and 12 cm.
6 Tape.
7 Scissors.

Bandaging a leg and the toes

Action	Rationale
1 Explain and discuss the procedure with the patient.	To ensure that the patient understands the procedure and gives his/her valid consent (NMC 2006: C; NMC 2008: C).
2 If possible, the patient should be seated upright on a bed or treatment couch. Raise the bed or couch to a comfortable height.	To ensure the comfort of both the patient and nurse (C).
3 Cut a length of tubular stockinette long enough to fit the patient's leg. Slip over the leg.	To protect the skin from chafing (Williams & Keller 2005: E).

4 If the toes are swollen or have a tendency to swell they must be bandaged. The little toe can be omitted. Using a narrow light retention bandage anchor the bandage around the foot and bring across the top of the foot to the big toe (see Action figure 4a). Bandage around the toe from the tip downwards (start at the level of the nail bed). Do not pull the bandage tight, but gently and firmly. Take the bandage under the foot and back over the top of the foot to the next toe (see Action figure 4b). Repeat the same procedure for each toe that needs to be bandaged. Finish by tucking in the end of the bandage (see Action figure 4c).

To reduce or prevent swelling (Williams & Keller 2005: E). To prevent friction to and around the little toe (Williams & Keller 2005: E).

5 Cut the foam into pads to fit over the dorsum of the foot, around the ankle and behind the knee (see Action figures 5a, b).

To protect bony prominences and joint flexures (Williams & Keller 2005: E).

6 Secure the pads firmly in place with light retention bandages.

7 Using foam and padding even out any exaggerated contours of the limb.

To create a smooth profile on which to apply the bandages (Williams & Keller 2005: E).

8 Using a 10 cm roll of padding, apply firmly in a spiral up the leg, starting around the foot. Use the 20 cm padding over the thigh (see Action figure 8).

To protect the skin and create a smooth profile on which to bandage (Williams & Keller 2005: E).

9 Take an 8 cm compression bandage and start by anchoring it loosely at the ankle. Advise the patient to hold their foot at a 90° angle whilst it is bandaged and take the bandage across the dorsum of the foot to wrap it around the foot close to the base of the toes (see Action figure 9). Continue bandaging the foot firmly, forming a figure of eight to cover the heel and ankle without leaving any gaps. Any surplus bandage should be taken up the leg in a spiral.

To avoid constriction at the ankle. Fluid will accumulate in any unbandaged areas (Williams & Keller 2005: E).

10 Using a 10 cm bandage, continue from where the first bandage finished, using a spiral up the leg and covering half of the bandage with each turn. Remember to bandage firmly. Use the widest bandage over the thigh. Secure the end of the last bandage with tape.

The bandage width must relate to the circumference of the limb with the narrowest bandage used on the smallest circumference (Thomas 2003: R 5).

11 Apply a second layer of bandage, from ankle to thigh, using a figure of eight. Secure the end with tape (see Action figure 11).

To keep the bandages in place and provide additional pressure along the length of the leg (Williams & Keller 2005: E).

12 Check the colour and temperature of the patient's toes. It may be difficult for the patient to flex the knee at first but this should get easier as the bandages loosen slightly.

To check that the blood flow is not compromised (Partsch 2003: E).

13 Remind the patient to use the limb as normally as possible, to exercise as advised and to remove the bandages if any pain, tingling or numbness is experienced.

To ensure good lymph flow and to prevent complications developing (Partsch 2003: E).

14 Record the details of the procedure followed in the patient's relevant documentation.

To maintain accurate records and provide a point of reference for subsequent treatment (NMC 2005: C).

Procedure guidelines *(cont.)*

Action 4(a) A narrow light retention bandage is anchored around the foot and brought across the foot to the big toe.

Action 4(b) The toes are bandaged in turn from the nail bed along the length of the toe.

Action 4(c) The bandage is taken under the foot and back over the top of the foot to bandage the next toe.

Action 5(a) Foam is used to cover dorsum of foot and around ankle.

Action 5(b) A foam pad is bandaged into position behind knee.

Action 8 Rolls of padding are applied firmly in a spiral up leg, starting around foot.

Action 9 Bandaging foot using an 8 cm compression bandage and starting close to toes.

Action 11 Applying a second layer of bandage, from ankle to thigh.

References and further reading

Aslem, M., Tierney, S. & Grace, P. (1996) Swollen leg or just big? *European Journal of Lymphology*, **6**(Suppl), 21.

Asmussen, P. & Strossenreuther, R. (2003) Compression therapy. In: *Textbook of Lymphology for Physicians and Lymphoedema Therapists* (eds M. Foldi, E. Foldi & S. Kubik). Urban Fischer, Munich, Germany, pp. 527–88.

Badger, C. (1993) Guidelines for the calculation of limb volume based on surface measurements. *British Lymphology Interest Group Newsletter*, Issue 7, Sir Michael Sobell House, Oxford.

Badger, C., Peacock, J. & Mortimer, P. (2000) A randomised, controlled parallel-group clinical trial comparing multilayer bandaging followed by hosiery versus hosiery alone in the treatment of patients with lymphoedema of the limb. *Cancer*, **88**(12), 2832–7.

Benner, P. (1984) *From Novice to Expert*. Addison-Wesley, California.

Bernas, M., Witte, M. & Witte, C. (1996) Limb volume measurements in lymphoedema. *Lymphology*, **29**(Suppl), 199–202.

Boland, R. & Adams, R. (1998) The effects of arm elevation and overnight head-up tilt on forearms and hand volume. *J Hand Ther*, **11**, 180–90.

Callam, M.J. *et al.* (1997) Hazards of compression treatment of the leg: an estimate from Scottish surgeons. *BMJ*, **295**, 1382.

Clark, M. (2003) Compression bandages: principles and definitions. In: *European Wound Management Association (EWMA) Position Document.Understanding Compression Therapy*. Medical Educational Partnership, London, pp. 5–7.

Doherty, D., Morgan, P. & Moffatt, C. (2006) Role of hosiery in lower limb lymphoedema. In: *Lymphoedema Framework; Template for Practice; Compression Hosiery in Lymphoedema*. Medical Educational Partnership, London, pp. 10–21.

Eagle, M. (2001) Compression bandaging. *Nurs Stand*, **15**(38), 47–52.

Engler, H. & Sweat, R. (1962) Volumetric arm measurements: techniques and results. *Am Surg*, **28**, 465–8.

Foldi, E., Junger, M. & Partsch, H. (2005) The science of lymphoedema bandaging. In: *European Wound Management Association (EWMA) Focus Document: Lymphoedema Bandaging in Practice*. Medical Educational Partnership, London, pp. 2–4.

Hampton, S. (1998) Bandage application. In: *Compression Therapy: A Complete Guide*. Journal of Wound Care/EMAP Healthcare Ltd, London, pp. 5–8.

Jenns, K. (2000) Management strategies. In: *Lymphoedema* (eds R. Twycross, K. Jenns & J. Todd). Radcliffe Medical Press, Oxford, pp. 97–117.

Juzo (2006) *Application of Compression Stockings*. Juzo UK, Dundee, Scotland.

Keeley, V. (2000) Classification of lymphoedema. In: *Lymphoedema* (eds R. Twycross, K. Jenns & J. Todd). Radcliffe Medical Press, Oxford, pp. 22–43.

Kettle, J., Rundle, F. & Oddie, T. (1958) Measurement of upper limb volumes: a clinical method. *Aust N Z J Surg*, **27**, 263–70.

Mason, W. (2000) Exploring rehabilitation within lymphoedema management. *Int J Palliat Nurs*, **6**(6), 265–73.

Moffatt, C., Doherty, D. & Morgan, P. (eds) (2006a) Assessment. In: *Lymphoedema Framework; Best Practice for the Management of Lymphoedema; International Consensus*. Medical Educational Partnership, London, pp. 6–14.

Moffatt, C., Doherty, D. & Morgan, P. (eds) (2006b) Compression garments. In: *Lymphoedema Framework; Best Practice for the Management of Lymphoedema; International Consensus*. Medical Educational Partnership, London, pp. 39–46.

Moffatt, C., Doherty, D. & Morgan, P. (eds) (2006c) Multi-layer inelastic lymphoedema bandaging. In: *Lymphoedema Framework; Best Practice for the Management of Lymphoedema; International Consensus*. Medical Educational Partnership, London, pp. 32–8.

Mortimer, P. (2003a) Differential diagnosis of chronic swelling of the limbs. In: *Diseases of the Lymphatics* (eds N. Browse, K. Burn & P. Mortimer). Arnold Publishers, London, pp. 157–66.

Mortimer, P. (2003b) Principles of medical and physical treatment. In: *Diseases of the Lymphatics* (eds N. Browse, K. Burn & P. Mortimer). Arnold Publishers, London, pp. 167–78.

Mortimer, P. *et al.* (1996) The prevalence of arm oedema following treatment for breast cancer. *Q J Med*, **89**, 377–80.

NMC (2005) *Guidelines for Records and Record Keeping*. Nursing and Midwifery Council, London.

NMC (2006) *A–Z Advice Sheet Consent*. www.nmc.org.

NMC (2008) *The Code: Standards of Conduct, Performance and Ethics for Nurses and Midwives*. Nursing and Midwifery Council, London.

Partsch, H. (2003) Understanding the pathophysiological effects of compression. In: *European Wound Management Association (EWMA) Position Document. Understanding Compression Therapy*. Medical Educational Partnership, London, pp. 2–7.

Piller, N. (1999) Gaining an accurate assessment of the stages of lymphoedema subsequent to cancer: the role of objective and subjective information, when to make measurements and their optimal use. *European Journal of Lymphology*, **7**(25), 1–9.

Ryan, M. *et al.* (2003) Aetiology and prevalence of lower limb lymphoedema following treatment for gynaecological cancer. *Aust N Z J Obstet Gynaecol*, **43**(2), 148–51.

Sitzia, J. (1995) Volume measurement in lymphoedema treatment: examination of the formulae. *Eur J Cancer Care*, **4**, 11–16.

Stanton, A. *et al.* (1997) Validation of an optoelectronic limb volumeter (Perometer). *Lymphology*, **30**, 77–97.

Stanton, A., Badger, C. & Sitzia, J. (2000) Non-invasive assessment of the lymphoedematous limb. *Lymphology*, **33**, 122–35.

Stillwell, G. (1973) The Law of Laplace: some clinical applications. *Mayo Clin Proc*, **48**, 863–9.

Taylor, R. *et al.* (2006) Reliability and validity of arm volume measurements for assessment of lymphoedema. *Physical Therapy*, **86**(2), 205–14.

Thomas, S. (2003) The use of the Laplace equation in the calculation of sub-bandage pressure. *European Wound Management Association (EWMA) Journal*, **3**(1), 21–3.

Thomas, S. & Nelson, A. (1998) Graduated external compression in the treatment of venous disease. In: *Compression Therapy: A Complete Guide*. Journal of Wound Care/EMAP Healthcare Ltd, London, pp. 1–4.

Tobin, M. *et al.* (1993) The psychological morbidity of breast cancer related arm swelling. *Cancer*, **72**(11), 3348–52.

Todd, J. (2000) Containment in the management of lymphoedema. In: *Lymphoedema* (eds R. Twycross, K. Jenns & J. Todd). Radcliffe Medical Press, Oxford, pp. 165–202.

Williams, A. & Keller, M. (2005) Practical guidance on lymphoedema bandaging of the upper and lower limbs. In: *European Wound Management Association (EWMA) Focus Document: Lymphoedema Bandaging in Practice*. Medical Educational Partnership, London, pp. 10–14.

Woods, M. (1993) Patients' perceptions of breast-cancer related lymphoedema. *Eur J Cancer Care*, **2**, 125–8.

Woods, M. (1994) An audit of swollen limb measurements. *Nurs Stand*, **9**(5), 24–6.

Woods, M. (2000a) Psychosocial aspects of lymphoedema. In: *Lymphoedema* (eds R. Twycross, K. Jenns & J. Todd). Radcliffe Medical Press, Oxford, pp. 89–96.

Woods, M. (2000b) Lymphoedema. In: *Stepping into Palliative Care: A Handbook for Community Professionals* (ed. J. Cooper). Radcliffe Medical Press, Oxford, pp. 81–8.

Woods, M. (2002) Using philosophy, knowledge and theory to assess a patient with lymphoedema. *Int J Palliat Nurs*, 8(4), 176–81.

Woods, M., Tobin, M. & Mortimer, P. (1995) The psychological morbidity of breast cancer patients with lymphoedema. *Cancer Nurs*, 18(6), 467–71.

Chapter 10

Discharge planning

Reference material **188**
Procedure guidelines: Discharge planning **196**
References and further reading **200**

Definition

Discharge planning is a process and not an isolated event. It should involve the development and implementation of a plan to facilitate the transfer of an individual from hospital to an appropriate setting and include the multidisciplinary team, the patient and their carers. Furthermore, it involves building on, or adding to, any assessments undertaken prior to admission (DH 2003a).

Reference material

One of the key elements of the Clinical Governance agenda is improved quality and effectiveness (DH 1998a). Good quality discharge should reduce delayed discharges (Tarling & Jauffur 2006) and facilitate meeting the targets set by The NHS Plan (DH 2000a), National Service Framework for Older People (DH 2002) and commissioning a patient-led National Health Service (NHS) (DH 2004a).

Therefore all hospitals should have a discharge policy which is developed, agreed and ideally jointly published with all the relevant local health and social service agencies. Standards should be applicable to the planning and delivery of care at all stages: preadmission and admission; the period as an inpatient; predischarge; the discharge process and postdischarge (Health Services Accreditation 1996). Patient preadmission clinics are an ideal opportunity to assess care required on discharge (DH 2003a).

Your Guide to the National Health Service (NHSE 2001) states that from the moment a patient arrives:

> Arrangements for discharging you from hospital will begin, and your discharge plan will be agreed with you, taking account of your needs. When you are ready to leave hospital, the nurses and doctors will talk to you about what will happen to you during your recovery and you will be told who to contact in an emergency.
>
> If you need ongoing care at home, your GP, midwife, health visitor, community nurse or social services department will be there to help you.
>
> If you need any medical equipment for your return home, the NHS and your social services department will aim to provide it promptly. If you need your home to be adapted in any way, your social services department will assess your needs.
>
> (NHSE 2001, p. 30)

All patients, whether short- or long-stay, those with few needs or those with complex needs, should receive comprehensive discharge planning. Some patients may have particular care needs on discharge; examples are listed in Box 10.1.

Aims of discharge planning

- To ensure patients have a safe discharge from hospital to the community.

> **Box 10.1 Patients who may have particular care needs on discharge***
>
> The following patients were identified as having particular care needs:
>
> - Live alone.
> - Are frail and/or elderly.
> - Have care needs which place a high demand on carers.
> - Have a limited prognosis.
> - Have serious illnesses and will be returning to hospital for further treatments.
> - Have continuing disability.
> - Have learning difficulties.
> - Have mental illness or dementia.
> - Have dependents.
> - Have limited financial resources.
> - Are homeless or live in poor housing.
> - Do not have English as their first language.
> - Have been in hospital for an 'extended stay'.
> - Require aids/equipment at home.
>
> *DH 1989; DH 2004b.

- To ensure patients and carers are involved throughout the discharge planning process.
- To provide patients and carers with written and verbal information to meet their needs on discharge.
- To provide continuity of care between the hospital and the agreed environment by facilitating effective communication. (Adapted from DH 2004b.)

Principles of discharge planning

The key principles for effective discharge planning are that:

- Unnecessary admissions are avoided and discharge is facilitated by a whole system approach to care planning.
- Patients and carers should be actively involved in the process (DH 1995; DH 2004c).
- Discharge planning should commence on the initial contact with patients.
- Discharge should be co-ordinated by a named person.
- Discharge planning should be a multidisciplinary process by which resources to meet the needs of patients and carers are put in place (Salter 1996).
- Effective use is made of transitional and intermediate care services, so that patients achieve their optimal outcome and acute hospital beds are used appropriately.
- Patients and carers understand the discharge planning process, their rights and receive appropriate information to enable them to make informed decisions about their future care. (Adapted from DH 2003a.)

The discharge planning process and the primary/secondary care interface

The discharge planning process can be initiated by a member of the primary health care team (PHCT) or social services

staff in the patient's home, prior to admission, in preadmission clinics or on hospital admission (Health Services
Accreditation 1996). Importance is attached to developing
a primary care-led NHS, reinforced by the government's
white paper, 'The New NHS: Modern, Dependable' (DH
1998b). The focus on quality, patient-centred care and services closer to where people live will be dependent on primary, secondary and tertiary professionals working together
(Davis 1998).

However, it is important to note that the Community Care
(Delayed Discharges) Act (DH 2003b) introduced a system of reimbursement to NHS bodies from social services
departments for delays caused by the failure of social services departments to provide timely assessment and/or services for a patient being discharged from an acute hospital
bed.

The discharge planning process takes into account a patient's physical, psychological, social, cultural and economic
needs. It involves not only patients but can involve families,
friends, carers, the hospital multidisciplinary team and the
community health/social services teams (Nixon *et al.* 1998),
with the emphasis on health and social services departments
working jointly.

In recent years the reduction in hospital beds has resulted in an increasing emphasis on shorter inpatient stays
(Stewart 2000). However, the notion of a seamless service
may be idealistic because of increasing time constraints and
the complex care needs of high-dependency patients (Smith
1996).

Occasionally the discharge process may not proceed as
planned; a discharge may be delayed for a number of reasons and a system should be in place to record this (for example see Figure 10.1). Patients may take their own discharge
against medical advice and this should be documented accordingly (for example see Box 10.2). Some patients receiving news of a poor prognosis may prefer to go home
to die and plans would need to be set up at short notice
(Figure 10.2).

The role of informal carers

Engaging and involving patients and carers as equal partners is central to successful discharge planning (DH 2003a).
The hospital discharge process is a critical time for carers. It
may be the first time they are confronted with the reality of
their role, the effect it may have on their relationship with
the person needing care, their family and their employment
(Hill & Macgregor 2001). Research suggests that if carers
are unsupported it can result in early readmission of the
patient (Holzhausen 2001). Recent government policy (DH
2004c) builds on existing legislation to support carers in a
practical way by providing information, helping carers to
remain at work and by helping carers to care for themselves.
Throughout discharge planning, carers' needs should be acknowledged. Carers may have different needs from patients
and they are entitled to a separate assessment (DH 2004c).
Health care professionals should allow carers sufficient time

---

> **Box 10.2**   Patients taking discharge against medical advice*
>
> ### Nursing staff responsibility
>
> If a patient wishes to take his/her own discharge the ward
> sister/co-ordinator should contact:
>
> 1 A member of the medical team.
> 2 The manager on call.
> 3 The Complex Discharge Co-ordinator.
>
> The Complex Discharge Co-ordinator will inform social ser-
> vices if appropriate. Out of hours, following a risk assessment,
> the manager on call will contact the local social services de-
> partment, if felt appropriate, and inform the hospital social ser-
> vices department the following day.
>
> ### Medical staff responsibility
>
> The doctor, following consultation with the patient, should
> complete the appropriate form prior to the patient leaving
> the hospital. The form must be signed by the patient and
> the doctor and filed in the medical notes. The doctor must
> immediately contact the patient's general practitioner (GP).
>   *Source: Royal Marsden NHS Foundation Trust 2006.

189

and information to make decisions, provide written information on the discharge plan and ensure adequate support is in
place before discharge (Hill & Macgregor 2001). This will
promote a successful and seamless transfer from hospital to
home.

Communication and discharge planning

Effective, safe discharge planning needs to be patient and
carer focused. Therefore it is dependent on a multidisciplinary approach and the sharing of good practice (Martin
2001). There is consistent evidence to suggest that best practice in hospital discharge involves multidisciplinary teamwork throughout the process (Borill *et al.* 2001). The multidisciplinary approach, where all staff have a clear understanding of their roles and responsibilities (for example see
Box 10.3), will also help to prevent inappropriate readmissions and delayed discharges (Stewart 2000). This approach
also promotes the highest possible level of independence for
the patient, their partner and family by encouraging appropriate self-care activities.

Ineffective discharge planning has been shown to have
detrimental effects on a patient's psychological and physical
well being and their illness experience (Smith 1996; Nazarko
1998). Planning care, providing adequate information and
involving patients, families and health care professionals will
keep disruption to a minimum.

Discharge Co-ordinators are health or social care professionals who have both hospital and community experience.
Their role is to advise and help with planning the care patients may need when leaving hospital, particularly when the

DISCHARGE DELAY MONITORING FORM
Please refer to accompanying guidelines

Ward
Week commencing

Were there any delayed discharges this week (please tick) YES ☐   NO ☐

If yes please complete form fully.

Please complete this form for patients who no longer need clinical care in a comprehensive cancer centre, but who stay in the hospital because of 'delayed or lack of appropriate Community/Social Services or internal failures to plan the discharge properly'

Patient's Details: (Give full address inc. postcode)   **Hospital No:** _____

Name: _____   **Consultant:** _____

Address: _____

_____

_____   **Postcode:** _____

Expected Date of Discharge: _____   **Actual Date of Discharge:** _____

Reason for Delay in Discharge: (Please tick the appropriate boxes)

Royal Marsden NHS Trust Failure   ☐   Other Hospital Failure   ☐

Hospice Failure   ☐   Transport failure   ☐

                                                           Internal Social Services failure   ☐

Community Health Service Failure e.g. D/N, Macmillan ☐   External Social Services failure   ☐

*Identify Health Authority*_____   *Identify Social Services Dept.* _____

Patient/Relative choice   ☐   Other   ☐

(Don't count if 24 hour's notice given to relatives)   Please specify _____

Full details of delay: Please complete
_____
_____
_____
_____

Signature: _____   **Print Name:** _____

Please send completed forms to Complex Discharge Co–Ordinator / Tracking Officer

Figure 10.1   Example of discharge delay monitoring form. Source: Royal Marsden NHS Foundation Trust (2006).

Name:	Hospital No:

Checklist for Discharge

This form should be used to assist with planning an urgent discharge home for a patient with terminal care needs. It should be used in conjunction with the discharge policy.

Sign and date to confirm when arranged and equipment given. Document relevant information in the discharge planning section of the nursing documentation. Document if item or care is not applicable.

Appoint a designated ward based discharge lead:

Name:.. Designation:... Contact No:............

	Date & Time	Signature, Print Name & Job Title
Patient / Family issues		
Meeting with patient/family to discuss: patient's condition and prognosis		
Plan agreed and discussed with patient and carers. Explain the level of care that will be provided in the community. Ensure an understanding that there will not be 24-hour nursing presence.		
Communication with District Nurse and Community Palliative Care Team		
Discuss • Patient and family needs • The role of each service and the timing and frequency of visits • Community Service cover at night (to support family) e.g. Marie Curie or other local services • The need to complete the Continuing Care Application Form, if necessary		
Agreed planned date and time of district nurses first visit..................................		
Agreed planned date and time of community palliative care team first visit..................................		
Night nursing service Start date..................................		
Communication with GP and Community Palliative Care Medical Team - Medical Responsibilities **(Hospital medical team to organize – the nurse to confirm when arranged)**		
Registrar to discuss with GP the patient needs and their prognosis, medication and the need to review the patient in the community for death certification purposes.		
Oxygen cylinder/ concentrator (delete as appropriate) ordered through GP and delivery date organized for..................................		
Medical summary faxed to GP ☐ copy with patient ☐		
Registrar to discuss with the Palliative Care Medical team the patient's needs and proposed plan of care		
Adequate supply of drugs prescribed for discharge (TTOs) including crisis drugs, i.e. Midazolam and morphine sulphate		
Medical letter or authorization for drugs to be administered by community nurses.		
'Do Not Attempt Resuscitation' letter for Community Staff		
'Do Not Attempt Resuscitation' letter for Ambulance Crew		

Figure 10.2   Checklist for patients being discharged home for urgent palliative care (*continued on p. 192*).

	Date & Time	Signature, Print Name & Job Title
Equipment – confirm delivery of equipment		
Hospital bed (electric/manual – please circle)		
Pressure relieving equipment		
Commode/urinal		
Hoist		
Backrest/mattress variator		
Other, please state..		
Provide 7 days supply of:		
Dressings		
If patient is being discharged with a syringe driver in situ then complete the syringe driver discharge checklist		
Sharps bin		
Continence aids		
Transport (confirm by ticking appropriate boxes) CHECK OTHER DISCHARGE DOCUMENTATION		
Transport booked: Date and Time...................................... Oxygen/suction ☐ Stretcher ☐ Paramedic crew ☐		
Escort (family/nurse)		
'Do Not Attempt Resuscitation' letter given to ambulance crew		
Family informed and aware that the patient may not survive the transfer journey and that the ambulance crew will not attempt resuscitation		
Written Information and Documentation		
Community Care Referral form completed and faxed for the attention of..		
Community Care Referral form and medical summary given to patient or relative (specify)		
Community Palliative Care Team form completed and faxed for the attention of..		
Patient/carer given list of contact numbers of community services **(including night service)**		
Medication list, stating reasons for drugs, given and explained to patient/relative		
Confirm with the Hospital Consultant whether a bed should be held for this patient for 24/48 hrs (delete as appropriate)		

Signature/print name of designated ward based discharge lead:...

Date/Time..

File this form in the patient's records on discharge.

Figure 10.2 (*cont.*)

Box 10.3   Guide to discharge planning for nursing staff

YOUR RESPONSIBILITIES:
The aim of this guide is to make discharge planning more effective. It should be used in conjunction with the Royal Marsden's *Discharge Policy and Procedure* (Royal Marsden NHS Foundation Trust 2006).

- Within 24 hours of each admission, make every effort to complete the full nursing assessment and discharge planning section of the care plan.
- On admission a provisional discharge date should be discussed with patients, carers and the medical team and documented. This must be reviewed daily.
- Be aware: if patients require a care package on discharge, social services require a minimum of 3 days to assess their needs under the Community Care (Delayed Discharges) Act 2003 (DH 2003b).
- Discharge date should be set in negotiation with the multidisciplinary team and discussed with the patient and carers.
- Please ensure that all complex discharges are discussed at ward multidisciplinary meetings.

AS APPROPRIATE:
- Refer to other members of the multidisciplinary team.
- If a social services care package is essential on discharge, forward Section 2/Section 5 Notification Forms to the Tracking Officer.
- For information regarding social services or carers support please complete a Trigger Form only and forward to the social services department.
- Refer to district nursing/specialist community services (try to give 48 hours notice). Complete the Community Care Referral Form and fax.
- Request nursing equipment for use in the community (it can take a week to obtain).
- Complete the NHS Continuing Healthcare assessment form if the patient may meet the criteria for NHS funded care, due to prognosis or complexity of need.
- Refer to Community Palliative Care Team and specify if urgent. Document all referrals made to community services with **DATE, CONTACT NAME, TELEPHONE AND FAX NUMBERS.**
- Give written details of services arranged to patient and/or carer.

DISCHARGE DELAYS:
For a definition of a delayed discharge at the Royal Marsden, please refer to the Discharge Policy.

- All delayed discharges must be discussed at ward multidisciplinary meetings and highlighted to the Complex Discharge Co-ordinators.
- Discharge Delay Monitoring Form to be completed for every delay by the ward manager or designated deputy and forwarded to the site-specific Tracking Office, Chelsea or Sutton.

For further information or advice on discharge planning please contact the Complex Discharge Co-ordinator or social services department.

nursing and care needs are complex. McKenna *et al.* (2000) cite poor communication between hospital and community, and to this end Nixon *et al.* (1998) have endorsed the value of co-ordination in a climate of shorter hospital stays and timely patient discharge.

For complex discharges, it is helpful if a key worker is appointed to manage the discharge (DH 2003a), the Discharge Co-ordinator for example, and, where appropriate, for family meetings/case conferences to take place and include the patient/carer, multidisciplinary team and PHCT and representatives (Health Services Accreditation 1996; Salter 1996). Additionally a guide to planning a complex discharge (Box 10.4) can highlight the communication required by the multidisciplinary team.

Nurse-led discharge

In The NHS Plan (DH 2000a) the Chief Nursing Officer identified 10 key roles for nurses, one being admitting and discharging patients with specific conditions using agreed protocols. Nurse discharge protocols can assist hospitals in reducing length of stay, reducing delays associated in waiting for a doctor to review a patient for discharge or to prescribe medication to take home, and also avoids unnecessary delays at weekends and evenings (NHS Modernisation Agency 2003).

Single Assessment Process

Referred to in The NHS Plan (DH 2000a) and reinforced in The National Service Framework for Older People (DH 2001a), the Single Assessment Process is designed to replace fragmented assessments carried out by different agencies with one seamless procedure (Hunter 2001). The aim is to produce a single, centrally held, electronic summary/tool containing all the information needed to assess, and in turn provide for, an older person's health and social care needs. The end result will be a comprehensive 'individual care plan' that will lay out their full needs and entitlements (Hunter 2001). Examples of health care professionals who may be involved in contributing to the Single Assessment Process are nurses and doctors, occupational therapists, physiotherapists, dietitians and speech therapists.

Although there has been a high level of commitment to the Single Assessment Process from both health and social care professionals, implementation has occurred at different rates. It appears that more progress has been made in the community rather than hospitals and general practitioner practices (NHS Connecting for Health 2005).

Intermediate care

The National Bed Enquiry (DH 2000b), The NHS Plan (DH 2000a) and The National Service Framework for Older People (DH 2001a) signalled the development of intermediate care as one of the major initiatives for services in the future. It is recognized that older people are best cared for at home

Box 10.4   Guide to arranging a complex discharge home

Helpful hints on arranging a complex discharge home

NB: This is not an exhaustive list and MUST BE DISCUSSED with the Complex Discharge Co-ordinator/ Specialist Sister, Discharge Planning, Palliative Care.

Complex discharge definition:

- A large package of care involving different agencies.
- The patient's needs have changed since admission, with different services requiring co-ordination.
- The family/carer requires intensive input into discharge planning considerations (e.g. psychological interventions):
    - Patients who are entitled to Continuing NHS Funded Care and who require a package of care on discharge.
    - Patients for repatriation.

1 **Comprehensive assessment by nurse on admission and document care accordingly.**

(a) Provisional discharge date set.
- This will only be an approximate date, depending on care needs, equipment, etc.
- It should be reviewed regularly with multidisciplinary team.
- Discharge should **not** be arranged for a Friday or weekend.

(b) Referrals to relevant members of multidisciplinary team.
e.g. Occupational therapist, physiotherapist, social services.

(c) Referral to Community Health Services (in liaison with multidisciplinary team).
e.g. District nurse (who may be able to arrange for night sitters), Community Palliative Care Team.

(d) Request equipment from district nurse and discuss with family.
e.g. Hoist, hospital bed, pressure-relieving mattress/cushion, commode, nebulizer.
- **If oxygen is required,** medical team to complete Home Oxygen Ordering Form (HOOF) and Home Oxygen Consent Form (HOCF) forms for oxygen cylinders and concentrators at home. Fax to relevant oxygen supplier.

2 **Discuss at ward multidisciplinary meeting, arrange family meeting/case conference as required**, and invite all appropriate health care professionals, including community staff.

(a) Appoint discharge co-ordinator at the multidisciplinary meeting.
- To act as co-ordinator for referrals and point of contact for any discharge concerns.
- To plan and prepare the family meeting/case conference and to arrange a chairperson and minute-taker for the meeting.
- Primary Team Nurse to liaise with discharge co-ordinator.

(b) Formulate a discharge plan at meeting.
- At the meeting, formulate a discharge plan in conjunction with patient, carers, and all hospital and community personnel involved and agree a discharge date: an occupational therapist home visit may be required.

(c) Ascertain discharge address.
- Liaise with services accordingly.
- It is important to agree who will care for patient/where the patient will be cared for, e.g. ground/first floor.
- Ascertain type of accommodation patient lives in so that the equipment ordered will fit in appropriately.
- NB. IF NOT RETURNING TO OWN HOME, A GP WILL BE REQUIRED TO TAKE PATIENT ON AS A TEMPORARY RESIDENT.

(d) Confirm PROVISIONAL discharge date.
- This will depend on when community services and equipment can be arranged.
- This must be agreed with the patient and family/informal carer/s.

Box 10.4 *(cont.)*

3 **Ascertain whether district nurse is able to undertake any necessary clinical procedures** in accordance with their Primary Care Trust policy, e.g. care of skin-tunnelled catheters. Consider alternative arrangements if necessary.

  (a) Confirm equipment agreed and delivery date.

    NB. Family must be informed of delivery date and also requested to contact ward to inform that this has been received.

  (b) Confirm **start date** for care.
  (c) Confirm with patient/family agreed discharge date.

    e.g. Social services/district nurse/community palliative care.
    ■ Liaise with Complex Discharge Co-ordinator for 'Community Services Arrangements' Form
    ■ Check community services able to enter patient home as necessary.

4 **Forty-eight hours prior to discharge,** Fax and telephone district nurse with Community Care Referral Form and discuss any special needs of patient, e.g. syringe driver, oxygen, wound care, intravenous therapy, methicillin-resistant *Staphylococcus aureus* (MRSA) or other infection status. Give written information and instructions.

  (a) Arrange transport and assess need for escort/oxygen during transport.
  (b) Ongoing review.

    ■ Should be in place for any change in patient's condition/treatment plan.
    ■ IF THERE IS A CHANGE, notify/liaise with MultidisciplinaryTeam and Community Services

  (c) If NO change within 24 hours of discharge, confirm that:

    ■ Patient is medically fit for discharge
    ■ All Community Services are in place as agreed above

    Patient has drugs to take out (TTO) and next appointment.

    ■ Ensure patient has drugs TTO with written and verbal instructions.
    ■ Next in/out-patient appointment as required.

    Access to home, heating and food are checked.

    ■ Check arrangements for patient to get into home (front door key), heating, food and someone there to welcome them home, as appropriate.

5 **Hospital equipment:** e.g. syringe drivers: ensure clearly marked and arrangements made for return.

6 **After discharge,** follow-up phone call to patient by ward nurse/Complex Discharge Co-ordinator as agreed to ensure all services in place.

if at all possible. To aid the transition period from hospital to home, intermediate care teams may provide a period of intensive care/rehabilitation following a hospital stay. It may be provided in a care home or in the individual's own home. It is likely to be limited to a maximum of 6 weeks; however, there are local variations in practice. Intermediate care needs to have a person centred approach involving patients and carers in all aspects of assessment, goal setting and discharge planning. Its success depends on local knowledge of the service and interagency collaboration (Hancock 2003). There is growing evidence that supports intermediate care initiatives reducing admissions to acute hospitals and reducing residential/nursing home placements (DH 2002).

Discharge to a care home

Discharge to a care home (whether it be in the form of a residential or nursing home) requires careful thought as for many patients the concept and planning of giving up their own home is one of the most traumatic events that a person has to consider. A thorough multidisciplinary assessment is essential, taking into account the individual needs of the patient and carer and exploring all the options before agreeing on a care home. Placements can be delayed while waiting for a vacancy and it may be necessary to consider an interim placement (DH 2003a).

In 2001 there were important changes in the funding arrangement for adults requiring registered nursing care in nursing homes in England (DH 2001b). All adults needing the skills and knowledge of a registered nurse to meet all or certain elements of their care needs have that care paid for by the NHS. The amount of funding, paid directly to the nursing home, is dependent on a comprehensive assessment of the patient's care needs by a registered nurse, who will usually be employed by the local Primary Care Trust. NHS-funded nursing care was provided via payment 'bands', which relate to the level of nursing care required. However, the National Framework (DH 2006), which came into effect in October 2007, replaced the banding system with a weekly rate for NHS-funded nursing care.

NHS Continuing Healthcare

NHS Continuing Healthcare is a general term that describes the care that people need over an extended period of time as the result of disability, accident or illness to address both physical and mental health needs. It may require services from the NHS and/or social care. It can be provided in a range of settings, for example, from a care home to care in people's own homes. NHS Continuing Healthcare describes a package of care arranged and funded solely by the NHS. NHS Continuing Healthcare should be awarded when it is established (through multidisciplinary assessment) that an individual's overall care needs are such that their primary need is a health need. There has been inconsistency in applying the criteria nationally (House of Commons Health Committee 2005) resulting in the Department of Health producing a National Framework for NHS Continuing Healthcare (DH 2006). This aims to establish a single policy on who should receive NHS funding and a standard process for assessing eligibility.

Discharge delays

A discharge delay is when a patient remains in hospital beyond the date agreed by the multidisciplinary team and beyond the time they are medically fit to leave (DH 2003a). For every patient who is 'delayed' the ward nurse should complete a form, similar to that in Figure 10.1, highlighting the reasons for the delay. It is the responsibility of health authorities, in collaboration with social services departments, to monitor the way in which discharges from hospitals are being undertaken and, if problems occur, to establish the reasons, so that any necessary changes are made to address the local needs (DH 1989). Each hospital should have at least a basic system of audit and quality control of discharge practice and procedures.

Conclusion

From the patient's and carer's perspective, discharge may be one of the most important events of the hospital stay (Holzhausen 2001). Planning for hospital discharge is an integral part of care and an ongoing process that should start prior to admission for planned admissions and as soon as possible for all other admissions (DH 2003a). It should involve the assessment and implementation of a multidisciplinary plan to facilitate the transfer of the patient from hospital to an appropriate setting and patients and carers should be involved at all stages.

Procedure guidelines   Discharge planning

Procedure

Action	Rationale
Initial assessment (at preadmission clinic or within first 24–48 hours of admission)	
1 The admitting nurse is responsible for ensuring that an initial assessment is completed when the patient is admitted and is documented in the patient's care plan. Assessment should be ongoing and regularly reviewed with the multidisciplinary team.	To enable the physical, psychological and social care needs of the patient and carers to be identified at an early stage (Biddington 2000: C; DH 2000c: C).
2 An expected date of discharge should be established.	To ensure planning for discharge commences (Biddington 2000: C).
3 Clarify whether the patient has dependants, e.g. elderly relatives, children or a disabled partner who is unwell. If so, establish who is looking after them and whether they receive any services.	Arrangements may need to be made for alternative carer or an increase in services. Notification may need to be made, e.g to school nurse/teacher if patient has children at school (E).
4 Establish who else is involved in giving care/support and the type of help given, e.g. local support group, voluntary agency, church.	To assess the support that the patient and carers may require at home so that appropriate services can be mobilized. To establish social network in order to co-ordinate care between voluntary and statutory agencies (E).
5 Ascertain the type of accommodation the patient is living in, e.g. house, bungalow (council or privately owned), residential or nursing home, sheltered housing.	To identify any potential accommodation needs which may entail social work intervention (E).

6 Ensure that the home address and telephone number of the patient are documented accurately in the care plan. Establish where the patient will be going on discharge and document the discharge address if different from the permanent address.

Personal information may not have been updated on previous nursing or medical records. It is crucial that this information is accurate when making referrals to community services, to ensure appropriate service provision (E).

7 Ensure that the patient is registered permanently with a GP, and with a GP on a temporary basis if going to a different address on discharge. Check the names, addresses and telephone numbers with the patient.

Community nursing services are unable to accept the patient without medical support. Accurate information is required to establish which district nurse will have responsibility for patient care. It is important for the patient that medical care can be provided at home (E).

8 Establish whether any statutory community health or social services have been involved before the patient's admission. Include the health visitor when the patient has children under the age of 5 years.

To enable contact for exchange of information. Valuable information can be obtained from community services to assist in assessing potential needs on discharge (DH 2003a: C).

Referrals for discharge planning

9 Assess the patient's ability to carry out activities of daily living at home prior to admission, e.g. was she/he able to climb stairs? Consider patient's current level of functioning and whether this will change as a result of treatment and/or rehabilitation.

To establish at an early stage whether an occupational therapy/physiotherapist assessment is required. Home assessment may be required by occupational therapy prior to discharge, which may involve complex planning and preparation (Kumar 2000; DH 2001c: C).

10 Refer to other hospital personnel as soon as potential needs are recognized, e.g. occupational therapist, physiotherapists, dietitian. Referral as soon as possible after admission is essential: do not wait until treatment is completed and discharge is imminent.

To ensure multidisciplinary planning and co-ordination. Considerable time may be needed to arrange community services and early referral helps to prevent discharge delays (E).

11 Patients identified as requiring local authority social services support are referred to the social services department. Some hospitals use a 'trigger' form as an aid to assessment, an example of which can be found in Box 10.1.

To ensure early and appropriate referral to the social services department for assessment (E).

12 A discharge planning care plan should be commenced. All members of the multidisciplinary team should document in the care plan their assessment, plans and action taken.

To facilitate multidisciplinary planning, co-ordination and communication (E).

13 Where there is a designated discharge co-ordinator s/he can act as a resource offering support and education to the ward team in the preparation of discharge plans, especially for those patients requiring a complex package of care.

To facilitate effective discharge planning and utilize expertise appropriately (E).

14 Formulate a discharge plan in conjunction with patient and carers and all involved hospital and community personnel and agree a discharge date.

To collate information and co-ordinate planning (DH 2004b: C).

15 For complex discharges a discharge planning meeting should be held.

To co-ordinate continuity of care planning (E).

Procedure guidelines *(cont.)*

16 The ward-based nurse is responsible for arranging and co-ordinating community nursing services (including the Community Palliative Care Team) in consultation with the discharge co-ordinator, if applicable.

To facilitate continuity of care between hospital and community (E).

17 Refer to the community nursing services with a minimum of 48 hours' notice. If a complex package of care is being organized more notice will be required. Invite community nurses to visit the ward where appropriate.

Community nurses may wish to assess the patient's nursing care needs and ensure preparation of the home prior to discharge. They need time to liaise with other agencies to co-ordinate care and to obtain any equipment required (E).

18 Ascertain whether district nurses are able to carry out necessary clinical procedures in accordance with their Trust policy, e.g. care of skin-tunnelled catheters. Consider alternative arrangements if necessary. Give written information and instructions.

District nurses may not have been trained in certain procedures or may be unfamiliar with particular equipment (E).

19 Details of patient's MRSA status (or other infections) must be given to community personnel and written in requirements.

To reduce risk of cross-infection. Community staff require full knowledge of the patient's history and nursing referral details (Halm *et al.* 2003: E; Smith 2003: E, C).

20 Complete the community care referral form or update letter.
   The form/letter should be completed and signed and a copy provided for all community services.

Provide information for community staff to ensure that they have accurate information (Halm *et al.* 2003: E).

21 Ensure any essential medical/nursing aids or equipment have been obtained before discharge by community services, e.g. oxygen, nebulizers, commode, pressure-relieving mattress, hoist.
   Home assessment may be required by occupational therapy prior to discharge.

Some equipment may not be available or may take some time to obtain. Equipment may be loaned from the community and appropriate legislation procedures must be followed for safety reasons (DH 2001c: C).

22 Patients requiring community nursing, physiotherapy, occupational therapy, stoma care, speech therapy and/or dietetic support on discharge will be referred by the appropriate hospital-based health care professional to their equivalent in the community.

To ensure continuity of specialist care (E).

Leaving the hospital on discharge

23 Medical staff are responsible for assessing the patient's medical fitness for discharge and for liaising with other members of the multidisciplinary team regarding arrangements for meeting the patient's care needs in the community.

To ensure that both health and social care needs are taken into consideration when formulating discharge plans (DH 2003a: C).

24 Ensure that patient and, with his/her agreement, carers have full information regarding the patient's medical condition and care required.

To prepare carers and to enable patient/carer support (E).

25 Teach the patient and carers any necessary skills, allowing sufficient time to practise before discharge. This should include information on the safe use of equipment, e.g. a hoist.

To enable the patient to be as independent as possible and promote an understanding of self-care techniques (E).

26 Ensure that the patient has a door key and can gain entrance to their residence. Wherever possible, ensure that someone is at home to receive the patient.

The patient may have left their key with a neighbour. It is helpful for someone to be available to welcome the patient and attend to any immediate needs (E).

27 Book transport if required with 48 hours' notice, using relevant form. Specify if patient needs a stretcher or chair, or requires escort. Ensure that transport is also booked for return clinic appointment if necessary.
   Cancel transport if discharge date or out-patients department appointment is altered.

The patient may not have private transport facilities and may be too weak to use public transport (E).

To prevent a waste of resources (E).

28 Patients should be given an appropriate supply of medication and, where necessary, a supply of wound dressings or medical equipment.

To ensure the safe and continuous administration of medication and use of equipment at home. Time is needed to obtain supplies in the community (E).

29 Discharge plans should not be altered without consultation with all the hospital personnel who have been involved in the planning, e.g. occupational therapist, social worker, Discharge Co-ordinator and also patient/family carers.

If there is no consultation this causes considerable confusion and stress for the patient/carers, and all involved services. It may result in the patient being unsupported at home (E).

30 If discharge is cancelled or postponed, or if the patient dies, ensure that all relevant community services are informed.

To avoid distress to relatives. To avoid wasted visits and promote good community relations (E).

31 Weekend discharge: patients who require a high level of health and social services support should not be discharged home on a Friday or Saturday or a public holiday. This applies particularly to patients who were previously unknown to community services. (NB. it may be appropriate, under the Community Care (Delayed Discharges) Act, 2003, to discharge patients if agreement has been obtained with Local Authority social services.) *Note*: assessment and planning for weekend leave are as important as for final discharge.

All community services will be operating at a reduced level and emergency medical back-up may be difficult to obtain (E).

Patient information on hospital discharge

32 Inform the patient and carers of potential side-effects of treatment and management.

To alleviate anxiety and to promote patient comfort, knowledge and safety (E).

33 Ensure that patient and carers have information on local support groups or national specialist organizations as appropriate.

Some patients may benefit from the kind of support offered by the organizations (E).

34 Reinforce any special instructions with written information or by giving an approved patient education booklet, e.g. one of the Royal Marsden Hospital series.

To promote an understanding of disease and treatment. To confirm arrangements made. To enable the patient to contact the appropriate services (E).

35 Information on community services arranged, including names and telephone numbers and expected date of first visit, should be given to the patient and carers prior to discharge. This information should also be documented in the patient's care plan.

To confirm arrangements made. To enable the patient to contact the appropriate services (E).

Procedure guidelines *(cont.)*

36 Ensure that arrangements have been made to provide patient with food at home on discharge and that there will be adequate heating.

To supply immediate needs (E).

37 Ensure that the patient and carers are given verbal and written information on the dosage, route, frequency and side-effects of any medication and how to obtain further supplies.

Lack of information makes it difficult for the GP to provide the medical care required (DH 2003a: C).

After discharge from hospital
38 A follow-up phone call should be made to establish how the patient is managing.

To ensure services are in place (E).

References and further reading

Biddington, W. (2000) Reviewing discharge planning processes and promoting good practice. *JCN*, **14**(5), 4–6.

Borill, C. *et al.* (2001) *Team Working and Effectiveness in Health Care*. Aston Centre for Health Service Organisation Research, Aston, Yorkshire.

Davis, S. (1998) *Primary Secondary Care Interface*. Proceedings of conference, 25 March. NHS Executive, June, Issue 2.

DH (1989) *Discharge of Patients from Hospital*. Health Circular (89) 5. HMSO, London.

DH (1995) *Carer's (Recognition and Services) Act*. HMSO, London.

DH (1998a) *A First Class Service: Quality in the New NHS*. NHSE, London.

DH (1998b) *The New NHS: Modern, Dependable*. HMSO, London.

DH (2000a) *The NHS Plan. A Plan for Investment, a Plan for Reform*. HMSO, London.

DH (2000b) *Shaping the Future NHS: Long Term Planning for Hospitals and Related Services. Consultation Document on the Findings of the National Bed Enquiry*. HMSO, London.

DH (2000c) *Patient and Public Involvement in the NHS*. HMSO, London.

DH (2001a) *The National Service Framework for Older People*. HMSO, London.

DH (2001b) *NHS Funded Nursing Care in Nursing Homes: What It Means for You*. HMSO, London.

DH (2001c) *Guide to Integrating Community Equipment Services*. HMSO, London.

DH (2002) *National Service Framework for Older People – Intermediate Care: Moving Forward*. HMSO, London.

DH (2003a) *Discharge from Hospital: Pathway, Process and Practice*. HMSO, London.

DH (2003b) *Delayed Transfers of Care: Planning for Implementation of Reimbursement and Improving Hospital Discharge Practice*. HMSO, London.

DH (2004a) *The NHS Improvement Plan: Putting People at the Heart of Public Services*. HMSO, London.

DH (2004b) *Achieving Timely 'Simple' Discharge from Hospital – a Toolkit for the Multi-disciplinary Team*. HMSO, London.

DH (2004c) *Carers and Disabled Children Act 2000 and Carers (Equal Opportunities) Act 2004. Combined Policy Guidance*. HMSO, London.

DH (2004d) *National Standards, Local Action: Health and Social Care Standards and Planning Framework*. Department of Health Publications, London (www.dh.gov.uk).

DH (2005/6–2007/8) *National Standards, Local Action; Health and Social Care Standards and Planning Framework*. Department of Health Publications, London (www.dh.gov.uk).

DH (2006) *National Framework for NHS Continuing Healthcare and NHS-funded Nursing Care in England. Consultation Document*. HMSO, London.

Halm, J. *et al.* (2003) Interdisciplinary rounds: impact on patients, family and staff. *Clin Nurse Spec*, **17**(3), 133–42.

Hancock, S. (2003) Intermediate care and older people. *Nurs Stand*, **17**(48), 45–51.

Health Services Accreditation (1996) *Service Standards for Discharge Care*. NHS, East Sussex.

Hill, M. & Macgregor, G. (2001) *Health's Forgotten Partners? How Carers are Supported Through Hospital Discharge*. Carers UK, London (www.carershealthmatters.org.uk).

Holzhausen, F. (2001) *'You Can Take Him Home Now'. Carers' Experiences of Hospital Discharge*. Carers National Association, London.

House of Commons Health Committee (2005) *NHS Continuing Care, Sixth Report of Session 2004–2005*, Vol. 1. House of Commons, Norwich, pp. 399–1.

Hunter, M. (2001) Will social services suffer in new regime? *Commun Care*, **13**(87), 10–11.

Kumar, S. (2000) *Multidisciplinary Approach to Rehabilitation*. Butterworth Heinemann, London.

Martin, J. (2001) Benchmarking – how do you do it? *Nurs Times*, **97**(42), 30–1.

McKenna, H. *et al.* (2000) Discharge planning: an exploratory study. *J Adv Nurs*, 9, 594–601.

Nazarko, L. (1998) Improving discharge: the role of the discharge co-ordinator. *Nurs Stand*, **12**(49), 35–7.

NHS Connecting for Health (2005) *CRDB SAP Action Team Output V1.0*. Crown Copyright.

NHSE (2001) *Your Guide to the National Health Service*. HMSO, London.

NHS Modernisation Agency (2003) *National Institute for Clinical Excellence: Protocol Based Care*. Department of Health, London.

Nixon, A., Whitter, M. & Stitt, P. (1998) Audit in practice: planning for discharge from hospital. *Nurs Stand*, **12**(26), 35–8.

Royal Marsden NHS Foundation Trust (2006) *Discharge Policy and Procedure*, Internal Document, The Royal Marsden NHS Foundation Trust, London.

Salter, M. (1996) Nursing the patient in the community. In: *Nursing the Patient with Cancer* (ed. V. Tschudin). Prentice Hall, Hemel Hempstead, pp. 438–51.

Smith, A. (2003) Antibiotic resistance. In: *Infection Control in the Community* (eds J. Lawrence & D. May). Churchill Livingstone, London, pp. 319–32.

Smith, S. (1996) Discharge planning: the need for effective communication. *Nurs Stand*, **10**(38), 39–41.

Stewart, W. (2000) Development of discharge skills: a project report. *Nurs Times*, **96**(41), 37.

Tarling, M. & Jauffur, H. (2006) Improving team meetings to support discharge planning. *Nurs Times*, **26**, 32–5.

Chapter 11

Drug administration: general principles

203 Reference material
212 Injections and infusions
219 Summary
220 *Procedure guidelines:* Self-administration of drugs
221 *Procedure guidelines:* Oral drug administration
224 *Procedure guidelines:* Injections: administration
231 *Procedure guidelines:* Rectal medication administration
231 *Procedure guidelines:* Vaginal medication administration
232 *Procedure guidelines:* Topical applications of medication
233 *Procedure guidelines:* Administration of medication in other forms
235 *Procedure guidelines:* Continuous infusion of intravenous drugs
238 *Procedure guidelines:* Intermittent infusion of intravenous drugs
241 *Procedure guidelines:* Injection (bolus or push) of intravenous drugs
244 *Problem solving:* Injection and infusion of intravenous fluids and drugs
251 References and further reading

Definition

Drug administration can be defined as the way medicines are selected, procured, delivered, prescribed, administered and reviewed to optimize the contributions that medicines make to producing informed and desired outcomes of patient care (Audit Commission 2001). The professional role of the nurse in medicines management is the safe handling and administration of medicines, including a responsibility for making sure that patients understand what medicines they are taking and why, including the likely side-effects (Luker & Wolfson 1999). Medicinal products are defined, according to the Medicines Act 1968, as, 'substances sold or supplied for administration to humans (or animals) for medicinal purposes' (HMSO 1968).

Indications

Drugs can be administered for the following purposes.

- Diagnostic purposes, e.g. assessment of liver function or diagnosis of myasthenia gravis.
- Prophylaxis, e.g. heparin to prevent thrombosis or antibiotics to prevent infection.
- Therapeutic purposes, e.g. replacement of fluids or vitamins, supportive purposes (to enable other treatments, such as anaesthesia), palliation of pain and cure (as in the case of antibiotics).

Reference material

Drug administration has been one of the most common clinical procedures a nurse has undertaken for at least the past 50 years (Shepherd 2002a). With changes in legal, professional and cultural boundaries in health care, the role of the nurse has broadened to one of medicines management.

The legal and professional context

Medicines management and specifically drug administration require thought and professional judgement (Luker & Wolfson 1999; NMC 2008a). All aspects of a medicine's use must be managed with a multidisciplinary approach to ensure it is supported by a strong evidence base and that the safety and well being of the patient remain paramount (Shepherd 2002a; NMC 2008b).

Legislation

Legislative frameworks, government guidelines and professional regulations govern medicines management in the UK. The two pieces of primary legislation of importance are the Medicines Act 1968 and the Misuse of Drugs Act 1971 (HMSO 1971).

The Medicines Act 1968

The Medicines Act 1968 (HMSO 1968) establishes a licensing system for medicines for human use, controlling the manufacture and distribution, regulating who can lawfully supply and be in possession of medicines and how they should be packaged and labelled. The Medicines and Health Care Products Regulatory Agency (MHRA) in the UK and the European Medicines Evaluation Agency (EMEA) are responsible for issuing the product licences. The availability of products is restricted by defining which of the following legal categories they are in:

- Prescription-only medicines (POM).
- Pharmacy only medicines (P).
- General sales list medicines (GSL).

Different requirements apply to the sale, supply and labelling of medicines in each category. In National Health Service (NHS) hospitals, adherence to the Act means that a pharmacist supervises the purchasing and supply of medicines, and that supply or administration to a patient is only on a doctor's prescription. Sections 9, 10 and 11 of the Act exempt doctors, dentists, pharmacists and nurses, respectively, from many restrictions otherwise imposed by the Act on the general public, and thus allow them to supply and use drugs in the practice of their respective professions.

Unlicensed medicines

An unlicensed medicine is a term used to refer to a medicine with no product licence. 'Off label' medicines refer to drugs which are licensed but used outside of the licensed indications. If a medicine is unlicensed, it should only be administered to a patient/client with their informed consent against a patient-specific direction not against a patient group direction (PGD) (NMC 2008a). However, 'off label' medicines, 'may be administered under a PGD if such use is exceptional, justified by best practice and the staus of the product clearly described' (NMC 2008a). The use of unlicensed and 'off label' medicines is common in hospitals, particularly in oncology and palliative care for clinical trials and symptom control. If an unlicensed medicine is administered to a patient/client, the manufacturer has no liability for any harm which may ensue (NMC 2008a). Therefore, it is very important that all prescribers, dispensing pharmacists and administering nurses are aware of their responsibilities with these medicines, and that the associated medico-legal implications are encompassed within organizations' clinical governance arrangements.

The Misuse of Drugs Act 1971

For reasons of public safety the Misuse of Drugs Act (1971) controls the import, export, production, supply, possession and manufacture of controlled drugs to prevent abuse as most are potentially addictive or habit forming. Other regulations of the Act govern safe storage, destruction and supply to known addicts.

The level of control to be exercised is related to the potential for abuse or misuse of the substances concerned. Under the current 2001 Misuse of Drugs regulations, controlled drugs are classified into five schedules, each representing a different level of control (HMSO 2001). The requirements of the Act as they apply to nurses working in a hospital with a pharmacy department are described in Table 11.1.

Implications of the Act for nursing practice

Hospital wards and departments are authorized to hold a stock of controlled drugs. These should be stored in a suitably secure cupboard, which is kept locked and to which access is restricted to registered nurses and pharmacy staff. Controlled drugs are obtained by the use of a special duplicate order form signed by the nurse in charge who is then responsible for them. The order forms must be stored in a locked cupboard when not in use.

Controlled drugs may be administered only to a patient in that ward or department when prescribed by an authorized medical or non-medical prescriber. A prescription must be written in the prescriber's handwriting. To write a prescription for a controlled drug, a prescriber must be resident in the UK and the pharmacist must know and have a record of his/her signature. In the hospital setting this excludes locum doctors from writing prescriptions for controlled drugs. The Aitken report (Central Health Services Council 1958) recommends that two nurses check all controlled drug entries. Appropriate records of their use must be maintained. There is no legal requirement for the nurse in charge or acting in charge of a ward or department to keep a record of Schedule 1 or 2 controlled drugs obtained or supplied. However, the Aitken report (Central Health Services Council 1958) recommended that this should be done and in practice a controlled drug register is usually kept according to the following guidelines:

- Each page should be clearly headed to indicate the drug and preparation to which it refers.
- Entries should be made as soon as possible after the relevant transaction has occurred and always within 24 hours.
- No cancellations or obliteration of an entry should be made. Corrections should be made by means of a note in the margin or at the foot of the page and this should be signed, dated and cross-referenced to the relevant entry.
- All entries should be indelible.
- The register should be used for controlled drugs only and for no other purposes and be stored in a locked cupboard when not in use.
- Completed registers and copies of orders should be kept for 2 years.

Unwanted drugs should normally be destroyed in the pharmacy but may, under some circumstances, be disposed of on the ward under the supervision of a pharmacist. An appropriate entry should then be made in the ward register.

In response to seven case reports, published between 2000 and 2005, regarding deaths due to the administration of high-dose (30 mg or greater) morphine or diamorphine

to patients who had not previously received doses of opiates, the National Patient Safety Agency (NPSA) released a safer practice notice in 2006, *Ensuring Safer Practice with High Dose Ampoules of Morphine and Diamorphine* (NPSA 2006). In line with this safer practice notice the following guidance should be adhered to:

- High-strength preparations of morphine or diamorphine (30 mg or above) should be stored in a separate location from lower-strength preparations (10 mg) within the controlled drugs cupboard.
- Awareness should be raised of the similarities of drug packaging, and consider use of alert stickers being attached to high-strength preparations by pharmacy.
- A review of stock levels should be taken in all clinical areas where morphine and diamorphine are stored to assess if high-strength preparations need to be kept on a permanent basis or whether they could be ordered according to specific patient requirements.
- Clear guidance should be provided to ensure the correct doses of diamorphine and morphine are prepared in the appropriate clinical situation. For example, diamorphine 5-mg and 10-mg ampoules could be used for both bolus administration and patients newly commenced on diamorphine infusions; diamorphine 30-mg ampoules could be reserved for patients already receiving diamorphine infusions and who require higher daily doses.
- Patients should be observed for the 1st hour after receiving their first dose of diamorphine or morphine injection.
- Naloxone injections should be available in all clinical areas where morphine and diamorphine is stored.

Storage of medicines

The Duthie Report (DH 1988) requires NHS Trusts to establish, document and maintain procedures to ensure and demonstrate that medicines are stored and handled in a safe and secure manner. Under the Duthie Report the nurse in charge of a ward or clinical area is responsible for the safe storage of all medicines. Some of these duties may be delegated, such as the ordering of additional medicines, but the responsibility remains with the nurse in charge. He/she is also responsible for controlling access (by keys or other means) to the medicines cupboards even if he/she decides to delegate this duty.

The storage of medicines is governed by the following principles.

Security

All drugs should be stored in locked cupboards with separate storage for internal medicines, external medicines, controlled drugs and medicines needing refrigeration or storage in a freezer.

Table 11.1   Summary of legal requirements for handling of controlled drugs (CDs) as they apply to nurses in hospitals with a pharmacy.

	Schedule 1: CDs Home Office Licence	Schedule 2: CDs subject to full controls	Schedule 3: CDs with no register entry	Schedule 4: CDs anabolic steroids/ benzodiazepines	Schedule 5: CDs needing invoice retention
Drugs in the schedule	Cannabis + derivatives but excluding nabilone, LSD (lysergic acid diethylamide)	Most opioids in common use including: alfentanyl; amphetamines; cocaine; diamorphine; methadone; morphine papaveretum; fentanyl; phenoperidine. Pethidine; codeine; Dihydrocodeine injections; Pentazocine	Minor stimulants Barbiturates (but excluding hexobarbitone, thiopentone) Diethylpropion Buprenorphine Temazepam†	Part 1: anabolic steroids Part 2: benzodiazepines	Some preparations containing very low strengths of: cocaine; codeine; morphine; pholcodine; and some other opioids
Ordering	Possession and supply permitted only by special licence from the Secretary of State issued (to a doctor only) for scientific or research purposes	A requisition must be signed in duplicate by the nurse in charge. The requisition must be endorsed to indicate that the drugs have been supplied. Copies should be kept for 2 years	As Schedule 2	No requirement*	No requirement*
Storage	Must be kept in a suitable locked cupboard to which access is restricted	As Schedule 1	Buprenorphine and diethylpropion: as Schedule 1 drugs All other drugs no requirement	No requirement*	No requirement*
Record keeping	Controlled drug register must be used	As Schedule 1	No requirement	No requirement*	No requirement*
Prescription	Prescription must include: ■ the name and address of patient ■ the drug, the dose, the form of preparation ■ the total quantity of drug or the total number of dosage units to be supplied. This quantity must be stated in words and figures The prescription must be written indelibly in the prescriber's own handwriting	As Schedule 1	As Schedule 1 Except for phenobarbitone (this includes all preparations of phenobarbitone and phenobarbitone sodium). Because of its use as an antiepileptic, it does not need to be written in the prescriber's own handwriting	No requirement*	No requirement*
Administration to patients	Under special licence only A doctor or dentist or anyone acting on their instructions may administer these drugs to anyone for whom they have been prescribed	A doctor or dentist or anyone acting on their instructions may administer these drugs to anyone for whom they have been prescribed	A doctor or dentist or anyone acting on their instructions may administer these drugs to anyone for whom they have been prescribed	No requirement*	No requirement*

* 'No requirement' indicates that the Misuse of Drugs Act 1971 imposes no legal requirements additional to those imposed by the Medicines Act 1968 (HMSO 1968).
† Temazepam preparations are exempt from record keeping and prescription requirements, but are subject to storage requirements.

Diagnostic reagents, intravenous and topical agents should also be kept separately.

Stability

No medicinal preparation should be stored where it may be subject to substantial variations in temperature, e.g. not in direct sunlight. The normal temperature ranges for storage are 'a cool place', normally interpreted as meaning between 1 and 15°C; 'refrigerated' at a temperature between 2 and 8°C; 'room temperature' between 15 and 25°C. Refrigerators must have their temperatures monitored and recorded daily and appropriate action taken if the recordings are not within 2 and 8°C.

Labelling

The wording of labels is chosen carefully to convey clearly all essential information. Printed labels should always be used.

Containers

The type of container used may have been chosen for specific reasons. Therefore all medicines should be stored in the containers in which they were supplied by pharmacy. Medicinal preparations should never be transferred (in bulk) from one container to another except in the pharmacy.

Stock control

A system of stock rotation must be operated (e.g. first in, first out) to ensure that there is no accumulation of old stocks. Only one pack/container of a named medicine should be in use at any one time.

Storage requirements of specific preparations

- *Aerosol containers* should not be stored in direct sunlight or over radiators: there is a risk of explosion if they are heated.
- *Creams* may deteriorate rapidly if subjected to extremes of temperature.
- *Eye drops and ointments* may become contaminated with micro-organisms during use and thus pose a danger to the recipient. Therefore in hospitals, eye preparations should be discarded 7 days after they are first opened. For use at home this limit is extended to 28 days.
- *Mixtures* may have a relatively short shelf-life. Most antibiotic mixtures require refrigerated storage and even then have a shelf-life of only 7–14 days. Always check the label for details.
- *Tablets and capsules* are relatively stable but are susceptible to moisture unless correctly packed. They should be stored only in the containers in which they were supplied by the pharmacy.
- *Vaccines* and similar preparations usually require refrigerated storage and may deteriorate rapidly if exposed to heat.

Patient's own drugs

Patients are encouraged to bring their medication into hospital with them to facilitate the collection of a comprehensive and accurate medication history. These medicines remain the patient's property and should either be stored securely in the ward's drug cupboard until discharge or sent home with a relative or carer. These medicines should neither be disposed of without the patient's consent nor used for other patients.

Types of medicinal preparations of drugs

Preparations for oral administration

Tablets

These come in a great variety of shapes, sizes, colours and types. The formulation may be very simple and result for instance in a plain, white, uncoated tablet, or complex and designed with specific therapeutic aims. Sugar coatings are used to improve appearances and palatability. In cases where the drug is a gastric irritant or is broken down by gastric acid, an enteric coating may be used. This is designed to allow the tablet to remain intact in the stomach and to pass unchanged into the small bowel where the coating dissolves and hence the drug is released and absorbed. Tablets may be formulated specifically to achieve control of the rate of release of drug from the tablet as it passes through the alimentary tract. Terms such as 'sustained-release', 'controlled-release' and 'modified-release' are used by manufacturers to describe these preparations. Tablets may also be formulated specifically to dissolve readily ('soluble' or 'effervescent'), to be chewed or to be held under the tongue ('sublingual') or placed between the gum and inside of the mouth ('buccal'). Unscored or coated tablets should not be crushed or broken, nor should most 'slow-release' or 'sustained action' tablets, since this can alter the rate of release of drug from the tablet.

Capsules

These offer a useful method of formulating drugs which are difficult to make into a tablet or are particularly unpalatable.

The capsule shells are usually made of gelatin and the contents of the capsules may be solid, liquid or of a paste-like consistency. The contents do not cause deterioration of the shell. The shell, however, is attacked by the digestive fluids and the contents are then released. Delayed-release capsule formulations also exist. Gastro-resistant capsules are delayed-release capsules that are intended to resist the gastric fluid and to release their active substance or substances in the intestinal fluid (British Pharmacopoeia 2007). If for any reason the capsule is unsuitable, the contents should not routinely be removed from the shell without first seeking advice from a pharmacist. Removing contents from the capsule could destroy their properties and cause gastric irritation or premature release of the drug into an incompatible pH (Downie *et al.* 2000).

Lozenges and pastilles

Lozenges and pastilles are solid, single-dose preparations intended to be sucked to obtain a local or systemic effect to the mouth and/or throat (British Pharmacopoeia 2007).

Elixirs, linctuses and syrups

Elixirs These are clear, flavoured oral liquids containing one or more active ingredients dissolved in a vehicle that usually contains a high proportion of sucrose.

Linctuses These are viscous oral liquids that may contain one or more active ingredients; the solution usually contains a high proportion of sucrose. Linctuses are intended for use in the treatment or relief of cough (British Pharmacopoeia 2007).

Syrups These do not contain active ingredients and many are used as vehicle ingredients for their flavouring and sweetening.

Mixtures

These are flavoured solutions or suspensions of drugs used mainly when patients cannot swallow a tablet or the drug is not available as a tablet. It is particularly important that suspensions are thoroughly mixed by shaking before each dose is measured. This ensures that the measured volume always contains the correct amount of drug.

Rectal and vaginal preparations

Enemas

These are solutions which are instilled into the rectum as laxatives or to obtain other localized therapeutic effects, or for diagnostic purposes.

Suppositories

These are solid wax pellets for rectal administration. They may either melt at body temperature or dissolve or disperse in the mucous secretions of the rectum. They may be used to obtain local effect (e.g. as laxatives) or for systemic therapy. Many drugs, such as the opioids, are well absorbed when administered this way. Suppositories sometimes offer a useful alternative to injections for very sick patients unable to take drugs orally. They must be administered according to the manufacturer's recommendations.

Pessaries

These are solid pellets for vaginal administration and are usually designed to have a local therapeutic action.

Topical preparations

Creams

Creams are emulsions of oil and water and are generally well absorbed into the skin. They are usually more cosmetically acceptable than ointments because they are less greasy and easy to apply (BNF 2008). They may be used as a 'base' in which a variety of drugs may be applied for local therapy (BNF 2008).

Ointments

Ointments are greasy preparations, which are normally anhydrous and insoluble in water, and are more occlusive than creams (BNF 2008). They are absorbed more slowly into the skin and leave a greasy residue. They have similar uses to creams, and are particularly suitable for dry, scaly lesions (BNF 2008).

Transdermal patches

A number of drugs such as hyoscine to prevent motion sickness, oestrogens for hormone replacement therapy and fentanyl for pain control are now available in 'transdermal patches'. A very small volume of drug solution is contained in a reservoir which is stuck on the skin. Drug molecules diffuse at a constant rate through a semipermeable membrane which is in direct contact with the skin when the patch is applied. The drug is absorbed through the skin and into the capillary blood supply from where it enters the systemic circulation. Advantages include a constant rate of drug administration over several days which may reduce the incidence of side-effects and improve patient compliance.

Wound products

See Chapter 48.

Injections

Injections are sterile solutions, emulsions or suspensions. They are prepared by dissolving, emulsifying or suspending the active ingredient and any added substances in water for injections, in a suitable non-aqueous liquid or in a mixture of these vehicles (British Pharmacopoeia 2007).

Single-dose preparations

The volume of the injection in a single-dose container is sufficient to permit the withdrawal and administration of the nominal dose using a normal technique.

Multidose preparations

Multidose aqueous injections contain a suitable antimicrobial preservative at an appropriate concentration except when the preparation itself has adequate antimicrobial properties. When it is necessary to present a preparation for parenteral use in a multidose container, the precautions to be taken for its administration and more particularly for its storage between successive withdrawals are given.

Parenteral infusions

Parenteral infusions are sterile, aqueous solutions or emulsions with water; they are free from pyrogens and are usually made isotonic with blood. They are principally intended for administration in large volume. Parenteral infusions do not contain any added antimicrobial preservative (British Pharmacopoeia 2007).

207

Inhalations

Two techniques, nebulization and aerosolization, permit the inhalation of a range of drugs with the aim of a localized therapeutic effect.

Nebulization involves the passage of air or oxygen driven through a solution of a drug. The resulting fine mist is then inhaled via a face mask (Trounce & Gould 2000). Some antibiotics and bronchodilators may be given in this way.

Aerosolization involves the use of a solution of drug in an inert diluent. Passing a metred volume of this solution through a valve under pressure allows the delivery to the patient of a measured dose of drug in a very fine spray of controlled particle size. Bronchodilators and steroids are administered commonly in this way. Although a very small total dose of drug is administered, the concentration achieved at the site of action is high. Rapid and effective control of symptoms is achieved but without the side-effects commonly associated with an equivalent systemic (oral or parenteral) dose of the drug(s).

Many patients can be taught to use aerosol inhalers effectively but some patients, particularly the elderly and small children, may find it difficult to use them. Spacer devices can help such patients because they remove the need to co-ordinate actuation with inhalation (BNF 2008). For those who cannot co-ordinate aerosol inhalation, alternative methods of administration include breath-actuated inhalers or dry powder inhalers which merely require the patient to breathe in. No co-ordination of hand movement and breathing is required. Some dry powder inhalers occasionally cause coughing due to irritation of the throat and trachea by the dry powder (Downie *et al.* 2000).

Administration

The effective and safe administration of drugs to patients demands a partnership between the various health professionals concerned, i.e. doctors, pharmacists and nurses. A medicine is an active chemical or biological substance with diagnostic, curative or preventive purposes. The manner in which it is administered determines the extent to which a patient gains any clinical benefit and whether any adverse effect is experienced. One of the main factors that determine whether or not a medicine will reach its intended site of action in the body is how it is given (Shepherd 2002a). Nurses are responsible for the correct administration of prescribed drugs to patients in their care at all times, being guided by the Nursing and Midwifery Council (NMC) *Standards for Medicines Management* (NMC 2008a).

All medicines administered in hospital must be considered prescription only. This is because administration, whether by a nurse or by a patient to themselves, may only take place in accordance with one or more of the following processes:

- patient specific direction (PSD)
- patient medicines administration chart (MAR)
- patient group directive (PGD)
- medicines act exemplar
- standing orders
- homely remedy protocol
- prescription form

(NMC 2008a, pp. 13–16).

'Verbal orders'

The NMC clearly states that the instruction by telephone to administer a previously unprescribed medicine is unacceptable. In exceptional circumstances, where the medication has been previously prescribed and the prescriber is unable to issue a new prescription, but where changes to the dose are considered necessary, the use of information technology (such as fax or e-mail) is the preferred method. This should be followed up by a new prescription confirming the changes . . . within a maximum of 24 hours. In any event the changes must be authorized before the new dosage is administered (NMC 2008a.)

Medicine administration should ensure that the correct patient receives:

- the appropriate medicine;
- in the appropriate formulation;
- by the appropriate route;
- at the appropriate dose;
- at the appropriate time;
- at the appropriate rate;
- for the appropriate duration of therapy;
- with the appropriate monitoring to ensure safety and efficacy of therapy;
- with the appropriate reporting of adverse drug reactions (Sexton 1999, p. 240).

To achieve this, the nurse must have a sound knowledge of the use, action, usual dose and side-effects of the drugs being administered. Institutional policies and procedures also assist the nurse to administer drugs safely and a sound knowledge of local procedures is essential. The importance of reporting errors to the appropriate authority should never be underestimated as research suggests that many undeclared medication errors are made by nurses. The immediate and honest disclosure that an error has occurred results in the patient receiving the required emergency treatment. Organizational policies therefore need to reflect a culture that encourages disclosure and in which the management of medication errors is viewed as a learning process as opposed to a punitive act (Martin 1994; Gladstone 1995). The NMC states that all errors and incidents require a thorough and careful investigation at a local level, taking full account of the context, circumstances and position of the practitioner involved. Such incidents require a sensitive management and a comprehensive assessment of all the circumstances before a professional and managerial decision is reached on the appropriate way to proceed (NMC 2008a.)

It must be recognized, however, that errors in drug administration can have traumatic consequences for the individual nurse involved and that disciplinary procedures invoke fear in most nurses (Arndt 1994).

Single nurse administration of medicines

In the majority of hospitals it is policy that medicines administration is carried out by a single qualified nurse. It is thought that single nurse administration of medicines will result in greater care being given since the nurse will be aware that she or he is solely responsible and accountable.

Those nurses who wish or need to have their administration supervised will retain the right to do so until such time as all parties agree that the requested level of proficiency has been achieved. The nurse checking the medicine must be able to justify any action taken and be accountable for the action taken. This is in keeping with the principles of *The Code* (NMC 2008b).

Self-administration of medicines

With evidence that between 30 and 70% of patients are non-compliant with taking prescribed medication (Royal Pharmaceutical Society 1997), the self-administration of medicines in hospitals is encouraged. Non-adherence to medication regimens is a significant problem in older patients (McGraw & Drennan 2001). Self-administration of medicines is recommended by the *National Service Framework for Older People* (Pratt *et al.* 2007) as a strategy to address this major issue. All patients benefit significantly from the opportunity to adjust to the responsibility of self-administration while still having access to professional support (NMC 2008a). It has also been found that patients who had administered their own medications in hospital were more likely to report that their overall care was excellent and that they were satisfied with the discharge process than patients who had not (Deeks & Byatt 2000). Bird (1990) suggests that for the majority of hospital patients, self-administration of drugs would appear to be a more appropriate method than the conventional system. Self-administration is not merely the process of patients taking their own drugs; it can also help clients retain or regain control over their health.

The safety and success of a self-administration system in hospital are based upon the nursing assessment of the patient and the subsequent teaching (Shepherd 2002b). The nursing assessment should include a measure of the patient's ability to interpret and participate in the prescribed treatment regimen and seek to determine whether the patient already takes prescribed treatment at home and how they manage that and whether they can understand the medicine labels and the dosage instructions (Shepherd 2002b). Teaching patients to take their own medication correctly forms part of their programme of rehabilitation, which should begin with the first multidisciplinary assessment on their arrival in hospital. Patients taught to self-administer their drugs in hospital are encouraged to regain independence and to participate in their own care. Self-administration also provides an opportunity to identify additional education needs and improve compliance. Importantly, it also raises awareness of those patients who are unable to self-administer and will need additional support on discharge (Shepherd 2002b).

Although, by definition, self-administration of medicines shifts the balance of responsibility for this part of care towards the patient, it in no way diminishes the fundamental professional duty of care. It is therefore essential that local policies, procedures and records are adequate to ensure that this duty is, and can be shown to be, discharged.

Even if a patient is self-administering their medication, continual assessment of this aspect of their care while they are in hospital is important. The nurse must continually be aware of the patient's capability to self-administer and the action of the drugs the patient is taking. No drug produces a single effect. The combined effect of two or more drugs taken together may be different from the effects when taken separately. The effectiveness of any drug should be noted and any signs of resistance or dependence reported.

Provision must be made for the patients to have access to their own lockable cupboard, usually at the bedside, for the specific purpose of allowing the safe storage of medicines.

209

Covert drug administration

The NMC recognizes that 'this a complex issue', as covert drug administration 'involves the fundamental principles of patient and client autonomy and consent to treatment, which are set out in common law and statute and underpinned by the Human Rights Act 1998' (NMC 2008a). The covert administration of medicines 'should not be confused with the administration of medicines against someone's will, which in itself may not be deceptive, but may be unlawful' (NMC 2008a).

Some vulnerable groups of patients, for example those who are confused, may refuse to take medication. Traditionally, in some places, medication has therefore been hidden or disguised in food. The NMC (2001a, b; 2008a) offered the following position statement:

> As a general principle, by disguising medication in food or drink, the patient or client is being led to believe that they are not receiving medication when in fact they are. The registered nurse, midwife or health visitor will need to be sure that what they are doing is in the best interests of the patient or client and be accountable for this decision.
>
> (NMC 2001a; NMC 2008a.)

Disguising medication in food and drink is acceptable under exceptional circumstances in which covert administration may be considered to prevent a patient, who is incapable of informed consent, from missing out on essential treatment (NMC 2001b; NMC 2008a). The following principles should be followed when making such a decision.

- The medication must be considered essential for the patient's health and well-being.

- The decision to administer medication covertly should be considered only as a contingency in an emergency, not as regular practice.
- The registered practitioner must make the decision only after discussion and with the support of the multiprofessional team and, if appropriate, the patient's relatives, carers or advocates.
- The pharmacist must be involved in these decisions as adding medication to food or drink can alter its pharmacological properties and thereby affect its performance.
- The decision and action taken must be fully documented in the patient's care plan and regularly reviewed.
- Regular attempts should continue to be made to encourage the patient to take the medication voluntarily (Treloar *et al.* 2000; NMC 2001b; NMC 2008a).

Nurse prescribing and Patient Group Directions

As nurses have undertaken increasingly specialized roles the need for them to have powers to prescribe has become more apparent. The Report of the Advisory Committee on Nurse Prescribing (DH 1989) initially recommended a limited nurses' formulary for District Nurses and Health Visitors. The Medicinal Products: Prescription by Nurse etc. Act (1992) granted the statutory authority for this to occur. The Crown Report (DH 1989) also recommended that doctors and nurses collaborate in drawing up local protocols for the administration of medicines in situations that would benefit specific groups of patients, for example those requiring vaccinations.

The practice of prescribing under group protocols became widespread across the NHS, and they were used to support initiatives such as nurse-led clinics (Laverty *et al.* 1997; Mallett *et al.* 1997). The legality of this practice was then questioned. Section 58 of the Medicines Act (1968) states that no one should administer any medication (other than to himself) unless he is the appropriate practitioner or a person who is acting according to directions from an appropriate practitioner. The terms *direction* and *administration* were open to interpretation and how they were used varied across the country (McHale 2002).

Nurse prescribing was therefore reviewed and two further reports were published:

- *Review of Prescribing, Supply and Administration of Medicines. A Report on the Supply and Administration of Medicines under Group Protocols* (DH 1998).
- *Review of Prescribing, Supply and Administration of Medicines. Final Report* (DH 1999).

The first specifically offered guidance about group protocols, including changing the name to patient group directions (PGDs).

- *Patient Group Directions.* This is defined as a specific written instruction for the supply or administration by nurses, pharmacists or other authorized named professionals of named medicines in an identified clinical situation, in the absence of a prescription. It is drawn up locally by doctors, pharmacists and other appropriate professionals and must be approved by the employer, advised by the relevant professional advisory committee. It applies to groups of patients or other service users who may not be individually identified before presentation for treatment (DH 2004). The Health and Safety Commission (HSC) advised that the majority of medication 'should be prescribed and administered on an individual patient specific basis', but that it is appropriate to use PGDs for the supply and administration of medicines in situations where this offers an advantage for patient care (DH 2000). Shepherd suggests that this means, 'where medical staff are either inaccessible or unavailable' (Shepherd 2002b, p. 44). The flowchart in Figure 11.1 aims to assist practitioners in deciding the appropriate system for the prescription, supply or administration of medicines.

The second report looked at the existing arrangements for prescribing, supply and administration of medicines and suggested the introduction of a new form of prescribing to be undertaken by non-medical health professionals (DH 2003a). Independent nurse prescribing was initially allowed from an extremely limited formulary (Shuttleworth 2005). It was then extended a number of times until finally appropriately qualified nurses were allowed to prescribe from the whole *British National Formulary*.

There are now two categories of prescriber:

1   *Independent prescribing:* This allows nurses who are registered as independent prescribers to prescibe any licensed medicine for any medical condition (this also includes some controlled drugs) but only within their own level of experience and competence, and acting in accordance with the NMC's Code (NMC 2008b). Only those who have undergone appropriate training and are registered with the NMC as an independent prescriber can prescribe (NMC 2006). It must also be judged that it is part of the nurse's role.

2   *Supplementary prescribing* has been defined as:

> A voluntary prescribing partnership between an independent prescriber and a supplementary prescriber to implement an agreed patient specific clinical management plan with the patient's agreement' (DH 2003b). Amendments to the Prescription Only Medicines Order and the NHS regulations allowed supplementary prescribing by suitably trained nurses from April 2003. Supplementary prescribers prescribe in partnership with a doctor or dentist (the independent prescriber) and are able to prescribe any medicine including controlled drugs and unlicensed medicines that are listed in an agreed Clinical Management Plan. The plan is drawn up with the patient's agreement, following diagnosis of the patient by an independent prescriber and following consultation and agreement between the independent and supplementary prescribers.

(DH 2003b, p. 6 and 7)

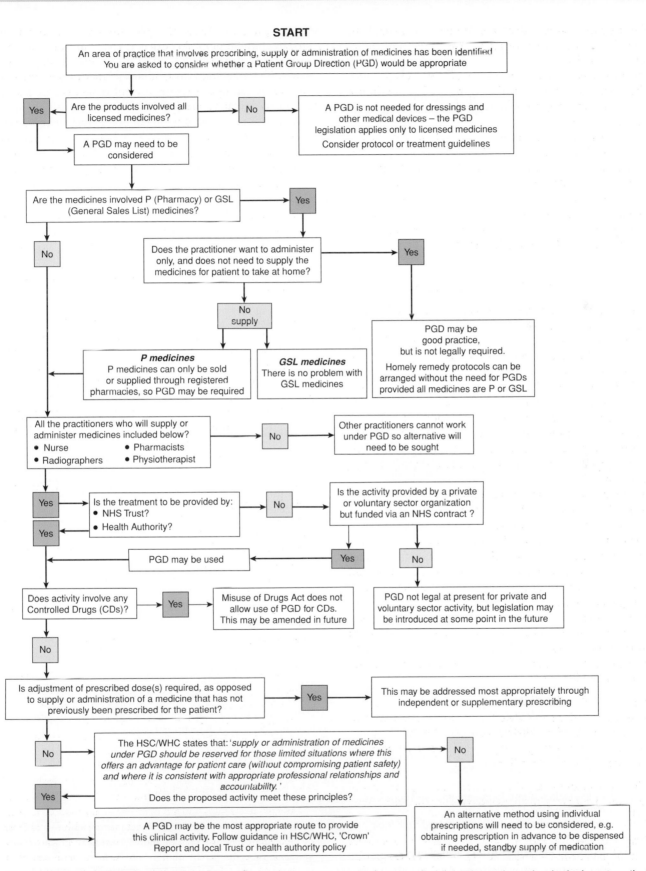

START

An area of practice that involves prescribing, supply or administration of medicines has been identified
You are asked to consider whether a Patient Group Direction (PGD) would be appropriate

Are the products involved all licensed medicines?

Yes — A PGD may need to be considered

No — A PGD is not needed for dressings and other medical devices – the PGD legislation applies only to licensed medicines

Consider protocol or treatment guidelines

Are the medicines involved P (Pharmacy) or GSL (General Sales List) medicines?

Yes — Does the practitioner want to administer only, and does not need to supply the medicines for patient to take at home?

No / **No supply**

Yes — PGD may be good practice, but is not legally required.

Homely remedy protocols can be arranged without the need for PGDs provided all medicines are P or GSL

P medicines
P medicines can only be sold or supplied through registered pharmacies, so PGD may be required

GSL medicines
There is no problem with GSL medicines

No

All the practitioners who will supply or administer medicines included below?
• Nurse   • Pharmacists
• Radiographers • Physiotherapist

No — Other practitioners cannot work under PGD so alternative will need to be sought

Yes — Is the treatment to be provided by:
• NHS Trust?
• Health Authority?

No — Is the activity provided by a private or voluntary sector organization but funded via an NHS contract ?

Yes

Yes — PGD may be used ← **Yes**

No — PGD not legal at present for private and voluntary sector activity, but legislation may be introduced at some point in the future

Does activity involve any Controlled Drugs (CDs)?

Yes — Misuse of Drugs Act does not allow use of PGD for CDs. This may be amended in future

No

Is adjustment of prescribed dose(s) required, as opposed to supply or administration of a medicine that has not previously been prescribed for the patient?

Yes — This may be addressed most appropriately through independent or supplementary prescribing

No

The HSC/WHC states that: 'supply or administration of medicines under PGD should be reserved for those limited situations where this offers an advantage for patient care (without compromising patient safety) and where it is consistent with appropriate professional relationships and accountability.'
Does the proposed activity meet these principles?

No — An alternative method using individual prescriptions will need to be considered, e.g. obtaining prescription in advance to be dispensed if needed, standby supply of medication

Yes — A PGD may be the most appropriate route to provide this clinical activity. Follow guidance in HSC/WHC, 'Crown' Report and local Trust or health authority policy

211

Figure 11.1   Patient group directions (PGDs) flowchart. The diagram above takes the practitioner through a logical process that aims to assist decision making. **The majority of clinical care should still be provided on an individual, patient-specific basis.**

The key principles that underpin supplementary prescribing are:

- The importance of communication between prescribing partners.
- The need for access to shared patient records.
- The patient is treated as a partner in their care and is involved at all stages in decision making, including whether part of their care is delivered via supplementary prescribing (NPC 2003a).

Preparation for both independent nurse prescribing and supplementary prescribing is at least 26 days in length and must follow the standards set out in NMC's *Circular 25/2002* (NMC 2001c). Any preparation must enable independent and supplementary non-medical prescribers to reach the competencies outlined in *Maintaining Competency in Prescribing: An Outline Framework to Help Nurse Prescribers* (NPC 2001) and the additional guidance in *Maintaining Competency in Prescribing: An Outline Framework to Help Nurse Supplementary Prescribers* (NPC 2003b).

The addition of prescriptive authority to the nurse role has been a positive way of making a service not only more responsive for service users, but also has helped to resource increasing demands on health services (Bridge *et al.* 2005). In 2005 it was estimated that there were 28 000 nurses who were able to prescribe from the limited formulary and 4000 extended prescribers (MHRA 2005). In a national survey of 246 nurse prescribers they concluded that nurse prescribing is largely successful in both practice and policy terms (Latter *et al.* 2005): this is discussed in more detail in Table 11.2.

Intravenous administration

Intravenous therapy is now an integral part of the majority of nurses' professional practice (RCN 2005). The nurse's role has progressed considerably from being able to add drugs to infusion bags (DHSS 1976) to now assessing patients and inserting the appropriate vascular access devices (VAD) prior to drug administration (Gabriel 2005).

Any nurse administering intravenous drugs must be competent in all aspects of intravenous therapy and act in accordance with the NMC Code (2008b), i.e. to maintain knowl-

Table 11.2 An evaluation of nurse prescribing. Source: Latter *et al.* 2005 (cited in Shuttleworth 2005).

- Most nurse prescribers were confident in their prescribing practice
- Most felt extended prescribing had a positive impact on patient care and enabled them to make better use of their skills
- Most felt that the limited nurse formulary imposed unhelpful limitation on their practice
- Nurses were satisfied with the support received from their medical practitioner
- Patients are positive about their experience of nurse prescribing
- Doctors were positive about the development of nurse prescribers in their teams

edge and skills (RCN 2005; Hyde 2008). Training and assessment should comprise both a theoretical and practical component and include legal and professional issues, fluid balance, pharmacology, drug administration, local and systemic complications, infection control issues, use of equipment and risk management (RCN 2005; Hyde 2008).

The nurse's responsibilities in relation to intravenous drug administration include:

1 Knowing the therapeutic use of the drug or solution, its normal dosage, side-effects, precautions and contraindications.
2 Preparing the drug aseptically and safely, checking the container and drug for faults, using the correct diluent and only preparing it immediately prior to administration.
3 Identifying the patient and checking allergy status.
4 Checking the prescription chart.
5 Checking and maintaining patency of the VAD.
6 Inspecting the site of the VAD and managing/reporting complications where appropriate.
7 Controlling the flow rate of infusion and/or speed of injection.
8 Monitoring the condition of the patient and reporting changes.
9 Make clear and immediate records of all drugs administered (RCN 2005; Finlay 2008; NMC 2008a, b).

The NMC Standards for Medicines Management states that 'wherever possible two registrants should check medication to be administered intravenously, one of whom should also be the registrant who then administers the intravenous medication (NMC 2008a, p. 31).

Injections and infusions

Injections can be described as the act of giving medication by use of a syringe and needle, and an infusion is defined as an amount of fluid in excess of 100 ml designated for parenteral infusion because the volume must be administered over a long period of time. However, medications may be given in small volumes (50–100 ml) or over a shorter period (30–60 minutes) (Weinstein 2007).

There are a number of routes for injection or infusion. The selection may be predetermined, e.g. intra-arterial, intracardiac or intrathecal injections. The choice of other routes will normally depend on the desired therapeutic effect and the patient's safety and comfort.

The NMC clearly states that:

It is unacceptable to prepare substances for injection in advance of their immediate use or to administer medication drawn into a syringe or container by another registrant when not in their presence. An exception of this is an already established infusion which has been instigated by another registrant following the principles set out above, or medication prepared under the direction of a pharmacist from a central intravenous additive service and clearly labelled for that patient/client.

(NMC 2008a.)

However, the NMC acknowledges that a registrant 'may be required in an emergency to prepare substances for other professionals' (NMC 2008a).

Intra-arterial

This special technique allows the delivery of a high concentration of drug to the tissues supplied by a particular artery. This route can be used for the administration of chemotherapy and vasodilators and for diagnostic purposes. Injection of drugs into an artery is a rare and hazardous procedure. The introduction of the cannula or catheter must be performed with care as the vessel may go into spasm, causing pain and occlusion. This could result in necrosis of an organ or part of a limb. Injection of irritant chemicals increases the risk of spasm and its sequelae (see Chapter 45); however, arterial catheterization is occasionally performed when it is desirable to deliver a high concentration of a drug to a tumour mass (see Chapter 12). The most common procedures are catheterization of the hepatic artery and isolated limb perfusion.

Intra-articular

In inflammatory conditions of the joints, corticosteroids are given by intra-articular injection to relieve inflammation and increase joint mobility (Downie *et al.* 2000).

Intrathecal

It may be necessary to administer some drugs intrathecally if they have poor lipid solubility and, as a result, do not pass the blood–brain barrier (Downie *et al.* 2000). A drug specially prepared for the intrathecal route should be used; doses should be carefully calculated and are usually much smaller than would be given by intramuscular or intravenous injection. In the treatment of meningitis, water-soluble antibiotics are administered by the intrathecal route to achieve adequate concentrations in the cerebrospinal fluid (CSF). In addition, antifungal agents, opioids, cytotoxic therapy and radio-opaque substances (used in the diagnosis of spinal lesions) are sometimes administered by this route (Downie *et al.* 2000) (see Chapter 12).

Intradermal

The intradermal route provides a local, rather than systemic effect, and is used primarily for diagnostic purposes such as allergy or tuberculin testing. It can also be used for the administration of local anaesthetics (Workman 1999). Observation of an inflammatory reaction is a priority, so the best sites are those that are lowly pigmented, thinly keratinized and hairless. Chosen sites are the inner forearms and

the scapulae. The injection site most commonly used is the medial forearm area. The injections are best performed using a 25 G needle inserted at a 10–15° angle, bevel up, just under the epidermis. Volumes of 0.5 ml or less should be used (Workman 1999).

Subcutaneous

Subcutaneous injections

These are given beneath the epidermis into the fat and connective tissue underlying the dermis. Injections are usually given using a 25 G needle, at a 45° angle. With the introduction of shorter length needles it is recommended that insulin injections be given at an angle of 90° (King 2003). The skin should be gently pinched into a fold to elevate the subcutaneous tissue which lifts the adipose tissue away from the underlying muscle (Workman 1999). The practice of aspirating to ensure a blood vessel has not been pierced is no longer recommended as it has been shown that this is unlikely to occur (Peragallo-Dittko 1997). The maximum volume tolerable using this route for injection is 2 ml and drugs should be highly soluble to prevent irritation (Workman 1999). Administration of infusions of drugs or fluids requires the insertion of a 25 G winged infusion set or a 24 G cannula. These should be inserted at an angle of 45° and secured with a transparent dressing to enable inspection of the site. This may also be appropriate for patients not receiving a continuous infusion but requiring frequent subcutaneous injections; this is common practice in palliative care in order to reduce the number of needlesticks injuries.

Injection sites

Sites recommended are the abdomen in the umbilical region, the lateral or posterior aspect of the lower part of the upper arm, the thighs (under the greater trochanter rather than mid-thigh) and the buttocks. It has been found that the amount of subcutaneous tissue at sites varies more than was previously thought; this is particularly significant for administration of insulin as inadvertent intramuscular administration can result in rapid absorption and hypoglycaemic episodes (King 2003). Rotation of sites can decrease the likelihood of irritation and ensure improved absorption.

Subcutaneous infusions of fluids (hypodermoclysis)

Subcutaneous fluids can be given to maintain adequate hydration in patients with mild or moderate dehydration (Sasson & Shvartzman 2001). The use of this route is generally limited to palliative care or elderly patients. It is not recommended for patients needing rapid administration of fluids, it is also contraindicated in patients with clotting disorders or who have problems with fluid overload (such as patients with cardiac failure).

A volume of 1000–2000 ml can be given over 24 hours; this can be given as a continuous infusion, over a number of hours (such as overnight) or as intermittent boluses (Moriarty & Hudson 2001). It is recommended that

213

electrolyte containing fluids such as sodium chloride 0.9% or dextrose saline be used although 5% glucose has also been used (Noble-Adams 1995). More than one site can be used to allow administration of a greater volume of fluid.

Advantages of this route include:

- Side effects are few and not generally significant.
- As it is a relatively easy procedure it can be carried out at home, reducing the need for hospitalization.
- Intravenous access can be problematic in elderly or debilitated patients; avoidance of this can reduce anxiety and distress (Noble-Adams 1995).

Research has shown that the use of peripheral cannulae rather than steel winged infusion devices results in sites remaining viable for longer (Torre 2002). Incidence of needle-stick injuries may also be reduced (Dawkins et al. 2000). It is now recommended that subcutaneous infusion be given via a plastic cannula (e.g. Insyte 24 G; 0.7 × 19 mm).

Side-effects of subcutaneous fluid administration include pain, bruising, local oedema, erythema and local infection.

Hyaluronidase is an enzyme which increases the rate of subcutaneous absorption of fluids. It can be given as a subcutaneous injection before commencing fluids. A randomized study compared absorption and side effects of administration of subcutaneous fluids with or without hyaluronidase. No significant differences were found although patients not receiving hyaluronidase showed an increase in size of the limb in which the fluid had been administered, but no differences in pain or local discomfort were found; so no clear benefit to use of hyaluronidase was demonstrated (Constans et al. 1991). It is currently unclear from the evidence available whether hyaluronidase should routinely be used (Rochon et al. 1997). Rarely severe allergic reactions have been reported.

There is a lack of clear evidence regarding the use of hydration in dying patients. It has been suggested that incidence of delirium may be reduced. It has also been suggested that administration of fluids can reduce feelings of thirst; studies have shown that this is not the case and it may be that a variety of factors play a part, for example certain drugs can cause a dry mouth (Viola et al. 1997). Currently practice varies but the risks and benefits for each patient should be carefully considered before a decision is made bearing in mind that issues of nutrition and hydration are particularly sensitive when the patient is dying.

Subcutaneous infusions of drugs

This may be the route of choice in patients with problems such as vomiting, diarrhoea or dysphagia and who are unable to tolerate drugs by the oral route; patients in bowel obstruction whose gut absorption may be impaired may also benefit. It is also commonly used for patients who are dying and no longer able to manage medication orally. Continuous subcutaneous infusion of insulin is used in a small number of diabetic patients; this may be used when adequate control cannot be achieved with multiple daily insulin doses. Such patients need to be under the care of a multidisciplinary team familiar with the use of such infusions (NICE 2003).

Infusions of a single drug, such as an antiemetic or analgesic, do not generally cause problems with stability. The drug should be diluted with a suitable diluent, sodium chloride is recommended for most drugs, and given over 12–24 hours (Dickman et al. 2005). The use of a combination of drugs can be problematic; there is anecdotal evidence regarding combinations of drugs but not many pharmaceutical studies confirming compatibility. Combinations of up to four drugs have been reported, but if compatibility is uncertain it may be best to use a second syringe pump. It is also important to ensure that the diluent used is compatible with all the drugs in the infusion. It is recommended that infusions are not exposed to direct sunlight or to increased temperatures as drug instability may result (Dickman et al. 2005).

Infusion sites

Choice of site should be based both on thickness of subcutaneous tissue and patient convenience. Sites recommended for subcutaneous infusion of drugs or fluids are the lateral aspects of the upper arms and thighs, the abdomen, the chest and the scapula (Mitten 2001). The following areas should not be used:

- Lymphoedematous areas, as absorption may be impaired and infection may be introduced.
- Sites over bony prominences, as there may be insufficient subcutaneous tissue.
- Previously irradiated skin areas, as absorption may be impaired.
- Sites near a joint, as movement may cause the cannula to become dislodged.
- Any areas of inflamed, infected or broken skin (Mitten 2001).

Care of the site

The site should be assessed regularly for patency; redness, leakage of fluid, bleeding, pain or swelling at the site can be signs of irritation and poor absorption. The time a site can be used for can vary from 1 to 14 days (Kain et al. 2006). The syringe should also be inspected for precipitation or cloudiness which may indicate imcompatibility. Some drugs are particularly likely to cause irritation and may need to be diluted in a greater volume of diluent; cyclizine and levomepromazine are among these.

If skin sites break down rapidly, suggestions include:

- Check compatibility of drugs and diluents.
- Consider increasing the amount of diluent or changing the diluent.
- Change the infusion device.
- Use a different site cleanser.
- Change the dressing used.
- Consider adding dexamethasone 1 mg to the driver; this may be helpful but is not currently recommended for routine use, care should also be taken as dexamethasone is incompatible with a number of drug combinations (Dickman et al. 2005).

Intramuscular

Intramuscular injections should be given into the densest part of the muscle. The injectable volume will depend on the muscle bed. In children, injectable volumes should be halved because muscle mass is less (Workman 1999). Current research evidence suggests that there are five sites that can be utilized for the administration of intramuscular injections (Workman 1999; Rodger & King 2000). These sites (Figure 11.2) are described below.

1 The mid-deltoid site (Figure 11.2a). This site has the advantage of being easily accessible whether the patient is standing, sitting or lying down. Owing to the small area of this site, the number and volume of injections which can be given into it are limited. Drugs such as narcotics, sedatives and vaccines, which are usually small in volume, tend to be administered into the deltoid site (Workman 1999). Rodger and King (2000) state that the maximum volume that should be administered at this site is 1 ml.

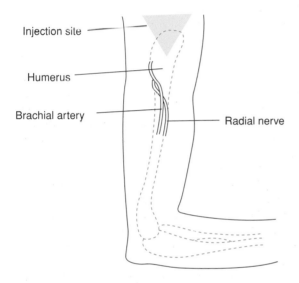

(a) The deltoid injection site

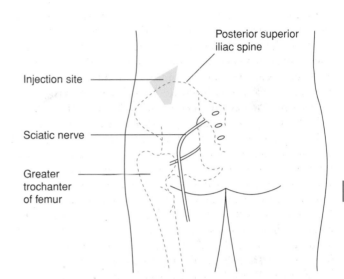

(b) The dorsogluteal injection site

215

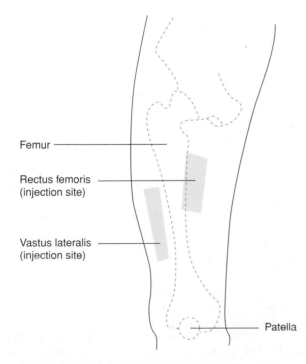

(c) The rectus femoris and vastus lateralis injection sites

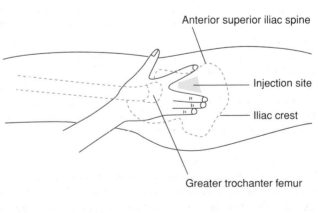

(d) The ventrogluteal injection site

Figure 11.2   Intramuscular injection sites. From Rodger and King (2000).

2 The dorsogluteal site (Figure 11.2b) is used for deep intramuscular and Z-track injections. The gluteus muscle has the lowest drug absorption rate. The muscle mass is also likely to have atrophied in elderly, non-ambulant and emaciated patients. This site carries with it the danger of the needle hitting the sciatic nerve and the superior gluteal arteries (Workman 1999). The Z-track method involves pulling the skin downwards or to one side of the injection site and inserting the needle at a right angle to the skin, which moves the cutaneous and subcutaneous tissues by approximately 1–2 cm (Workman 1999). The injection is given and the needle withdrawn, while releasing the retracted skin at the same time. This manoeuvre seals off the puncture tract. In adults up to 4 ml can be safely injected into this site (Rodger & King 2000).

3 The rectus femoris site (Figure 11.2c) is used for antiemetics, narcotics, sedatives, injections in oil, deep intramuscular and Z-track injections. The rectus femoris is the anterior quadriceps muscle, which is rarely used by nurses, but is easily accessed for self-administration of injections or for infants (Workman 1999).

4 The vastus lateralis site (Figure 11.2c) is used for deep intramuscular and Z-track injections. One of the advantages of the vastus lateralis site is its ease of access but more importantly, there are no major blood vessels or significant nerve structures associated with this site. Up to 5 ml can be safely injected (Rodger & King 2000).

5 The ventrogluteal site (Figure 11.2d) is used for antibiotics, antiemetics, deep intramuscular and Z-track injections in oil, narcotics and sedatives. This is the site of choice for intramuscular injections (Rodger & King 2000). Up to 2.5 ml can be safely injected into the ventrogluteal site (Rodger & King 2000).

Skin preparation

There are many inconsistencies regarding skin cleaning prior to subcutaneous or intramuscular injections. Previous studies have suggested that cleaning with an alcohol swab is not always necessary, does not result in infections and may predispose the skin to hardening (Dann 1969; Koivistov & Felig 1978; Workman 1999).

Dann (1969), in a study over a period of 6 years involving more than 5000 injections, found no single case of local and/or systemic infection. Koivistov and Felig (1978) concluded that whilst skin preparations did reduce skin bacterial count, they are not necessary to prevent infections at the injection site. Some trusts accept that if the patient is physically clean and the nurse maintains a high standard of hand hygiene and asepsis during the procedure, skin disinfection is not necessary (Workman 1999).

In the immunosuppressed patient, the skin should be cleaned as such patients may become infected by inoculation of a relatively small number of pathogens (Downie et al. 2000). The practice at The Royal Marsden Hospital is to continue to clean the skin prior to injection in order to reduce the risk of contamination from the patient's skin flora.

The skin should be cleaned using an 'alcohol swab' (containing 70% isopropyl alcohol) for 30 seconds and then allowed to dry. If the skin is not dry before proceeding, skin cleaning is ineffective and the antiseptic may cause irritation by being injected into the tissues (Downie et al. 2000).

Needle bevel

Three categories of needle bevel are available:

1 *Regular*: for all intramuscular and subcutaneous injections.
2 *Intradermal*: for diagnostic injections and other injections into the epidermis.
3 *Short*: rarely used.

Intramuscular needle gauge size and length

Needles should be long enough to penetrate the muscle and still allow a quarter of the needle to remain external to the skin (Workman 1999). The most common sizes are 21 or 23 G and 2.5–5.0 cm long. Lenz (1983) states that when choosing the correct needle length for intramuscular injections it is important to assess the muscle mass of the injection site, the amount of subcutaneous fat and the weight of the patient. Without such an assessment, most injections intended for gluteal muscle are deposited in the gluteal fat. The following are suggested by the author as ways of determining the most suitable size of needle to use.

Deltoid and vastus lateralis muscles
The muscle to be used should be grasped between the thumb and forefinger to determine the depth of the muscle mass or the amount of subcutaneous fat at the injection site.

Gluteal muscles
The layer of fat and skin above the muscle should be gently lifted with the thumb and forefinger for the same reasons as before. Use the patient's weight to calculate the needle length required. Lenz (1983) recommends the following guide:

31.5–40.0 kg:	2.5 cm needle.
40.5–90.0 kg:	5.0–7.5 cm needle.
90 kg:	10–15 cm needle.

Intramuscular injections and pain

Patients are often afraid of receiving injections because they perceive the injection will be painful (Workman 1999). Torrence (1989) listed a number of factors that cause pain:

- The needle.
- The chemical composition of the drug/solution.
- The technique.
- The speed of the injection.
- The volume of drug.

Workman (1999) listed a number of techniques that could be utilized to reduce pain and discomfort experienced by the patient such as adequate preparation of the patient, using ice or freezing spray to numb the skin, correct choice of site and technique and positioning of the patient so that the muscles are relaxed. Field (1981) attempts to answer the question of what it is like to give an injection, and goes on to explore the meaning and use of language relating to injections, the feelings involved in preparing and administering injections, and the meaning of the patient's response to the nurse.

Intravenous

Advantages of using the intravenous route

1 An immediate, therapeutic effect is achieved owing to rapid delivery of the drug to its target site, which allows a more precise dose calculation and therefore more reliable treatment.
2 Pain and irritation caused by some substances when given intramuscularly or subcutaneously are avoided.
3 The vascular route affords a route of administration for the patient who cannot tolerate fluids or drugs by the gastrointestinal route or is unable to take them by mouth.
4 Some drugs cannot be absorbed by any other route; the large molecular size of some drugs prevents absorption by the gastrointestinal route, while other drugs, unstable in the presence of gastric juices, are destroyed.
5 The intravenous route offers the facility for control over the rate of administration of drugs; prolonged action can be provided by administering a dilute infusion intermittently or over a prolonged period of time (Weinstein 2007; Whittington 2008).

Disadvantages of using the intravenous route

1 There is an inability to recall the drug and reverse its action. This may lead to increased toxicity or a sensitivity reaction.
2 Insufficient control of administration may lead to speed shock or circulatory overload.
3 Additional complications may occur, such as the following:
    (a) microbial contamination (extrinsic or intrinsic);
    (b) vascular irritation, e.g. chemical phlebitis;
    (c) drug incompatibilities and interactions if multiple additives are prescribed (Weinstein 2007).
4 Needle phobia.
5 Altered body image, especially with central vascular access devices (Dougherty 2008).
6 Time taken for administration (Hockley et al. 1995).

Principles to be applied throughout preparation and administration

Asepsis and reducing the risk of infection

Microbes on the hands of health care personnel contribute to hospital-associated infection (Weinstein 2007). Therefore aseptic technique must be adhered to throughout all intra-

venous procedures (see Chapter 5). The nurse must employ good hand washing and drying techniques using a bactericidal soap or a bactericidal alcohol handrub. If asepsis is not maintained, local infection, septic phlebitis or septicaemia may result (RCN 2005; Hart 2008; Pratt et al. 2007).

The insertion site should be inspected at least once a day for complications such as infiltration, phlebitis or any indication of infection, e.g. redness at the insertion site of the device or pyrexia (RCN 2005). These problems may necessitate the removal of the device and/or further investigation (Finlay 2008).

It is desirable that a closed system of infusion is maintained wherever possible, with as few connections as is necessary for its purpose (Finlay 2008; Hart 2008). This reduces the risk of bacterial contamination. Any extra connections within the administration system increase the risk of infection. Three-way taps have been shown to encourage the growth of micro-organisms. They are difficult to clean due to their design, as micro-organisms can become lodged and are then able to multiply in the warm, moist environment (Finlay 2008; Hart 2008). This reservoir for micro-organisms may then be released into the circulation.

The injection sites on administration sets or injection caps should be cleaned using an alcohol-based antiseptic, allowing time for it to dry (Pratt et al. 2007). Connections should be cleaned before changing administration sets and manipulations kept to a minimum. Administration sets should be changed according to use (intermittent/continuous therapy), type of device and type of solution, and the set must be labelled with the date and time of change (RCN 2005; NPSA 2007).

To ensure safe delivery of intravenous fluids and medication:

- Replace all tubing when the vascular device is replaced (Pratt et al. 2007).
- Replace solution administration sets and stopcocks used for continuous infusions every 72 hours unless clinically indicated, e.g. if drug stability data indicate otherwise (RCN 2005; Pratt et al. 2007). Research has indicated that routine changing of administration sets (used for infusing solutions) every 48–72 hours instead of every 24 hours is not associated with an increase in infection and could result in considerable savings for hospitals (RCN 2005; Pratt et al. 2007).
- Replace solution administration sets used for lipid emulsions and parenteral nutrition at the end of the infusion or within 24 hours of initiating the infusion (RCN 2005; Pratt et al. 2007). Certain intravenous fluids including lipid emulsions, blood and blood products are more likely than other parenteral fluids to support microbial growth if contaminated and therefore replacement of the intravenous tubing is required more frequently than 48–72 hours (Pratt et al. 2007).
- Replace blood administration sets at least every 12 hours and after every second unit of blood (McClelland 2007; RCN 2005; Pratt et al. 2007).

217

■ All solution sets used for intermittent infusions, e.g. antibiotics, should be discarded immediately after use and not allowed to hang for reuse (RCN 2005).

Inspection of fluids, drugs, equipment and their packaging must be undertaken to detect any points where contamination may have occurred during manufacture and/or transport. This intrinsic contamination may be detected as cloudiness, discoloration or the presence of particles (Perucca 2001; Weinstein 2007; BMA & RPS 2008). Infusion bags should not be left hanging for longer than 24 hours. In the case of blood and blood products this is reduced to 5 hours (McClelland 2007; RCN 2005).

Safety
All details of the prescription and all calculations must be checked carefully in accordance with hospital policy in order to ensure safe preparation and administration of the drug(s).

Drug calculations
The following formulas can be applied to calculate dose, volume or rate of infusion, as illustrated in Higgins (2005).

The drug volume required from stock strength

$$\frac{\text{Strength required}}{\text{Stock strength}} \times \text{Volume of stock solution}$$

$$= \text{Volume required}$$

What you want/What you have got

$$\times \text{Volume of stock solution}$$

Infusion rates   *Gravitational flow administration:*

Volume required/Duration (hour)

$\times$ Set value (drops/ml)/Minutes (60) = Drops per minute

Volumetric infusion pumps:

Volume to be infused/Duration of infusion

$$= \text{Volume per hour}$$

Weight-related doses

Prescribed volume $\times$ Body weight

$$= \text{volume, e.g. ml per weight, e.g. kg}$$

Prescribed dose $\times$ Body weight

$$= \text{dose, e.g. mg per weight, e.g. kg}$$

It is important to note that the 'use of calculators to determine the volume or quantity of medication should not act as a substitute for arithmatical knowledge and skill' (NMC 2008a).

The nurse must also check the compatibility of the drug with the diluent or infusion fluid. The nurse should be aware of the types of incompatibilities, and the factors which could influence them. These include pH, concentration, time, temperature, light and the brand of the drug. If insufficient information is available, a reference book (e.g. *British National Formulary* [BMA & RPS 2008]) or the product data sheet must be consulted (NPSA 2007; Whittington 2008). If the nurse is unsure about any aspect of the preparation and/or administration of a drug, they should not proceed and should consult with a senior member of staff (NMC 2008a). Constant monitoring of both the mixture and the patient is important. The preferred method and rate of intravenous administration must be determined.

Drugs should never be added to the following: blood; blood products, i.e. plasma or platelet concentrate; mannitol solutions; sodium bicarbonate solution, etc. Only specially prepared additives should be used with fat emulsions or amino acid preparations.

Accurate labelling of additives and records of administration are essential (RCN 2005; NPSA 2007).

Any protective clothing which is advised should be worn, and vinyl gloves should be used to reduce the risk of latex allergy (Hart 2008). Health care professionals who use gloves frequently or for long periods face a high risk of allergy from latex products. All health care facilities should develop policies and procedures that determine measures to protect staff and patients from latex exposure and outline a treatment plan for latex reactions (Dougherty 2002).

It has been suggested that needle-free systems can increase the risk of bloodstream infections (Danzig *et al.* 1995). However, most studies have found no difference in microbial contamination when comparing conventional and needle-free systems (Brown *et al.* 1997; Luebke *et al.* 1998; Mendelson *et al.* 1998). It appears that an increased risk is only associated where there is lack of compliance with cleaning protocols or changing of equipment (Pratt *et al.* 2007).

Preventing needlestick injuries should be key in any health and safety programme and organizations should introduce safety devices and needle-free systems wherever possible (NHS Employers 2005). Basic rules of safety include not resheathing needles, disposal of needles immediately after use into a recognized sharps bin and convenient location of sharps bins in all areas where needles and sharps are used (MHRA 2004; RCN 2005; Hart 2008).

Comfort
Both the physical and psychological comfort of the patient must be considered. Comprehensive explanation of the practical aspects of the procedure together with information about the effects of treatment will contribute to reducing anxiety and will need to be tailored to each patient's individual needs.

Methods of administering intravenous drugs

There are three methods of administering intravenous drugs: continuous infusion, intermittent infusion and intermittent injection.

Continuous infusion
Continuous infusion may be defined as the intravenous delivery of a medication or fluid at a constant rate over a prescribed time period, ranging from 24 hours to days to achieve a controlled therapeutic response. The greater

dilution also helps to reduce venous irritation (Weinstein 2007; Whittington 2008).

A continuous infusion may be used when:

- The drugs to be administered must be highly diluted.
- A maintenance of steady blood levels of the drug is required.

Preprepared infusion fluids with additives such as those containing potassium chloride should be used whenever possible. This reduces the risk of extrinsic contamination, which can occur during the mixing of drugs (Weinstein 2007). Only one addition should be made to each bottle or bag of fluid after the compatibility has been ascertained. More additions can increase the risk of incompatibility occurring, e.g. precipitation (Weinstein 2007; Whittington 2008). The additive and fluid must be mixed well to prevent a layering effect which can occur with some drugs (Whittington 2008). The danger is that a bolus injection of the drug may be delivered. To safeguard against this, any additions should be made to the infusion fluid and the container inverted a number of times to ensure mixing of the drug and prevent a bolus of the drug being infused, before the fluid is hung on the infusion stand (NPSA 2007). The infusion container should be labelled clearly after the addition has been made. Constant monitoring of the infusion fluid mixture (Weinstein 2007; Whittington 2008) for cloudiness or presence of particles should occur, as well as checking the patient's condition and intravenous site for patency, extravasation or infiltration.

Intermittent infusion

Intermittent infusion is the administration of a small-volume infusion, i.e. 50–250 ml, over a period of between 20 minutes and 2 hours. This may be given as a specific dose at one time or at repeated intervals during 24 hours (Pickstone 1999).

An intermittent infusion may be used when:

- A peak plasma level is required therapeutically.
- The pharmacology of the drug dictates this specific dilution.
- The drug will not remain stable for the time required to administer a more dilute volume.
- The patient is on a restricted intake of fluids (Whittington 2008).

Delivery of the drug by intermittent infusion may utilize a system such as a 'Y' set, if the primary infusion is of a compatible fluid, or a burette set with a chamber capacity of 100 or 150 ml. This is when the drug can be added to the burette and infused while the primary infusion is switched off. A small-volume infusion may also be connected to a cannula specifically to keep the vein open, and maintain patency.

All the points considered when preparing for a continuous infusion should be taken into account here, e.g. preprepared fluids, single additions of drugs, adequate mixing, labelling and monitoring.

Direct intermittent injection

Direct intermittent injection (also known as intravenous push or bolus) involves the injection of a drug from a syringe into the injection port of the administration set or directly into a vascular access device. Most are administered anywhere from 3 to 10 minutes depending upon the drug (Weinstein 2007; Whittington 2008).

A direct injection may be used when:

- A maximum concentration of the drug is required to vital organs. This is a 'bolus' injection which is given rapidly over seconds, as in an emergency, e.g. adrenaline.
- The drug cannot be further diluted for pharmacological or therapeutic reasons or does not require dilution. This is given as a controlled 'push' injection over a few minutes.
- A peak blood level is required and cannot be achieved by small-volume infusion.

Rapid administration could result in toxic levels and an anaphylactic-type reaction. Manufacturers' recommendations of rates of administration (i.e. millilitres or milligrams per minute) should be adhered to. In the absence of such recommendations, administration should proceed slowly, over 5–10 minutes (Dougherty 2002).

Delivery of the drug by direct injection may be via the cannula through a resealable needleless injection cap, extension set or via the injection site of an administration set.

- If a peripheral device is in situ the bandage and dressing must be removed to inspect the insertion of the cannula, unless a transparent dressing is in place (Finlay 2008).
- Patency of the vein must be confirmed prior to administration and the vein's ability to accept an extra flow of fluid or irritant chemical must also be checked (Dougherty 2008).

Administration into the injection site of a fast-running drip may be advised if the infusion in progress is compatible in order to dilute the drug further and reduce local chemical irritation (Dougherty 2002). Alternatively, a stop–start procedure may be employed if there is doubt about venous patency. This allows the nurse to constantly check the patency of the vein and detect early signs of extravasation. If the infusion fluid is incompatible with the drug, the administration set may be switched off and a compatible solution may be used as a flush (NPSA 2007).

If a number of drugs are being administered, 0.9% sodium chloride must be used to flush in between each drug to prevent interactions. In addition, 0.9% sodium chloride should be used at the end of the administration to ensure that all of the drug has been delivered. The device should then be flushed to ensure patency is maintained (see Chapter 45) (Dougherty 2008).

Summary

The nurse is responsible for the administration of drugs by a variety of methods. The NMC's *Standards for Medicines Management* emphasizes that this 'is not solely a mechanistic task to be performed in strict compliance with the written prescription of a medical practitioner (now independent supplementary prescriber)' (NMC 2008a, p. 6). Shepherd (2002b) maintains that the administration of a medicine is arguably the most common clinical procedure that a nurse will undertake. He goes on to state that it is the manner in which a medicine is administered that determines to some extent whether or not the patient gains any clinical benefit and whether any adverse effect is experienced.

The nurse is accountable for the safe administration of drugs. In order to do this the nurse requires a thorough knowledge of the principles and their application, and a responsible attitude, which ensures that medications are not given without full knowledge of immediate and late effects, toxicities and nursing implications. The nurse must also be able to justify any actions taken and be accountable for the action taken (NMC 2008b).

Procedure guidelines   Self-administration of drugs

Equipment

1 Drugs to be administered.
2 Recording sheet or book as required by law or hospital policy.

3 Patient's prescription chart, to check dose, route, etc.
4 Any protective clothing required by hospital policy for specified drugs, such as antibiotics or cytotoxic drugs (see Chapter 12).

Procedure

Action	Rationale
1 Discuss medication history with the patient on his/her admission. This should include an assessment of the patient's ability to self-administer medication using the following criteria. ■ Is the patient willing to participate in self-administration? ■ Is the patient confused or forgetful? ■ Does the patient have a history of drug/alcohol abuse/self-harm? ■ Does the patient self-administer medicines at home? ■ Can the patient read the labels on the medicines? ■ Can the patient open the medicine containers? ■ Can the patient open the locker where the medicines are stored while they are in hospital? ■ Does the patient know what his/her medicines are for, their dosage, instructions and potential side-effects (Shepherd 2002b)? Document this assessment in the patient's nursing records.	To ensure an accurate record of: all medicines being taken (prescribed or otherwise); dietary supplements, e.g. multivitamins, herbal remedies, complementary therapies; allergies or hypersensitivities; understanding of current medicines; possible problems with self-administration (Shepherd 2002b: E; Jordan *et al*. 2003: E; NMC 2005: C; NMC 2008a: C). If frequent changes of drug or dose are expected, immediate self-administration may be undesirable and/or impractical. Appropriate medicines already in the patient's possession may be used, subject to local policy and agreement with the pharmacist (Shepherd 2002b: E; NMC 2008a: C).
2 Review proposed (inpatient) prescription in liaison with pharmacist and compare with details given by patient and medicines in his/her possession.	
3 Consider whether there are any constraints on self-administration, and if so, how they might be overcome. Discuss this with appropriate members of the multidisciplinary team.	To promote successful and safe self-administration and ensure that medicines are dispensed and labelled appropriately for the patient's needs (Shepherd 2002a: E; DH 2003d: C; NMC 2008a: C). Constraints such as physical or visual handicap must be addressed. Changes in performance status may result from the underlying condition or its treatment, and must be allowed for (Shepherd 2002a: E; NMC 2008a: C). If a compliance aid such as a 'dosette' box is to be used, responsibility for filling and labelling the aid, especially whilst used on the ward, must be agreed and documented in local policies (Shepherd 2002a: E; NMC 2008a: C).

4 Regularly discuss with the patient his/her medication and any problems they may be having with the regimen. Document discussions in the care plan. Teach any special skills required, e.g. correct use of aerosol inhalers.

To promote the informed commitment and involvement of patients in their own care, where appropriate. To ensure that treatment is received as intended (Shepherd 2002b: E; NMC 2008a: C).

5 Check that drugs are taken as intended, and that the necessary records are kept.

To discharge the nurse's overall responsibility for patient care and well being. To maintain a record of responsibilities undertaken (NMC 2005: C; NMC 2008a: C; NMC 2008b: C).

Particular care with record keeping is needed in the period of gradual transition from nurse administration to self-administration. Any problems encountered must be addressed (NMC 2005: C; NMC 2008a: C; NMC 2008b: C).

The detail and format of the record may vary according to: the patient's needs and performance status; the complexity of treatment; and local circumstances and policy (NMC 2005: C; NMC 2008a: C; NMC 2008b: C).

6 Monitor changes in the patient's prescription.

To ensure that: changes are put into effect promptly; drugs are properly relabelled or redispensed; any discontinued drugs are retrieved from the patient (Shepherd 2002b: E; DH 2003d: C; NMC 2008a: C).

7 Check when drug supplies are expected to run out and make arrangements for resupply. Order drugs to take out (TTO) as far in advance as possible.

To ensure that drugs are represcribed and dispensed in time to allow uninterrupted treatment and to facilitate planned discharge (Shepherd 2002b: E; DH 2003d: C; NMC 2008a: C).

8 Evaluate the effectiveness of the self-administration teaching programme and record any difficulties encountered and interventions made.

To identify further learning and teaching needs and modify care plan accordingly (Shepherd 2002b: E; NMC 2005: C; NMC 2008a: C; NMC 2008b: C).

Procedure guidelines   Oral drug administration

Equipment

1 Refer to Procedure guidelines: Self-administration of drugs.

2 Medicine container (disposable if possible).

Procedure

Action

1 Wash hands with bactericidal soap and water or bactericidal alcohol handrub.

Rationale

To minimize the risk of cross-infection (DH 2007: C).

2 Before administering any prescribed drug, check that it is due and has not already been given. Check that the information contained in the prescription chart is complete, correct and legible.

To protect the patient from harm (DH 2003d: C; NMC 2008a: C).

Procedure guidelines *(cont.)*

3 Before administering any prescribed drug, consult the patient's prescription chart and ascertain the following: (a) Drug. (b) Dose. (c) Date and time of administration. (d) Route and method of administration. (e) Diluent as appropriate. (f) Validity of prescription. (g) Signature of doctor. (h) The prescription is legible.	To ensure that the patient is given the correct drug in the prescribed dose using the appropriate diluent and by the correct route (DH 2003d: C; NMC 2008a:C). To protect the patient from harm (DH 2003d: C; NMC 2008a: C). To protect the patient from harm (DH 2003d: C; NMC 2008a: C). To protect the patient from harm (DH 2003d: C; NMC 2008a: C). To protect the patient from harm (DH 2003d: C; NMC 2008a: C).
4 Select the required medication and check the expiry date.	Treatment with medication that is outside the expiry date is dangerous. Drugs deteriorate with storage. The expiry date indicates when a particular drug is no longer pharmacologically efficacious (DH 2003d: C; NMC 2008a: C).
5 Empty the required dose into a medicine container. Avoid touching the preparation.	To minimize the risk of cross-infection. To minimize the risk of harm to the nurse (DH 2007: C).
6 Take the medication and the prescription chart to the patient. Check the patient's identity by asking the patient to state their full name and date of birth. If patient unable to confirm details then check patient identity band against prescription chart.	To ensure that the medication is administered to the correct patient (NPSA 2005: C).
7 Evaluate the patient's knowledge of the medication being offered. If this knowledge appears to be faulty or incorrect, offer an explanation of the use, action, dose and potential side-effects of the drug or drugs involved.	A patient has a right to information about treatment (NMC 2008a: C; NMC 2008b: C).
8 Administer the drug as prescribed.	To meet legal requirements and hospital policy (DH 2003d: C; NMC 2005: C; NMC 2008a: C; NMC 2008b: C).
9 Offer a glass of water, if allowed.	To facilitate swallowing the medication (Jordan *et al.* 2003: E).
10 Record the dose given in the prescription chart and in any other place made necessary by legal requirement or hospital policy.	To meet legal requirements and hospital policy (DH 2003d: C; NMC 2005: C; NMC 2008a: C; NMC 2008b: C).
11 Administer irritant drugs with meals or snacks.	To minimize their effect on the gastric mucosa (Shepherd 2002a: E; Jordan *et al.* 2003: E).
12 Administer drugs that interact with food, or that are destroyed in significant proportions by digestive enzymes, between meals or on an empty stomach.	To prevent interference with the absorption of the drug (Shepherd 2002a: E; Jordan *et al.* 2003: E).

13 Do not break a tablet unless it is scored and appropriate to do so. Break scored tablets with a file or a tablet cutter. Wash after use.	Breaking may cause incorrect dosage, gastrointestinal irritation or destruction of a drug in an incompatible pH. To reduce risk of contamination between tablets (Shepherd 2002a: E; Jordan *et al.* 2003: E; DH 2003d: C; NMC 2008a: C).
14 Do not interfere with time-release capsules and enteric coated tablets. Ask patients to swallow these whole and not to chew them.	The absorption rate of the drug will be altered (Shepherd 2002a: E; Jordan *et al.* 2003: E).
15 Sublingual tablets must be placed under the tongue and buccal tablets between gum and cheek.	To allow for correct absorption (Shepherd 2002a: E).
16 When administering liquids to babies and young children, or when an accurately measured dose in multiples of 1 ml is needed for an adult, an oral syringe should be used in preference to a medicine spoon or measure.	An oral syringe is much more accurate than a measure or a 5 ml spoon. Use of a syringe makes administration of the correct dose much easier in an uncooperative child. Oral syringes are available and are designed to be washable and reused for the same patient. However, in the immunocompromised patient single use only is recommended. Oral syringes must be clearly labelled for oral or enteral use only (DH 2003d: C).
17 In babies and children especially, correct use of the syringe is very important. The tip should be gently pushed into and towards the side of the mouth. The contents are then *slowly* discharged towards the inside of the cheek, pausing if necessary to allow the liquid to be swallowed. If children are uncooperative it may help to place the end of the barrel between the teeth.	To prevent injury to the mouth and eliminate the danger of choking the patient (Watt 2003: E). To get the dose in and to prevent the patient spitting it out (Watt 2003: E).

Controlled drug administration

Equipment
1 Refer to Procedure guidelines: Self-administration of drugs or Procedure guidelines: Injections: administration.

Action	Rationale
1 Consult the patient's prescription chart, and ascertain the following: (a) Drug. (b) Dose. (c) Date and time of administration. (d) Route and method of administration. (e) Diluent as appropriate. (f) Validity of prescription. (g) Signature of doctor.	To ensure that the patient is given the correct drug in the prescribed dose using the appropriate diluent and by the correct route (DH 2003d: C; NMC 2008a: C).
2 Select the correct drug from the controlled drug cupboard.	
3 Check the stock against the last entry in the ward record book. (At The Royal Marsden Hospital, a second person is required to check the stock level and both nurses are required to sign the controlled drugs book.)	To comply with hospital policy (DH 2003d: C; NMC 2008a: C; NPSA 2006: C).

223

Procedure guidelines *(cont.)*

4 Check the appropriate dose against the prescription chart.

5 Return the remaining stock to the cupboard and lock the cupboard.

6 Enter the date, dose and the patient's name in the ward record book.

7 Take the prepared dose to the patient, whose identity is checked.

To prevent error and confirm patient's identity (NPSA 2005: C).

8 Administer the drug after checking the prescription chart again. Once the drug has been administered, the prescription chart is signed by the nurse responsible for administering the medication.

9 Record the administration on appropriate charts.

To maintain accurate records, provide a point of reference in the event of any queries and prevent any duplication of treatment (DH 2003d: C; NMC 2005: C; NMC 2008a: C; NMC 2008b: C).

224

Procedure guidelines Injections: administration

Equipment

1 Clean tray or receiver in which to place drug and equipment.
2 21 G needle(s) to ease reconstitution and drawing up, 23 G if from a glass ampoule.
3 21, 23 or 25 G needle, size dependent on route of administration.
4 Syringe(s) of appropriate size for amount of drug to be given.
5 Swabs saturated with isopropyl alcohol 70%.
6 Sterile topical swab, if drug is presented in ampoule form.
7 Drug(s) to be administered.
8 Patient's prescription chart, to check dose, route, etc.
9 Recording sheet or book as required by law or hospital policy.
10 Any protective clothing required by hospital policy for specified drugs, such as antibiotics or cytotoxic drugs (see Chapter 12).

Procedure

Action	Rationale
1 Collect and check all equipment.	To prevent delays and enable full concentration on the procedure (E).
2 Check that the packaging of all equipment is intact.	To ensure sterility. If the seal is damaged, discard (NPSA 2007:C).
3 Wash hands with bactericidal soap and water or bactericidal alcohol handrub.	To prevent contamination of medication and equipment (DH 2007: C).
4 Prepare needle(s), syringe(s), etc., on a tray or receiver.	To contain all items in a clean area (E).

Action	Rationale
5 Inspect all equipment.	To check that none is damaged; if so, discard or report to Medicines and Health Care Products Regulatory Agency (MHRA) (C).
6 Consult the patient's prescription chart, and ascertain the following: (a) Drug. (b) Dose. (c) Date and time of administration. (d) Route and method of administration. (e) Diluent as appropriate. (f) Validity of prescription. (g) Signature of doctor.	To ensure that the patient is given the correct drug in the prescribed dose using the appropriate diluent and by the correct route (NMC 2008a: C; NPSA 2007: C).
7 Check all details with another nurse if required by hospital policy.	To minimize any risk of error (NMC 2008a: C).
8 Select the drug in the appropriate volume, dilution or dosage and check the expiry date.	To reduce wastage. Treatment with medication that is outside the expiry date is dangerous. Drugs deteriorate with storage. The expiry date indicates when a particular drug is no longer pharmacologically efficacious (NPSA 2007: C).
9 Proceed with the preparation of the drug, using protective clothing if advisable.	To protect practitioner during preparation (NPSA 2007: C).
10 Take the prepared dose to the patient, whose identity is checked.	To prevent error and confirm patient's identity (NPSA 2005: C).
11 Evaluate the patient's knowledge of the medication being offered. If this knowledge appears to be faulty or incorrect, offer an explanation of the use, action, dose and potential side-effects of the drug or drugs involved.	A patient has a right to information about treatment (NMC 2008a: C).
12 Close room door or curtains if appropriate.	To ensure patient privacy and dignity (E).
13 Administer the drug as prescribed.	To ensure patient receives treatment (E).
14 Record the administration on appropriate charts.	To maintain accurate records, provide a point of reference in the event of any queries and prevent any duplication of treatment (NMC 2005: C; NMC 2008a: C; NPSA 2007: C).

225

Single-dose ampoule: solution preparation

Action	Rationale
1 Inspect the solution for cloudiness or particulate matter. If this is present, discard and follow hospital guidelines on what action to take, e.g. return drug to pharmacy.	To prevent the patient from receiving an unstable or contaminated drug (NPSA 2007: C).
2 Tap the neck of the ampoule gently.	To ensure that all the solution is in the bottom of the ampoule (NPSA 2007: C).
3 Cover the neck of the ampoule with a sterile topical swab and snap it open. If there is any difficulty a file may be required.	To minimize the risk of contamination. To prevent aerosol formation or contact with the drug which could lead to a sensitivity reaction. To reduce the risk of injury to the nurse (NPSA 2007: C).

Procedure guidelines *(cont.)*

Action	Rationale
4 Inspect the solution for glass fragments; if present, discard.	To minimize the risk of injection of foreign matter into the patient (NPSA 2007: C).
5 Withdraw the required amount of solution, tilting the ampoule if necessary.	To avoid drawing in any air (NPSA 2007: C).
6 Replace the sheath on the needle and tap the syringe to dislodge any air bubbles. Expel air. *Note*: replacing the sheath should **not** be confused with resheathing used needles. An alternative to expelling the air with the needle sheath in place would be to use the ampoule or vial to receive any air and/or drug.	To prevent aerosol formation (NPSA 2007: C). To ensure that the correct amount of drug is in the syringe (NPSA 2007: C).
7 Attach a new needle if required (and discard used needle into appropriate sharps container) or attach a plastic end cap.	To reduce the risk of infection. To avoid tracking medications through superficial tissues. To ensure that the correct size of needle is used for the injection. To reduce the risk of injury to the nurse (NPSA 2007: C).

Single-dose ampoule: powder preparation

Action	Rationale
1 Tap the neck of the ampoule gently.	To ensure that any powder lodged here falls to the bottom of the ampoule (NPSA 2007: C).
2 Cover the neck of the ampoule with a sterile topical swab and snap it open. If there is any difficulty a file may be required.	To minimize the risk of contamination. To prevent contact with the drug which could cause a sensitivity reaction. To prevent injury to the nurse (NPSA 2007: C).
3 Inject the correct diluent slowly into the powder within the ampoule.	To ensure that the powder is thoroughly wet before agitation and is not released into the atmosphere (NPSA 2007: C).
4 Agitate the ampoule.	To dissolve the drug (NPSA 2007: C).
5 Inspect the contents.	To detect any glass fragments or any other particulate matter. If present, continue agitation or discard as appropriate (NPSA 2007: C).
6 When the solution is clear withdraw the prescribed amount, tilting the ampoule if necessary.	To ensure the powder is dissolved and has formed a solution with the diluent. To avoid drawing in air (NPSA 2007: C).
7 Replace the sheath on the needle and tap the syringe to dislodge any air bubbles. Expel air.	To prevent aerosol formation. To ensure that the correct amount of drug is in the syringe (NPSA 2007: C).
8 Attach a new needle if required (and discard used needle into appropriate sharps container) or attach a plastic end cap.	To reduce the risk of infection. To avoid tracking medications though superficial tissues. To ensure that the correct size of needle is used for the injection. To reduce the risk of injury to the nurse (NPSA 2007: C).

Multidose vial: powder preparation

Action	Rationale
1 Remove the tamper evident seal and clean the rubber septum with the chosen antiseptic and let it air dry for at least 30 seconds.	To prevent bacterial contamination of the drug, as the plastic lid prevents damage and does not ensure sterility (NPSA 2007: C).

Use either of these methods for reconstitution:

Reconstitution method (a): 2–6

2 Insert a 21 G needle into the cap to vent the bottle (see Action figure 2a).	To prevent pressure differentials, which can cause separation of needle and syringe (NPSA 2007: C).
3 Inject the correct diluent slowly into the powder within the ampoule.	To ensure that the powder is thoroughly wet before it is shaken and is not released into the atmosphere (NPSA 2007: C).
4 Remove the needle and the syringe.	To enable adequate mixing of the solution (E).
5 Place a sterile topical swab over the venting needle (see Action figure 2b) and shake to dissolve the powder. *Note*: the nurse may encounter other presentations of drugs for injection, e.g. vials with a transfer needle, and should follow the manufacturer's instructions in these instances.	To prevent contamination of the drug or the atmosphere. To mix the diluent with the powder and dissolve the drug (NPSA 2007: C).
6 Inspect the solution for cloudiness or particulate matter. If this is present, discard. Follow hospital guidelines on what action to take, e.g. return drug to pharmacy.	To prevent patient from receiving an unstable or contaminated drug (NPSA 2007: C).

Reconstitution method (b): 7–13

7 With the needle sheathed draw into the syringe a volume of air equivalent to the required volume of solution to be drawn up.	To prevent bacterial contamination of the drug (NPSA 2007: C).
8 Remove the needle cover and insert the needle into the vial through the rubber septum.	To gain access to the vial (E).
9 Invert the vial. Keep the needle in the solution and slowly depress the plunger to push the air into the vial.	To create an equilibrium in the vial (NPSA 2007: C).
10 Release the plunger so that the solution flows back into the syringe (if a large volume of solution is to be withdrawn use a push pull technique).	To create an equilibrium in the vial (NPSA 2007: C).
11 Inject the diluent into the vial. Keeping the tip of the needle above the level of the solution in the vial, release the plunger. The syringe will fill with the air which has been displaced by the solution.	This 'equilibrium method' helps to minimize the build up of pressure in the vial.
12 With the needle and syringe in place, gently swirl the vial to dissolve all the powder.	To mix the diluent with the powder and dissolve the drug (NPSA 2007: C).
13 Inspect the solution for cloudiness or particulate matter. If this is present, discard. Follow hospital guidelines on what action to take, e.g. return drug to pharmacy.	To prevent patient from receiving an unstable or contaminated drug (NPSA 2007: C).

Continue from 14

Withdrawal of medication from vial

14 Withdraw the prescribed amount of solution, and inspect for pieces of rubber which may have 'cored out' of the cap (see Action figure 2c). *Note*: coring can be minimized by inserting the needle into the cap, bevel up, at an angle of 45° to 60°. Before complete insertion of the needle tip, lift the needle to 90° and proceed (see Action figure 14).	To ensure that the correct amount of drug is in the syringe (NPSA 2007: C). To prevent the injection of foreign matter into the patient (NPSA 2007: C).

Procedure guidelines *(cont.)*

15 Remove air from syringe without spraying into the atmosphere by injecting air back into the vial (see Action figure 2d) or replace the sheath on the needle and tap the syringe to dislodge any air bubbles. Expel air.

To reduce risk of contamination of practitioner. To prevent aerosol formation (NPSA 2007: C).

16 Attach a new needle if required (and discard used needle into appropriate sharps container) or attach a plastic end cap.

To reduce the risk of infection. To avoid possible trauma to the patient if the needle has barbed. To avoid tracking medications through superficial tissues. To ensure that the correct size of needle is used for the injection (NPSA 2007: C).

Fluid level

Sterile swab

Second needle tip above fluid level

(a)   (b)   (c)   (d)

Action 2   Suggested method of vial reconstitution to avoid environmental exposure. (a) When reconstituting vial, insert a second needle to allow air to escape when adding diluent for injection. (b) When shaking the vial to dissolve the powder, push in second needle up to Luer connection and cover with a sterile swab. (c) To remove reconstituted solution, insert syringe needle and then invert vial. Ensuring that tip of second needle is above fluid, withdraw the solution. (d) Remove air from syringe without spraying into the atmosphere by injecting air back into vial.

45–60°

Action 14   Method to minimize coring.

Subcutaneous injection administration

Action	Rationale
1 Explain and discuss the procedure with the patient.	To ensure that the patient understands the procedure and gives his/her valid consent (Griffith & Jordan 2003: E; NMC 2006: C; NMC 2008b: C).
2 Consult the patient's prescription chart, and ascertain the following: (a) Drug. (b) Dose. (c) Date and time of administration. (d) Route and method of administration. (e) Diluent as appropriate. (f) Validity of prescription. (g) Signature of doctor.	To ensure that the patient is given the correct drug in the prescribed dose using the appropriate diluent and by the correct route (NMC 2008a: C; NPSA 2007: C).
3 Assist the patient into the required position.	To allow access to the appropriate injection site (Workman 1999: E).
4 Remove appropriate garments to expose the injection site.	To gain access for injection (Workman 1999: E).

5 Assess the injection site for signs of inflammation, oedema, infection and skin lesions.	To promote effectiveness of administration (Workman 1999: E).
	  To reduce the risk of infection (Workman 1999: E).
	  To avoid skin lesions and avoid possible trauma to the patient (Workman 1999: E).

6 Choose the correct needle size.	To minimize the risk of missing the subcutaneous tissue and any ensuing pain (Workman 1999: E).
7 Clean the injection site with a swab saturated with isopropyl alcohol 70%.	To reduce the number of pathogens introduced into the skin by the needle at the time of insertion. (For further information on this action see Skin preparation section, above.)
8 Gently pinch the skin up into a fold.	To elevate the subcutaneous tissue, and lift the adipose tissue away from the underlying muscle (Workman 1999: E).
9 Insert the needle into the skin at an angle of 45° and release the grasped skin (unless administering insulin when an angle of 90° should be used). Inject the drug slowly.	Injecting medication into compressed tissue irritates nerve fibres and causes the patient discomfort. The introduction of shorter insulin needles makes 90° the more appropriate angle (Trounce & Gould 2000: E).
10 Withdraw the needle rapidly. Apply pressure to any bleeding point.	To prevent haematoma formation (E).
11 Record the administration on appropriate sheets.	To maintain accurate records, provide a point of reference in the event of any queries and prevent any duplication of treatment (NMC 2005: C; NPSA 2007: C; NMC 2008a: C).

229

Procedure guidelines *(cont.)*

Action	Rationale
12 Ensure that all sharps and non-sharp waste are disposed of safely and in accordance with locally approved procedures. For example, sharps into sharps bin and syringes into yellow clinical waste bag.	To ensure safe disposal and to avoid laceration or other injury to staff (MHRA 2004: C; DH 2005b: C).

Intramuscular injection administration

Action	Rationale
1 Explain and discuss the procedure with the patient.	To ensure that the patient understands the procedure and gives his/her valid consent (Griffith & Jordan 2003: E; NMC 2006b: C; NMC 2008b: C).
2 Consult the patient's prescription sheet, and ascertain the following: (a) Drug. (b) Dose. (c) Date and time of administration. (d) Route and method of administration. (e) Diluent as appropriate. (f) Validity of prescription. (g) Signature of doctor.	To ensure that the patient is given the correct drug in the prescribed dose using the appropriate diluent and by the correct route (NMC 2008a: C; NPSA 2007: C).
3 Assist the patient into the required position.	To allow access to the injection site and to ensure the designated muscle group is flexed and therefore relaxed (Workman 1999: E).
4 Remove the appropriate garment to expose the injection site.	To gain access for injection (Workman 1999: E).
5 Assess the injection site for signs of inflammation, oedema, infection and skin lesions.	To promote effectiveness of administration (Workman 1999: E). To reduce the risk of infection (Workman 1999: E). To avoid skin lesions and avoid possible trauma to the patient (Workman 1999: E).
6 Clean the injection site with a swab saturated with isopropyl alcohol 70% for 30 seconds and allow to dry for 30 seconds (Workman 1999).	To reduce the number of pathogens introduced into the skin by the needle at the time of insertion, to prevent stinging sensation if alcohol is taken into the tissues upon needle entry (Workman 1999: E). (For further information on this action see Skin preparation section, above.)
7 Stretch the skin around the injection site.	To facilitate the insertion of the needle and to reduce the sensitivity of nerve endings (Workman 1999: E).
8 Holding the needle at an angle of 90°, quickly plunge it into the skin.	To ensure that the needle penetrates the muscle (Workman 1999: E).
9 Pull back the plunger. If no blood is aspirated, depress the plunger at approximately 1 ml every 10 seconds and inject the drug slowly. If blood appears, withdraw the needle completely, replace it and begin again. Explain to the patient what has occurred.	To confirm that the needle is in the correct position and not in a vein (Workman 1999: E). This allows time for the muscle fibres to expand and absorb the solution (Workman 1999: E). To prevent pain and ensure even distribution of the drug.
10 Wait 10 seconds before withdrawing the needle.	To allow the medication to diffuse into the tissue (Workman 1999: E).

11 Withdraw the needle rapidly. Apply pressure to any bleeding point.	To prevent haematoma formation (E).
12 Record the administration on appropriate charts.	To maintain accurate records, provide a point of reference in the event of any queries and prevent any duplication of treatment (NMC 2005: C; NMC 2008a: C; NPSA 2007: C).
13 Ensure that all sharps and non-sharp waste are disposed of safely and in accordance with locally approved procedures, e.g. put sharps into sharps bin and syringes into yellow clinical waste bag.	To ensure safe disposal and to avoid laceration or other injury to staff (MHRA 2004: C; DH 2005b: C).

Procedure guidelines   Rectal medication administration

Rectal preparations
For further information about the administration of rectal medication see the relevant sections in Chapter 15.

Procedure guidelines   Vaginal medication administration

Equipment

1 Disposable gloves.
2 Topical swabs.
3 Disposable sanitary pad.
4 Lubricating jelly.
5 Prescription chart.

Vaginal pessary insertion

Action	Rationale
1 Explain and discuss the procedure with the patient.	To ensure that the patient understands the procedure and gives her valid consent (Griffith & Jordan 2003: E; NMC 2006b: C; NMC 2008b: C).
2 Consult the patient's prescription sheet and ascertain the following: (a) Drug. (b) Dose. (c) Date and time of administration. (d) Route and method of administration. (e) Validity of prescription. (f) Signature of doctor.	To ensure that the patient is given the correct drug in the prescribed dose and by the correct route (NMC 2008a: C).
3 Select the appropriate pessary and check it with the prescription chart.	To ensure that the correct medication is given to the correct patient at the appropriate time (NMC 2008a: C; NPSA 2007: C).
4 Close room door or curtains keeping the patient covered as much as possible.	To ensure patient privacy and dignity (E).
5 Assist the patient into the appropriate position, either left lateral with buttocks to the edge of the bed or supine with the knees drawn up and legs parted.	To facilitate easy access to the vaginal canal and correct insertion of the pessary (Manufacturer's instruction: C).
6 Wash hands with bactericidal soap and water or bactericidal alcohol handrub, and put on gloves.	To minimize the risk of cross-infection (DH 2007: C).

231

Procedure guidelines *(cont.)*

7 Apply lubricating jelly to a topical swab and from the swab on to the pessary.	To facilitate insertion of the pessary and ensure the patient's comfort (Manufacturer's instruction: C).
8 Insert the pessary along the posterior vaginal wall and into the top of the vagina. *Note*: This procedure is best performed late in the evening when the patient is unlikely to get out of bed.	To ensure that the pessary is retained and that the medication can reach its maximum efficiency (Manufacturer's instruction: C).
9 Wipe away any excess lubricating jelly from the patient's vulval and/or perineal area with a topical swab.	To promote patient comfort (E).
10 Make the patient comfortable and apply a clean sanitary pad.	To absorb any excess discharge (E).
11 Remove and dispose of gloves safely and in accordance with locally approved procedures.	To ensure safe disposal (DH 2005b: C; MHRA: C).
12 Record the administration on appropriate charts.	To maintain accurate records, provide a point of reference in the event of any queries and prevent any duplication of treatment (NMC 2005: C; NMC 2008a: C; NPSA 2007: C).

Procedure guidelines   Topical applications of medication

Equipment

1 Clean non-sterile gloves.
2 Sterile topical swabs.

3 Applicators.

Procedure

Action	Rationale
1 Explain and discuss the procedure with the patient.	To ensure that the patient understands the procedure and gives his/her valid consent (Griffith & Jordan 2003: E; NMC 2006b: C; NMC 2008b: C).
2 Check the patient's prescription chart.	To ensure that the patient is given the correct drug and dose (NMC 2008a: C).
3 Assist the patient into the required position.	To allow access to the affected area of skin (E).
4 Close room door or curtains if appropriate.	To ensure patient privacy and dignity (E).
5 Use aseptic technique if the skin is broken.	To prevent local or systemic infection (DH 2007: C).
6 If the medication is to be rubbed into the skin, the preparation should be placed on a sterile topical swab. The wearing of gloves may be necessary.	To minimize the risk of cross-infection. To protect the nurse (DH 2007: C).
7 If the preparation causes staining, advise the patient of this.	To ensure that adequate precautions are taken beforehand and to prevent unwanted stains (NMC 2008b:C).
8 Record the administration on appropriate charts.	To maintain accurate records, provide a point of reference in the event of any queries and prevent any duplication of treatment (NMC 2005: C; NMC 2008a: C; NPSA 2007: C).

Procedure guidelines   Administration of medication in other forms

Procedure

Inhalation of medication

Action	Rationale
1 Explain and discuss the procedure with the patient.	To ensure that the patient understands the procedure and gives his/her valid consent (Griffith & Jordan 2003: E; NMC 2006b: C; NMC 2008b: C).
2 Seat the patient in an upright position if possible.	To permit full expansion of the diaphragm (E).
3 Consult the patient's prescription chart, and ascertain the following: (a) Drug. (b) Dose. (c) Date and time of administration. (d) Route and method of administration. (e) Diluent as appropriate. (f) Validity of prescription. (g) Signature of doctor.	To ensure that the patient is given the correct drug in the prescribed dose using the appropriate diluent and by the correct route (NMC 2006b: C).
4 Administer only one drug at a time unless specifically instructed to the contrary.	Several drugs used together may cause undesirable reactions or they may inactivate each other (Jordan *et al.* 2003: E).
5 Measure any liquid medication with a syringe.	To ensure the correct dose (DH 2003d: C).
6 Clean any equipment used after use, and discard all disposable equipment in appropriate containers.	To minimize the risk of infection (DH 2007: C; MHRA: C).
7 Correct use of inhalers is essential (see manufacturer's information leaflet) and will be achieved only if this is carefully explained and demonstrated to the patient. If further advice is required, contact the hospital pharmacist.	Incorrect use may result in most of the dose remaining in the mouth and/or being expelled almost immediately. This renders treatment ineffective (Watt 2003: C; Manufacturer's instructions: C).
8 Record the administration on appropriate charts.	To maintain accurate records, provide a point of reference in the event of any queries and prevent any duplication of treatment (NMC 2005: C; NMC 2008a: C; NPSA 2007: C).

233

Gargling medication

Action	Rationale
1 Throat irrigations should not be warmer than body temperature.	Liquid warmer than body temperature may cause discomfort or damage tissue (E).

Nasal drop administration

Action	Rationale
1 Explain and discuss the procedure with the patient.	To ensure that the patient understands the procedure and gives his/her valid consent (Griffith & Jordan 2003: E; NMC 2006b: C; NMC 2008b: C).

Procedure guidelines *(cont.)*

2 Consult the patient's prescription sheet, and ascertain the following: (a) Drug. (b) Dose. (c) Date and time of administration. (d) Route and method of administration. (e) Validity of prescription. (f) Signature of doctor.	To ensure that the patient is given the correct drug in the prescribed dose and by the correct route (NMC 2006b: C).
3 Have paper tissues available.	To wipe away secretions and/or medication (E).
4 Ask the patient to blow their nose to clear the nasal passages if appropriate.	To ensure maximum penetration for the medication (E).
5 Hyperextend the patient's neck (unless clinically contraindicated, e.g. cervical spondylosis).	To obtain a safe optimum position for insertion of the medication (E).
6 Avoid touching the external nares with the dropper.	To prevent the patient from sneezing (E).
7 Request the patient to maintain his/her position for 1 or 2 minutes.	To ensure full absorption of the medication (E).
8 Each patient should have his/her own medication and dropper.	To minimize the risk of cross-infection (DH 2007: C).
9 Record the administration on appropriate charts.	To maintain accurate records, provide a point of reference in the event of any queries and prevent any duplication of treatment (NMC 2005: C; NMC 2008a: C; NPSA 2007: C).

Eye medications

For information on administering eye medications see Chapter 31.

Ear drop administration

Action	Rationale
1 Explain and discuss the procedure with the patient.	To ensure that the patient understands the procedure and gives his/her valid consent (Griffith & Jordan 2003: E; NMC 2006b: C; NMC 2008b: C).
2 Consult the patient's prescription chart and ascertain the following: (a) Drug. (b) Dose. (c) Date and time of administration. (d) Route and method of administration. (e) Validity of prescription. (f) Signature of doctor.	To ensure that the patient is given the correct drug in the prescribed dose using the appropriate diluent and by the correct route (NMC 2008a: C).
3 Ask the patient to lie on his/her side with the ear to be treated uppermost.	To ensure the best position for insertion of the drops (E).
4 Warm the drops to body temperature if allowed.	To prevent trauma to the patient (E).
5 Pull the cartilaginous part of the pinna backwards and upwards.	To prepare the auditory meatus for instillation of the drops (E).

6 Allow the drop(s) to fall in direction of the external canal.	To ensure that the medication reaches the area requiring therapy (E).
7 Request the patient to remain in this position for 1 or 2 minutes.	To allow the medication to reach the eardrum and be absorbed (E).
8 Record the administration on appropriate charts.	To maintain accurate records, provide a point of reference in the event of any queries and prevent any duplication of treatment (NMC 2005: C; NMC 2008a: C; NPSA 2007: C).

Procedure guidelines   Continuous infusion of intravenous drugs

This procedure may be carried out by the infusion of drugs from a bag, bottle or burette.

Equipment

1 Clinically clean receiver or tray containing the prepared drug to be administered.
2 Patient's prescription chart.
3 Recording chart or book as required by law or hospital policy.
4 Protective clothing as required by hospital policy for specific drugs.
5 Container of appropriate intravenous infusion fluid.
6 Swab saturated with isopropyl alcohol 70%.
7 Drug additive label.

Procedure

Action	Rationale
1 Explain and discuss the procedure with the patient.	To ensure that the patient understands the procedure and gives his/her valid consent (Griffith & Jordan 2003: E; NMC 2006b: C; NMC 2008b: C).
2 Inspect the infusion in progress.	To check it is the correct infusion being administered at the correct rate and that the contents are due to be delivered on time in order for the next prepared infusion bag to be connected. To check whether the patient is experiencing any discomfort at the site of insertion, which might indicate the peripheral device needs to be resited (NPSA 2007: C).
3 Before administering any prescribed drug check that it is due and has not already been given.	To protect the patient from harm (NPSA 2007: C).
4 Before administering any prescribed drug, consult the patient's prescription chart and ascertain the following: (a) Drug. (b) Dose. (c) Date and time of administration. (d) Route and method of administration. (e) Diluent as appropriate. (f) Validity of prescription. (g) Signature of doctor. (h) The prescription is legible.	To ensure that the patient is given the correct drug in the prescribed dose using the appropriate diluent and by the correct route. To protect the patient from harm (NMC 2008a: C; NPSA 2007: C). To comply with NMC (2008a) *Standards for Medicines Management.*

235

Procedure guidelines *(cont.)*

5 Wash hands with bactericidal soap and water or bactericidal alcohol handrub, and assemble the necessary equipment.	To minimize the risk of infection (DH 2007: C).
6 Prepare the drug for injection described in the Procedure guidelines: Injections: administration.	To ensure the drug is prepared (NPSA 2007: C).
7 Check the name, strength and volume of intravenous fluid against the prescription chart.	To ensure that the correct type and quantity of fluid are administered (NMC 2008a: C; NPSA 2007: C).
8 Check the expiry date of the fluid.	To prevent an ineffective or toxic compound being administered to the patient (NPSA 2007: C).
9 Check that the packaging is intact and inspect the container and contents in a good light for cracks, punctures, air bubbles.	To check that no contamination of the infusion container has occurred (NPSA 2007: C).
10 Inspect the fluid for discoloration, haziness and crystalline or particulate matter.	To prevent any toxic or foreign matter being infused into the patient (NPSA 2007: C).
11 Check the identity and amount of drug to be added. Consider: (a) Compatibility of fluid and additive. (b) Stability of mixture over the prescription time. (c) Any special directions for dilution, e.g. pH, optimum concentration. (d) Sensitivity to external factors such as light. (e) Any anticipated allergic reaction. If any doubts exist about the listed points, consult the pharmacist or appropriate reference works.	To minimize any risk of error. To ensure safe and effective administration of the drug. To enable anticipation of toxicities and the nursing implications of these (NPSA 2007: C).
12 Any additions must be made immediately before use.	To prevent any possible microbial growth or degradation (NPSA 2007: C).
13 Wash hands thoroughly using bactericidal soap and water or bactericidal alcohol handrub.	To minimize the risk of cross-infection (DH 2007: C).
14 Place infusion bag on flat surface.	To prevent puncturing the side of the infusion bag when making additions (NPSA 2007: C).
15 Remove any seal present.	To expose the injection site on the container (E).
16 Clean the site with the swab and allow it to dry.	To reduce the risk of contamination (NPSA 2007: C).
17 Inject the drug using a new sterile needle into the bag, bottle or burette. A 23 or 25 G needle should be used.	To minimize the risk of contamination. To enable resealing of the latex or rubber injection site (NPSA 2007: C).

236

18 If the addition is made into a burette at the bedside:
   (a) Avoid contamination of the needle and inlet port.
   (b) Check that the correct quantity of fluid is in the chamber.
   (c) Switch the infusion off briefly.
   (d) Add the drug.

To minimize the risk of contamination (NPSA 2007: C).
To ensure the correct dilution (NPSA 2007: C).

To ensure a bolus injection is not given (NPSA 2007: C).

19 Invert the container a number of times, especially if adding to a flexible infusion bag.

To ensure adequate mixing of the drug (NPSA 2007: C).

20 Check again for haziness, discoloration and particles. This can occur even if the mixture is theoretically compatible, thus making vigilance essential.

To detect any incompatibility or degradation (NPSA 2007: C).

21 Complete the drug additive label and fix it on the bag, bottle or burette.

To identify which drug has been added, when and by whom (NPSA 2007: C).

22 Place the container in a clean receptacle. Wash hands and proceed to the patient.

To minimize the risk of contamination (DH 2007: C).

23 Check the identity of the patient with the prescription chart and infusion bag.

To minimize the risk of error and ensure the correct infusion is administered to the correct patient (NPSA 2007: C).

24 Check that the contents of the previous container have been delivered.

To ensure that the preceding prescription has been administered (NPSA 2007: C).

25 Switch off the infusion. Place the new infusion bag on a flat surface and then disconnect empty infusion bag.

To ensure that the administration set spike will not puncture the side wall of the infusion bag (NPSA 2007: C; Finlay 2008: E).

26 Push the spike in fully without touching the spike and hang the new infusion bag on the infusion stand.

To reduce the risk of contamination (DH 2007: C).

27 Restart the infusion and adjust the rate of flow as prescribed.

To ensure that the infusion will be delivered at the correct rate over the correct period of time (NPSA 2007: C).

28 If the addition is made into a burette, the infusion can be restarted immediately following mixing and recording and the infusion rate adjusted accordingly.

To ensure that the infusion will be delivered correctly (NPSA 2007:C).

29 Ask the patient whether any abnormal sensations, etc., are experienced.

To ascertain whether there are any problems that may require nursing care and refer to medical staff where appropriate (E).

30 Discard waste, making sure that it is placed in the correct containers, e.g. sharps into a designated receptacle.

To ensure safe disposal and avoid injury to staff. To prevent reuse of equipment (MHRA 2004: C; DH 2005b: C).

31 Complete the patient's recording chart and other hospital and/or legally required documents.

To maintain accurate records. To provide a point of reference in the event of any queries. To prevent any duplication of treatment (NMC 2005: C).

237

Procedure guidelines   Intermittent infusion of intravenous drugs

Equipment

Equipment for this procedure is as described for the previous procedure (i.e. items 1–7), together with the following:

8 Intravenous administration set.
9 Intravenous infusion stand.
10 Clean dressing trolley.
11 Clinically clean receiver or tray.
12 Sterile needles and syringes.
13 20 ml for injection of a compatible flush solution, e.g. 0.9% sodium chloride or 5% dextrose.

14 Flushing solution to maintain patency plus sterile injection cap.
15 Alcohol-based lotion for cleaning injection site, e.g. chlorhexidine in 70% alcohol.
16 Alcohol-based hand wash solution or rub.
17 Sterile dressing pack.
18 Hypoallergenic tape.

Procedure

Action	Rationale
1 Explain and discuss the procedure with the patient.	To ensure that the patient understands the procedure and gives his/her valid consent (Griffith & Jordan 2003: E; NMC 2006c: C; NMC 2008b: C).
2 Before administering any prescribed drug, check that it is due and has not been given already. Check that the information contained in the prescription chart is complete, correct and legible.	To protect the patient from harm (NPSA 2007: C; NMC 2008a: C).
3 Before administering any prescribed drug, consult the patient's prescription chart and ascertain the following: (a) Drug. (b) Dose. (c) Date and time of administration. (d) Route and method of administration. (e) Diluent as appropriate. (f) Validity of prescription. (g) Signature of doctor. (h) The prescription is legible.	To ensure that the patient is given the correct drug in the prescribed dose using the appropriate diluent and by the correct route (NMC 2008a: C; NPSA 2007: C). To protect the patient from harm. To comply with NMC (2008a) *Standards for Medicines Management.*
4 Prepare the intravenous infusion and additive as described for the previous procedure (i.e. items 2–13).	To ensure the drug is prepared correctly (NPSA 2007: C).
5 Prime the intravenous administration set with infusion fluid mixture and hang it on the infusion stand.	To ensure removal of air from set and check that tubing is patent. To prepare for administration (NPSA 2007: C).
6 Draw up 10 ml of compatible flush solution for injection in two separate syringes, using an aseptic technique.	To ensure sufficient flushing solution is available (E).
7 Draw up solution (as per hospital policy) to be used for maintaining patency, e.g. 0.9% sodium chloride.	To prepare for administration (E).
8 Place the syringes in a clinically clean receiver or tray on the bottom shelf of the dressing trolley.	To ensure top shelf is used for sterile dressing pack in order to minimize the risk of contamination (E).
9 Collect the other equipment and place it on the bottom shelf of the dressing trolley.	To ensure all equipment is available to commence procedure (E).
10 Place a sterile dressing pack on top of the trolley.	To minimize risk of contamination (E).

11 Check that all necessary equipment is present.	To prevent delays and interruption of the procedure (E).
12 Wash hands thoroughly using bactericidal soap and water or bactericidal alcohol handrub before leaving the clinical room.	To minimize the risk of cross-infection (DH 2007: C).
13 Proceed to the patient. Check patient's identity with prescription chart and prepared drugs.	To minimize the risk of error and ensure the correct drug is given to the correct patient (NMC 2008a; NPSA 2007: C).
14 Open the sterile dressing pack.	To minimize the risk of cross-infection (DH 2007: C).
15 Add lotion for cleaning the injection cap to the gallipot in order to wet the low-linting swabs.	To ensure the swabs can be used for cleaning when sufficient alcohol-based lotion is applied (E).
16 Wash hands with bactericidal soap and water or with a bactericidal alcohol handrub.	To minimize the risk of cross-infection. (DH 2007:C)
17 If peripheral device is in situ remove the patient's bandage and dressing.	To observe the insertion site (Dougherty 2008: E).
18 Inspect the insertion site of the device.	To detect any signs of inflammation, infiltration, etc. If present, take appropriate action (DH 2003c: C).
19 Wash hands as above (see item 16).	To minimize the risk of contamination (DH 2007: C).
20 Put on gloves, if appropriate.	To protect against contamination with hazardous substances, e.g. cytotoxic drugs (NPSA 2007: C).
21 Place a sterile towel under the patient's arm.	To create a sterile area on which to work (E).
22 (a) If using a needleless injection system, clean the cap with alcohol-soaked swabs. (b) If using a non-injectable cap, clean the connection between the cap and the device/extension set then remove the cap while applying digital pressure at the point in the vein where the cannula tip rests.	To minimize the risk of contamination and maintain a closed system (Pratt et al. 2007: C). To minimize the risk of contamination and to prevent blood spillage (E).
23 Inject gently 10 ml of 0.9% sodium chloride for injection.	To confirm the patency of the device (E).
24 Check that no resistance is met, no pain or discomfort is felt by the patient, no swelling is evident, no leakage occurs around the device and there is a good back-flow of blood on aspiration.	To ensure the device is patent (Dougherty 2008: E).
25 Connect the infusion to the device.	To commence treatment (E).
26 Open the roller clamp.	To check the infusion is flowing freely (E).
27 Check the insertion site and ask the patient if he/she is comfortable.	To confirm that the vein can accommodate the extra fluid flow and that the patient experiences no pain, etc. (E).
28 Adjust the flow rate as prescribed.	To ensure that the correct speed of administration is established (NPSA 2007: C).

239

Procedure guidelines *(cont.)*

29	Tape the administration set in a way that places no strain on the device, which could in turn damage the vein.	To reduce the risk of mechanical phlebitis or infiltration (Dougherty 2008: E).
30	If peripheral device is in situ cover it with a sterile topical swab and tape it in place.	To maintain asepsis (Dougherty 2008: E).
31	Remove gloves, if used.	To ensure disposal (E).
32	If the infusion is to be completed within 30 minutes, bandaging is unnecessary and the patient may be instructed to keep the arm resting on the sterile towel. Otherwise reapply bandage.	To reduce the risk of dislodging the device (E).
33	The equipment must be cleared away and new equipment only prepared when required at the end of the infusion.	To ensure that the equipment used is sterile prior to use (E).
34	Monitor flow rate and device site frequently.	To ensure the flow rate is correct and the patient is comfortable, and to check for signs of infiltration (NPSA 2007: C).
35	When the infusion is complete, wash hands using bactericidal soap and water or bactericidal alcohol handrub, and recheck that all the equipment required is present.	To maintain asepsis and ensure that the procedure runs smoothly (DH 2007: C; Finlay 2008: E).
36	Stop the infusion when all the fluid has been delivered.	To ensure that all of the prescribed mixture has been delivered and prevent air infusing into the patient (NPSA 2007: C).
37	Put on non-sterile gloves, if appropriate.	To protect against contamination with hazardous substances (E).
38	Disconnect the infusion set and flush the device with 10 ml of 0.9% sodium chloride or other compatible solution for injection. (A 'minibag' may be used to flush the drug through the tubing but the cost implications of this as well as the risk to patients on restricted intake should be considered before this is adopted routinely.)	To flush any remaining irritating solution away from the cannula (E).
39	Attach a new sterile injection cap if necessary.	To maintain a closed system (Hart 2008: E).
40	Flushing must follow.	To maintain the patency of the device (Dougherty 2008: E).
41	Clean the injection site of the cap with a swab saturated with chlorhexidine in 70% alcohol.	To minimize the risk of contamination (Hart 2008: E).
42	Administer flushing solution (using a 23 or 25 G needle if necessary) using the push pause technique and ending with positive pressure.	To maintain the patency of the device and if needle used enable reseal of the injection site (Dougherty 2008: E).
43	If a peripheral device is in situ cover the insertion site and cannula with a new sterile low-linting swab. Tape it in place. Apply a bandage.	To minimize the risk of contamination of the insertion site. To reduce the risk of dislodging the cannula (E).

44 Remove gloves, if used.	To ensure disposal (E).
45 Assist the patient into a comfortable position.	To ensure the patient is comfortable (E).
46 Record the administration on appropriate charts.	To maintain accurate records, provide a point of reference in the event of any queries and prevent any duplication of treatment (NMC 2005: C).
47 Discard waste, placing it in the correct containers, e.g. sharps into a designated container.	To ensure safe disposal and avoid injury to staff (MHRA 2004; DH 2005b; NHS Employers 2005).

Procedure guidelines   Injection (bolus or push) of intravenous drugs

This procedure may be carried out via any of the following:

1 The injection or Y site of an intravenous administration set.
2 An injection cap attached to any vascular access device.
3 An extension set, multiple adaptor or stopcock (one-, two- or three-way).

Equipment

1 Clinically clean receiver or tray containing the prepared drug(s) to be administered.
2 Patient's prescription chart.
3 Protective clothing as required by hospital policy or specific drugs.
4 Clean dressing trolley.
5 Clinically clean receiver or tray.
6 Sterile needles and syringes.
7 0.9% sodium chloride, 20 ml for injection or compatible solution.
8 Flushing solution, in accordance with hospital policy.
9 Alcohol-based solution for cleaning injection site, e.g. chlorhexidine in 70% alcohol.
10 Sterile dressing pack.
11 Hypoallergenic tape.
12 Sharps container.

Procedure

Action	Rationale
1 Explain and discuss the procedure with the patient.	To ensure that the patient understands the procedure and gives his/her valid consent (Griffith & Jordan 2003: E; NMC 2006c: C; NMC 2008b: C).
2 Before administering any prescribed drug, check that it is due and has not been given already. Check that the information contained in the prescription chart is complete, correct and legible.	To protect the patient from harm (NMC 2008b: C).
3 Before administering any prescribed drug, consult the patient's prescription sheet and ascertain the following: (a) Drug. (b) Dose. (c) Date and time of administration. (d) Route and method of administration. (e) Diluent as appropriate. (f) Validity of prescription. (g) Signature of doctor. (h) The prescription is legible	To ensure that the patient is given the correct drug in the prescribed dose using the appropriate diluent and by the correct route (NMC 2008a: C; NPSA 2007:C). To protect the patient from harm. To comply with NMC (2008a) *Standards for Medicines Management.*

241

Procedure guidelines *(cont.)*

4 Select the required medication and check the expiry date.	Treatment with medication that is outside the expiry date is dangerous. Drugs deteriorate with storage. The expiry date indicates when a particular drug is no longer pharmacologically efficacious (NPSA 2007: C).
5 Wash hands with bactericidal soap and water or bactericidal alcohol handrub, and assemble necessary equipment.	To minimize the risk of infection (DH 2007: C).
6 Prepare the drug for injection as per procedure described earlier.	To prepare the drug correctly (E).
7 Prepare a 20 ml syringe of 0.9% sodium chloride (or compatible solution) for injection, as described, using aseptic technique.	To use for flushing between each drug (NPSA 2007: C).
8 Draw up flushing solution, as required by hospital policy.	To prepare for administration (E).
9 Place syringes in a clinically clean receptacle on the bottom shelf of the dressing trolley, along with the receptacle containing any drug(s) to be administered.	To ensure top shelf is used for sterile dressing pack in order to minimize the risk of contamination (E).
10 Collect the other equipment and place it on the bottom of the trolley.	To ensure all equipment is available to commence procedure (E).
11 Place a sterile dressing pack on top of the trolley.	To minimize the risk of contamination (E).
12 Check that all necessary equipment is present.	To prevent delays and interruption of the procedure (E).
13 Wash hands thoroughly.	To minimize the risk of infection (DH 2007: C).
14 Proceed to the patient and check identity with prescription chart and prepared drug.	To minimize the risk of error and ensure the correct patient (NPSA 2007: C).
15 Open the sterile dressing pack. Add lotion to wet the low-linting swab.	To gain access to equipment and to ensure the swab is soaked with cleaning solution (E).
16 Wash hands with bactericidal soap and water or with bactericidal alcohol handrub.	To reduce the risk of infection (DH 2007: C).
17 If a peripheral device is in situ, remove the bandage and dressing (if appropriate).	To observe the insertion site (E).
18 Inspect the insertion site of the device.	To detect any signs of inflammation, infiltration, etc. If present, take appropriate action (see Problem solving, below) (DH 2003c: C).
19 Observe the infusion, if in progress.	To confirm that it is infusing as desired (NPSA 2007: C) To prevent drug interaction. Some manufacturers may recommend that the drug is given into the injection site of a rapidly running infusion (NPSA 2007: C).

20	Check whether the infusion fluid and the drugs are compatible. If not, change the infusion fluid to 0.9% sodium chloride to flush between the drugs.	
21	Wash hands or clean them with an alcohol handrub.	To minimize the risk of infection (DH 2007: C).
22	Place a sterile towel under the patient's arm.	To create a sterile field (E).
23	Clean the injection site with a swab saturated with chlorhexidine in 70% alcohol and allow to dry.	To reduce the number of pathogens introduced by the needle at the time of the insertion. To ensure complete disinfection has occurred (Pratt *et al.* 2007: C).
24	Switch off the infusion or close the fluid path of a tap or stopcock.	To prevent excessive pressure within the vein. To prevent contact with an incompatible infusion fluid. To allow the nurse to concentrate on the site of insertion and injection (NPSA 2007: C).
25	If a peripheral device is in situ use a sterile 23 or 25 G needle if the injection is made through a resealable site and gently inject 0.9% sodium chloride. This may not be necessary if the patient has a 0.9% sodium chloride infusion in progress.	To enable resealing of the site at the end of the injection. To confirm patency of the vein. To prevent contact with an incompatible infusion solution (NPSA 2007: C).
26	Open the roller clamp of the administration set fully. Inject the drug at a speed sufficient to slow but not stop the infusion and inject the drug smoothly in the direction of flow at the specified rate.	To prevent a back-flow of drug up the tubing. To prevent excessive pressure within the vein. To prevent speed shock (NPSA 2007: C).
27	Ensure used needles and syringes are disposed of immediately into appropriate sharps container (or are returned to tray). Do not leave any sharps on opened sterile pack.	To reduce the risk of needlestick injury and to prevent contamination of pack (RCN 2005: C).
28	Observe the insertion site of the device throughout.	To detect any complications at an early stage, e.g. extravasation or local allergic reaction (Dougherty 2008: E).
29	Blood return and/or 'flashback' must be checked frequently throughout the injection (i.e. every 3–5 ml).	To confirm that the device is correctly placed and that the vein remains patent (Weinstein 2007: E).
30	Consult the patient during the injection about any discomfort, etc.	To detect any complications at an early stage, and ensure patient comfort (Dougherty 2008: E).
31	If more than one drug is to be administered, flush with 0.9% sodium chloride between administrations by restarting the infusion or changing syringes.	To prevent drug interactions (NPSA 2007: C).
32	At the end of the injection, flush with 0.9% sodium chloride by restarting the infusion or attaching a syringe containing 0.9% sodium chloride.	To flush any remaining irritant solution away from the device site (NPSA 2007: C).
33	Observe the insertion site of the cannula carefully.	To detect any complications at an early stage. Extra pressure within the vein caused by both fluid flow and injection of the drug may cause rupture of the vessel (Dougherty 2008: E).

243

Procedure guidelines (cont.)

34 After the final flush of 0.9% sodium chloride adjust the infusion rate as prescribed or open the fluid path of the tap/stopcock or use flushing solution.	To continue delivery of therapy. To maintain the patency of the cannula (Finlay 2008: E).
35 If a peripheral device is in situ cover the insertion site with new sterile low linting swab and tape it in place.	To minimize the risk of contamination of the insertion site (E).
36 Apply a bandage.	To reduce the risk of dislodging the cannula (E).
37 Assist the patient into a comfortable position.	To ensure the patient is comfortable (E).
38 Record the administration on appropriate charts.	To maintain accurate records, provide a point of reference in the event of any queries and prevent any duplication of treatment (NMC 2005: C).
39 Dispose of used syringes with needles, unsheathed, directly into a sharps container during procedure or place back on to plastic tray and then dispose of in a sharps container as soon as possible. *Do not* disconnect needle from syringe prior to disposal. Other waste should be placed into the appropriate plastic bags.	To avoid needlestick injury (MHRA 2004: C; NHS Employers 2005: C).

244

Problem solving: Injection and infusion of intravenous fluids and drugs

The problems associated with injection and infusion of intravenous fluids and drugs fall into two categories:

1 Local venous complications associated with the cannula insertion site.
2 Systemic problems which affect the whole patient, exerting effects on vital organs and their functions.

The nurse must regularly observe the insertion site, the infusion and the patient to detect any complications at the earliest possible moment and to prevent progression to more serious conditions. Early detection is aided by paying attention to the patient's comments of discomfort or pain. The patient's symptoms and physical signs both constitute reasons for resiting of the peripheral device or discontinuation of the infusion (Lamb & Dougherty 2008). Signs and symptoms are used as problem headings.

Problem	Possible causes	Preventive nursing measures	Suggested action
Infusion slows or stops.	Change in position of the following:		
	(a) Patient.	Check the height of the fluid container if the patient is active and receiving an infusion using gravity flow.	Adjust the height of the container accordingly. But the infusion should not hang higher than 1 m (above the patient) as the increased height will result in increased pressure and possible rupture of the vessel/device (Quinn 2008).
	(b) Limb.	Prevent by avoiding use of joints when inserting peripheral devices. Instruct the patient on the amount of movement permitted. Continued movement could result in mechanical phlebitis (Lamb & Dougherty 2008).	Move the arm or hand until infusion starts again. Secure the device, then bandage or splint the limb again carefully in the desired position. Take care not to cause damage to the limb.

Problem	Possible causes	Preventive nursing measures	Suggested action
	(c) Administration set.	Tape the administration set so that it cannot become kinked or occluded.	Check for kinks and/or compression if the patient is active or restless and correct accordingly.
	(d) Cannula.	Secure the cannula firmly to prevent movement. It may come into contact with the vein wall or a valve. Infusions sited in small veins are prone to this problem.	Remove the bandage and dressing and manoeuvre the peripheral device gently, without pulling it out of the vein, until the infusion starts again. Secure adequately.
Technical problems:			
	(a) Negative pressure prevents flow of fluid.	Ensure that the container is vented using an air inlet.	Vent if necessary, using venting needle.
	(b) Empty container.	Check fluid levels regularly.	Replace the fluid container before it runs dry.
	(c) Venous spasm due to chemical irritation or cold fluids/drugs.	Dilute drugs as recommended. Remove solutions from the refrigerator a short time before use.	Apply a warm compress to soothe and dilate the vein, increase the blood flow and dilute the infusion mixture.
	(d) Injury to the vein.	Detect any injury early as it is likely to progress and cause more serious conditions (see below).	Stop the infusion and request resiting of the cannula.
	(e) Occlusion of the device due to fibrin formation.	Maintain a continuous, regular fluid flow or ensure that patency is maintained by flushing. Instruct the patient to keep arm below the level of the heart if ambulant and attached to a gravity flow infusion.	**If peripheral device**: remove extension set/injection cap and attempt to flush the cannula gently using a 10 ml syringe of 0.9% sodium chloride. If resistance is met, stop and request a resiting of the peripheral device (see Chapter 45). **If central venous access device (CVAD)**: remove injection cap and attempt to flush the cannula gently using a 10 ml syringe of 0.9% sodium chloride. If resistance is met attempt to instil antifibrinolytic agent such as urokinase (see Chapter 45).

245

Problem solving *(cont.)*

Problem	Possible causes	Preventive nursing measures	Suggested action
	(f) The cannula has become displaced either completely or partially, i.e. fluid or drug has leaked into the surrounding tissues (infiltration). If the drugs were vesicant in nature this would then be defined as extravasation.	Secure the cannula and tape the administration set so that no stress is placed on them. Instruct the patient on the amount of movement permitted (Fabian 2000).	Confirm that infiltration of drugs has/has not occurred by: (i) inspecting the site for leakage, swelling, etc.; (ii) testing the temperature of the skin: it will be cooler if infiltration has occurred; (iii) comparing the size of the limb with the opposite limb. (iv) Once infiltration has been confirmed, stop the infusion and request a resiting of the device. If the infusion is allowed to progress, discomfort and tissue damage will result. Apply cold or warm compresses to provide symptomatic relief, whichever provides the most comfort for the patient. Reassure the patient by explaining what is happening. Document in care plan and monitor site (Lamb & Dougherty 2008). (v) If extravasation, follow hospital policy and procedure (see Chapter 12).
Erythema (inflammation) around the insertion site, and/or pain and swelling.	Phlebitis due to:	Observe the site regularly and use an assessment tool such as the VIP Scale to assess the site (Jackson 1998; DH 2003c). (See Figure 11.3.)	Failure to detect and act when phlebitis is at an early stage, for whatever reason, will result in painful and incapacitating thrombophlebitis. Dislodgement of a thrombus could cause a pulmonary embolus (Lamb & Dougherty 2008; Weinstein 2008).
	(a) Sepsis.	Adhere to aseptic techniques when performing all intravenous procedures (RCN 2005)	Stop the infusion, remove the device and resite the device. Follow hospital policy about sending cannula tip for bacterial analysis. Clean the area and apply a sterile dressing. Check regularly. Document.

Problem	Possible causes	Preventive nursing measures	Suggested action
	(b) Chemical irritation.	Dilute drugs according to instructions. Check compatibilities carefully to reduce the risk of particulate formation. Administer the drugs as an infusion instead of a bolus injection. Be aware of the factors involved, e.g. pH (Lamb & Dougherty 2008). Apply local heat above the cannula site (Lamb & Dougherty 2008). Apply a glycerol trinitrate (GTN) patch to aid vasodilatation (Wright *et al.* 1985).	Stop the infusion and resite the device. If the infusion is allowed to progress, tissue damage and severe pain will result. Apply warm compresses to provide symptomatic relief. Encourage movement of the limb. Reassure the patient by explaining what has happened. Document.
	(c) Mechanical irritation.	Secure the device and then bandage or splint the limb if the infusion is sited at a point of flexion. Use an extension set to minimize manipulation of the device. Instruct the patient on the amount of movement permitted (Campbell 1996; Jackson 1998; Taylor 2000).	Stop the infusion and remove the device. Resite the device. Although inflammation of this type progresses more slowly, it will cause discomfort. Provide symptomatic relief as above. Encourage movement and reassure the patient by explaining what has happened. Document.
	Infection with or without discharge.	Adhere to aseptic techniques when performing all intravenous procedures. Observe all recommendations for equipment changes, etc.	Stop the infusion, remove the peripheral device. Resite the peripheral device in opposite arm if possible. Follow hospital policy about sending device tip for bacterial analysis. If CVAD take a swab from exit site then clean the area and apply a sterile dressing. Check regularly. Observe the patient for signs of systemic infection.
	Cellulitis due to: (a) Sepsis. (b) Non-specific sterile inflammation.	As above.	As above. Due to the nature of the connective tissue any infection or inflammation spreads quickly, especially if the limb is oedematous.
	Local allergic reaction, e.g. flare reaction which occurs with anthracyclines such as doxorubicin.	Ask whether the patient has any allergies before administration of any drugs or fluids, including sensitivities to topical solutions, which may cause erythema at the site (NMC 2008a). Check whether the particular medication is commonly associated with local or venous flushing.	Observe the patient for systemic reaction. Treat the local area symptomatically. Reassure the patient. Inform medical staff. Document patient reaction.

Problem solving (cont.)

Problem	Possible causes	Preventive nursing measures	Suggested action
Local oedema.	During infusion or injection: (a) Infiltration. (b) Phlebitis. (c) Extravasation of medication (see Chapter 12).	Secure the device and tape the administration set so that no stress is placed on the cannula. Use an extension set. Instruct the patient on the amount of movement permitted. Check regularly for swelling, e.g. tightness of bandages or around rings. Observe the patient carefully throughout drug administration.	Stop the infusion, remove the peripheral device then resite the device in opposite arm if possible. Apply warm compresses to provide symptomatic relief. Reassure the patient by explaining what is happening. Stop the injection immediately extravasation is suspected. Act in accordance with hospital policy. Some drugs may cause inflammation and supportive, symptomatic relief will be required. Others may have the potential to cause necrosis of tissue and further action may be necessary. Document.
Oedema of the limb.	Infiltration.	Tape the device and administration set so that no stress is placed on the device, which in turn can lead to damage of the vein. Use an extension set. Instruct the patient on the amount of movement permitted. Check regularly for swelling, as above.	Stop the infusion, remove the peripheral device then resite the device in opposite arm if possible. Provide symptomatic relief and support. Reassure the patient.
	Circulatory overload.	Administer infusion fluids at the prescribed rate and do not make sudden alterations of flow. Use infusion equipment wherever possible and administration set with anti-free-flow systems. Be aware of the patient's renal and cardiac status. Monitor intake and output routinely (Lamb & Dougherty 2008; Weinstein 2007).	Slow the infusion. Monitor vital signs for increase in blood pressure and respirations. Place the patient in an upright position and keep him/her warm to promote peripheral circulation and relieve stress on the central veins. Reassure the patient. Notify a doctor immediately.
	Thrombosis.	Ensure the tip is located in correct position.	The patient may require ultrasound to diagnose a clot in the arm. If confirmed then the patient will require anticoagulation. The device may be removed.
Pain at the insertion site.	All of the previous listed conditions may be accompanied by soreness or pain.	As previously listed.	Provide local symptomatic relief, e.g. warmth, as required. Administer systemic analgesia, as prescribed, if necessary.

Problem	Possible causes	Preventive nursing measures	Suggested action
Pyrexia, rigors, tachycardia.	Septicaemia.	Adhere to aseptic techniques when performing all intravenous procedures. Inspect all equipment, infusion fluids, etc., before use. Observe recommendations for additives, equipment changes and general management. Avoid the use of equipment that can increase the risk of contamination, e.g. stopcocks (Finlay 2008; Lamb & Dougherty 2008).	Notify a doctor immediately. Follow hospital policy about sending equipment for bacterial analysis.
Decrease in blood pressure, tachycardia, cyanosis, unconsciousness.	Embolism: (a) Air.	Check the containers and change before they run through, especially bottles. Clear all air from tubing before commencing infusion. Check all connections regularly and make sure they are secure. Use infusion equipment with air in line detectors.	Turn the patient onto left side and lower the head of the bed to prevent air from entering the pulmonary artery. Notify a doctor immediately. Administer oxygen (RCN 2005; Lamb & Dougherty 2008; Weinstein 2007). Reassure the patient.
	(b) Particle.	Check all infusion fluids before and after any additions have been made. Check drug compatibility and stability. Flush adequately between solutions. Observe the solution throughout the infusion for precipitate formation (Finlay 2008).	As above, but also change the container and administration set. Replace with new equipment and 0.9% sodium chloride infusion from a different batch. Follow hospital policy about sending contaminated fluid and equipment for bacterial analysis.
Itching, rash, shortness of breath.	Allergic reaction due to sensitivity to an intravenous fluid, additive or drug.	Ask the patient whether he/she has any allergies before administration of any drugs or fluids. Check whether the particular medication is commonly associated with any allergic reactions and observe the patient during treatment.	Stop drug infusion or injection and maintain the patency of the vascular access device using 0.9% sodium chloride. Notify a doctor immediately. Reassure the patient. Ensure that hydrocortisone and epinephrine are available. Document.
Flushed face, headache, congestion of the chest, possibly progressing to loss of consciousness.	Speed shock due to too rapid administration of drugs. May be a small volume (Lamb & Dougherty 2008; Weinstein 2007).	Administer drugs and infusion at the correct rate. Check the flow rate frequently. Use infusion equipment with anti-free-flow administration sets if the delivery rate is crucial.	As above.

249

Problem solving *(cont.)*

Figure 11.3 Vein infusion phlebitis scale (VIP Scale) (Jackson 1998)

References and further reading

Arduino, M.J. *et al.* (1997) Microbiological evaluation of needle-less and needle access devices. *Am J Infect Control*, **25**(5), 377–80.

Arndt, M. (1994) Research and practice: how drug mistakes affect self-esteem. *Nurs Times*, **90**(15), 27–31.

Audit Commission (2001) *A Spoonful of Sugar: Medicines Management in NHS Hospitals*. Audit Commission, London.

Beyea, S.C. & Nicholl, L.S.H. (1995) Administration of medications via the intramuscular route: an integrative review of the literature and research based protocol for the procedure. *Appl Nurs Res*, **5**(1), 23–33.

Bird, C. (1990) A prescription for self-care. *Nurs Times*, **86**(43), 52–5.

BNF (2008) *British National Formulary*. BMJ Publishing Group Ltd, London.

Brenneis, C. *et al.* (1987) Local toxicity during subcutaneous infusion of narcotics. *Cancer Nurs*, **10**(4), 172–6.

Bridge, J., Hemingway, S. & Murphy, K. (2005) Implications of non medical prescribing of controlled drugs. *Nurs Times*, **101**(44), 32–3.

British Pharmacopoeia (2007) *British Pharmacopoeia*, The Stationary Office, London.

Brock, A.M. (1979) Self-administration of drugs in the elderly. *Nurs Forum*, **18**(4), 340–57.

Brown, J., Moss, H. & Elliot, T. (1997) The potential for catheter microbial contamination from a needleless connector. *J Hosp Infect*, **36**(3), 181–9.

Campbell, J. (1996) Intravenous drug therapy. *Prof Nurse*, **11**(7), 437–42.

Central Health Services Council (1958) *Report of Joint Sub-Committee on the Control of Dangerous Drugs and Poisons in Hospitals* (Chairman J.K. Aitken). HMSO, London.

Cole, D. (1999) Selection and management of central venous access devices in the home setting. *J Intraven Nurs*, **22**(6), 315–19.

Constans, T. *et al.* (1991) Hypodermoclysis in dehydrated elderly patients – local effects with and without hyaluronidase. *J Palliat Care*, **7**(2), 10–12.

Cookson, S. *et al.* (1998) Increased blood stream infection rates in surgical patients associated with variation from recommended use and care following implementation of a needleless device. *Infect Control Hosp Epidemiol*, **19**(1), 23–7.

Cresswell, J. (1999) *Nurse Prescribing Handbook*. Association of Nurse Prescribing and Community Nurse, UK.

Dann, T.C. (1969) Routine skin preparation before injection: an unnecessary procedure. *Lancet*, ii, 96–7.

Danzig, L.E. *et al.* (1995) Bloodstream infections associated with a needleless intravenous infusion system in patients receiving home infusion therapy. *JAMA*, **273**(23), 1862–4.

Dawkins, L. *et al.* (2000) A randomised trial of winged Vialon cannulae and metal butterfly needles. *Int J Palliat Nurs*, **6**(3), 110–16.

Deeks, P. & Byatt, K. (2000) Are patients who self-administer their medicines in hospital more satisfied with their care? *J Adv Nurs*, **31**(2), 395–400.

DH (1988) *Guidelines for the Safe and Secure Handling of Medicines (The Duthie Report)*. HMSO, London.

DH (1989) *Report of the Advisory Group on Nurse Prescribing*. Crown One. HMSO, London.

DH (1998) *Review of Prescribing, Supply and Administration of Medicines. A Report on the Supply and Administration of Medicines under Group Protocols*. Crown Two. HMSO, London.

DH (1999) *Review of Prescribing, Supply and Administration of Medicines. Final Report*. Crown Three. HMSO, London.

DH (2000) Patient Group Directions (HSC 2000/026) Health and Safety Commission London.

DH (2001a) Guidelines for preventing infections associated with the insertion and maintenance of central venous catheters. *J Hosp Infect*, **47**(Suppl), S47–67.

DH (2001b) *National Service Framework for Older People*. HMSO, London.

DH (2003a) *Supplementary Prescribing*. National Health Service, London. (www.doh. gov.uk/supplementary prescribing).

DH (2003b) *Supplementary Prescribing by Nurses and Pharmacists within the NHS in England: a guide for implementation*. National Health Service, London.

DH (2003c) *Winning Ways: Working Together to Reduce Healthcare-Associated Infection in England*. Department of Health, London.

DH (2003d) *Building a Safer NHS for Patients: Improving Medication Safety*. Department of Health, London.

DH (2004) *Extending Independent Nurse Prescribing within the NHS in England: a Guide to Implantation*. Department of Health, London.

DH (2005a) *Saving Lives: A Delivery Programme to Reduce Healthcare-associated Infection including MRSA*. Department of Health, London.

DH (2005b) *Hazardous waste (England) regulations*. Department of Health, London.

DH (2006) *Improving Patients Access to Medicines – a Guide to Implementing Nurse and Pharmacist Independent Prescribing within the NHS in England*. Department of Health, London.

DHSS (1976) *Health Services Development, Addition of Drugs to Intravenous Fluids, HC(76)9 (Breckenridge Report)*. HMSO, London.

Dickman, A., Schneider, J. & Varga, J. (2005) *The Syringe Driver: Continuous Infusions in Palliative Care*, 2nd edn. Oxford University Press, Oxford.

Dorr, T. & Von Hoff, D. (1993) *Cancer Chemotherapy Handbook*, 2nd edn. Appleton & Lange, Hemel Hempstead.

Dougherty, L. (2002) Delivery of intravenous therapy. *Nurs Stand*, **16**(16), 45–52.

Dougherty, L. (2008) Obtaining peripheral access. In: *Intravenous Therapy in Nursing Practice* (eds L. Dougherty & J. Lamb), 2nd edn. Blackwell Publishing, Oxford.

Downie, G., MacKenzie, J. & Williams, A. (Eds) (2000) Administration of medicines. In: *Pharmacology and Drugs Management for Nurses*, 2nd edn. Churchill Livingstone, London, pp. 495–557.

Epperson, E.L. (1984) Efficacy of 0.9% sodium chloride injection with and without heparin for maintaining indwelling intermittent injection sites. *Clin Pharm*, 3, 626–9.

Fabian, B (2000) IV complications: Infiltration. *J Intraven Nurs*, **23** (4), 229–31.

Field, P.A. (1981) A phenomenological look at giving an injection. *J Adv Nurs*, **6**(4), 291–6.

Finlay, T. (2008) Safe administration of IV therapy. In: *Intravenous Therapy in Nursing Practice* (eds L. Dougherty & J. Lamb), 2nd edn. Blackwell Publishing, Oxford.

Gabriel, J. (2005) Vascular access: Indications and implications for patient care. *Nursing Standard*, **19** (26) 45–52.

Gatford, J. & Anderson, R. (1998) *Nursing Calculations*, 5th edn. Churchill Livingstone, Edinburgh.

Gladstone, J. (1995) Drug administration errors: a study into the factors underlying the occurrence and reporting of drug errors in a district general hospital. *J Adv Nurs*, **22**(4), 628–37.

251

Glynn, A. *et al.* (1997) *Hospital Acquired Infection – Surveillance Policies and Practice*. Central Public Health Laboratory, London.

Griffith, R. & Jordan, S. (2003) Administration of medicines part 1: the law and nursing. *Nurs Stand*, **18**(2), 47–53.

Hanchett, M. & Kung, L.Y. (1999) Do needleless intravenous systems increase the risk of infection? *J Intraven Nurs*, **22**(6), 117–21.

Hart, S. (2008) Infection control in IV therapy. In: *Intravenous Therapy in Nursing Practice* (eds L. Dougherty & J. Lamb), 2nd edn. Blackwell Publishing, Oxford.

Higgins, D. (2005) Drug Calculations. *Nurs Times*, **101**(46), 24–5.

HMSO (1968) *Medicines Act*. HMSO, London.

HMSO (1971) *Misuse of Drugs Act*. HMSO, London.

HMSO (2001) *Misuse of Drugs Regulations*. HMSO, London.

Hockley, J. *et al.* (1995) Audit to pinpoint IV drug administration pitfalls. *Nurs Times*, **91**(51), 33–4.

Hutton, M. (1998) Numeracy skills for IV calculations. *Nurs Stand*, **12**(43), 49–56.

Hyde, L. (2002) Legal and professional aspects of intravenous therapy. *Nurs Stand*, **16**(26), 39–42.

Hyde, L. (2008) Legal and professional aspects of IV therapy. In: *Intravenous Therapy in Nursing Practice* (eds L. Dougherty & J. Lamb), 2nd edn. Blackwell Publishing, Oxford.

Jackson, A. (1998) A battle in vein infusion phlebitis. *Nurs Times*, **94**(4), 68–71.

Jordan, S., Griffiths, H. & Griffith, R. (2003) Administration of medicines part 2: pharmacology. *Nurs Stand*, **18**(3), 45–54

Kain, V. *et al.* (2006) Developing guidelines for syringe driver management. *Int J Palliat Nurs*, **12**(2), 60–8.

King, L. (2003) Subcutaneous insulin injection technique. *Nurs Stand*, **17**(34), 45–52.

Koivistov, V.A. & Felig, P. (1978) Is skin preparation necessary before insulin injection? *Lancet*, **i**, 1072–3.

Kuhn, M.M. (1989) *Pharmacotherapeutics. A Nursing Process Approach*, 2nd edn. F.A. Davis, Philadelphia.

Lamb, J. & Dougherty, L. (2008) Local and systemic complications of intravenous therapy. In: *Intravenous Therapy in Nursing Practice* (eds L. Dougherty & J. Lamb), 2nd edn. Blackwell Publishing, Oxford.

Latter, S. *et al.* (2005) *An Evaluation of Extended Formulary Independent Nurse Prescribing: Executive Summary of Final Report*. University of Southampton, Southampton.

Laverty, D., Mallett, J. & Mulholland, J. (1997) Protocols and guidelines for managing wounds. *Prof Nurse*, **13**(2), 79–80.

Lenz, C.L. (1983) Make your needle selection right to the point. *Nursing*, **13**(2), 50–1.

Luebke, M.A. *et al.* (1998) Comparison of the microbial barrier properties of a needleless and conventional needle based intravenous access system. *Am J Infect Control*, **26**, 437–41.

Luker, K. & Wolfson, D. (1999) Introduction. In: *Medicines Management for Clinical Nurses* (eds K. Luker & D. Wolfson). Blackwell Science, Oxford.

Luker, K.A. *et al.* (1998) Nurse–patient relationships: the context of nurse prescribing. *J Adv Nurs*, **28**, 235–42.

Mallett, J. *et al.* (1997) Nurse prescribing by protocol. *Nurs Times*, **93**(8), 50–2.

Martin, P.J. (1994) Professional updating through open learning as a method of reducing errors in the administration of medicines. *J Nurs Manage*, **2**(5), 209–12.

McClelland, B. (2007) *Handbook of Transfusion Medicine*, 3rd edn. HMSO, London.

McGraw, C. & Drennan, V. (2001) Self administration of medicine and older people. *Nurs Stand*, **15**(18), 33–6.

McHale, J. (2002) Extended prescribing: the legal implications. *Nurs Times*, **98**(32), 36–8.

Mendelson, M.H. *et al.* (1998) Study of a needleless intermittent intravenous access system for peripheral infusions: analysis of staff, patient and institutional outcomes. *Infect Control Hosp Epidemiol*, **19**(6), 401–6.

MHRA (2004) *Reducing Needlestick and Sharps Injuries*. Medicines and Healthcare Products Regulatory Agency, London.

MHRA (2005) *Consultation on Options for the Future of Independent Prescribing by Extended Formulary Nurse Prescribers*. Medicines and Healthcare Products Regulatory Agency, London.

Mitten, T. (2001) Subcutaneous drug infusions: a review of problems and solutions. *Int J Palliat Nurs*, **7**(2), 75–85.

Moriarty, D. & Hudson, E. (2001) Hypodermoclysis for rehydration in the community. *Br J Community Nurs*, **6**(9), 437–43.

NHS Employers (2005) *The Management of Health, Safety and Welfare Issues for NHS Staff*. NHS Confederation (Employers) Company, London.

NHS Executive (2000) *Health Service Circular HSC 2000/26. Patient Group Directions (England Only)*. SI 2000, No. 1919. NHS Executive, Leeds.

NHSE (1998a) *Nurse Prescribing. A Guide for Implementation*. HMSO, London.

NHSE (1998b) *Nurse Prescribing. Implementing the Scheme across England*. HSC 1998/232. HMSO, London.

NICE (2003) *Technology Appraisal Guidance No 57. Guidance on the Use of Continuous Subcutaneous Insulin Infusion for Diabetes*. National Institute for Health and Clinical Excellence, London.

Nicolson, H. (1986) The success of the syringe driver. *Nurs Times*, **82**, 49–51.

NMC (2001a) *Covert Administration of Medicines can be Justified*. Press statement, 5th September. Nursing and Midwifery Council, London.

NMC (2001b) *UKCC Position Statement on the Covert Administration of Medicines – Disguising Medicine in Food and Drink*. Nursing and Midwifery Council, London.

NMC (2001c) *Circular 25/2002*. Nursing and Midwifery Council, London.

NMC (2005) *Guidelines for Records and Record Keeping*. Nursing and Midwifery Council, London.

NMC (2006a) *Standards of Proficiency for Nurse and Midwife Prescribers*. Nursing and Midwifery Council, London.

NMC (2006b) *A–Z Advice Sheet Consent*. www.nmc.org.

NMC (2008a) *Standards for Medicines Management*. Nursing and Midwifery Council, London.

NMC (2008b) *The Code: Standards of Conduct, Performance and Ethics for Nurses and Midwives*. Nursing and Midwifery Council, London.

Noble-Adams, R. (1995) Dehydration: subcutaneous fluid administration. *Br J Nurs*, **4**(9), 488–94.

NPC (2001) *Maintaining Competency in Prescribing: an Outline Framework to Help Nurse Prescribers*. National Health Service, London.

NPC (2003a) *Supplementary Prescribing. A Resource to Help Healthcare Professionals to Understand the Framework and Opportunities*. National Health Service, London.

NPC (2003b) *Maintaining Competency in Prescribing: an Outline Framework to Help Nurse Supplementary Prescribers*. National Health Service, London.

NPSA (2005) *Wristbands for Hospital Inpatients Improves Safety (Safer Practice Notice 11)*. NPSA, London.

NPSA (2006) *Ensuring Safer Practice with High Dose Ampoules of Morphine and Diamorphine, Alert No. 2006/12, 25th May.* NPSA, London.

NPSA (2007) *Promoting Safer Use of Injectable Medicines, Alert No. 2007/20, 28th March.* NPSA, London.

Osbourne, J., Blais, K. & Hayes, J.S. (1999) Nurses' perceptions: when is it a medication error? *J Nurs Admin*, **29**(4), 33–8.

Peragallo-Dittko, V. (1997) Rethinking subcutaneous injection technique. *Am J Nurs*, **97**(5), 71–2.

Perdue, L. (2001) Intravenous complications. In: *Intravenous Therapy: Clinical Principles and Practices* (eds J. Hankins *et al.*), 2nd edn. W.B. Saunders, Philadelphia, pp. 418–45.

Perucca, R. (2001) Obtaining vascular access. In: *Intravenous Therapy: Clinical Principles and Practices* (eds J. Hankins *et al.*), 2nd edn. W.B. Saunders, Philadelphia, pp. 375–88.

Pickstone, M. (1999) *A Pocketbook for Safer IV Therapy.* Medical Technology and Risk Series. Scitech Educational Ltd, Kent.

Pratt, R.J. *et al.* (2007) Epic 2: national evidence-based guidelines for preventing healthcare-associated infections in NHS hospitals in England. *J Hosp Infect*, **65**(1)(Suppl), S1–S12.

Quinn, C. (2008) Flow control. In: *Intravenous Therapy in Nursing Practice* (eds L. Dougherty & J. Lamb), 2nd edn. Blackwell Publishing, Oxford.

RCN (2005) *Standards for Infusion Therapy.* Royal College of Nursing, London.

Regnard, C.F. & Davies, A. (1986) *A Guide to Symptom Relief in Advanced Cancer.* Haigh and Hochland, Manchester.

Rochon, P. *et al.* (1997) A systematic review of the evidence for hypodermoclysis to treat dehydration in older people. *J Gerontol*, **52A**(3), M169–76.

Rodger, M.A. & King, L. (2000) Drawing up and administering intra-muscular injection: a review of the literature. *J Adv Nurs*, **31**(3), 574–82.

Royal Pharmaceutical Society of Great Britain (1997) *From Compliance to Concordance.* Royal Pharmaceutical Society of Great Britain, London.

Sasson, M. & Shvartzman, P. (2001) Hypodermoclysis: an alternative infusion technique. *Am Fam Physician*, **64**(9), 1575–8.

Sexton, J. (1999) The nurse's role in medicines administration – legal and procedural framework. In: *Medicines Management for Clinical Nurses* (eds K. Luker & D. Wolfson). Blackwell Science, Oxford.

Shepherd, M. (2002a) Medicines 2. Administration of medicines. *Nurs Times*, **98**(16), 45–8.

Shepherd, M. (2002b) Medicines 3. Managing medicines. *Nurs Times*, **98**(17), 43–6.

Shuttleworth, A. (2005) Are nurses ready to take on the BNF? *Nurs Times*, **101**(48), 29–30.

Simmonds, B.P. (1983) CDC guidelines for the prevention and control of nosocomial infections: guidelines for prevention of intravascular infections. *Am J Infect Control*, **11**(5), 183–9.

Taxis, K. & Barber, N. (2003) Ethnographic study on the incidence and severity of intravenous drug errors. *BMJ*, **326**, 684–7.

Taylor, N.J. (2000) Fascination with phlebitis. *Vasc Access Devices*, **5**(3), 24–8.

The Medicinal Products: Prescription by Nurse etc Act (1992)

Torre, M. (2002) Subcutaneous infusion: non-metal cannulae vs metal butterfly needles. *Br J Community Nurs*, **7**(7), 365–9.

Torrence, C. (1989) Intramuscular injection, part 1 and 2. *Surg Nurses*, **2**(5), 6–10; **2**(6), 24–7.

Treloar, A., Beats, B. & Philpot, M. (2000) A pill in the sandwich: covert medication in food and drink. *J R Soc Med*, **93**, 408–11.

Trissel, L.A. (2003) *Handbook on Injectable Drugs*, 12th edn. American Society of Health System Pharmacists, Bethesda, MD.

Trounce, J. & Gould, D. (2000) *Clinical Pharmacology for Nurses*, 16th edn. Churchill Livingstone, London.

Viola, R., Wells, G. & Peterson, J. (1997) The effects of fluid status and fluid therapy on the dying: a systematic review. *J Palliat Care*, **13**(4), 41–52.

Watt, S. (2003) Safe administration of medines to children: part 2. *Paediatr Nurs*, **15**(5), 40–4.

Weinstein, S.M. (2007) *Plumer's Principles and Practices of Intravenous Therapy*, 8th edn. Lippincott, Philadelphia.

Whittington, Z. (2008) Pharmacological aspects of IV therapy. In: *Intravenous Therapy in Nursing Practice* (eds L. Dougherty & J. Lamb), 2nd edn. Blackwell Publishing, Oxford.

Workman, B. (1999) Safe injection techniques. *Nurs Stand*, **13**(39), 47–52.

Wright, A. *et al.* (1985) Use of transdermal glyceryl trinitrate to reduce failure of intravenous infusion due to phlebitis and extravasation. *Lancet*, **ii**, 1148–50.

253

Chapter 12

Drug administration: cytotoxic drugs

255 Reference material
257 *Procedure guidelines:* Cytotoxic drugs: environmental precautions
261 *Procedure guidelines:* Cytotoxic drugs: accidental exposure
262 **Routes of administration**
262 **Intravenous administration**
262 Reference material
264 *Procedure guidelines:* Cytotoxic drugs: intravenous administration
266 **Extravasation of vesicant drugs**
266 Reference material
272 *Procedure guidelines:* Extravasation management: peripheral cannula
274 **Oral administration**
274 Reference material
275 **Intramuscular and subcutaneous injection**
275 Reference material
275 **Topical application**
275 Reference material
276 **Intrathecal administration**
277 Reference material
278 **Intrapleural instillation**
278 Reference material
279 *Procedure guidelines:* Cytotoxic drugs: intrapleural administration
280 *Problem solving:* Intrapleural cytotoxic drug administration
280 **Intravesical instillation**
280 Reference material
281 *Procedure guidelines:* Cytotoxic drugs: intravesical instillation
282 *Problem solving:* Intravesicular instillation of cytotoxic drugs
283 **Intraperitoneal administration**
283 Reference material
284 *Procedure guidelines:* Cytotoxic drugs: intraperitoneal instillation
285 *Problem solving:* Intraperitoneal instillation of cytotoxic drugs
285 **Intra-arterial administration**
285 Reference material
287 *Problem solving:* Intra-arterial administration of cytotoxic drugs
288 References and further reading

Definition

The term cytotoxic literally translated means 'toxic to cells'. Hence these drugs are those which kill cells (malignant or non-malignant).

Reference material

Cancer chemotherapy has its origins from observations of the effects of sulphur mustard gas during World War 1. There are now many drugs licensed for the treatment of cancer and most of these drugs (with the exception of anti-hormonal drugs used to treat breast and prostate cancers) target rapidly dividing cells either through the effects on DNA or factors involved in mitosis (Kelland 2005).

Cancer drugs can be classified into the following categories: alkylating agents; antimetabolites; antimicrotubule agents; topoisomerase inhibitors and anti-hormonal agents. An understanding of the cell cycle is important when considering the use of anti-cancer drugs because the drugs can either act on the phases of the cell cycle or act independently of the cell cycle (Kelland 2005). Chemotherapy can be administered as single agent or in combination regimens. The use of chemotherapy does have health and safety implications for health care personnel.

Cytotoxic drug handling by nursing, pharmacy and other health care professionals is an occupational hazard (Weinstein 2007). Cytotoxic drugs have been shown to be mutagenic, teratogenic and carcinogenic when given at therapeutic levels to animals and humans to destroy malignant cells (MARCH guidelines 2007; Weinstein 2007). Patients have been shown to develop secondary cancers as a result of treatment with cytotoxic drugs and such risks may be acceptable when patients have a life-threatening illness (Ferguson & Wright 2003). However, these effects are not acceptable to personnel involved in the reconstitution and administration of cytotoxic drugs and the handling of waste and spills. The risk to health associated with exposure is measured by the time, dose and routes of exposure. Since safe levels of exposure to hazardous agents cannot be determined because of the lack of a reliable monitoring method to measure exposure risks, the need for personal protective equipment is vital for the protection of health care workers. Cytotoxic drugs can be absorbed through the skin (although with the majority of the compounds there is little or no absorption through intact skin, the exceptions are those which are lipid soluble) (Weinstein 2007). Skin exposure can be by contact with contaminated equipment used in preparing or administering the drugs or during the handling and disposal of waste. A study by Pethran *et al.* (2003) demonstrated that antineoplastic drugs were found in the urine of nurses and pharmacy personnel who were involved in the handling of cytotoxic drugs (Pethran *et al.* 2003). On the basis of the evidence available at present, risks to personnel involved in the reconstitution and administration of cytotoxic drugs fall into three categories: short-term effects; reproductive risks; and systemic effects:

- Short-term effects are usually caused by direct contact with the skin, eyes and mucous membranes, e.g. dermatitis, inflammation of mucous membranes, excessive lacrimation, pigmentation, blistering (associated with mustine) and other miscellaneous, allergic reactions (Dranitsaris *et al.* 2005; Weinstein 2007). Cytotoxic drugs may also have harmful short- or long-term systemic effects if inhaled or ingested during preparation. These effects include light-headedness, dizziness, nausea, headache, rashes and skin discoloration (Hayden & Goodman 2005).

- Reproductive risks include the inability to conceive following exposure to a cytotoxic drug. A number of experimental studies have suggested that serious long-term effects may result from exposure to cytotoxic drugs during pregnancy. Effects include chromosomal abnormalities (Harrison 2001) and reproductive function disorders including infertility (Valanis *et al.* 1997). It has been shown that although alterations in cell structure have been detected, they appear to be transient and of a low level. It has yet to be demonstrated whether these changes in cell structure are harmful and whether this level of mutagenesis can be equated with more serious consequences. There are also many limitations in testing blood and urine due to the range of agents which cannot be detected, low levels of drugs and metabolites and reduced sensitivity of the tests (Ferguson & Wright 2003). This has led to difficulties when offering staff monitoring and surveillance and it is less common to do extensive biological testing as there are no data to support a cause and effect in cell structure.

- The hazards of handling cytotoxic drugs are well recognized along with the requirement to adhere to safety measures recommended in order to protect all staff who prepare, administer and handle cytotoxic drugs or waste products. Control of Substances Hazardous to Health (COSHH) Regulations were introduced and updated in 2002 (DH 2002b). Employers are obliged to: identify substances that are a hazard to staff and others who may be exposed; manage how the drugs should be handled; and what to do in the event of a spill or accident. The regulations state that health care personnel should have access to the ideal environment, protective clothing, policies and procedures, a system of monitoring and recording effects, and any necessary equipment such as spill kits. This includes consideration of the following:

1 The environment: the most effective means of minimizing the hazard is to arrange for all cytotoxic drugs to be prepared on a named patient basis by trained pharmacy staff in a specially equipped area (MARCH 2003; Polovich *et al.* 2005). Chemotherapy should be reconstituted in a vertical class II or III biological safety cabinet with laminar flow or an isolator if drugs are prepared on the ward (Ferguson & Wright 2003; Hayden & Goodman 2005; Weinstein 2007). Cabinets should be situated

Figure 12.1 Protective clothing required when dealing with a spillage.

in a specified or dedicated area with access restricted to trained or supervised personnel.

2 Protective clothing: protective clothing should always be worn during all types of cytotoxic drug handling. There are minimum requirements for the type and degree of protective clothing which are based on possible exposure and type of environment.

(a) Gloves: disposable gloves should be worn at all times and appear to be the only type of protective clothing which most practitioners consistently wear when handling cytotoxic drugs. Polovich *et al.* (2005) cites

94–99% of nurses routinely wearing gloves when handling hazardous materials. No type of glove is completely impermeable to every cytotoxic agent and there is no consensus as to which glove material offers the best protection (Hayden & Goodman 2005; Weinstein 2007; Gabriel 2008). The key points to consider when selecting gloves are thickness and integrity as the main factors which affect permeation rates include glove thickness, lipophilicity, the nature of the solvent in which the cytotoxic drug is dissolved and glove material composition (Ferguson & Wright 2003; Polovich *et al.* 2005). Using poor-quality low-cost gloves is neither safe nor cost effective. The risk of allergic reactions in health care workers to latex and powdered medical gloves has been well documented in recent years. The National Health Service Executive (NHSE) issued a Health Service Circular (HSC) (DH 1999) which recommended that health care organizations limit their use of these types of gloves. Powder-free gloves should be used for handling cytotoxic drugs and should be inspected for any defects before use. Gloves should be changed regularly (every 1 hour) during each work session or at the end of a work session, and immediately if contaminated with cytotoxic agent or punctured (Polovich 2003; Polovich *et al.* 2005). The use of gloves made of other material such as nitrile provides protection when dealing with a cytotoxic spill. Double gloving is recommended when reconstituting cytotoxic drugs (Polovich 2003; Polovich *et al.* 2005; Weinstein 2007).

(b) Gowns: the literature supports the use of a disposable gown for both reconstitution and administration. It has been suggested that a long-sleeved, non-absorbent gown made of a low-linting, low-permeability material such as Tyvek is used (Cass *et al.* 1997; Weinstein 2007). Armlets and plastic aprons can be used as a substitute for long-sleeved gowns during administration (HSE 2003; Polovich *et al.* 2005).

(c) Goggles: goggles are used to protect the eyes from splashes and particles; they should fully cover the eyes of the handler. Goggles should meet BS EN 166–8 requirements and be worn whenever reconstituting chemotherapy, where there is a possibility of splashing, or dealing with a spill (Ferguson & Wright 2003) (see Figure 12.1).

(d) Masks: these should be worn whenever there is a possibility of inhalation or the drug is being prepared in an uncontrolled environment. Masks should conform to BS EN 149 : 1992 standard. The key factor with regard to requirements for respiratory protective equipment is that it fits well and is sealed properly to the wearer's face. A range of different sizes of disposable masks should be made available to health care workers (Ferguson & Wright 2003). A suitable dust mask or particulate respirator, such as the 3M 8810, affords the best protection.

There is no doubt that the existence of a formal hospital policy for handling has been shown to have a positive influence in the use of personal protective equipment. Minimizing occupational exposure to hazardous drugs, and therefore reducing health risks for personnel, can only be achieved by the strict adherence to policies and procedures regarding the safe handling of cytotoxic drugs (Ferguson & Wright 2003; Polovich 2003; Polovich *et al.* 2005).

Risk assessment

A full risk assessment under the COSHH Regulations must be made by all departments and wards handling, preparing or administering cytotoxics (DH 2002b). The assessment should identify all appropriate procedures for the safety of staff. A generic COSHH assessment form for the administration and reconstitution of chemotherapy out of hours should be kept in all ward COSHH assessment files. Ward sisters/charge nurses have a duty to ensure that all staff on the ward are made aware of the COSHH assessment procedures. The questionnaire should include details of the individual performing the procedure, patient's details and the reason for which the reconstitution was performed. Information from the questionnaires can then be collated and passed to the safety committee, e.g. the Safe Handling of Hazardous Therapeutic Substances (SHOHTS) Committee, which should include the consultant occupational health doctor and representatives from pharmacy, clinical divisions, wards and Health and Safety. All cases of reconstitution out of hours should be reviewed and procedures that do not comply with the Safe Handling Policy investigated. Recommendations can then be proposed to the Health and Safety Committee.

Occupational health offers staff protection by monitoring. Routine health surveillance should be carried out for staff directly involved in handling cytotoxics on a regular basis, e.g. certain staff working in the pharmacy (Box 12.1). The Cytotoxic Health Surveillance Programme comprises of regular general health screening as well as specific tests to determine if an individual has been exposed to harmful levels of cytotoxic substances.

Box 12.1 Cytotoxic health questionnaires

1 Annual 'cytotoxic health questionnaires' which cover:
   - Detailed medical history of the individuals.
   - Exposure record.
   - Personal protective equipment used.
   - Control measures in place.
   - Symptoms which may be attributed to the effects of harmful levels of cytotoxic drugs, e.g. headache, dizziness, eye or skin irritation.
2 Six-monthly blood tests are taken, which include full blood count, urea and electrolytes and liver function tests.
3 Six-monthly urinalysis is performed to detect raised protein, presence of glucose, blood and bilirubin and to detect any abnormal cytology.
4 In the event that any abnormalities are present, the individual is referred to the occupational health doctor.

The Health and Safety Executive (HSE 2003) have produced a document on the safe handling of cytotoxic drugs. National evidence-based guidelines have been implemented in an attempt to reduce exposure, provide adequate protective equipment, ensure regular staff monitoring and provide effective written procedures for dealing with preparation, administration, disposal and dealing with spills and accidents. In order to limit exposure, cytotoxic drugs should be prepared only by skilled, knowledgeable and experienced health care professionals (Polovich *et al.* 2005; RCN 2005).

257

Procedure guidelines Cytotoxic drugs: environmental precautions

The safest method of reconstituting cytotoxic drugs outside a pharmacy department is to use an isolator (Figure 12.2). There is a variety of systems and each will have specific instructions for its use. The following procedure is for the Envair 'Mini-Iso' isolator. The system creates a negative pressure in the isolator by drawing air out by a fan and passing it through a HEPA filter, which will trap any cytotoxic drug powder or aerosol which may escape from the drug vial during reconstitution (Polovich *et al.* 2005).

When used as instructed the isolator will minimize the risk to nurses when reconstituting any dose of cytotoxic drugs, but it will not protect the drug from the risk of microbial contamination so aseptic technique must always be used.

Nursing staff should not be involved in the routine reconstitution of cytotoxic drugs, as this is the function of the pharmacy department. However, there may be emergency situations when the nurse is requested to prepare chemotherapy and it is essential that this is performed safely. It should only be undertaken by competent, confident staff who have received appropriate training and have previous experience in the procedures required. The following procedure should be used for guidance. Protective clothing is absolutely vital when using the isolator.

. . . .

Cytotoxic reconstitution using an isolator

Equipment

1 One pair of disposable non-sterile gloves.
2 Syringes, needles.

3 Drug to be reconstituted and appropriate diluent.
4 Appropriate cleaning solution.

. . . .

Procedure guidelines *(cont.)*

Procedure

Action	Rationale
1 Prior to commencing reconstitution carefully check the gauntlets, especially the fingers and at the point of attachment to the isolator.	The gauntlets are designed for prolonged use, they need to be changed when torn or punctured (Manufacturer's instructions: C).
2 Place hand through slot on right of the top cover of the isolator and press the green button.	To enable the isolator to be switched on (Manufacturer's instructions: C).
3 Allow the isolator to run for 3–4 minutes and ensure that the gauge needle is reading over 50 pascals before use.	To ensure that the isolator is prepared to be operated safely (E).
4 Assemble all equipment required.	To avoid interruption of work (E).
5 Put on two pairs of non-sterile gloves, which should be worn under the isolator gloves and when passing equipment into or out of the isolator.	To provide extra operator protection in case of damage to the gauntlets while preparing the drug (E).
6 Open the door on the right side of the isolator by turning the handle anticlockwise through 180°.	To allow equipment to be placed inside the isolator (E).
7 Place equipment into the isolator and close and lock the door (by turning 180° clockwise).	To ensure doors are securely closed so that negative pressure can be achieved (Manufacturer's instructions: C).
8 Place hands into gauntlets.	
9 Reconstitute the dose in the usual way (see Chapter 11) using aseptic technique.	To minimize the risk of contamination (E).
10 Move everything to the right prior to removing hands from gauntlets.	To enable easy removal of the prepared drug and waste (E).
11 Leave the isolator fan on.	To ensure any spills/aerosols are contained within the isolator (E).
12 Open the isolator door and remove all equipment.	
13 Dispose of waste in usual way.	To reduce the risk of contamination and needlestick injury (DH 2005: C; HSE Guidelines 2003: C).
14 Moisten a sheet of paper with cleaning spray provided and wipe inside of isolator.	To maintain equipment in good clean working order (Manufacturer's instructions: C).
15 Turn off isolator by pushing green button.	
16 Complete cytotoxic reconstitution surveillance form and send to occupational health department.	To ensure follow-up and health surveillance check (E).

Cytotoxic spillage management

Equipment

1 Two plastic overshoes.
2 Two disposable armlets.
3 Two clinical waste bags.
4 Two pairs of disposable non-sterile latex or nitrile gloves.
5 Goggles (non-disposable): EN 166–8.
6 Particulate respirator mask.
7 Plastic apron.
8 Gown.
9 Paper towels.
10 Plastic bucket.
11 Copy of spillage procedure.

Procedure

Action	Rationale
1 Act immediately. Assess the level of exposure of any individual and isolate them from the spill.	Any spillage may become a health hazard (Polovich et al. 2005:C).
2 Collect spillage kit.	It contains all necessary equipment (Polovich et al. 2005: C).
3 Put on both pairs of gloves, goggles and a gown and then a disposable plastic apron over the gown (see Figure 12.1).	To provide personal protection (E).
4 If there is visible powder spill, put on a good-quality particulate respirator mask.	To prevent inhalation of powder (E).
5 If spillage is on the floor, put on overshoes.	For protection and to minimize the spread of contamination (E).
6 Wipe up powder spillage quickly with well dampened paper towels, starting at the outer edge of the spill area and working in a circular motion towards the middle to contain spill (Weinstein 2007) and dispose of them as 'high-risk' waste.	To prevent dispersal of powder. To prevent spread of contamination to a wider area. To protect others and ensure safe disposal by incineration (DH 2005: C; Weinstein 2007: E).
7 Mop up liquids which have been spilled on a hard surface with paper towels, starting at the outer edge of the spill area and working in a circular motion towards the middle to contain spill (Cass et al. 1997), and dispose of them as 'high-risk' waste.	To prevent spread of contamination to a wider area. To protect others and ensure safe disposal by incineration (DH 2005: C; E).
8 Wash hard surfaces at least twice with copious amounts of cold, soapy water and dry with paper towels. The floor should then be given a routine clean as soon afterwards as possible. If spillage has occurred on a carpet it will require cleaning as soon as possible.	To remove residual contamination (E).
9 If spillage is on clothing, remove it as soon as possible and treat as 'soiled linen'.	To decontaminate clothing without hazard to laundry staff (E).
10 If spillage has penetrated clothing, wash contaminated skin liberally with soap and cold water.	To decontaminate skin and prevent drug absorption (E).
11 If spillage is on bed linen put on gloves and an apron, change it immediately and treat as 'soiled linen'.	To protect the patient. To protect the laundry staff (E).

Procedure guidelines *(cont.)*

12 If an accident or spillage involving direct skin contact occurs, the area should be washed thoroughly with soapy water as soon as possible. In the event of a cytotoxic splash to the eye, irrigate thoroughly with 0.9% sodium chloride or tap water for at least 15 minutes.	To decontaminate the area and minimize the risk of drug absorption and damage (Weinstein 2007: E).
13 Any accident or spillage by nursing staff involving direct skin contact with a cytotoxic drug must be reported to the occupational health department and manager as soon as possible after the first aid is performed and appropriate documentation completed (see Guidelines below).	To ensure that details of accidental contact are entered in the nurse's health record, and appropriate follow-up is initiated (Polovich *et al.* 2005: C).

Cytotoxic spillage: health surveillance

Action

1 Complete cytotoxic incident investigation form:
   - Full details of the incident.
   - Details of the immediate first aid provided, e.g. washing and removal of contaminated clothing.
   - Details of personal protective equipment worn at the time.
   - The full name of the drug involved and the individual components of the constituent, including diluents.
2 A risk assessment is performed using the information provided. The risk assessment evaluates the health association with the exposure which itself is measured by the time, dose and routes of exposure.
3 Completion of the Cytotoxic Health Questionnaire which includes a detailed medical history of the individual and examination. Details of immediate effects are noted, e.g. skin effects, headaches, dizziness, and if changes are present the employee is referred to the occupational health doctor for further assessment, advice and treatment.
4 Blood tests are taken which include routine blood count and biochemistry and liver function tests.
5 Urinalysis is performed and details of protein, glucose, blood, bilirubin and bladder cytology are noted.
6 The occupational health nurse will contact the Health and Safety Team to obtain details of risk assessments performed on the ward.
7 Repeat bloods should be taken on day 7 and day 28 following the incident and any health effects noted. If there are any changes, the employee should be referred to the occupational health doctor.

Cytotoxic waste disposal

Action	**Rationale**
1 'Sharps' should be placed in the special container provided.	To ensure incineration and to prevent laceration and/or inoculation during transit and disposal (DH 2005: C; E).
2 Dry waste, intravenous administration sets and other contaminated material should be placed in 'high-risk' waste disposal bags. The practitioner should wear gloves and an apron.	To ensure careful handling and disposal by incineration and prevent practitioner from surface contamination (DH 2005: C; Polovich *et al.* 2005: C).
3 Any part dose of a drug remaining should be placed in a special waste container.	
4 Reusable trays and other equipment should be washed with copious amounts of water followed by the usual procedure for disinfection.	To reduce the risk of cross-contamination and cross-infection (E).
5 Unused doses of cytotoxics should be returned, unopened, to the pharmacy.	To enable them to be relabelled and reissued, stability permitting, or to be destroyed safely (E).

Cytotoxic drugs: disposal of excreta
Universal protective clothing should always be worn when handling patient's body fluids, for example disposable gloves and gown. Goggles should be worn if there is any risk of splashing, thus minimizing risk to all staff (RCN 2005).

Figure 12.2   An isolator.

Procedure guidelines   Cytotoxic drugs: accidental exposure

Action	Rationale
1 Contamination of the skin, mucous membranes and eyes should be treated promptly. All areas should be washed with copious amounts of tap water or 0.9% sodium chloride for at least 15 minutes (Polovich 2003). Eye wash may be available.	To minimize the risk of any local damage to tissue (Polovich *et al.* 2005: C; Weinstein 2007: E).
2 Accidental infiltration of the skin with a vesicant drug should be treated as an extravasation and the appropriate procedure followed (see Management of extravasation section, below).	To minimize the risk of any local damage to tissue (E).
3 If erythema and/or other local reaction occurs in any circumstances, contact the occupational health unit or a member of the medical staff so that appropriate treatment may be advised.	To prevent further damage and/or complications (E).
4 It is essential after any accident involving direct contact with a cytotoxic drug, or if any local or systemic symptoms occur after handling such a drug, that the occupational health unit should be contacted.	To assist with recording and monitoring of staff exposure (Polovich *et al.* 2005: C).
5 If pregnancy is suspected or intended, the occupational health unit should be contacted.	To discuss future work patterns and any anxiety that may be felt (E).

Routes of administration

Cytotoxic drugs can be administered via a variety of routes (see Chapter 11). However, regardless of the route used there are certain preadministration principles which the nurse should apply. The nurse should remember that the administration of medicines is a collaborative process which involves the nurse, doctor and pharmacist (NMC 2008a). The nurse must identify and remedy any knowledge or practice deficit and operate within the limit of his/her competence (NMC 2008b). Cytotoxic drugs should be administered by a knowledgeable and skilled practitioner.

1 *Provision of information*: The provision of patient information is an integral part of the care pathway. The patient should be fully informed of all the possible side-effects of chemotherapy, how to cope with any side-effects at home, types of supportive therapy they may receive, as well as where and how they are to receive the drugs. Patients should then receive written information, which can be used to reinforce verbal explanation and will enable patients to spend time reading and formulating any questions about treatments (van der Molen 2005; Infusion Nurses Society 2006; NMC 2008b). The main aim of providing information is to help the patient and their family to: gain control, reduce anxiety, improve compliance, develop realistic expectations, promote self-care, enhance participation, and generate feelings of safety and security (van der Molen 2005). The nurse should consider barriers to effective communication, for example hearing difficulties, sight difficulties, culture and language difficulties, and plan realistic interventions in respect of such barriers.

2 *Gaining the patient's consent*: Patients have a fundamental and ethical right to determine what happens to their bodies, and consent is central to all aspects of health care delivery. The nurse when gaining valid consent must be sure that: the patient is a legally competent person, and gives consent voluntarily after being fully informed of what they are consenting to (NMC 2008b). Written consent must be obtained before chemotherapy is commenced and every time the patient is changed from one protocol/regimen to another. The standard National Health Service (NHS) consent form dictates the amount of information necessary in order to obtain valid consent. For example, if there is a possibility that the patient may require a blood transfusion then the patient and the doctor must sign to state that this has been discussed with the patient. One copy of the consent form is kept in the medical notes whilst the other is given to the patient (DH 2002a).

3 *Ascertaining whether the patient is fit for treatment*, e.g. full blood count, renal function: certain blood results are required in order to:
   (a) Calculate the dose of drug, e.g. in the case of platinum-based drugs, ethylenediaminetetra-acetic

acid (EDTA), or if 24-hour urine collection for creatinine is required (Polovich *et al.* 2005).
   (b) Ensure that the patient is fit enough to receive the treatment. If any of the blood results are too low, then supportive therapy may be prescribed.

4 *Calculating body surface area*: This is done by using the patient's height and weight and should be performed everytime a cycle or dose of chemotherapy is given. The patient's height and weight should be recorded on the prescription chart, ideally by the person who performed the recording. The surface area is then determined, and this will be used to calculate the dose of chemotherapy drug.

Knowledge of the chemotherapy regimen

The nurse should ensure that he/she has checked the five rights:

- The right patient.
- The right drug chemotherapy regimen (many chemotherapy prescriptions are computer-generated to reduce the risk of error).
- The right dose.
- The right time.
- The right route of administration. (NMC 2008a; Finlay 2008.)

The prescription should be signed by the medical practitioner and verified by a pharmacist. Electronic prescribing and the use of computer-generated prescriptions may reduce the risk of medication error.

Intravenous administration

Definition

This is the administration of cytotoxic drugs via a peripheral or central vein and is the most commonly used route for the administration of cytotoxic drugs.

Indications

Intravenous administration enables:

- Rapid and reliable delivery of a cytotoxic drug to the tumour site.
- Rapid dilution of a drug which reduces local irritation and the risk of tissue damage.
- Accurate titration of drug to achieve desired effect.

Reference material

Choosing the appropriate device

Cytotoxic drugs may be administered via a winged infusion device, a peripheral cannula or a central venous access

Table 12.1   Arguments for using either a large- or small-gauge peripheral vascular access device.

Larger	Smaller
1 Enables irritant drugs to reach general circulation quickly, without irritating peripheral veins	1 Less chance of puncturing the posterior vein wall
2 Administration time is decreased and therefore patient does not need to spend as much time in a stressful environment	2 Less likely to cause trauma and result in scar formation
	3 Less pain on needle insertion
	4 Increased blood flow around small needle increases dilution of drug and reduces risk of chemical phlebitis

device (CVAD). A winged infusion device is used mainly for bolus injections of non-vesicant drugs, due to the potential risk of infiltration associated with steel needles (Gabriel 2008). A peripheral cannula is used for bolus injections and short or intermittent infusions of both vesicant and non-vesicant drugs (Table 12.1). However, this device is associated with phlebitis and requires repeated resiting every 72–96 hours (Scales 2005; Infusion Nurses Society 2006; Gabriel 2008). A central venous catheter is useful for patients with poor venous access, those at high risk of extravasation and for those undergoing long-term, high-dose or continuous infusional chemotherapy (Weinstein 2007; Gabriel 2008). These devices are associated with infection and thrombosis (Dougherty 2006).

When the peripheral route is used a winged infusion device or cannula may be used. The insertion site of choice should be the large veins of the forearm (cephalic or basilic) as these are easier to access, reduce the risk of chemical phlebitis and result in fewer problems if extravasation should occur (Weinstein 2007). The next area of choice would be the dorsum of the hand, then the wrist. The antecubital fossa should only be used as the last resort as it can limit movement and is associated with problems if extravasation occurs in this area (Weinstein 2007; Gabriel 2008). The general rule is to start distally and proceed proximally where possible and also to alternate the arms (Weinstein 2007) to ensure that the same veins are not being used and damaged by chemical and mechanical irritation (Scales 2005).

When using the peripheral intravenous route the following should be adhered to:

- Patency should be checked at the start of administration by achieving a blood return and then flushing with 10 ml of 0.9% sodium chloride to ensure there is no resistance, swelling or pain. Blood return should then be checked after every 2–4 ml of drug is administered (Weinstein 2007; Gabriel 2008).
- The site should be assessed for signs of phlebitis.
- The site should be observed when a bolus injection is administered, particularly if a vesicant drug, for signs of infiltration or extravasation.
- Certain vesicants must not be administered as infusions into a peripheral vein as the risk of extravasation and

damage is greater than via the central venous route (Weinstein 2007).

In addition, where possible a new site should be used for vesicants, to ensure the vein is healthy and patent, although this may not always be possible. There are some controversial issues related to peripheral intravenous cytotoxic drug administration (Table 12.2).

CVADs have the advantage of providing a more reliable form of vascular access. This is because the problems associated with peripheral devices such as phlebitis, venous irritation and pain are eliminated as central venous access enables rapid dilution and circulation of the drug. However, extravasation can still occur as a result of: catheter tip malposition, catheter malfunction, a damaged catheter, port needle dislodgement or fibrin sheath formation along the length of the catheter, faulty equipment, human error and system problems (Mayo 1998; Dougherty 2006).

Methods

Cytotoxic drugs may be administered as a direct bolus injection, a bolus via the side arm of a rapid infusion of 0.9% sodium chloride or a continuous infusion. The choice is dependent on:

- The type of cytotoxic drug, e.g. etoposide is only given as an infusion.
- Pharmacological considerations, e.g. stability, need for dilution.
- Degree of venous irritation, e.g. vinorelbine is a highly irritant drug.
- Whether the drug is a vesicant.
- The type of device in situ (Gabriel 2008).

The advantage of the bolus injection is that the integrity of the vein and any early signs of extravasation can be observed more easily than during an infusion. However, bolus injections can increase the risk of venous irritation due to the

Table 12.2   Controversial issues: use of antecubital fossa.

For	Against
1 Larger veins permit rapid infusion of drug	1 Mobility is restricted
2 Larger veins allow irritant drugs to reach general circulation more quickly and with less irritation than small veins	2 Risk of extravasation is increased if patient tends to be mobile
3 Easier to palpate and therefore increases successful insertion of device	3 Early recognition of extravasation is difficult due to the deep veins. This means there is less chance of observing swelling which could go undetected. The patient may also have a delayed reaction to pain
	4 Damage can result in loss of structure and function, ulceration and fibrosis

263

constant contact of the drug with the intima of the vein, resulting in pain, which make it difficult to differentiate between venous spasm and extravasation (Gabriel 2008). It could also lead to inappropriate rapid administration of the drug (Weinstein 2007).

Bolus injections administered via the side arm of a rapid infusion of solution ensure greater dilution of potentially irritating drugs and enable rapid removal of the drug from the insertion site and smaller vessels. The disadvantages are that a small vein may not allow rapid flow of the infusate and this may result in the drug backing up the tubing, causing the practitioner to clamp the tubing whilst checking for blood return and flow rate of the infusate, there-fore interrupting constant observation of the site (Gabriel 2008).

Adding the drug to an infusion bag allows for greater dilution, thus reducing the possibility of chemical irritation. Some drugs may only be administered as infusions owing to the type of side-effects associated with them (e.g. hypotension with etoposide) and long-term continuous infusions, e.g. 5-fluorouracil (5-FU), may also be necessary to reduce the risk of side-effects such as diarrhoea. Patency and device position cannot be easily assessed and the longer the infusion, the greater the possibility of device dislodgement, extravasation or infiltration and general complications associated with the device (Weinstein 2007).

Procedure guidelines   Cytotoxic drugs: intravenous administration

The aim of the procedure for administration of chemotherapy intravenously is to protect both nurse and patient from contamination and also to prevent extravasation of drugs which could result in local tissue damage. The large majority of cytotoxic agents will be delivered to the ward/unit individually packaged for delivery to a named patient, by injection or infusion. If this is not so, specific guidelines should be followed (see Procedure guidelines: Cytotoxic drugs: environmental precautions, above). Equipment such as Luer-lok syringes and needle-free administration sets help protect the nurse and patient from contamination.

Procedure

Action	Rationale
1 Explain and discuss the procedure with the patient. Evaluate the patient's knowledge of cytotoxic therapy. If this knowledge appears to be inadequate, offer an explanation of the use, action, dose and potential side-effects of the drug or drugs involved.	To ensure that the patient understands the procedure and gives his/her valid consent. The patient has a right to information (DH 2002a: C; van der Molen 2005; NMC 2008b: C).
2 Put on gloves and an apron before commencing the procedure.	To protect the nurse from local contamination of skin or clothing (Polovich 2003; Polovich *et al.* 2005: E). *Note*: with careful handling technique, this risk is minimal but splashes can occur when changing syringes or infusion containers. Always change infusion bags over a deep plastic tray to contain any splashes.
3 Prepare necessary equipment for an aseptic administration procedure.	To minimize the risk of local and/or systemic infection. Patients are frequently immunosuppressed and at greater risk of hospital-acquired infection.
4 Check that all details on the syringe or infusion container are correct when compared with the patient's prescription, before opening the sterile packaging.	To ensure the patient is given the correct drug which has been dispensed for him/her. To prevent wastage.
5 Be aware of the immediate effects of the drug.	To observe the patient during administration. To be prepared to manage any side-effects that occur.
6 Take the medication and the prescription chart to the patient. Check the patient's identity, drug, dose, route and timing of administration.	To prevent error and comply with professional guidelines (NMC 2008a: C).
7 Inspect the device site, and consult the patient about sensation around the device insertion site.	To detect any problems, e.g. phlebitis, which would render the device unusable (Dougherty 2006; Lavery & Ingram 2006: P).

8 Check the patency of the vein for blood return and then flush using 0.9% sodium chloride.	To determine whether the vein will accommodate the extra fluid flow and irritant drugs and remain patent.
9 Protect the patient from contact with the drugs by: (a) Ensuring the needle (if used) is inserted or a syringe (if using a needle-less injection system) is attached carefully into the injection site of the administration set, extension set or injection cap.	To prevent exiting on the other side of the intravenous equipment and contaminating or inoculating the patient.
(b) Take care when removing the blind hub, changing needles/syringes, and inserting the administration set into the infusion container or changing bags (which must be done with the bag lying flat on a hard surface).	To avoid leakage or splashes and contamination of the nurse or patient. To prevent mis-spiking the bag and puncturing it.
(c) Secure a good connection between needle and syringe by always using Luer–Lok syringes.	To prevent leakage or separation, which may occur due to pressure during administration, resulting in spray and contamination.
(d) Checking the injection site or injection cap at the end of the procedure.	To ensure that there is no leakage.
(e) Act promptly if any contamination of an individual is noted by washing the area with soap and water.	To prevent any local skin reaction (itchiness, redness or inflammation of the skin). To prevent absorption on skin, mucous membranes, etc (Polovich 2003; Polovich *et al.* 2005: C).
10 Administer drugs in the correct order, antiemetics then cytotoxic drugs, i.e. vesicants first.	To ensure that those agents likely to cause tissue damage are given when venous integrity is greatest, i.e. at the beginning of the administration process (Gabriel 2008: E).
11 Ensure the correct administration rate.	To prevent 'speed shock'. To prevent extra pressure and irritation within the vein.
12 Observe the vein throughout for signs of infiltration or extravasation, e.g. swelling or leakage at the site of injection. Note the patient's comments about sensation at the site, e.g. pain.	To detect any problems at the earliest moment. To prevent any damage to soft tissue, and to enable the remainder of the drug(s) to be given correctly at another site. To enable prompt treatment to be given, thus minimizing local damage, and possibly preserving venous access for future treatment. (For further information see Management of extravasation section, below.)
13 Flush the device with 5–10 ml 0.9% sodium chloride between drugs and after administration.	To prevent drug interaction. To prevent leakage of drug from the puncture site, on removal of the device.
14 Be aware of the patient's comfort throughout the procedure.	To minimize trauma to the patient. To involve the patient in treatment and detect any side-effects and/or problems that may then be avoided at the next treatment.
15 Record details of the administration in the appropriate documents.	To prevent any duplication of treatment and to provide a point of reference in the event of queries and adhere to professional guidelines (*Guidelines for Records and Record Keeping*) (NMC 2005: C).

Extravasation of vesicant drugs

Definition

Extravasation is the inadvertent administration of vesicant solution or medication into surrounding tissues which can lead to tissue necrosis, while infiltration is the inadvertent administration of non-vesicant solutions/medications into the surrounding tissues (Polovich *et al.* 2005; RCN 2005; Infusion Nurses Society 2006). A vesicant is any solution or medication that causes the formation of blisters with subsequent tissue necrosis (Polovich *et al.* 2005; Hayden & Goodman 2005). Vesicants can be DNA and non-DNA binding, with DNA binding not only causing tissue injury but resulting in a far more prolonged course (Goolsby & Lombardo 2006). Irritants are drugs capable of causing inflammation and irritation but if these drugs infiltrate they rarely cause any tissue breakdown (Stanley 2002; Polovich *et al.* 2005; Hayden & Goodman 2005). Flare reaction is a local inflammatory reaction to an agent manifested by red tracking along the vein or red blotches but without pain (although the area may feel itchy) (Polovich *et al.* 2005). It occurs in 3–6% of patients (How & Brown 1998). It is caused by a venous inflammatory response to histamine release, is characterized by redness and blotchiness and may result in the formation of small weals, having a similar appearance to a nettle rash. It usually subsides in 30–60 minutes, with 86% resolving within 45 minutes (How & Brown 1998; Hayden & Goodman 2005), but it responds well within a few minutes to the application of a topical steroid (Weinstein 2007).

Reference material

Extravasation is a well-recognized complication of intravenous (IV) chemotherapy administration, but in general is a condition that is often under-diagnosed, undertreated and under-reported (Stanley 2002). The incidence of extravasation is estimated to be between 0.5 and 6.0% of cytotoxic drug administration (Kassner 2000; Khan & Holmes 2002; Lawson 2003; Masoorli 2003; Goolsby & Lombardo 2006) with some estimates for peripheral extravasation between 23 and 25% (Roth 2003). CVADs have decreased the incidence

Table 12.3   Drug sequencing – rationale for administering vesicant drugs first or last (Stanley 2002; Weinstein 2007).

Vesicants first	Vesicants last
1 Vascular integrity decreases over time	1 Vesicants are irritating and increase vein fragility
2 Vein is most stable and least irritated at start of treatment	2 Venous spasm may occur and mask signs of extravasation
3 Initial assessment of vein patency is most accurate	
4 Patient's awareness of changes more acute	

of extravasation but it can still occur, usually as a result of a leaking or damaged catheter, fibrin sheath formation (Mayo 1998) or a port needle dislodgement (Schulmeister 1998). The incidence estimated is up to 6% with ports (Masoorli 2003). However, whilst the incidence is lower, the severity of the injuries is far greater as detection tends to occur later (Kassner 2000; Stanley 2002; Polovich *et al.* 2005). Even when practitioners have many years of experience, extravasation of vesicant agents can occur and is an extremely stressful event, but is not in itself an act of negligence (Weinstein 2007). Early detection and treatment are crucial if the consequences of an untreated or poorly managed extravasation are to be avoided (Figure 12.3). These may include:

- Pain from necrotic areas.
- Physical defect.
- The cost of hospitalization and plastic surgery.
- Delay in the treatment of disease.
- Psychological distress.
- Litigation: nurses are now being named in malpractice allegations, and extravasation injuries are an area for concern (Dougherty 2003; Masoorli 2003; Roth 2003; Weinstein 2007).

Prevention of extravasation

The nurse's focus should be on safe intravenous technique and implementing strategies to minimize the risk (Weinstein 2007). This includes the following strategies.

Monitoring the site

Confirming venous patency by flushing with 0.9% sodium chloride solution with at least 5–10 ml prior to administration of vesicants and frequent monitoring thereafter (Goolsby & Lombardo 2006; Weinstein 2007). Checking blood return after every 2–5 ml is recommended but cannot be relied upon as the key sign when giving a bolus injection, and monitoring the site every 5–10 minutes for any swelling (Weinstein 2007).

Location of the device

The most appropriate site for the location of a peripheral cannula is considered to be the forearm (Schrijvers 2003; Weinstein 2007). However, a large straight vein over the dorsum of the hand is preferable to a smaller vein in the forearm (Weinstein 2007). Siting over joints should be avoided as tissue damage in this area may limit joint movement in the future. It is also recommended that the antecubital fossa should never be used for the administration of vesicants because of the risk of damage to local structures such as nerves and tendons (Hayden & Goodman 2005; Weinstein 2007; Gabriel 2008). Avoid venepuncture sites in limbs with impaired circulation, sclerosis, thrombosis or scar formation. Also avoid cannulation below a recent venepuncture site (Goolsby & Lombardo 2006).

Figure 12.3   Extravasation.

Patients at risk

Patients who are at increased risk of extravasation (Box 12.2) should be observed more closely and cared for with extra caution.

Sequence of drugs (Table 12.3)

Vesicants should be given first (Kassner 2000; Hayden & Goodman 2005; Goolsby & Lombardo 2006). Reasons for this include:

1 Vascular integrity decreases over time.
2 Vein is most stable and least irritated at start of treatment.

Box 12.2   Patients at risk of extravasation*

- Infants and young children.
- Elderly patients.
- Those who are unable to communicate, e.g. sedated, unconscious, confused, language issues.
- Those with chronic diseases, e.g. cancer, peripheral vascular disease, superior vena cava (SVC) syndrome, lymphoedema.
- Those on medications: anticoagulants, steroids.
- Those who have undergone repeated intravenous cannulation/venepuncture.
- Those with fragile veins or who are thrombocytopenic.

*Polovich *et al.* 2005; Hayden & Goodman 2005; Sauerland *et al.* 2006.

---

3 Initial assessment of vein patency is most accurate.
4 Patient's awareness of changes more acute (Weinstein 2007).

Types of devices

The use of steel needles is associated with a greater risk of extravasation and should be discouraged and a plastic cannula should be used instead (Schrijvers 2003; Polovich *et al.* 2005; Sauerland *et al.* 2006). Vesicants should be given via a newly established cannula wherever possible (Dougherty 2005; Goolsby & Lombardo 2006) and consideration should be given to changing the cannula site after 24 hours (Hayden & Goodman 2005). However, if the fluid runs freely, there is good blood return and there are no signs of erythema, pain or swelling at the site, there is no reason to inflict a second cannulation on the patient (Weinstein 2007). Consideration should be given to a CVAD if peripheral access is difficult.

Method of administration

Many vesicants must be given as a slow bolus injection, often via the side arm of a fast-running intravenous infusion of a compatible solution, e.g. doxorubicin or epirubicin via an infusion of 0.9% sodium chloride. If repeated infusions are to be given then a CVAD may be more appropriate (Stanley 2002; Weinstein 2007).

Table 12.4   Nursing assessment of extravasation versus other reactions (Polovich *et al.* 2005; Weinstein 2007).

Assessment parameter	Flare reaction	Venous irritation	Extravasation — Immediate manifestations, i.e. during drug administration	Extravasation — Delayed manifestations, i.e. from 24 hours after extravasation
Pain	None	Aching, throbbing sensation along vein and in the limb	Severe stinging or burning pain (not always present). This can last from minutes to hours and will eventually subside. Occurs during drug administration at the device site and surrounding areas	Can continue following extravasation or start within 48 hours
Redness	Immediate blotches or tracking along the vein. This will subside within 30–45 minutes with or without treatment (usually steroid cream)	Vein may become red or darkened	Not always present immediately: more likely to see blanching of the skin. As area becomes inflamed redness will appear around the device site	Later occurrence
Swelling	Unlikely	Unlikely	May occur immediately but may not always be easy to identify immediately	Usually within 48 hours
Blood return	Usually present	Usually present but may require application of heat to improve blood return	Inability to obtain blood return (peripheral or central) but blood return may be present throughout	
Ulceration	Unlikely	Unlikely	Unlikely	Can occur within 48–96 hours but may take 3–4 weeks to develop
Others	Urticaria	None	Change in quality of the infusion or pressure on the syringe	Local tingling and sensory deficits

Skill of the practitioner

Correct choice of device and location, the ability to use the most appropriate vasodilatation techniques, early recognition of extravasation and prompt action come from ensuring only skilled and knowledgeable practitioners administer vesicant drugs and/or insert the vascular access device (Schrijvers 2003; Dougherty 2005; Goolsby & Lombardo 2006; Sauerland *et al.* 2006). Successful cannulation at the first attempt is ideal, as vesicants have been known to seep into tissues at a vein entry site of a previous cannulation (Gault & Challands 1997; Perdue 2001). This also includes accessing a port as it is vital that the correct selection of needle is made and that the device is secured adequately (Camp Sorrell 2005).

Patient information

Patients should be informed of the potential problems of administering vesicants and the possible consequences of extravasation (Stanley 2002; Sauerland *et al.* 2006; Weinstein 2007). Adequate information given to patients will ensure early recognition and co-operation as patients are the first to notice pain. The patient should be urged to report immediately any change in sensation such as burning or stinging (Goolsby & Lombardo 2006).

Drugs capable of causing tissue necrosis

Before administration of vesicant cytotoxic drugs the nurse should know which agents are capable of producing tissue necrosis. The following is a list of examples of those in common use:

Group A drugs	Group B drugs
Vinca alkaloids	Amsacrine
Vinblastine	Carmustine (concentrated solution)
Vindesine	Dacarbazine (concentrated solution)
Vinorelbine	Dactinomycin
Vincristine	Daunorubicin
Vinflunine	Doxorubicin
Paclitaxel	Epirubicin
	Idarubicin
	Mithramycin
	Mitomycin C
	Mechlorethamine
	Streptozocin

If in any doubt, the drug data sheet should be consulted or reference made to a research trial protocol. Drugs should not be reconstituted to give solutions which are higher than the manufacturer's recommended concentration, and the method of administration should be checked, e.g. infusion, injection.

A variety of vesicant non-cytotoxic agents in frequent use are also capable of causing severe tissue damage if extravasated. Examples include:

Group A drugs	Group B drugs
Calcium chloride	Aciclovir
Calcium gluconate	Amphotericin
Phenytoin	Cefotaxime
Hypertonic solutions, e.g.	Diazepam
sodium chloride >0.9%	Ganciclovir
Sodium bicarbonate (>5%)	Potassium chloride
	(>40 mmol/l)
Glucose 50%	Mannitol

This potential hazard should always be remembered. The actions listed in this procedure may not be appropriate in all these instances. Drug data sheets should always be checked and the pharmacy departments should be consulted if the information is insufficient, regarding action to take if a vesicant drug extravasates.

Signs and symptoms of extravasation (see Table 12.4)

Extravasation should be suspected if:

1 The patient complains of burning, stinging pain or any other acute change at the injection site, although this is not always present (Hayden & Goodman 2005). This should be distinguished from a feeling of cold, which may occur with some drugs, or venous spasm which can be caused by irritation usually accompanied by pain described as an achiness or tightness (Hayden & Goodman 2005). Any change of sensation warrants further investigation (Goolsby & Lombardo 2006).
2 Swelling is the most common symptom (Polovich et al. 2005). Induration or leakage may also occur at the injection site. Swelling may not always be immediately obvious if the patient has the cannula sited in an area of deep subcutaneous fat, in a deep vein or if the leak is via the posterior vein wall (Dougherty 2005).
3 Blanching of the skin occurs (Comerford et al. 2002). Erythema can occur around the injection site but this is not usually present immediately (Hayden & Goodman 2005). It is important that this is distinguished from a 'flare' reaction (Polovich et al. 2005).
4 Blood return is one of the most misleading of all signs particularly related to peripheral devices. In peripheral devices, if blood return is sluggish or absent this may indicate lack of patency or incorrect position of the device. However if no other signs are apparent this should not be regarded as an indication of a non-patent vein, as a vein may not bleed back for a number of reasons and extravasation may occur even in the event of good blood return (Hayden & Goodman 2005). Any change in blood flow should be investigated (Hayden & Goodman 2005; Weinstein 2007). In CVADs there should always be blood return and if this is absent steps should be followed in or-

der to be able to verify correct tip and needle position or resolve a fibrin sheath (see Figure 45.1).
5 A resistance is felt on the plunger of the syringe if drugs are given by bolus (Vandergrift 2001; Stanley 2002).
6 There is absence of free flow when administration is by infusion, once other reasons have been excluded, e.g. position (Vandergrift 2001; Stanley 2002).

Note: one or more of the above may be present. If extravasation is suspected or confirmed, the injection or infusion must be stopped immediately and action must be taken (Polovich et al. 2005; Infusion Nurses Society 2006; Weinstein 2007).

Management of extravasation

The management of extravasation of chemotherapy agents is controversial and there is little documented evidence of efficacy. Until recently, no antidote has received clear validation in controlled clinical trials and no randomized trials managing cytotoxic extravasation in humans have been completed (Bertolli 1995). Some studies performed on animals have demonstrated both effective and ineffective treatments but extrapolation from animals to humans is limited (Polovich et al. 2005; Wickham et al. 2006). Other studies have been small with low numbers of patients. Another problem is that it is often difficult to ascertain whether any extravasation has actually occurred (Weinstein 2007). Therefore recommendations are based on more consistent experimental evidence, cumulative clinical experience from available case reports and uncontrolled studies and empirical guidelines (Bertolli 1995). Drugs where there is evidence of effective management include: anthracyclines (Rudolph & Larson 1987), vinca alkaloids (Bertolli 1995), computed tomography (CT) contrast media (Federle et al. 1998) and paclitaxel (Bertolli et al. 1997).

The management of extravasation involves several stages including the following.

Stage 1: stopping infusion/injection and aspirating the drug

It appears that most authors are agreed that aspirating as much of the drug as possible, as soon as extravasation is suspected, is beneficial (Rudolph & Larson 1987; Vandergrift 2001; Polovich et al. 2005; Weinstein 2007) and can help lower the concentration of the drug in the area (Goolsby & Lombardo 2006). However, withdrawal is only immediately possible during bolus injections, as an infusion would need to be stopped and a syringe attached in an attempt to aspirate. Aspiration may be successful if extravasation presents itself as a raised blister, but may be unsuccessful if tissue is soft and soggy (CP Pharmaceuticals 1999; Stanley 2002). It may help to reduce the size of the lesion (Vandergrift 2001). In practice it may achieve little and often distresses the patient (Gault & Challands 1997). The likelihood of withdrawing blood (as suggested by Ignoffo & Friedman 1980) is small and the practitioner may waste valuable time attempting this which could lead to delay in the rest of the management procedure.

269

Stage 2: removing device

Some clinicians advocate that the peripheral vascular access device be left in situ in order to instil the antidote via the device and into the affected tissues (Kassner 2000; Stanley 2002; Weinstein 2007). However, others recommend that the peripheral device should be removed to prevent any injected solution increasing the size of the affected area (Rudolph & Larson 1987; CP Pharmaceuticals 1999; Vandergrift 2001). There appears to be no research evidence to support either practice.

Stage 3: applying hot or cold packs

Cooling appears to be a better choice, with the exception of the vinca alkaloids and some non-cytotoxic drugs, than warming (Bertolli 1995; CP Pharmaceuticals 1999). Cold causes vasoconstriction, localizing the extravasation and perhaps allowing time for local vascular and lymphatic systems to contain the drug. It should be applied for 15–20 minutes, 3–4 times a day for up to 3 days (Gault & Challands 1997; CP Pharmaceuticals 1999; Polovich et al. 2005). Heat promotes healing after the first 24 hours by increasing the blood supply (Polovich et al. 2005; Weinstein 2007). It also decreases local drug concentration, increasing the blood flow which results in enhanced resolution of pain and reabsorption of local swelling.

Stage 4: use of antidotes

A number of antidotes are available, but again there is a lack of scientific evidence to demonstrate their value and so the role of antidotes is still not clear (Polovich et al. 2005). There appear to be two main methods: (i) localize and neutralize (using hyaluronidase) (CP Pharmaceuticals 1999); and (ii) spread and dilute (using an antidote) (Stanley 2002). Administration of antidotes if not via the cannula is by the pincushion technique; that is, instilling small volumes around and over the areas affected using a small gauge (25) needle towards the centre of a clock face. The procedure causes considerable discomfort to patients, and if large areas are to be tackled analgesia should be considered (Stanley 2002).

Hyaluronidase is an enzyme which breaks down hyaluronic acid, a normal component of tissue 'cement' and helps to reduce or prevent tissue damage by allowing rapid diffusion of the extravasated fluid and promoting drug absorption (Few 1987). The usual dose is 1500 IU (Bertolli 1995; Vandergrift 2001). It should be injected within 1 hour of extravasation, ideally through the intravenous device delivering the enzyme to the same tissue (Gault & Challands 1997; Vandergrift 2001; Stanley 2002; Weinstein 2007). NB. Hyaluronidase increases the absorption of local anaesthetic. Therefore if local anaesthetic has been applied to the area, e.g. Ametop gel prior to cannulation, within 6 hours of extravasation, then the patient should be monitored for signs and symptoms of systemic anaesthesia such as increased pulse rate and decreased respirations and the doctor informed immediately (BMA/RPSGB 2008).

Corticosteroids have long been advocated as a treatment for anthracycline extravasation in reducing inflammatory components, although inflammation is not a prominent feature of tissue necrosis (Camp Sorrell 1998) and they appear to have little benefit. Data now discourages the use of locally injected steroids, as there is little evidence to support their use (Bertolli 1995; Gault & Challands 1997; Wickham et al. 2006). However, given as a cream they can help to reduce local trauma and irritation (Stanley 2002).

Dimethyl sulfoxide (DMSO) is a potent free radical scavanger that rapidly penetrates tissues when applied topically (Bertolli 1995). Reports on the clinical use of topical DMSO show it is effective and well tolerated in extravasation (Bertolli 1995). However, this is based on a high dose (95%) and only 50% is easily available in the UK (Stanley 2002). Side-effects from DMSO include itching, erythema, mild burning and a characteristic breath odour (Bertolli 1995).

Recently Dexrazoxane, a topoisomerase II catalytic inhibitor, used clinically to minimize the cardiotoxicity of doxorubicin, has been tested in animal models and a small number of patients for its use in extravasation. It is given IV 3–6 hours after the extravasation and it appears to reduce the wound size and duration with anthracyclines. The triple dosage appears to be more effective than a single dose (Langer et al. 2000; El Saghir et al. 2004). A consensus group (Jackson et al. 2006) have developed recommendations for the use of Dexrazoxane:

1 For anthracycline extravasations resulting from peripheral administration, the site expert or team should be consulted in order to determine whether the use of Dexrazoxane is indicated.
2 Absolute indications are if the peripherally extravasated volume exceeds 15 ml and in the event of a central venous extravasation.

Finally, granulocyte macrophage-colony stimulating factor (GM-CSF) is a growth factor and has been found effective in accelerating wound healing and inducing formation of granulation of tissue (Ulutin et al. 2000; El Saghir et al. 2004).

Stage 5: elevation of limb

This is recommended as it minimizes swelling (Rudolph & Larson 1987) and movement should be encouraged to prevent adhesion of damaged areas to underlying tissue (Gabriel 2008).

Stage 6: surgical techniques

Some centres suggest that a plastic surgery consultation be performed as part of the management procedure in order to remove the tissue containing the drug. Surgical intervention is recommended, especially if the lesion is greater than 2 cm; there is significant residual pain 1–2 weeks after extravasation, or there is minimal healing 2–3 weeks after injury despite local therapeutic measures (Goolsby & Lombardo 2006). Liposuction or a flush-out technique can remove extravasated drug without resorting to excision and skin grafting. A liposuction cannula can be used to aspirate extravasated material and subcutaneous fat. If there is little subcutaneous fat, e.g. preterm infants, then the saline flush-out technique is recommended, particularly if done within the first 24 hours. It has been suggested as a less traumatic and cheaper procedure than surgery. Four small stab incisions are made and large volumes of 0.9% sodium chloride are administered which flush out the extravasated drug (Gault & Challands 1997). Management of large extravasations from CVADs is usually by surgical intervention and washout of affected tissues.

Extravasation kits

The use of extravasation kits has been recommended in order to provide immediate management (Khan & Holmes 2002; Hayden & Goodman 2005). Kits should be assembled according to the particular needs of individual institutions. They should be kept in all areas where staff are regularly administering vesicant drugs, so staff have immediate access to equipment (Gabriel 2008). The kit should be simple to avoid confusion, but comprehensive enough to meet all reasonable needs (Stanley 2002) (see Procedure guidelines: Extravasation management: peripheral cannula, below). Instructions should be clear and easy to follow, and the use of a flow chart enables staff to follow the management procedure in easy steps (Figure 12.4).

Mixed vesicant extravasation

Consideration should be given to the management of mixed vesicant drug extravasation in terms of which drug to treat with which antidote. It has been recommended to act in accordance with the drug which possesses the most deleterious properties (How & Brown 1998).

Informing the patient

Patients should always be informed when an extravasation has occurred and be given an explanation of what has happened and what management has been carried out (McCaffrey Boyle & Engelking 1995). An information sheet should be given to patients with instructions of what symptoms to look out for and when to contact the hospital during the follow-up period (Gabriel 2008).

Wound management

Damage will be affected by the site, amount of drug, concentration of the agent and if it binds to DNA or not (Polovich et al. 2005). Ulceration may occur over a period of days to weeks and extravasation wounds may be complicated by tissue ischaemia related to endothelial damage (Naylor

Suspect an extravasation if:

1 Patient complains of burning or stinging pain *or*
2 There is evidence of swelling, induration, leakage at the site *or*
3 There is resistance on plunger of syringe or absence of free flow of infusion *or*
4 There is no blood return (if found in isolation, this should not be regarded as an indication of a non-patent vein)

Stop the injection/infusion
Withdraw as much of the drug as possible
Remove the cannula
Collect the extravasation pack

Group A drugs

Inject 1500 IU hyaluronidase subcutaneously around site.
Apply warm pack to aid absorption of hyaluronidase.
Warm pack to remain in situ for 2–4 hours

Group B drugs

Apply cold pack to cause vasoconstriction.
Apply cold packs for 15–20 minutes, 3–4 times for at least 24 hours.
However if extravasation is with any of the following category B drugs: mitomycin C; doxorubicin; idarubicin; epirubicin; actinomycin D then:

• Draw around area of extravasation with indelible pen
• Put on gloves
• Apply thin layer of DMSO topically to the marked area using the small plastic spatula in lid of the bottle
• Allow it to dry
• Apply gauze
• This should be applied within 10–25 minutes

Consider the administration of dexrazoxane

Elevate the limb

Apply hydrocortisone cream to reduce local inflammation (twice daily)

Where appropriate, apply DMSO every 2 hours on day 1 and then every 6 hours for up to 7 days

Inform medical staff

Document in duplicate – one copy in patient's notes and one to IV team

Give patient a patient information sheet

Figure 12.4   Treatment of extravasation.

271

2005). The type of injury will dictate the type of dressing. Assessment of the wound should include position and size of the wound, amount and type of tissue present, amount and type of exudate, and extent and spread of erythema (Naylor 2005).

Documentation and follow up

An extravasation must be reported and fully documented as it is an accident and the patient may require follow-up care. (NMC 2005; RCN 2005). Information may also be used for statistical purposes, for example collation and analysis using the green card scheme devised by St. Chad's Hospital, Birmingham (Stanley 2002). Statistics on the incidence, degree, causes and corrective action should be monitored and analysed (Infusion Nurses Society 2006). Finally, it may be required in case of litigation, which is now on the increase (Dougherty 2003; Masoorli 2003).

The procedure detailed here represents the policy of The Royal Marsden Hospital for the management by nursing staff of extravasation injury, drawn up with the assistance of pharmacist and medical colleagues. It relates specifically to the management of extravasation of a drug from a peripheral cannula.

Procedure guidelines   Extravasation management: peripheral cannula

Equipment

To assist the nurse, an extravasation kit should be assembled and should be readily available in each ward/unit. It contains:

1 Gel packs × 2 : one to be kept in the fridge and one available for heating (an electric heating blanket can be used whilst pack is heating).
2 Hyaluronidase 1500 IU/2 ml sterile water.
3 Hydrocortisone cream 1% 15 g tube × 1.
4 2 ml syringes × 1.

5 25 G needles × 2.
6 Alcohol swabs.
7 Documentation forms.
8 Copy of extravasation management procedure.
9 Patient information leaflet.

Procedure

Action	Rationale
1 Explain and discuss the procedure with the patient.	To ensure that the patient understands the procedure and gives his/her valid consent (DH 2002a: C; NMC 2008b: C).
2 Stop injection or infusion *immediately*, leaving the cannula in place.	To minimize local injury. To allow aspiration of the drug to be attempted (Polovich *et al.* 2005: C; RCN 2005: C).
3 Aspirate any residual drug from the device and suspected extravasation site.	To minimize local injury by removing as much drug as possible and only attempt if appropriate. Subsequent damage is related to the volume of the extravasation, in addition to other factors (Polovich *et al.* 2005: C; RCN 2005: C).
4 Remove the cannula.	To prevent the device from being used for antidote administration (Rudolph & Larson 1987: E).
5 Collect the extravasation pack and take it to the patient.	It contains all the equipment necessary for managing extravasation (Stanley 2002: E; Dougherty 2005: E).
6 **Group A drugs:** Draw up hyaluronidase 1500 IU in 1 ml water for injection and inject volumes of 0.1–0.2 ml subcutaneously at points of the compass around the circumference of the area of extravasation. Apply warm pack.	This is the recommended agent for group A drugs. The warm pack speeds up absorption of the drug by the tissues (Bertolli 1995: C).

272

Group B drugs:
Apply cold pack or ice instantly.

To localize the area of extravasation, slow cell metabolism and decrease the area of tissue destruction. To reduce local pain (Polovich *et al.* 2005: C).

However, if extravasation is with any of the following category B drugs: mitomycin C; doxorubicin; idarubicin; epirubicin; actinomycin D then:

- Draw around area of extravasation with indelible pen.
- Put on gloves.
- Apply thin layer of DMSO topically to the marked area using the small plastic spatula in lid of the bottle.
- Allow it to dry.
- Apply gauze.
- This should be applied within 10–25 minutes.

This is the recommended agent for these anthracyclines and helps to reduce local tissue damage (Bertolli 1995: C).

7 Where possible elevate the extremity and/or encourage movement.

To minimize swelling and to prevent adhesion of damaged area to underlying tissue, which could result in restriction of movement (Rudolph & Larson 1987: E).

8 Inform a member of the medical staff at the earliest opportunity and administer any other prescribed antidotes, e.g. dexrazoxane.

To enable actions differing from agreed policy to be taken if considered in the best interests of the patient. To notify the doctor of the need to prescribe any other drugs (E).

9 Apply hydrocortisone cream 1% twice daily, and instruct the patient how to do this. Continue as long as erythema persists.

To reduce local inflammation and promote patient comfort (Stanley 2002: E).

10 Where appropriate, apply DMSO every 2 hours on day 1 and then every 6 hours for up to 7 days (patients will need to have this prescribed as a to take out [TTO] and continue treatment at home where necessary).

To help reduce local tissue damage (Bertolli 1995: C).

11 Heat packs (group A drugs) should be reapplied after initial management for 2–4 hours. Cold packs (group B drugs) should be applied for 15–20 minutes, 3–4 times a day for up to 3 days.

To localize the steroid effect in the area of extravasation. To reduce local pain and promote patient comfort (Bertolli 1995: C).

12 Provide analgesia as required.

To promote patient comfort. To encourage movement of the limb as advised (E).

13 Document the following details, in duplicate, on the form provided:
   (a) Patient's name/number.
   (b) Ward/unit.
   (c) Date, time.
   (d) Signs and symptoms.
   (e) Venepuncture site (on diagram).
   (f) Drug sequence.
   (g) Drug administration technique, i.e. 'bolus' or infusion.
   (h) Approximate amount of the drug extravasated.
   (i) Diameter, length and width of extravasation area.
   (j) Appearance of the area.

Procedure guidelines *(cont.)*

(k) Step-by-step management with date and time of each step performed and medical officer notification. (l) Patient's complaints, comments, statements. (m) Indication that patient's information sheet given to patient. (n) Follow-up section. (o) Whether photograph was taken. (p) If required, when patient referred to plastic surgeon. (q) Signature of the nurse.	To provide an immediate full record of all details of the incident, which may be referred to if necessary. To provide a baseline for future observation and monitoring of patient's condition. To comply with NMC guidelines (Kassner 2000: E; NMC 2005: C; RCN 2005: C; Weinstein 2007: E).
14 Explain to the patient that the site may remain sore for several days.	To reduce anxiety and ensure continued co-operation (P: E).
15 Observe the area regularly for erythema, induration, blistering or necrosis. *Inpatients*: monitor daily. Where appropriate, take photograph.	To detect any changes at the earliest possible moment (RCN 2005: C).
16 All patients should receive written information explaining what has occurred, what management has been carried out, what they need to look for at the site and when to report any changes. For example, increased discomfort, peeling or blistering of the skin should be reported immediately.	To detect any changes as early as possible, and allow for a review of future management. This may include referral to a plastic surgeon (Gault & Challands 1997: E; Polovich et al. 2005: C; RCN 2005: C).
17 If blistering or tissue breakdown occurs, begin dressing techniques and seek advice regarding wound management.	To minimize the risk of a superimposed infection and sterile increase healing (Naylor 2005: E).
18 Depending on size of lesion, degree of pain, type of drug, refer to plastic surgeon.	To prevent further pain or other complications as chemically induced ulcers rarely heal spontaneously (Polovich et al. 2005: C; Dougherty 2005: E).

Oral administration

Definition

The administration of cytotoxic drugs via the oral route.

Indications

The oral route is convenient, economical, non-invasive and sometimes less toxic than the other routes (Hayden & Goodman 2005). The oral route can be beneficial when chronic exposure to a drug is important; for example, cell-cycle specific drugs (Scurr et al. 2005). Most oral drugs are absorbed well if the gastrointestinal tract is functioning normally. However, the oral route can be unreliable for a number of reasons, including:

- Patients may not comply with therapy, or forget to take their medication or may feel the side-effects associated are too unpleasant, e.g. nausea and vomiting, hot flushes (Hayden & Goodman 2005). However, the use of antiemetics as well as rescheduling the timing of the dose administered may prove beneficial.
- Patients may not take medications as instructed; for example, continuing to take the medication despite side-effects since they believe the medication is helping. However, it is imperative that the nurse ensures that the patient understands the importance of timing and schedule of the medication prescribed and when to stop medication if side-effects become too severe. The use of medication cards can assist the patient to record the doses of medication that have been taken. Patients should be advised to wear gloves when handling oral chemotherapy tablets or to use a non touch approach by tipping the tablets into a plastic medication container.
- Some patients may experience difficulty taking tablets or capsules and therefore attempt to crush them, which could result in changes to the tablets' disposition and effectiveness.
- There is the potential loss of the drug if emesis occurs.
- Concomitant medications can affect the absorption of oral chemotherapy (Scurr et al. 2005).

Reference material

Nurses administering tablets or capsules should use a non-touch technique to avoid damage and contamination of the tablets or capsules and contamination of themselves (Polovich *et al.* 2005). If tablets have to be counted, this should be done using a triangle, which should be washed and dried after use. Many tablets are coated and this protects the drug in its inner core. There is no risk of contamination if these coatings remain in tact. A small number of tablets are compressed powders, but there appears to be no risk of contamination where there is no free powder visible. It is important that these tablets are not crushed because they will then release powder which could be inhaled. Capsules are also not a risk if they have not been opened or broken or have not leaked. They should not be crushed or opened and the powder tipped out (Polovich *et al.* 2005). Any visible spillage should be dealt with as previously directed (see Procedure guidelines: Cytotoxic drugs: environmental precautions, above). Patients should receive counselling regarding how to take their oral chemotherapy (see Box 12.3 for an example of a checklist).

Intramuscular and subcutaneous injection

Definition

The administration of cytotoxic drugs by injection into the muscle or subcutaneous tissues.

Indications

Intramuscular and subcutaneous injections are a useful route:

- When administering therapy in the community.
- For patient convenience.
- When regular administration is required and journeys to the hospital are impractical, e.g. younger or elderly patients on maintenance therapy.

It is also useful if venous access is limited, although only small volumes (up to 3 ml) are recommended using this route (Sewell *et al.* 2002; Polovich 2003; Polovich *et al.* 2005).

Reference material

Only a few cytotoxic drugs can be administered via these routes due to a number of factors:

- The irritant nature of the drugs and/or tissue damage.
- Incomplete absorption may occur.
- Bleeding as a result of thrombocytopenia.
- Discomfort of regular injections (Polovich 2003; Polovich *et al.* 2005).

Cytotoxic and biological agents administered in this way are:

- Methotrexate.
- Bleomycin.

- Cytosine arabinoside.
- L-Asparaginase.
- Ifosfamide.
- Interferon.
- Colony stimulating factor (Stanley 2002; Weinstein 2007).

Although the volume of drug and diluent handled is less than for the intravenous route, preparation and reconstitution of the agents should be commensurate with the information listed under Procedure guidelines: Cytotoxic drugs: accidental exposure. The nurse should continue to wear gloves during administration. Spillage and disposal of equipment should be dealt with as previously directed (see Procedure guidelines: Cytotoxic drugs: environmental precautions) and systems of work modified to ensure these guidelines are followed. Where community nurses are to be responsible for administration, they must be supplied with adequate information when the patient is discharged.

Recommendations about administration should be followed carefully, e.g. deep intramuscular injection using a Z-track technique to prevent leakage onto the skin (Hayden & Goodman 2005) and rotation of sites to prevent local irritation developing. The skin should be cleaned with antiseptic prior to injection (Sansivero & Barton-Burke 2001) and the smallest needle used, the gauge of which will allow passage of the solution to minimize discomfort and scarring (Weinstein 2007).

Topical application

Definition

Topical application is the application of cream or ointments containing cytotoxic agents.

Indications

Topical application is only suitable for superficial lesions and has been found to be useful in the treatment of cutaneous malignant lesions, e.g. cutaneous T-cell lymphomas, basal cell carcinoma, squamous cell carcinoma and Kaposi's sarcoma (Hayden & Goodman 2005).

Reference material

Topical agents include mustine and 5-FU (Hayden & Goodman 2005). The most widely used is 5% 5-FU cream for the treatment of basal and squamous cell carcinomas, which is usually applied once or twice daily until significant penetration of the damaged or diseased skin can be achieved, and a typical response pattern has been observed. This can take

---

Box 12.3 Procedure and checklist for teaching patients on oral anti-cancer chemotherapy

1 Prior to the **first cycle** of treatment all patients should be seen and taught by an appropriately trained pharmacist, pharmacy technician or nurse using the checklist below.
2 All outpatients should be taught by an appropriately trained pharmacist, pharmacy technician or nurse. Inpatients should be taught by an appropriately trained nurse.
3 Before **every treatment cycle**, all patients should be seen by an appropriately trained pharmacist, pharmacy technician or nurse (out-patients) or nurse (in-patients) to ensure:
  (a) They were seen and taught as described above on their first cycle of treatment.
  (b) They had no problems taking their first cycle of treatment, e.g. they understood how to take their tablets, they had no problems with vomiting.
  (c) If a dose reduction has been made, the patient is aware why their dose has been changed and how many tablets/capsules they should take.
4 After teaching the patient using the checklist below, the pharmacist, pharmacy technician or nurse should sign the appropriate section on the Oral Chemotherapy Prescription Proforma.

Teaching points prior to the first cycle of chemotherapy

1 The patient understands that the medicine has been prescribed only for them and should not be given to anyone else.
2 They understand that the medicine should be stored in a safe place away from children and should not be handled by anyone else (unless it is being given by a carer, see point 3).
3 If a carer is administering the medicine, they are aware that they should not handle the tablets or capsules directly (they should be tipped or pushed out from the blister pack directly into a medicine pot).
4 The patient (or relative/carer) understands how and when to take their medicine (in particular, if there are breaks in treatment they know when this should be and how long it should be for).
5 The patient understands any specific directions (usually identified by the directorate pharmacist on the proforma) relating to taking their medicine.
6 They know what they should do if they miss a dose. (If they miss a dose they should not try and catch up or double the next dose. They should take the next dose as prescribed. Missed doses should be recorded on patient treatment diaries where applicable.)
7 They understand what to do if they vomit a dose. (If they vomit a dose they should only repeat the dose if they can see all the tablets whole in their vomit. If they cannot see the tablets or are uncertain they should not repeat the dose, they should wait and take the next dose as prescribed.)
8 They understand what the side-effects of treatment are and what they should do if they experience them. In particular they know who they should contact.
9 They know how to obtain further supplies. (All supplies of oral chemotherapy should be obtained from the hospital pharmacy.)
10 They understand what they should do with left-over tablets. (All left-over tablets should be returned to the hospital pharmacy. They should not be disposed of in household refuse or flushed down the toilet.)
11 They understand the role of their general practitioner and the role of the hospital multiprofessional team. (Any side-effects of treatment should be reported to the hospital team. The hospital doctors are responsible for prescribing the chemotherapy.) In case of chest pain during treatment, the patient should contact 999 as an emergency.
12 A factsheet, such as 'Taking oral chemotherapy' has been given to the patient.
13 They are able to take their medicine in the dosage form supplied.
14 If the patient is unable to swallow tablets or capsules, they have been given the appropriate factsheet such as 'Crushing oral chemotherapy tablets safely', 'Dissolving oral chemotherapy tablets safely', 'Opening oral chemotherapy capsules safely' or 'Giving chemotherapy by mouth or through a feeding tube using a syringe'.
15 If applicable they have been given a patient treatment diary which has been completed by a nurse or pharmacist.

---

up to 4 weeks when local erythema, blistering and ulceration occur. Once the affected skin starts sloughing, regranulization of normal tissue will begin to occur (Sewell *et al.* 2002).

Considerations include safe handling when applying the cream by wearing gloves and using low-linting swabs or non-metal applicators (Hayden & Goodman 2005; Weinstein 2007). It is important to protect the normal skin and avoid the eyes and other mucous membranes. The affected area should not be washed vigorously during the treatment (Hayden & Goodman 2005). The area should be observed for any adverse reactions such as pain, pruritus and hyperpigmentation, which may result in discontinuation and subsequent dose reduction.

Intrathecal administration

Definition

Intrathecal administration is the administration of cytotoxic drugs into the central nervous system (CNS) via the cerebrospinal fluid. This is usually achieved using a lumbar puncture (Stanley 2002; Polovich *et al.* 2005; Hayden & Goodman 2005).

Indications

Intrathecal administration has proved to be of benefit in prophylactic treatment in cases of leukaemias and some lymphomas, where the CNS may provide a sanctuary site for tumour cells not reached during systemic chemotherapy (Hayden & Goodman 2005). It has no place in the treatment of CNS metastases of solid tumours (Stanley 2002).

Reference material

Intrathecal administration is only appropriate for a limited number of drugs:

- Thiotepa.
- Cytarabine.
- Methotrexate (Scurr *et al.* 2005).

Chemotherapy administered using this route has the potential to cause great harm (Sewell *et al.* 2002) and has been associated with the deaths of at least 13 patients since 1985. The risks of intrathecal chemotherapy have been well documented in *An Organization with a Memory* (DH 2000) and the government set a target to eliminate the incidents of patients dying or being paralysed by maladministered intrathecal injections by the end of 2001 (DH 2000). Two reports on injection errors (Toft 2001) gave rise to the publication of the national guidance for the safe administration of intrathecal chemotherapy. All Trusts which administer intrathecal chemotherapy have been required to comply with the guidance since the end of 2001.

The key requirements of the guidance are noted in Box 12.4.

The advantage of this route is that it allows the direct access to the CNS of drugs which do not normally cross the blood–brain barrier in sufficient amounts and thus ensures constant levels of the drug in this area. The main disadvantage is that it requires a standard lumbar puncture before the drug can be injected, and this may need to be performed on a daily to weekly basis (Stanley 2002; Hayden & Goodman 2005). Although this can be quick and easy to perform it can be distressing for the patient, and could even result in CNS trauma and infection. It may also only reach the epidural or subdural spaces and therefore the concentrations in the ventricles may not be therapeutic (Hayden & Goodman 2005). However, central instillation of the drug into the ventricle can be achieved via an Ommaya reservoir, which is surgically implanted through the cranium (Sewell *et al.* 2002; Hayden & Goodman 2005; Weinstein 2007). It carries more risks but provides permanent access and can be inserted under local or general anaesthetic (Sansivero & Barton-Burke 2001; Hayden & Goodman 2005).

The preparation of the drug must be performed using aseptic technique to reduce the risk of infection. The drug should be free from preservatives to reduce neurotoxicity. Cerebrospinal fluid removal and volumes of medications should not be more than 2 ml/min. Expected side-effects of

---

Box 12.4 Key requirements for the safe administration of intrathecal chemotherapy*

- The Chief Executive, who has overall responsibility for ensuring compliance with the guidance, should identify a 'designated lead' to oversee compliance within the Trust.
- A register must be established and maintained which lists designated personnel who have been trained and authorized to prescribe, dispense, issue, check or administer intrathecal chemotherapy.
- A formal induction programme must be provided for all new staff including training that is appropriate to their role in prescribing, dispensing, checking, issuing or administering of chemotherapy.
- Annual reviews of competence are required for all professional staff (nurses, doctors, pharmacy) who remain on the register.
- All staff involved with chemotherapy must be provided with a written protocol, which reflects both the national guidance and additional local information.
- Intrathecal chemotherapy must only be prescribed by a Medical Consultant, Associate Specialist or Specialist Registrar whose name is on the register. Senior house officers (SHOs) must never prescribe.
- A purpose-designed intrathecal chemotherapy chart must be used.
- Intrathecal chemotherapy drugs must only be dispensed and issued by pharmacy staff on the register. These drugs must only be transported from the pharmacy by the administering doctor or pharmacy staff on the register.
- Intrathecal chemotherapy drugs must be administered after intravenous chemotherapy drugs and should only be issued following written confirmation that any intravenous chemotherapy drugs have already been administered. The only exception is where intrathecal chemotherapy is being given to a child under general anaesthesia.
- Intrathecal chemotherapy must be administered in a designated, separate area and under normal circumstances only within normal working hours.
- The administering doctor must use a formal checking procedure to ensure that the right drug is given to the right patient. These checks must be completed with a chemotherapy-trained nurse (or a nurse trained and deemed competent to carry out this check if a chemotherapy-trained nurse is not available), the patient and, if appropriate, a relative or guardian. The nurse checking must be on the designated register. The checks made by the administering doctor and nurse must be recorded on the prescription chart prior to administration.

* DH HSC 2003/10.

neurotoxicity related to the drugs include headache, nausea and vomiting, drowsiness, fever, stiff neck, ataxia and blurred vision (Sansivero & Barton-Burke 2001). Neurological and vital signs checks should be obtained at least every 1–2 hours initially, and then on a scheduled frequency. Observations should include signs of infection, headache and signs of increasing intracranial pressure, and monitoring the function of the pump or reservoir (Polovich *et al.* 2005; Hayden & Goodman 2005).

Intrapleural instillation

Definition

Introduction of cytotoxic drugs, or other substances, into the pleural cavity.

Indications

Pleural effusion is a common complication of malignant disease and may pose a considerable management problem. Instillation should occur following drainage of an effusion to prevent or delay a recurrence caused by malignant cells, as after aspiration alone 60% of patients would present with pleural malignant recurrence (Hayden & Goodman 2005).

The most common neoplasms associated with the development of malignant pleural effusions are those of the:

■ Breast.
■ Lung.
■ Gastrointestinal tract.
■ Prostate.
■ Ovary (Hayden & Goodman 2005).

Such effusions can be very distressing to the patient, causing progressive discomfort, dyspnoea and death from respiratory insufficiency.

The alteration in normal anatomy due to the pressure of an effusion is illustrated in Figure 12.5. In health less than 5 ml of transudate fluid is present between the visceral and parietal pleurae. This fluid acts as a lubricant and hydraulic seal (see Chapter 21). Infections and malignancies disrupt this mechanism, often repeatedly. Patients may survive for months or years, therefore effective palliation is important in maintaining or improving their quality of life. Administering chemotherapy via this route may alleviate symptoms and also has the potential for delivering the drugs to a site of poor systemic penetration (Sewell *et al.* 2002). A recent study using intrapleural hypotonic cisplatin for malignant pleural effusion demonstrated encouraging results. Eighty patients were observed during the study of which 27 (34%) and 39 (49%) achieved a complete response and partial response respectively (Seto *et al.* 2006).

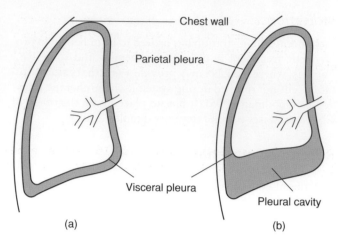

Figure 12.5 Lung anatomy. (a) Normal lung anatomy showing pleura. (b) Lung demonstrating presence of pleural effusion.

Reference material

Several methods have been used to treat pleural effusions, including:

■ Surgical techniques, such as ablation of the pleural space.
■ Radiotherapy.
■ Systemic chemotherapy.
■ The insertion of a small-bore catheter placement and the installation of a pleural shunt (Sewell *et al.* 2002) to deliver cytotoxic agents.

In addition, instillation of sclerosing agents into the pleural space has been used and been reported to have highly variable success rates of 20–88% (Sewell *et al.* 2002). Cytology may show the presence of tumour cells in effusion fluid, but even when these are absent, instillation of drugs may be effective in preventing recurrence due to the inflammatory reaction which obliterates the pleural space.

These agents have included talc, radioactive phosphorus, bacille Calmette-Guérin (BCG), tetracycline and, more recently, cytotoxic drugs. The drug most frequently instilled is bleomycin, but others include mitozantrone, doxorubicin, mustine and thiotepa (Sewell *et al.* 2002; Hayden & Goodman 2005).

Improvements in equipment used, for example flexible cannulae or catheters, and lengthening of both the initial drainage period and that following instillation of the drug have contributed to increased patient comfort and greater effectiveness (Hayden & Goodman 2005). The insertion of small-bore percutaneously placed catheters or ports, as well as pleuroperitoneal shunts (Hayden & Goodman 2005), has been found to be useful for recurrent effusions.

The literature recommends that the patient should be turned regularly following instillation of the drug to facilitate its complete distribution over the pleural surfaces. It has been recommended that the timing for turning should be every 10–15 minutes for between 2 and 6 hours (Quan 1999). The rationale for such turning is based on clinical observation and there is a lack of work comparing patients who are turned with those who are not.

Local pleural pain and inflammation can last for 24–48 hours after instillation. Good symptom management should focus upon emesis control, adequate analgesia and emotional support and chest tube security to ensure patient comfort (Hayden & Goodman 2005).

Procedure guidelines   Cytotoxic drugs: intrapleural administration

The procedure and problem solving related to intrapleural drainage (see Chapter 21) should be consulted for all aspects of thoracic drainage. The following information covers specific points regarding drug instillation.

Procedure
Instillation of intrapleural cytotoxic drugs

Action	Rationale
1 Explain and discuss the procedure with the patient.	To ensure that the patient understands the procedure and gives his/her valid consent (DH 2002a: C; NMC 2008b: C).
2 Administer premedication to patients if prescribed.	To relax the patient (E).
3 Prepare the required equipment (see Chapter 11, Procedure guidelines: Injections: administration) and cytotoxic drug. Wear protective clothing.	To ensure the procedure goes smoothly without interruption. Protect practitioner from exposure (HSE 2003: C).
4 Assist the doctor with the instillation and provide support for the patient.	To increase the efficiency of the procedure and reduce discomfort for the patient (E).
5 At the end of the procedure clamp the drainage tube and leave for the desired period.	To prevent back-flow of the drug (Weinstein 2007: E).

Rotation of patient receiving intrapleural cytotoxic drugs

Action	Rationale
1 Assess the clinical status of the patient and ability to tolerate the desired rotation.	To prevent discomfort the patient may feel and to ensure that the doctor is informed of the patient's inability to comply (E).
2 Turn the patient in the following rotation: (a) Left side. (b) Supine. (c) Right side. (d) Prone.	To ensure that the drug coats and washes the pleural cavity completely (E).
3 Carry out the rotations as instructed. Examples are as follows: (a) 5 minutes in each position, repeated once, equals 20 minutes. (b) 30 minutes in each position, repeated once, equals 2 hours. (c) 1 hour in each position equals 4 hours.	As above (E).
4 Observe regularly for patient comfort. Administer analgesic as required.	To keep the patient comfortable and free from pain (E).
5 Record the patient's respirations and colour at least every 15 minutes for 1 hour, then every hour until stable, then 4-hourly, or as frequently as the patient's condition dictates. Record temperature at least 4-hourly.	To ensure there is no change in respiratory function following the procedure (E). To observe for pyrexia, a common side-effect that may indicate a developing infection or a reaction to chemotherapy (E).

279

Procedure guidelines *(cont.)*

Drainage of intrapleural cytotoxic drugs

Action	Rationale
1 Ensure the patient is in a comfortable position, and is aware of any limitations about movement.	To prevent discomfort or dislodgement of the drainage tube (E).
2 Unclamp the chest tube.	To allow drainage of the drug instilled (E).
3 Maintain the underwater seal until a volume of less than 50 ml is drained during 24 hours for 2 consecutive days or for a maximum of 7 days, or in consultation with medical staff.	To allow complete drainage of the drug instilled, and any additional fluid (E).
4 Record the colour and amount of fluid drained.	To monitor the immediate effectiveness of therapy (E).

Problem solving: Intrapleural cytotoxic drug administration

Problem	Cause	Suggested action
Local or systemic effects associated with specific cytotoxic drugs, e.g. rigors due to bleomycin.	Absorption of the drug into circulation in sufficient quantities to cause toxicity.	Be aware that this can occur. Initiate preventive action, e.g. obtain a prescription for corticosteroid cover to prevent rigors, or observe for a reaction and treat symptomatically.

Intravesical instillation

Definition

Intravesical instillation is the instillation of cytotoxic drugs directly into the bladder, via a urinary catheter.

Indications

Intravesical instillation has been shown to be effective in the treatment of small, multiple, superficial, well-differentiated, non-invasive papillomatous carcinomas, as high drug concentrations can be achieved using this route, because there is limited penetration of the drug into normal and malignant tissue. This method is only of benefit when treating small and superficial disease (Scurr *et al.* 2005). It also minimizes recurrence in patients with a history of multiple tumours known to readily seed locally (Stanley 2002). Intravesical instillation also reduces cytotoxic exposure to patients and their carers because excretion of the drug is quicker than when administered systemically (Washburn 2007).

Reference material

Instillation of cytotoxic agents, and immunotherapy, into the bladder via a urinary catheter has been used for many years in selected cases and has proven to be an effective and simple method of controlling and treating superficial bladder cancer (Scurr *et al.* 2005). In measurable disease, average response rates are 60%. Approximately 30% of patients experience a complete response. Cytotoxic drugs found to be effective include:

- Thiotepa.
- Mitomycin C.
- Doxorubicin.
- Epirubicin.
- Mitoxantrone.
- BCG (Washburn 2007).

Intravesical instillation allows a high concentration of drug to bathe the endothelium, which enables localized treatment to the tumour and limits the systemic absorption so toxicity is reduced. Systemic toxicity is a problem with thiotepa, but otherwise the main problems are local inflammation, pain, burning on urination, frequency and occasional haematuria. The procedure should be performed using an aseptic technique as there is an increased risk of urinary tract infection.

Treatment protocols vary. Instillation first involves the insertion of a urinary catheter, drainage of the bladder, then the instillation of the drug. This usually takes about 50–60 minutes; it is retained for 1–2 hours with frequent movement by the patient to disperse the drug through the bladder (Sewell *et al.* 2002; Hayden & Goodman 2005). Therapy may be repeated on alternating days for three doses or weekly for varying lengths of time (4–12 weeks).

Patients should be instructed in good personal hygiene such as washing hands and genitalia thoroughly after void-ing, and the toilet should be flushed at least twice after void-ing. An increase in oral intake while the treatment is being given will increase the dilution of medication required and may reduce side-effects (Hayden & Goodman 2005).

Procedure guidelines   Cytotoxic drugs: intravesical instillation

Refer also to the Procedure guidelines for urinary catheterization (see Chapter 18) and bladder lavage and irrigation (see Chapter 14). The following guidelines and problem solving relate to specific chemotherapy administration.

Equipment

1 Urotainer containing prescribed drug in clinically clean tray (delivered from pharmacy reconstitution unit).
2 Sterile gloves.
3 Disposable apron and eye protection.
4 Gate clip or equivalent clamp for catheter.
5 Catheter drainage bag, if catheter is to remain in position.
6 10 or 20 ml sterile syringe.
7 Small dressing pack, that includes a sterile field.

Procedure

Action	Rationale
1 Explain and discuss the procedure with the patient.	To ensure that the patient understands the procedure and gives his/her valid consent (DH 2002b: C; NMC 2008b: C).
2 Check the patient's full blood count, as instructed by the medical staff, and inform them of any deficit before administration.	Absorption of the drug through the bladder wall may cause some myelosuppression. However, there are differing opinions as to whether regular checks are necessary (E).
3 Check all the details on the container of cytotoxic drug against the patient's prescription chart.	To minimize the risk of error and comply with legal requirements (NMC 2008a: C).
4 Assemble all necessary equipment, including the cytotoxic drug container, and proceed to the patient.	To ensure that the instillation proceeds smoothly and without interruption (E).
5 Screen the patient's bed/couch.	To ensure privacy during the procedure (E).
6 Check that the patient's identity matches the patient's details on the prescription chart.	To ensure that the correct patient has been identified. To reduce the risk of error (NMC 2008a: C).
7 If patient does not have a catheter in situ, then pass a catheter (see Chapter 14).	
8 Ensure the bladder is empty of urine.	To prevent dilution of the drug (E). (Washburn 2007)
9 Put on gloves, apron and eye protection.	To protect the nurse from contact with the cytotoxic drugs. With correct technique the risk of contamination is minimal, but splashes can occur (Hayden & Goodman 2005: E).
10 Using aseptic technique and sterile gloves, place a receiver under the end of the catheter to catch any urine and disconnect the drainage bag.	To protect the patient from infection. To protect the nurse from drug spillage. To gain access to the catheter. To prevent urine from soiling the bed (E).
11 Remove the cover from the urotainer, connect to the catheter and release the clamp on urotainer.	To facilitate drug instillation (E).

281

Procedure guidelines *(cont.)*

12 Using gravity to create pressure instil the cytotoxic drug into the bladder. Gentle squeezing may be needed to assist this process.	Rapid instillation would be uncomfortable for the patient, especially if the bladder is small or scarred from previous treatment or disease (E).
13 When the correct prescribed volume has been instilled, slide urotainer clamp over filling port.	To prevent drainage of drug from the bladder (Weinstein 2007: E).
14 When the drug has been in the bladder for 1 hour, request the patient to micturate or slide clamp across filling port and place receiver under connectors. Disconnect urotainer and connect new drainage bag.	One hour is the usual time specified for intravesical drugs to ensure the maximum therapeutic effect with minimum toxicity. To prevent contamination of bed linen (E).
15 If the catheter is to be removed, withdraw the water from the catheter balloon (if appropriate – some catheters do not have a balloon: see Chapter 18) using the sterile syringe and remove the catheter using gentle traction. Dispose of equipment into yellow clinical waste bag and seal.	The catheter may not be required for continued urinary drainage, and may have been inserted to facilitate drug administration, particularly in the outpatient department. The risk of infection is greater if the catheter remains in situ (E).
16 Make the patient comfortable.	
17 Provide outpatients with information about the amount of movement required.	Following outpatient instillation, the journey home is usually sufficient to coat the bladder mucosa (E).
18 Advise the patient on fluid intake, suggesting ways in which he or she may increase it in the following 24-hour period.	To provide a good fluid output, washing out the bladder and reducing the likelihood of local irritation or difficulty in urination due to debris from the tumour. To make patients aware of this side-effect (E).
19 Patient should be made aware that their urine may be cloudy. Instruct the patient to report any discomfort or inability to pass urine immediately to ward staff or general practitioner/district nurse, or to telephone the hospital if anxious.	To detect and resolve any problems at the earliest moment. To reduce anxiety experienced by the patient (E).

282

Problem solving: Intravesicular instillation of cytotoxic drugs

Problem	Cause	Suggested action
No drainage of urine when the catheter is inserted.	Bladder is empty or the catheter is in the wrong place, e.g. in the urethra or in a false track. False tracks may develop after repeated cystoscopy or bladder surgery.	Do not inflate the balloon but tape the catheter to the skin to keep it in position. Check when the patient last micturated. Encourage the patient to drink a few glasses of fluid. Do not give the drug until urine flow is seen or correct positioning of the catheter is established. Inform a doctor if no urine has drained during the next 30 minutes.
Haematuria (within 24–48 hours)	Trauma of catheterization or loosening of blood clots following cystoscopy by fluid injected into the bladder.	Inform a doctor. Observe the patient for signs of clot retention, shock, haemorrhage or fluid retention. Encourage the patient to drink fluids.

Problem	Cause	Suggested action
Leakage from around the catheter following administration of the drug.	Catheter slipping out of the bladder or bladder spasm caused by the drug.	Check the position of the catheter. Inform a doctor if leakage persists. Protect the patient's skin by wrapping sterile topical swabs around the catheter (Polovich *et al.* 2005: C). Estimate the volume lost by leakage. Wash contaminated skin thoroughly.
Patient unable to retain the requisite drug volume in the bladder for the time required.	Low bladder capacity; weak sphincter muscles; unstable detrusor muscle causing uncontrolled bladder contractions.	Note actual duration of the drug in the bladder and inform a doctor.
Patient has pain during instillation of the drug or while the drug is in the bladder.	Following resection of mucosa, the bladder can become acutely sensitive to irritants, thus causing painful spasm resulting in possible expelling of the cytotoxic agent.	Allow the drug to drain out and/or stop instillation if the pain is severe. Inform a doctor. Administer Entonox if appropriate (see Chapter 28, Pain management: Entonox administration) and have analgesics prescribed for subsequent administration.
Patient unable to pass urine after the drug has been in situ for the required length of time.	Anxiety; poor bladder tone; prostatism.	Reassure the patient. Encourage the patient to drink fluids.
Urine does not drain from the catheter when the clamp is released.	Catheter wrongly placed. Catheter blocked with clots and/or debris.	Check the position of the catheter. Perform bladder lavage.

283

Intraperitoneal administration

Definition

Intraperitoneal administration is the introduction of cytotoxic drugs into the peritoneal cavity following drainage of ascites to prevent or delay a recurrence.

Indications

Treatment failures of primary malignant tumours of the colon and rectum as well as ovary occur most frequently as local regional disease. Extensive tumours may be present intra-abdominally without evidence of disease at other sites in the body. In view of this, chemotherapy treatment given intraperitoneally has been shown to be effective in treating locally recurrent ovarian and colon cancer (Sewell *et al.* 2002; Hayden & Goodman 2005).

Reference material

The peritoneal space is semi-permeable, which allows high concentrations of the drugs to be achieved at the site of the tumour throughout the peritoneal space, but with lower concentrations entering the bloodstream thus reducing the toxicity (Sewell *et al.* 2002). Therefore, increased dosages of drug can be delivered to the tumour site than could be delivered systemically.

Large volumes of fluid containing chemotherapy agents should be administered intermittently. The chemotherapy agents used include:

- Cisplatin.
- Carboplatin.
- Bleomycin.
- Paclitaxel.
- Mitoxantrone.
- Mitomycin C.
- 5-FU (Sewell *et al.* 2002).

There are three methods of accessing the peritoneal space:

1 Intermittent placement of a temporary indwelling catheter into the peritoneal cavity. This is used for a short time such as for symptom relief or palliation.
2 Placement of an external catheter such as a Tenckhoff. This is surgically placed through the anterior abdominal wall and the catheter exits through the skin on the abdomen. This is the most widely used method and the Tenckhoff catheter has the advantages of allowing a high

flow rate (2 litres in 10–15 minutes) and also allows for manipulation to dislodge fibrin deposits (Hayden & Goodman 2005). Problems include occlusion infection, leakage around the catheter and body image problems.

3 Placement of an implantable peritoneal port. The port is internal with no care required when not accessed and therefore has a lower rate of infection and may be more acceptable to the patient. However, ports tend to provide a slower flow rate than a catheter (Hayden & Goodman 2005).

General complications of intraperitoneal chemotherapy include respiratory distress, abdominal pain and distension, discomfort and diarrhoea (which all result in increased abdominal pressure) (Polovich *et al.* 2005). Other problems include mechanical difficulties with the catheter (inflow and outflow obstructions), electrolyte imbalance and peritonitis caused by chemical irritation of the peritoneal space, or by infection or both. In general, intraperitoneal chemotherapy is usually tolerated well by patients and provides a safe and effective treatment in the management of peritoneal disease.

Procedure guidelines Cytotoxic drugs: intraperitoneal instillation

Refer also to the procedure for ascitic drainage (Procedure guidelines: Abdominal paracentesis) in Chapter 4. The following guidelines and problem solving deal with specific aspects of chemotherapy administration.

Equipment

1 Syringe or infusion bag containing prescribed drug in clinically clean tray (delivered from pharmacy reconstitution unit).
2 Sterile gloves.
3 Disposable apron and goggles.

4 Gate clip or equivalent clamp for catheter.
5 Catheter drainage bag, if catheter is to remain in position.
6 Small dressing pack, containing sterile field.

Procedure

Action	Rationale
1 Explain and discuss the procedure with the patient.	To ensure that the patient understands the procedure and gives his/her valid consent (DH 2002a: C; NMC 2008b: C).
2 Administer premedication to patient if prescribed.	To ensure the patient is relaxed during the procedure (E).
3 Check all the details on the container of the cytotoxic drug against the patient's prescription chart.	To minimize the risk of error and comply with legal requirements (NMC 2008a: C).
4 Assemble all necessary equipment, including the cytotoxic drug container, and proceed to the patient.	To ensure that the instillation proceeds smoothly and without interruption (E).
5 Prior to instillation, prewarm infusion to body temperature (Hayden & Goodman 2005; Polovich *et al.* 2005).	To prevent cramping (E).
6 Use a Y-tube irrigation set. The catheter is attached by this Y-tube to a bottle of dialysate and a drainage bag.	To ensure minimum intervention in draining peritoneal cavity (E).
7 Instill fluid at prescribed rate, usually 1–2 litres over 10–15 minutes, but can be extended to 30–60 minutes (Hayden & Goodman 2005).	To ensure the correct instillation at the correct rate (NMC 2008a: C)
8 Wait prescribed period of time after administration prior to draining off excess fluid. This may be from 1 to 3 hours.	To ensure fluid has coated all parts of peritoneal cavity (E).
9 Observe regularly for patient comfort and intervene as appropriate. If the patient experiences any discomfort or pain, administer prescribed analgesia.	To keep patient comfortable and pain free (E).

10	Record temperature 4-hourly.	To observe for pyrexia, a common side-effect that may indicate a developing infection or a reaction to chemotherapy (E).
11	Unclamp drainage tube and, where necessary, flush port or pump using appropriate flushing solution. The catheter may be removed after drainage is complete.	To allow drainage of drug (E).
	Note: if there is leakage around drain site or a drainage bag is attached, nurses must remember that the fluid may still contain cytotoxic drug and should therefore take the same precautions as when handling any cytotoxic waste.	To reduce the risk of contamination to the patient and staff (HSE 2003: C).
12	Record accurate fluid balance.	To assess amount of drug received by patient (NMC 2005: C).

Problem solving: Intraperitoneal instillation of cytotoxic drugs

Problem	Cause	Suggested action
Abdominal pain or discomfort.	Peritoneal irritation following placement of catheter. Incomplete drainage of the dialysate solution. Failure to warm dialysate solution to body temperature. Chemical peritonitis resulting from chemotherapeutic agent. Bacterial peritonitis.	Observe for a reaction and treat symptomatically.
Leakage from around the catheter following administration of the drug.	Peritoneum is not intact or catheter is not entirely within peritoneal cavity.	Strict aseptic technique required. Dressings to be changed frequently. When skin around the catheter has healed, there should be no further leakage.

Intra-arterial administration

Definition

Intra-arterial administration is the delivery of a cytotoxic drug to the tumour site by catheterization of the artery providing the blood supply to the affected organ. This allows a high concentration of drug to be delivered.

Indications

Intra-arterial chemotherapy has been used to treat a variety of malignancies at a number of different sites. These include:

- Head and neck lesions.
- Liver metastases from colorectal cancer.
- Sarcomas/melanomas of upper and lower limb (including isolated limb perfusion).
- Carcinoma of the stomach.
- Carcinoma of the breast.
- Carcinoma of the cervix.

The tumour site determines which artery will be used to deliver the chemotherapy since it is the artery supplying the tumour which is cannulated. The commonest route is the hepatic artery (Weinstein 2007).

Reference material

The advantage of the route is that it facilitates the delivery of high concentrations of drug to the primary or secondary tumour mass (Sewell *et al.* 2002). A reduction in systemic circulating levels of drugs has been shown to occur in many circumstances resulting in a corresponding reduction in side-effects to the patient (Hayden & Goodman 2005). The cytotoxic drugs used vary with the histology and site of the tumour. All of the following have been administered via the intra-arterial route:

- Actinomycin D.
- BCNU (carmustine).
- Bleomycin.
- Cisplatin.
- Doxorubicin.
- 5-FU (5-fluorouracil).
- 5-FUDR.
- Methotrexate.
- Melphalan.
- Mitomycin C.
- Vincristine (Weinstein 2007).

The main disadvantage of this route is that very high levels of drug in a perfused organ may result in excessive tissue damage (Sewell *et al.* 2002). It also requires the insertion of an arterial device and specialized nursing skill to operate the arterial pump (Weinstein 2007). Two main methods are used for infusional chemotherapy; these are termed external and internal arterial infusions.

The external method involves radiographic placement of an arterial catheter and attachment to an external infusion pump (Hayden & Goodman 2005). Temporary catheter placement is used for short-term therapies, i.e. from hours up to 5 days. Therapy can be given intermittently for several courses. This method is unsuitable for long-term use (6 months or longer) as it is uncomfortable, inconvenient and expensive, although a subcutaneous implanted port increases the patient's comfort and freedom (Hayden & Goodman 2005).

Once the catheter is in place and secured, cytotoxic drugs may be administered by:

- Injection, using a syringe.
- Small volume infusion, using a syringe pump.
- Large volume infusion, using a volumetric pump.

Internal or implantable methods involve the surgical placement of a totally implantable pump and appear to have a lower complication rate than the external method. The catheter is inserted into an appropriate artery and attached to the pump, which is filled with chemotherapy. This approach is more frequently used for colorectal cancer metastases to the liver.

Confirmation that the artery supplies the desired area can be achieved by instillation of yellow fluorescent dye if the tumour site is visible, or contrast medium if an internal organ such as the liver is the target area.

All delivery systems must provide adequate pressure to combat arterial pressure, i.e. 300 mmHg (Hayden & Goodman 2005). The majority of infusion pumps meet this requirement. Patient education is very important as the patient may have to maintain the implantable pump and be able to recognize any complications or malfunctions.

Principles of nursing care

Insertion is an operative procedure and consent must be obtained. Adequate explanation to the patient is essential, especially what to expect on return to the ward.

The catheter is inserted in theatre or in the X-ray department and its position checked at that time. The catheter is then secured and an occlusive dressing applied. This should *not* be touched as it is essential that the catheter is *not* displaced.

A three- or one-way tap is connected to the catheter and it is at this point that all manipulations take place. An extension set should be connected to this at the time of insertion or on return to the ward to prevent unnecessary handling near the skin exit site.

The system will consist of: catheter/tap/extension set/administration set and infusion device.

Certain general rules apply:

1 The dressing must not be touched but should be observed regularly for signs of bleeding. This should be reported immediately to the medical staff, including the radiologist.
2 All procedures or manipulations must be performed using aseptic technique.
3 All connections must be Luer locking to prevent exsanguination, air embolism or disconnection under pressure.
4 The catheter must be clamped securely or switched off closing the tap in situ before any equipment changes.
5 A positive pressure greater than arterial pressure must be maintained at all times.
6 When chemotherapy is not being infused, the flushing solution must be used to maintain patency. This should be via a syringe or syringe pump during transfer between wards or departments, or via a syringe pump or infusion pump in the ward. A nurse escort may be necessary for transfers. It should be delivered at the minimum rate sufficient to combat arterial pressure and maintain patency, approximately 3–5 ml per hour or 10 drops per minute, dependent on the device used. If a specialist delivery system is used, then manufacturers' instructions should be followed.
7 The patient must be instructed how often they are allowed to move and mobilize. This may vary depending on the site of the catheter. Assistance may be needed to maintain personal hygiene and relieve pressure in order to prevent the development of pressure ulcers on all points of contact.
8 The position of the catheter may be checked daily by X-ray, which will be performed on the ward. Fluoroscopy and instillation of dye are other methods of confirming position.
9 At the end of treatment, the patency of the arterial catheter should be maintained using an appropriate flushing solution until a decision has been made about removal. Instructions for this and the amount of heparin to be used should be prescribed in advance to enable the nurse to initiate the procedure when appropriate.

10 Before removal, the tap may be switched off and the catheter allowed to clot. The catheter should be removed by a doctor and firm pressure applied for at least 5 minutes or until all bleeding has ceased. A dressing should be applied to the site. Pressure dressings are not indicated if bleeding has ceased as they can obscure the formation of a haematoma.

Complications associated with intra-arterial chemotherapy

1 Arterial occlusion and thrombosis: the literature indicates that thrombosis occurs in over 40% of arteries catheterized for over 48 hours. However, this is dependent on the vessel used. Most catheters used for chemotherapy delivery pose no problem and will remain patent for the treatment period. However, a thrombus may embolize causing vascular insufficiency, distal or central embolism (Weinstein 2007). When occlusion occurs due to thrombus formation or spasm, blood flow is usually maintained by the collateral circulation until the vessel recovers. Presence of a pulse and the colour of the area should be checked daily or a Doppler flow meter may be used. Any abnormality should be reported to the medical staff and radiologist. The catheter should be removed by the doctor using firm, steady traction, in an attempt to prevent dislodging any thrombus present. The condition of the patient and the limb/area should be observed carefully at the time that vital signs are measured.

2 Damage to the artery, arteriovenous fistula, aneurysm formation: the incidence of these is low and the likelihood of problems occurring can be minimized by gentle handling of the catheter and immobilization of the limb/area as soon as appropriate.

3 Chemical hepatitis and biliary sclerosis: the occurrence of these will be evident from elevated liver enzymes. Therefore, monitoring of liver function tests is important. Any elevation is usually transient.

4 Exsanguination/air embolism: the seriousness of an air embolus depends on the siting of the arterial catheter and whether it is a direct route to the carotid artery and so to the brain. Luer–Lok connections must be used throughout the pathway. These should be checked at regular intervals, and continuous flow maintained. Care must be taken when changing equipment to prevent blood loss occurring, or air entering the catheter, e.g. shut off the tap, firm clamping, if necessary.

Problem solving: Intra-arterial administration of cytotoxic drugs

287

Problem	Cause	Suggested action
Haemorrhage.	Excessive movement. Insufficient pressure on site following removal of catheter.	Observe the dressing at regular intervals. Monitor pulse and blood pressure at least 4 hourly. Instruct the patient on the amount of movement permitted and to report any feeling of faintness, or oozing noted on dressing. After removal of the catheter, vital signs and the dressing should be observed at least every 15 minutes for 2 hours. Whether the patient should remain on bedrest for 24 hours is dependent on the site where the patient has been catheterized. If bleeding occurs, pressure should be applied immediately and a member of the medical staff contacted.
Displacement of the catheter.	Dressing disturbed. Excessive movement by patient.	Do not disturb the dressing. Instruct the patient on amount of movement permitted. Check position daily.
Infection.	Poor aseptic technique.	Strict asepsis must be maintained for all procedures and manipulations of the arterial catheter (Weinstein 2007). Temperature must be taken at least every 4 hours and any pyrexia investigated.
Extravasation of drugs/failure of drug to reach target area (both rare).	Incorrect placement of catheter.	If there is any doubt concerning the placement of the catheter the doctor and radiologist should be notified, as extravasation of the drug may lead to ulceration and necrosis.

References and further reading

Bertolli, G. (1995) Prevention and management of extravasation of cytotoxic drugs. *Drug Saf*, **12**(4), 245–55.

Bertolli, G., Cafferata, M. & Ardizzoni, A. (1997) Skin ulceration potential of paclitaxel in a mouse skin model in vivo. *Cancer*, **79**, 2266–9.

British Medical Association/Royal Pharmaceutical Society of Great Britain (BMA/RPSGB) (2008) *British National Formulary*. The Pharmaceutical Press, London.

Camp Sorrell, D. (2005) *Oncology Nursing Society Access Device Guidelines; Recommendations for Nursing Practice and Education*. Oncology Nursing Society, Pittsburgh, PA.

Camp Sorrell, D. (1998) Developing extravasation protocols and monitoring outcomes. *J Intraven Nurs*, **21**(4), 232–9.

Cass, Y. *et al.* (1997) Health and safety aspects of cytotoxic services. In: *The Cytotoxic Handbook* (eds M. Allwood, A. Stanley & P. Wright), 3rd edn. Radcliffe Medical Press, Oxford, pp. 35–54.

Comerford, K., Eggenberger, T. & Robinson, K. (2002) Chemotherapy infusions. In: *Intravenous Therapy Made Incredibly Easy* (ed A.T. McPhee). Springhouse Corporation, Philadelphia, pp. 239–68.

Cox, K. *et al.* (1988) The management of cytotoxic drug extravasation: guidelines drawn up by a working party for the Clinical Oncological Society of Australia. *Med J Aust*, **148**, 185–9.

CP Pharmaceuticals (1999) *How Quickly Could You Act?* CP Pharmaceuticals, Wrexham.

DH (1999) HSC 1999/186. *Latex medical gloves and powdered latex medical gloves: reducing the risk of allergic reaction to latex and powdered medical gloves*. HMSO, London.

DH (2000) *An Organisation with a Memory*. HMSO, London.

DH (2002a) *Reference Guide to Consent for Examination or Treatment*. HMSO, London.

DH (2002b) *The Control of Substances Hazardous to Health Regulations 2002 (COSHH)*. HMSO, London.

DH (2003) HSC 2003/10. *Updated National Guidance on the Safe Administration of Intrathecal Chemotherapy*. Department of Health, London.

DH (2007) *Handling Needles in the Waste and Recycling Industry*. HMSO, London.

Dougherty, L. (2003) An expert witness working within the legal system in the United Kingdom. *J Vas Ass Net*, **8**(2), 29–37.

Dougherty, L. (2005) Intravenous management. In: *The Royal Marsden Hospital Handbook of Cancer Chemotherapy* (eds D. Brigthon & M. Wood). Elsevier Churchill Livingstone, Edinburgh, pp. 93–108.

Dougherty, L. (2006) *Central Venous Access Devices*. Blackwell Publishing, Oxford.

Dranitsaris, G. *et al.* (2005) Are health care providers who work with cancer drugs at an increased risk for toxic events? A systematic review and meta-analysis of the literature. *J Oncol Pharm Pract*, **11**, 69–78.

El Saghir, N. *et al.* (2004) Dexrazoane for anthracycline extravasation and GM-SCF for skin ulceration and wound healing. *Lancet Oncol*, **5**, 320–1.

Federle, M., Chang, P.J. & Confer, S. (1998) Frequency and effects of extravasation of non isotonic CT contrast media during rapid bolus injection. *Radiology*, **206**, 637–40.

Ferguson, L. & Wright, P. (2003) Health and Safety aspects of cytotoxic services. In: *The Cytotoxic Handbook* (eds M. Alwood *et al.*), 4th edn. Radcliffe Medical Press, Oxford, pp. 35–61.

Few, B.J. (1987) Hyaluronidase for treating intravenous extravasations. *MCN Pharmacopoeia*, **12**, 23.

Gabriel, J. (2008) Safe administration of intravenous cytotoxic drugs In: *Intravenous Therapy in Nursing Practice* (eds L. Dougherty & J. Lamb), 2nd edn. Blackwell Publishing, Oxford (in press).

Gault, D.T. (1993) Extravasation injuries. *Br J Plast Surg*, **46**(2), 91–6.

Gault, D. & Challands, J. (1997) Extravasation of drugs. *Anaesth Rev*, **13**, 223–41.

Goolsby, T.V. & Lombardo, F.A. (2006) Extravasation of chemotherapeutic agents: prevention and treatment. *Semin Oncol*, **33**, 139–43.

Hayden, B.K. & Goodman, M. (2005) Chemotherapy: principles of administration. In: *Cancer Nursing – Principles and Practice* (eds C. Henke Yarbro *et al.*), 6th edn. Jones and Bartlett, Boston, MA, pp. 351–411.

Harrison, B. (2001) Risks of handling cytotoxic drugs: A review. In: *The Chemotherapy Source Book* (ed. M.C. Perry), 3rd edn. Lippincott Williams & Wilkins, Philadelphia, pp. 566–82.

HSE (2003) *Safe Handling of Cytotoxic Drugs*. Health and Safety Executive, London.

How, C. & Brown, J. (1998) Extravasation of cytotoxic chemotherapy from peripheral veins. *Eur J Oncol Nurs*, **2**(1), 51–8.

Ignoffo, R.J. & Friedman, M.A. (1980) Therapy of local toxicities caused by extravasation of cancer chemotherapeutic drugs. *Cancer Treat Rev*, **7**, 17–27.

Infusion Nurses Society (2006) *Infusion Nursing Standards of Practice*. JIN, 29 (1S). Lippincott Williams & Wilkins, Philadelphia.

Irving, V. (2001) Managing extravasation injuries in preterm infants. *NT Plus*, **97**(35), 40–6.

Jackson, G. *et al.* (2006) *Consensus opinion on the use of dexrazoxane (Savene^{TM}) in the treatment of anthracycline extravasation*. Topotarget, UK.

Kassner, E. (2000) Evaluation and treatment of chemotherapy extravasation injuries. *J Pediatric Oncol Nurs*, **17**, 135–48.

Kelland, L. (2005) Cancer cell biology, drug action and resistance. In: *The Royal Marsden Hospital Handbook of Cancer Chemotherapy* (eds D. Brigthon & M. Wood). Elsevier Churchill Livingstone, Edinburgh, pp. 3–15.

Khan, M.S. & Holmes, J.D. (2002) Reducing morbidity from extravasation injuries. *Ann Plast Surg*, **48**(6), 628–32.

Langer S.W., Sehested, M. & Buhl Jensen, P. (2000) Treatment of antracycline extravasation with dexrazoxane. *Clin Cancer Res*, **6**, 3680–6.

Lavery, I. & Ingram, P. (2006) Prevention of infection in peripheral intravenous devices. *Nurs Stand*, **20**, 49–56.

Lawson, T. (2003) A legal perspective on CVC-related extravasation. *Journal of Vascular Access Devices*, **8**(1), 25–7.

MARCH (Management and Awareness of the Risks of Cytotoxics Handling) (2007). Guidelines available on the website: www.marchguidelines.com. Accessed on 16/8/07.

Masoorli, S. (2003) Extravasation injuries associated with the use of central vascular access devices. *JVAD*, **8**(1), 21–3.

Mayo, D.J. (1998) Fibrin sheath formation and chemotherapy extravasation: a case report. *Supp Care Cancer*, **6**, 51–6.

McCaffrey Boyle, D. & Engelking, C. (1995) Vesicant extravasation: myths and realities. *Oncol Nurs Forum*, **22**(1), 57–65.

Naylor, W (2005) Extravasation wounds; aetiology and management. In: *The Royal Marsden Hospital Handbook of Cancer Chemotherapy* (eds D. Brigthon & M. Wood). Elsevier Churchill Livingstone, Edinburgh, pp. 109–12.

NMC (2005) *Guidelines for Records and Record Keeping*. Nursing and Midwifery Council, London.

NMC (2008a) *Standards for Medicines Management*. Nursing and Midwifery Council, London.

NMC (2008b) *The Code: Standards of Conduct, Performance and Ethics for Nurses and Midwives*. Nursing and Midwifery Council, London.

Perdue, M.B. (2001) Intravenous complications. In: *Infusion Therapy in Clinical Practice* (eds J. Hankin *et al.*), 2nd edn. W.B. Saunders, Philadelphia, pp. 418–45.

Pethran, A. *et al.* (2003) Uptake of antineoplastic agents in pharmacy and hospital personnel. Part 1: monitoring of urinary concentrations. *Int Arch Occup Environ Health*, **76**, 5–10.

Polovich, M. (2003) *Oncology Nursing Society. Safe Handling of Hazardous Drugs*, 2nd edn. Oncology Nursing Press, Pittsburgh, PA.

Polovich, M., White, J.M. & Kelleher, L.O. (2005) *Oncology Nursing Society. Chemotherapy and Biotherapy Guidelines and Recommendations for Practice*, 2nd edn. Oncology Nursing Press, Pittsburgh, PA.

Quan, W. (1999) Malignant, pleural, peritoneal and pericardial effusions and meningeal infiltrates. In: *Handbook of Chemotherapy* (ed. R.T. Skeet), 5th edn. Lippincott, Williams & Wilkins, Philadelphia, pp. 279–81.

RCN (2005) *Standards for Infusion Therapy*. Royal College of Nursing, London.

Roth, D. (2003) Extravasation injuries of peripheral veins: a basis for litigation. *JVAD*, **8**(1), 13–20.

Rudolph, R. & Larson, D.L. (1987) Etiology and treatment of chemotherapeutic agent extravasation injuries: a review. *J Clin Oncol*, **5**(7), 1116–26.

Sansivero, G. & Barton-Burke, M. (2001) Chemotherapy administration: general principles for vascular access. In: *Cancer: A Nursing Process Approach* (eds M. Barton-Burke, G. Wilkes & K. Ingwerson), 3rd edn. Jones and Bartlett, Sudbury Massachusetts, pp. 645–70.

Sauerland, C. *et al.* (2006) Vesicant extravasation part 1: mechanisms, pathogenesis and nursing care to reduce risks. *ONF*, **33**(6), 1134–41.

Scales, K. (2005) Vascular access: a guide to peripheral venous cannulation. *Nurs Stand*, **19**(49), 48–52.

Scurr, M. *et al.* (2005) Combination chemotherapy and chemotherapy principles. In: *The Royal Marsden Hospital Handbook of Cancer Chemotherapy* (eds D. Brigthon & M. Wood). Elsevier Churchill Livingstone, Edinburgh, pp. 17–29.

Schrijvers, D.L. (2003) Extravasation: the dreaded complication of chemotherapy. *Ann Oncology*, **14**(Suppl 3), 26–30.

Schulmeister, L. (1989) Needle dislodgement from implanted venous access devices – inpatients and outpatient experiences. *J Intraven Nurs*, **12**, 90–2.

Schulmeister, L. (1998) A complication of vascular access device insertion. *J Intraven Nurs*, **21**(4), 197–202.

Seto, T. *et al.* (2006) Intrapleural hypotonic cisplatin treatment for malignant pleural effusion in 80 patients with non-small-cell lung cancer: a multi institutional phase II trial. *Br J Cancer*, **95**(6), 717–21.

Sewell, G., Summerhayes, M. & Stanley, A. (2002) Administration of chemotherapy. In: *The Cytotoxics Handbook* (eds M. Allwood *et al.*), 4th edn. Radcliffe Medical Press, Oxford, pp. 85–115.

Shulman, R. *et al.* (1998) Management of extravasation of IV drugs. In: *UCL Injectable Drug Administration*. Blackwell Science, Oxford, pp. 13–18.

Stanley, A. (2002) Managing complications of chemotherapy administration. In: *The Cytotoxic Handbook* (eds M. Allwood *et al.*), 4th edn. Radcliffe Medical Press, Oxford, pp. 119–92.

Toft, B. (2001) *External Inquiry into the Adverse Incident that Occurred at the Queen's Medical Centre, Nottingham, on 4th January 2001*. Department of Health, London.

Ulutin, H.C. *et al.* (2000) Comparison of granulocyte-colony stimulating factor and granulocyte macrophage-colony stimulating factor in the treatment of extravasation ulcers. *Eur J Gynaecol Oncol*, **21**, 613–15.

Valanis, B. *et al.* (1997) Occupational exposure to antineoplastic agents and self reported infertility among nurses and pharmacists. *J Occup Environ Med*, **39**(6), 574–80.

Vandergrift, K.V. (2001) Oncologic therapy. In: *Infusion Therapy in Clinical Practice* (eds J. Hankin *et al.*), 2nd edn. W.B. Saunders, Philadelphia, pp. 248–75.

van der Molen, B. (2005) Patient information and education. In: *The Royal Marsden Hospital Handbook of Cancer Chemotherapy* (eds D. Brigthon & M. Wood). Elsevier Churchill Livingstone, Edinburgh, pp. 49–59.

Washburn, D. (2007) Intravesical antineoplastic therapy following transurethral resection of bladder tumors: nursing implications from the operating room to discharge. *Clinical Journal of Oncology Nursing*, **11**(4), 553–9.

Weinstein, S. (2007) Antineoplastic therapy. In: *Plumer's Principles and Practices of Intravenous Therapy*, 8th edn. Lippincott, Williams & Wilkins, Philadelphia, pp. 486–573.

Wickham, R. *et al.* (2006) Vesicant extravasation part II: evidence based management and continuing controversies. *ONF*, **33**(6), 1143–50.

289

Chapter 13

Drug administration: delivery (infusion devices)

291 Reference material
296 **Infusion devices**
296 Gravity infusion devices
298 Infusion pumps
301 Summary
302 *Procedure guidelines:* Subcutaneous administration of drugs using a syringe driver (e.g. Sims (Graseby) Medical MS26)
303 *Procedure guidelines:* Syringe driver: preparation of the syringe and priming the infusion set for 24-hour drug administration using the Sims (Graseby) Medical MS26
304 *Procedure guidelines:* Syringe driver: inserting the winged infusion set or cannula and connecting syringe
307 *Problem solving:* Syringe drivers
309 References and further reading

Definition

An infusion device is designed to accurately deliver measured amounts of fluid or drug via a number of routes (e.g. intravenous, subcutaneous or epidural) over a period of time. The infusion device is set at an appropriate rate to achieve the desired therapeutic response and prevent complications (Quinn 2000; Dougherty 2002; Medical Devices Agency 2003).

Indications

The nurse has a responsibility to determine when and how to use an infusion device to deliver hydration, drugs, transfusions and nutritional support, and how to select the appropriate device in order to manage the needs of the patient. Common types of infusion devices include: gravity infusion devices, gravity drip rate controllers, infusion pumps, syringe pumps, specialist pumps (e.g. patient controlled analgesia pumps, epidurals). The following factors should be considered when selecting an appropriate infusion delivery system (Quinn 2008):

1 Risk to the patient of:
   (a) Overinfusion.
   (b) Underinfusion.
   (c) Uneven flow.
   (d) Inadvertent bolus.
   (e) High pressure delivery.
   (f) Extravascular infusion.
2 Delivery parameters:
   (a) Infusion rate and volume required.
   (b) Accuracy required (over a long or short period of time).
   (c) Alarms required.
   (d) Ability to infuse into site chosen (venous, arterial, subcutaneous).
   (e) Suitability of device for infusing drug (e.g. ability to infuse viscous drugs).
3 Environmental features:
   (a) Ease of operation.
   (b) Frequency of observation and adjustment.
   (c) Type of patient (neonate, child, critically ill).
   (d) Mobility of patient.

Reference material

Infusion devices enable the delivery of a drug or fluid to a patient at a constant rate over a set period of time to achieve the desired therapeutic response. The process for infusional therapy includes:

- Prescription of the fluid or drug.
- Preparation of the infusion solution.
- Selection of the appropriate infusion device.
- Calculation and setting of the rate of infusion.
- Administration of the fluid to the patient.
- Monitoring and recording of the actual delivery.
- Disposal. (Medical Devices Agency 2003, p. 6.)

Box 13.1 Groups at risk of complications associated with flow control (adapted from Quinn 2008).

- Infants and young children.
- The elderly.
- Patients with compromised cardiovascular status.
- Patients with impairment or failure of organs, e.g. kidneys.
- Patients with major sepsis.
- Patients suffering from shock, whatever the cause.
- Postoperative or post-trauma patients.
- Stressed patients, whose endocrine homeostatic controls may be affected.
- Patients receiving multiple medications, whose clinical status may change rapidly.

The nurse must have knowledge of the solutions, their effects, rate of administration, factors that affect flow of infusion, as well as the complications which could occur when flow is not controlled (Weinstein 2007). The nurse should have an understanding of which groups require accurate flow control in order to prevent complications (Box 13.1) and how to select the most appropriate device for accuracy of delivery to best meet the patient's flow control needs (according to age, condition, setting and prescribed therapy) (Weinstein 2007).

The identification of risks is crucial, e.g. complex calculations, prescription errors (Dougherty 2002; Weinstein 2007) and the risks associated with the infusions, i.e. neo-natal risk infusions, high-risk infusion, low-risk infusions and ambulatory infusions (Quinn 2000; Medical Devices Agency 2003). The early detection of errors and infusion-related complications, e.g. over and underinfusion (Box 13.2) is imperative in

---

Box 13.2 Complications of inadequate flow control (Quinn 2008, p. 195).

Complications associated with overinfusion

- Fluid overload with accompanying electrolyte imbalance.
- Metabolic disturbances during parenteral nutrition, mainly related to serum glucose levels.
- Toxic concentrations of medications, which may result in a shock-like syndrome ('speed shock').
- Air embolism, due to containers running dry before expected.
- An increase in venous complications, e.g. chemical phlebitis, caused by reduced dilution of irritant substances (Weinstein 2007).

Complications associated with underinfusion

- Dehydration.
- Metabolic disturbances.
- A delayed response to medications or below therapeutic dose.
- Occlusion of a cannula/catheter due to slow flow or cessation of flow.

---

order to instigate the appropriate interventions in response to an error or to manage any complications, as serious errors or complications can result in patient death (Quinn 2000; Dougherty 2002; NPSA 2003). Overinfusion accounts for about half of the reported errors involving infusion pumps with 80% due to user error rather than a fault with the device (Medical Devices Agency 2000). The use of infusion devices, both mechanical and electronic, has increased the level of safety in intravenous therapy. However, it is recommended that a clearly defined structure for management of infusion systems must exist within a hospital (Medical Devices Agency 2003; NPSA 2004; Department of Health, Social Services and Public Safety 2006; Health Care Standards Unit 2007a, b; NHS Litigation Authority 2007).

Criteria for selection of an infusion device:

- Rationalization of devices.
- Clinical requirement.
- Education.
- Compatibility with other equipment.
- Disposables.
- Product support.
- Costs.
- Service and maintenance.
- Regulatory issues, e.g. compliance with European Community Directives (Quinn 2000; Medical Devices Agency 2003; Department of Health, Social Services and Public Safety 2006; Health Care Standards Unit 2007a, b; NHS Litigation Authority 2007).

Strategies need to be developed for replacement of old, obsolete or inappropriate devices (Quinn 2000; Medical Devices Agency 2003; Department of Health, Social Services and Public Safety 2006; Health Care Standards Unit 2007a, b; NHS Litigation Authority 2007), planned service mainte-

nance programmes and acceptance testing (Medical Devices Agency 2003).

'Fifteen million infusions are performed in the NHS every year and 700 unsafe incidents are reported each year with 19% attributed to user error' (NPSA 2004, p. 1). Between 1990 and 2000 there were 1485 incidents reported to the Medical Devices Agency which involved infusion pumps (Medical Devices Agency 2003). In 50% of incidents no cause was established. However, of the remaining incidents, 27% were attributed to user error (e.g. misloading of the administration set or syringe, setting the wrong rate, confusing pump type) and 20% to device-related issues (e.g. poor maintenance, cleaning) (Williams & Lefever 2000; Medical Devices Agency 2003). Syringe pumps have given rise to the most significant problems in terms of patient mortality and morbidity (Fox 2000; Medical Devices Agency 2003; NPSA 2003).

The high frequency of human error has highlighted the need for more formalized, validated, competency-based training and assessment (Pickstone 2000; Quinn 2000; Medical Devices Agency 2003; NPSA 2003, 2004). They must be familiar with the device they are using and not attempt to operate any device that they have not been fully trained to use (Murray & Glenister 2001; NPSA 2003). As a minimum, the training should cover the device, drugs and solutions, and the practical procedures related to setting up the device and problem solving (Medical Devices Agency 2000, 2003). Staff should also be made aware of the mechanisms for reporting faults with devices and procedures for adverse incident reporting within their trust and to the Medicines and Healthcare Products Regulatory Agency (MHRA) and the National Patient Safety Agency (NPSA) (MHRA 2006b).

A useful checklist (Table 13.1) has been produced by the Medical Devices Agency for staff to follow prior to using

Table 13.1 Checklist: How safe is your practice? Adapted from Medical Devices Agency (2000, p. 10; 2001, pp. 8 & 9).

- Have I been trained in the use of the infusion device?
- Was the training formalized and recorded or did I just pick it up as I went along?
- How was my competency in relation to the infusion device assessed?
- Have I read the user instructions on how to use the infusion device and am I familiar with any warning labels?
- When was the infusion device last serviced?
- Are there any signs of wear, damage or faults?
- Do I know how to set up and use the infusion device?
- Is the infusion device and any additional equipment in good working order?
- Do I know how the infusion device should perform and the monitoring that needs to be done to check its performance?
- Am I using the correct additional equipment, e.g. the appropriate disposable administration set for the infusion pump?
- Do I know how to recognize whether the infusion device has failed?
- Do I know what to do if the infusion device fails?
- Do I know how and to whom to report an infusion device-related adverse incident?
- Does checking the infusion device indicate it is functioning correctly and to the manufacturer's specification?
- What action should be taken if the infusion device is not functioning properly?
- Is there up-to-date documentation to record regular checking of the infusion device?
- What are the details (name and serial number) of the infusion device being used?
- What is the cleaning and/or decontamination procedure for the infusion device and what are my responsibilities in this process?
- Do I know how to report an adverse incident?
- Do I have access to MHRA Device Bulletins of relevance to my area of practice and do I read and take note of Hazard and Safety Notices?

a medical device to ensure safe practice (Medical Devices Agency 2000, 2003).

Factors influencing flow rates

Once an infusion device is set up, the nurse should check the patient and the infusion rate regularly to ensure the prescribed flow rate is maintained (Medical Devices Agency 2003). The following factors may increase or decrease intravenous flow rates, particularly with mechanical devices using gravity flow, and should be taken into account when setting up an infusion device.

Type of fluid

The composition, viscosity and concentration of the fluid affects flow (Pickstone 1999; Quinn 2000; Springhouse 2005; Weinstein 2007). Irritating solutions may result in venospasm and impede the flow rate, this may be resolved by use of a warm pack over the cannula site and the limb (Springhouse 2005; Weinstein 2007).

Height of the infusion container

Intravenous fluids run by gravity and so any changes in the height of the container will alter the flow rate. The height of the container can be hung up to 1.5 m above the infusion site which will provide a hydrostatic pressure of 110 mmHg (Medical Devices Agency 2003; Springhouse 2005). One metre above the infusion site would create 70 mmHg of pressure, which is adequate to overcome venous pressure (normal range in an adult is 25–80 mmHg) (Pickstone 1999). Therefore any alterations in the patient's position may alter the flow rate and necessitate a change in the speed of the infusion to maintain the appropriate rate of flow (Perucca 2001; Weinstein 2007). Positioning of the patient will affect flow and patients should be instructed to keep the arm lower than the infusion, if the infusion is reliant on gravity (Quinn 2008).

Administration set

The flow rate of the infusion may be affected in several ways:

- Roller clamps or screw clamps, used to adjust and maintain rates of flow on gravity infusions, vary considerably in their efficiency and accuracy which is often dependent on a number of variables such as patient movement and height of infusion container (Perucca 2001). Roller clamps should be positioned on the upper third of the tubing near the fluid container, making access convenient for staff and out of the way of the patient to avoid accidental handling (Perucca 2001). The clamp should be repositioned periodically to prevent the tubing developing a memory (cold creep) where the tubing tries to retain its round shape and pushes the clamp open or where pinched tubing does not reopen (Perucca 2001; Medical Devices Agency 2003). The roller clamp should be used as the primary means of occluding the tubing even if

there is an anti-free-flow device (Medical Devices Agency 2003).
- The inner diameter of the lumen and the length of tubing will also affect flow. Microbore sets have a narrow lumen, therefore flow is restricted to some degree. However, these sets may be used as a safeguard against 'runaway' or bolus infusions by either an integrated anti-siphon valve or anti-free-flow device (Quinn 2000; Perucca 2001; Weinstein 2007).
- Inclusion of other in-line devices, e.g. filters, may also affect the flow rate (Perucca 2001; Medical Devices Agency 2003).

Vascular access device

The flow rate may be affected by any of the following:

- The condition and size of the vein, e.g. phlebitis can reduce the lumen size and decrease flow (Weinstein 2007).
- The gauge of the cannula/catheter (Medical Devices Agency 2003; Springhouse 2005; Weinstein 2007).
- The position of the device within the vein, i.e. whether it is up against the vein wall.
- The site of the vascular access device, e.g. the flow may be affected by the change in position of a limb: such as a decrease in flow when a patient bends their arm if a cannula is sited over the elbow joint (Springhouse 2005).
- Kinking, pinching or compression of the cannula/catheter or tubing of the administration set may cause variation in the set rate (Medical Devices Agency 2003; Springhouse 2005).
- Restricted venous circulation, e.g. blood pressure cuff or the patient lying on the limb increases the risk of an occlusion of the device and may result in clot formation (Gabriel 1999; Quinn 2008).

The patient

Patients occasionally adjust the control clamp or other parts of the delivery system, for example, changing the height of the container, thereby making flow unreliable. Some pumps have tamper-proof features to minimize the risk of accidental manipulation of the infusion device (Perucca 2001) or unauthorized changing of infusion device controls (Amoore & Adamson 2003).

Infusion-related complications

Circulatory overload (isotonic fluid expansion)

A critical and common complication of intravenous therapy is circulatory overload, which is *isotonic fluid expansion*. It is caused by infusion of fluids of the same tonicity as plasma into the vascular circulation, for example sodium chloride 0.9%. As isotonic solutions do not affect osmolarity, water does not flow from the extracellular to the intracellular compartment. The result is that the extracellular compartment expands in proportion to the fluid infused (Weinstein 2007). Because of the electrolyte concentration, no extra water is

293

available to enable the kidneys selectively to excrete and re-store the balance.

If circulatory overload is detected early, treatment consists of withholding all fluids until excess water and electrolytes have been eliminated by the body and/or administration of diuretics to promote rapid diuresis (Weinstein 2007). How-ever, careful monitoring should continue to prevent isotonic contraction occurring (where there is loss of fluid and elec-trolytes isotonic to the extracellular fluid such as blood and large volumes of fluid from diarrhoea and vomiting; Weinstein 2007). If fluid administration is allowed to con-tinue unchecked, it can result in left-sided heart failure, circu-latory collapse and cardiac arrest (Edwards 2001; Dougherty 2002).

Dehydration

Dehydration may be categorized either as hypertonic or hy-potonic contraction and may be caused by underinfusion. Hypertonic contraction occurs when water is lost without corresponding loss of salts (Weinstein 2007) and occurs in patients unable to take sufficient fluids (elderly, unconscious or incontinent patients) or who have excess insensible water loss via skin and lungs or as a result of certain drugs in ex-cess. Hypotonic contraction occurs when fluids containing more salt than water are lost and this results in a decrease in osmolarity of the extracellular compartment (Weinstein 2007).

It is important that the nurse recognizes the symptoms of overinfusion or underinfusion and certain factors should be considered when monitoring patients (Weinstein 2007) (Table 13.2).

Speed shock

Speed shock is a systemic reaction that occurs when a sub-stance foreign to the body is rapidly introduced into the cir-culation (Weinstein 2007). This complication can manifest following administration of intravenous bolus injections or when large volumes of fluid are given too rapidly. This should not be confused with pulmonary oedema, which relates to the volume of fluid infused into the patient. Rapid, uncon-trolled administration of drugs will result in toxic concen-trations reaching vital organs. Toxicity may be manifested by an exaggeration of the usual pharmacological actions of the drug or by signs and symptoms specific for that drug or class of drugs. The most extreme toxic response which can occur if a drug is given at a dose or rate exceeding that recommended is termed the lethal response.

Signs of speed shock may include:

- Flushed face.
- Headache and dizziness.
- Congestion of the chest.
- Tachycardia and fall in blood pressure.
- Syncope.
- Shock.
- Cardiovascular collapse. (Perdue 2001; Weinstein 2007.)

Prevention of speed shock involves the nurse having knowl-edge of the drug and the recommended rate of adminis-tration. When commencing an infusion using gravity flow, check that the solution is flowing freely before adjusting the rate. Movement of the patient or the device within the ves-sel can cause the infusion to flow more or less freely after a few minutes of setting the rate (Weinstein 2007). For high-risk medications an electronic flow control device is recom-mended (RCN 2005). Although most pumps have an anti-free-flow mechanism, always close the roller clamp prior to removing the set from the pump (Pickstone 1999; MHRA 2006a). If speed shock occurs, the infusion must be slowed down or discontinued. Medical staff should be notified im-mediately and the patient's condition treated as clinically indicated (Perdue 2001).

Siphonage

Uncontrolled flow from a syringe is called siphonage; this is a result of gravity or leakage of air into the syringe and ad-ministration set. Siphonage can occur whether or not the sy-ringe is fixed into an infusion device (Pickstone 1999; Quinn 2000). It has been reported that, 'in practice, a 50 ml syringe attached to a length of administration set with an internal diameter of 3 mm has been shown to empty by siphonage in less than 1 minute' (Pickstone 1999, p. 57).

To minimize the risk of siphonage the following safe prac-tice should be taken:

- The syringe (plunger and barrel) should be correctly lo-cated and secured.
- Intravenous administration extension sets should always be micro/narrow bore in diameter to increase the re-sistance to flow; wide-bore extension sets should be avoided.
- Position of the syringe pump should always be the same level as the infusion site (Medical Devices Agency 2003).
- The use of extension sets with an integral anti-siphonage valve (Quinn 2000; Medical Devices Agency 2003).

Paediatric considerations

The MHRA classify infusion devices into categories of infu-sion risk. Neonatal infusions are the highest risk category, high-risk infusions are typically the infusion of fluids in chil-dren where accuracy of the flow rate is essential (Medical Devices Agency 2003). Infusion therapy within the paedi-atric setting requires very specific skills (Sundquist 2001). Competency in calculation of paediatric dosages, maintain-ing a stringent fluid balance, use of paediatric-specific devices and management of complications are paramount.

Principles of equipment selection and application

The MHRA, formerly the Medical Devices Agency, has made recommendations on the safety and performance of infusion

Table 13.2 Monitoring overinfusion and underinfusion.

Type of fluid/ electrolyte imbalance	Patients at risk	Signs and symptoms	Treatment
Circulatory overload (isotonic fluid expansion)	Early postoperative or post-trauma patients, older people, those with impaired renal and cardiac function and children	■ Weight gain ■ A relative increase in fluid intake compared to output ■ A high bounding pulse pressure, indicating a high cardiac output ■ Raised central venous pressure measurements ■ Peripheral hand vein emptying time longer than normal. (Peripheral veins will usually empty in 3–5 seconds when the hand is elevated and will fill in the same length of time when the hand is lowered to a dependent position) ■ Peripheral oedema ■ Hoarseness ■ Dyspnoea, cyanosis and coughing due to pulmonary oedema and neck vein engorgement	If detected early: withholding all fluids until excess water and electrolytes have been eliminated by the body and/or administration of diuretics to promote rapid diuresis
Dehydration **(hypertonic contraction or hypotonic contraction)**	**Hypertonic** Elderly, unconscious or incontinent patients **Hypotonic** Infants are at greatest risk, especially if they have diarrhoea Loss of salt from various sources: excess diuresis, fistula drainage, burns, vomiting or sweating	**Hyper/Hypotonic contraction** ■ Weight loss **Hypercontraction** ■ Thirst (although this may be absent in the elderly) ■ Irritability and restlessness and possible confusion ■ Diminished skin turgor ■ Dry mouth and furred tongue **Hypocontraction** ■ Negative fluid balance ■ Weak, thready, rapid pulse rate ■ Increased 'hand filling time' ■ Increased skin turgor	Replacement of fluids and electrolytes

295

devices in order to enable users to make the appropriate choice of equipment to suit most applications (Medical Devices Agency 2003). The classification system is divided into three major categories according to the potential risks involved. These are shown in Table 13.3. A pump suited to the most risky category of therapy (A) can be safely used for the other categories (B and C). A pump suited to category B can be used for B and C, whereas a pump with the lowest specification (C) is suited only to category C therapies (Medical Devices Agency 2003) (Figure 13.1). Hospitals are required to label each infusion pump with its category and it is necessary to know the category of the proposed therapy and match it with a pump of the same or better category. A locally produced list of drugs/fluids by their categories will need to be provided to all device users (Medical Devices Agency 2003).

Requirements of devices
Accuracy of delivery

In order to meet requirements for high-risk and neonatal infusions, pumps must be accurate to within ±5% of the set rate when measured over a 60-minute period (Perucca 2001; Medical Devices Agency 2003). They also have to satisfy short-term, minute-to-minute accuracy requirements, which determine smoothness and consistency of output (Medical Devices Agency 2003).

Occlusion response and pressure

Flow will occur if the pressure at the tip of an intravascular device is just fractionally above the pressure in the vein; the pressure does not need to be excessive. In an adult

Table 13.3 Therapy categories and performance parameters.

Therapy category	Therapy description	Patient group	Critical performance parameters
A	Drugs with narrow therapeutic margin	Any	Good long-term accuracy Good short-term accuracy
	Drugs with short half-life	Any	Rapid alarm after occlusion Small occlusion bolus
	Any infusion given to neonates	Neonates	Able to detect very small air embolus (volumetric pumps only) Small flow rate increments Good bolus accuracy Rapid start-up time (syringe pumps only)
B	Drugs, other than those with a short half-life	Any except neonates	Good long-term accuracy Alarm after occlusion
	Total parenteral nutrition Fluid maintenance Transfusions	Volume sensitive except neonates	Small occlusion bolus Able to detect small air embolus (volumetric pumps only) Small flow rate increments
	Diamorphine	Any except neonates	Bolus accuracy
C	Total parenteral nutrition Fluid maintenance Transfusions	Any except volume sensitive or neonates	Long-term accuracy Alarm after occlusion Small occlusion bolus Able to detect air embolus (volumetric pumps only) Incremental flow rates

Crown copyright material is reproduced with the permission of the Controller of HMSO and Queen's Printer for Scotland. Medical Devices Agency (2003).

peripheral vein pressure is approximately 25 mmHg, while in a neonate it measures 5 mmHg (Quinn 2000). Most pumps have a variable pressure setting which allows the user to use their own judgement about the pressure needed to deliver therapy safely. It can be set as low as 100–250 mmHg (2–5 psi) for infusions of vesicants or routine infusions via healthy veins (Perucca 2001) or a maximum of 500 mmHg (10 psi) in positional central venous catheters. Flow is dependent upon pressure divided by resistance. If long extension sets of small internal bore are used, the resistance to flow will increase (Pickstone 1999; Quinn 2000). If an administration set occludes the resistance increases and the infusion will not flow into the vein. The longer the occlusion occurs, the greater the pressure and the pump will continue to pump until an occlusion alarm is activated. There are two types of occlusions defined: upstream, between the pump and the container, and downstream, which is between the pump and the patient. An upstream occlusion alarms when a vacuum is created in the upstream tubing or full reservoir, due to collapsed or empty plastic fluid container or clamped/kinking tubing. A downstream occlusion is when the pressure required by the pump exceeds a certain psi limit (Perucca 2001).

Pumps alarm at a pressure termed 'occlusion alarm pressure' and many pumps allow the user to set the pressure within a range (Medical Devices Agency 2003). Therefore the time it takes to alarm depends on the rate of flow: high rates alarm more quickly. When the alarm is activated, a certain amount of stored bolus will be present and it is important that what could be a potentially large bolus is not released into the vein. The release of the stored bolus could lead to rupture of the vein or constitute overinfusion, which may be detrimental to the patient particularly if it is a critical medication (Amoore & Adamson 2003; Medical Devices Agency 2003). For a syringe pump, to prevent a bolus being delivered to the patient, the clamp should not be opened as this will release the bolus: the first action is to remove the pressure by opening the syringe plunger clamp and then deal with the occlusion.

Air-in-line detectors are designed to detect only visible or microscopic 'champagne' bubbles. They should not create anxiety over small particles of air but alert the nurse to the integrity of the system. Most air bubbles detected are too small to have a harmful effect; however, the nurse should clarify the cause of any alarms (Perucca 2001; Medical Devices Agency 2003).

The Medical Devices Agency (2003) has set performance criteria for infusion pumps (see Table 13.3).

Infusion devices

Gravity infusion devices

Gravity flow

Gravity infusion devices depend entirely on gravity to deliver the infusion. The system consists of an administration set

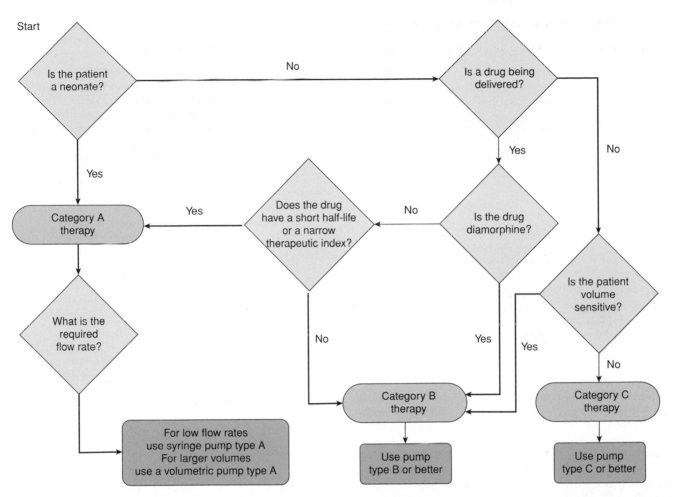

Figure 13.1   Decision tree for selection of infusion device. Crown copyright material is reproduced with the permission of the Controller of HMSO and Queen's Printer for Scotland. Medical Devices Agency (2003).

297

containing a drip chamber and a roller clamp to control the flow, which is usually measured by counting drops (Pickstone 1999). The indications for use are:

- Administration of drugs or fluids where adverse effects are not anticipated and which do not need to be infused with absolute precision.
- Where the patient's condition does not give cause for concern and no complication is predicted.

The flow rate is calculated using a formula that requires the following information: the volume to be infused; the number of hours the infusion is running over; and the drop rate of the administration set (which will differ depending on type of set). The number of drops per millilitre is dependent on the type of administration set used and the viscosity of the infusion fluid. Increased viscosity causes the size of the drop to increase. For example, crystalloid fluid administered via a solution set is delivered at the rate of 20 drops/ml; the rate of packed red cells given via a blood set will be calculated at 15 drops/ml.

The rate of administration of a continuous or intermittent infusion may be calculated from the following equation (Pickstone 1999):

$$\frac{\text{Volume to be infused}}{\text{Time in hours}} \times \frac{\text{Drop rate}}{60\ \text{minutes}} = \text{Drops per minute}$$

In this equation, 60 is a factor for the conversion of the number of hours to the number of minutes.

Advantages and disadvantages

The advantages of the gravity flow system are that it is simple to set up. It is low cost and the infusion of air is less likely than with electronic devices (Pickstone 1999). However, the system does require frequent observation and adjustment due to:

- The tubing changing shape over time.
- Creep or distortion of tubing made of polyvinyl chloride (PVC).

- Fluctuations of venous pressure which can affect the flow of the solution.
- The roller clamp can be unreliable, leading to inconsistent flow rates.

There can also be variability of drop size, and if the roller clamp is inadvertently left open free flow will occur. Infusion rates with viscous fluids can be reduced (particularly if administered via small cannulae) and there is a limitation on the type of infusion as it is not suitable for arterial infusions: this is because viscosity and arterial flow offer a high resistance to flow which cannot be overcome by gravity flow (Pickstone 1999; Quinn 2008).

Gravity drip rate controllers

A controller is a mechanical device that operates by gravity. These devices use standard solution sets and although they look much like a pump, they have no pumping mechanism. The desired flow rate is set in drops per minute and controlled by battery or mains powered occlusion valves (Medical Devices Agency 2003).

Advantages and disadvantages

Although they can maintain a drip rate within 1%, volumetric accuracy is not guaranteed and many of the disadvantages associated with gravity flow still remain. The main advantages are they are relatively inexpensive and can usually use standard gravity sets. They also incorporate some audible and visual alarm systems (Medical Devices Agency 2003).

Infusion pumps

These devices pump fluid from an infusion bag or bottle via an administration set (Quinn 2008).

Volumetric pumps

A volumetric pump works by calculating the volume delivered. This is achieved when the pump measures the volume displaced in a 'reservoir'. The reservoir is an integral component of the administration set. The pump calculates that every fill and empty cycle of the reservoir delivers a given amount of solution (Perucca 2001). The mechanism of action may be piston generated or linear peristaltic: where fingers in the pump move in a wave-like manner pushing the fluid out of the chamber (Pickstone 1999). The indications for use are all large volume infusions, both venous and arterial.

Most volumetric pumps have a linear peristaltic pumping mechanism, although some use cassettes. All are mains and battery powered, with the rate selected in millilitres per hour. The accuracy of flow is usually within 5% when measured over a period of time, which is more than adequate for most clinical applications (Pickstone 1999; Medical Devices Agency 2003).

Advantages and disadvantages

These pumps are able to overcome resistance to flow by increased delivery pressure and do not rely on gravity. This generally makes the performance of pumps predictable and capable of accurate delivery over a wider range of flow rates (Medical Devices Agency 2003).

The pumps also incorporate a wide range of features including air-in-line detectors, variable pressure settings and comprehensive alarms such as end of infusion, keep vein open (KVO, where the pump switches to a low flow rate, e.g. 5 ml/h, in order to continue flow to prevent occlusion of the device) and low battery. Many have a secondary infusion facility, which is to allow for intermittent therapy, e.g. antibiotics. The pump is programmed to switch to a secondary set and, when completed, it reverts back to the primary infusion at the previously set rate. The changing hospital environment has led to an increased demand on volumetric pumps, which in turn has resulted in the development of multichannel and dual-channel infusion pumps. These pumps may consist of two devices with an attached housing or of several infusion channels within a single device (Perucca 2001).

The disadvantages are that these are usually relatively expensive and often dedicated administration sets are required. The use of the wrong set could result in error even if the pump appears to work. Some are complicated to set up, which can also lead to errors (Medical Devices Agency 2003).

Syringe pumps

Syringe pumps are low-volume, high-accuracy devices designed to infuse at low flow rates. The plunger of a syringe containing the substance to be infused is driven forward by the syringe pump at a controlled rate to deliver it to the patient (Medical Devices Agency 2003).

Syringe pumps are useful where small volumes of highly concentrated drugs need to be infused (Pickstone 1999). The volume for infusion is limited to the size of the syringe used in the device, which is usually a 60-ml syringe, but most pumps will accept different sizes and brands of syringe. These devices are calibrated for delivery in millilitres per hour (Weinstein 2007).

Advantages and disadvantages

Syringe pumps are mains and/or battery powered, are usually easy to operate, and tend to cost less than volumetric pumps. The alarm systems are becoming more comprehensive but include low battery, end of infusion and syringe clamp open alarm. Most of the problems associated with the older models, for example free flow, mechanical backlash (slackness which delays the start-up time of the infusion) and incorrect fitting of the syringe, have been eliminated in the newer models (Pickstone 1999; Medical Devices Agency 2003). The risk of free flow is minimized by the use of an anti-siphonage valve which may be integral to the administration set (Pickstone 1999). Despite the use of an anti-siphonage valve, the

298

clamp of the administration set must still be used (Medical Devices Agency 2003). Where mechanical backlash is an issue and there is a prime or purge option, this should be used at the start of the infusion to take up the mechanical slack (Amoore *et al.* 2001).

Specialist pumps

Patient-controlled analgesia pumps

Patient-controlled analgesia (PCA) devices are typically syringe pumps (although some are based on volumetric designs) (Medical Devices Agency 2003). The syringe pump forces down on the syringe piston, collapsing the syringe at a preset rate, but the distinguishing feature is the ability of the pump to deliver doses on demand, which occurs when the patient pushes a button (Perucca 2001). Whether or not the dose is delivered is determined by preset parameters in the pump. That is, if the maximum amount of drug over a given period of time has already been delivered, a further dose cannot be delivered.

PCA pumps are useful for patients who require analgesia. PCA pumps are used more in the acute setting, but are also useful in ambulatory situations.

Infusion options of a PCA pump are usually categorized into three types:

- Basal: a 'baseline' rate can be accompanied by intermittent doses requested by patients. This aims to achieve pain relief with minimal medication, but not necessarily to achieve a pain-free state (Perucca 2001).
- Continuous: designed for the patient who needs maximum pain relief without the option of demand dosing, e.g. epidural.
- Demand: drug delivered by intermittent infusion when button is pushed and can be used alone or supplemented by the basal rate. Doses can be limited by a designated maximum amount (Perucca 2001).

The PCA pump can dispense a bolus dose, with an initial bolus dose being called a loading dose. This may benefit patients as the one time dose is significantly higher than a demand dose in order to achieve immediate pain relief.

Advantages and disadvantages

These devices offer a 'lock-out' feature (when a key or a combination of numbers is necessary to gain access to pump controls), which is designed for patient safety. These pumps have an extensive memory capability which can be accessed through the display via a printer or computer (Medical Devices Agency 2003). This facility is critical for the pump's effective use in pain relief (Perucca 2001), as it enables the clinician to determine when and how often demand is made by a patient and what total volume has been infused (Perucca 2001). It has also been shown that they increase patient satisfaction, patients require less sedation, their anxiety is reduced and so are their nursing needs and time in hospital (Ripamonti & Bruera 1997).

Anaesthesia pumps

These are syringe pumps designed for delivery of anaesthesia or sedation and must only ever be used for that purpose. They should be restricted to operating theatres or critical care units and should be clearly labelled. They infuse at a very high flow rate and have a high-rate bolus facility in order to deliver the induction dose of anaesthesia quickly (Dolan 1999). There are new types of anaesthesia pumps that are available, total intravenous anaesthesia (TIVA) and target controlled infusion (TCI), which have been designed to control the induction, maintenance and reversal phases of anaesthesia (Absalom & Struys 2006).

Epidural pumps

These pumps are a method of providing analgesia (most commonly a combination of opioids and anaesthetic agents) via a fine catheter inserted directly into the epidural space. As a form of analgesia delivery, the efficacy of the epidural route has been well highlighted (Wheatley *et al.* 2001; Block *et al.* 2003; Werawatganon & Charuluxanun 2005).

Ambulatory infusion devices

Ambulatory devices are small devices which were developed to allow patients more freedom and to enable the patient to continue with normal activities or to move unencumbered by a large infusion device (Perucca 2001). Ambulatory devices range in size and weight and are used for small volumes of drugs and are mainly designed for patients to wear and use when ambulant. The solution containers are often more cumbersome than the actual pump itself. Due to their size, the number of alarms may be more limited. Considerations for selection of an ambulatory device include the following:

- Type of therapy.
- Patient's ability to understand how to manage the infusion device.
- Drug stability.
- Frequency of doses.
- Reservoir volumes required.
- Control of flow/flow rates.
- Type of access.
- Cost effectiveness.
- Portability.
- Convenience.

Ambulatory pumps fall into two categories: mechanical and battery-operated infusion devices.

Mechanical infusion devices

These are simple and compact but may not necessarily be cost effective as they are usually disposable. The mechanism for delivery is by balloon or simple spring, or they may be gas-powered.

Elastomeric balloons

These are made of a soft rubberized material capable of being inflated to a predetermined volume and the drug is then administered over a very specific infusion time. The balloon is encapsulated inside a rigid transparent container which may be round or cylindrical. The rate of infusion is not controlled by the balloon but by the diameter of the restricting outlet located in the preattached tubing. It is designed for single use that supplies the patient's need for a single dose infusion of drugs, e.g. intermittent small volume parenteral therapies such as delivery of antibiotics. Its small size causes little disruption to the patient's daily activities and it tends to be well tolerated (Perucca 2001).

Spring mechanism

Spring coil piston syringes have a spring which powers the plunger of a syringe in the absence of manual pressure. The volume is restricted by the size of the syringe, which is usually prefilled. The spring coil container tends to be a multidose, small-volume administration device and is a combination of a spring coil in a collapsible flattened disk. Its shape can accommodate many therapies and volumes (Perucca 2001).

Battery-operated infusion devices

Battery-operated pumps are small and light enough to be carried around by the patient without interfering with most everyday activities. They are operated using rechargeable or alkaline batteries but, owing to their size, the available battery capacity tends to be low. The length of time the battery lasts is often dependent on the rate the pump is set at. Most give an output in the form of a small bolus delivered every few minutes. Most devices have an integral case or pouch which allows the pump and the reservoir/syringe to be worn with discretion by the patient. There are two types: ambulatory volumetric infusion pumps and syringe drivers.

Ambulatory volumetric infusion/syringe pumps

An ambulatory volumetric infusion/syringe pump is an infusion device which pumps in the same way as a large volumetric pump, but by nature of its size it is portable and useful in the ambulatory setting (hospital or home care).

This pump is suitable for patients who have been prescribed continuous infusional treatment for a period of time,

for example from 4 days to 6 months, and enables the patients, where appropriate, to receive treatment at home, because it is small and portable.

The advantages of the ambulatory pump are:

- Able to deliver drugs continuously or intermittently.
- Infusion routes: central, peripheral venous, epidural, intra-arterial, intrathecal and subcutaneous.
- Delivery of drugs accurately over a set period of time.
- Improving potential outcomes of treatment by delivering treatment continuously.
- Heightening the patient's independence and control by allowing them to be at home and participate in their own care.
- Is compact, light and easy to use.
- Has audible alarm systems.

The disadvantages are:

- It may require the insertion of a central venous access device, which has associated complications and problems.
- It could malfunction at home, which could be distressing and dangerous for the patient.
- In spite of its ease of use, some patients may not be able to cope with it at home.
- Patients may have to adapt their lifestyle to cope with living with a pump continuously.

Syringe drivers

A syringe driver is a portable battery-operated infusion device. It is used to deliver drugs at a predetermined rate via the appropriate parenteral route and is suited for symptom management, and palliative care (Dickman *et al.* 2005). The syringe driver should be used for patients who are unable to tolerate oral medication, for example, in nausea and vomiting, dysphagia, intestinal obstruction, local disease or sometimes in intractable pain which is unrelieved by oral medications and where rapid dose titration is required. Drugs administered by subcutaneous infusion include opioid analgesics, antiemetics, anxiolytic sedatives, corticosteroids, non-steroidal anti-inflammatory drugs and anticholinergic drugs (Dickman *et al.* 2005).

The Sims (Graseby) Medical MS16A and MS26 syringe drivers are typical examples of the drivers in use; however, other types are available and nurses should follow the manufacturer's instruction manual for details of their use. The MS16A allows drug administration on an hourly rate. This driver is clearly marked with a pink '1 h' in the bottom right hand corner of the driver. The MS26 delivers drugs on a 24-hourly rate. This driver is clearly marked with a yellow '24 h' in the bottom right hand corner of the driver (Figure 13.2). It is important that users are aware that the MS16A syringe driver is calibrated in millimetres per hour, and the MS26 is calibrated in millimetres per day. Confusion between the two drivers in relation to rate settings has resulted in fatal errors

Figure 13.2   Sims (Graseby) Medical MS26 daily rate syringe driver.

(Dickman *et al.* 2005; MHRA 2006b). Most sizes and brands of plastic syringes can be used with these drivers; however, it is recommended to use Luer–Lok syringes to avoid leakage or accidental disconnection.

The advantages of the syringe driver are:

- It avoids the necessity of intermittent injections.
- Mixtures of drugs may be administered.
- Infusion timing is accurate, which is particularly advantageous in the community where the ability to constantly monitor the rate is not feasible.
- The device is lightweight and compact, allowing mobility and independence.
- Rate can be increased.
- Simple calculations of dosage are required over a 12- or 24-hour period.
- It allows patients to spend more time at home with their symptoms managed effectively.

The disadvantages are:

- The patient may become psychologically dependent on the device.
- Inflammation or infection may occur at the insertion site of the subcutaneous cannula.
- The rate calculation differs between the Sims (Graseby) Medical MS16A and MS26 syringe drivers and this can be confusing for the nurse.
- The alarm system of some syringe drivers, e.g. the Sims (Graseby), operates only if the plunger is obstructed. It does not alert the nurse if the flow is too rapid or is too slow.

Improving infusion device safety

A high frequency of human error is reported in the use of infusion device systems, so competence-based training in the use of devices is advocated for users of infusion device systems (Medical Devices Agency 2003; NPSA 2004). By rationalizing the range of infusion device types within organizations and the establishment of a centralized equipment library, the number of patient safety incidents will be reduced (Medical Devices Agency 2003; NPSA 2004). Smart infusion pumps reduce pump programming errors by the setting of pre-programmed upper and lower dose limits for specific drugs. The pump will alert the nurse when setting the infusion device if the pump has been set outside of the pre-set dose limits (Wilson & Sullivan 2004; Keohane *et al.* 2005; Weinstein 2007). Whatever infusion device is used, the need to monitor the patient and the device remain paramount for patient safety.

Summary

There are many infusion control devices available ranging from the simple to the complex and nurses should have a sound knowledge of how the device works or seek assistance from a colleague. Careful calculation and control of flow rates are essential as delivery of fluids and medications are critical for patient safety. Standardization of equipment reduces confusion and therefore reduces the risk of user error (Medical Devices Agency 2003; NPSA 2003, 2004; Department of Health, Social Services and Public Safety 2006; MHRA 2006b; Health Care Standards Unit 2007a, b; NHS Litigation Authority 2007).

Procedure guidelines   Subcutaneous administration of drugs using a syringe driver (e.g. Sims (Graseby) Medical MS26)

Equipment

1 Clinically clean receiver or tray containing the prepared drug to be administered.
2 Syringe driver MS26.
3 Battery (PP3 size, 9 volt alkaline).
4 Plastic peripheral cannulae (e.g. Insyte 24 G) and microbore driver set (100 cm) with needle-free Y connector injection site (or 100 cm winged infusion set).
5 Luer–Lok syringe of suitable size (e.g. 10 ml).
6 Swab saturated with isopropyl alcohol 70%.
7 Transparent adhesive dressing.
8 Drugs and diluent.
9 Needle (to draw up drug).
10 Drug additive label.
11 Patient's prescription chart.
12 Recording chart or book as required by law or hospital policy.
13 Sharps box.

Calculating the rate setting for administration of drugs using a syringe driver (e.g. Sims (Graseby) Medical MS26) over a 24-hour period (using a BD Plastipak Luer–Lok syringe)

1 Measure stroke length in millimetres. The stroke length is the *length* of fluid to be infused, i.e. the distance the plunger has to travel (irrespective of the number of millilitres) (see Action figure 1).

Example:
Stroke length = 48 mm
Delivery time = 1 day
Rate setting = 48 mm

2 Check the delivery time (previously prescribed) in days.

Set rate using screwdriver provided (see Action figure 2).

3 Calculate:

$$Rate = \frac{Fluid\ length}{Infusion\ period\ in\ days}$$

See instruction booklets provided with individual syringe driver.

Action 1   Measuring stroke length.

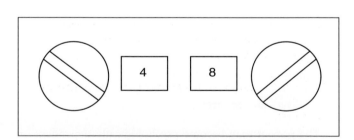

Action 2   Setting the rate.

Procedure guidelines   **Syringe driver: preparation of the syringe and priming the infusion set for 24-hour drug administration using the Sims (Graseby) Medical MS26**

Action	Rationale
1 Explain and discuss the procedure with the patient.	To ensure that the patient understands the procedure and gives his/her valid consent (Griffith & Jordan 2003: E; NMC 2006b: C; NMC 2008b: C).
2 Before administering any prescribed drug check that it is due and has not already been given.	To protect the patient from harm (NPSA 2007: C).
3 Before administering any prescribed drug, consult the patient's prescription chart and ascertain the following: (a) Drug. (b) Dose. (c) Date and time of administration. (d) Route and method of administration. (e) Diluent as appropriate. (f) Validity of prescription. (g) Signature of doctor. (h) The prescription is legible.	To ensure that the patient is given the correct drug in the prescribed dose using the appropriate diluent and by the correct route. To protect the patient from harm (NMC 2008a: C; NPSA 2007: C). To comply with NMC (2006a: C, 2008a: C).
4 Calculate and check dosage of drugs required over a 24-hour period.	To establish correct dosages of drugs (Pickstone 1999: E).
5 Wash hands with bactericidal soap and water or bactericidal alcohol handrub, and assemble the necessary equipment.	To minimize the risk of infection (Pratt *et al.* 2007: C).
6 Check the name, strength and volume of subcutaneous drug(s) against the prescription chart.	To ensure that the correct type and quantity of fluid are administered (NMC 2008a: C; NPSA 2007: C).
7 Check the expiry date of the drug(s).	To prevent an ineffective or toxic compound being administered to the patient (NPSA 2007: C).
8 Check that the packaging is intact and inspect the container and contents in a good light for cracks, punctures, air bubbles.	To check that no contamination of the infusion container has occurred (NPSA 2007: C).
9 Check the identity and amount of drug to be prepared. Consider: (a) Compatibility of drugs. (b) Stability of mixture over the prescription time. (c) Any special directions for dilution, e.g. pH, optimum concentration. (d) Sensitivity to external factors such as light. (e) Any anticipated allergic reaction. If any doubts exist about the listed points, consult the pharmacist or appropriate reference works.	To minimize any risk of error. To ensure safe and effective administration of the drug. To enable anticipation of toxicities and the nursing implications of these (NPSA 2007: C).

303

Procedure guidelines *(cont.)*

10 Using a 10 ml BD Plastipak Luer–Lok syringe, draw up drugs required with diluent to measure a total volume of 7.8 ml. Refer to Procedure guidelines: Injections: administration in Chapter 11.

To ensure accuracy and avoid any infusion errors. To ensure the drug is prepared correctly (NPSA 2007: C).

11 Inspect the fluid for discoloration, haziness and crystalline or particulate matter. If this occurs, discard and re-evaluate drug compatability.

To prevent any toxic or foreign matter being infused into the patient (NPSA 2007: C).
To detect any incompatibility or degradation (NPSA 2007: C).

12 This can occur even if the mixture is theoretically compatible, thus making vigilance essential.

13 Establish the correct rate setting of the driver using the correct calculation.

To monitor rate and ensure drug is infused safely (Pickstone 1999: E; Dickman *et al*. 2005: E).

14 Complete the drug additive label and fix it on the syringe.

To identify which drug has been added, when and by whom (NPSA 2007: C).

15 Wash hands with bactericidal soap and water or bactericidal alcohol handrub.

To minimize the risk of infection (Pratt *et al*. 2007: C).

16 Connect prepared syringe to a 100 cm microbore driver set with needle-free Y connector injection site.

This length of tubing allows patient greater freedom of movement (E).

17 Prime the infusion by gently depressing the plunger of the syringe until the fluid is visible at the end of the infusion set.

This removes extraneous air from the system (E). Ensures patient receives drugs immediately and accurately (E).

Additional note

Priming the infusion set after calculation will reduce the delivery time by approximately half an hour for the first infusion.
Do not alter previously calculated rate setting despite volume reduction in barrel of syringe.

Procedure guidelines Syringe driver: inserting the winged infusion set or cannula and connecting syringe

Action

Rationale

1 Place the syringe and infusion set in a clean receptacle. Wash hands and proceed to the patient.

To minimize the risk of contamination (Pratt *et al*. 2007: C).

2 Check the identity of the patient against the prescription chart, syringe drug additive label and with the patient if possible.

To minimize the risk of error and ensure the correct drug is administered to the correct patient (NMC 2006a: C; NMC 2008a: C; NPSA 2007: C).

3 Explain and discuss the procedure with the patient.

To ensure that the patient understands the procedure and gives his/her valid consent (Griffiths & Jordan 2003: E; NMC 2006b: C).

4 Assist the patient into a comfortable position.

5 Expose the chosen site for infusion (see Infusion sites in the Subcutaneous infusion drugs section in Chapter 11).

6 Clean the chosen site with a swab saturated with 70% isopropyl alcohol. Wait until the alcohol evaporates.	To reduce the risk of infection (Pratt *et al*. 2007: C).
7 Grasp the skin firmly.	To elevate the subcutaneous tissue.
8 Insert the infusion needle into the skin at an angle of 45° and release the grasped skin. (If using a cannula, remove the stylet and connect the extension set.)	Positioning shallower than 45° may shorten the life of the infusion site.
9 Apply transparent dressing to secure infusion needle.	To prevent movement and reduce the risk of mechanical phlebitis and infection (Weinstein 2007: E; Pratt *et al*. 2007: C).
10 Check that the infusion set and syringe are securely connected.	To ensure that there is no disconnection so that the drug(s) are administered correctly (E).
11 Connect the syringe to the syringe driver.	To ensure the syringe is connected correctly to the syringe driver (E).
12 Place the syringe on the syringe driver along the grooved lines, with barrel clamp firmly in position.	To ensure the syringe is in the correct position (C).
13 Secure in place with rubber strap.	To ensure the syringe is securely clamped to the barrel (C).
14 Slide the actuator assembly along the lead screw by pressing white release button, as shown in Action figure 14, until it rests against the end of the plunger.	To enable the pump mechanism to operate correctly (C).
15 Secure plunger with additional safety clamp (see Action figure 15) and clear perspex container.	To ensure extra security and minimize the risk of errors in infusional rates (C).
16 Fit the battery ensuring contact by flashing light on front of syringe driver.	
17 Press start/test button to commence infusion. The indicator light should flash to indicate functioning syringe pump.	To check the infusion device is operating correctly (C).
18 Complete the patient's prescription chart and other hospital and/or legally required documents.	To comply with local drug administration policies and ensure the safe administration and monitoring of the infused drug and accurate records. To provide a record in the event of any queries (NMC 2005: C). To prevent any duplication of treatment (NMC 2005: C).
19 Monitor the patient for any infusion related complications.	To detect complications promptly (Pickstone 1999: E; Quinn 2000: E; Dougherty 2002: E; Medical Devices Agency 2003: C; Dickman *et al*. 2005).

Procedure guidelines *(cont.)*

20 Record the infusion device serial number, the infusion device and infusion site checks.

Frequency of checks:
- At start of infusion – record date, time, start volume, infusion rate setting, name of person setting up infusion.
- Based upon the type of infusion and patient's condition; however at a minimum these should be carried out 15 minutes and 1 hour after the initial set up and thereafter a minimum of every 4 hours.
- Device must be checked at the start of each shift and/or when setting up an infusion.

Infusion device and infusion checks:
- Check and record the date, time, rate and volume remaining and that the battery/syringe driver is working.
- Record any reasons for changing of the drug, dose, rate setting of syringe driver or site.
- Check subcutaneous site for:
  (a) Pain/discomfort.
  (b) Swelling/induration.
  (c) Erythema.
  (d) Leakage of fluid.
  (e) Bleeding.

To provide a record in the event of any queries (NMC 2005: C).
To detect any errors and infusion related complications (Pickstone 1999: E; Quinn 2000: E; Dougherty 2002: E; Medical Devices Agency 2003: C; Dickman *et al*. 2005: E).

21 Ask the patient to report any complaints of pain and tenderness at the infusion site and if they experience any change in their symptoms or have new symptoms.

To ascertain whether there are any problems that may require nursing care and refer to medical staff where appropriate (E).

22 Discard waste, making sure that it is placed in the correct containers, e.g. sharps into a designated receptacle.

To ensure safe disposal and avoid injury to staff. To prevent reuse of equipment (MHRA 2004: C; DH 2005: C).

Additional notes

1 Different manufacturers of syringes have different barrel sizes, e.g. 7.8 ml in a 10-ml syringe made by one company may yield a different stroke length to 7.8 ml in a 10-ml syringe made by another (Dickman *et al*. 2005: E).

2 If more than one drug is to be administered, for example analgesic and antiemetic, it is important not to increase the rate of the syringe driver to yield more pain relief, as this will increase the antiemetic dose (Dickman *et al*. 2005: E).

3 If 'breakthrough' analgesia is required, it is preferable to administer the equivalent of a 4-hourly dose as an injection using the needle-free Y connector injection site or as a separate extra statim subcutaneous injection (when a winged infusion set is in use). Bolus pushes using the boost button are not recommended, for the following reasons:
  (a) Those outlined in point 2 above.
  (b) A 'boost' push yields only 0.23 mm of extra analgesia (C).
  (c) Pain assessment is more difficult and evaluation of pain control is hindered.
  (d) Inaccuracies of infusion time may occur as a result.

4 Accurate documentation of the site, rate, flow, start time and drugs used is imperative in order to avoid confusion and errors among staff (Quinn 2000: E; Dougherty 2002: E; Medical Devices Agency 2003: C; Dickman *et al*. 2005: E; NMC 2005: C; NMC 2006a: C; NMC 2008a: C).

5 Appropriate education/teaching material, e.g. syringe driver instruction manual and guidelines on problem solving, is required for both the patients and staff (Medical Devices Agency 2003: C).

Action 14   Connecting syringe to syringe driver.

Action 15   Securing the plunger.

Problem solving: Syringe drivers

Problem	Possible causes	Preventive nursing measures	Suggested action
Infusion pump alarming:			
(a) Air detected	Air bubbles in administration set.	Ensure all air is removed from all equipment prior to use.	Remove all air from the administration set and restart the infusion.
(b) Tube misload	Administration set has been improperly loaded.	Ensure set is loaded correctly.	Check that the set is loaded correctly and reload if necessary.
(c) Upstream occlusion	Closed clamp, obstruction or kink in the administration set is preventing fluid flow.	Ensure the container/fluid bag has been adequately pierced by the administration spike. Ensure that the tubing is taped to prevent kinking. Ensure the regulating (roller) clamp is open.	Inspect the administration set and restart the infusion. If tubing is kinked, reposition, tape and restart infusion. Check the administration set and open the clamp; restart the infusion.
(d) Downstream occlusion	Phlebitis/infiltration or extravasation.	Observe site regularly for signs of swelling, pain and erythema.	Remove peripheral device, provide symptomatic relief where appropriate. Initiate extravasation procedure. Resite as appropriate.
	Closed distal clamp.	Ensure clamps are open.	Locate distal occlusion, restart infusion.

Problem solving (cont.)

Problem	Possible causes	Preventive nursing measures	Suggested action
(e) KVO alert (keep vein open)	The volume infused is complete and the device is infusing at the KVO rate.	Programme in a new volume as appropriate.	Do not turn the device off. Allow KVO mode to run to maintain patency of device. Prepare new infusion or discontinue as appropriate.
Infusion devices malfunctioning (electrical/mechanical)	Not charging at mains.	Ensure that the device is kept plugged in where appropriate.	Change device and remove device from use until fully charged. Send to works department to check plug.
	Low battery.	Check lead is pushed in adequately.	
	Batteries keep requiring replacement.	Do not use small rechargeable batteries in ambulatory devices.	
	Technical fault.	Ensure all infusion devices are serviced regularly.	Remove infusion device from use and contact biomedical engineering (BME) department or relevant personnel.
	Device soiled inside mechanism.	Maintain equipment and keep clean and free from contamination.	Remove administration set, wipe pump, reload. Do not use alcohol-based solutions on internal mechanisms.
Unstable infusion device	Mounted on old, poorly maintained stands.	Ensure that stands are maintained and kept clean. Replace old stands.	Remove device from stand. Remove stand and send to works department for repair.
	Mounted on incorrect stands.	Ensure the correct stands are used.	Check the stand and change to appropriate stand.
	Equipment not balanced on stand.	Ensure that all equipment is balanced around the stand.	Remove devices and attach to two stands if necessary. Balance equipment.
Under/overinfusion	Technical fault with equipment.	Ensure regular servicing of devices.	Remove device from use immediately and label to prevent further use. Report incident to medical staff and nursing staff. Report to appropriate person, e.g. nurse specialist or an electro-biomedical engineer for checking. Complete an incident form. Inform head of risk management and MHRA as appropriate.
	Incorrect rate setting.	Ensure that the rate is calculated prior to commencing infusion. Check infusion rate regularly within the first hour and at start of each shift to ensure correct rate is set.	Check patient's condition. Inform medical staff and senior member of nursing staff.

References and further reading

Absalom, A. & Struys, M. (2006) *An Overview of TCI & TIVA*. Academia Press, Ghent, Belgium.

Amoore, J. et al. (2001) Syringe pumps and start up time: ensuring safe practice. *Nurs Stand*, 15(17), 43–5.

Amoore, J. & Adamson, L. (2003) Infusion devices: characteristics, limitations and risk management. *Nurs Stand*, 17(28), 45–52.

Block, B.M. *et al.* (2003) Efficacy of postoperative analgesia: a meta-analysis. *JAMA*, 290, 2455–63.

Department of Health, Social Services and Public Safety (2006) *Controls Assurance Standards: Medical Devices and Equipment Management*. www.dhsspsni.gov.uk/medical_devices_06_pdf. Accessed 27/11/06.

DH (2003) *Building a Safer NHS for Patients: Improving Medication Safety*. Department of Health, London.

DH (2005) *Hazardous waste (England) regulations*. Department of Health London.

Dickman, A., Schneider, J. & Varga, J. (2005) *The Syringe Driver: Continuous Subcutaneous Infusions in Palliative Care*, 2nd edn. Oxford University Press, Oxford.

Dougherty, L. (2002) Delivery of intravenous therapy. *Nurs Stand*, 16(16), 45–56.

Edwards, S. (2001) Regulation of water, sodium and potassium: implications for practice. *Nurs Stand*, 15(22), 36–45.

Fox, N. (2000) Armed and dangerous. *Nurs Times*, 96(44), 24–6.

Gabriel, J. (1999) Long term central venous access. In: *Intravenous Therapy in Nursing Practice* (eds L. Dougherty & J. Lamb). Churchill Livingstone, Edinburgh, pp. 301–31.

Griffith, R. & Jordan, S. (2003) Administration of medicines part 1: the law and nursing. *Nurs Stand*, 18(2), 47–53.

Health Care Standards Unit (2007a) *First Domain – Safety (Info Bank) C4b*. www.hcsu.org.uk/index.php?option=com_content&task=view&id=197&Itemid=109. Accessed 28/08/07.

Health Care Standards Unit (2007b) *Updated signpost C4b*. www.hcsu.org.uk/index.php?option=com_content&task=view&id=309&Itemid=111. Accessed 28/03/07.

Keohane, C.A. *et al.* (2005) Intravenous medication safety and smart infusion systems. *J Infus Nurs*, 28(5), 321–8.

Lamb, J. (1999) Local and systemic complications of intravenous therapy. In: *Intravenous Therapy in Nursing Practice* (eds L. Dougherty & J. Lamb). Churchill Livingstone, Edinburgh, pp. 163–93.

Medical Devices Agency (2000) *Equipped to Care*. Medical Devices Agency, London. www.mhra.gov.uk/home/idcplg?IdcService=SS_GET_PAGE&useSecondary=true&ssDocName=CON007425&ssTargetNodeId=575. Accessed 28/3/07.

MDA (2001) *Devices in Practice – guide for health and social care professionals*. www.mhra.gov.uk/home/idcplg?IdcService=SS_GET_PAGE&useSecondary=true&ssDocName=CON007423&ssTargetNodeId=575. Accessed 28/3/07.

Medical Devices Agency (2003) *Infusion Systems Device Bulletin*. DB 9503. Medical Devices Agency, London. www.mhra.gov.uk/home/idcplg?IdcService=SS_GET_PAGE&useSecondary=true&ssDocNameCON007321&ssTargetNodeId=572. Accessed 23/03/07.

MHRA (2004) *Reducing Needlestick and Sharps Injuries*. Medicines and Healthcare Products Regulatory Agency, London.

MHRA (2006a) *Free-flow situations*. www.mhra.gov.uk/home/idcplg?IdcService=GET_FILE&dID=20057&noSaveAs=0&Rendition=WEB. Accessed 03/06.

MHRA (2006b) *Reporting adverse incidents and disseminating medical device alerts*. DB2006 (01). www.mhra.gov.uk/home/idcplg?IdcService=SS_GET_PAGE&useSecondary=true&ssDocName=CON007304&ssTargetNodeId=572. Accessed 27/11/06.

Murray, W. & Glenister, H. (2001) How to use medical devices safely. *Nurs Times*, 97(43), 36–8.

NHS Litigation Authority (2007) *NHSLA Risk Management Standards for Acute Trusts*. www.nhsla.com/NR/rdonlyres/F9DA791B-AF6D-4198-AC49-EE9B81A91B17/0/NHSLARiskManagementStandardsforAcuteTrusts200708website.doc. Accessed 28/08/07.

NMC (2005) *Guidelines for Records and Record Keeping*. Nursing and Midwifery Council, London.

NMC (2006a) *Medicines Management A–Z Advice Sheet*. Nursing and Midwifery Council. www.nmc-uk.org/aFrameDisplay.aspx?DocumentID=1801. Accessed 27/11/06.

NMC (2006b) *A–Z Advice Sheet Consent*. www.nmc.org.

NMC (2008a) *Standards for Medicines Management*. Nursing and Midwifery Council, London.

NMC (2008b) *The Code: Standards of Conduct, Performance and Ethics for Nurses and Midwives*. Nursing and Midwifery Council, London.

NPSA (2003) *Risk Analysis of Infusion Devices*. National Patient Safety Agency, London.

NPSA (2004) *Safer Practice Notice 01: Infusion Devices*. National Patient Safety Agency. www.npsa.nhs.uk/site/media/documents/526_npsa_saferpractice_01.pdf. Accessed 27/11/06.

NPSA (2007) *Promoting Safer Use of Injectable Medicines, Alert no.2007/20*. www.npsa.nhs.uk/site/media/documents/2602_0434_injectables_meds_alert_v20.pdf. Accessed 28/03/07.

Perdue, M.B. (2001) Intravenous complications. In: *Infusion Therapy in Clinical Practice* (eds J. Hankin *et al.*), 2nd edn. W.B. Saunders, Philadelphia, pp. 418–45.

Perucca, R. (2001) Types of infusion therapy equipment. In: *Infusion Therapy in Clinical Practice* (eds J. Hankin *et al.*), 2nd edn. W.B. Saunders, Philadelphia, pp. 300–33

Pickstone, M. (1999) *A Pocketbook for Safer IV Therapy*. Medical Technology and Risk Series. Scitech, Kent.

Pickstone, M. (2000) Using the technology triangle to assess the safety of technology-controlled clinical procedures in critical care. *Int J Intens Care*, 7(2), 90–6.

Pratt, R.J. *et al.* (2007) Epic 2: National evidence-based guidelines for preventing healthcare-associated infections in NHS hospitals in England. *J Hosp Infect*, 65(Suppl), S2–12.

Quinn, C. (2000) Infusion devices: risks, functions and management. *Nurs Stand*, 14(26), 35–41.

Quinn, C. (2008) Intravenous flow control and infusion devices. In: *Intravenous Therapy in Nursing Practice*, 2nd edn (eds L. Dougherty & J. Lamb). Blackwell Publishing, Oxford, pp. 197–224.

RCN (2005) *Standards for Infusion Therapy. RCN IV: Therapy Forum November 2005*. Royal College of Nursing, London.

Ripamonti, C. & Bruera, E. (1997) Current status of patient controlled analgesia in cancer patients. *Oncology*, 11(3), 373–80.

Springhouse (2005) *Intravenous Therapy Made Incredibly Easy*, (ed. L. Bruck), 3rd edn. Lippincott, Williams & Wilkins, Philadelphia.

Sundquist, S.B. (2001) Didactic components of a comprehensive paediatric competency programme. *J Infus Nurs*, 24(6), 367–74.

Weinstein, S. (2007) *Plumer's Principles and Practices of Intravenous Therapy*, 8th edn. Lippincott, Williams & Wilkins, Philadelphia.

Werawatganon, T. & Charuluxanun, S. (2005) Patient controlled intravenous opioid analgesia versus continuous epidural analgesia for pain after intra-abdominal surgery. *Cochrane Database of Systematic Reviews* 2005, Issue 1. CD004088.

Wheatley, R., Schug, S. & Watson, D. (2001) Safety and efficacy of postoperative epidural analgesia. *Br J Anaesth*, 87(1), 47–61.

Williams, C. & Lefever, J. (2000) Reducing the risk of user error with infusion pumps. *Prof Nurse*, 15(6), 382–4.

Wilson, K. & Sullivan, M. (2004) Preventing medication errors with smart infusion technology. *Am J Health Syst Pharm*, 61(2), 177–83.

309

Chapter 14

Elimination: bladder lavage and irrigation

311 Reference material
314 *Procedure guidelines:* Bladder lavage
316 *Procedure guidelines:* Urinary catheter: maintenance solution administration
318 *Procedure guidelines:* Continuous bladder irrigation
319 **Bladder irrigation recording chart**
321 *Problem solving*
321 References and further reading

Definitions

Lavage

Bladder lavage is the manual washing out of the bladder with sterile fluid (Evans & Godfrey 2000).

Catheter maintenance solution

Catheter maintenance solution is a prepacked sterile reagent (usually 50 ml) that is allowed to drain into the bladder under gravity. The fluid is retained in the bladder (by clamping sterile reagent tube) for a specified time (usually 15 minutes) and then allowed to drain out under gravity (Evans & Godfrey 2000).

Irrigation

Bladder irrigation is the continuous washing out of the bladder with sterile fluid, usually 0.9% normal saline (Ng 2001).

Indications

Bladder lavage, catheter maintenance solutions and irrigation are indicated for the following reasons:

Lavage

- To clear an obstructed catheter.
- To remove the potential sources of obstruction, e.g. blood clots or sediment from infection (Evans & Godfrey 2000).

Catheter maintenance solutions

- To minimize recurrent catheter blockage due to encrustation.
- Reduce urethral trauma from encrustation on catheter removal (Getliffe 1996a).

Irrigation

- To prevent the formation and retention of blood clots, e.g. following prostatic surgery.
- On rare occasions to remove heavily contaminated material from a diseased urinary bladder (Scholtes 2002; Fillingham & Douglas 2004; Cutts 2005).

Reference material

Solutions used for lavage and irrigation

A number of prepacked sterile washout solutions or, as they are now commonly called, catheter maintenance solutions are available for cleaning the bladder; these include the following:

- 0.9% sodium chloride: used for mechanical flushing to remove tissue debris and small blood clots.
- Chlorhexidine 0.02%: used to prevent or reduce bacterial growth, in particular *Escherichia coli* and *Klebsiella*.

- Mandelic acid (1%): used to prevent the growth of urease-producing bacteria by acidifying the urine.
- 6% citric acid solution, 'solution R': used to dissolve persistent crystallization in the catheter or bladder.
- 3.23% citric acid and magnesium oxide solution, 'Suby G': used to prevent and/or dissolve crystallization in the catheter or bladder (Rew & Woodward 2001).

The selection of a particular solution will depend on its therapeutic properties in relation to the patient's needs.

The agent most commonly recommended for lavage and irrigation is 0.9% sodium chloride and should be used in every case unless an alternative solution is prescribed. 0.9% sodium chloride is isotonic; consequently it does not affect the body's fluid or electrolyte levels, enabling large volumes of the solution to be used as necessary (Cutts 2005). In particular, 3-litre bags of 0.9% sodium chloride are available for irrigation purposes.

Although not a common complication, absorption of irrigation fluid can occur during bladder irrigation. This can produce a potentially critical situation, as absorption leads to electrolyte imbalance and circulatory overload (Getliffe 1996a). Absorption is most likely to occur in theatre where glycine irrigation fluid, devoid of sodium or potassium, is forced under pressure into the prostatic veins (Forristal & Maxfield 2004). The 0.9% sodium chloride can not be used during surgery as it contains electrolytes which interfere with diathermy (Gilbert & Gobbi 1989). However, the risk of absorption still remains while irrigation continues postoperatively. For this reason it is important that fluid balance is monitored carefully during irrigation (Scholtes 2002).

Sterile water should never be used to irrigate the bladder as it will be readily absorbed by osmosis; however, it may be used as a purely mechanical means to flush out catheters for patients at home (Addison 2000).

Bladder lavage has been used in the management of catheter associated infections, catheter encrustation and blockage (Getliffe 1996a). However, potential risks to the bladder arise from the procedure itself and/or the solution used and there is considerable confusion and controversy surrounding its use in practice (Getliffe 1994b, 1996a; Rew 1999; Pomfret *et al.* 2004). Varying levels of knowledge have been found among nurses with regard to the type of washout fluid to use in specific circumstances and also the frequency of administration (Bailey 1991; Castledine 2001; Pomfret *et al.* 2004; Castledine 2006).

Catheter-associated infection

Catheter-associated urinary tract infections are a common complication occurring in over 90% of patients within 4 weeks of catheterization (Jewes *et al.* 1988). The risk of catheter-associated bacteriuria increases by 5–8% a day during catheterization (Mulhall *et al.* 1988) and is inevitable in long-term patients (Getliffe 1996b). Antibiotics will not prevent infection in long-term catheterized patients and their use

311

is not recommended unless systemic symptoms are present (Simpson 2001). Bladder lavage using antibiotic or antiseptic solutions (chlorhexidine, noxythiolin, povidone iodine and acetic acid) have been commonly used to prevent, reduce or treat urinary tract infections (Getliffe, 2004). However, studies have shown that chlorhexidine may in fact remove sensitive bacteria in the normal urethral flora, allowing subsequent colonization by resistant organisms (Davies *et al.* 1987; Stickler *et al.* 1987; King & Stickler 1992). Furthermore, reviews of alternative solutions (noxythiolin, povidone iodine and acetic acid) and various antibiotics have been shown to be ineffective against a number of commonly occurring pathogens; therefore their use in long-term catheterized patients is not advocated (Stickler & Chawla 1987; Stickler 1990).

Catheter-associated urinary infections are difficult to treat as bacteria adhere to the surface of the catheter in the form of a biofilm (Costerton *et al.* 1999; Trautner & Darouiche 2004). Whilst antimicrobials may successfully kill bacteria in the urine, bacteria in the biofilm are generally less susceptible to these agents; consequently, they may still persist following treatment and potentially restart the cycle of infection (Gristina *et al.* 1987; Stickler *et al.* 1987).

Three theories have been suggested to explain why this may happen:

- Microbial secretions 'bind' the biofilm to the surface, making it difficult to remove and for antibiotic and antiseptic agents to penetrate (Getliffe 1996b; Liedl 2001).
- Cells in the biofilm exist in a slow-growing or starved state and are therefore not very susceptible to many antimicrobial agents (Getliffe 1996b; Liedl 2001).
- The micro-organisms in the biofilm undergo cellular changes so they develop into a different phenotype that has different sensibility to antibiotic agents from their free-living counterparts (Liedl 2001).

As yet there is no catheter material that resists biofilm formation in the clinical setting (Getliffe 1996b; Morris *et al.* 1997; Rew & Woodward 2001); however, all-silicone catheters have been found to take longer to become encrusted than the silicone-coated, Teflon and latex catheters (Kunin *et al.* 1987) (see Chapter 18).

Catheter encrustations and blockages

Recurrent catheter encrustation and blockage is a common problem with approximately 50% of catheterized patients being susceptible (Kohler-Ockmore 1992; Getliffe 1994a). Catheter blockage may occur as the result of detrusor spasm, twisted drainage tubing or constipation, but the most common reason is the formation of encrustation on the catheter surface and within its lumen with deposits of mineral salts from the urine (Getliffe 1996a; Godfrey & Evans 2000; Rew & Woodward 2001). Catheter encrustations form on any catheter surface in contact with urine, including the catheter tip and balloon, as well as the catheter lumen (Getliffe *et al.* 2000).

Several studies have shown that catheter encrustations are caused by the interaction of bacteria and urinary pH (Burr & Nusbeibeh 1995; Choong *et al.* 1999; Mathur *et al.* 2006). Catheter encrustations commonly consist of magnesium, ammonium phosphate (struvite) and calcium phosphate (apatite) deposits (Getliffe 1996b; McCarthy & Hunter 2001), which precipitate from urine when it becomes alkaline during infection from urease-secreting micro-organisms (Mobley & Warren 1987; Getliffe 1996a; Evans & Godfrey 2000). The urease producers implicated most commonly in catheter encrustations are of the *Proteus* species, in particular *Proteus mirabilis* (Getliffe 1996b; Stickler & Hughes 1999; Liedl 2001).

The development of catheter encrustations may lead to:

- Blockage of the catheter lumen.
- Bypassing of urine.
- Retention of urine.
- Pain and patient distress.
- Unnecessary catheter changes (Rew 1999; Getliffe 2004).

Getliffe's (1994a) study attempted to identify characteristics of patients who were at greater risk of obstructing their catheters. Patients who 'blocked' their catheters were found to have high urinary pH and ammonia concentrations. High ammonia concentration and alkaline urine are found when urine is infected with urease producing micro-organisms, such as *P. mirabilis*. Significantly more females were classed as 'blockers'; this may be due to the greater risks females have of developing catheter-associated urinary infections (Kennedy *et al.* 1983), as the shorter female urethra may allow more rapid colonization. 'Blockers' were also found to be significantly less mobile than 'non-blockers'. There was no significant relationship noted between non-blockers and high average daily fluid intake; this study therefore does not support the advice conventionally given to 'drink plenty' to reduce mineral precipitation.

There have been very few clinical studies about the use of bladder maintenance solutions to dissolve the minerals which cause encrustation and increase catheter life. The 0.9% sodium chloride has been shown to have no effect in dissolving encrustations, but it may, through the mechanical effect of flushing, dislodge debris (Flack 1993).

A study carried out by Kennedy *et al.* (1992) showed that citric acid solution with (Suby G) and without magnesium oxide (solution R) administered twice weekly for 3 weeks did not have a demonstrable effect in preventing crystal formation. However, 6% citric acid solution R has been shown to dissolve fragments of struvite renal calculi following lithotripsy (Holden & Rao 1991). Catheter encrustations may be dissolved using this solution but potential inflammatory tissue reactions of the urothelium limit its use (Getliffe 1996a). Getliffe (1996a) suggests it may be used prior to catheter removal to dissolve external encrustations, which cause pain and tissue trauma on withdrawal of the catheter. Getliffe's (1994b) in vitro study suggested that mandelic acid solution may be particularly effective in reducing encrustation.

Mandelic acid 1% has been shown to be effective in removing *Pseudomonas* species from the urine of catheterized patients, although it needs to be used twice a day for a long period (on average 19 days). It has also shown to be a biocidal agent against some biofilms of single or mixed bacterial species (Stickler & Hewitt 1991). This agent is thought to have a dual role, first in reducing urinary pH and second in dissolving struvite and calcium phosphate deposits. However, tissue reactions to mandelic acid 1% in clinical situations have yet to be demonstrated, as does its efficacy in the presence of urinary elements such as mucin and organic debris (Getliffe 1996a; Rew 1999).

Potential risks to the bladder urothelium associated with bladder maintenance solutions have raised concerns (Getliffe 1996a). Dilute acid solutions have been shown to remove the surface layer of mucus in the bladder (Parsons *et al.* 1970) and an increased shedding of urothelial cells has been observed following washouts with both acidic and neutral pH solutions (Elliot *et al.* 1989; Kennedy *et al.* 1992). This infers that both chemical irritation and physical force of instillation can be potential risk factors in disrupting bladder urothelium (Getliffe 2004). This highlights the importance of administering prepackaged maintenance solutions by gravity and not manually using a bladder syringe in order to minimize mechanical damage (Gates 2000).

There have been few clinically-based studies of the use of catheter maintenance solutions on which to base decisions on the optimum volume and frequency of bladder washouts. As the aim of a bladder washout is to remove encrustation from the catheter and not (as is commonly thought) the bladder, it has been suggested that 'mini' washouts regularly performed would be effective at reducing encrustations and minimizing irritant effects on the bladder (Getliffe 1994a; Getliffe & Dolman 2003; Yates 2004). A catheter lumen holds 4–5 ml of fluid; therefore, smaller volumes of 10–20 ml would still completely fill the catheter lumen and bathe the catheter tip. Therefore the bladder mucosa would not be exposed to large volumes of washout solution (Getliffe 2004). Getliffe (1994a) suggests that washouts could then be performed more frequently without increasing the risk of tissue damage. This suggestion has been supported by an in vitro study by Getliffe *et al.* (2000). Two sequential washouts with 50 ml of Suby G retained for 15 minutes were found to be significantly better at removing encrustations than a single washout of 100 ml; however, this theory is yet to be tested in a clinical setting. Despite the controversy surrounding the use of bladder maintenance solutions, an audit undertaken by several Primary Care Trusts and reported by Pomfret *et al.* (2004) showed that they are still widely used, although practice is varied and inconsistent. These findings highlight the need for researchers to undertake clinical-based studies in order that specific bladder lavage guidelines can be established to guide nursing practice (NICE 2003; Yates 2004; Pomfret & Mackenzie 2005; McNulty *et al.* 2006).

Patient assessment

There are a number of risks associated with bladder lavage (including introducing infection) and the procedure should not be undertaken lightly (McCarthy & Hunter 2001; NICE 2003). Prior to taking a decision to use bladder maintenance solutions, patients should be assessed and a catheter history should be noted (Rew 1999). The guiding principle for effective catheter management always involves addressing the individual needs of the patient (Godfrey & Evans 2000). Assessment of all aspects of catheter care should be taken, including:

- Patient activity and mobility (catheter positioning, catheter kinking).
- Diet and fluid intake.
- Standards of patient hygiene.
- Patients' and/or carers' ability to care for the catheter (Getliffe 1996a; Rew 1999; Ng 2001; Rew 2005).

Newly catheterized patients should be monitored to ascertain how long the catheter remains in situ before showing signs of blockage, without any interference with prophylactic washouts. A catheter history should be established, and documented, to enable future care to be planned (Rew 1999). In order to develop a distinct pattern of catheter history, Norberg *et al.* (1983) suggest that 3–5 consecutive catheters should be observed before treatment, if needed, is instigated. For patients with a history of encrustation, the use of pH indicator papers is also recommended to assist in the assessment of urine alkalinity. This can be used in conjunction with the collection of a urine specimen for microbiological analysis to identify any specific organisms, which may require systemic antibiotics (Rew 2005). To minimize the risk of introducing infection and to ensure the urine sample is fresh, the aforementioned investigations should be collected directly from the catheter at weekly catheter bag changes and where possible taken at the same time of day each week considering that urinary pH changes throughout the day (Rew 2005) (see Chapter 18).

An important aspect of management, for patients where a clear pattern of catheter history can be established, is the scheduling of catheter changes prior to likely blockages (Getliffe 1996b; Yates 2004). In patients where no clear pattern emerges, or for whom frequent catheter changes are traumatic, acidic bladder washouts can be beneficial in reducing catheter encrustations (Getliffe 1996a; Rew 1999; McCarthy & Hunter 2001; Yates 2004). The administration of catheter maintenance solutions to eliminate catheter encrustation can also be timed to coincide with catheter bag changes (every 5–7 days) so that the catheter system is not opened more than necessary (Yates 2004).

Cytotoxic agents given intravesically

For details on the administration of cytotoxic agents, (see Chapter 12, Procedure guidelines: Cytotoxic drugs: intravesical instillation).

Irrigating solution

Y giving set

Clamp

Access point for
inflating balloon

Catheter drainage bag

Figure 14.1   Closed urinary drainage system with provision for intermittent or continuous irrigation.

Catheters used for irrigation

A three-way urinary catheter must be used for irrigation in order that fluid may simultaneously be run into, and drained out from, the bladder (Getliffe 1996a; Ng 2001; Cutts 2005). A large-gauge catheter (16–24) is often used to accommodate any clot and debris which may be present. This catheter is commonly passed in theatre when irrigation is required, e.g. after prostatectomy (Forristal & Maxfield 2004). Occasionally if a patient is admitted with a heavily contaminated bladder, e.g. blood clots, bladder irriga-

tion may be started on the ward. If the patient has a two-way catheter, this must be replaced with a three-way type (Scholtes 2002) (Fig. 14.1).

It is recommended that a three-way catheter is passed if frequent intravesical instillations of drugs or antiseptic solutions are prescribed and the risk of catheter obstruction is not considered to be very great. In such cases the most important factor is minimizing the risk of introducing infection and maintaining a closed urinary drainage system, for which the three-way catheter allows.

Procedure guidelines   Bladder lavage

. . . .

Equipment

1 Sterile dressing pack.
2 Sterile catheter tip syringe, 60 ml.
3 Sterile jug.
4 Antiseptic solution.
5 Bactericidal alcohol handrub.
6 Clamp.

7 New catheter bag (for balloon two-way catheter) or sterile spigot (for three-way catheter).
8 Sterile receiver.
9 Sterile solution for lavage.
10 Absorbent sheet.

. . . .

Procedure

Action	Rationale
1 Explain and discuss the procedure with the patient.	To ensure that the patient understands the procedure and gives his/her valid consent (P; NMC 2006: C).
2 Screen the bed. Ensure that the patient is in a comfortable position allowing access to the catheter.	For the patient's privacy and to reduce the risk of cross-infection. Curtains are drawn at this stage so that dust and airborne organisms disturbed by the curtains do not settle on the sterile field (DH 2005a: C).
3 Perform the procedure using an aseptic technique.	To minimize the risk of infection (DH 2005a: C). (For further information on aseptic technique see Chapter 5.)
4 If necessary, draw up solutions using a 60-ml syringe, preferably with needle adapter. Cap the syringe and place it in a sterile receiver.	It is easier to draw up solutions from vials in the clinical area than at the bedside (E).
5 Take the trolley to the bedside, disturbing the screens as little as possible. Open the outer wrappings of packs and put them on the top shelf of the trolley.	To minimize airborne contamination. To begin to prepare equipment for procedure (E).
6 Prepare the sterile field. Pour the lavage solution into the sterile jug.	To prepare equipment for procedure (E).
7 Place absorbent sheet under the catheter junction and clamp the catheter. Wash hands with bactericidal alcohol handrub.	To prevent leakage when the catheter is disconnected. To reduce the risk of infection (DH 2005a: C).
8 Put on sterile gloves, place sterile towel under the junction of the catheter and the tubing of the drainage bag and disconnect them.	To create a sterile field and reduce the risk of cross-infection (DH 2005a: C). When the patient has a three-way catheter the drainage bag will not need disconnecting as the washout fluid is injected through the side-arm of the catheter. This should be spigotted off after use and the fluid remaining in the bladder will drain into the catheter bag (E).
9 Clean gloved hands with a bactericidal alcohol handrub. Clean around the end of the catheter with sterile low-linting gauze and an antiseptic solution.	To remove surface organisms from gloves and catheter and thus reduce the risk of introducing infection into the catheter (DH 2005a: C).
10 Draw up the irrigating fluid into the bladder syringe and insert the nozzle into the end of the catheter.	To prepare syringe for lavage (E).
11 Release the clamp on the catheter and gently inject the contents of the syringe into the bladder, trying not to inject air.	Rapid injection of fluid could be uncomfortable for the patient. Large volumes of air in the bladder cause distension and discomfort (Getliffe 1994a: R 5).
12 Remove the syringe and allow the bladder contents to drain by gravity into a receiver placed on a sterile towel.	To allow catheter to drain gently (E). To reduce risk of cross-infection (DH 2005a: C).
13 Repeat steps 11 and 12 of the procedure until the washout is complete or the returning fluid is clear.	To ensure the bladder is free of contaminants (Getliffe 1994a: R 5).

Procedure guidelines *(cont.)*

14 If the fluid does not return naturally, aspirate gently with the syringe.	Gentle suction is sometimes required to remove obstructive material from the catheter. If suction is applied too forcefully the urothelium may be sucked into the eyes of the catheter, preventing drainage and causing pain and trauma which may predispose to infection (Lowthian 1991: R 5; Macaulay 2004: R 5).
15 Connect a new catheter bag or sterile spigot if a three-way catheter is in place, and allow the remaining fluid to drain out.	A closed drainage system must be re-established as soon as possible to reduce the risk of bacterial invasion through the catheter (E).
16 If the solution is to remain in the bladder, the catheter should be clamped when all the fluid has been injected and the clamp released after the desired period.	To allow solution to act on bladder mucosa/catheter (E).
17 Measure the volume of washout fluid returned and compare it with the volume of fluid injected. Record any discrepancies of volume in the appropriate documents.	To keep an accurate record of urinary output and to observe for catheter obstruction (E).
18 Make the patient comfortable, remove equipment, clean the trolley, and wash hands.	To reduce the risk of cross-infection (DH 2005a: C).

Procedure guidelines   Urinary catheter: maintenance solution administration

Equipment

1 Sterile dressing pack.
2 Antiseptic solution.
3 Bactericidal alcohol handrub.

4 Absorbent sheet.
5 New catheter bag.
6 Catheter maintenance solution.

Procedure

Action	Rationale
1 Explain and discuss the procedure with the patient.	To ensure that the patient understands the procedure and gives his/her valid consent (P; NMC 2006: C).
2 Screen the bed. Ensure that the patient is in a comfortable position, allowing the nurse access to the catheter.	For the patient's privacy and to reduce the risk of cross-infection (DH 2005a: C). Curtains are drawn at this stage so that dust and airborne organisms disturbed by the curtains do not settle on the sterile field (DH 2005a: C).
3 Perform the procedure using aseptic technique.	To minimize the risk of infection (DH 2005a: C). (For further information on aseptic technique see Chapter 5.)
4 Take the trolley to the bedside, disturbing the screens as little as possible. Open the outer wrappings of packs and put them on the top shelf of the trolley.	To minimize airborne contamination (DH 2005a: C). To begin to prepare the equipment for the procedure.

5 Remove outer packaging from catheter maintenance solution and place both 50 ml sterile solution containers on to the sterile field. Warm solution to body temperature by immersing package in water.

To prepare equipment for the procedure. Two 50 ml maintenance solution containers have been found to be the most effective way of treating encrustation (Getliffe *et al*. 2000: R 2b).
Warm solutions to prevent bladder spasm (Rew 1999: R 5).

6 Expose the whole length of the catheter and observe for any signs of discharge, meatal problems and length of catheter in patient. (If patient is using a leg bag, remove straps and place bag on the bed before exposing the catheter.) Place the absorbent pad under catheter drainage bag junction.

To prepare patient for procedure (P). To detect for signs of infection, skin excoriation or displacement of catheter. If any signs noted report to medical staff as appropriate (C).

7 Wash hands with bactericidal rub and put on sterile gloves. Place sterile towel under catheter junction.

To reduce the risk of infection (DH 2005a: C).

8 Slide clamp on solution container tubing to closed, remove the security ring on the solution container connection port and loosen cover from the connection port.

To prevent fluid loss when connection port is opened (C). To prepare equipment (C).

9 Squeeze the end of the catheter together just above the connection to the drainage bag. Disconnect the drainage bag, keeping the catheter squeezed. Remove the cover from the connecting port on the solution container and insert it into the catheter. Release the catheter.

To prevent urine leaking from the catheter (E).

10 Slide the clamp open on the solution container, raise the bag slightly above the level of the bladder and allow the required amount of the solution to flow into the bladder. Gentle pressure may be needed initially to start the flow.

Rapid instillation of fluid could be uncomfortable for the patient (P). Administering maintenance solution via gravity and not physical force will reduce the risk of damage to the bladder mucosa (Getliffe *et al*. 2000: R 2b; Rew 2005: R 5).

Instil maximum of 50 ml solution or to bladder capacity.

To avoid by-passing (Getliffe & Dolman 2003: R 2b).

Where instillation is being used to dissolve encrustation, a second instillation may be performed.

This is more effective in dissolving encrustation (Getliffe *et al*. 2000: R 2b).

11 If the fluid is to be retained for a period of time close the clamp and place the bag on the bed. Reposition the covers and ensure the patient is comfortable for the required time (P).

To allow the solutions time to act on the catheter encrustations (Evans & Godfrey 2000: R 5). For the patient's privacy and comfort (P).

12 When the solution is to be removed, ensure the bag is below the level of the bladder, open the clip and allow the solution to drain back.

For gravity to help facilitate drainage (E).

13 When all the solution has drained back out of the bladder, close the clamp, disconnect the solution container and connect a new drainage bag. Note the amount of fluid returned.

To prevent spillage of solution. To re-establish closed drainage system (E).

317

Procedure guidelines *(cont.)*

14 Make the patient comfortable, remove and dispose of equipment, clean the trolley and wash hands.	To reduce risk of cross-infection (DH 2005a: C).
15 Sign prescription chart. Document that catheter maintenance solution has been administered and note any complication or problems encountered with the procedure.	To maintain accurate records. Provide a point of reference in the event of any queries and prevent duplication of treatment (E).

Procedure guidelines   Continuous bladder irrigation

Equipment

1 Sterile dressing pack.
2 Antiseptic solution.
3 Bactericidal alcohol handrub.
4 Clamp.
5 Sterile irrigation fluid.

6 Disposable irrigation set.
7 Infusion stand.
8 Sterile jug.
9 Absorbent sheet.

Procedure

Commencing bladder irrigation

Action	Rationale
1 Explain and discuss the procedure with the patient.	To ensure that the patient understands the procedure and gives his/her valid consent (NMC 2006: C; NMC 2008: C).
2 Screen the patient and ensure that he/she is in a comfortable position allowing access to the catheter.	For the patient's privacy and to reduce the risk of cross-infection. Curtains are drawn at this stage so that dust and airborne organisms disturbed by the curtains do not settle on the sterile trolley (DH 2005a: C).
3 Perform the procedure using an aseptic technique.	To minimize the risk of infection (DH 2005a: C). (For further information on aseptic technique see Chapter 18.)
4 Open the outer wrappings of the pack and put it on the top shelf of the trolley.	To prepare equipment (E).
5 Insert the end of the irrigation giving set into the fluid bag and hang the bag on the infusion stand. Allow fluid to run through the tubing so that air is expelled.	To prime the irrigation set so that it is ready for use. Air is expelled in order to prevent discomfort from air in the patient's bladder (E).
6 Clamp the catheter and place absorbent sheet under the catheter junction.	To prevent leakage of urine through the irrigation arm when the spigot is removed (E). To contain any spillages.
7 Clean hands with a bactericidal alcohol handrub. Put on gloves.	To minimize the risk of cross-infection (DH 2005a: C).
8 Place a sterile paper towel under the irrigation inlet of the catheter and remove the spigot.	To create a sterile field. To prepare catheter for connection to irrigation set (Scholtes 2002: R 5).
9 Discard the spigot and gloves.	To prevent reuse and reduce risk of cross-infection (DH 2005a: C).

318

10 Put on sterile gloves. Clean around the end of the irrigation arm with sterile low-linting gauze and an antiseptic solution.

To remove surface organisms from gloves and catheter and to reduce the risk of introducing infection into the catheter (DH 2005a: C).

11 Attach the irrigation giving set to the irrigation arm of the catheter. Keep the clamp of the irrigation giving set closed.

To prevent overdistension of the bladder, which can occur if fluid is run into the bladder before the drainage tube has been unclamped (Scholtes 2002: R 5).

12 Release the clamp on the catheter tube and allow any accumulated urine to drain into the catheter bag. Empty the urine from the catheter bag into a sterile jug.

Urine drainage should be measured before commencing irrigation so that the fluid balance may be monitored more accurately (Scholtes 2002: R 5).

13 Discard the gloves.

These will be contaminated, having handled the cathether bag (DH 2005a, b: C).

14 Set irrigation at the required rate and ensure that fluid is draining into the catheter bag.

To check that the drainage system is patent and to prevent fluid accumulating in the bladder (C).

15 Make the patient comfortable, remove unnecessary equipment and clean the trolley.

To reduce the risk of cross-infection (DH 2005a: C).

16 Wash hands.

To reduce the risk of cross-infection (DH 2005a: C).

Care of the patient during bladder irrigation

Action

Rationale

1 Adjust the rate of infusion according to the degree of haematuria. This will be greatest in the first 12 hours following surgery (average fluid input is 6–9 litres during the first 12 hours, falling to 3–6 litres during the next 12 hours). The aim is to obtain a drainage fluid which is rosé in colour.

To remove blood from the bladder before it clots and to minimize the risk of catheter obstruction and clot retention. (Scholtes 2002: R 5.)

2 Check the volume in the drainage bag frequently when infusion is in progress, e.g. half-hourly or hourly, or more frequently as required.

To ensure that fluid is draining from the bladder and to detect blockages as soon as possible, also to prevent overdistension of the bladder and patient discomfort (E, P). To empty catheter drainage bags before they reach capacity.

3 Using rubber-tipped 'milking' tongs, 'milk' the catheter and drainage tube, as required.

To remove clots from within the drainage system and to maintain an efficient outlet (Lowthian 1991: R 5).

4 Record the fluid balance chart accurately. The fluid balance of all patients having bladder irrigation must be monitored.

So that urine output is known and any related problems, e.g. renal dysfunction, may be detected quickly and easily (E).

Bladder irrigation recording chart

The bladder irrigation recording chart (Figure 14.2) is designed to provide an accurate record of the patient's urinary output during the period of irrigation.

Procedure for use of chart

Record the time (column A) and the fluid volume in each bag of irrigating solution (column B) as it is put up.

When the irrigating fluid has all run from the first bag into the bladder, record the original volume in the bag in

319

Patient name:			Hospital no:		
(A) Date and time	(B) Volume put up	(C) Volume run in	(D) Total volume out	(E) Urine	(F) Urine running total
10/7/06 10.00 10.30 11.10 11.40	2000	2000	700 850 600		
			2150	150	150
11.45 12.30 13.15 14.20	2000	2000	500 700 800		
			2400	400	550
14.25 15.30 17.00	2000 Irrigation stopped	1200	850 800		
			1650	450	1000

Figure 14.2   Bladder irrigation recording chart.

column C. Record the corresponding time in column A. Do not attempt to estimate the fluid volume run-in while a bag is in progress as this will be inaccurate. If, however, a bag is discontinued, the volume run-in can be calculated by measuring the volume left in the bag and deducting this from the original volume. This should be recorded in column C (Scholtes 2002).

The catheter bag should be emptied as often as is necessary, the volume being recorded in column D and the corresponding time in column A. The catheter bag must also be emptied whenever the bag of irrigating fluid is empty, and the volume recorded in column D.

When each bag of fluid has run through, add up the total volume drained by the catheter in column D, and write this in red. Subtract from this the total volume run-in (column C) to find the urine output (D − C = E). Write this in column E. Draw a line across the page to indicate that this calculation is complete and continue underneath for the next bag.

Problem solving

Problem	Cause	Suggested action
Fluid retained in the bladder when the catheter is in position.	Fault in drainage apparatus, e.g.:	
	Blocked catheter	'Milk' the tubing. Wash out the bladder with 0.9% sodium chloride (E).
	Kinked tubing	Straighten the tubing (E).
	Overfull drainage bag	Empty the drainage bag (E).
	Catheter clamped off	Unclamp the catheter (E).
Distended abdomen related to an overfull bladder during the irrigation procedure.	Irrigation fluid is infused at too rapid a rate.	Slow down the infusion rate (E).
	Fault in drainage apparatus.	Check the patency of the drainage apparatus (E).
Leakage of fluid from around the catheter.	Catheter slipping out of the bladder.	Insert the catheter further in (E). Decompress balloon fully to assess the amount of water necessary. Refill balloon until it remains in situ, taking care not to overfill beyond safe level (see manufacturer's instructions) (E).
	Catheter too large or unsuitable for the patient's anatomy.	If leakage is profuse or catheter is uncomfortable for the patient, replace the catheter with one of smaller size (E).
Patient experiences pain during the lavage or irrigation procedure.	Volume of fluid in the bladder is too great for comfort.	Reduce the fluid volume within the bladder (E).
	Solution is painful to raw areas in the bladder.	Inform the doctor. Administer analgesia as prescribed (E).
Retention of fluid with or without distended abdomen, with or without pain.	Perforated bladder.	Stop irrigation. Maintain in recovery position. Call medical assistance (E). Monitor vital signs. Monitor patient for pain, tense abdomen (E).

For further details, see Chapter 18, Problem solving: Urinary catheter.

321

References and further reading

Addison, R. (2000) *Bladder Washout/Irrigation/Instillations. A Guide for Nurses*. Braun Medical, Sheffield.

Bailey, S. (1991) Using bladder washouts. *Nurs Times*, 87(24), 75–6.

Burr, R.G. & Nusbeibeh, I. (1995) The blocking urinary catheter: the role of variation in urine flow. *Br J Urol*, 76, 61–5.

Castledine, G. (2001) Case 42: Bladder washout – Staff nurse who carried out a bladder washout using Diet Coke. *Br J Nurs*, 10(3), 144.

Castledine, G. (2006) Nurse whose inexperience and negligence in bladder washout put her patient at risk. *Br J Nurs*, 15(3), 141.

Choong, S.K.S. *et al.* (1999) The physicochemical basis of urinary catheter encrustation. *Br J Urol*, 83, 770–5.

Costerton, J.W. *et al.* (1999) Bacterial biofilms: a common cause of persistent infections. *Science*, 284, 1318–22.

Cox, A.J. *et al.* (1987) Calcium phosphate in catheter encrustation. *Br J Urol*, 59, 159–63.

Cutts, B. (2005) Developing and implementing a new bladder irrigation chart. *Nurs Stand*, 20(8), 48–53.

Davies, A.J. *et al.* (1987) Does instillation of chlorhexidine into the bladder of catheterised geriatric patients help reduce bacteriuria? *J Hosp Infect*, **9**, 72–5.

DH (2005a) *Saving Lives: A Delivery Programme to Reduce Healthcare Infection including MRSA*. Department of Health, London.

DH (2005b) *Hazardous waste (England) regulations*. Department of Health, London.

Dudley, M.N. & Barriere, S.L. (1981) Antimicrobial irrigations in the prevention and treatment of catheter-related urinary tract infections. *Am J Hosp Pharm*, **38**, 59–65.

Elliot, T.S. (1990) Disadvantages of bladder irrigation in catheterized patients. (Brief research report.) *Nurs Times*, **86**, 52.

Elliot, T.S. *et al.* (1989) Bladder irrigation or irritation? *Br J Urol*, **64**, 391–4.

Evans, A. & Godfrey, H. (2000) Bladder washouts in the management of long-term catheters. *Br J Nurs*, **9**(14), 900–4.

Ferrie, B.G., Glen, E.S. & Hunter, B. (1979) Long-term urethral catheter drainage. *Br Med J*, **2**(6197), 1046–7.

Fillingham, S. & Douglas, J. (2004) *Urological Nursing*, 3rd edn. Bailliere Tindall, Edinburgh.

Flack, S. (1993) Finding the best solution. *Nurs Times*, **11**, 68–74.

Forristal, H. & Maxfield, J. (2004) Prostatic problems. In: *Urological Nursing* (eds S. Fillingham & J. Douglas), 3rd edn. Bailliere Tindall, London, pp. 161–84.

Gates, A. (2000) The benefits of irrigation in catheter care. *Prof Nurse*, **16**(1), 835–8.

Getliffe, K.A. (1994a) The characteristics and management of patients with recurrent blockage of long-term urinary catheters. *J Adv Nurs*, **20**, 140–9.

Getliffe, K.A. (1994b) The use of bladder wash-outs to reduce urinary catheter encrustation. *Br J Urol*, **73**, 696–700.

Getliffe, K.A. (1996a) Bladder instillations and bladder washouts in the management of catheterized patients. *J Adv Nurs*, **23**, 548–54.

Getliffe, K.A. (1996b) Care of urinary catheters. *Nurs Stand*, **11**(11), 47–54.

Getliffe, K.A. (2004) The effect of acidic maintenance solutions on catheter longevity. *Nurs Times*, **100**(16), 32–4.

Getliffe, K.A. & Dolman, M. (2003) *Promoting Continence: A Clinical and Research Resource*, 2nd edn. Bailliere Tindall, London.

Getliffe, K., Hughes, S.C. & Le Claire, M. (2000) The dissolution of urinary catheter encrustation. *Br J Urol*, **85**(1), 60–4.

Gilbert, V. & Gobbi, M. (1989) Bladder irrigation (principles and methods). *Nurs Times*, **85**, 40–2.

Godfrey, H. & Evans, H. (2000) Management of long-term urethral catheters: minimizing complications. *Br J Nurs*, **9**(2), 74–80.

Griffith, D.P. & Musher, O.N. (1976) Urease: the primary cause of infection induced urinary stones. *Invest Urol*, **13**(5), 346–82.

Gristina, A.G. *et al.* (1987) Adhesive colonisation of biomaterials and antibiotic resistance. *Biomaterials*, **8**, 423–6.

Hedelin, H. *et al.* (1984) The composition of catheter encrustations, including the effects of allopurinol treatment. *Br J Urol*, **56**, 250–4.

Holden, D. & Rao, P.N. (1991) Management of staghorn stones using a combination of lithotripsy, percutaneous nephrolithotomy and solution R irrigation. *Br J Urol*, **67**, 13–17.

Jewes, L.A. *et al.* (1988) Bacteriuria and bacteraemia in patients with long-term indwelling catheters: a domiciliary study. *J Med Microbiol*, **26**, 61–5.

Kennedy, A.P. *et al.* (1983) Factors relating to the problems of long-term catheterization. *J Adv Nurs*, **8**, 207–12.

Kennedy, A.P. *et al.* (1992) Assessment of the use of bladder washouts/instillations in patients with long term indwelling catheters. *Br J Urol*, **70**, 610–15.

King, J.B. & Stickler, D.J. (1992) The effects of repeated instillations of antiseptics on catheter-associated urinary tract infections. *Urol Res*, **20**, 403–7.

Kohler-Ockmore, J. (1992) Urinary catheter complications. *J District Nurs*, **10**(8), 18–20.

Kunin, C.M., Chin, Q.A. & Charnbers, S. (1987) Formation of encrustation on in-dwelling urinary catheters in the elderly. *J Urol*, **77**(3), 347–51.

Liedl, B. (2001) Catheter-associated urinary tract infections. *Curr Opin Urol*, **11**(1), 75–9.

Lowthian, P. (1991) Using bladder syringes sparingly. *Nurs Times*, **87**(10), 61–4.

Macaulay, D. (2004) Urinary drainage systems. In: *Urological Nursing* (eds. S. Fillingham & J. Douglas), 2nd edn. Bailliere Tindall, London, pp. 90–130.

Mathur, S. *et al.* (2006) Prospective study of individuals with long-term urinary catheters colonized with *Proteus* species. *Br J Urol*, **97**, 121–8.

McCarthy, K. & Hunter, I. (2001) Importance of pH monitoring in the care of long-term catheters. *Br J Nurs*, **10**(19), 1240–6.

McNulty, C.A.M. *et al.* (2006) Urinary catheterization in care homes for older people; self-reported questionnaire audit of catheter management by care home staff. *J Hosp Infect*, **26**, 29–36.

Mobley, H.L.T. & Warren, J.W. (1987) Urease positive bacteriuria and obstruction of long-term urinary catheters. *J Clin Microbiol*, **25**, 2216–17.

Morris, N.S., Stickler, D.J. & Winters, C. (1997) Which indwelling urethral catheters resist encrustations by *Proteus mirabilis* biofilms? *Br J Urol*, **80**, 58–63.

Mulhall, A.B., Chapman, R.G. & Crow, R.A. (1988) Bacteriuria during indwelling urethral catheterisation. *J Hosp Infect*, **11**(3), 253–62.

Ng, C. (2001) Assessment and intervention knowledge of nurses in managing catheter patency in continuous bladder irrigation following TURP. *Urol Nurs*, **21**(2), 97–108.

NICE (2003) *Infection Control. Prevention of Health Care-associated Infection in Primary and Community Care. Clinical Guidance 2*. National Institute for Health and Clinical Excellence, London.

NMC (2005) *Guidelines for Records and Record Keeping*. Nursing and Midwifery Council, London.

NMC (2006) *A–Z Advice Sheet Consent*. www.nmc.org.

NMC (2008) *The Code: Standards of Conduct, Performance and Ethics for Nurses and Midwives*. Nursing and Midwifery Council, London.

Norberg, B., Norberg, A. & Parkhede, U. (1983) The spontaneous variation in catheter life in long-stay geriatric patients with indwelling catheters. *Gerontology*, **29**, 332–5.

Parsons, C.L., Mulholland, S.G. & Anwar, H. (1970) Antibacterial activity of bladder surface mucin duplicated by exogenous glycosaminoglycan (heparin). *Infect Immun*, **25**, 552–4.

Pomfret, I. & Mackenzie, R. (2005) Questioning practice – the need for research in continence care. *J Comm Nurs*, **19**(11), 32–5.

Pomfret, I. *et al.* (2004) Using bladder instillations to manage indwelling catheters. *Br J Nurs*, **13**(5), 261–7.

Rao, G.G. & Elliott, T.S.J. (1988) Bladder irrigation. *Age Ageing*, **17**(6), 373–8.

Rew, M. (1999) Use of catheter maintenance solutions for long-term catheters. *Br J Nurs*, **8**(11), 708–15.

Rew, M. (2005) Caring for catheterized patients: urinary catheter maintenance. *Br J Nurs*, **14**(2), 87–92.

Rew, M. & Woodward, S. (2001) Troubleshooting common problems associated with long-term catheters. *Br J Nurs*, **10**(12), 764–74.

Roe, B.H. (1989) Use of bladder washouts: a study of nurses' recommendations. *J Adv Nurs*, **14**(6), 494–500.

Roe, B.H. (1990) The basis for sound practice. *Nurs Stand*, **4**, 25–7.

Scholtes, S. (2002) Management of clot retention following urological surgery. *Nurs Times*, **98**(28), 48–50.

Simpson, L. (2001) Indwelling urethral catheters. *Nurs Stand*, **15**(46), 47–54.

Stickler, D.J. (1990) The role of antiseptics in the management of patients undergoing short term indwelling bladder catheterisation. *J Hosp Infect*, **16**, 89–108.

Stickler, D.J. & Chawla, J.C. (1987) The role of antiseptics in the management of patients with long term indwelling bladder catheters. *J Hosp Infect*, **10**, 219–28.

Stickler, D.J. & Hewitt, P. (1991) Activity of antiseptic against biofilms of mixed bacterial species growing on silicone surfaces. *Eur J Microbiol Infect*, **10**, 416–21.

Stickler, D.J. & Hughes, G. (1999) Ability of *Proteus mirabilis* to swarm over urethral catheters. *Eur J Clin Microbiol Infect Dis*, **18**(3), 206–8.

Stickler, D.J. et al. (1981) Some observations on the activity of three antiseptics used as bladder irrigants in the treatment of UTI in patients with indwelling catheters. *Paraplegia*, **19**, 325–33.

Stickler, D.J., Clayton, C.L. & Chawla, J.C. (1987) The resistance of urinary tract pathogens to chlorhexidine bladder washouts. *J Hosp Infect*, **10**, 28–39.

Trautner, B.W. & Darouiche, R.O. (2004) Role of biofilm in catheter-associated urinary tract infection. *Am J Inf Con*, **32**(3), 177–83.

Yates, A. (2004) Crisis management in catheter care. *J Comm Nurs*, **18**(5), 28–30.

323

Chapter 15

Elimination: bowel care

325 Reference material
325 *Procedure guidelines:* Bedpan use: assisting a patient
326 *Procedure guidelines:* Commode use: assisting a patient
335 **Enemas**
335 Reference material
336 *Procedure guidelines:* Enema administration
338 *Problem solving:* Enema administration
338 **Suppositories**
338 Reference material
339 *Procedure guidelines:* Suppository administration
340 **Digital rectal examination**
341 *Procedure guidelines:* Digital rectal examination
342 **Manual evacuation**
343 *Procedure guidelines:* Manual evacuation of faeces
344 **Rectal irrigation**
345 Reference material
345 References and further reading

Definitions

Diarrhoea

Diarrhoea results when the balance between absorption, secretion and intestinal motility is disturbed (Hogan 1998). It has been defined as an abnormal increase in the quantity, frequency and fluid content of stool and associated with urgency, perianal discomfort and incontinence (Basch 1987), and is characterized by at least three loose, liquid stools per day (Bell 2004; NANDA-I 2007).

Constipation

Constipation results when there is a delayed movement of intestinal content through the bowel (Walsh 1997). It has been defined as persistent, difficult, infrequent or incomplete defecation, which may or may not be accompanied by hard, dry stools (Norton 2006; NANDA-I 2007).

Reference material

Bowel elimination is a sensitive issue and providing effective care and management for problems associated with it can be problematic. The difficulties associated with this can be minimized if the nurse seeks to respect the patient's dignity when carrying out procedures such as assisting them with using a bedpan or a commode.

Procedure guidelines   Bedpan use: assisting a patient

Equipment

1 Disposable apron and gloves.
2 Slipper bedpan and paper cover.
3 Toilet paper.
4 Manual handling equipment as appropriate.
5 Additional nurse if required.
6 Wash bowl, warm water, disposable wipes and a towel.

Procedure

Action	Rationale
1 Carry out appropriate manual handling assessment prior to commencing procedure and establish whether an additional nurse or equipment such as a hoist are necessary.	To maintain a safe environment.
2 Take the equipment to the bedside and explain the procedure to the patient.	To ensure that the patient understands the procedure and gives his/her valid consent (NMC 2006: C; NMC 2008b: C).
3 Close door/draw curtains around the patient's bed area.	To maintain privacy and dignity and avoid any unnecessary embarrassment for the patient (P).
4 Remove the bedclothes and, providing there are no contra-indications (e.g. if patient is on flat bed rest), assist the patient into an upright sitting position.	An upright, 'crouch like' posture is considered anatomically correct for defecation and poor posture adopted while using a bedpan has been shown to cause extreme straining during defecation. Patients should therefore be supported with pillows in order to achieve an upright position on the bedpan (Taylor 1997: E).
5 Ask the patient to raise their hips/buttocks and insert the bedpan beneath the patient's pelvis, ensuring that the wide end of the bedpan is between the legs, and the narrow is beneath the buttocks.	A slipper bedpan provides more comfort for a patient who is unable to sit upright on a conventional bedpan (Nicol *et al.* 2004: E).
6 Offer patients the use of pillows and encourage them to lean forward slightly.	To provide support and optimize positioning for defecation (Taylor 1997: E).

325

Procedure guidelines *(cont.)*

7 If the patient is unable to adopt a sitting/upright position, then roll them onto one side, using appropriate manual handling equipment, and insert a slipper bedpan with the narrow/flat end underneath their buttocks and wide end between their legs. Then roll the patient onto their back and so onto the bedpan.

8 Once the patient is on the bedpan, encourage them to move their legs slightly apart and check to ensure that their positioning is correct.

To avoid any spillage onto the bed clothes and reduce risk of contamination and cross-infection.

9 Cover the patient's legs with a sheet.

To maintain privacy and dignity (P).

10 Ensure that toilet paper and call bell are within patient's reach and leave the patient, but remain nearby.

To maintain privacy and dignity (P).

11 When the patient has finished using the bedpan, bring washing equipment to the bedside, remove the bedpan, and replace paper cover. Assist patient with cleaning perianal area using warm water and soap. Apply a small amount of barrier cream to the perineal/buttock area if appropriate.

Talcum powder should not be used and barrier creams should be applied sparingly, gently layered on in the direction of the hair growth rather than rubbed into the skin (Le Lievre 2002: E).

12 Offer a bowl of water for the patient to wash their hands.

For infection control and patient's comfort (P).

13 Ensure bedclothes are clean, straighten sheets and rearrange pillows, assisting patient to a comfortable position. Ensure call bell is within reach of the patient.

For patient comfort (P).

14 Take bedpan to the dirty utility (sluice) room and where necessary, measure urine output and note characteristics (see Bristol Stool Form Chart: Figure 15.1) and amount of faeces.

To monitor and evaluate patient's elimination patterns (E).

15 Dispose of contents safely and place bedpan in the washer/disposal unit.

To reduce any risk of contamination or cross-infection.

16 Remove disposable apron and gloves. Wash hands using soap and water/alcohol handrub.

For infection control.

17 Record any urine output/bowel action in patient's documentation.

To maintain accurate documentation.

Procedure guidelines   Commode use: assisting a patient

Equipment

1 Disposable apron and gloves.
2 Commode with conventional bedpan inserted below seat.
3 Toilet paper.
4 Manual handling equipment as appropriate.
5 Additional nurse if required.
6 Wash bowl, warm water, disposable wipes and a towel.

Procedure

Action	Rationale
1 Carry out appropriate manual handling assessment prior to commencing procedure and ensure that patient's weight does not exceed the maximum recommended for commode (see manufacturer's guidelines).	To maintain a safe environment.
2 Take the equipment to the bedside and explain the procedure to the patient.	To ensure that the patient understands the procedure and gives his/her valid consent (NMC 2006: C; NMC 2008b: C).
3 Close door/draw curtains around the patient's bed area.	To maintain privacy and dignity and avoid any unnecessary embarrassment for the patient (P).
4 Remove the commode cover. Assist the patient out of the bed/chair and onto the commode.	
5 Ensure the patient's feet are positioned directly below their knees and flat on the floor. The use of a small footstool and/or pillows may help to achieve a comfortable position.	An upright, crouching posture is considered anatomically correct for defecation. Pillows and a footstool can provide support and optimize positioning for defecation (Taylor 1997: E).
6 Once the patient is on the commode, encourage them to move their legs slightly apart and check to ensure that their positioning is correct.	To avoid any spillage and reduce risk of contamination and cross-infection.
7 Cover the patient's knees with a towel or sheet.	To maintain privacy and dignity (P).
8 Ensure that toilet paper and call bell are within patient's reach and leave the patient, but remain nearby.	To maintain privacy and dignity (P).
9 When the patient has finished using the commode, bring washing equipment to the bedside. Assist patient with cleaning perianal area using toilet paper and, where necessary, warm water and soap. Apply a small amount of barrier cream to the perineal/buttock area if appropriate.	Talcum powder should not be used and barrier creams should be applied sparingly, gently layered on in the direction of the hair growth rather than rubbed into the skin (Le Lievre 2002: E).
10 Offer a bowl of water for the patient to wash their hands.	For infection control and patient's comfort (P).
11 Assist the patient to stand and walk to bed/chair, ensuring that they are comfortably positioned. Ensure call bell is within reach of the patient.	For patient comfort (P).
12 Replace cover on the commode and return to the dirty utility (sluice) room.	To reduce any risk of contamination or cross-infection and to avoid patient embarrassment.
13 Remove pan from underneath the commode and where necessary, measure urine output, and note characteristics (see Bristol Stool Form Chart: Figure 15.1) and amount of faeces.	To monitor and evaluate patient's elimination patterns (E).
14 Dispose of contents safely and place pan in the washer/disposal unit. Clean commode using warm, soapy water.	For infection control.
15 Remove disposable apron and gloves. Wash hands using soap and water/alcohol hand rub.	For infection control.
16 Record any urine output/bowel action in patient's documentation.	To maintain accurate documentation.

Many patients are too embarrassed to discuss bowel function and will often delay reporting problems, despite the sometimes severe impact these symptoms have on their quality of life (Cadd *et al.* 2000). Generally complaints will be either that the patient has diarrhoea or is constipated. These should be seen as symptoms of some underlying disease or malfunction and managed accordingly.

The nurse's priority is to effectively assess the nature and cause of the problem, to help find appropriate solutions and to inform and support the patient. This requires sensitive communication skills to dispel embarrassment and ensure a shared understanding of the meanings of the terms used by the patient (Smith 2001).

Anatomy and physiology

This section will consider the normal structure and function of the bowel, which includes the small and large intestine. The small intestine begins at the pyloric sphincter of the stomach, coils through the abdomen and opens into the large intestine at the ileocaecal junction. It is approximately 6 m in length and is divided into three segments: the duodenum (25 cm), jejunum (2.5 m) and ileum (3.5 m) (Thibodeau & Patton 2007). The mucosal surface of the small intestine is covered with finger-like processes called villi, which increase the surface area available for absorption and digestion. A number of digestive enzymes are also secreted by the small intestine (Tortora & Derrickson 2008).

Movement through the small bowel is divided into two types, namely segmentation and peristalsis, and is controlled by the autonomic nervous system. Segmentation refers to the localized contraction of the intestine, which mixes the intestinal contents and brings particles of food into contact with the mucosa for absorption. Once the majority of a meal has been absorbed through this process, intestinal content is then pushed along the small intestine by repeated peristaltic wave-like actions. Intestinal content usually remains in the small bowel for 3–5 hours (Tortora & Derrickson 2008).

The total volume of fluid, including ingested liquids and gastrointestinal secretions, that enters the small intestine daily is about 9.3 litres. The small intestine is responsible for absorbing around 90% of the nutrients, electrolytes and water within this volume by diffusion, facilitated diffusion, osmosis and active transport (Tortora & Derrickson 2008). Water is able to move across the intestinal mucosa in both directions, but is influenced by the absorption of nutrients and electrolytes. As various electrolytes and nutrients are actively transported out of the lumen, they create a concentration gradient, promoting water absorption, via osmosis, in order to maintain an osmotic balance between intestinal fluid and blood. This ultimately leads to only about 1 litre of effluent passing through into the colon (Wood 1996; Thibodeau & Patton 2007; Tortora & Derrickson 2008).

From the ileocaecal sphincter to the anus the colon is approximately 1.5–1.8 m in length. Its main function is to eliminate the waste products of digestion by the propulsion of faeces towards the anus. In addition, it produces mucus to lubricate the faecal mass, thus aiding its expulsion. Other functions include the absorption of fluid and electrolytes, including sodium and potassium, the storage of faeces and the synthesis of vitamins B and K by bacterial flora (Thibodeau & Patton 2007; Tortora & Derrickson 2008).

Faeces consist of the unabsorbed end products of digestion, bile pigments, cellulose, bacteria, epithelial cells, mucus and some inorganic material. They are normally semi-solid in consistency and contain about 70% water (Tortora & Derrickson 2006). The colon absorbs about 2 litres of water in 24 hours, so if faeces are not expelled they will gradually become hard due to dehydration and more difficult to expel. If there is insufficient roughage (fibre) in the faeces, colonic stasis occurs, which leads to continued water absorption and further hardening of the faeces. The movement of faeces through the colon towards the anus is by mass peristalsis, a gastro colic reflex initiated by the presence of food in the stomach, which begins at the middle of the transverse colon and quickly drives the colonic contents into the rectum. This mass peristaltic movement generally occurs 3–5 times a day (Perdue 2005). In response to this stimulus, faeces move into the rectum (Norton 1996b; Taylor 1997; Tortora & Derrickson 2008). The rectum is very sensitive to rises in pressure, even of 2–3 mmHg, and distension will cause a perineal sensation with a subsequent desire to defecate. A co-ordinated reflex empties the bowel from mid-transverse colon to the anus. During this phase the diaphragm, abdominal and levator ani muscles contract and the glottis closes. Waves of peristalsis occur in the distal colon and the anal sphincter relaxes, allowing the evacuation of faeces (Tortora & Derrickson 2008). The stimulus to defecate varies in individuals according to habit, and if a decision is made to delay defecation, the stimulus disappears and a process of retroperistalsis occurs whereby the faeces moves back into the sigmoid colon (Perdue 2005). If these natural reflexes are inhibited on a regular basis they are eventually suppressed and reflex defecation is inhibited, resulting in such individuals becoming severely constipated.

Diarrhoea

The term diarrhoea originates from the Greek for 'to flow through' (Bell 2004) and can be characterized according to its onset and duration (acute or chronic) or by type (e.g. secretory, osmotic or malabsorptive). Sudden onset acute diarrhoea is very common, usually self-limiting, lasts less than 2 weeks and often requires no investigation or treatment (Shepherd 2000). The causes of acute diarrhoea include:

- Dietary indiscretion (eating too much fruit, alcohol misuse).
- Allergy to food constituents.
- Infective (King 2002):
  (a) Travel-associated.
  (b) Viral.
  (c) Bacterial (usually associated with food).
  (d) Antibiotic-related.

■ Contrast media for screening purposes (Taylor 1997; Campbell & Lunn 1999).

Chronic diarrhoea generally lasts longer than 2 weeks and may have more complex origins (Hogan 1998). Chronic causes include (Taylor 1997; Fallon & O'Neill 1997):

■ Inflammatory bowel disease, e.g. ulcerative colitis, Crohn's disease.
■ Malabsorption, e.g. coeliac disease, tropical sprue.
■ Organic disease, e.g. neoplasms, diverticulitis.
■ Endocrine disorders, e.g. thyrotoxicosis, diabetes, carcinoid tumours.
■ Intestinal obstruction including faecal obstruction.
■ Miscellaneous colitis including pseudomembranous colitis, radiation enteritis, gut reaction and drug therapy, e.g. laxatives, antibiotics, chemotherapy.

Diarrhoea can have profound physiological and psychosocial consequences on a patient. Severe or extended episodes of diarrhoea may result in dehydration, electrolyte imbalance and malnutrition. Patients not only have to cope with increased frequency of bowel movement but may have abdominal pain, cramping, proctitis and anal or perianal skin breakdown. Food aversions may develop or patients may stop eating altogether as they anticipate subsequent diarrhoea following intake. Consequently this may lead to weight loss and malnutrition. Fatigue, sleep disturbances, feelings of isolation and depression are all common consequences for those experiencing diarrhoea (Hogan 1998). Patients with a stoma may also need to change their appliances more frequently and skin excoriation may occur which can exacerbate distress (Campbell & Lunn 1999). The impact of severe diarrhoea should not be underestimated; it is highly debilitating and may cause patients on long-term therapy to be non-compliant resulting in a potentially life-threatening problem (Kornblau et al. 2000).

Assessment

The cause of diarrhoea needs to be identified before effective treatment can be instigated. This may include clinical investigations such as stool cultures for bacterial, fungal and viral pathogens or a more formal medical evaluation of the gastrointestinal tract (Kornblau et al. 2000).

Ongoing nursing assessment is essential for ensuring individualized management and care. The lack of a systematic approach to assessment and poor documentation causes problems in effective management of diarrhoea (Cadd et al. 2000; Smith 2001). Nurses need to be aware of contributing factors and be sensitive to patients' beliefs and values in order to provide holistic care. A comprehensive assessment is therefore essential and should include:

1 History of onset, frequency and duration of diarrhoea.
2 Consistency, colour and form of stool including the presence of blood, fat, mucus. Stools can be graded using a scale such as the Bristol Stool Form Chart (Figure 15.1), where diarrhoea would be classified as types 6 or 7 (Longstreth et al. 2006).
3 Symptoms associated with diarrhoea, e.g. pain, nausea, vomiting, fatigue, weight loss, fever.
4 Recent lifestyle changes, emotional disturbances, or travel abroad.
5 Fluid intake and dietary history including any cause and effect relationships between food consumption and bowel action.
6 Normal medication, including recent antibiotics, laxatives or chemotherapy.
7 Effectiveness of antidiarrhoeal medication (dose and frequency).
8 Significant past medical history, e.g. bowel resection, pancreatitis, pelvic radiotherapy.
9 Hydration status (e.g. evaluation of mucous membranes and skin turgor).
10 Perianal or peristomal skin integrity.
11 Stool cultures for bacterial, fungal and viral pathogens.
12 Patient's preferences and own coping strategies including non-pharmacological interventions and their effectiveness.
(Taylor 1997; Hogan 1998; Cadd et al. 2000; Kornblau et al. 2000; King 2002; Chelvanayagam & Norton 2004.)

Management

Once the cause of diarrhoea has been established, management should be focused on resolving the cause of the diarrhoea and providing physical and psychological support for the patient. Most cases of chronic diarrhoea will resolve once the underlying condition is treated, e.g. drug therapy for Crohn's disease, or with dietary management for coeliac disease. Episodes of acute diarrhoea, usually caused by bacteria or viruses, generally resolve spontaneously and are managed by symptom control and the prevention of complications (Shepherd 2000).

All episodes of acute diarrhoea must be considered potentially infectious until proved otherwise. The risk of spreading the infection to others can be reduced by adopting universal precautions such as wearing of gloves, aprons and gowns, disposing of all excreta immediately and, ideally, nursing the patient in a side room with access to their own toilet (King 2002). Advice should always be sought from infection control teams.

The prevention and/or correction of dehydration is the first step in managing an episode of diarrhoea. Simple steps to encourage patients to drink include:

■ Providing drinks to suit individual taste preferences.
■ Adding ice to drinks.
■ Ice-lollies.
■ Using china cups or glass instead of plastic or polystyrene cups.

Dehydration can be corrected by using oral rehydration solutions, or by intravenous fluids and electrolytes.

329

THE BRISTOL STOOL FORM SCALE

Type 1	Separate hard lumps, like nuts (hard to pass)
Type 2	Sausage-shaped but lumpy
Type 3	Like a sausage but with cracks on its surface
Type 4	Like a sausage or snake, smooth and soft
Type 5	Soft blobs with clear-cut edges (passed easily)
Type 6	Fluffy pieces with ragged edges, a mushy stool
Type 7	Watery, no solid pieces ENTIRELY LIQUID

Figure 15.1   Bristol Stool Form Chart. Reproduced by kind permission of Dr K.W. Heaton, Reader in Medicine at the University of Bristol. © 2000 Norgine Ltd.

Antimotility drugs such as loperamide or codeine phosphate may be useful in some cases, for example in blind loop syndrome and radiation enteritis. These drugs reduce gastrointestinal motility to relieve the symptoms of abdominal cramps and reduce the frequency of diarrhoea (Shepherd 2000). It is important to rule out any infective agent as the cause of diarrhoea before using any of these drugs as they may make the situation worse by slowing the clearance of the infective agent (Taylor 1997). Occasionally intractable diarrhoea may be reduced by a subcutaneous infusion of octreotide, but this is more commonly indicated in patients with a high output of diarrhoea from a stoma (Fallon & O'Neill 1997).

Preserving the patient's privacy and dignity is essential during episodes of diarrhoea. The nurse has an important role in minimizing the patient's distress by adjusting language and using terms that are appropriate to the individual to reduce embarrassment (Smith 2001) and by listening to the patient's preference for care (Cadd et al. 2000).

It is important that the patient has easy access to clean toilet and washing facilities and that requests for assistance are answered promptly. Skin care is also essential to prevent bacteria present in faecal matter from destroying the skin's cellular defences and causing skin damage. This is particularly important with diarrhoea since it has high levels of faecal enzymes that come into contact with the perianal skin (Le Lievre 2002). The anal area should be gently cleaned with warm water immediately after every episode of diarrhoea (Taylor 1997). Soap should be avoided, unless it is an emollient, to avoid excessive drying of the skin and gentle patting of the skin is preferred for drying to avoid friction damage. Talcum powder should not be used and barrier creams should be applied sparingly, gently layered on in the direction of the hair growth rather than rubbed into the skin (Le Lievre 2002).

Constipation

Constipation occurs when there is either a failure of colonic propulsion (slow colonic transit), or a failure to evacuate the rectum (rectal outlet delay) or a combination of these problems (Norton 1996a; Teahon 1999; Norton 2006). The management of constipation depends on the cause and there are numerous possible causes, with many patients being affected by more than one causative factor (Figure 15.2). While constipation is not life-threatening it does cause a great deal of distress and discomfort. Particularly, constipation can be associated with abdominal pain or cramps, feelings of general malaise or fatigue and feelings of bloatedness. Nausea, anorexia, headaches, confusion, restlessness, retention of urine, faecal incontinence and halitosis may also be present in some cases (Norton 1996b; Maestri-Banks 1998).

It has been estimated that up to 27% of a given population experience constipation (Cook et al. 1999; Longstreth et al. 2006). There is a lack of consensus amongst both health care professionals and the general public as to what actually constitutes constipation (Perdue 2005; Norton 2006). Over

recent years a set of international criteria (Rome Criteria) have been developed and recently revised (Longstreth et al. 2006) which can help to more accurately and consistently define constipation. According to the new Rome III Criteria an individual who is diagnosed with constipation should report having at least two of the following symptoms within the last 3 months where those symptoms began at least 6 months prior to diagnosis (Longstreth et al. 2006; Norton 2006.):

- Straining for at least 25% of the time.
- Lumpy or hard stool for at least 25% of the time.
- A sensation of incomplete evacuation for at least 25% of the time.
- A sensation of anorectal obstruction or blockage for at least 25% of the time.
- Manual manoeuvres used to facilitate defecation at least 25% of the time (e.g. manual evacuation).
- Less than three bowel movements a week.
- Also, in such patients loose stools are rarely present without the use of laxatives.

The myth of daily bowel evacuation being essential to healthy living has persisted through the centuries. It is thought that less than 10% of the population has a bowel evacuation daily (Edwards et al. 2003). This myth has resulted in laxative abuse becoming one of the commonest types of drug abuse in the Western world. The annual cost to the National Health Service (NHS) of prescribing medications to treat constipation is in the region of $45 million (DH 2005a). An individual's bowel habit is dictated by their diet, lifestyle and environment, and the notion of what is a 'normal' bowel habit varies considerably. Studies have revealed that in the USA and UK 95–99% of people pass at least three stools per week (Ehrenpreis, 1995) and normal bowel movement has been defined as ranging between three times a day and three times a week (Nazarko 1996). Given that there is such a wide normal range it is important to establish the patient's usual bowel habit and the changes that may have occurred.

Assessment

It is of vital importance that nurses adopt a proactive preventative approach to the assessment and management of constipation. Kyle et al. (2005a) have recently developed the Eton Scale, a constipation risk assessment tool. Whilst testing of the tool's sensitivity and reliability is still being carried out, it highlights the key risk factors that should be considered and provides advice and suggested actions according to the individual's level of risk. There are a variety of factors that may affect normal bowel functioning which should be considered within an assessment, including:

- Nutritional intake/recent changes in diet.
- Fluid intake.
- Mobility, e.g. lack of exercise.
- Medication, e.g. analgesics, antacids, iron supplements, tricyclic antidepressants.

331

Pain

Psychological

Ignoring urge to defecate
Emotional disturbances
Unfavourable lavatory
   conditions, e.g. bedpans,
   commodes

Psychiatric

Dementia
Depression
Chronic psychoses
Anorexia nervosa

Endocrine/metabolic

Dehydration
Hypothyroidism
Hypercalcaemia
Lead poisoning
Acute porphyria

Diet and laxatives

Inadequate bulk
Illicit use of laxatives
Inadequate fluid intake

Drug-induced

Opiates
Antidepressants
Diuretics
Aluminium antacids
Codeine
Hypotensives
Anticholinergics
Iron supplements
Overuse of laxatives

Exercise immobility

Temporary, e.g. hospitalization
Permanent, e.g.
paraplegia, hemiplegia

Obstruction

Tumours
Hirschsprung's disease
Chagas' disease
Megacolon
Sigmoid volvulus
Faecal impaction

Muscular deficiencies

Dysmotility
Hypomotility
Idiopathic slow bowel
Pregnancy
Ageing process
Slow transit syndrome

Neurological deficiencies

Paraplegia
Multiple sclerosis

Constipation

Infrequent or difficult and/or
   painful passage of small
   hard stools

Figure 15.2   Classification of constipation: combined sources.

332

- Lack of privacy, e.g. having to use shared toilet facilities, commodes or bedpans.
- Medical condition, including disease process or symptoms, e.g. cancer, vomiting.
- Radiological investigations of the bowel involving the use of barium.
- Change in patient's normal routine/lifestyle/home circumstances.
- Change in psychological status, e.g. depression.

(Fallon & O'Neill, 1997; Maestri-Banks 1998; Christer *et al.* 2003; Edwards *et al.* 2003; Thompson *et al.* 2003; Kyle *et al.* 2005a.)

In addition to the identification of these risk/contributing factors, it is important to take a careful history of a patient's bowel habits, taking particular note of the following:

1 Any changes in the patient's usual bowel activity. How long have these changes been present and have they occurred before?
2 Frequency of bowel action.
3 Volume, consistency and colour of the stool. Stools can be graded using a scale such as the Bristol Stool Form Chart (see Figure 15.1) where constipation would be classified as types 1 or 2 (Longstreth *et al.* 2006).
4 Presence of mucus, blood, undigested food or offensive odour.
5 Presence of pain or discomfort on defecation.
6 Use of oral or rectal medication to stimulate defecation and its effectiveness.

A digital rectal examination can also be performed, providing the nurse has received suitable training or instruction, to assess the contents of the rectum and to identify conditions which may cause discomfort such as haemorrhoids or anal fissures (Winney 1998; Hinrichs & Huseboe 2001; Peate 2003; RCN 2006).

Management

The effective treatment of constipation relies on the cause being identified by thorough assessment, as described above. Constipation can be categorized as primary, secondary or iatrogenic (Perdue 2005). Factors that lead to the development of primary constipation are extrinsic or lifestyle-related and include:

- An inadequate diet (low fibre).
- Poor fluid intake.
- A lifestyle change.
- Ignoring the urge to defecate.

Constipation that is attributed to an intrinsic, disease process or conditions such as anal fissures, colonic tumours or hypercalcaemia is classified as secondary constipation, whereas iatrogenic constipation generally results from treatment or medication (Perdue 2005). Constipation of unknown cause must be investigated in order to ensure that appropriate treatment is instigated (Taylor 1997; Teahon 1999).

Dietary manipulations may help to resolve mild constipation, although it is much more likely to help prevent constipation from recurring. Increasing dietary fibre increases stool bulk, which in turn improves peristalsis and stool transit time. This results in a softer stool being delivered to the rectum (Norton 1996b). The Government's strategy on food and health (DH 2005b) aims to increase the UK average daily fibre intake from the current 13.8 g to 18.0 g (this recommended amount is based on the Englyst method [DH 1998; British Nutrition Foundation 2004]). There are two types of fibre: insoluble is contained in foods such as wholegrain bread, brown rice, fruit and vegetables and soluble is contained in foods such as oats, pulses, beans and lentils. It is recommended that fibre should be taken from a variety of both soluble and insoluble foods and eaten at times spread throughout the day (Teahon 1999; Edwards *et al.* 2003; British Nutrition Foundation 2004; Food Standards Agency 2006). Care should be taken to increase dietary fibre intake gradually as bloating and abdominal discomfort can result from a sudden increase, particularly in the older person and those with slow-transit constipation (Cummings 1994; Norton 1996a; Bush 2000; Edwards *et al.* 2003). Other sources of dietary laxatives can be encouraged with care, for example prunes contain diphenylisatin and onions contain indigestible sugars (Norton 1996a).

Dietary changes need to be taken in combination with other lifestyle changes. Daily fluid intake should be between 2.0 and 2.5 litres (Taylor 1997; Teahon 1999; Day 2001). Fruit juices such as orange and prune juice can help stimulate bowel activity (Winney 1998) and coffee has been shown to stimulate colonic motor and bowel activity (Brown *et al.* 1990; Addison 1999a). The motor response takes place within minutes of drinking coffee and can last for up to 90 minutes (Addison 2000a). There is a need for further studies to examine the role of dietary manipulations in the management of constipation, particularly the function of dietary fibre and fluid intake (Addison 2000b).

Patients should be advised not to ignore the urge to defecate and to allow sufficient time for defecation (Norton 1996a). It is important that the correct posture for defecation is adopted; crouching or a 'crouch like' posture is considered anatomically correct (Taylor 1997) and the use of a foot stool by the toilet may enable patients to adopt a better defecation posture (Norton 1996a; Taylor 1997; Edwards *et al.* 2003). The use of the bedpan should always be avoided if possible as the poor posture adopted while using a bedpan has been shown to cause extreme straining during defecation (Taylor 1997). Patients should be supported with pillows to enable them to achieve an upright position if the use of a bedpan is unavoidable.

Where possible patients should be encouraged to increase their level of exercise; physical activity has been found to have a positive effect on peristalsis, particularly after eating (Thompson *et al.* 2003). Therapies such as homeopathy and reflexology can also be utilized (Emly *et al.* 1997; Rankin-Box 2000; Edwards *et al.* 2003). However, overall laxatives are the most commonly used treatment for constipation

Table 15.1 Types of laxative.

Type of laxative	Example	Brand names and sources
Bulk producers	Dietary fibre Mucilaginous polysaccharides Methylcellulose	Bran, wholemeal bread, Fybogel (ispaghula), Normacol (sterculia)
Stool softeners	Synthetic surface active agents, liquid paraffin	Agarol, Dioctyl, Petrolager, Milpar
Osmotic agents	Sodium, potassium and magnesium salts	Magnesium sulphate, milk of magnesia, lactulose
Stimulant laxatives	Sodium picosulphate, glycerin	Senna, Senokot, bisacodyl, Dulcolax, co-danthrusate, Picolax, glycerol

(Table 15.1). In general they should be used as a short-term measure to help relieve an episode of constipation as long-term use can perpetuate constipation and a dependence on laxatives can develop (Butler 1998).

Laxatives

Laxatives can be defined simply as substances that cause evacuation of the bowel by a mild action (Mosby 2006). A laxative with a mild or gentle effect is also known as an aperient and one with a strong effect is referred to as a cathartic or a purgative. Purgatives should be used only in exceptional circumstances, i.e. where all other interventions have failed, or when they are prescribed for a specific purpose. The aim of laxative treatment is to achieve comfortable rather than frequent defecation and, wherever possible, the most natural means of bowel evacuation should be employed with preference given to use of oral laxatives where appropriate (Fallon & O'Neill 1997; Perdue 2005). The many different types of laxatives available may be grouped into four types according to the action they have (see Table 15.1).

Bulking agents

Bulking agents are usually the first line of laxative treatment and work by retaining water and promoting microbial growth in the colon, increasing faecal mass and stimulating peristalsis (Peate 2003). Ispaghula husk (Isogel, Regulan) and sterculia (Normacol) both trap water in the intestine by the formation of a highly viscous gel which softens faeces, increases weight and reduces transit time (Butler 1998). These agents need plenty of fluid in order to work (2–3 litres per day), so their appropriateness should be questioned for those with advanced cancer, or for the older patient (Maestri-Banks 1998; Hinrichs & Huseboe 2001; Perdue 2005). They also take a few days to exert their effect (Maestri-Banks 1998) and so are not suitable to relieve acute constipation. Also, they are contraindicated in some patients, including those who have bowel obstruction, faecal impaction, acute abdominal pain, reduced muscle tone, or those who have had recent bowel surgery. Increasing the bulk may worsen impaction, lead to increased colonic faecal loading or even intestinal obstruction (Norton 1996a), and in some cases may increase the risk of faecal incontinence. Other potentially harmful effects include malabsorption of minerals, calcium,

iron and fat-soluble vitamins, and reduced bioavailability of some drugs (Taylor 1997). Another problem initially is that bulk laxatives tend to distend the abdomen, often making the individual feel full and uncomfortable. Sometimes this leads to temporary anorexia (Taylor 1997).

Stool softeners

Stool softening preparations, such as docusate sodium and glycerol (glycerin) suppositories act by lowering the surface tension of faeces which allows water to penetrate and soften the stool (Hinrichs & Huseboe 2001; Peate 2003). They may also have a weak stimulatory effect (Barrett 1992), but drugs of this type are often given in combination with a chemical stimulant (Shepherd 2000). Softening agents usually take 1–3 days to work (Day 2001).

Liquid paraffin acts as a lubricant as well as a stool softener by coating the faeces and allowing easier passage. However, its use should be avoided as there are a number of problems associated with this preparation. The use of liquid paraffin interferes with the absorption of fat-soluble vitamins and can also cause skin irritation, changes to the bowel mucosa and accidental inhalation of droplets of liquid paraffin may result in lipoid pneumonia (Maestri-Banks 1998; Peate 2003; BNF 2007).

Osmotic agents

These may be divided into two subgroups: lactulose and magnesium preparations. Lactulose is a synthetic disaccharide which exerts an osmotic effect in the small bowel. Distension of the small bowel induces propulsion which in turn reduces transit time. Colonic bacteria metabolize lactulose into a short chain organic salt which is then absorbed; therefore the osmotic effect does not continue throughout the colon (Barrett 1992). This process of metabolism also produces gas which in turn stimulates colonic movements and increases bacterial growth. This results in increased stool weight and thus colonic transit time is shortened (Spiller 1994). However, bowel action may still take up to 3 days to occur following administration (Shepherd 2000) and flatulence, cramps and abdominal discomfort are associated with high dosages. Magnesium preparations also exert an osmotic effect on the gut and additionally they stimulate the release of cholecystokinin. This encourages intestinal motility and fluid secretion (Nathan 1996). They have a rapid effect, working within 2–6 hours, so fluid intake is important with these preparations as patients may experience diarrhoea and dehydration (Hinrichs & Huseboe 2001). These preparations should be avoided in patients with renal or hepatic impairment (Taylor 1997).

Stimulant laxatives

Laxatives including bisacodyl, danthron and senna stimulate the nerve plexi in the gut wall increasing peristalsis and promoting the secretion of water and electrolytes in the small and large bowel (Maestri-Banks 1998; Shepherd 2000; Peate 2003). Abdominal cramping may be increased if the stool is hard and a stool softener may be used in combination with this group of drugs (Taylor 1997; ABPI 1999). Long-term use of these laxatives should be avoided, except for patients on long-term opiates, as they may lead to impaired bowel function such as atonic non-functioning (cathartic) colon (Taylor 1997; ABPI 1999; Hinrichs & Huseboe 2001).

Preparations containing danthron are restricted to certain groups of patients, i.e. the elderly, the terminally ill and some cardiac patients, as some studies on rodents have indicated a potential carcinogenic risk (Taylor 1997; ABPI 1999; Shepherd 2000). Danthron preparations should not be used for incontinent patients, especially those with limited mobility, as prolonged skin contact will colour the skin pink or red and superficial sloughing of the discoloured skin will occur (Taylor 1997; ABPI 1999).

Enemas

Definition

An enema is the administration of a substance in liquid form into the rectum, either to aid bowel evacuation or to administer medication (Higgins 2006). Administration requires skill and knowledge from the practitioner and adherence to the Nursing and Midwifery Council (NMC) (2008a) *Standards for Medicines Management*.

Indications

Enemas may be prescribed for the following reasons:

- To clean the lower bowel before surgery; X-ray examination of the bowel using contrast medium or before endoscopy examination.
- To treat severe constipation when other methods have failed.
- To introduce medication into the system.
- To soothe and treat irritated bowel mucosa.
- To decrease body temperature (due to contact with the proximal vascular system).
- To stop local haemorrhage.
- To reduce hyperkalaemia (calcium resonium).
- To reduce portal systemic encephalopathy (phosphate enema).

Contraindications

Enemas are contraindicated under the following circumstances:

- In paralytic ileus.
- In colonic obstruction.
- Where the administration of tap water or soap and water enemas may cause circulatory overload, water intoxication, mucosal damage and necrosis, hyperkalaemia and cardiac arrhythmias.
- Where the administration of large amounts of fluid high into the colon may cause perforation and haemorrhage.
- Following gastrointestinal or gynaecological surgery, where suture lines may be ruptured (unless medical consent has been given).
- Frailty.
- Proctitis.
- The use of micro-enemas and hypertonic saline enemas in patients with inflammatory or ulcerative conditions of the large colon.
- Recent radiotherapy to the lower pelvis unless medical consent has been given (Davies 2004).

Reference material

Types of enemas

Evacuant enemas

An evacuant enema is a solution introduced into the rectum or lower colon with the intention of it being expelled, along with faecal matter and flatus, within a few minutes. The osmotic activity increases the water content of the stool so that rectal distension follows and induces defecation by stimulating rectal motility (Barrett 1992; Roe 1994).

The following solutions are often used:

- Phosphate enemas with standard or long rectal tubes in single-dose disposable packs. Although these are often used for bowel clearance before X-ray examination and surgery, there is little evidence to support their use due to the associated risks and contraindications. Davies (2004) and Bowers (2006) highlight the risk of phosphate absorption resulting from pooling of the enema due to lack of evacuation and also the risk of rectal injury caused by the enema tip. Studies have found that if evacuation does not occur, patients may suffer from hypovolaemic shock, renal failure and oliguria. When using this type of enema it is vital that good fluid intake is encouraged and maintained.
- Dioctyl sodium sulphosuccinate 0.1%, sorbitol 25% in single-dose disposable packs, are used to soften impacted faeces.
- Sodium citrate 450 mg, sodium alkylsulphoacetate 45 mg, sorbic acid 5 mg in single-dose disposable packs.

335

Retention enemas

A retention enema is a solution introduced into the rectum or lower colon with the intention of being retained for a specified period of time. Two types of retention enema are in common use:

- Arachis oil (may be obtained in a single-dose disposable pack). This needs to be used cautiously as it is contra-indicated in patients with peanut allergies (Day 2001).
- Prednisolone.

Enemas containing arachis oil enhance the lubricating process, as well as softening impacted faeces (Butler 1998). These work by penetrating faeces, increasing the bulk and softness of stools. They work most effectively when warmed to body temperature and retained for as long as possible (Clarke 1988).

All types of enemas need to be prescribed and checked against the prescription before administration. It is essential that the implications and procedure are fully explained to the patient, so as to relieve anxiety and embarrassment.

Procedure guidelines   Enema administration

Equipment

1 Disposable incontinence pad.
2 Disposable gloves.
3 Topical swabs.
4 Lubricating jelly.
5 Rectal tube and funnel (if not using a commercially prepared pack).
6 Solution required or commercially prepared enema.

Procedure

Action	Rationale
1 Explain and discuss the procedure with the patient.	To ensure that the patient understands the procedure and gives his/her valid consent (NMC 2006: C; NMC 2008b: C).
2 Ensure privacy.	To avoid unnecessary embarrassment to the patient (P).
3 Allow patient to empty bladder first if necessary.	A full bladder may cause discomfort during the procedure (Higgins 2006: E).
4 Ensure that a bedpan, commode or toilet is readily available.	In case the patient feels the need to expel the enema before the procedure is completed (P).
5 Warm the enema to room temperature by immersing in a jug of hot water.	Heat is an effective stimulant of the nerve plexi in the intestinal mucosa. An enema at room temperature or just above will not damage the intestinal mucosa. The temperature of the environment, the rate of fluid administration and the length of the tubing will all have an effect on the temperature of the fluid in the rectum (E).
6 Assist the patient to lie on the left side, with knees well flexed, the upper higher than the lower one, and with the buttocks near the edge of the bed.	This allows ease of passage into the rectum by following the natural anatomy of the colon. In this position gravity will aid the flow of the solution into the colon. Flexing the knees ensures a more comfortable passage of the enema nozzle or rectal tube (Higgins 2006: E).
7 Place a disposable incontinence pad beneath the patient's hips and buttocks.	To reduce potential infection caused by soiled linen. To avoid embarrassing the patient if the fluid is ejected prematurely following administration (P).
8 Wash hands with bactericidal soap and water or bactericidal alcohol handrub, and put on disposable gloves.	To minimize the risk of cross-infection (DH 2005c: C).

9 Place some lubricating jelly on a topical swab and lubricate the nozzle of the enema or the rectal tube.

This prevents trauma to the anal and rectal mucosa which reduces surface friction (Higgins 2006: E).

10 Expel excessive air from enema and introduce the nozzle or tube slowly into the anal canal while separating the buttocks. (A small amount of air may be introduced if bowel evacuation is desired.)

The introduction of air into the colon causes distension of its walls, resulting in unnecessary discomfort to the patient. The slow introduction of the lubricated tube will minimize spasm of the intestinal wall (evacuation will be more effectively induced due to the increased peristalsis) (C).

11 Slowly introduce the tube or nozzle to a depth of 10.0–12.5 cm.

This will bypass the anal canal (2.5–4.0 cm in length) and ensure that the tube or nozzle is in the rectum (C).

12 If a retention enema is used, introduce the fluid slowly and leave the patient in bed with the foot of the bed elevated by 45° for as long as prescribed.

To avoid increasing peristalsis. The slower the rate at which the fluid is introduced the less pressure is exerted on the intestinal wall. Elevating the foot of the bed aids in retention of the enema by the force of gravity (C).

13 If an evacuant enema is used, introduce the fluid slowly by rolling the pack from the bottom to the top to prevent backflow, until the pack is empty or the solution is completely finished.

The faster the rate of flow of the fluid the greater the pressure on the rectal walls. Distension and irritation of the bowel wall will produce strong peristalsis which is sufficient to empty the lower bowel (Higgins 2006: E).

14 If using a funnel and rectal tube, adjust the height of the funnel according to the rate of flow desired.

The forces of gravity will cause the solution to flow from the funnel into the rectum. The greater the elevation of the funnel, the faster the flow of fluid (E).

15 Clamp the tubing before all the fluid has run in.

To avoid air entering the rectum and causing further discomfort (E).

16 Slowly withdraw the tube or nozzle.

To avoid reflex emptying of the rectum (E).

17 Dry the patient's perineal area with a gauze swab.

To promote patient comfort and avoid excoriation (P).

18 Ask the patient to retain the enema for 10–15 minutes before evacuating the bowel.

To enhance the evacuant effect (C).

19 Ensure that the patient has access to the nurse call system, is near to the bedpan, commode or toilet, and has adequate toilet paper.

To enhance patient comfort and safety. To minimize the patient's embarrassment (P).

20 Remove and dispose of equipment.

To minimize risk of cross-infection (DH 2005c: C).

21 Wash hands.

To minimize risk of cross-infection (DH 2005c: C)

22 Record in the appropriate documents that the enema has been given, its effects on the patient and its results (colour, consistency, content and amount of faeces produced, using the Bristol Stool Form Chart [see Figure 15.1]).

To monitor the patient's bowel function (Gill 1999: C).

23 Observe patient for any adverse reactions (Peate 2003).

To monitor the patient for complications (Peate 2003: C).

Problem solving: Enema administration

Problem	Cause	Suggested action
Unable to insert the nozzle of enema pack or rectal tube into the anal canal.	Tube not adequately lubricated. Patient in an incorrect position. Patient apprehensive and embarrassed about the situation. Patient unable to relax anal sphincter.	Apply more lubricating jelly. Ask the patient to draw knees up further towards the chest. Ensure adequate privacy and give frequent explanations to the patient about the procedure. Ask the patient to take deep breaths and 'bear down' as if defecating (E).
Unable to advance the tube or nozzle into the anal canal.	Spasm of the canal walls.	Wait until spasm has passed before inserting the tube or nozzle more slowly, thus minimizing spasm. Ask patient to take slow deep breaths to help to relax (E).
Unable to advance the tube or nozzle into the rectum.	Blockage by faeces. Blockage by tumour.	Withdraw tubing slightly and allow a little solution to flow and then insert the tube further. If resistance is still met, stop the procedure and inform a doctor (E).
Patient complains of cramping or the desire to evacuate the enema before the end of the procedure.	Distension and irritation of the intestinal wall produce strong peristalsis sufficient to empty the lower bowel.	Stop instilling the enema fluid and wait with the patient until the discomfort has subsided (E).
Patient unable to open bowels after an evacuant enema.	Reduced neuromuscular response in the bowel wall.	Inform the doctor that the enema was unsuccessful and reassure the patient (E).

Suppositories

Definition

A suppository is a medicated solid formulation that melts at body temperature when inserted into the rectum (Moppett & Parker 1999).

Indications

The use of suppositories is indicated under the following circumstances:

- To empty the bowel prior to certain types of surgery and investigations.
- To empty the bowel to relieve acute constipation or when other treatments for constipation have failed.
- To empty the bowel before endoscopic examination.
- To introduce medication into the system.
- To soothe and treat haemorrhoids or anal pruritus.

Contraindications

The use of suppositories is contraindicated when one or more of the following pertain:

- Chronic constipation, which would require repetitive use.

- Paralytic ileus.
- Colonic obstruction.
- Malignancy of the perianal region.
- Low platelet count.
- Following gastrointestinal or gynaecological operations, unless on the specific instructions of the doctor.

Reference material

Administration of suppositories

The use of suppositories dates back to about 460 BC. Hippocrates recommended the use of cylindrical suppositories of honey smeared with ox gall (Hurst 1970). The torpedo-shaped suppositories commonly used today came into being in 1893, when it was recommended that they were inserted apex (pointed end) first (Moppett 2000).

This practice has been questioned by Abd-el-Maeboud *et al.* (1991) who suggest that suppositories should be inserted blunt end first. This advice is based on anorectal physiology; if a suppository is inserted apex first the circular base distends the anus and the lower edge of the anal sphincter fails to close tightly. The normal squeezing motion (reverse vermicular contraction) of the anal sphincter therefore fails to drive the suppository into the rectum. These factors can lead to anal irritation and expulsion of the suppository (Moppett 2000). The study by Abd-el-Maeboud et al. (1991) remains the only research evidence supporting this practice. Whilst their work demonstrated that patients found insertion and retention of suppositories much easier and more comfortable using the base-first method, the isolated nature of this research means that manufacturers' instructions continue to recommend apex end first. Therefore this area of practice remains somewhat unclear: the Abd-el-Maeboud et al. (1991) study, coupled with the anatomical and physiological rationale would imply that blunt end first is preferential.

There are several different types of suppository available. Retention suppositories are designed to deliver drug therapy, e.g. analgesia, antibiotic, non-steroidal anti-inflammatory drug (NSAID). Those designed to stimulate bowel evacuation include glycerine, bisacodyl and sodium bicarbonate. Lubricant suppositories, e.g. glycerine, should be inserted directly into the faeces and allowed to dissolve. They have a mild irritant action on the rectum and also act as faecal softeners (BNF 2007). However, stimulant types, such as bisacodyl, must come into contact with the mucous membrane of the rectum if they are to be effective as they release carbon dioxide causing rectal distension and thus evacuation.

Procedure guidelines   Suppository administration

Equipment

1 Disposable incontinence pad.
2 Disposable gloves.
3 Topical swabs or tissues.
4 Lubricating jelly.
5 Suppository(ies) as required (check prescription before administering a medicinal suppository, e.g. aminophylline).

Procedure

Action	Rationale
1 Explain and discuss the procedure with the patient. If you are administering a medicated suppository, it is best to do so after the patient has emptied his/her bowels.	To ensure that the patient understands the procedure and gives his/her valid consent (NMC 2006: C; NMC 2008b: C). To ensure that the active ingredients are not impeded from being absorbed by the rectal mucosa or that the suppository is not expelled before its active ingredients have been released (Moppett 2000: E).
2 Ensure privacy.	To avoid unnecessary embarrassment to the patient (P).
3 Ensure that a bedpan, commode or toilet is readily available.	In case of premature ejection of the suppositories or rapid bowel evacuation following their administration (P).
4 Assist the patient to lie on the left side, with the knees flexed, the upper higher than the lower one, with the buttocks near the edge of the bed.	This allows ease of passage of the suppository into the rectum by following the natural anatomy of the colon. Flexing the knees will reduce discomfort as the suppository is passed through the anal sphincter (Moppett 2000: E).
5 Place a disposable incontinence pad beneath the patient's hips and buttocks.	To avoid unnecessary soiling of linen, leading to potential infection and embarrassment to the patient if the suppositories are ejected prematurely or there is rapid bowel evacuation following their administration (E).
6 Wash hands with bactericidal soap and water or bactericidal alcohol handrub, and put on gloves.	To reduce the risk of cross-infection (DH 2005c: C).
7 Place some lubricating jelly on the topical swab and lubricate the blunt end of the suppository if it is being used to obtain systemic action. Separate the patient's buttocks and insert the suppository blunt end first, advancing it for about 2–4 cm. Repeat this procedure if a second suppository is to be inserted.	Lubricating reduces surface friction and thus eases insertion of the suppository and avoids anal mucosal trauma. Research has shown that the suppository is more readily retained if inserted blunt end first (Abd-el-Maeboud et al. 1991). (For further information, see Suppositories section, above.) The anal canal is approximately 2–4 cm long. Inserting the suppository beyond this ensures that it will be retained (Abd-el-Maeboud et al. 1991: R 2b).

339

Procedure guidelines *(cont.)*

8 Once suppository(ies) has been inserted, clean any excess lubricating jelly from the patient's perineal area.	To ensure the patient's comfort and avoid anal excoriation (Moppett 2000: E).
9 Ask the patient to retain the suppository(ies) for 20 minutes, or until he/she is no longer able to do so. If a medicated suppository is given, remind the patient that its aim is not to stimulate evacuation and to retain the suppository for at least 20 minutes or as long as possible.	This will allow the suppository to melt and release the active ingredients. Inform patient that there may be some discharge as the medication melts in the rectum (Henry 1999: E).
10 Remove and dispose of equipment. Wash hands.	To reduce risk of infection (DH 2005c: C).
11 Record that the suppository(ies) have been given, the effect on the patient and the result (amount, colour, consistency and content, using the Bristol Stool Chart [see Figure 15.1]) in the appropriate documents.	To monitor the patient's bowel function (Gill 1999: C).
12 Observe patient for any adverse reactions.	To monitor for any complictions (Peate 2003: E).

Digital rectal examination

A digital rectal examination (DRE) is an invasive procedure that can be carried out, as part of a nursing assessment, by a qualified nurse who has received suitable education and training (RCN 2006). The procedure involves the nurse inserting a lubricated gloved finger into the rectum. This examination should only be performed in the following circumstances (RCN 2006):

- To establish whether faecal matter is present in the rectum and if so, to assess the amount and consistency.
- To assess the need for rectal medication and to evaluate its efficacy in certain circumstances, e.g. in patients who have diminished anal/rectal sensation.
- For digital stimulation to trigger defecation by stimulating the recto-anal reflex (Weisner & Bell 2004; RCN 2006).
- To assess anal sphincter function and tone.
- To assess anal/rectal sensation.

This examination should not be a primary investigation for constipation but should only be performed after a full assessment. Discussion with medical staff should occur to confirm diagnosis and jointly plan appropriate interventions to treat the constipation (RCN 2006).

Before carrying out a DRE the perineal and perianal area should be checked for signs of rectal prolapse, haemorrhoids, anal skin tags or lesions, foreign bodies or infestations. The condition of the skin should be noted, as should the type and amount of any discharge or leakage. If any of these

abnormalities are seen, a DRE should not be carried out until advice is taken from a specialist nurse or medical practitioner (RCN 2006).

As nursing roles develop, clinical nurse specialists and nurse practitioners may be increasingly involved in areas of care that may involve undertaking DRE as part of a physical assessment or procedure. Such instances may include:

- The assessment of prostate size, consistency, mobility and anatomical limits.
- During procedures such as the placement of a rectal probe/sensor prior to urodynamic studies or the placement of catheters used in the treatment of constipation or anismus (RCN 2006).

Precautions

Special care should be used in performing DRE in patients when disease processes or treatments in particular affect the anus or the bowel mucosa. These conditions include (RCN 2006):

- Active inflammation of the bowel, e.g. ulcerative colitis.
- Recent radiotherapy to the pelvic area.
- Rectal/anal pain.
- Rectal surgery or trauma to the anal/rectal area.
- Obvious rectal bleeding.
- Spinal injury patients, because of autonomic dysreflexia.
- Patients with known allergies, e.g. latex.
- Patients with a history of abuse.

Procedure guidelines   Digital rectal examination

Equipment

1 Disposable incontinence pad.
2 Disposable gloves (check if patient allergic to latex).
3 Lubricating gel.
4 Tissues or topical swabs.

Procedure

Action	Rationale
1 Explain and discuss procedure with the patient.	To ensure that the patient understands the procedure and gives his/her valid consent (NMC 2006: C; NMC 2008a: C).
2 Ensure privacy.	To avoid unnecessary embarrassment to the patient.
3 Ensure that a bedpan, commode or toilet is readily available.	DRE can stimulate the need for bowel movement (Weisner & Bell 2004: E).
4 Assist the patient to lie in the left lateral position with knees flexed, the upper knee higher than the lower knee, with the buttocks towards the edge of the bed.	This allows ease of digital examination into the rectum by following the natural anatomy of the colon. Flexing the knees reduces discomfort as the examining finger passes the anal sphincter (Kyle *et al.* 2005b: C).
5 Place a disposable incontinence pad beneath the patient's hips and buttocks.	To reduce potential infection caused by soiled linen. To avoid embarrassing the patient if faecal staining occurs during or after the procedure (E).
6 Wash hands with bactericidal soap and water or bactericidal alcohol handrub and put on disposable gloves.	To minimize the risk of cross-infection (DH 2005c: C).
7 Place some lubricating gel on a swab and gloved index finger. Inform patient you are about to proceed.	To minimize discomfort as lubrication reduces friction and to ease insertion of the finger into the anus/rectum. Lubrication also helps minimize anal mucosal trauma (Kyle *et al.* 2005b: C). Assists with patient co-operation with the procedure (NMC 2008b: C).
8 Observe anal area prior to the insertion of the finger into the anus for evidence of skin soreness, excoriation, swelling, haemorrhoids, rectal prolapse and infestation. Proceed to insert finger into the anus/rectum.	May indicate incontinence or pruritus. Swelling may be indicative of possible mass or abscess. Abnormalities such as bleeding, discharge or prolapse should be reported to medical staff before any examination is undertaken (RCN 2006: C).
9 On insertion of finger assess anal sphincter control; resistance should be felt.	Digital insertion with resistance indicates good internal sphincter tone, poor resistance may indicate the opposite (Addison 1999b: E).
10 Digital examination may feel faecal matter within the rectum; note consistency of any faecal matter.	May establish loaded rectum and indicate constipation and the need for rectal medication (RCN 2006: C).
11 Clean anal area after the procedure.	To prevent irritation and soreness occurring. Preserves patient dignity and personal hygiene.

341

Procedure guidelines *(cont.)*

12 Remove gloves and dispose of equipment in appropriate clinical waste bin. Wash hands with bactericidal soap and water.	To minimize the risk of cross-infection (DH 2005c: C).
13 Assist patient into a comfortable position and offer toilet facilities as appropriate.	To promote comfort (P).
14 Document findings and report to medical team.	To ensure continuity of care and assist in nursing diagnosis so appropriate corrective action may be initiated (RCN 2006: C).

Manual evacuation

Manual evacuation of the rectum is an invasive procedure involving digital removal of faeces, which should only be performed when necessary, generally as a last resort, and after individual assessment (Rigby 2003; RCN 2006). Advances in oral, rectal and surgical treatments have reduced the need for manual evacuations to be performed; however, for certain groups of patients, such as those with spinal injuries, spina bifida or multiple sclerosis, this procedure may be the only suitable bowel-emptying technique forming a long-standing, integral part of their bowel routine (Kyle *et al.* 2005b).

Nurses who have received appropriate training may perform manual evacuation and, in addition, they should ensure that their employer has defined policies and procedure for undertaking this role (Withell 2000; RCN 2006). If appropriate, the patient and their personal carer may wish for the carer to maintain their established programme of bowel management (Harrison 2000).

Indications for assisted evacuation of bowels (manual evacuation or digital stimulation) include (RCN 2006):

- Faecal impaction/loading.
- Incomplete defecation.
- Inability to defecate.
- If other bowel-emptying techniques have failed.
- Neurogenic bowel dysfunction.
- Patients with spinal injury.

Patients are at risk of rectal trauma if these procedures are not performed with care or knowledge. The nurse should be aware of any conditions that may contraindicate performance of these procedures (see Precautions in the Digital rectal examination section, above). Manual evacuation of faeces can be distressing, it may be painful and it can be a dangerous procedure. In particular, stimulation of the vagus nerve in the rectal wall can slow the patient's heart, in addition to the risk of bowel perforation and bleeding (Powell & Rigby 2000; Kyle *et al.* 2005b).

If this procedure is used as an acute intervention the patient's pulse rate should be recorded before and during the process. Patients with a spinal injury should also have their blood pressure measured before, during and at the end of the procedure. A baseline blood pressure measurement should be available for comparison (RCN 2006). Every time the procedure is performed the consistency of the stool should be noted before continuing. If the stool is hard and dry, lubricant suppositories should be inserted and left for 30 minutes before commencing. If the stool is too soft to remove effectively, consider delaying the procedure for 24 hours to allow further water reabsorption to occur. During the procedure the nurse should observe the patient for signs of:

- Distress, pain or discomfort.
- Bleeding.
- Autonomic dysreflexia: hypertension, bradycardia, headache, flushing above the level of the spinal injury, sweating, pallor below the level of spinal injury, nasal congestion (Harrison 2000).
- Collapse (RCN 2006).

Autonomic dysreflexia is unique to patients with spinal cord injury. It is an abnormal response from the autonomic nervous system to a painful (noxious) stimulus perceived below the level of spinal cord injury (Harrison 2000; Powell & Rigby 2000). Distended bowel caused by constipation or impaction can lead to autonomic dysreflexia and therefore it is important that an effective programme of bowel management is established and followed (Harrison 2000).

Managing bowel problems such as constipation and prolonged bowel evacuation in patients following spinal cord injury requires a multimodality approach. This includes dietary fibre, digital stimulation, enemas, suppositories, stool softeners and abdominal massage (Amir *et al.* 1998; Addison & White 2002). Digital stimulation is a method of initiating the defecation reflex by dilating the anus, by either a finger or an anal dilator (Weisner & Bell 2004) but is only useful if the rectum is full.

Procedure guidelines   Manual evacuation of faeces

Equipment

1 Disposable incontinence pad.
2 Disposable gloves (check if patient is allergic to latex).
3 Lubricating gel.
4 Tissues or topical swabs.

5 Receiver and/or yellow bag.
6 Specimen pot (if required).
7 Bedpan or commode (if appropriate).

Procedure

Action	Rationale
1 Explain and discuss procedure with the patient.	To ensure that the patient understands the procedure and gives his/her valid consent (NMC 2006: C; NMC 2008b: C).
2 Ensure privacy.	To avoid unnecessary embarrassment to the patient.
3 Take the patient's pulse. In spinal injury patients a blood pressure reading should also be taken (RCN 2006: C).	Provides a baseline measurement. Stimulation of the vagus nerve in the rectal wall can lead to a reduction in pulse rate (Powell & Rigby 2000: E). In spinal cord injury, stimulus below the level of injury may result in symptoms of autonomic dysreflexia including hypertension (Kyle *et al.* 2005b: C).
4 Assist the patient to lie in the left lateral position with knees flexed, the upper knee higher than the lower knee, with the buttocks towards the edge of the bed.	This allows ease of digital insertion into the rectum, by following the natural anatomy of the colon. Flexing the knees reduces discomfort as the finger passes the anal sphincter (Kyle *et al.* 2005b: C).
5 Place a disposable incontinence pad beneath the patient's hips and buttocks.	To reduce potential infection caused by soiled linen. To avoid embarrassing the patient if faecal staining occurs during or after the procedure.
6 Wash hands with bactericidal soap and water or bactericidal alcohol handrub and put on disposable gloves.	To minimize the risk of cross-infection (DH 2005c: C).
7 Place some lubricating gel on a swab and gloved index finger.	To minimize discomfort as lubrication reduces friction and to ease insertion of the finger into the anus/rectum. Lubrication also helps minimize anal mucosal trauma (Kyle *et al.* 2005b: C).
8 Inform patient you are about to proceed.	Assists with patient co-operation with the procedure (NMC 2008b: C).
9 Observe anal area prior to the insertion of the finger into the anus for evidence of skin soreness, excoriation, swelling, haemorrhoids or rectal prolapse.	May indicate incontinence or pruritus. Swelling may be indicative of possible mass or abscess. Abnormalities such as bleeding, discharge or prolapse should be reported to medical staff before any examination is undertaken (RCN 2006: C).
10 Proceed to insert finger into the anus/rectum. Proceed with caution in those patients with spinal cord injury.	The majority of spinal cord injury patients will not experience any pain (Kyle *et al.* 2005b: C).

343

Procedure guidelines *(cont.)*

11 If the stool is type 1 (see Bristol Stool Form Chart: Figure 15.1), remove one lump at a time until no more faecal matter is felt.	To relieve patient's discomfort (Kyle *et al.* 2005b: C).
12 If a solid faecal mass is felt, split it and remove small pieces with hooked finger until no more faecal matter is felt.	To relieve patient discomfort (Kyle *et al.* 2005b: C).
13 Check the patient's pulse at least once during the procedure. In spinal injury patients a blood pressure reading should also be taken at least once during the procedure or at any sign of distress (RCN 2006: C). If the patient is displaying a reduction in pulse rate or change in rhythm, or in the spinal cord injury patient, a raised blood pressure, STOP the procedure and if possible sit the patient up and administer appropriate medications as prescribed (Kyle *et al.* 2005b: C).	Stimulation of the vagus nerve in the rectal wall can lead to a reduction in pulse rate (Powell & Rigby 2000). In spinal cord injury, stimulus below the level of injury may result in symptoms of autonomic dysreflexia including hypertension (Kyle *et al.* 2005b: C).
14 If faecal mass is too hard to break up, or more than 4 cm across, stop the procedure and discuss with the multidisciplinary team.	To avoid unnecessary pain and damage to the anal sphincter the patient may require the procedure to be carried out under anaesthetic (Kyle *et al.* 2005b: C).
15 As faeces is removed it should be placed in an appropriate receiver.	To assist in appropriate disposal and reduce contamination or cross-infection risk.
16 Encourage patients who receive this procedure on a regular basis to have a period of rest or, if appropriate, to assist using the Valsalva manoeuvre.	Patient and nurse education is required to use this technique safely and so further guidance should be sought before introducing this manoeuvre as it may lead to complications such as haemorrhoids (Kyle *et al.* 2005b: C).
17 Wash and dry the patient's anal region and buttocks.	To ensure patient feels comfortable and clean (P).
18 Remove gloves and dispose of equipment in appropriate clinical waste bin. Wash hands with bactericidal soap and water.	To minimize the risk of cross-infection (DH 2005d: C).
19 Assist patient into a comfortable position.	To promote comfort (P).
20 Document findings and report to medical team.	To ensure continuity of care and assist in nursing diagnosis so appropriate actions may continue (RCN 2006: C).

344

Rectal irrigation

Definition

Rectal irrigation, or lavage, involves washing out the rectum using large volumes of non-sterile fluid. It is a method of achieving rectal emptying without the need for medication, by distending the rectal wall progressively, which stimulates the stretch receptors to initiate the urge to defecate. The patient then empties the fluid and any stool in the rectum (Gardiner 2004).

Historically, this invasive method was used routinely to cleanse the bowel prior to investigations such as a barium enema, to improve the image obtained, or before major abdominal surgery, to reduce the risk of infection and improve healing. Whilst there may still be an occasional need to carry out such a procedure intraoperatively (e.g. if preoperative bowel cleansing methods have been unsuccessful), the method of choice for bowel preparation prior to such invasive procedures is now oral bowel-cleansing solutions, such as Citramag and Picolax (BNF 2007). While such oral preparations are much easier to administer, they are not without complications, as patients are at risk of dehydration, fatigue, electrolyte imbalance and excoriation of perianal area. It is therefore recommended that patients are well hydrated during administration of such preparations and that manufacturer's guidelines are followed.

Rectal irrigation may therefore be performed in the following circumstances:

- For bowel cleansing, only in exceptional circumstances, where oral preparations have proved to be ineffective.
- As a method for symptomatic relief of functional bowel disorders.

Contraindications

Rectal irrigation is contraindicated in patients who have a history of any one of the following:

- Severe or prolapsed haemorrhoids.
- Anal fissure.
- Inflammatory bowel disease.
- Large tumour in the rectum or sigmoid colon.
- Post-radiation proctitis.
- Internal fistulae.
- Pelvic radiotherapy.
- Recent bowel surgery.
- Congestive cardiac failure.
- Impaired renal function.

In the first eight of the contraindications listed above, the reason for employing caution is because of the damage that could be inflicted by the mechanical aspects of rectal irrigation. When the bowel has already been traumatized there is a greater potential risk of causing irritation or, in extreme cases, perforation while inserting the catheter and running large volumes of fluid in and out of the rectum.

With the last two contraindications the potential risk lies with the possibility of large amounts of fluid and/or electrolytes becoming absorbed through the bowel. (Generally speaking, with the amounts and type of fluid used and the relatively short time that it stays in the bowel, this should not present a major problem.)

Reference material

Choice of fluid

Rectal lavage/irrigation requires a simple, non-sterile solution that can be used with relative safety in large volumes to wash out the residual faecal matter. The solution which fulfils these criteria ideally is tap water. Rectal lavage using tap water is not without risk as large volumes of this hypotonic solution can upset the patient's electrolyte balance. Water is drawn by osmosis into the intestinal cells and water intoxication can result, with symptoms of weakness, sweating, pallor, vomiting, coughing and dizziness. However, this is a relatively rare complication and generally tap water is very well tolerated.

The other advantages of tap water are as follows:

- It is cheap and easily available.
- It can be easily warmed to the correct temperature (37°C).
- It is non-irritant to the bowel mucosa.
- It does not cause excessive peristalsis with resulting cramps and colic.

References and further reading

Abd-el-Maeboud, K.H., El-Naggar, T. & El-Hawi, E.M.M. (1991) Rectal suppositories: commonsense mode of insertion. *Lancet*, **338**, 798–800.

ABPI (1999) *ABPI Compendium of Data Sheets and Summaries of Product Characteristics 1999–2000*. Datapharm Publications, Leatherhead, Surrey.

Addison, R. (1999a) Practical procedures for nurses No. 37.1. Fluid intake and continence care. *Nurs Times*, **95**(49).

Addison, R. (1999b) Practical procedures for nurses No. 33.1. Digital rectal examination 1. *Nurs Times*, **95**(40).

Addison, R. (2000a) Fluid intake: how coffee and caffeine affect continence. *Nurs Times*, **96**(40) (Suppl), 7–8.

Addison, R. (2000b) Fluids, fibre and constipation. *Nurs Times*, **96**(31) (Suppl), 11–12.

Addison, R. & White, M. (2002) Spinal injury and bowel management. *Nurs Times*, **98**(4), 61.

Amir, I. *et al.* (1998) Bowel care for the individual with spinal cord injury: comparison of four approaches. *Spinal Med*, **21**(1), 21–4.

Barrett, J.A. (1992) Faecal incontinence. In: *Clinial Nursing Practice. The Promotion and Management of Continence* (ed. B. Roe). Prentice Hall, New York, pp. 196–219.

Basch, A. (1987) Symptom distress changes in elimination. *Semin Oncol Nurs*, **3**(4), 287–92.

Bell, S. (2004) Investigations and management of chronic diarrhoea in adults. In: *Bowel Continence Nursing* (eds C. Norton & S. Chelvanayagam). Beaconsfield Publishers, Beaconsfield, Bucks, pp. 92–102.

BNF (2007) *British National Formulary Volume 54; 1.6.3: Faecal Softeners*. BMJ Publishing and the Royal Pharmaceutical Society of Great Britain, London.

Bowers, B. (2006) Evaluating the evidence for administering phosphate enemas. *Br J Nurs*, **15**(7), 378–81.

British Nutrition Foundation (2004) Dietary fibre. www.nutrition. org.uk. Accessed 9/8/06.

Brown, S.R., Cann, P.A. & Read, N. (1990) Effect of coffee on distal colon function. *Gut*, **31**, 450–53.

Bush, S. (2000) Fluids, fibre and constipation. *Nurs Times*, **96**(31) (Suppl), 11–12.

Butler, M. (1998) Laxatives and rectal preparations. *Nurs Times*, **94**(3), 56–8.

Cadd, A. *et al.* (2000) Assessment and documentation of bowel care management in palliative care: incorporating patient preferences into the care regimen. *J Clin Nurs*, **9**, 228–35.

Campbell, T. & Lunn, D. (1999) Colorectal cancer. Part 3 patient care. *Prof Nurse*, **15**(2), 117–21.

Chelvanayagam, S. & Norton, C. (2004) Nursing assessment of adults with faecal incontinence. In: *Bowel Continence Nursing* (eds C. Norton & S. Chelvanayagam). Beaconsfield Publishers, Beaconfield, Bucks, pp. 45–62.

Christer, R., Robinson, L. & Bird, C. (2003) Constipation: causes and cures. *Nurs Times*, **99**(25), 26–7.

Clarke, B. (1988) Making sense of enemas. *Nurs Times*, **84**(30), 40–4.

Cook, T. *et al.* (1999) The conservative management of constipation in adults. *J Assoc Chart Physiother Women's Health*, **85**, 24–8.

Crawshaw, A. (2004) How to establish a rectal irrigation service. *Gastrointest Nurs*, **2**(2), 29–31.

Cummings, J.H. (1994) Non-starch polysaccharides (dietary fibre) including bulk laxatives in constipation. In: *Constipation* (eds M.A. Kamm & J.E. Lennard-Jones). Wrightson Biomedical, Petersfield, Hampshire, pp. 307–314.

Davies, C. (2004) The use of phosphate enemas in the treatment of constipation: use of laxatives. *Br J Nurs*, **12**(19), 1130–6.

Day, A. (2001) The nurse's role in managing constipation. *Nurs Stand* **16**(8), 41–4.

DH (1998) *Nutritional Aspects of the Development of Cancer. Report on Health and Social Subjects 48.* HMSO, London.

DH (2005a) *Prescription Cost Analysis: England 2004.* HMSO, London.

DH (2005b) *Choosing a Better Diet: A Food and Health Action Plan.* HMSO, London.

DH (2005c) *Saving Lives: Delivery Programme to Reduce Healthcare Associated Infection including MRSA.* Department of Health, London.

DH (2005d) *Hazardous waste (England) regulations.* Department of Health, London.

Edwards, C., Dolman, M. & Horton, N. (2003) Down, down and away! An overview of adult constipation and faecal incontinence. In: *Promoting Continence. A Clinical and Research Resource* (eds K. Getliffe & E. Dolman), 2nd edn. Bailliere Tindall, London, pp. 185–226.

Ehrenpreis, E.D. (1995) Definitions and epidemiology of constipation. In: *Constipation. Etiology, Evaluation and Management* (eds S.D. Wexner & D.C.C. Bartolo). Butterworth Heinemann, Philadelphia, pp. 3–8.

Emly, M., Wilson, L. & Darby, J. (1997) Abdominal massage for adults with learning disabilities. *Nurs Times*, **97**(30) (Suppl), 61–2.

Fallon, M. & O'Neill, B. (1997) Clinical review. ABC of palliative care: constipation and diarrhoea. *BMJ*, **315**, 1293–6.

Food Standards Agency (2006) Starchy foods – fibre. www.eatwell. gov.uk/healthydiet/nutritionessentials/starchfoods/. Accessed 9/8/06.

Gardiner, A. (2004) Rectal irrigation for relief of functional bowel disorders. *Nurs Stand*, **19**(9), 39–42.

Gill, D. (1999) Practical procedures for nurses. Stool specimen assessment, Part 1: Assessment. *Nurs Times*, **96**, 26.

Harrison, P. (2000) *HDU/ICU Managing Spinal Injury: Critical Care.* Spinal Injuries Association, London.

Henry, C. (1999) The advantages of using suppositories. *Nurs Times*, **95**(17), 50–51.

Higgins, D. (2006) How to administer an enema. *Nurs Times*, **102**(20), 24–5.

Hinrichs, M. & Huseboe, J. (2001) Research-based protocol: management of constipation. *J Gerontol Nurs*, **27**(2), 17–28.

Hogan, C.M. (1998) The nurse's role in diarrhoea management. *Oncol Nurs Forum*, **25**(5), 879–86.

Hurst, A. (1970) *Selected Writings of Sir Arthur Hurst (1989–1944).* Ballantyne, Spottiswode.

King, D. (2002) Determining the cause of diarrhoea. *Nurs Times*, **98**(23) (Suppl), 47–8.

Kornblau, A. *et al.* (2000) Management of cancer treatment-related diarrhea: issues and therapeutic strategies. *J Pain Symptom Manage*, **19**(2), 118–29.

Kyle, G. *et al.* (2005a) The Eton Scale: a tool for risk assessment for constipation. *Nurs Times*, **101**(18 Suppl), 50–1.

Kyle, G., Oliver, H. & Prynn, P. (2005b) *The Procedure for the Digital Removal of Faeces. Guidelines 2005.* Norgine, Uxbridge, UK.

Le Lievre, S. (2002) An overview of skin care and faecal incontinence. *Nurs Times,*, **98**(4) (Suppl), 58–9.

Longstreth, G.F. *et al.* (2006) Functional bowel disorders. *Gastroenterology*, **130**, 1480–91.

Maestri-Banks, A. (1998) An overview of constipation – causes and treatment. *Int J Palliat Nurs*, **4**(6), 271–5.

Moppett, S. (2000) Which way is up for a suppository? *Nurs Times*, **96**(19 Suppl), 12–13.

Moppett, S. & Parker, M. (1999) Insertion of a suppository. (Practical procedures for nurses, part 29). *Nurs Times*, **95**(23), supplement.

Mosby (2006) *Mosby's Dictionary of Medicine, Nursing and Health Professions.* Mosby Elsevier, St. Louis, MO.

NANDA-I (2007) *Nursing Diagnoses: Definitions and Classifications 2007–2008.* North American Nursing Diagnosis Association International, Philadelphia.

Nathan, A. (1996) Laxatives. *Pharm J*, **257**, 52–5.

Nazarko, L. (1996) Preventing constipation in older people. *Prof Nurse*, **11**(12), 816–18.

Nicol, M., Barin, C., Bedford-Turner, S. (2000) *Essential Nursing Skills.* Mosby International, Edinburgh.

NMC (2006) *A–Z Advice Sheet Consent.* www.nmc.org.

NMC (2008a) *Standards for Medicines Management.* Nursing and Midwifery Council, London.

NMC (2008b) *The Code: Standards of Conduct, Performance and Ethics for Nurses and Midwives.* Nursing and Midwifery Council, London.

Norton, C. (1996a) The causes and nursing management of constipation. *Br J Nurs*, **5**(20), 1252–8.

Norton, C. (1996b) *Nursing for Continence*, 2nd edn. Beaconsfield Publishers, Beaconsfield, Bucks.

Norton, C. (2006) Constipation in older patients: effects on quality of life. *Br J Nurs*, **15**(4), 188–92.

Peate, I. (2003) Nursing role in the management of constipation: use of laxatives. *Br J Nurs*, **12**(19), 1130–6.

Perdue, C. (2005) Managing constipation in advanced cancer care. *Nurs Times*, **101**(21), 36–40.

Petticrew, W. (1997) Treatment of constipation in older people. *Nurs Times*, **93**(48), 55–6.

Powell, M. & Rigby, D. (2000) Management of bowel dysfunction: evacuation difficulties. *Nurs Stand*, **14**(47), 47–54.

Rankin-Box, D. (2000) An alternative approach to bowel disorders. *Nurs Times*, **96**(19 Suppl), 24–5.

RCN (2006) *Digital Rectal Examination and Manual Removal of Faeces: Guidance for Nurses.* Royal College of Nursing, London.

Rigby, D. (2003) Manual evacuation of faeces. *Nurs Times*, **99**(1) (Suppl), 48.

Roe, B. (1994) *Clinical Nursing Practice: The Promotion and Management of Continence.* Prentice Hall, New York.

Shepherd, M. (2000) Treating diarrhoea and constipation. *Nurs Times*, **96**(6) (Suppl), 15–16.

Smith, S. (2001) Evidence-based management of constipation in the oncology patient. *Eur J Oncol Nurs*, **5**(1), 18–25.

Spiller, R.C. (1994) *Diarrhoea and Constipation.* Libra Pharmaceuticals, Petroc Press, Reading, Berks.

Taylor, C. (1997) Constipation and diarrhoea. In: *Nursing in Gastroenterology* (eds L. Bruce & T.M.D. Finlay). Churchill Livingstone, Oxford, pp. 27–54.

Teahon, E. (1999) Constipation. In: *Essential Coloproctology for Nurses* (eds T. Porret & N. Daniel). Whurr, London, pp. 206–221.

Thibodeau, G. & Patton, K.T. (2007) *Anatomy and Physiology*, 6th edn. Mosby Elsevier, St Louis, MO.

Thompson, M.J. *et al.* (2003) Management of constipation. *Nurs Stand*, 18(14–16), 41–2.

Tortora, G.A. & Derrickson, B. (2008) *Principles of Anatomy and Physiology*, 12th edn. John Wiley & Sons, New York.

Walsh, M. (1997) *Watson's Clinical Nursing and Related Sciences*, 5th edn. Bailliere Tindall, London.

Weisner, P. & Bell, S. (2004) Bowel dysfunction: assessment and management in the neurological patient. In: *Bowel Continence Nursing* (eds C. Norton & S. Chelvanayagam). Beaconsfield Publishers, Beaconsfield, Bucks.

Weller, B. (1989) *Encyclopaedic Dictionary of Nursing and Health Care*. Bailliere Tindall, Eastbourne.

Winney, J. (1998) Constipation. *Nurs Stand*, 13(11), 49–56.

Withell, B. (2000) A protocol for treating acute constipation in the community setting. *Br J Community Nurs*, 5(3), 110–17.

Wood, S. (1996) Nutrition and the short bowel syndrome. In: *Stoma Care Nursing: A Patient-Centred Approach* (ed. C. Myres). Edward Arnold, London, pp. 79–89.

Chapter 16

Elimination: continent urinary diversions

349 Reference material
355 **Teaching intermittent self-catheterization of a continent urinary diversion stoma**
355 Reference material
355 *Procedure guidelines:* Continent urinary diversion stoma: self-catheterization
357 *Procedure guidelines:* Continent urinary diversion stoma drainage tubes: flushing
358 *Problem solving:* Continent urinary diversion stoma
359 Useful addresses
359 References and further reading

Definition

A urinary diversion is a surgically created system for removing urine from the body when either the bladder or urethra is either non-existent or no longer viable. There are two main types: a urostomy (see Chapter 17) and continent urinary diversions. Continent urinary diversions differ in that a system is created to collect and store urine before it is removed from the body.

Indications for formation of a continent urinary diversion

A continent urinary diversion may be formed to:

- Store and expel urine from the body if the lower urinary tract is defective or absent.
- Offer patients a choice of urinary diversion.
- Improve or maintain the individual's body image, psychological and social well-being by removing the necessity of wearing external devices, e.g. urostomy pouch or incontinence pads (Randles 1990; Leaver 2002).

Continent urinary diversions are increasingly available as an alternative to the conventional ileal conduit (see Chapter 17).

Reference material

Principles of a continent urinary diversion

A continent urinary diversion is surgically constructed to replace a defective or non-existent lower urinary tract. It consists of three components:

- A reservoir to store urine.
- A continence mechanism to retain urine in the reservoir.
- A channel or tunnel to let the urine out (Leaver 1996, 2002).

The reservoir can be the bladder itself, an augmented bladder, or made completely of ileum, colon or a combination of the two. The continence mechanism may be constructed during the operation using the same tissues used to construct the reservoir or an existing valve or sphincter may be utilized (Leaver 2002). Five types of continence system have been identified:

- The flutter valve, created by the intussusception of a segment of bowel, usually ileum, e.g. Kock nipple.
- The flap valve, created by tunnelling a narrow tube between the muscle and mucosal layers of the reservoir, e.g. Mitrofanoff valve.
- The ileocaecal valve.
- The urethral sphincter.
- The anal sphincter.

The channel or tunnel component can be formed by utilizing other tube/tunnel-like structures such as the appendix, ureter or fallopian tube. Alternatively, a segment of ileum or colon can be used (Leaver 1996).

There are a number of different types of continent diversions performed today; these include those with catheterizable stomas, rectal bladders and orthotopic neobladders. The aim of these diversions is to mimic, as far as possible, the normal bladder function. The goals are:

- To create a pouch with the ability to hold an adequate volume of urine at low pressure.
- To preserve and protect the upper tract by preventing reflux.
- To prevent or minimize the absorption of urine, thus avoiding metabolic disturbances.
- To control urine voiding by sphincter control or self-catheterization (Razor 1993; Leaver 1996).

Indications for surgical formation of a continent urinary diversion

The indications for the formation of a continent urinary diversion and an ileal conduit are similar (see Chapter 17). These include:

- Congenital abnormalities, e.g. bladder extrophy.
- Pelvic cancers, e.g. bladder, cervical.
- Neuropathic bladder: a condition where the nerve impulses do not reach the bladder as the result of an underlying disease or injury, e.g. myelomeningocoele.
- Trauma.
- Incontinence.
- Interstitial cystitis.
- Radiation fibrosis.
- Irreparable fistula.
- An existing diversion, e.g. ileal conduit (Woodhouse 1991; Leaver 1994; Dixon et al. 2001).

Continent urinary diversions with catheterizable stomas

There are a number of different types of continent urinary diversions with catheterizable stomas performed today (Box 16.1). These procedures differ in construction, using different structures to form the reservoir and tunnel and different techniques to create the continence mechanism. The

---

Box 16.1 Types of continent urinary diversion with catheterizable stomas

1 Mitrofanoff pouch
2 Kock pouch
3 Benchekroun pouch
4 Mainz pouch
5 Indiana pouch
6 Le bag
7 Miami

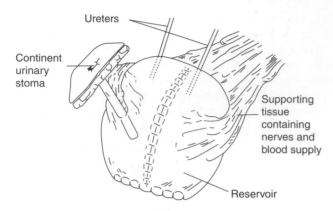

Figure 16.1   Continent urinary diversion.

outcomes for patients and the nursing care involved are essentially similar in most cases. The most commonly performed procedure of this type in the UK is arguably the Mitrofanoff (Leaver 1996) (Figure 16.1).

This type of diversion involves the patient having two admissions into hospital. The first is to form the continent urinary diversion. Following the operation, a sterile fine-bore tube is left in the continent urinary stoma to keep it patent and allow the urine to drain into a catheter bag. After recovering from the operation, patients are taught how to take care of the tubing, leg bags and night drainage systems. Patients are then discharged home to be readmitted 6 weeks after the operation to be taught self-catheterization. This admission lasts between 24 and 48 hours. During this time, patients are taught self-catheterization and encouraged to practise the technique. Nursing staff are available to detect and rectify any problems. This allows patients time to gain confidence in self-catheterization before they return home.

In a continent urinary diversion the urine drains into the urinary reservoir or bladder through the ureters. Patients can self-catheterize into the continent urinary stoma every 4–6 hours to empty the urine reservoir (Figure 16.2). This is achieved by the patient adjusting any restrictive clothing and inserting a special tube into the continent urinary stoma, pointing the other end into the toilet. When urine has drained out the tube is removed, washed with water and replaced in its container (usually a plastic bag, spectacle case or cosmetic bag).

Before each discharge, patients are given verbal and written advice (Horn 1990), and can contact the hospital 24 hours a day.

The Mitrofanoff pouch was devised in the late 1970s/early 1980s by Paul Mitrofanoff (1980) in France. Initially, it was devised for patients with bladder neck obstruction or incompetence. The bladder was preserved and the appendix was used as the continent urinary stoma. One end of the appendix is buried in a submuscular tunnel in the bladder, forming an obstructing flap valve. The other end is brought to the surface of the abdominal wall to form a continent stoma. As the bladder fills with urine more pressure is put on the valve, causing it to become even more obstructed. A

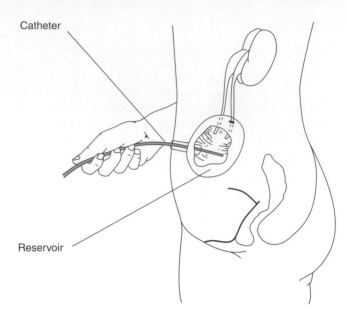

Figure 16.2   Self-catheterization into the continent urinary stoma.

catheter is passed into the stoma along the channel, through the valve and into the bladder when the patient wants to empty their bladder (Leaver 1996).

Mitrofanoff's principle can be adapted to suit each individual patient taking into account their underlying condition and the available body tissues (Duckett & Snyder 1985; Leaver 1994). For example, patients with urinary incontinence may have their bladder preserved and urethra oversewn; a tunnel may then be fashioned using their appendix. Other patients with bladder cancer following cystectomy may have a new 'bladder' constructed from a segment of ileum and, in the absence of an appendix, another segment of ileum may be used to construct the tunnel.

Rectal bladder

A type of rectal bladder, the ureterosigmoidostomy, is the oldest known continent urinary diversion (Fisch & Hohenfellner 1992). In this procedure the ureters are directly implanted into the sigmoid colon, where the urine and faeces mix and are evacuated via the anus. This procedure became unpopular because of continual complications of infection, electrolyte imbalance, loss of renal function, renal calculi, the high rate of incontinence, especially at night, and its poor reputation for morbidity and mortality (Leaver 2002).

Improved understanding of how some complications arise, development in surgical techniques and greater ability to manage electrolyte imbalances have all led to renewed interest in the rectal bladder (Woodhouse & Christofides 1998; Leaver 2002; D'Elia et al. 2004). High-pressure peristalsis in the bowel has been shown to cause the reflux of faeces into the kidneys (Coffey 1911). If the bowel is detubularized this high pressure can be overcome. To detubularize the rectum,

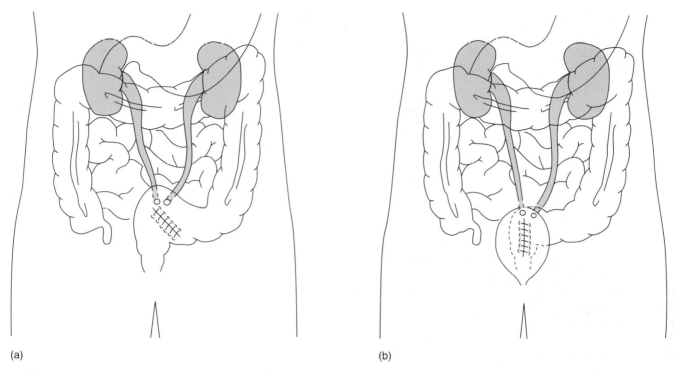

Figure 16.3 (a) Mainz Sigma II or rectal bladder. (b) Orthotopic neobladder.

it is opened longitudinally and closed transversely to form a pouch, which remains continuous with the sigmoid colon (Figure 16.3a). The ureters are implanted in a serous lined extramural tunnel into this pouch. This pouch is called the sigma-rectum pouch or Mainz Sigma II (D'Elia *et al.* 2004). This modified pouch acts as a reservoir for urine until the patient is ready to void. The patient can, in time, distinguish between needing to void urine and opening their bowels even though both events take place via the rectum (Leaver 2002).

Orthotopic neobladder

In this type of diversion the neobladder is constructed by using the ileum or a section of the large colon and then it is anastomosed to the urethra to allow voiding in the conventional way (Pontieri-Lewis & Vates 1993) (Figure 16.3b). Therefore this procedure is only suitable for patients where the urethra is left intact. As a radical cystectomy for female patients typically involves a total urethrectomy, the orthotopic neobladder is more commonly indicated for men (Pontieri-Lewis & Vates 1993) although this procedure is beginning to be offered more frequently to women (Stein *et al.* 1996; Dixon *et al.* 2001).

The ability to pass urine naturally via the urethra and maintaining a normal anatomical appearance are the major advantages of this procedure. Patients need to use the Valsalva manoeuvre to empty the neobladder and some may find this difficult and may need to perform clean intermittent self-catheterization to achieve this. Pelvic floor exercises should be taught preoperatively and performed on a daily basis. Continence can be problematic; most patients (83–96%) achieve continence during the day (Arai *et al.* 1999; Crivellaro *et al.* 2004), but may experience night-time incontinence.

Patient selection

Patients are selected carefully for this type of surgery. They must be physically and psychologically able to undergo a lengthy major procedure and to comply with regular lifelong follow-up (Matthews & Courts 2001; Varol & Studer 2004; Perimenis & Koliopanou 2004). Patients need to have an adequate renal function and a healthy bowel, particularly if the bladder is to be replaced with a reservoir constructed from a segment of bowel (Leaver 1996; Matthews & Courts 2001; Varol & Studer 2004; Perimenis & Koliopanou 2004).

It is important to ensure that patients undergoing the formation of a rectal bladder have good anal sphincter control. This can be established with the porridge test. A sloppy porridge enema is instilled into the patient's rectum and the patient needs to hold 300–350 ml for 3–4 hours without leaking. It is important that during this time the patient performs as many usual activities as possible, i.e. walking, climbing stairs, etc. The porridge imitates the contents of the rectum postoperatively (Leaver 2002).

Patients undergoing catheterizable continent diversions must be motivated towards self-catheterization and be dextrous enough to manipulate a nelaton catheter. Patients undergoing orthotopic reconstruction must be continent and have an intact pelvic floor.

351

Specific preoperative preparation

Patients undergo the usual preparation for anaesthesia (see Chapter 30). Only the specific preparation is discussed here although physical preparation may vary according to the individual surgeon's preference.

Preoperative counselling

Once patients have been selected as suitable candidates, psychological preparation should begin as soon as possible. Boore (1978), Hayward (1978), Roberts (1991), Matthews and Courts (2001) and Varol and Studer (2004) have illustrated the importance of preoperative information and explanation in reducing postoperative physical and psychological stress to the individual following the formation of a stoma (ileal conduit or colostomy). Their research is also applicable to patients receiving continent urinary diversion stomas. This is discussed in Chapter 17.

Patients should receive a full explanation of their operation and the type or types of urinary diversion which are available for them, including all the advantages and disadvantages of each diversion. The amount and type of information should be adapted to the individual's requirements. The stoma nurse or specialist is valuable in the preoperative stage (Varol & Studer 2004). Many patients focus on the lack of appliance wearing in these types of surgery and are blind to the complications of the surgery itself (Leaver 2002). They should be shown pictures of the appropriate urinary diversion and encouraged to familiarize themselves with the equipment: pouches, wafers, catheterization tubes and bladder syringes. Patients undergoing orthotopic reconstruction should be taught pelvic floor exercises (Kegel exercises) and voiding strategies (Matthews & Courts 2001; Varol & Studer 2003; Perimenis & Koliopanou 2004). All patients should be aware that they will need to work towards increasing the capacity of their new reservoirs in the weeks and months post surgery.

Useful aids

Useful aids for teaching patients and helping them to understand the procedure and the implications it may have on their lives include the following:

- Information booklets.
- Videos.
- Diagrams/photographs.
- Samples of equipment.
- Contact with others who have the same type(s) of continent diversion, ideally of a similar age, sex and background to the patient.

Bowel preparation

Patients need to commence a regimen to evacuate all faecal matter from the intestine 2–3 days before surgery. Patients may be admitted for all of this preparation or they may start the regimen at home. The regimen used depends on the surgeon's preference. It is necessary to clear the bowel to:

- Prevent hard faecal masses from impacting proximal to an anastomosis.
- Prevent faeces spilling from the cut ends of the bowel during the operation.
- Reduce bacterial contamination when the bowel is opened (Alexander-Williams 1980).

Patients undergoing this procedure are at risk of developing hypovolaemia and electrolyte imbalance. Therefore, it is important that the fluid loss is replaced orally or intravenously (Skinner & Lieskovsky 1988; Woodhouse 1989).

Sexual dysfunction

Following the formation of a continent urinary diversion possible sexual impairment for both men and women may occur. This is the same as for other stoma patients and is discussed in Chapter 17.

Pre- and postoperative counselling is given to each patient and partner. Each person's potential sexual dysfunction should be discussed and treated individually.

Specific postoperative care

Reconstruction of the lower urinary tract is a lengthy procedure and has a significant complication rate (Leaver 1996; Varol & Studer 2004). Patients may require a short stay in a high dependency unit after surgery. Postoperative care is similar to that for major abdominal surgery, with special attention to urinary output and the patency of the many drainage tubes (Figure 16.4). Extensive experience has shown that to allow healing of the continent diversion and to reduce the risk of urine leaking into the peritoneum it is important that the reservoir is kept empty for 4–8 weeks depending on the type of diversion that has been performed.

The drains and catheters used are unique to the type of diversion and determined by the surgeon's preference. They can often be overwhelming for the patient so each tube should be explained and an anticipated date for its removal should be given to reduce anxiety (Dixon et al. 2001). There will often be one or two fine-bore catheters placed in the ureters (ureteric stents) which will initially drain most of the urine. One or two catheters may be present in the new reservoir to keep it drained; these can become blocked with debris or mucus (which is produced by the bowel) so they should be flushed with sterile 0.9% sodium chloride four times daily starting from day 1 postoperatively. Initially only 20 ml should be used, but this should increase to 50–100 ml on day 4 postoperatively. If the catheters do block there is a high risk that the new reservoir will become distended and anastamotic leaks may occur (Perimenis & Koliopanou 2004). After the first week the emphasis of the procedure changes from maintaining the patency of the catheters to

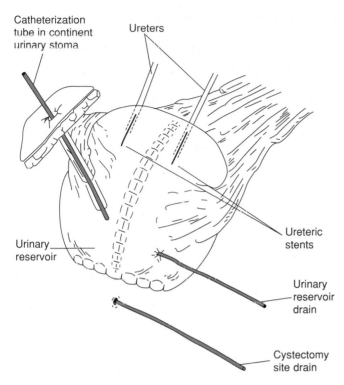

Catheterization tube in continent urinary stoma

Ureters

Ureteric stents

Urinary reservoir

Urinary reservoir drain

Cystectomy site drain

Figure 16.4 Siting of wound drains to reduce risk of haematoma and abscess formation.

removal of *all* mucus present in the reservoir. Fifty-millilitres of sterile 0.9% sodium chloride should be gently instilled and drawn back. The solution and mucus removed is then discarded, and the process is repeated until no further mucus is obtained. This may require a total of 400–600 ml of sterile 0.9% sodium chloride. It is important that no force is used to draw back the flush solution; if resistance is felt the bladder syringe should be removed and the solution allowed to drain. It is important that mucus is removed as it is implicated in the formation of stones (Hensle *et al.* 2004).

Patients who have undergone a catheterizable continent diversion or orthotopic neobladder should be taught how to perform this procedure, as it will have to be maintained following their discharge home.

The ureteric stents, if present, are gently pulled on day 7 after the operation to remove them. If resistance is felt the stents should be left in and the procedure repeated on a daily basis, until the stents slide out. Generally the stents are totally removed by day 10. By this time wound drains, the nasogastric tube or gastrostomy tube and all intravenous catheters should also have been removed. After this time the patient may have a cystogram or 'pouchogram' performed to check that the reservoir is intact. If there are no leaks detected on this examination the pouch catheter is removed. Patients with a catheterizable continent diversion are left with one catheter, which is on free drainage. Patients with a neobladder may also be discharged home with a catheter in situ depending on the surgeon's preference. Patients with

catheters in situ are discharged home for 3–6 weeks with this catheter in place on free drainage and with instructions to carry out at least twice daily washouts. This is to ensure that the urine drains and the reservoirs are not stretched at any time. Some patients prefer to be discharged with both the stoma catheter and pouch catheter in place, although only one is usually on free drainage.

Patients with a rectal bladder will now start voiding via the anus. The new bladder will start to stretch and its volume capacity will increase. Voiding will eventually be every 2–4 hours, often emptying once at night (Leaver 2002).

Patient education before discharge

All patients who have undergone continent urinary diversion have similar discharge needs. They are taught how to recognize a urinary tract infection and advised to drink at least 2–3 litres of fluid daily to reduce the risk of this happening. All patients undergoing continent diversion are advised to wear a medical alert bracelet, so that if they are found unconscious at any time a doctor or nurse will be aware of the surgery that has been performed.

Patients with an orthotopic neobladder are advised to undertake pelvic floor muscle exercises (Kegel exercises) 4–6 times a day to promote continence (Razor 1993). They should also be seen by a specialist nurse to be taught voiding techniques and instructed regarding toileting regimens. These neobladders are generally constructed to hold a capacity of 500 ml but it will take time for the patient to build up to this capacity (Perimenis & Koliopanou 2004).

Patients who have a diversion with a catheterizable stoma are taught how to flush their catheters and wash out their reservoirs to prevent blockages and mucus build-up. These patients are then readmitted in 3–4 weeks to have their catheters removed and reservoirs activated and to be taught self-catheterization.

Patients should be seen by the nurse specialist before discharge and a request for community nurses to continue support at home should be made. An explanatory letter and the relevant literature are supplied. Patients are encouraged to seek advice from the ward staff at any time.

Second admission

Patients with catheterizable stomas are readmitted 6 weeks after the operation to expand the pouch and to be taught intermittent self-catheterization. The stoma catheter is clamped and patients are encouraged to drink fluids. This allows the pouch to fill up with urine and helps the patient establish what sensation is experienced as this happens. Patients have described this sensation as a feeling of fullness, bloated feeling, discomfort or an ache. However, some patients experience no sensations at all when the pouch is full and have to establish a voiding programme to avoid overfilling of the pouch. The stoma catheter is released after

2–3 hours, depending on how the patient tolerates the sensation and on the amount of fluid drunk. This process is repeated 1–2 times more, during the day, to continue expanding the pouch. Experience has shown that at this stage the average pouch capacity is 250–300 ml. The pouches are generally constructed to hold 500 ml and it may take several weeks to reach this target. Patients continue to expand their pouch at their own pace once they are discharged.

Once the pouch has been initially stretched, the catheter is removed and the catheterization procedure is explained and demonstrated (see the Teaching intermittent self-catheterization of a continent urinary diversion stoma section, below). Patients should be supervised during the catheterization process until they are competent and confident with the procedure. Generally, patients remain in hospital for 1–2 days.

Patients with a neobladder should be advised to expect some urinary incontinence in the first few days after the catheter is removed; it usually happens just before the next void. As the neobladder capacity expands continence will improve (Varol & Studer 2004). Patients should be taught voiding techniques and advised to continue performing pelvic floor (Kegel) exercises. They should also be given equipment and advised on how to manage their incontinence during the time whilst their bladder compliance improves.

Discharge advice

Once proficient with the new continent diversion patients are discharged home with a 2–4 week outpatient clinic appointment to see the surgeon and nurse specialist. Before patients are discharged they should be informed about the following:

- To empty pouch every 4–6 hours to prevent overdistension and to always empty pouch before participating in strenuous activities to minimize the pressure put on the pouch. If the pouch becomes too full there is a risk of trauma to, or rupture of, the pouch, leakage of urine via the tunnel or, because of increased pressure on the valve, it may make catheterization difficult or impossible (Busuttil-Leaver 2004).
- To ensure an undisturbed sleep by reducing the amount of fluid the patient drinks 3 hours before going to sleep. The patient should catheterize or void before going to sleep and on waking.
- To keep a catheter available at all times (in suit, car, handbag, at work and at home), in case the patient needs to empty the urine.
- A small amount of mucus may leak from the continent urinary stoma and a piece of gauze can be worn to protect clothing.

Patients should be informed that it could take time to become accustomed to and gain confidence in their new continent urinary diversion. They should be given contact details of appropriate nursing staff that may be called for advice and reassurance.

Long- and short-term problems

A number of complications have been identified; these may be short-term 'teething' problems while the pouch settles down and the patient becomes familiar with it. However, some patients require further surgery or treatment to rectify problems to ensure their pouch function is acceptable. The most common complications are:

- Infection.
- Stenosis of the stoma.
- Leakage via the stoma.
- Inability to empty pouch.
- Loss of tunnel.
- High-pressure bladder system.
- Stone formation. A number of factors have been implicated in this process: these include urinary stasis, increased mucus production from the intestinal segment and colonization with urea splitting bacteria.
- Metabolic acidosis.
- Renal damage.
- Pouch rupture.
- Incontinence.
- Skin irritation with Mainz II if anal sphincter leaks.
- Secondary malignancy following Mainz II due to the high risk posed by the mixture of urine and faeces in the bowel. Neoplasms usually are seen 20–30 years after surgery (Stewart 1986). Yearly endoscopic follow-up should be carried out from the 12th post-operative year in order to detect any tumours early (Wagstaff et al. 1991; McCahill et al. 1992; Woodhouse 1994; Woodhouse & Christofides 1998). As the formation of a continent urinary diversion is a relatively new surgical technique, the long-term complications (other than those listed above) are unknown. Therefore patients remain on long-term follow-up at those centres where these procedures are performed.

Psychological effects

Several surveys have been undertaken to compare ileal conduits with different types of continent urinary diversions in terms of social and sexual effects, and to assess the effect on the patient of converting an ileal conduit to a continent urinary diversion (Mansson et al. 1988, 1991; Oishi et al. 1993; McGuire et al. 2000). Each examined the effect of cystectomy and investigated issues such as depression, adjustment to the new skills required for self-catheterization or use of stoma appliances, and changes in social, sports and sexual activity. The evidence suggests that patients are able to learn the manual skills required of them, but that all experience some degree of depression and altered body image. Patients with ileal conduits reported a more negative body image and a higher incidence of depression compared with the other two groups. Patients with a primary continent urinary diversion also exhibited depression and altered body image. Patients whose ileal conduit was converted to a continent urinary diversion experienced less depression and fewer negative changes in body image. It is conjectured that this is because these patients perceive a definite improvement in their situation when the conversion is carried out (Mansson *et al.* 1988, 1991; Oishi *et al.* 1993; Sullivan *et al.* 1998; McGuire *et al.* 2000).

These studies did not investigate altered body image or psychological morbidity in patients whose ileal conduits or continent urinary diversions were performed for non-malignant disease. Kennedy *et al.* (1993), however, describe the experiences of four women who had successful pregnancies following continent urinary diversions for non-malignant disease.

The importance of the role of stoma therapists and nursing staff in providing information tailored for the individual and in teaching new skills is recognized by patients, and it is suggested that these functions play a part in adjustment to changes brought about by surgery (Boyd *et al.* 1987; Mansson *et al.* 1988, 1991; Oishi *et al.* 1993).

Teaching intermittent self-catheterization of a continent urinary diversion stoma

Definition

Intermittent self-catheterization is when patients insert a self-catheterization (nelaton type) catheter into the urinary reservoir via the continent urinary stoma using a clean technique (for further information see Chapter 18). It is performed to evacuate or instil fluids, after which the tube is removed.

Indications

Intermittent self-catheterization may be carried out for the following reasons:

- To empty the contents of the urinary reservoir every 4–6 hours. If the reservoir is left too long between emptying it can become overstretched and lose its elasticity.
- To allow irrigation of the urinary reservoir for the removal of mucus which may occlude the continent urinary stoma and potentially lead to stone formation.

Reference material

The following research has been gathered from urethral self-catheterization. However, the same principles would apply to a continent urinary stoma.

Intermittent self-catheterization is intended to make life easier and not more complicated. It is associated with a lower incidence of urinary tract infection than long-term indwelling catheters (Lapides 1971; Lapides *et al.* 1974; Diokno *et al.* 1983; Lindenhall *et al.* 1994).

Types of tubing used for intermittent self-catheterization

Catheters used for intermittent self-catheterization should be smooth-surfaced and flexible. The nelaton-type of catheter, which is made of soft plastic and has two drainage eyes at one end and a funnel at the other, is most commonly used for patients with continent diversions. The smallest size of catheter which will drain the reservoir at an acceptable speed should be used (Busuttil-Leaver 2004). If the continent stoma and tunnel has been constructed from a fine tube-like structure, such as a ureter or fallopian tube, a small gauge catheter (6–10 CH) may be needed. Fine-bore feeding tubes have been used in some instances (Horn 1990; see Chapter 18).

Teaching self-catheterization

Intermittent self-catheterization should be taught in a place that offers privacy, with a good clear light and a mirror (bathroom, toilet or at the patient's bedside) (Horn 1990). It is a clean and not a sterile procedure. Patients can learn self-catheterization with the aid of a mirror or by touch, and are observed and assisted by a nurse until they are proficient (see Procedure guidelines: Continent urinary diversion stoma: self-catheterization, below).

During the day patients are encouraged to drink 2–3 litres of fluid to reduce the risk of any urinary tract infection and to catheterize every 4–6 hours to prevent the reservoir becoming distended and losing its elasticity. However, patients can reduce their fluid intake during the evening so that they need catheterize only before they go to sleep and again when they get up in the morning.

Procedure guidelines   Continent urinary diversion stoma: self-catheterization

This procedure should always be performed aseptically in hospital. At home it is performed as a clean technique.

Equipment

1 Catheters for catheterization depending upon the size of the stoma.
2 Tissues.
3 Clean jug or bowl.
4 Low-linting gauze and non-allergenic skin protective tape to cover stoma if it oozes mucus.

Procedure guidelines *(cont.)*

Procedure

Action	Rationale
1 Explain and discuss the procedure with the patient.	To ensure that the patient understands the procedure and gives his/her valid consent (NMC 2006: C; NMC 2008: C).
2 Collect all equipment necessary for the procedure.	To ensure all the equipment required is easily available (E).
3 Take the equipment to the toilet, bathroom or screened bed area. Ensure there is a good light and a full-length mirror.	To ensure the patient's privacy. To ensure patient can see the stoma clearly (E).
4 The equipment should be arranged on a clean surface and within easy reach for the procedure.	To reduce the risk of contamination by surface bacteria. So that equipment is easily available (E).
5 The patient needs to remove any inhibiting clothing.	To ensure the patient can examine the stoma (E).
6 The patient should wash their hands with soap and water, then dry them.	To ensure the hands are clean (DH 2005a: C).
7 The patient should look at the stoma, if necessary with the aid of a hand or full-length mirror.	To look for mucus and swelling around the stoma (E).
8 The patient should wipe away any mucus with a tissue soaked in warm water and gently pat dry.	To ensure the opening of the stoma is clear and mucus does not block the catheter during insertion into stoma (E).
9 If a lubricated catheter is to be used follow manufacturers' guidelines. If it is not, lubricate tip of catheter with water-soluble lubricant.	To act as a lubricant to allow the catheter to enter the urinary reservoir without causing internal trauma (E).
10 Ensure the untipped end of the catheter is in a receiver, i.e. jug, bowl or toilet.	To ensure the urine goes into a bowl and not onto the patient (E).
11 The patient can either use a mirror to guide the tube into the opening of the stoma or feel the opening with two fingers slightly apart with the stoma between.	To act as a guide to pass the catheter into the continent urinary stoma (E).
12 Insert the catheter gently into the stoma following the pathway inside (usually towards the middle of the abdomen) until urine starts to flow, then insert tube a further 4–6 cm to reduce risk of contamination.	The direction of insertion and the diameter of catheter inserted depend on the type, size and shape of continent urinary stoma (E). To negotiate continence device (E).
13 When all the urine has stopped flowing advance the catheter to ensure the bladder is completely empty. Slowly remove the catheter using a rotating action. If urine starts flowing again wait until it stops before removing the catheter any further.	To ensure complete emptying of the urinary reservoir. The rotating action reduces the suction effect and pain due to friction (Leaver 1996: C). It may dislodge any debris or mucus blocking the tube and allow the urine to flow (Leaver 1996).

14 Remove the tube.
  Cover the end of the catheter with a finger just before it is removed from the tunnel. Hold the catheter over the recepticle before removing the finger.
	To trap urine in catheter and stop it leaking on to the patient (Colley 1998).
	  To allow complete drainage of the tube.

15	If single-use catheter is used dispose of catheter in yellow bin.	To ensure safe disposal (DH 2005b: C).
	If a reusable catheter used rinse tubing through with lukewarm tap water and dry with a tissue.	To rinse out any urine (Colley 1998).
	Replace the catheter in its plastic container.	To keep the catheter clean.
16	Cover the stoma with a non-adherent dressing and secure with skin-protective tape.	To prevent mucus staining the patient's clothing (E).
17	The patient should wash their hands with soap and water, and then dry them.	To remove any urine on the hands.
18	The patient can then dress, collect equipment and dispose of any soiled dressings.	To prevent cross-infection (DH 2005a: C).

Procedure guidelines   Continent urinary diversion stoma drainage tubes: flushing

This procedure should always be performed aseptically in hospital. At home it is performed as a clean technique.

Equipment

1 Syringe with appropriate tip to engage tube.
2 Sterile 0.9% sodium chloride or water sufficient to perform procedure 20–100 ml.
3 Gloves.
4 Antiseptic solution.

5 Sterile dressing pack.
6 Sterile field.
7 Sterile receiver.
8 New drainage bag.

Procedure

Action	Rationale
1 Explain and discuss the procedure with patient.	To ensure that the patient understands the procedure and gives his/her valid consent (NMC 2006: C; NMC 2008: C).
2 Screen the bed. Ensure that the patient is in a comfortable position allowing access to the drainage tube.	For the patient's privacy and to reduce the risk of cross-infection. Curtains are drawn at this stage so that dust and airborne organisms disturbed by the curtains do not settle on the sterile field (DH 2005a: C).
3 Perform the procedure using aseptic technique.	To minimize the risk of cross-infection (for further information on aseptic technique see Chapter 5).
4 Move trolley to the bedside, disturbing the curtains as little as possible.	To minimize airborne contamination. To commence preparation of equipment for procedure (DH 2005a: C).
5 Open the outer wrappings of the packs and put them on the top shelf of the trolley. Prepare fluid to carry out the flush by decanting it into a sterile receiver ready to be drawn into a syringe.	To minimize airborne contamination. To commence preparation of equipment for procedure (DH 2005a: C).
6 Prepare the sterile field.	To prepare the equipment for procedure (E).
7 Wash hands with bactericidal alcohol handrub.	To reduce risk of infection (DH 2001: C).
8 If possible, clamp drainage tube.	To prevent leakage, if possible, when the drainage tube is disconnected (E).

Procedure guidelines *(cont.)*

9	Place a sterile towel under the junction of the drainage tube and drainage bag and disconnect.	To create a sterile field and reduce the risk of cross-infection.
10	Clean hands with a bactericidal alcohol handrub and put on gloves.	To remove organisms from the surface of the gloves and so reduce the risk of introducing infection into the drainage tube (DH 2005a: C).
11	Clean around drainage tube entrance with sterile low-linting gauze and antiseptic solution.	To reduce the risk of introducing infection into the drainage tube (DH 2005a: C).
12	Draw up correct volume of irrigation fluid. Introduce catheter tip into drainage tube, release clamp if applied previously, and gently inject the sterile water into the drainage tube.	To flush the possible blockage from the tube (E).
13	Remove syringe. Allow drainage tube to drain into sterile receptacle.	To assess the presence of a blockage in the drainage tube (E).
14	Connect new drainage bag.	To prevent introduction of bacteria into the drainage tube via the original bag.
15	Measure fluid collected from drainage tube, subtracting the volume of fluid used to flush tube.	To accurately record drainage from tube. Observe for further blockages (E).
16	Make the patient comfortable, remove equipment, clean trolley and wash hands. Repeat steps 13 and 14 as often as necessary to remove debris.	To reduce the risk of cross-infection.

Problem solving: Continent urinary diversion stoma

Problem	Cause	Suggested action
Unable to flush drainage tube using moderate amount of force.	Severe blockage. Displaced tube.	Inform medical staff of situation, suggest investigation to determine the position of the tube.
No fluid drainage from tube after flushing.	Dehydration. Displaced tube. Reblocked tube.	Assess the patient's nutritional state: skin turgor, fluid balance chart, mucous membranes. Review patient with medical team. If good fluid intake has been established and the tube is in position, repeat process.
Cannot insert the catheter into the stoma.	Using too large a catheter. Unable to locate opening. Opening occluded, e.g. due to swelling.	Advise the patient to try a smaller sized catheter, and to use a magnifying mirror to find the opening. Advise the patient to rest for 10 minutes to let the stoma relax and then to insert catheter. A warm bath may help to dilate the opening. If still unable to catheterize, then patient should contact the hospital.

Problem	Cause	Suggested action
		Doctor may give subcutaneous injection of steroid to reduce swelling. A needle and syringe may be used to draw off a quantity of urine to take pressure off the valve and thus allow the catheter to be inserted. If the opening remains occluded, a suprapubic catheter may be inserted to allow the swelling to subside and drain the urine from the reservoir. The stoma may need to be dilated by a doctor.
Partial insertion only of catheter is possible.	Tubing kinked. Stricture in the stoma.	Remove tubing and try with fresh tubing of the same size. Or try with a size smaller tubing. If unable to catheterize, contact the hospital.
Patient has not catheterized for 4 hours and feels distended; is easily catheterized but no urine is passed.	Tubing not reaching the reservoir. Tubing kinked. Tube is double-backing on itself. Tube blocked with mucus.	Insert tubing further. Do not use force. If there is resistance then stop. Contact the hospital. Cough. The increased intra-abdominal pressure may dislodge the plug of mucus. While the tube is inserted, flush it with tap water. Remove tubing, examine for mucus and reinsert once it is clear. Flush the urinary reservoir.
Stoma leaks urine between catheterizations.	Reservoir not emptied regularly. Plug blocking tubing, preventing complete drainage. Stoma failure.	Mucus catheterize every 3–4 hours. If the patient has drunk large amounts, or alcohol (a diuretic), or is taking diuretic medication, it may be necessary to catheterize more frequently. Flush reservoir at least twice a day. If still leaking inform the hospital. Surgical fashioning of the stoma may be necessary.
Staining of blood during catheterization.	Trauma due to rough technique. Using wrong type of self-catheterization catheter.	Lubricate the tube well with water and insert gently into stoma. Use lubricating jelly. If blood staining continues or increases in amount then inform the hospital. Use low-friction self-catheterization catheter.

359

Useful addresses

Medic-Alert Foundation, 1 Bridge Wharf, 156 Caledonian Road, London N1 9UU (Tel. 020 7833 3034), website: www.medicalert.org.uk.

Royal Marsden Hospital (The), Fulham Road, London SW3 6JJ (Tel. 0207 3528171).

Sexual Dysfunction Association, Windmill Place Business Centre, 2–4 Windmill Lane, Southall, Middlesex UB2 4NJ (Tel. 0870 7743571), www.sexualdysfunctionassociation.com.

Urostomy Association (The), Central Office, Foxglove Avenue, Uttoxeter, Staffs ST14 8UN (Tel. 08452412159), website: wwwuagbi.org.

References and further reading

Alexander-Williams, J. (1980) Cleaning the gut for colonic surgery. *World Med*, 15(10), 18–19.

Arai, Y. *et al.* (1999) Voiding function of orthotopic neobladder in women. *Urology*, 54(1), 44–9.

Boore, J.R.P. (1978) *A Prescription for Recovery: The Effects of Pre-operative Preparation of Surgical Patients on Post-operative Stress, Recovery and Infection*. Royal College of Nursing, London.

Boyd, S.D. *et al.* (1987) Quality of life survey of urinary diversion patients: comparison of ileal conduits versus continent urinary reservoirs. *J Urol*, 138, 1386–9.

Busuttil-Leaver, R.B. (2004) Reconstructive surgery for the promotion of continence. In: *Urological Nursing* (eds S. Fillingham & J. Douglas), 3rd edn. Bailliere Tindall, London, pp. 135–59.

Coffey, R.C. (1911) Physiologic implantation of the severed ureter or common bile duct into the intestine. *JAMA*, 5, 97–103.

Colley, W. (1998) Intermittent self catheterisation (2). *Nurs Times*, 94(23), 33a-33b.

Colpman, D. & Welford, K. (2004) Urinary drainage systems. In: *Urological Nursing* (eds S. Fillingham & J. Douglas), 3rd edn. Bailliere Tindall, London, pp. 67–92.

Crivellaro, S., Michaels, M.J., Kocjancic, E. & Libertino, J.A. (2004) The Lahey clinic experience with continent urinary diversion. *Br J Urol Int*, 94(7), 1087–91.

D'Elia, G. *et al.* (2004) Mainz Pouch II technique: 10 year experience. *BJU Int*, 93, 1037–42.

DH (2001) Standard principles for preventing hospital acquired infection. *J Hosp Infec*, 47 (suppl), 521–37.

DH (2005a) *Saving Lives: A Delivery Programme to Reduce Healthcare Infection including MRSA*. Department of Health, London.

DH (2005b) *Hazardous waste (England) regulations*. Department of Health, London.

Diokno, A.C. *et al.* (1983) Fate of patients started on clean intermittent self-catheterisation therapy 10 years ago. *J Urol*, 3(2), 191–3.

Dixon, L., Wasson, D. & Johnson, V. (2001) Urinary diversions: a review of nursing care. *Urol Nurs*, 21(5), 337–46.

Duckett, J.W. & Snyder, H.M. (1985) Use of the Mitrofanoff principle in urinary reconstruction. *World J Urol*, 3, 191–3.

Fisch, M. & Hohenfellner, R. (1992) The sigma-rectum pouch (Mainz II pouch). In: *Continent Urinary Diversion* (eds R. Hohenfellner & R. Wammeck). Churchill Livingstone, Edinburgh.

Hayward, J. (1978) *Information – A Prescription Against Pain*. Royal College of Nursing, London.

Hensle, T.W., Bingham, J., Lam, J. & Shabsigh, A. (2004) Preventing reservoir calculi after augmentation cystoplasty and continent urinary diversion: the influence of an irrigation protocol. *Br J Urol Int*, 93(4), 585–7.

Horn, S.A. (1990) Nursing patients with a continent urinary diversion. *Nurs Stand*, 4(21), 24–6.

Kennedy, W.A. *et al.* (1993) Pregnancy after orthotopic continent urinary diversion. *Surg Gynaecol Obstet*, 177(4), 405–9.

Lapides, J. *et al.* (1974) Follow-up on unsterile intermittent self-catheterisation. *J Urol*, 111(2), 184–7.

Lapides, S. (1971) Clean intermittent self-catheterization in the treatment of urinary tract disease. *Trans Am Assoc Genitourin Surg*, 63, 92–96.

Leaver, R.B. (1994) The Mitrofanoff pouch: a continent urinary diversion. *Prof Nurse*, 9(11), 748–53.

Leaver, R.B. (1996) Continent urinary diversions – the Mitrofanoff principle. In: *Stoma Care Nursing – A Patient-Centred Approach* (ed. C. Myers). Edward Arnold, London, pp. 166–79.

Leaver, R.B. (2002) Continent urinary diversions and rectal bladders. In: *The Essentials of Pouch Care Nursing* (ed. J. Williams). Whurr Publishing, London, pp. 128–42.

Lindenhall, B. *et al.* (1994) Long-term intermittent catheterisation: the experience of teenagers and young adults with myelomeningocele. *J Urol*, 152(1), 187–9.

Mansson, A. *et al.* (1988) Quality of life after cystectomy. *Br J Urol*, 62(4), 240–5.

Mansson, A. *et al.* (1991) Psychological adjustment to cystectomy for bladder carcinoma and effects on interpersonal relationships. *Scand J Caring Sci*, 5(3), 129–34.

Matthews, S. & Courts, N.F. (2001) Orthotopic neobladder surgery: nursing care promotes independence in patients with bladder cancer. *Am J Nurs*, 101(7), 24AA–GG.

McCahill, P.D. *et al.* (1992) Toxic shock syndrome: a complication of continent urinary diversion. *J Urol*, 147(3), 681–7.

McGuire, M.S. *et al.* (2000) The type of urinary diversion after radical cystectomy significantly impacts on the patient's quality of life. *Ann Surg Oncol*, 7(1), 4–8.

Mitrofanoff, P. (1980) Cystomie continente trans appendiclaire dans le traitment des vessies neurologiques. *Chirurgie Pediatr*, 21, 297–305.

Morris, J. *et al.* (1989) *The Benefits of Providing Information to Patients*. Centre for Health Economics, University of York, York.

NMC (2006) *A–Z Advice Sheet Consent*. www.nmc.org.

NMC (2008) *The Code: Standards of Conduct, Performance and Ethics for Nurses and Midwives*. Nursing and Midwifery Council, London.

Oishi, K. *et al.* (1993) Quality of life of patients with a continent urinary reservoir. *Hinyokika-kiyo*, 39(1), 7–14.

Perimenis, P. & Koliopanou, E. (2004) Postoperative management and rehabilitation of patients receiving an ileal orthotopic bladder substitution. *Urol Nurs*, 24(5), 383–6.

Pontieri-Lewis, V. & Vates, T.S. (1993) Post-operative management of patients undergoing radical cystectomy and urinary diversion. *Medsurg Nurs*, 2(5), 369–74.

Raleigh, E.H. *et al.* (1990) Significant others benefit from preoperative information. *J Adv Nurs*, 15(8), 941–5.

Randles, J. (1990) The Mitrofanoff pouch. *Nursing*, 4(18), 20–2.

Randles, J. (1992) An alternative to urinary conduit. *Nurs Stand*, 6(42), 33–6.

Razor, B.R. (1993) Continent urinary reservoirs. *Semin Oncol Nurs*, 9(4), 272–85.

Roberts, S. (1991) Theatre nursing operation reassurance, preoperative visiting. *Nurs Times*, 87(41), 70–1.

Skinner, D.G. & Lieskovsky, D. (1988) Technique of radical cystectomy. In: *Diagnosis and Management of Genitourinary Cancer* (eds D.G. Skinner & D. Lieskovsky). W.B. Saunders, Philadelphia, pp. 607–22.

Stein, J.P. *et al.* (1996) The use of orthotopic neobladders in women undergoing cystectomy for pelvic malignancy. *World J Urol*, 14(1), 9–14.

Stewart, M. (1986) Urinary diversions and bowel cancer. *Ann R Coll Surg Eng*, 68, 98–102.

Sullivan, L.D. *et al.* (1998) An evaluation of quality of life in patients with continent urinary diversions after cystectomy. *Br J Urol*, 81, 699–704.

Varol, C. & Studer, U.E. (2004) Managing patients after ileal orthotopic bladder substitution. *BJU Int*, 93, 266–70.

Wagstaff, K.E. *et al.* (1991) Blood and urine analysis in patients with intestinal bladders. *J Urol*, 68, 311–16.

Woodhouse, C.R.J. (1989) The Mitrofanoff principle for continent urinary diversions. *Br J Urol*, 63(1), 53–7.

Woodhouse, C.R.J. (1991) *Long-term Paediatric Urology*. Blackwell Scientific, Oxford.

Woodhouse, C.R.J. (1994) *The Infective Metabolic and Histological Consequences of Enterocystoplasty*. European Board of Urology, European Urology Update Series, Vol. 3. Union European des Medecins Specialistes.

Woodhouse, C.R.J. & Christofides, M. (1998) Modified ureterosigmoidostomy (Mainz II): technique and early results. *Br J Urol*, 81(2), 247–52.

Zeimer, M.M. (1983) Effects of information on post-surgical coping. *Nurs Res*, 32(5), 282–7.

Chapter 17

Elimination: stoma care

Reference material **362**
Procedure guidelines: Stoma care **370**
Procedure guidelines: Urine specimen collection (ileal conduit or urostomy) **372**
Procedure guidelines: Stoma bridge or rod removal **373**
Problem solving: Stoma care **374**
Useful addresses **375**
References and further reading **375**

Definition

'Stoma' is a word of Greek origin meaning 'mouth' or 'opening' (Taylor 2005). A bowel or urinary stoma is usually created by bringing a section of bowel out on to the abdominal wall as a diversionary procedure because the urinary or colonic tract beyond the position of the stoma is no longer viable.

Indications

Stoma care is required for the following purposes:

- To collect urine or faeces in an appropriate appliance.
- To achieve and maintain patient comfort and security.
- To maintain good skin and stoma hygiene (Black 1997).

Reference material

Types of stoma

Colostomy

A colostomy may be formed from any section of the large bowel (sigmoid, descending, transverse or ascending). Its position in the colon will dictate the output and consistency of faeces. Stomas formed in the sigmoid colon produce a semi-formed or formed stool; stoma formed higher in the colon will produce a more liquid stool. Colostomies may be permanent or temporary and either an 'end' or 'terminal' (Figure 17.1) or a defunctioning or loop colostomy (Figure 17.2). Temporary colostomies may be raised to divert the faecal output, either to allow healing of an anastomosis further along the colon, to relieve a distal obstruction or bowel injury, or to allow healing of colonic or rectoanal disease (Taylor 2005). With a defunctioning loop colostomy

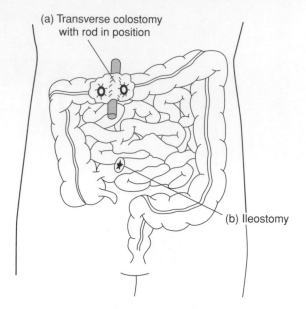

Figure 17.2 (a) Transverse colostomy and (b) ileostomy.

the colon is exteriorized; a rod or bridge may be used to maintain a hold on the abdominal surface then the bowel is opened and mucocutaneous sutures are inserted to form the stoma (Black 2000b). Such a rod or bridge is usually removed 5–10 days after insertion (Figure 17.2). A further operation will be required to close this stoma when it is no longer needed, i.e. when the anastomosed bowel has healed. The term 'defunctioning' is used to indicate that the bowel distal to the stoma is being rested (Borwell 1994; Myers 1996; Black 2000b; Taylor 2000).

Ileostomy

An ileostomy is formed when a section of ileum, usually the last 20 cm, is brought out onto the abdominal wall, the ileum is everted to form a spout which allows the effluent to drain into an appliance (Black 2000a) (Figure 17.2). Ileostomies may be permanent (usually end) or temporary (usually loop). Temporary ileostomies are often formed to allow healing of an anastomosis lower down in the bowel; to allow healing of an ileo-anal pouch or to aid healing of diseased bowel (Taylor 2005). It is important that the proximal (active) side of a loop ileostomy has a spout to enable the effluent to drain into an appliance. Rods or bridges may be used as with loop colostomies. In some cases of ulcerative colitis, the whole colon (total colectomy) may be removed; these patients may have an ileal–anal pouch constructed. To form these pouches the terminal ileum is fashioned into a reservoir and brought down and attached to the anus.

Urostomy (ileal loop, ileal conduit, colonic conduit)

A urostomy is formed when the bladder is removed or diseased. A section of ileum is isolated, along with its mesentery

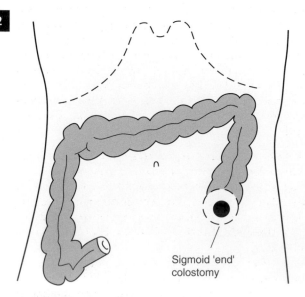

Figure 17.1 Sigmoid 'end' colostomy.

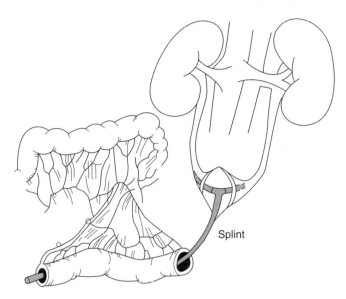

Figure 17.3 Urostomy.

vessels, the remaining ends of the ileum are anastamosed to restore continuity. The isolated section is mobilized, the proximal end is closed and the ureters, once resected from the bladder, are implanted at this end. The distal end is brought out on to the surface of the abdominal wall and everted to form a spout (Figure 17.3) as in an ileostomy (Fillingham & Fell 2004; Black 2000b). Although urostomies are usually formed from ileum, the colon may also be utilized (Fillingham & Fell 2004). Urine from a urostomy will contain mucus from the bowel used in its construction (Taylor 2005).

Other types of urinary diversion

Other types of urinary diversion include ureterostomy, a procedure that brings the ureters out onto the abdominal wall together (one stoma) or separately (two stomas). This may be a permanent or temporary procedure, it may be used for ill patients with poor renal function and when less extensive abdominal surgery is indicated. Stomas formed in this way are often small and flush to the abdomen. They are prone to stenosis and it is often difficult to maintain a leak-proof appliance (Fillingham & Fell 2004). It may be possible for some patients with bladder disease to have a continent diversion. For further information on these continent urinary diversions, see Chapter 16.

Indications for bowel stoma

- Cancer of the bowel.
- Cancer of the pelvis.
- Trauma.
- Neurological damage.
- Congenital disorders.
- Ulcerative colitis.
- Crohn's disease.

- Diverticular disease.
- Familial polyposis coli.
- Intractable incontinence.
- Fistula.
- Radiation enteritis.

Indications for urinary stoma

- Cancer of the bladder.
- Cancer of the pelvis.
- Trauma.
- Congenital disorders.
- Neurological damage.
- Fistula.
- Intractable incontinence (Black 1994a; Taylor 2005).

Preoperative preparation, assessment and care

Physical preparation of the patient will vary according to the type of operation and the policies of individual surgeons and hospitals. This will involve the usual preparation for anaesthesia (see Chapter 30), preparation of the area of the body involved and of the bowel. Other specific procedures may also be included (Winkley 1998).

Psychological preparation of the individual facing stoma surgery should begin as soon as surgery has been considered, preferably by utilizing the skills of a trained stoma care nurse. Boore (1978), Hayward (1978), Ivimy (1997) and Beddows (1997) have illustrated the importance of preoperative information and explanation in reducing postoperative physical and psychological stress. It is important that the information and discussions are tailored to the individual's needs, taking into account their level of anxiety and distress (Borwell 1997c). Ongoing assessment of the patient's understanding of the information given should be carried out and documented.

Information-giving and discussion with patients about their stoma and lifestyle start preoperatively and continue throughout the patient's stoma experience. Preoperatively patients want information about the proposed surgical procedure and on a number of practical issues about living with a stoma including diet; lifestyle and work; appearance of stoma; stoma appliances and how to obtain them; relationships and sexual function (Kelly & Henry 1992). The aims of these interactions are as follows:

1 To help the individual with a stoma to return to his/her previous place in society whenever possible.
2 To help in the process of adapting to a changed body image. Patients' involvement with preoperative decision making positively influences their postoperative adjustment (Price 1990; Salter 1997; Black 2000a; Brown & Randle 2005).
3 To reduce anxiety. The patient's perception of life with a stoma may have a positive or detrimental influence on rehabilitation. Exploration of their understanding of stomas may reveal misunderstandings and commonly

held myths which can be corrected. Patients may be aware of others in their social network who have a stoma: it is important to discuss their perceptions of these ostomates (Salter 1992; Bryant 1993; Brown & Randle 2005).

4 To explain that the presence of a stoma itself need not adversely affect any previous quality of life such as hobbies, work, social life or any other interests, although the underlying disease which has led to the stoma might (Salter 1992).

5 To prepare the patient for the appearance and likely behaviour pattern of the stoma (Pullen 1998; Cronin 2005).

6 To reassure patients that they will be able to manage an appliance whatever the environment (Salter 1995).

7 To assure patients that they will be supported fully while in hospital and that continuing support will be available in the community (Salter 1995; Pullen 1998).

Such preoperative education has been shown to increase cooperation and trust and reduce anxiety, the length of time the patient remains in hospital and the amount of postoperative analgesia required (Wade 1989). Family and/or close friends may also be involved, when appropriate, on agreement with the patient (Price 1996).

It is important to determine whether a patient will be able to manage a stoma by assessing the following:

- Visual capability.
- Manual dexterity.
- Physical limitations/disabilities, e.g. Parkinson's disease, arthritis, loss of an upper limb.
- Skin conditions.
- Abnormal contours, e.g. the changes that occur with spina bifida.
- Mental state, including previous psychiatric disorders, coping strategies, attitudes to body/stoma, memory.
- Sociocultural, e.g. occupation, social and sporting activities, family and social support, culture and religion.

Siting of the stoma is one of the most important preoperative tasks to be carried out by the doctor, stoma care nurse or ward nurse with appropriate knowledge and skills (Figures 17.4 & 17.5). This minimizes future difficulties such as interference by the stoma with clothes, or skin problems caused by leakage of the appliance due to a badly sited stoma (e.g. on the waistline or in a body crease) (Bass *et al.* 1997; Erwin-Toth & Barrett 1997; Qin & Bao-Min 2001). When siting the stoma, consideration should be given to the following:

1 A flat area of the skin to facilitate safe adhesion of the appliance.

2 Avoidance of bony prominences such as hips and ribs which may interfere with the adhesion of the appliance, or pendulous breasts which may obscure the stoma from the patient's view, making self-care impossible.

3 Avoidance of skin creases, especially in the region of the groin or the umbilicus, to avoid urine or faecal matter tracking along the skin creases.

4 Avoidance of scars, which may cause skin creases that may lead to leakages.

Figure 17.4 Position of stoma.

5 Avoidance of waistline or belt areas, as patient's clothing may put pressure on the stoma which may lead to leaks or trauma.

6 Maintenance of the stoma within the rectus sheath, as this reduces the risk of herniation later (Myers 1996; Erwin-Toth & Barrett 1997; Sjodahl *et al.* 1998). The muscle may be identified by asking the patient to lie flat, then to raise the head. The muscle may also be palpated and easily felt when the patient coughs.

7 Ideally, the patient should be able to see the stoma site (Blackley 1998).

The patient must be observed while lying, sitting in a comfortable chair, with the abdominal muscles relaxed, and standing (Erwin-Toth & Barrett 1997). Consideration must be given to any bending or lifting involved with the patient's

Figure 17.5 Site of urostomy.

work and any other activities in which the patient partakes. Account must also be taken of any weight gain or loss in the postoperative period, as this may change the contours of the abdomen and hence the position of the stoma.

Personnel who may be expected to provide information

- Medical staff.
- Stoma care nurse.
- Nursing staff on ward.
- Primary health care team.
- Another suitable ostomate. 'Visitors' are trained by the voluntary associations and, ideally, should be of similar age, sex and background to the patient to enable the patient to discuss problems of adapting to life with a stoma (Rheaume & Gooding 1991; Mowdy 1998).

Useful aids

- Information booklets.
- Samples of the various appliances.
- Diagrams.
- Audio tapes.
- DVDs.

These aids are valuable to reinforce and clarify the verbal information.

Postoperative period

Stoma function

Colostomy function

In the first few days a sigmoid colon stoma will produce haemaserous fluid and wind. By day 5 there should be some faecal fluid and then by day 7–14 semi-formed stool (Cottam 1999). A closed appliance may be used. In the case of a stoma formed in the transverse colon, only a small amount of water will be reabsorbed from the faecal matter, so the faecal matter will be unformed. This means a drainable pouch will need to be used.

Patients with a sigmoid colostomy may find that wholemeal foods assist in producing a formed stool once or twice daily (Myers 1996; Black 1998). Medications that reduce peristaltic action, e.g. codeine phosphate, may also be used to control diarrhoea. The only means of controlling a sigmoid colostomy, however, is by regular irrigation or by use of a Conseal plug system. Stoma care nurses will need to assess patients before teaching them how to perform the irrigation procedure or to use Conseal plugs.

Ileostomy function

For the first few days the stoma will produce haemaserous fluid and wind. By days 5–10 there will be brown faecal matter (Cottam 1999). The fluid output after surgery can be as much as 1500 ml/24 hours but this will gradually reduce to 500–850 ml/24 hours as the bowel settles down (Black

2000a). Sometimes the output from a stoma remains high (>1000 ml/24 hours), which may be due to the amount of small bowel removed at surgery or an underlying bowel condition; these patients require careful management. It is important that fluid balance recordings are made and serum electrolyes are measured as they are at risk of sodium and/or magnesium depletion (Burch 2004). Patients with high output stoma may need to be managed by specialist teams which include gastroenterologists, dietitians and stoma care nurses. The effluent takes on a porridge-like consistency when a normal intake of food is established. A drainable appliance is therefore used. The effluent contains enzymes, which will excoriate the skin, therefore if the pouch leaks it must be changed promptly to prevent skin breakdown. The effluent cannot be controlled and is often more active after meals (Myers 1996; Black 1997). Sometimes medication, e.g. codeine or loperamide, which reduces peristaltic action, may be used to control excessive watery output.

Urostomy/ileal conduit function

Urine will dribble from the stoma every 20–30 seconds and it starts draining immediately. Normal output is 1500 ml/24 hours (Cottam 1999), but may be less after periods of reduced fluid intake, e.g. at night. Urinary stents (fine-bore catheters) may be in place from the ureters past the anastomosis and out of the stoma. They are placed to maintain patency and protect the suturing until primary healing is completed (Black 2000b). Stents are left in situ for 7–10 days.

Irrigation

Irrigation is a method of controlling the output of a colostomy by means of washing out the stoma with warm tap water (with the use of a coned irrigation set), every 24–48 hours.

The advantage of successful colostomy irrigation is that there is no stool leakage between irrigations (Davis 1996; Black 2000b). Patients who wish to use irrigation will be taught how to do it by their stoma care nurses.

Postoperative stages

Stage I

In theatre, an appropriately sized transparent drainable appliance should be applied, which should be left on for approximately 2 days. For the first 48 hours postoperatively, the stoma should be observed for signs of ischaemia or necrosis, the stoma colour (a pink and healthy appearance indicates a good blood supply), size and stoma output should be noted, as should the presence of any devices, i.e. ureteric stents, or bridge with a loop stoma (Kirkwood 2006). The drainable appliance should always be emptied frequently, gas should be allowed to escape and the appliance should not be allowed to get more than half full with effluent. If the appliance becomes too full, leaks may occur and the weight from the effluent or the pressure from gas may cause the appliance to fall off (Black 1997). A leak-proof, odour resistant well-fitted appliance at this time does much to promote patient confidence (Kirkwood 2006). The first time a bowel stoma acts the type, appearance, quantity and consistency of the matter passed should be recorded; this includes any flatus that may be passed (Kirkwood 2006).

Immediately postoperatively patients would not be expected to perform their own stoma care but would be encouraged to observe the nurse caring for them and discuss it with the nurse. During appliance changes observations should be made of:

■ Stoma: colour, size and general appearance, i.e. oedematous, flush with abdomen, retracted.
■ Peri-stomal skin: presence of any erythema, broken areas, rashes.
■ Stoma/skin margin (mucocutaneous margin): sutures intact, tension on sutures, separation of stoma edge from skin (mucocutaneous separation).

Any abnormalities should be reported to the stoma care nurse and medical staff (Black 2000b; Burch 2004; Kirkwood 2006).

Viewing the stoma may be difficult for the patient, who may be very aware of other people's reaction to it (Price 1993). The patient's reaction to their stoma should be observed and recorded.

Stage II

As the patient's condition improves they should be encouraged to participate in the care of their stoma. A demonstration change of the appliance should be given with a full explanation of the principles of stoma care. This will be followed by further opportunities to discuss any problems or raise new queries. Care procedures should be divided into small successive stages and patients should be given support to work through these stages until they are able to take on the care of their stoma. Provided the patient agrees, it is useful to involve the patient's partner or close friends or relatives at this stage. Their acceptance of the stoma may encourage the patient and help to restore the patient's self-esteem (Salter 1995). They may now be ready to discuss appliances and choose the one that they wish to use at home. Preparation for discharge will be discussed (Black 1994b; Heywood Jones 1994).

Stage III

Ideally, the patient should now be independent, eating a normal diet, be ready for discharge and should be competent in stoma care.

If the family or close friends are closely involved during all stages and are supportive, patients are better able to adapt to the threat of mutilating surgery and altered pattern of elimination (Price 1993). The family or close friends are also likely to require support and information so that they are in a position to help the ostomate. Acceptance of the stoma is a gradual process and, on discharge from hospital, patients may only be beginning to adapt to life with a stoma (Salter 1997).

Specific discharge plans

Follow-up support

The patient is discharged with adequate supplies until a prescription is obtained from the general practitioner. Written reminders are provided of how to care for the stoma, how to obtain supplies of appliances, and any other information that may be required. The patient should have details of non-medical stoma clinics, details about the relevant agencies and information about voluntary associations. Arrangements should also have been made for a home visit from the stoma care nurse and/or the community nurse (Blackley 1998; Cronin 2005).

Obtaining supplies

All National Health Service (NHS) patients with a permanent stoma are entitled to free prescriptions for their stoma care products, and should complete the relevant forms for exemption from payment. Appliances can then be obtained from the local chemist, free home delivery services or directly from the appropriate manufacturers.

Diet

All patients should be encouraged to eat a wide variety of foods. Our digestive system reacts in an individual way to different foods and so it is important that patients try a wide range of foods on several occasions and that none should be specifically avoided (Bridgewater 1999). Patients can then make decisions about different foods based on their own experience of their own reaction. Explanations of how the gut functions, how it has been changed since surgery and the effects certain foodstuffs may cause should be given.

Colostomy and ileostomy formation means the loss of the anal sphincter so passage of wind cannot be controlled. High-fibre foods such as beans and pulses produce wind as they are broken down in the gut; hence individuals who eat large quantities of these foodstuffs may be troubled by wind. There are several non-food causes of wind, such as chewing gum, eating irregularly and drinking fizzy drinks, which should be considered before blaming a particular food (Bridgewater 1999). Eating yoghurt or drinking buttermilk may help reduce wind for these patients. Green vegetables, pulses and spicy food are examples of foods that may cause colostomy and ileostomy output to increase or become watery. Boiled rice, smooth peanut butter, apple sauce and bananas are some of the foods that may help thicken stoma output (Bridgewater 1999; Black 2000b).

Some foods, e.g. tomato skin and pips, may be seen unaltered in the output from an ileostomy (Hulten & Palselius 1996; Black 1997; Blackley 1998). Celery, dried fruit, nuts and potato skins are some of the foods which can temporarily block ileostomies (Bridgewater 1999; Black 2000b). The blockage is usually related to the amount eaten (Wood 1998). The offending food can be tried at another time in small quantities, ensuring it is chewed well and not eaten in a hurry (Bridgewater 1999).

There are no dietary restrictions with a urostomy. It must be stressed, however, that an adequate fluid intake must be maintained to minimize the risk of urinary tract infection. The recommended fluid intake for all individuals is 1.5–2.0 litres per day (Bridgewater 1999). Fluid intake should be increased in hot weather or at times when there is an increase in sweating, e.g. exercise, fever. Beetroot, radishes, spinach and some food dye may discolour urine; some drugs may also have this effect, e.g. metronidazole, nitrofurantoin. Urine may develop a strong odour following consumption of asparagus or fish (Bridgewater 1999).

Fear of malodour

This is a common fear for patients with bowel stomas, often based on hearsay or experience with other ostomists in hospital or the community. Appliances are odour free when fitted correctly. Flatus may be released via charcoal filters and deodorizers are available. The individual must be reassured, however, that any problems that occur postoperatively will be investigated, with a good possibility of their being solved by such means as the use of alternative appliances (Black 2000b; Burch 2004).

Sex and the ostomate

The possibility of sexual impairment for both men and women after stoma surgery depends on the nature of the operation, and the ensuing damage to the nerves and tissues involved. The psychological impact of the surgery and its effect on the individual's body image must also be taken into consideration. Surgery that results in physical sexual disability will have psychological repercussions, while some sexual difficulties may be of psychological origin (Salter 1996; Borwell 1997c; Black 2004). Impairment may be permanent or temporary. In the latter case, resolution of the difficulty may take anything up to 2 years. Pre- and postoperative counselling should be offered for both patient and partner.

All patients may experience loss of libido and sexual desire. Ejaculatory disturbances occur following cystectomy so men facing this surgery should be offered sperm banking prior to surgery. Erectile dysfunction is a common complication of pelvic surgery and there are a number of treatment options available. These include oral medications (sildenafil, tadalafil, vardenafil), sublingual apomorphine, intraurethral and intracavernosal aprosdadil, vacuum devices and penile implants (Ashford 1998; Newey 1998; Kirby et al. 1999).

Female patients may experience dyspareunia; this may be due to narrowing or shortening of the vagina, a reduction in the volume of vaginal secretions or changes in genital sensations (Schover 1986; Borwell 1999; Black 2004). The use of a lubricant, adopting different positions during lovemaking or encouraging greater relaxation by extending foreplay may help resolve painful intercourse (Bryant 1993; Borwell 1999; Black 2004).

Useful references on the psychological and sexual aspects of care may be found in Borwell (1997b, c), Huish et al. (1998), Wells (2000) and Heath and White (2001).

Stoma appliances and accessories

Many of the appliances now available are very similar in style, colour and efficiency and often there is very little to choose between them when the time comes for the ostomate to decide what to wear.

The aim of good stoma care is to return patients to their place in society (Black 1994b). One of the ways in which this can be facilitated is to provide them with a safe, reliable appliance. This means that there should be no fear of leakage or odour and the appliance should be comfortable, unobtrusive, easy to handle and disposable. The ostomate should be allowed a choice from the management systems available. It is also important to identify and manage problems with the stoma or peristomal skin early. When choosing the appropriate management system for the new ostomate, factors which need to be considered include:

- Type of stoma.
- Type of effluent.
- Patient's cognitive ability.
- Manual dexterity.
- Lifestyle.
- Condition of peristomal skin.
- Siting of stoma.
- Patient preference (Black 2000a; Kirkwood 2006).

Management systems available: pouches, plugs and irrigation

Pouches

Although some people whose stomas were created several years ago are wearing non-disposable rubber bags, most appliances used today are made from an odour-proof plastic film. These pouches usually adhere to the body by a hydrocolloid wafer or flange (Taylor 2000). Pouches may be opaque or clear and often have a soft backing to absorb perspiration. They usually have a built-in integral filter containing charcoal to neutralize any odour.

Choosing the right size

It is important that the flange of the appliance fits snugly around the stoma within 0.3 cm of the stoma edge (Kirkwood 2006). This narrow edge is left exposed so that the appliance does not rub on the stoma. Stoma appliances usually come with measuring guides to allow for choice of size. During the initial weeks following surgery the oedematous stoma will gradually reduce in size and the appliances will have to be changed accordingly.

Fear of malodour

Pouches usually have a built-in integral filter containing charcoal to neutralize any odour when flatus is released;

Figure 17.6 Stoma equipment. (a) Drainable bowel stoma pouch; (b) urostomy pouch; (c) closed bag.

therefore, smell is only noticeable when emptying or changing an appliance (Rudoni & Sica 1999). There are also various deodorizers available. These come in the form of drops or powders that may be put into the pouch or sprays, which can be sprayed into the air just before changing or emptying the pouch (Burch & Sica 2005). The individual should be reassured that any problems with odour or leakage will be investigated and that in most circumstances the problem will be solved with alternative appliances or accessories (Bryant 1993; Black 1997).

Types of pouch

The type of pouch used will depend on the type of stoma and effluent expected.

Closed pouches are mainly used when formed stool is expected, e.g. sigmoid colostomy (Figure 17.6c). These pouches have a flatus filter and need to be changed once or twice a day.

Drainable pouches are used when the effluent is fluid or semi-formed, i.e. ileostomy or transverse colostomy (Figure 17.6a). These pouches have specially designed filters, which are less likely to become blocked or leak faecal fluid. These pouches need to be emptied regularly and the outlet rinsed carefully and then closed with a clip or 'roll-up' method. They may be left on for up to 3 days.

Urostomy pouches have a drainage tap for urine and should be emptied regularly (Figure 17.6b). They can be attached to a large bag and tubing for night drainage. These pouches can remain on for up to 3 days.

One- or two-piece systems

All types of pouch (closed, drainable or with a tap) as described above fall into one of two broad categories: one-piece or two-piece systems.

- **One-piece.** This comprises a pouch attached to an adhesive wafer that is removed completely when the pouch is changed. This is an easy system for an ostomate with dexterity problems, e.g. arthritis, peripheral neuropathy, to handle.
- **Two-piece.** This comprises a wafer onto which a pouch is clipped or stuck. It can be used with sore and sensitive skin because when the pouch is removed the flange is left intact and so the skin is left undisturbed.

Plug system

Patients with colostomies may be able to stop the effluent by inserting a plug into the stoma lumen. This plug swells in the moist environment and behaves as a seal. This system should only be introduced by a stoma nurse specialist (Taylor 2000).

Accessories

The specific products in this section have been mentioned as examples of what aids are available and reference to them is not necessarily intended as a recommendation.

Solutions for skin and stoma cleaning

Mild soap and water, or water only, is sufficient for skin and stoma cleaning. It is important that all soap residues are removed as they may interfere with pouch adhesion. Detergents, disinfectants and antiseptics cause dryness and irritation and should not be used. The stoma is not a wound or a lesion and should be regarded as a resited urethra or anus.

Skin barriers

1 **Creams:**
   Unless made specifically for use on peristomal skin, creams should not be used, as the residual surface film of grease prevents adherence of the appliance. Creams usually have a soothing and moisturizing effect.
   Use: For sensitive skin, as a protective measure.
   Method: Use sparingly; massage gently into the skin until completely absorbed; excess grease may be wiped off with a soft tissue.
   Example: Chiron barrier cream (aluminium chlorohydrate 2% in an emulsified base) (ABPI 1999).
   Precaution: Not to be used on broken or sore skin.

2 **Protective films:**
   Use: Act as a film on the skin, first to prevent irritation and, second, to give protection as it is removed with the adhesive of the bag, thus preventing removal of the stratum corneum of the skin. Most of the newer films do not contain alcohol so may be used on broken skin, although some of the older preparations do.
   Method: Swab impregnated wipe or foam applicator on to skin; dries quickly. There is also a spray available.
   Examples: Cavilon no sting barrier film, LBF, Skinsafe non-sting protective film.
   Precaution: If preparation contains alcohol do not use on broken skin as it will cause stinging (ABPI 1999).

3 **Protective wafers:**
   Use: These are hypoallergenic and are designed to cover and protect skin, and allow healing if the skin is sore or broken. They may be useful in cases of skin reaction or allergy to the adhesive or an appliance.
   Method: The wafers may be cut with the aid of a template (pattern) to the required shape and fitted on to the skin. The appliances are then attached to the wafer. The rim of the wafer should not press against the stoma but should fit to 0.5 cm around it.
   Examples: Stomahesive or Comfeel type of wafers. Stomahesive is composed of gelatin, pectin, sodium carboxymethylcellulose and polyisobutylene (Martindale 1993); it adheres painlessly to normal, erythematous, moist or broken skin; it is available in three sizes.
   Precautions: Allergy may occur, but rarely.

4 **Seals/washers:**
   Use: These are used to provide skin protection around the stoma; they will protect a smaller area than the wafers mentioned above. They are also useful to fill in 'dips' or 'gulleys' in the skin. They can be used to extend the wear time of an appliance when a stoma has a corrosive output which quickly breaks down the inner edge of a baseplate.
   Method: Like the wafers, they have an adhesive side and may be applied directly to the skin. They form an integral part of some of the appliances.
   Examples: Salts, cohesive seals, Dansac washers.
   Precautions: As for protective wafers above.

5 **Pastes:**
   Use: Useful to fill in crevices and 'gulleys' in the skin to provide a smooth surface for an appliance.
   Method: Stomahesive: a syringe may be used to apply paste. Either leave for 60 seconds after applying to the skin, when the surface will be dry, making the paste easier to mould into the skin contour, or apply with a spatula, or wet the finger first to prevent the paste sticking and mould the paste immediately. It will sting on raw areas as it contains alcohol. Apply a little Orahesive powder to these areas first.
   Examples: Stomahesive paste, soft paste.

6 **Protective paste:**
   Use: To protect raw areas. Does not contain alcohol so will not cause irritation (useful for fistula problems).
   Method: Orabase, similar to Stomahesive paste in composition but with the addition of liquid paraffin. Liquid paraffin will inhibit adhesives sticking so care must be taken to ensure Orabase paste is not applied under appliances.
   Example: Orabase paste.

7 **Powders:**
   Use: For protection of sore or raw areas without impeding adhesion of the appliance.
   Method: Sprinkle on affected areas.
   Example: Orahesive powder.

8 **Adhesive preparations:**
   Use: Only required when appliance does not adhere well to the skin, e.g. because of leakage, uneven site, or if abdominal fistulae present.
   Method: The individual products differ considerably in their method of application and it is recommended that the user consults the manufacturer's instructions.
   Example: Saltair solution.

9 **Adhesive removers:**
   Use: If patient finds removing stoma appliance uncomfortable or residue from a hydrocolloid appliance is left on the peristoma skin.
   Method: Swab skin with impregnate wipe at the edge of baseplate which should begin to lift; as baseplate lifts swab the skin under baseplate until baseplate has been removed or spray area.
   Examples: Appeel wipes and spray, Lift wipes and bottle, Ostoclear sachets or spray.

369

Precaution: Some adhesive removers contain alcohol and therefore should not be used on broken skin. Those listed in the example do not contain alcohol (there are other non alcohol containing products available).

10 **Stoma baseplate securing tape:**
Uses: Used when baseplate is having difficulty in adhering fully such as with parastoma hernia, prolapsed stomas and badly sited stomas such as those near bony prominences.
Method: Apply to edge of baseplate that is having difficulty adhering.
Examples: Hydroframe, SecuPlast, Ostofix flange security tape.

11 **Thickening agents:**
Uses: To help solidify loose stoma output and so reduce pouch noise (Burch & Sica 2005).
Method: Place sachets, capsules or gel in pouch.
Examples: Morform sachet, Gel-X capsules, OstoSorb gel.

12 **Convex devices:**
Use: These devices are designed to be used with retracted stomas. The convex shape allows a greater seal round the stoma by filling in any crevices caused by retraction, scars or skin creases. The convexity pushes the peristomal skin down and causes the stoma to protrude a little. There is now a wide range of convex products available which all apply different levels of pressure to the peristoma skin. These include inserts, seals, soft convex flanges and rigid convex flanges.
Examples: Adapt ring Convex inserts, soft seal range of appliances, impression range of appliances.
Precautions: Changes to peristomal skin can result due to the result of convexity and patients should be taught to observe for this (Burch & Sica 2005). Bruising and ulceration are signs of skin damage (Wyss 2004); pyoderma gangrenosum is also associated with pressure on the peristomal skin due to convex appliances (Lyon & Beck 2001).

Deodorants

1 **Aerosols:**
Use: To absorb or mask odour.
Method: One or two puffs into the air before emptying or removing appliance.
Examples: Limone, Naturcare, FreshAire.

2 **Drops and powders:**
Use: For deodorizing bag contents.
Method: Before fitting pouch or after emptying and cleaning drainable pouch, squeeze tube two or three times.
Examples: Ostobon deodorant powder, Nodor S drops, Saltair No-roma.

Procedure guidelines   Stoma care

These procedural guidelines contain the basic information needed for changing a stoma appliance. Modifications may be made according to the following factors:

1 The place of change, i.e. bathroom, bedside, availability of sink, etc.
2 The person changing the appliance, i.e. nurse, patient or carer.
3 Type of appliance used, e.g. one- or two-piece, closed or drainable.
4 Any accessories used, e.g. adhesive remover, barrier creams, seal/washer.

Equipment
1 Clean tray holding:
   (a) Tissues, wipes.
   (b) New appliance.
   (c) Measuring device/template.
   (d) Scissors.
   (e) Disposal bags for used appliances, tissues and wipes.
   (f) Relevant accessories, e.g. adhesive remover, protective film, seals/washers.
2 Bowl of warm water.
3 Soap (if desired).
4 Jug for contents of appliance.
5 Gloves. This practice should be explained to patients so that they do not feel it is just because they have a stoma that gloves are worn. (It is recognized that it could be difficult to attach an appliance with gloves in situ [due to adhesive], but once the stoma has been cleaned of excreta and blood, gloves may be removed to apply bag.)

Procedure

Action	Rationale
1 Explain and discuss the procedure with the patient.	To ensure that the patient understands the procedure and gives his/her valid consent (NMC 2006: C; NMC 2008: C). To familiarize the patient with the procedure.
2 Ensure that the patient is in a suitable and comfortable position where the patient will be able to watch the procedure, if well enough. A mirror may be used to aid visualization.	To allow good access to the stoma for cleaning and for secure application of the stoma bag. The patient will become familiar with the stoma and will also learn much about the care of the stoma by observation of the nurse (Bryant 1993: P).
3 Use a small protective pad to protect the patient's clothing from drips if the effluent is fluid and apply gloves for nurse's protection.	Avoids the necessity for renewing clothing or bedclothes and demoralization of the patient as a result of soiling (E).
4 If the bag is of the drainable type, empty the contents into a jug before removing the bag.	For ease of handling the appliance and prevention of spillage (E).
5 Remove the appliance. Peel the adhesive off the skin with one hand while exerting gentle pressure on the skin with the other.	To reduce trauma to the skin. Erythema as a result of removing the appliance is normal and quickly settles (Broadwell 1987: C).
6 Fold appliance in two to ensure no spillage and place in disposal bag.	To ensure safe disposal according to environmental policy (E; DH 2005b: C).
7 Remove excess faeces or mucus from the stoma with a damp tissue.	So that the stoma and surrounding skin are clearly visible (E).
8 Examine the skin and stoma for soreness, ulceration or other unusual phenomena. If the skin is unblemished and the stoma is a healthy red colour, proceed.	For the prevention of complications or the treatment of existing problems (E).
9 Wash the skin and stoma gently until they are clean.	To promote cleanliness and prevent skin excoriation (E).
10 Dry the skin and stoma gently but thoroughly.	The appliance will attach more securely to dry skin (E & C).
11 Measure the stoma, cut appliance leaving 3 mm clearance. Apply a clean appliance.	Appliance should provide skin protection. The aperture should be cut just a little larger than the stoma so that effluent can not cause skin damage This should be no more than 3 mm from the stoma (Kirkwood 2006: C).
12 Dispose of soiled tissues and the used appliance in a disposable bag and place it in an appropriate plastic bin. At home the bag should be placed in a plastic bag tied and disposed of in a rubbish bag.	To ensure safe disposal (E).
13 Wash hands thoroughly using bactericidal soap and water or bactericidal alcohol handrub.	To prevent spread of infection by contaminated hands.

371

Procedure guidelines   Urine specimen collection (ileal conduit or urostomy)

Equipment

1 Sterile dressing pack.
2 Soft catheter: Nelaton type, not larger than 12 or 14 Fr.
3 Disposable plastic apron.
4 Universal specimen container.

5 Skin-cleaning solution.
6 Bactericidal alcohol handrub.
7 Clean stoma appliance.

Procedure

Action	Rationale
1 Explain and discuss the procedure with the patient.	To ensure that the patient understands the procedure and gives his/her valid consent (NMC 2006: C; NMC 2008: C).
2 Ensure that the patient is in a comfortable position, e.g. sitting up, supported by pillows, and that the stoma is easily accessible.	For patient comfort and to allow access to the stoma (E).
3 Screen the bed, then wash hands using bactericidal soap and water or bactericidal alcohol handrub and dry them.	For the patient's privacy and to reduce the risk of cross-infection (see Chapter 5). Curtains are drawn at this stage so that dust and airborne organisms disturbed by the curtains do not settle on the sterile trolley (DH 2005a: C).
4 Prepare the trolley and take it to the patient's bedside.	To ensure equipment is easily available (E).
5 Put on a disposable plastic apron.	To reduce risk of cross-infection.
6 Remove the sterile dressing pack, catheter and receiver from their outer wrappings. Place them on the top shelf of the trolley.	To prepare equipment (E).
7 Remove the appliance from the stoma and cover the stoma with a clean topical swab.	To absorb any spillage from the stoma (E).
8 Clean hands with a bactericidal alcohol handrub, and put on clean disposable gloves before opening the sterile field on the trolley.	To reduce the risk of introducing infection into the stoma during the procedure (E).
9 Remove the non-linting gauze with forceps, check and discard it. Arrange a towel to absorb spillage from the stoma.	To keep the areas as clean as possible and to protect the patient and the bedclothes from spilled urine (E).
10 Clean around the stoma with water or saline, from the centre outwards.	Good cleaning of the area reduces the risk of introduction of surface pathogens into the ileal loop (E).
11 Apply gentle skin traction to allow stomal opening to be more visible. Insert the catheter tip gently to a depth of 2.5–5.0 cm only and wait for urine to drain through. Collect the sample in the specimen container. The recommended volume is 3–5 ml.	To avoid catheter coming into contact with external surfaces of stoma. Gentle handling reduces the risk of ileal perforation and is more comfortable for the patient (E). To ensure adequate sample of urine for bacteriological assessment (E).

12 Remove the catheter and seal in the specimen container. Remove gloves and attend to stoma care and apply a pouch as usual. Make the patient comfortable.	To prevent spillage of sample (E). To ensure patient comfort (E).
13 Dispose of equipment.	
14 Wash hands with bactericidal soap and water and dry.	To reduce risk of cross-infection (DH 2005a: C).
15 Check that the specimen is labelled correctly and dispatch it to the laboratory with the appropriate forms.	

Procedure guidelines   Stoma bridge or rod removal

Equipment

1 Clean tray holding:
  (a) Tissues.
  (b) New appliances.
  (c) Disposal bags for used appliances and tissues.
  (d) Relevant accessories, e.g. belt.

2 Bowl of warm water.
3 Soap if desired.
4 Jug for contents of appliance.
5 Gloves.

Procedure

Action	Rationale
1 Explain and discuss the procedure with the patient.	To ensure that the patient understands the procedure and gives his/her valid consent (NMC 2006: C; NMC 2008: C).
2 Ensure the patient is in a suitable and comfortable position.	To allow good access to the stoma for cleaning and for secure application of stoma bag (E).
3 Apply gloves.	To reduce risk of cross-infection (DH 2005a: C).
4 If the bag is of the drainable type, empty the contents into a jug before removing the bag.	For ease of handling the appliance and prevention of spillage (E).
5 Remove the appliance. Peel the adhesive off the skin with one hand while exerting gentle pressure on the skin with the other.	To reduce trauma to the skin. Erythema as a result of removing the appliance is normal and quickly settles (Broadwell 1987: C).
6 Remove excess faeces or mucus from the stoma with a damp tissue.	So that the stoma and surrounding skin are clearly visible (E).
7 (a) Slide the bridge gently to one side to ensure the mobile wing of the bridge is away from the stoma. Turn this wing so that it becomes flush with the bridge. Gently slide the bridge through the stoma loop (see Action figure 7). (b) Fold the bridge in half so that the bridge appears in a 'C' shape. Gently slide the bridge through the stomal loop (see Action figure 7).	To prepare bridge for removal (E).

373

Procedure guidelines (*cont.*)

8	Examine the skin and stoma for soreness, ulceration or other unusual phenomena. If the skin is unblemished and the stoma is a healthy red colour, proceed. If the skin is red and/or broken, treat as outlined in Problem solving, below. If the stoma is not a healthy red colour inform medical and/or stoma care nurse.	For the prevention of complications or the treatment of existing problems (see Problem solving, below) (E).
9	Wash the skin and stoma gently until they are clean.	To promote cleanliness and prevent skin excoriation (E).
10	Dry the skin and stoma gently but thoroughly.	The appliance will attach more securely to dry skin (E).
11	Apply a clean appliance.	To contain effluent from the stoma (E).
12	Dispose of soiled tissues, the bridge and the used bag.	To prevent environmental contamination (E).
13	Wash hands with bactericidal soap and water or bactericidal alcohol handrub.	To reduce risk of cross-infection (DH 2005a: C).

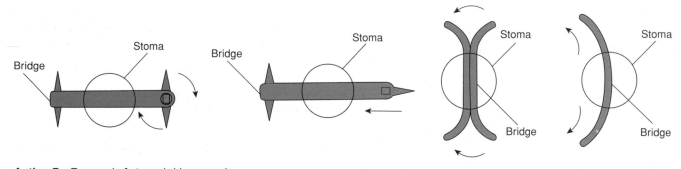

Action 7   Removal of stoma bridge or rod.

Problem solving: Stoma care

Stoma

Problem	Cause	Suggested action
Leakage of urine or faeces	Ill-fitting appliance.	Remeasure stoma and ensure a snug-fitting appliance. Prepare template for future use.
	Skin creases or 'gulleys' preventing correct application of adhesive. Infrequent emptying of drainable bag leading to stress on adhesion.	Build up indented areas and fill in gulleys to create a smooth surface, e.g. using paste. Drainable bags should be emptied frequently, e.g. 2–3-hourly if necessary.
Sore skin	Leakage.	As above.
	Skin reaction to adhesive.	Change to an appliance from another manufacturer or apply a protective square between skin and adhesive. Anti-inflammatory agents may be required for very severe reactions.
	Poor hygiene.	Improve the technique of nurses, patient or carers.

Problem	Cause	Suggested action
Odour	Ill-fitting appliance; lack of seal between skin and adhesive. Poor hygiene. Poor technique, e.g. when emptying drainable bag.	Fit the appliance with care. Consider a change of the type of appliance. Improve the technique of nurses, patient or carers. Empty the bag, then rinse the end with water to ensure that it is clean before closing.

Urostomy specimen

Stoma specimen of urine contaminated. Ileum perforated during specimen collection. Difficulty passing catheter into conduit.	Contaminants introduced during specimen collection. Catheter too hard or inserted too roughly. Small degree of retraction of ileum. Unpredictable direction of ileum.	Take a repeat specimen, observing aseptic procedure and cleaning the stoma well. Report to a doctor immediately. Apply gentle pressure to the area around the stoma to make it protrude. Gently insert your little (gloved) finger into the stoma to determine the direction of the conduit. Insert the catheter tip along this line.

Useful addresses

Association for Spina Bifida and Hydrocephalus (ASBAH), 42 Park Road, Peterborough PE1 2UQ (Tel. 01733 555988), website: www.asbah.org.

Colostomy Association, 15 Station Road, Reading, Berkshire RG1 1LG (Tel. 0118 9391537 or 0800 5876744), website: www.colostomyassociation.org.uk.

IA (Ileostomy and Internal Pouch Support Group), Peremill House, 1–5 Mill Road, Ballyclare, Co. Antrim BT39 9DR (Tel. 028 9334 4043 or 0800 01847244).

Urostomy Association (The), Central Office, Foxglove Avenue, Uttoxeter, Staffs ST14 8UN (Tel. 08452412159), www.uagbi.org.

References and further reading

ABPI (1999) *Compendium of Data Sheets and Summaries of Product Characteristics 1999–2000*. Datapharm Publications, London.

Ashford, L. (1998) Erectile dysfunction. *Prof Nurse*, **13**(9), 603–8.

Bass, E.M. *et al.* (1997) Does preoperative stoma marking and education by the enterostomal therapist affect outcome? *Dis Colon Rectum*, **40**(4), 440–2.

Beddows, J. (1997) Alleviating pre-operative anxiety in patients: a study. *Nurs Stand*, **11**(37), 35–8.

Black, P. (2000a) Practical stoma care. *Nurs Stand*, **14**(41), 47–55.

Black, P. (2000b) *Holistic Stoma Care*. Bailliere Tindall, London.

Black, P.K. (1994a) Stoma care: a practical approach. *Nurs Stand*, **8**(34), RCN Nurs Update, Learning Unit 045.

Black, P.K. (1994b) Choosing the correct stoma appliance. *Br J Nurs*, **3**(11), 545–6, 548, 550.

Black, P.K. (1997) Practical stoma care. *Nurs Stand*, **11**(47), 49–55.

Black, P.K. (1998) Update. Colostomy. *Prof Nurse*, **13**(12), 851–7.

Black, P.K. (2004) Osychological, sexual and cultural issues for patients with a stoma. *Br J Nurs*, **13**(12), 692–7.

Blackley, P. (1998) *Practical Stoma, Wound and Continence Management*. Research Publications, Australia.

Boore, J.R.P. (1978) *A Prescription for Recovery: The Effect of Preoperative Preparation of Surgical Patients on Postoperative Stress, Recovery and Infection*. Royal College of Nursing, London.

Borwell, B. (1994) Colostomies and their management. *Nurs Stand*, **8**(45), CE article 332, 49–55.

Borwell, B. (1997a) Ileo-anal pouch surgery and its after-care. *Community Nurse*, **3**(7) 15–20.

Borwell, B. (1997b) The psychosexual needs of a stoma patient. *Prof Nurse*, **12**(4), 250–5.

Borwell, B. (1997c) Psychological considerations of stoma care nursing. *Nurs Stand*, **11**(48), 49–55.

Borwell, B. (1999) Sexuality and stoma care. In: *Stoma Care in the Community. A Clinical Resource for Practitioners* (ed. P. Taylor). Nursing Times Books, London, pp. 110–135.

Bridgewater, S.E. (1999) Dietary considerations. In: *Stoma Care in the Community. A Clinical Resource for Practitioners* (ed. P. Taylor). Nursing Times Books, London, pp. 187–202.

Broadwell, D.C. (1987) Peristomal skin integrity. *Nurs Clin North Am*, **22**(2), 321–32.

Brown, H. & Randle, J. (2005) Living with a stoma: a review of the literature. *J Clin Nurs*, **14**.

Bryant, R.A. (1993) Ostomy patient management: care that engenders adaptation. *Cancer Invest*, **11**(5), 565–77.

Burch, J. (2004) The management and care of people with stoma complications. *Br J Nurs*, **13**(6), 307–18.

Burch, J. & Sica, J. (2005) Stoma care accessories: an overview of a crowded market. *Br J Community Nurs*, **10**(1), 24–31.

Cottam, J. (1999) Recovering after stoma surgery (Know How series). *Community Nurse*, **5**(9), 24–5.

Cronin, E. (2005) Best practice in discharging patients with a stoma. *Nurs Times*, **101**(47), 67–8.

Davis, K. (1996) Irrigation technique. In: *Stoma Care Nursing – A Patient-Centred Approach* (ed. C. Myers). Arnold, London, pp. 136–145.

DH (2005a) *Saving Lives: A Delivery Programme to Reduce Healthcare Infection including MRSA*. Department of Health, London.

DH (2005b) *Hazardous waste (England) regulations*. Department of Health, London.

Erwin-Toth, P. & Barrett, P. (1997) Stoma site marking: a primer. *Ostomy Wound Manag*, **43**(4), 18–25.

Fillingham, S. & Fell, S. (2004) Urological stomas. In: *Urological Nursing*, (eds S. Fillingham & J. Douglas), 2nd edn. Bailliere Tindall, London, pp. 207–225.

Hayward, J. (1978) *Information – A Prescription Against Pain*. Royal College of Nursing, London.

Heath, H. & White, I. (2001) *The Challenge of Sexuality in Health Care*. Blackwell Science, London.

Heenan, A.L.J. (1996) Two piece stoma systems. *Prof Nurse*, **11**(5), 313–14.

Heywood Jones, I. (1994) Skills update. Stoma care. *Community Outlook*, **4**(12), 22–3.

Horn, S. (1991) Nursing patients with a continent urinary diversion. *Nurs Stand*, **4**(21), 24–6.

Huish, M., Kumar, D. & Stones, C. (1998) Stoma surgery and sex problems in ostomates. *Sex Marital Ther*, **13**(3), 311–28.

Hulten, L. & Palselius, I. (1996) Are dietary restrictions necessary for ileostomy surgery? *Eurostoma*, **13**, 20.

Ivimy, A. (1997) Postoperative recovery is influenced by preoperative care. *Eurostoma*, **17**, 8–9.

Kelly, L. (1995) Patients becoming people. *J Community Nurs*, **9**(8), 12–16.

Kelly, M.P. & Henry, T. (1992) A thirst for practical knowledge: stoma patients' opinions of the services they receive. *Prof Nurse*, **7**(6), 350–6.

Kirby, R., Carson, C. & Goldstein, I. (1999) *Erectile Dysfunction: A Clinical Guide*. Isis Medical Media, Oxford.

Kirkwood, L. (2006) Postoperative stoma care and the selection of appliances. *J Community Nurs*, **20**(3), 12–18.

Leaver, R. (1996) Continent urinary diversions: the Mitrafanoff principle. In: *Stoma Care Nursing – A Patient-Centred Approach* (ed. C. Myers). Arnold, London, pp. 166–79.

Lyon, C.C. & Beck, M.H. (2001) Dermatitis. In: *Abdominal Stomas and their Skin Disorders* (eds C.C. Lyon & A.J. Smith). Martin Duntitz, London, pp. 41–96.

Martindale (1993) *The Extra Pharmacopoeia* (ed. J.E.F. Reynolds), 13th edn. Pharmaceutical Press, London.

Mowdy, S. (1998) The role of the WOC nurse in an ostomy support group. *J Wound Ostomy Continence Nurs*, **25**, 51–4.

Myers, C. (1996) *Stoma Care Nursing – A Patient-Centred Approach*. Arnold, London.

Newey, J. (1998) Causes and treatment of erectile dysfunction. *Nurs Stand*, **12**(47), 39–40.

NMC (2006) *A–Z Advice Sheet Consent*. www.nmc.org.

NMC (2008) *The Code: Standards of Conduct, Performance and Ethics for Nurses and Midwives*. Nursing and Midwifery Council, London.

Ortiz, H. *et al.* (1993) Does the frequency of colostomy hernia depend on the colostomy location in the abdominal wall? *World Council Enterost Ther J*, **13**(2), 13–14.

Price, B. (1990) *Body Image Nursing: Concepts and Care*. Prentice Hall, New York.

Price, B. (1993) Profiling the high risk altered body image patient. *Senior Nurse*, **13**(4), 17–21.

Price, B. (1996) Practical support roles for relatives of stoma patients. *Eurostoma*, **16**, 10–11.

Pullen, M. (1998) Support role. *Nurs Times*, **94**(47).

Qin, W. & Bao-Min, Y. (2001) The relationship between site selection and complications in stomas. *World Council Enterost Ther*, **21**(2), 10–12.

Rheaume, A. & Gooding, B.A. (1991) Social support, coping strategies, and long term adaptation to ostomy among self-help group members. *J Enterost Ther*, **18**, 11–15.

Rudoni, C. & Sica, J. (1999) NaturCare from AlphaMed: the non-scented ostomy deodorant. *Br J Nurs*, **8**(17), 1168–70.

Salter, M. (1992) Body image: the person with a stoma, Part 1. *Wound Manage*, **2**(2), 8–9.

Salter, M. (1995) Guest editorial: some observations on body image. *World Council Enterost Ther*, **15**(3), 4–7.

Salter, M. (1996) Sexuality and the stoma patient. In: *Stoma Care Nursing – A Patient-Centred Approach* (ed. C. Myers). Arnold, London, pp. 203–219.

Salter, M. (1997) *Altered Body Image: The Nurse's Role*. Bailliere Tindall, London.

Schover, L.R. (1986) Sexual rehabilitation of the ostomy patient. In: *Ostomy Care and the Cancer Patient* (eds D.B. Smith & D.E. Johnson). Grune & Stratton, Orlando, pp. 103–19.

Sjodahl, R. *et al.* (1998) Parastoma hernias in relation to site of abdominal stoma. *Br J Surg*, **75**, 569–72.

Taylor, P. (2000) Choosing the right stoma appliance for a colostomy. *Nurse Prescrib Commun Nurse*, **6**(9), 35–8.

Taylor, P. (2005) An introduction to stomas: reasons for their formation. *Nurs Times*, **101**(29), 63–4.

Topping, A. (1990) Sexual activity and the stoma patient. *Nurs Stand*, **4**(41), 24–6.

Wade, B. (1989) Nursing care of the stoma patient. *Surg Nurse*, **2**(5), Suppl, ix–xii.

Wells, D. (2000) *Caring for Sexuality in Health and Illness*. Churchill Livingstone, London.

Willis, J. (1995) Stoma care principles and product type. *Nurs Times*, **91**(2), 43–5.

Winkley, M. (1998) Pre-operative fasting. *Nurs Times*, **94**(40), 56.

Wood, S. (1998) Nutrition and stoma patients. *Nurs Times*, **94**(48), 65–67.

Wyss, H. (2004) Retracted stoma and the optimisation of convex ostomy products. *World Council Enterost Ther J*, **24**(3), 26–8.

Chapter 18

Elimination: urinary

Reference material 378
Procedure guidelines: Urinary catheterization 384
Procedure guidelines: Urinary catheterization: intermittent self-catheterization 388
Procedure guidelines: Urine specimen collection: catheter (CSU) 390
Procedure guidelines: Urinary catheter bag: emptying 392
Procedure guidelines: Urinary catheter removal 392
Problem solving: Urinary catheter 393
Penile sheaths 395
Reference material 395
Procedure guidelines: Penile sheath application 396
References and further reading 397

Definition

'A catheter is a hollow tube that is used to remove fluid from, or instil fluid into, a body cavity or viscus' (Pomfret 1996, p. 245). Urinary catheterization is the insertion of a specially designed tube into the bladder using aseptic technique, for the purpose of draining urine, the removal of clots/debris, and the instillation of medication.

Indications

Male

In the male, urinary catheterization may be carried out for the following reasons:

- To empty the contents of the bladder, e.g. before or after abdominal, pelvic or rectal surgery and before certain investigations.
- To determine residual urine.
- To allow irrigation of the bladder.
- To bypass an obstruction.
- To relieve retention of urine.
- To introduce cytotoxic drugs in the treatment of papillary bladder carcinomas.
- To enable bladder function tests to be performed.
- To measure urinary output accurately, e.g. when a patient is in shock, undergoing bone marrow transplantation or receiving high-dose chemotherapy.
- To relieve incontinence when no other means is practicable.

Female

In the female, urinary catheterization may be carried out for the nine reasons listed above and for two further reasons:

- To empty the bladder before childbirth, if thought necessary.
- To avoid complications during the insertion of radioactive material (e.g. caesium) into the cervix/womb.

Reference material

Catheter selection

A wide range of urinary catheters are available, made from a variety of materials and with different design features. Careful assessment of the most appropriate material, size and balloon capacity will ensure that the catheter selected is as effective as possible, that complications are minimized and that patient comfort and quality of life are promoted (Pomfret 1996; Robinson 2001). Types of catheter are listed in Table 18.1 and illustrated in Figure 18.1, together with their suggested use. Catheters should be used in line with the manufacturer's recommendations, in order to avoid product liability (RCN 1994).

Balloon size

In the 1920s, Fredrick Foley designed a catheter with an inflatable balloon to keep it positioned inside the bladder. Balloon sizes vary from 2.5 ml for children to 30 ml. The latter is used to aid haemostasis after prostatic surgery. Large balloon catheters (30 ml) weigh approximately 48 g, causing pressure on the bladder neck and pelvic floor and potential damage to these structures (Kristiansen *et al.* 1983; Pomfret 2000; Robinson 2001). These catheters are associated with leakage of urine, pain and bladder spasm as they can cause irritation to the bladder mucosa and trigone (Stewart 1998; Robinson 2001). Large balloons are inclined to sit higher in the bladder, allowing a residual pool of urine to collect below the balloon, providing a reservoir for infection (Getliffe 1996; Pomfret 2000).

Consequently, a 5–10 ml balloon is recommended for adults and a 3–5 ml balloon for children. Care should be taken to use the correct amount of water to fill the balloon because too much or too little may cause distortion of the catheter tip. This may result in irritation and trauma to the bladder wall consequently causing pain, spasm, bypassing and haematuria. If under inflated, one or more of the drainage eyes may become occluded or the catheter may

Table 18.1 Types of catheter.

Catheter type	Material	Uses
Balloon (Foley) two-way catheter: two channels, one for urine drainage; second, smaller channel for balloon inflation	Latex, PTFE coated latex, silicone elastomer coated, 100% silicone, hydrogel coated	Most commonly used for patients who require bladder drainage (short-, medium- or long-term)
Balloon (Foley) three-way irrigation catheter: three channels, one for urine; one for irrigation fluid; one for balloon inflation	Latex, PTFE coated latex, silicone, plastic	To provide continuous irrigation (e.g. after prostatectomy). Potential for infection is reduced by minimizing need to break the closed drainage system (Gilbert & Gobbi 1989; Mulhall *et al.* 1993)
Non-balloon (Nelaton) or Scotts, or intermittent catheter (one channel only)	PVC and other plastics	To empty bladder or continent urinary reservoir intermittently; to instil solutions into bladder

PTFE, polytetrafluoroethylene; PVC, polyvinylchloride.

become dislodged. Over inflation risks rupturing the balloon and leaving fragments of balloon inside the bladder (Pomfret 2000; Robinson 2001).

Catheter balloons ought to be filled only with sterile water. Tap water and 0.9% sodium chloride should not be used as salt crystals and debris may block the inflation channel, causing difficulties with deflation. Any micro-organisms which may be present in tap water can pass through the balloon into the bladder (Falkiner 1993; Stewart 1998).

Catheter size

Urethral catheters are measured in charrières (ch). The charrière is the outer circumference of the catheter in millimetres and is equivalent to three times the diameter. Thus a 12 ch catheter has a diameter of 4 mm.

Potential side-effects of large-gauge catheters include:

- Pain and discomfort.
- Pressure ulcers, which may lead to stricture formation.
- Blockage of paraurethral ducts.
- Abscess formation (Edwards *et al.* 1983; Crow *et al.* 1986; Roe & Brocklehurst 1987; Blandy & Moors 1989; Winn 1998).

The most important guiding principle is to choose the smallest size of catheter necessary to maintain adequate drainage (McGill 1982). If the urine to be drained is likely to be clear, a 12 ch catheter should be considered. Larger gauge catheters may be necessary if debris or clots are present in the urine (Pomfret 1996; Winn 1998).

Length of catheter

There are three lengths of catheter currently available:

- Female length: 23–26 cm.
- Paediatric: 30 cm.
- Standard length: 40–44 cm.

The shorter female length catheter is often more discreet and less likely to cause trauma or infections because movement in and out of the urethra is reduced. Infection may also be caused by the longer catheter looping or kinking (Pomfret 2000; Robinson 2001). In obese women or those in wheelchairs, however, the inflation valve of the shorter catheter may cause soreness by rubbing against the inside of the thigh, and the catheter is more likely to pull on the bladder neck; therefore, the standard length catheter should be used (Pomfret 2000; Godfrey & Evans 2000; Evans *et al.* 2001).

Tip design

Several different types of catheter tip are available in addition to the standard round tip (Figure 18.2). Each tip is designed to overcome a particular problem:

- The *Tieman-tipped catheter* has a curved tip with one to three drainage eyes to allow greater drainage. This

catheter has been designed to negotiate the membranous and prostatic urethra in patients with prostatic hypertrophy.

- The *whistle-tipped catheter* has a lateral eye in the tip and eyes above the balloon to provide a large drainage area. This design is intended to facilitate drainage of debris, e.g. blood clots.
- The *Roberts catheter* has an eye above and below the balloon to facilitate the drainage of residual urine.

Catheter material

A wide variety of materials are used to make catheters. The key criterion in selecting the appropriate material is the length of time the catheter is expected to remain in place. Three broad timescales have been identified:

- Short-term (1–14 days).
- Short- to medium-term (2–6 weeks).
- Medium- to long-term (6 weeks–3 months).

Patients should be assessed individually as to the ideal time to change their catheters. The use of a catheter diary will help to ascertain a pattern of catheter blockages so changes can be planned accordingly.

The principal catheter materials are as follows.

1 *Polyvinylchloride (PVC)*. Catheters made from PVC or plastic are quite rigid. They have a wide lumen, which allows a rapid flow rate; however, their rigidity may cause some patients discomfort. They are mainly used for intermittent catheterization or postoperatively. They are recommended for short-term use only (Pomfret 1996).

2 *Latex*. Latex is a purified form of rubber and is the softest of the catheter materials. It has a smooth surface, with a tendency to allow crust formation. Latex absorbs water and consequently the catheter may swell, reducing the diameter of the internal lumen and increasing its external diameter (Pomfret 2000; Robinson 2001). It has been shown to cause urethral irritation (Wilksch *et al.* 1983) and therefore should only be considered when catheterization is likely to be short-term. Hypersensitivity to latex has been increasing in recent years (Woodward 1997) and latex catheters have been the cause of some cases of anaphylaxis (Young *et al.* 1994). Woodward (1997) suggests that patients should be asked whether they have ever had an adverse reaction to rubber products before catheters containing latex are utilized.

3 *Teflon (polytetrafluoroethylene [PTFE])* or *silicone elastomer coatings*. A Teflon or silicone elastomer coating is applied to a latex catheter to render the latex inert and reduce urethral irritation (Slade & Gillespie 1985). Teflon or silicone elastomer coated catheters are recommended for short- or medium-term catheterization.

4 *All silicone*. Silicone is an inert material which is less likely to cause urethral irritation. Silicone catheters are not coated, and therefore have a wider lumen. The lumen of these catheters, in cross-section, is crescent or D-shaped, which may induce formation of encrustation (Pomfret

Inflation/deflation valve
Foley catheter
10 ml balloon

Nelaton catheter
Drainage eyelets

To drainage bag
Collapsible section
Balloon

From irrigation fluid
Catheter
Three-way catheter
30 ml balloon

Figure 18.1 Catheter types.

Tiemann tip
Whistle-tipped catheter
Roberts catheter
Standard tip

Figure 18.2 Catheter tips.

1996). Because silicone permits gas diffusion, balloons may deflate and allow the catheter to fall out prematurely (Studer 1983; Barnes & Malone-Lee 1986). These catheters may be more uncomfortable as they are more rigid than the latex-cored types (Pomfret 2000). All silicone catheters are suitable for patients with latex allergies. Silicone catheters are recommended for long-term use.

5 *Hydrogel coatings*. Catheters made of an inner core of latex encapsulated in a hydrophilic polymer coating have recently been developed. The polymer coating is well tolerated by the urethral mucosa, causing little irritation. Hydrogel coated catheters become smoother when rehydrated, reducing friction with the urethra. They are also inert (Nacey & Delahunt 1991), and are reported to be resistant to bacterial colonization and encrustation

(Roberts *et al.* 1990; Woollons 1996). Hydrogel coated catheters are recommended for long-term use.

6   The *conformable catheter* is designed to conform to the shape of the female urethra, and allows partial filling of the bladder. The natural movement of the urethra on the catheter, which is collapsible, is intended to prevent obstructions (Brocklehurst *et al.* 1988). They are made of latex and have a silicone elastomer coating. Conformable catheters are approximately 3 cm longer than conventional catheters for women.

Research into new types of catheter materials is ongoing, particularly examining materials that resist the formation of biofilms and reduce instances of urinary tract infections. Catheters coated with a silver alloy have been shown to prevent urinary tract infections (Saint *et al.* 1998). However, the studies that demonstrated this benefit were all small scale and a number of questions about the long-term effects of using such catheters, such as silver toxicity, need to be addressed. Argyria is a condition caused by the deposition of silver locally or systemically in the body, and can give rise to nausea, constipation and loss of night vision (Cymet 2001). As these catheters are much more expensive a cost-effectiveness analysis should also be carried out before they are used more widely (Best Practice 2000; Centre for Reviews and Dissemination Reviewers 2002). Further research in this area has implied that the use of these silver alloy catheters may be beneficial when catheterization is in high-risk patients, e.g. diabetic and intensive care patients (Saint *et al.* 2000), and used for short periods, 2–14 days, with particular regard to women (Saint *et al.* 2000; Lai & Fontecchio 2002). The Cochrane Collaboration analysed all the research trials on this issue and was fairly dismissive of the quality of the data achieved; however, the implication is that the financial cost may be worthwhile in specifically selected cases (Brosnahan *et al.* 2006). The Department of Health (DH), Rapid Review Panel has identified this product as being of potential value and it is under review.

Anaesthetic lubricating gel

The use of anaesthetic lubricating gels is well recognized for male catheterization, but there is some controversy in their use for female catheterization. In male patients the gel is instilled directly into the urethra and then external massage is used to move the gel down its length, unless a conforming gel such as instillagel is used and then this is not necessary. In female patients the anaesthetic lubricating gel or plain lubricating gel is applied to the tip of the catheter only, if it is used at all. It has been suggested that most of the lubricant is wiped off the catheter at the urethral introitus so therefore it fails to reach the urethral tissue (Muctar 1991).

These differences in practice imply that catheterization is a painful procedure for men but is not so for women. This assumption is not based on any empirical evidence or on any biological evidence. Other than the differences in length and route, the male and female urethra are very similar except for the presence of lubricating glands in the male urethra (Tortora & Derrickson 2008). The absence of these lubricating glands in the female urethra suggests that there is perhaps a greater need for the introduction of a lubricant. Women have complained of pain and discomfort during catheterization procedures (Mackenzie & Webb 1995), suggesting that the use of anaesthetic lubricating gels must be reconsidered (BAUN 2000; Woodward 2005). The literature does highlight a couple of issues on the use of lignocaine gel. Firstly where and how it is applied: if not instilled for long enough, i.e. more than 4 minutes, it will have only a lubricating affect (Association for Continence Advice 2003; Tanabe *et al.* 2004); and if the gel is not instilled up the urethra it will not dilate or anaesthetize it (NICE 2003; Bardsley 2005). There is a need for caution with the use of lignocaine in the elderly, those with cardiac dysrhythmias and those with sensitivity to the drug, as there is a danger of injury to the urothelial lining of the urethra during the procedure, allowing systemic absorption of the drug (BNF 2006).

Trauma can occur during catheterization, which in turn can increase the risk of infection. Using single use lubrication gels with antiseptic properties can reduce these risks (Pratt *et al.* 2001; BNF 2006). Since there is a lack of research to clarify the efficacy of lubricating gels, practice must be based on the research evidence that is available and the physiology and anatomy of the urethra.

Infections

Catheter-associated infections are the most common hospital-acquired infection, possibly accounting for up to 35–40% of all hospital infection (Roadhouse & Wellstead 2004). The maintenance of a closed drainage system is central in reducing the risk of catheter-associated infection. It is thought that micro-organisms reach the bladder by two possible routes: from the urine in the drainage bag or via the space between the catheter and the urethral mucosa (Gould 1994; Getliffe 1995). The most common sites where bacteria may enter the system are illustrated in Figure 18.2. To reduce the risk of infection it is important to keep manipulations of the closed system to a minimum; this includes unnecessary emptying, changing the drainage bags or taking samples. Before handling catheter drainage systems, hands must be decontaminated and a pair of clean non-sterile gloves should be worn (Pratt *et al.* 2001). All urine samples should only be obtained via the specially designed sampling ports using an aseptic technique.

Urine drainage bags should only be changed according to clinical need, i.e. when that catheter is changed or if the bag is leaking, or at times dictated by the manufacturer's instructions, for example every 5–7 days (Wilson 1998; Pratt *et al.* 2001). Urine drainage bags positioned above the level of the bladder and full bags cause urine to reflux which is associated with infection. Therefore bags should always be positioned below the level of the bladder to maintain an unobstructed flow and emptied appropriately. Urine drainage bags should be hung on suitable stands to avoid contact with the

Space between urethra and catheter

Poor technique obtaining specimens

Catheter detached from bag

(ii) (i)

(iii) Poor technique emptying catheter bag

Figure 18.3 Common sites of cross-infection in a catheterized patient. (i) On catheter tip during insertion. (ii) Migration on the inside of the catheter via biofilm. (iii) Connection points of linked systems.

floor. In situations when dependent drainage is not possible, the system should be clamped until dependent drainage can be resumed (Kunin 1997). When emptying drainage bags, clean separate containers should be used for each patient and care should be taken to avoid contact between the drainage tap and the container (Pratt *et al.* 2001) (see Figure 18.3).

Meatal cleaning

Cleaning the urethral meatus, where the catheter enters the body, is a nursing procedure intended to minimize infection of the urinary tract. Studies examining the use of a variety of antiseptic, antimicrobial agents or soap and water found that there was no reduction in bacteriuria when using any of these preparations for meatal cleaning compared to routine bathing or showering (Pratt *et al.* 2001). Further studies support the view that vigorous meatal cleaning is unnecessary and may increase the risk of infection (Saint & Lipsky 1999). Therefore it is recommended that routine personal hygiene is all that is needed to maintain meatal hygiene (Pratt *et al.* 2001).

Drainage bags

A wide variety of drainage systems are available. Selecting a system involves consideration of the reasons for catheterization, the intended duration, the wishes of the patient, and infection control issues (Wilson & Coates 1996).

Urine drainage bags are available in a wide selection of sizes ranging from the large 2 litre capacity bag, which is used more commonly in non-ambulatory patients and overnight, to 350–750 ml leg bags. There are also large drainage bags that incorporate urine-measuring devices, which are used when very close monitoring of urine output is required.

There are a number of different styles of body-worn or leg bags. They allow patients greater mobility; they can be worn under the patient's own clothes and therefore are much more discreet, helping to preserve the patient's privacy and dignity. Shapes vary from oblong to oval and some have cloth backing for greater comfort in contact with the skin. Others are ridged to encourage an even distribution of urine through the bag, resulting in better conformity to the leg. The length of the inlet tube also varies (direct, short, long and adjustable length) and the intended position on the leg, i.e. thigh, knee or lower leg, determines which length is used. The patient should be asked to identify the most comfortable position. Several different tap designs exist and patients must have the manual dexterity to operate the mechanism. Most leg bags allow for larger 1–2 litre bags to be connected via the outlet tap, to increase capacity for night-time use.

Leg drainage bags

A variety of supports are available for use with these bags, including sporran waist belts, leg holsters, knickers/pants and leg straps (Roe 1992).

Leg straps

The use of thigh straps (e.g. Simpla G-Strap) helps to immobilize the catheter and thus reduce the trauma potential to the bladder neck and urethra. It is particularly appropriate for men, due to the longer length and weight of the tube being used; however, some women may also find the extra support more comfortable.

Catheter valves

Catheter valves, which eliminate the need for drainage bags, are also available. The valve allows the bladder to fill and empty intermittently, and is particularly appropriate for patients who require long-term catheterization, as they do not require a drainage bag.

Catheter valves are only suitable for patients who have good cognitive function, sufficient manual dexterity to manipulate the valve and an adequate bladder capacity. It is important that catheter valves are released at regular intervals to ensure that the bladder does not become over distended. (These valves must not be used on patients following certain operations to the prostate or bladder, as pressure caused by the distending bladder may cause perforation or rupture; in most of these instances the urethral catheter is only required for a short period of time and free drainage is the preferred method.) As catheter valves preclude free drainage they are unlikely to be appropriate for patients with uncontrolled detrusor over-activity, ureteric reflux or renal impairment (Fader *et al.* 1997). Catheter valves are designed to fit with linked systems so it is possible for patients to connect to a drainage bag. This may be necessary when access to toilets may be limited, for example overnight or on long journeys.

Catheter valves are licensed by the DH to remain in situ for 5–7 days, and this corresponds with most manufacturers' recommendations (Pomfret 1996). Little research into the advantages and disadvantages of catheter valves has been completed.

Suprapubic catheterization

Suprapubic catheterization is the insertion of a catheter through the anterior abdominal wall into the dome of the bladder. The procedure is performed under general or local anaesthesia, using a percutaneous system (Kirkwood 1999). A number of different suprapubic catheters are available. A trocar is used with all types of catheters in order to make the tract through which the catheter is threaded. Specifically designed catheters incorporate a fixing plate, which requires sutures to secure the catheter to the skin of the abdomen. For long-term use a Foley catheter is adequate. Large charrière size (18–22 ch) hydrogel coated or 100% silicone catheters are recommended (Winder 1994).

Suprapubic catheterization does offer some advantages over urethral catheterization. There is a reduction in the risk of patients developing urinary tract infection, as the bacterial count on the abdominal skin is less than around the perineal and perianal areas, although bacteriuria and encrustation still occur in susceptible patients (Winn 1998; Simpson 2001). Urethral integrity is retained and it allows for the resumption of normal voiding after surgery. Clamping the suprapubic catheter allows urethral voiding to occur, and the clamp can be released if voiding is incomplete. Pain and catheter-associated discomfort are reduced. Patient satisfaction is increased as, for some, their level of independence is increased and sexual intercourse can occur with fewer impediments (Hammarsten & Lindquist 1992; Barnes *et al.* 1993; Fillingham & Douglas 2004; Wilson 1998).

There are a number of risks and disadvantages associated with suprapubic catheterization:

- Bowel perforation and haemorrhage at the time of insertion.
- Infection, swelling, encrustation and granulation at insertion site.
- Pain, discomfort or irritation for some patients.
- Bladder stone formation and possible long-term risk of squamous cell carcinoma.
- Urethral leakage (Addison & Mould 2000).

Caring for a suprapubic catheter is the same as for a urethral catheter. Immediately following insertion of a suprapubic catheter, aseptic technique should be employed to clean the insertion site. Dressings may be required if secretions soil clothing, but they are not essential. Once the insertion site has healed (7–10 days), the site and catheter can be cleaned during bathing using soap, water and a clean cloth (Fillingham & Douglas 2004).

Intermittent self-catheterization

Intermittent self-catheterization (ISC) is not a new technique, although it has become noticeably more popular in recent years.

The procedure involves the episodic introduction of a catheter into the bladder to remove urine. After this the catheter is removed, leaving the patient catheter-free between catheterizations. In hospital this should be a sterile procedure because of the risks of hospital-acquired infection. However, in the patient's home a clean technique may be used (Wilson 1998; Lapides *et al.* 2002). Catheterization should be carried out as often as necessary to stop the bladder becoming over-distended and to prevent incontinence (Bennett 2002). How frequent this is depends on the individual but may vary from once a week, to once a day, to 4–6 times a day.

The advantages of intermittent catheterization over indwelling urethral catheterizations include improved quality of life, as patients are free from bulky pads or indwelling catheters and drainage bags, greater patient satisfaction and greater freedom to express sexuality. In addition, urinary tract complications are minimized and normal bladder function is maintained (Webb *et al.* 1990; Bakke & Malt 1993; Chai *et al.* 1995; Bakke *et al.* 1997).

Patients suitable for intermittent self-catheterization include:

- Those with a bladder capable of storing urine without leakage between catheterizations.
- Those who can comprehend the technique.
- Those with a reasonable degree of dexterity and mobility to position themselves for the procedure and manipulate the catheter.
- Those who are highly motivated and committed to carry out the procedure (Colley 1998).
- Those who have a willing partner to perform the technique (i.e. if agreeable to both).
- This procedure may be required by patients who have undergone continent reconstruction to manage initial postoperative incontinence. Patients with a Mitrofanoff reconstruction will need to perform this procedure for life (see Chapter 16).

383

Nelaton catheters are generally used to carry out intermittent self-catheterizations. These catheters are available in standard, female and paediatric lengths and in charrière sizes 6–24; as they are not left in the bladder they do not have a balloon (Winder 1995). They are normally manufactured from plastic but there is also a non-PVC, chlorine-free catheter obtainable. Some Nelaton catheters are coated with a lubricant which is activated by soaking the catheter in water for a short while; others are packaged with a lubricant gel which coats the catheter as it slides out of the packaging. These catheters are for single use only. Uncoated catheters, which require separate lubrication, may be reused by a single patient for up to a week, but the catheter must be rinsed in running water and properly dried after use; between uses it should be kept in a clean bag or container (Lapides *et al.* 1972; Barton 2000).

Procedure guidelines   Urinary catheterization

Equipment

1 Sterile catheterization pack containing gallipots, receiver, low-linting swabs, disposable towels.
2 Disposable pad.
3 Sterile gloves.
4 Selection of appropriate catheters.
5 Sterile anaesthetic lubricating jelly.
6 Universal specimen container.

7 0.9% sodium chloride or antiseptic solution.
8 Bactericidal alcohol handrub.
9 Hypoallergenic tape or leg strap for tethering.
10 Sterile water.
11 Syringe and needle.
12 Disposable plastic apron.
13 Drainage bag and stand or holder.

Procedure

Urinary catheterization: male

Action	Rationale
1 Explain and discuss the procedure with the patient.	To ensure that the patient understands the procedure and gives his valid consent (NMC 2006: C; NMC 2008: C).
2 (a) Screen the bed.	To ensure patient's privacy. To allow dust and airborne organisms to settle before the field is exposed (DH 2005a: C).
(b) Assist the patient to get into the supine position with the legs extended.	To ensure the appropriate area is easily accessible (E).
(c) Do not expose the patient at this stage of the procedure.	To maintain patient's dignity and comfort (NMC 2008: C).
3 Wash hands using bactericidal soap and water or bactericidal alcohol handrub.	To reduce risk of infection (DH 2005a: C).
4 Put on a disposable plastic apron.	To reduce risk of cross-infection from micro-organisms on uniform (DH 2005a: C).
5 Prepare the trolley, placing all equipment required on the bottom shelf.	The top shelf acts as a clean working surface (E).
6 Take the trolley to the patient's bedside, disturbing screens as little as possible.	To minimize airborne contamination (DH 2005a: C).
7 Open the outer cover of the catheterization pack and slide the pack onto the top shelf of the trolley.	To prepare equipment (E).
8 Using an aseptic technique, open the supplementary packs.	To reduce the risk of introducing infection into the bladder (NICE 2003: C).
9 Remove cover that is maintaining the patient's privacy and position a disposable pad under the patient's buttocks and thighs.	To ensure urine does not leak onto bedclothes (E).
10 Clean hands with a bactericidal alcohol handrub.	Hands may have become contaminated by handling the outer packs (DH 2005a: C).
11 Put on sterile gloves.	To reduce risk of cross-infection (NICE 2003: C).

12 Place sterile towels across the patient's thighs and under buttocks.	To create a sterile field.
13 Wrap a sterile topical swab around the penis. Retract the foreskin, if necessary, and clean the glans penis with 0.9% sodium chloride or an antiseptic solution.	To reduce the risk of introducing infection to the urinary tract during catheterization (E).
14 Insert the nozzle of the lubricating jelly into the urethra. Squeeze the gel into the urethra, remove the nozzle and discard the tube. Massage the gel along the urethra.	Adequate lubrication helps to prevent urethral trauma. Use of a local anaesthetic minimizes the discomfort experienced by the patient (Bardsley 2005: P).
15 Squeeze the penis and wait approximately 5 minutes.	To prevent anaesthetic gel from escaping. To allow the anaesthetic gel to take effect (E).
16 Grasp the penis behind the glans, raising it until it is almost totally extended. Maintain grasp of penis until the procedure is finished.	This manoeuvre straightens the penile urethra and facilitates catheterization (Stoller 1995: P). Maintaining a grasp of the penis prevents contamination and retraction of the penis.
17 Place the receiver containing the catheter between the patient's legs. Insert the catheter for 15–25 cm until urine flows.	The male urethra is approximately 18 cm long (Bardsley 2005: P).
18 If resistance is felt at the external sphincter, increase the traction on the penis slightly and apply steady, gentle pressure on the catheter. Ask the patient to strain gently as if passing urine.	Some resistance may be due to spasm of the external sphincter. Straining gently helps to relax the external sphincter (E).
19 Either remove the catheter gently when urinary flow ceases, or:	
(a) When urine begins to flow, advance the catheter almost to its bifurcation.	Advancing the catheter ensures that it is correctly positioned in the bladder (E).
(b) Gently inflate the balloon according to the manufacturer's direction, having ensured that the catheter is draining properly beforehand.	Inadvertent inflation of the balloon in the urethra causes pain and urethral trauma (Getliffe 2003: E).
(c) Withdraw the catheter slightly and attach it to the drainage system.	
(d) Support the catheter, if the patient desires, either by using a specially designed support, e.g. Simpla G-Strap, or by taping the catheter to the patient's leg. Ensure that the catheter does not become taut when patient is mobilizing or when the penis becomes erect. Ensure that the catheter lumen is not occluded by the fixation device or tape.	To maintain patient comfort and to reduce the risk of urethral and bladder neck trauma. Care must be taken in using adhesive tapes as they may interact with the catheter material (Pomfret 1996: P; Fillingham & Douglas 2004: E).
20 Ensure that the glans penis is clean and then reduce or reposition the foreskin.	Retraction and constriction of the foreskin behind the glans penis (paraphimosis) may occur if this is not done (Pomfret 2003: E).
21 Make the patient comfortable. Ensure that the area is dry.	If the area is left wet or moist, secondary infection and skin irritation may occur (Pomfret 2003: E).
22 Measure the amount of urine.	To be aware of bladder capacity for patients who have presented with urinary retention. To monitor renal function and fluid balance. It is not necessary to measure the amount of urine if the patient is having the urinary catheter routinely changed (Pomfret 2003: E).

385

Procedure guidelines *(cont.)*

23 Take a urine specimen for laboratory examination, if required (see Chapter 40).	For further information, see the Procedure guidelines: Urine specimen collection: catheter (CSU), below.
24 Dispose of equipment in a yellow plastic clinical waste bag and seal the bag before moving the trolley.	To prevent environmental contamination. Yellow is the recognized colour for clinical waste (DH 2005b: C).
25 Draw back the curtains.	
26 Record information in relevant documents; this should include reasons for catheterization, date and time of catheterization, catheter type, length and size, amount of water instilled into the balloon, batch number, manufacturer, any problems negotiated during the procedure, and a review date to assess the need for continued catheterization or date of change of catheter.	To provide a point of reference or comparison in the event of later queries (NMC 2005: C; NMC 2008: C).

Urinary catheterization: female

Action	Rationale
1 Explain and discuss the procedure with the patient.	To ensure that the patient understands the procedure and gives her valid consent (NMC 2006: C; NMC 2008: C).
2 (a) Screen the bed.	To ensure patient's privacy. To allow dust and airborne organisms to settle before the sterile field is exposed (DH 2005a: C).
(b) Assist the patient to get into the supine position with knees bent, hips flexed and feet resting about 60 cm apart.	To enable genital area to be seen (E).
(c) Do not expose the patient at this stage of the procedure.	To maintain the patient's dignity and comfort (NMC 2008: C).
3 Ensure that a good light source is available.	To enable genital area to be seen clearly (E).
4 Wash hands using bactericidal soap and water or bactericidal alcohol handrub.	To reduce risk of cross-infection (DH 2005a: C).
5 Put on a disposable apron.	To reduce risk of cross-infection from micro-organisms on uniform (DH 2005a: C).
6 Prepare the trolley, placing all equipment required on the bottom shelf. (Also see Catheter selection section, above.)	To reserve top shelf for clean working surface (E).
7 Take the trolley to the patient's bedside, disturbing screens as little as possible.	To minimize airborne contamination (DH 2005a: C).
8 Open the outer cover of the catheterization pack and slide the pack on the top shelf of the trolley.	To prepare equipment (E).
9 Using an aseptic technique, open supplementary packs.	To reduce risk of introducing infection into the urinary tract (E).
10 Remove cover that is maintaining the patient's privacy and position a disposable pad under the patient's buttocks.	To ensure urine does not leak onto bedclothes (E).

11 Clean hands with a bactericidal alcohol handrub.	Hands may have become contaminated by handling of outer packs, etc (DH 2005a: C).
12 Put on sterile gloves.	To reduce risk of cross-infection (DH 2005a: C).
13 Place sterile towels across the patient's thighs.	To create a sterile field (E).
14 Using low-linting swabs, separate the labia minora so that the urethral meatus is seen. One hand should be used to maintain labial separation until catheterization is completed.	This manoeuvre provides better access to the urethral orifice and helps to prevent labial contamination of the catheter (E).
15 Clean around the urethral orifice with 0.9% sodium chloride or an antiseptic solution, using single downward strokes.	Inadequate preparation of the urethral orifice is a major cause of infection following catheterization. To reduce the risk of cross-infection (DH 2005a: C).
16 Insert the nozzle of the lubricating jelly into the urethra. Squeeze the gel into the urethra, remove the nozzle and discard the tube. Allow 5 minutes for the gel's antiseptic and anaesthetic effect to occur.	Adequate lubrication helps to prevent urethral trauma. Use of a local anaesthetic minimizes the patient's discomfort (Woodward 2005: P).
17 Place the catheter, in the receiver, between the patient's legs.	To provide a temporary container for urine as it drains (E).
18 Introduce the tip of the catheter into the urethral orifice in an upward and backward direction. If there is any difficulty in visualizing the urethral orifice due to vaginal atrophy and retraction of the urethral orifice, the index finger of the 'dirty' hand may be inserted in the vagina, and the urethral orifice can be palpated on the anterior wall of the vagina. The index finger is then positioned just behind the urethral orifice. This then acts as a guide, so the catheter can be correctly positioned (Jenkins 1998). Advance the catheter until 5–6 cm has been inserted.	The direction of insertion and the length of catheter inserted should bear relation to the anatomical structure of the area (E).
19 Either remove the catheter gently when urinary flow ceases, or:	
(a) Advance the catheter 6–8 cm.	This prevents the balloon from becoming trapped in the urethra.
(b) Inflate the balloon according to the manufacturer's directions, having ensured that the catheter is draining adequately.	Inadvertent inflation of the balloon within the urethra is painful and causes urethral trauma (Getliffe 2003: P).
(c) Withdraw the catheter slightly and connect it to the drainage system.	
(d) Support the catheter, if the patient desires, either by using a specially designed support, e.g. Simpla G-Strap, or by taping the catheter to the patient's leg. Ensure that the catheter does not become taut when patient is mobilizing. Ensure that the catheter lumen is not occluded by the fixation device or tape.	To maintain patient comfort and to reduce the risk of urethral and bladder neck trauma. Care must be taken in using adhesive tapes as they may interact with the catheter material (Pomfret 1996: P).
20 Make the patient comfortable and ensure that the area is dry.	If the area is left wet or moist, secondary infection and skin irritation may occur (E).

387

Procedure guidelines *(cont.)*

21 Measure the amount of urine.	To be aware of bladder capacity for patients who have presented with urinary retention. To monitor renal function and fluid balance. It is not necessary to measure the amount of urine if the patient is having the urinary catheter routinely changed (Fillingham & Douglas 2004: E).
22 Take a urine specimen for laboratory examination if required.	For further information, see the procedure on collection of a catheter specimen of urine, below.
23 Dispose of equipment in a yellow plastic clinical waste bag and seal the bag before moving the trolley.	To prevent environmental contamination. Yellow is the recognized colour for clinical waste (DH 2005b: C).
24 Draw back the curtains.	
25 Record information in relevant documents; this should include reasons for catheterization, date and time of catheterization, catheter type, length and size, amount of water instilled into the balloon, batch number, manufacturer, any problems negotiated during the procedure and a review date to assess the need for continued catheterization or date of change of catheter. *Note*: beware of patient having a vasovagal attack. This is caused by the vagal nerve being stimulated so that the heart slows down, leading to a syncope faint. If it happens, lie the patient down in the recovery position. Inform doctors.	To provide a point of reference or comparison in the event of later queries (NMC 2005: C).

Procedure guidelines Urinary catheterization: intermittent self-catheterization

Equipment

1 Mirror (for female patients).
2 Appropriately sized catheters for male/female patients.
3 Lubricating gel.
4 Clean container (e.g. plastic envelope) for catheter.

Procedure

Self catheterization: female

Action	Rationale
1 Wash hands using bactericidal soap and water or bactericidal alcohol handrub.	To reduce risk of cross-infection (DH 2005a: C).
2 Take up a comfortable position, depending on mobility (e.g. sitting on toilet; standing with one foot placed on toilet seat).	To facilitate insertion of intermittent catheter (E).
3 Spread the labia (the lips at the entrance to the vagina) and wash genitalia, from front to back, with soap and water, then dry.	To reduce the risk of introducing infection (DH 2005a: C).
4 Open catheter packaging or container. If using an uncoated catheter a water-soluble lubricating gel may be applied to the surface of the catheter. If using a coated catheter pre-soak it in water to activate the slippery coating (Barton 2000).	To prepare catheter and to ease insertion (E).

5 Find the urethral opening above the vagina. A mirror can be used to help identify the urethral opening. Gently insert the catheter into the urethra, taking care not to touch the part of the catheter entering the body.	To reduce risk of introducing an infection.
6 Drain the urine into the toilet or suitable container. When the urine stops flowing slowly remove the catheter, halting if more urine starts to flow.	To ensure that the bladder is completely emptied.
7 Before removing the catheter from the urethra put a finger over the funnel end of the catheter and then remove the catheter from the urethra.	To trap urine in the catheter and prevent spillage on to clothing or the floor (E).
8 Hold the catheter over the toilet or suitable container and remove finger from the funnel end to release the trapped urine.	To prevent spillage on to clothing or the floor.
9 If using a coated catheter dispose of the catheter in a suitable receptacle.	To prevent environmental contamination.
If the catheter is uncoated and is to be reused wash through with tap water.	To remove urine.
Allow to drain then dry the outside of the catheter. Store in a dry container (as per manufacturer's instructions). These catheters may be used for 5–7 days.	To reduce risk of infection.
NB: If carrying out this procedure in hospital a new catheter must be used every time.	To reduce the risk of hospital-acquired infections (DH 2005a: C).
10 Wash hands with soap and water.	To reduce the risk of infection.

Self catheterization: male

Action	Rationale
1 Wash hands using bactericidal soap and water or bactericidal alcohol handrub.	To prevent infection (DH 2005a: C).
2 Stand in front of a toilet or a low bench with a suitable container if it is easier.	To catch urine (E).
3 Clean glans penis with plain water. If the foreskin covers the penis it will need to be held back during the procedure.	To reduce risk of infection (DH 2005a: C).
4 Open catheter packaging or container. If using an uncoated catheter a water-soluble lubricating gel may be applied to the surface of the catheter. If using a coated catheter pre-soak it in water to activate the slippery coating.	To prepare catheter and to ease insertion (E).
5 Hold penis with the non-dominant hand upwards towards your stomach.	To prevent trauma to the penoscrotal junction (E).
6 Hold the catheter with the dominant hand, being careful not to touch the part of the catheter entering the body, and gently insert it into the opening of the urethra. Advance the catheter into the bladder.	To reduce the risk of introducing an infection (DH 2005a: C).
There will be a change of feeling as the catheter passes through the prostate gland and into the bladder. It may be a little sore on the first few occasions only.	The prostate gland surrounds the urethra just below the neck of the bladder and consists of much firmer tissue. This can enlarge and cause an obstruction, especially in older men (E).
If there is any resistance, do not continue. Withdraw the catheter and contact a nurse or doctor.	

389

Procedure guidelines *(cont.)*

7 Drain the urine into the toilet or suitable container. When the urine stops flowing slowly remove the catheter, halting if more urine starts to flow.	To ensure that the bladder is completely emptied.
8 Before removing the catheter from the urethra put a finger over the funnel end of the catheter and then remove the catheter from the urethra.	To trap urine in the catheter and prevent spillage on to clothing or the floor (E).
9 Hold the catheter over the toilet or suitable container and remove finger from the funnel end to release the trapped urine.	Hold the catheter over the toilet or suitable container and remove finger from the funnel end to release the trapped urine.
10 If using a coated catheter dispose of the catheter in a suitable receptacle.	To prevent environmental contamination.
If the catheter is uncoated and is to be reused wash through with tap water.	To remove urine.
Allow to drain then dry the outside of the catheter. Store in a dry container (as per manufacturer's instructions). These catheters may be used for 5–7 days.	To reduce risk of infection.
NB: If carrying out this procedure in hospital a new catheter must be used every time.	To reduce the risk of hospital-acquired infections (DH 2005a: C).
11 Wash hands with soap and water.	To reduce the risk of infection.
12 Standing in front of a mirror is helpful for patients with a large abdomen.	For ease of observation.

Procedure guidelines   Urine specimen collection: catheter (CSU)

Equipment

1 Swab saturated with isopropyl alcohol 70%.
2 Gate clip.
3 Sterile syringe and needle.
4 Universal specimen container.

Procedure

Action	Rationale
1 Explain and discuss the procedure with the patient.	To ensure that the patient understands the procedure and gives his/her valid consent (NMC 2006: C; NMC 2008: C).
2 Screen the bed.	To ensure the patient's privacy (NMC 2008: C).
3 Only if there is no urine in the tubing, clamp the tubing below the rubber cuff until sufficient urine collects. (An access point is now available on catheter bags.)	To obtain an adequate urine sample (E).
4 Wash hands using bactericidal soap and water or bactericidal alcohol handrub.	To reduce risk of infection (DH 2005a: C).
5 Clean the access point with a swab saturated with 70% isopropyl alchohol.	To reduce risk of cross-infection (DH 2005a: C).

6 Using a sterile syringe and needle (if necessary), aspirate the required amount of urine from the access point (see Action figure 6).

Needle sampling port: insert the needle into the port at an angle of 45° and aspirate the required amount of urine, withdraw the needle.
Needleless sampling port: insert the syringe firmly into the centre of the sampling port (following manufacturer's instructions). Aspirate the required amount of urine and disconnect the syringe.

If the catheter bag or tubing is punctured it causes leakage carrying organisms with it. Specimens collected from the catheter bag may give false results due to organisms proliferating there (E).
To reduce the risk of the needle going straight through the tubing (E).

To reduce the risk of needlestick injury (NMC 2008: C).

7 Reclean access point with a swab saturated with 70% isopropyl alchohol.

To reduce contamination of access point and to reduce risk of cross-infection (DH 2005a: C).

8 Place the specimen in a sterile container.

To ensure that only organisms for investigation are preserved (Fillingham & Douglas 2004: E).

9 Wash and dry hands with bactericidal soap and water.

To reduce risk of cross-infection (DH 2005a: C).

10 Unclamp if necessary.

To allow drainage to continue (E).

11 Make the patient comfortable.

12 Label the container and dispatch it (with the completed request form) to the laboratory as soon as possible after sample is taken to allow more accurate results from culture.

To ensure the best possible conditions for laboratory tests (Fillingham & Douglas 2004: E).

Action 6   Taking a specimen. Needle sampling port.

Procedure guidelines   Urinary catheter bag: emptying

Equipment

1 Swabs saturated with 70% isopropyl alcohol.
2 Sterile jug.

3 Disposable gloves.

Procedure

Action	Rationale
1 Explain and discuss the procedure with the patient.	To ensure that the patient understands the procedure and gives his/her valid consent (NMC 2006: C; NMC 2008: C).
2 Wash hands using bactericidal soap and water or bactericidal alcohol handrub, and put on disposable gloves.	To reduce risk of cross-infection (DH 2005a: C).
3 Clean the outlet valve with a swab saturated with 70% isopropyl alcohol.	To reduce risk of infection (DH 2005a: C).
4 Allow the urine to drain into the jug.	To empty drainage bag and accurately measure volume of contents (E).
5 Close the outlet valve and clean it again with a new alcohol-saturated swab.	To reduce risk of cross-infection (DH 2005a: C).
6 Cover the jug and dispose of contents in the sluice, having noted the amount of urine if this is requested for fluid balance records.	To reduce risk of environmental contamination (DH 2005b: C).
7 Wash hands with bactericidal soap and water.	To reduce risk of infection (DH 2005a: C).

Procedure guidelines   Urinary catheter removal

Equipment

1 Dressing pack containing sterile towel, gallipot, foam swab or non-linting gauze.
2 Disposable gloves.

3 Needle and syringe for urine specimen, specimen container.
4 Syringe for deflating balloon.

Procedure

Action	Rationale
1 Catheters are usually removed early in the morning.	So that any retention problems can be dealt with during the day (E).
2 Explain procedure to patient and inform him or her of potential post-catheter symptoms, i.e. urgency, frequency and discomfort, which are often caused by irritation of the urethra by the catheter.	So that patient knows what to expect, and can plan daily activity. For adequate flushing of bladder, especially to dilute and expel debris and infected urine, if present (Fillingham & Douglas 2004: C).

3 Clamp below the sampling port until sufficient urine collects. Take a catheter specimen of urine using the sampling port.

To obtain an adequate urine sample and to assess whether post-catheter antibiotic therapy is needed (DH 2005a: C).

4 Wearing gloves, use saline to clean the meatus and catheter, always swabbing away from the urethral opening.

To reduce risk of infection (DH 2005a: C).

In women, never clear from the perineum/vagina towards the urethra.

To help reduce the risk of bacteria from the vagina and perineum contaminating the urethra (E).

5 Release leg support.

For easier removal of catheter (E).

6 Having checked volume of water in balloon (see patient documentation), use syringe to deflate balloon.

To confirm how much water is in the balloon. To ensure balloon is completely deflated before removing catheter (E).

7 Ask patient to breathe in and then out; as patient exhales, gently (but firmly with continuous traction) remove catheter.

To relax pelvic floor muscles (E).

Male patients should be warned of discomfort as the deflated balloon passes through the prostate gland.

It is advisable to extend the penis as per the process for insertion to aid removal (E).

8 Clean meatus, tidy away equipment, and make the patient comfortable.
Symptoms should resolve over the following 24–48 hours. If not, further investigation may be needed.
Encourage patient to exercise and to drink 2–3 litres of fluid per day.

Problem solving: Urinary catheter

With catheter in place

Problem	Cause	Suggested action
Urinary tract infection introduced during catheterization.	Faulty aseptic technique. Inadequate urethral cleaning. Contamination of catheter tip.	Inform a doctor. Obtain a catheter specimen of urine.
Urinary tract infection introduced via the drainage system.	Faulty handling of equipment. Breaking the closed system. Raising the drainage bag above bladder level.	Inform a doctor. Obtain a catheter specimen of urine.
No drainage of urine.	Incorrect identification of external urinary meatus (female patients). Blockage of catheter.	Check that catheter has been sited correctly. In the female if catheter has been wrongly inserted in the vagina, leave the catheter in position to act as a guide, re-identify the urethra and catheterize the patient. Remove the inappropriately sited catheter.
Empty bladder.		Check patient's volaemic status. Increase fluid intake, whether oral or by other means to discount dehydration as the cause. On insertion of the new catheter, urine will drain.

Problem solving (cont.)

Problem	Cause	Suggested action
Urethral mucosal trauma.	Incorrect size of catheter. Procedure not carried out correctly or skilfully. Movement of the catheter in the urethra. Creation of false passage as a result of too rapid insertion of catheter.	Recatheterize the patient using the correct size of catheter. Check the catheter support and apply or reapply as necessary. Nurse may need to remove the catheter and wait for the urethral mucosa to heal.
Inability to tolerate indwelling catheter.	Urethral mucosal irritation.	Nurse may need to remove the catheter and seek an alternative means of urine drainage.
	Psychological trauma.	Explain the need for and the functioning of the catheter.
	Unstable bladder. Radiation cystitis.	
Inadequate drainage of urine.	Incorrect placement of a catheter. Kinked drainage tubing.	Resite the catheter. Inspect the system and straighten any kinks.
	Blocked tubing, e.g. pus, urates, phosphates, blood clots.	If a three-way catheter, such as a Foley, is in place, irrigate it. If an ordinary catheter is in use, milk the tubing in an attempt to dislodge the debris, then attempt a gentle bladder washout. Failing this, the catheter will need to be replaced; a three-way one should be used if the obstruction is being caused by clots and associated haematuria.
Fistula formation.	Pressure on the penoscrotal angle.	Ensure that correct strapping is used.
Penile pain on erection.	Not allowing enough length of catheter to accommodate penile erection.	Ensure that an adequate length is available to accommodate penile erection.
Paraphimosis.	Failure to retract foreskin after catheterization or catheter toilet.	Always retract the foreskin.
Formation of crusts around the urethral meatus.	Increased urethral secretions collect at the meatus and form crusts, due to irritation of urothelium by the catheter (Fillingham & Douglas 2004).	Correct catheter toilet.
Leakage of urine around catheter.	Incorrect size of catheter.	Replace with the correct size, usually 2 ch smaller.
	Incorrect balloon size. Bladder hyperirritability.	Select catheter with 10 ml balloon. Use Roberts tipped catheter. As a last resort, bladder hyperirritability can be reduced by giving diazepam or anticholinergic drugs.

Problem	Cause	Suggested action
Unable to deflate balloon.	Valve expansion. Valve displacement.	1 Check the non-return valve on the inflation/deflation channel. If jammed, use a syringe and needle to aspirate by means of the inflation arm above the valve.
	Channel obstruction.	2 Obstruction by a foreign body can sometimes be relieved by the introduction of a guidewire through the inflation channel. 3 Inject 3.5 ml of dilute ether solution (diluted 50/50 with sterile water or 0.9% sodium chloride) into the inflation arm. 4 Alternatively, the balloon can be punctured suprapubically using a needle under ultrasound visualization. 5 Following catheter removal the balloon should be inspected to ensure it has not disintegrated, leaving fragments in the bladder. *Note*: steps 2–4 should be attempted by or under the directions of a urologist. The patient may require cystoscopy following balloon deflation to remove any balloon fragments and to wash the bladder out.
Dysuria.	Inflammation of the urethral mucosa.	Ensure a fluid intake of 2–3 litres per day. Advise the patient that dysuria is common but will usually be resolved once micturition has occurred at least three times. Inform medical staff if the problem persists.
Retention of urine.	May be psychological.	Encourage the patient to increase fluid intake. Offer the patient a warm bath. Inform medical staff if the problem persists.
Urinary tract infection.		Encourage a fluid intake of 2–3 litres a day. Collect a specimen of urine. Inform medical staff if the problem persists. Administer prescribed antibiotics.

Penile sheaths

Definition

Penile sheaths are external devices applied over the penis that direct urine into a urinary drainage bag from where it can be conveniently emptied. They are used by men to manage urinary incontinence.

Indications

Penile sheaths may be used to relieve incontinence when no other means is practicable or when all other methods have failed.

Reference material

Penile sheaths (otherwise known as conveens) are only to be considered once other methods of promoting continence have failed, as the promotion and treatment of incontinence should be the primary concern of the nurse (Pomfret 2003). They should be considered as a preferable alternative to other methods of continence control, such as pads which quickly can become sodden (Pomfret 2003) and cause skin problems, and catheters, which have several potential complications (Fader *et al.* 2001).

The factors that are important in the selection of the sheath is that the sheath is comfortable to wear, adheres well to the skin, does not leak, and is easy to put on and take off (Continence Foundation 2005).

Size selection

Modern sheaths come in a variety of sizes and the correct size required can be determined by measuring the girth of the penile shaft. Some devices come with a handy guide with different diameters cut into it so that the correct size can be easily determined. They are available from the manufacturers in a variety of different sizes, which generally increase in increments of 5–10 mm (Continence Foundation 2005).

Fixation

Over the years there have been a number of ways that sheaths have been attached to the penis. However, the main methods in current use follow two different approachs. First, the sheaths can be self-adhesive, in which the sheath itself has a section along its length with adhesive on the internal aspect of it that sticks to the penile shaft as it is applied. The second method is a double-sided strip of hypoallergenic or foam material applied in a spiral around the penis (which increases the surface area of the conveen adhered to the penis) and then the sheath is applied over the top.

Procedure guidelines Penile sheath application

Equipment

1 Bowl of warm water and soap.
2 Non sterile gloves.
3 Selection of appropriate penile sheaths.
4 Bactericidal alcohol handrub.
5 Disposable plastic apron.
6 Drainage bag and stand or holder.
7 Hypoallergenic tape for tethering or leg strap.
8 Catheter leg bag.

Procedure

Action	Rationale
1 Explain and discuss the procedure with the patient.	To ensure that the patient understands the procedure and gives his valid consent (NMC 2006: C).
2 (a) Screen the bed.	To ensure patient's privacy. To allow dust and airborne organisms to settle before the field is exposed (NMC 2008: C).
(b) Assist the patient to get into the supine position with the legs extended.	To ensure the appropriate area is easily accessible (E).
(c) Do not expose the patient at this stage of the procedure.	To maintain patient's dignity and comfort (NMC 2008: C).
3 Wash hands using bactericidal soap and water or bactericidal alcohol handrub.	To reduce risk of infection (DH 2005a: C).
4 Put on a disposable plastic apron.	To reduce risk of cross-infection from micro-organisms on uniform (DH 2005a: C).
5 Prepare the trolley, placing all equipment required on the bottom shelf.	The top shelf acts as a clean working surface (E).
6 Take the trolley to the patient's bedside, disturbing screens as little as possible.	To minimize airborne contamination (DH 2005a: C).
7 Remove cover that is maintaining the patient's privacy and position a disposable pad under the patient's buttocks and thighs.	To ensure urine does not leak onto bedclothes (E).
8 Clean hands with a bactericidal alcohol handrub.	Hands may have become contaminated by handling the outer packs (DH 2005a: C).

9 Put on non-sterile gloves.	To reduce risk of cross-infection (DH 2005a: R).
10 Retract the foreskin, if necessary, and clean the penis with soap and water. Dry completely and reduce or reposition the foreskin.	To remove old adhesive and ensure sheath sticks to the skin and to prevent retraction and constriction of the foreskin behind the glans penis (paraphimosis) which may occur if this is not performed (Continence Foundation 2005: C).
11 Trim any excess pubic hair from around the base of the penis.	To prevent sheath from painfully pulling pubic hair when applied (Continence Foundation 2005: C).
12 Apply sheath following manufacturer's guidelines ensuring that there is a space between the glans penis and the sheath. Squeeze the sheath gently around the penile shaft.	To prevent the sheath from rubbing the glans penis and causing discomfort and potential skin irritation and to ensure sheath has adhered to penis (Pomfret 2003: C).
13 Connect catheter bag and ensure tubing is not kinked.	To facilitate drainage of urine into catheter bag (E).
14 Dispose of equipment in a yellow plastic clinical waste bag and seal the bag before moving the trolley.	To prevent environmental contamination. Yellow is the recognized colour for clinical waste (DH 2005b: C).
15 Draw back the curtains once the patient has been covered.	To maintain the patient's dignity (NMC 2008: C).
16 Record information in relevant documents; this should include reasons for applying penile sheath, date and time of application, sheath type, length and size, manufacturer, any problems negotiated during the procedure, and a review date to assess the need for reapplication.	To provide a point of reference or comparison in the event of later queries (NMC 2005b: C).

References and further reading

Addison, R. (2001) Intermittent self-catheterisation. *Nurs Times*, 97(20), 67–9.

Addison, R. & Mould, C. (2000) Risk assessment in suprapubic catheterization. *Nurs Stand*, 14(36), 43–6.

Association for Continence Advice (2003) *Notes on Good Practice*. Association for Continence Advice, London.

Bakke, A. & Malt, U.F. (1993) Social functioning and general well being in patients treated with clean intermittent catheterisation. *J Psychosom Res*, 37(4), 371–80.

Bakke, A., Digranes, A. & Hoisaeter, P.A. (1997) Physical predictors of infection in patients treated with clean intermittent catheterisation: a prospective 7-year study. *Br J Urol*, 79(1), 85–90.

Bardsley, A. (2005) Use of lubricant gels in urinary catheterisation. *Nurs Stand*, 20(8), 41–6.

Barnes, D.G. *et al.* (1993) Management of the neuropathic bladder by supra-pubic catheterisation. *Br J Urol*, 72, 169–72.

Barnes, K.E. & Malone-Lee, J. (1986) Long-term catheter management: minimising the problem of premature replacement due to balloon deflation. *J Adv Nurs*, 11, 303–7.

Barton, R. (2000) Intermittent self-catheterisation. *Nurs Stand*, 15(9), 1–9.

BAUN (2000) *Guidelines for Female Urethral Catheterisation using 2% Lignocaine Gel (Instillagel)*. British Association of Urological Nurses Fitwise, Bathgate, Scotland.

Bennett, E. (2002) Intermittent self-catheterisation and the female patient. *Nurs Stand*, 30(17), 37–42.

Best Practice (2000) Management of short term indwelling urethral catheters to prevent urinary tract infections. *Best Practice*, 4(1), 1–6.

Blandy, J.P. & Moors, J. (1989) *Urology for Nurses*. Blackwell Science, Oxford.

BNF (2006) *British National Formulary No 51*. British Medical Association and Royal Pharmaceutical Society of Great Britain, London.

Brocklehurst, J.C. *et al.* (1988) A new urethral catheter. *Br Med J*, 296, 1691–3.

Brosnahan, J., Jull, A. & Tracy, C. (2006) Types of urethral catheters for management of short-term voiding problems in hospitalised adults (review). The Cochrane Collaboration. *The Cochrane Library*, Issue 2. John Wiley & Sons, New York.

Centre for Reviews and Dissemination Reviewers (2002) *Management of Short Term Indwelling Urethral Catheters to Prevent Urinary Tract Infections: a Systematic Review*. Database of Abstracts of Reviews of Effectiveness. Centre for Reviews and Dissemination Reviewers, York.

Chai, T. *et al.* (1995) Compliance and complications of clean intermittent catheterisation in the spinal-cord injured patient. *Paraplegia*, 33(3), 161–3.

Colley, W. (1998) Catheter care 1. *Nurs Times*, 94(23), insert.

Continence Foundation (2005) Factsheet 2: penile sheaths. www.continence.foundation.org.uk. Accessed on 25/4/07.

Crow, R.A. *et al.* (1986) *A Study of Patients with an Indwelling Catheter and Related Nursing Practice*. Nursing Practice Unit, University of Surrey.

Cruickshank, J.P. & Woodward, S. (2001) *Management of Continence and Urinary Catheter Care.* Mark Allen, London.

Cymet, T. (2001) Do silver alloy catheters increase the risk of systemic argyria? *Arch Intern Med*, **161**(7), 1014–15.

DH (2005a) *Saving Lives: A Delivery Programme to Reduce Healthcare infection including MRSA.* Department of Health, London.

DH (2005b) *Hazardous waste (England) regulations.* Department of Health, London.

Doherty, W. (2000) Intermittent self-catheterisation: draining the bladder. *Nurs Times*, **96**(31), 13.

Edwards, L.E. *et al.* (1983) Post-catheterisation urethral strictures: a clinical and experimental study. *Br J Urol*, **55**, 53–6.

Evans, A., Painter, D. & Feneley, R. (2001) Blocked urinary catheters: nurses' preventive role. *Nurs Times*, **97**(1), 37–8.

Fader, M. *et al.* (1997) A multi-centre comparative evaluation of catheter valves. *Br J Nurs*, **6**(7), 359–67.

Fader, M. *et al.* (2001) Sheaths for urinary incontinence: a randomized trial. *Br J Urol*, **87**, 367–72.

Falkiner, F.R. (1993) The insertion and management of indwelling urethral catheters – minimising the risk of infection. *J Hosp Infect*, **25**, 79–90.

Fillingham, S. & Douglas, J. (2004) *Urological Nursing*, 3rd edn. Baillière Tindall, London.

German, K. *et al.* (1997) A randomized cross-over study comparing the use of a catheter valve and a leg-bag in urethrally catheterised male patients. *Br J Urol*, **79**(1), 96–8.

Getliffe, K. (1995) Care of urinary catheters. *Nurs Stand*, **10**(1), 25–31.

Getliffe, K. (1996) Care of urinary catheters. *Nurs Stand*, **11**(11), 47–54.

Getliffe, K. (2003) Catheters and catheterisation. In: *Promoting Continence: a Clinical and Research Resource* (eds K. Getliffe & M. Dolman). Baillière Tindall, London, pp. 259–301.

Gilbert, A. & Gobbi, M. (1989) Making sense of bladder irrigation. *Nurs Times*, **85**(16), 40–2.

Godfrey, H. & Evans, A. (2000) Management of long-term catheters: minimising complications. *Br J Nurs*, **9**(2), 74–81.

Gould, D. (1994) Keeping on tract. *Nurs Times* **90**(40), 58–64.

Hammarsten, J. & Lindquist, K. (1992) Supra-pubic catheter following transurethral resection of the prostate: a way to decrease the number of urethral strictures and improve the outcome of operation. *J Urol*, **147**, 648–52.

Jenkins, S.C. (1998) Digital guidance of female urethral catheterization. *Br J Urol*, **82**, 589–90.

Kirkwood, L. (1999) Taking charge. *Nurs Times*, **95**(6), 63–4.

Kristiansen, P. *et al.* (1983) Long-term urethral catheter drainage and bladder capacity. *Neurol Urodyn*, **2**, 135–43.

Kunin, C.M. (1997) *Urinary Tract Infections: Detection, Prevention and Management*, 5th edn. Williams and Wilkins, Baltimore.

Lai, K.K. & Fontecchio, S. (2002) Use of silver-hydrogel urinary catheters on the incidence of catheter-associated urinary tract infections in hospitalized patients. *Am J Infect Control*, **30**, 221–5.

Lapides, J. *et al.* (1972) Clean, intermittent self-catheterisation in the treatment of urinary tract disease. *J Urol*, **107**, 458–61.

Lapides, J. *et al.* (2002) Clean, intermittent self-catheterization in the treatment of urinary tract disease. *J Urol*, **167**(4), 1584–6.

Leaver, R. & Pressland, D. (2001) Intermittent self-catheterisation in urinary tract reconstruction. *Br J Community Nursing Nurs*, **6**(5), 253–8.

Mackenzie, J. & Webb, C. (1995) Gynopia in nursing practice: the case of urethral catheterization. *J Clin Nurs*, **4**, 221–6.

McGill, S. (1982) Catheter management: it's size that's important. *Nurs Mirror*, **154**, 48–9.

Milligan, F. (1999) Male sexuality and urethral catheterisations: a review of the literature. *Nurs Stand*, **13**(38), 43–7.

Moore, K. (1995) Intermittent self-catheterisation: research based practice. *Br J Nurs*, **4**(18), 1057–63.

Muctar, S. (1991) The importance of a lubricant in transurethral interventions. *Urologue (B)*, **31**, 153–5 [translation].

Mulhall, A.B. *et al.* (1993) Maintenance of closed urinary drainage systems: are practitioners aware of the dangers? *J Clin Nurs*, **2**, 135–40.

Nacey, J.N. & Delahunt, B. (1991) Toxicity study of first and second generation hydrogel-coated latex catheters. *Br J Urol*, **67**, 314–16.

NICE (2003) *Full Guidelines. Prevention of Healthcare Associated Infection in Primary and Community Care. Section 3. Urinary Catheterisation.* National Institute for Health and Clinical Excellence, London.

NMC (2005) *Guidelines for Records and Record Keeping.* Nursing and Midwifery Council, London.

NMC (2006) *A–Z Advice Sheet Consent.* www.nmc.org.

NMC (2008) *The Code: Standards of Conduct, Performance and Ethics for Nurses and Midwives.* Nursing and Midwifery Council, London.

Pomfret, I.J. (1996) Catheters: design, selection and management. *Br J Nurs*, **5**(4), 245–51.

Pomfret, I.J. (2000) Catheter care in the community. *Nurs Stand*, **22**(14), 46–51.

Pomfret, I.J. (2003) Back to basics: an introduction to continence issues. *J Community Nurs*, **16**(7), 36–41.

Pratt, R.J. *et al.* (2001) Guidelines for preventing infections associated with the insertion and maintenance of short-term indwelling urethral catheters in acute care. *J Hosp Infect*, **47**(Suppl), S39–46.

RCN (1994) *Guidelines on Male Catheterisation: the Role of the Nurse.* Royal College of Nursing, London.

Roadhouse, A.J. & Wellstead, A. (2004) The prevention of indwelling catheter related urinary tract infections – the outcome of a performance improvement project. *Br J Infection Control*, **5**(5), 22–3.

Roberts, J.A. *et al.* (1990) Bacterial adherence to urethral catheters. *J Urol*, **144**, 264–9.

Robinson, J. (2001) Urethral catheter selection. *Nurs Stand*, **25**(15), 39–42.

Roe, B.H. (1992) Use of indwelling catheters. In: *Clinical Nursing Practice: The Promotion and Management of Continence* (ed. B.H. Roe). Prentice Hall, Hemel Hempstead, pp. 177–191.

Roe, B.H. & Brocklehurst, J.C. (1987) Study of patients with indwelling catheters. *J Adv Nurs*, **12**, 713–18.

Ryan-Woolley, B. (1987) *Urinary Catheters: Aids for the Management of Incontinence.* King's Fund Project Paper No. 65. King's Fund, London.

Saint, S. (2002) How to prevent urinary catheter-related infections in the critically ill. *J Crit Illn*, **15**(8), 419–23.

Saint, S. & Lipsky, B.A. (1999) Preventing catheter-associated bacteriuria. Should we? Can we? How? *Arch Intern Med*, **159**, 800–8.

Saint, S. *et al.* (1998) The efficacy of silver alloy-coated urinary catheters in preventing urinary tract infection: a meta-analysis. *Am J Med*, **105**(3), 236–41.

Saint, S. *et al.* (2000) The potential clinical and economical benefits of silver alloy urinary catheters in preventing urinary tract infections. *Arch Intern Med*, **160**, 2670–5.

Simcare (1989) *Intermittent Self-Catheterization – A Guide for Patients' Families.* Simcare, Lancing.

Simpson, L. (2001) Indwelling urethral catheters. *Nurs Stand*, **15**(46), 47–54, 56.

Slade, N. & Gillespie, W.A. (1985) *The Urinary Tract and the Catheter: Infection and Other Problems.* John Wiley & Sons, Ltd, Chichester.

Stewart, E. (1998) Urinary catheters: selection, maintenance and nursing care. *Br J Nurs*, 7(19), 1152–61.

Stoller, M. (1995) Retrograde instrumentation of the urinary tract. In: *Smith's General Urology* (eds E.A. Tanagho & J.W. McAninch). Prentice-Hall, London, pp. 160–171.

Studer, U.E. (1983) How to fill silicone catheter balloons. *Urology*, 22, 300–2.

Tanabe, P. *et al.* (2004) Factors affecting pain scores during female urethral catheterization. *Acad Emerg Med*, 11(6), 699–702.

Thakar, R. & Stanton, S. (2000) Management of urinary incontinence in women. *BMJ*, 323(7272), 1326–31.

Tortora, G.A. & Derrickson, B. (2008) *Principles of Anatomy and Physiology*, 12th edn. John Wiley & Sons, Inc., New York.

Webb, R.J., Lawson, A.L. & Neal, D.E. (1990) Clean intermittent self-catheterisation in 172 adults. *Br J Urol*, 65(1), 20–3.

Wilksch, J. *et al.* (1983) The role of catheter surface morphology and extractable cytotoxic material in tissue reactions to urethral catheters. *Br J Urol*, 55, 48–52.

Wilson, M. (1998) Infection control. *Prof Nurse Study Suppl*, 13(5), S10–13.

Wilson, M. & Coates, D. (1996) Infection control and urine drainage bag design. *Prof Nurse*, 11(4), 245–52.

Winder, A. (1994) Suprapubic catheterisation. *Community Outlook*, 4(12), 25–6.

Winder, A. (1995) Intermittent self catheterisation. *Community Nurs*, 9(2), 24–8.

Winn, C. (1996) Catheterisation: extending the scope of practice. *Nurs Stand*, 10(52), 49–56.

Winn, C. (1998) Complications with urinary catheters. *Prof Nurse Study Suppl*, 13(5), S7–10.

Woodward, S. (1997) Complications of allergies to latex urinary catheters. *Br J Nurs*, 6(4), 786–93.

Woodward, S. (2005) Use of lubricant in female urethral catheterization. *Br J Nurs*, 14(19), 1022–3.

Woollons, S. (1996) Urinary catheters for long-term use. *Prof Nurse*, 11(12), 825–32.

Young, A.E. *et al.* (1994) A case of latex anaphylaxis. *Br J Hosp Med*, 52(11), 599–600.

Chapter 19

Gene therapy for the management of cancer

401 Reference material
405 *Procedure guidelines:* Gene therapy: patient care
410 Further advice
410 References and further reading

Definition

Gene therapy is defined as a therapeutic procedure in which genes are intentionally introduced into human somatic cells (Russell & Peng 2003). By the insertion, augmentation or substitution of a functioning gene into a cell it can provide the cell with a new function, which will correct a genetic disorder (O'Connor & Crystal 2006), e.g. cystic fibrosis (Anson *et al.* 2006), or correct a malformation, e.g. primary immunodeficiency disease (Bonilla & Geha 2006), or to achieve a therapeutic effect (Gale 2003). In the case of cancer, the aim of gene therapy is to eliminate the malignant cell (Freyta *et al.* 2004).

Reference material

Normal cells contain the mechanisms to repair damage to the genetic material. Cancer can occur when such mechanisms are absent or fail to protect against genetic error through cell division. This failure allows multiplication of abnormal cells, invasion of local tissue and ultimately distant metastases (Gabriel 2004). The overall goal of gene therapy is to improve health by correcting the gene alteration in affected cells in cancers for which conventional treatments are not effective (Vassaux & Martin-Duque 2004).

The process by which genes are inserted, augmented or substituted into a cell is termed genetic modification. Genetic modification in relation to an organism means the altering of the genetic material by a method which does not occur naturally. Essentially, this means that in order for genetic modification to have occurred, there must be a change to a micro-organism's genetic material using a method not based on mating or natural recombination (HSE 2000a). Genetic modification as part of human gene therapy activities takes the form of *ex vivo* (experiments conducted outside of living organisms, e.g. as in a laboratory) or *in vivo* (experiments performed in living organisms) therapy. *Ex vivo* gene therapy is achieved by introducing the gene into the patient's cells in the laboratory and reinfusing them into the patient. *In vivo* describes the direct administration of the genetic material into the patient using an appropriate delivery system such as a virus, by methods such as injections or infusion (Gallo *et al.* 2005).

Genetic modification involves the manipulation of nucleic acid and, in particular, DNA. Molecules of DNA contain information for cellular structure and function. Every cell in an organism contains a complete set of genes, 'the genome', which are found on chromosomes (Edmunds 2004). Gene therapy involves ascertaining which gene controls which inherited feature, and then introducing, deleting or enhancing a particular trait in an organism, by altering its genetic composition. In most cases this involves extracting DNA from one micro-organism, manipulating or restructuring it and then transferring it into another micro-organism. Transfer usually takes place by attaching the gene of interest to another DNA carrier called a vector (a carrier used to transport foreign DNA across the cell membrane into the cell). The most commonly used vectors are plasmids and genetically modified viruses (Russell & Peng 2003).

For example, one of the best viruses in terms of its potential ability to deliver therapeutic genes to cancer cells is the adenovirus (Tagawa *et al.* 2006). Other vectors that are currently being used include retroviruses, such as herpes simplex virus type 1 vaccine virus and Fowlpox virus (Liu 2003). The adenovirus contains DNA and can, therefore, be manipulated to transport a genetically modified gene into any cell it invades. The virus will do no harm as long as genes conferring virulence are removed when the new genes are inserted (Hull & Chester 2002). Genetic modification of the virus means its virulence is reduced and it can no longer replicate, which ensures viral infection cannot occur. The manipulated virus is called an 'attenuated' adenovirus (Kim *et al.* 2002). Viruses are useful as vectors as they are capable of invading living cells and replicating themselves only within the target cell. For example, an adenovirus can be genetically altered in such a way that it assumes command of tumour cells but not healthy ones. The virus replicates in the tumour causing cell death; however, healthy non-tumour cells remain unaffected (Liu 2003).

There are four potential uses for gene therapy:

1 Enhancement gene transfer, which involves transferring a gene that would enhance or improve a specific desirable trait.
2 Eugenics, which is genetic engineering of society to favour certain desirable human traits (Launis 2002).
3 Somatic cell gene transfer, which places a gene in a body cell other than an egg or sperm cell. Somatic cells are the cells which make up the body of an individual, excluding the egg or sperm cells. They are the targets for gene therapy, as they cannot pass on the new trait to the person's offspring (Nippert 2002).
4 Germline cell gene transfer. Germline cells are cells in embryonic life that become sperm in males and eggs in females and which transmit genetic information to the next generation. Germline cell gene transfer makes inheritable alterations to egg or sperm cells, which can be passed onto future children (Smith 2003).

Gene therapy has the potential to be used to treat disorders caused by a defect in a single gene. This may be inherited diseases such as cystic fibrosis, or diseases such as cancer (Freyta *et al.* 2004; Anson *et al.* 2006). Gene therapy is experimental and much is unknown about the immediate and future safety and toxicity effects. The only form of gene therapy currently being used is somatic cell therapy for human clinical trials in patients with incurable diseases (Cantore *et al.* 2003).

Gene therapy has the potential to enhance useful properties or reduce unwanted properties of the genes being used. There are many different approaches to the choice of the genes. Examples include:

■ Tumour suppressor genes: such genes produce proteins to regulate the rate at which cells devide. The absence or dysfunction of the tumour suppressor genes causes cell growth to become mutated; the cells may grow uncontrollably and become malignant (Libermann & Zerbini 2006).

- Tumour susceptibility genes: the tumour susceptibility genes are a class of genes which include oncogenes, tumour suppressor genes and DNA repair genes, which predispose an organism to the development of tumours (Liu 2003).

The goal of traditional cancer treatments is to eliminate cancer cells; however, during this process many normal cells may also be eliminated. Gene therapy is a novel therapeutic approach that targets disease directly at the molecular and cellular levels and is expected to be less toxic than traditional treatments such as chemotherapy and radiotherapy. Gene therapy allows for the modification of cancer cells using gene transfer, either to enhance host immunity or to act directly on cancer cells (Liu 2003). Gene therapy should therefore improve the quality of life for the patient with cancer. However, gene therapy research is still in its infancy and it is, therefore, too early to identify benefits (Kaneda & Tabata 2006) or to predict the possible consequences of gene therapy (Woods *et al.* 2006).

Regulatory controls for gene therapy

All work with genetically modified micro-organisms (GMM), including gene therapy, is controlled by the following regulations, the majority of which focus on safety. For example:

1 The Genetically Modified Organisms (Contained Use) Regulations (HSE 2000a). These regulations implement the requirements of the EC Directive 98/81/EC on the contained use of GMM. The regulations have been made under the powers of Health and Safety at Work Act (1974) and European Directive 98/81/EC (1998). The regulations are concerned with protecting both human health and the environment and are designed to ensure the safe use and handling of GMM under containment. 'Contained use' means any operation in which micro-organisms are genetically modified or in which such GMM are cultured, stored, used, transported, destroyed or disposed of and for which physical barriers, or a combination of physical barriers with chemical or biological barriers or both, are used to limit their contact with the general population and the environment (HSE 2000a).

2 ACGM Compendium of Guidance. Guidance from the Health and Safety Commission's Advisory Committee on Genetic Modification (HSE 2000b). This compendium represents what is considered good practice by the committee. It aims to provide detailed advice about assessing risk to human health and the environment, as well as the appropriate containment measures to ensure that any risks identified are controlled. Compliance with this document is not compulsory; however, complying with this guidance illustrates good practice, which is adequate to comply with the Genetically

Modified Organisms (Contained Use) Regulations (HSE 2000a, b).

3 The Control of Substances Hazardous to Health (COSHH) Regulations and associated Approved Codes of Practice (ACoP) (HSE 2002a). Within these regulations, the biological agents covered by the COSHH regulations are 'any that have been genetically modified' (HSE 2000a, p3). These regulations require formal risk assessments and appropriate control measures to be provided in order to reduce potential health risks to those working with the genetically modified organisms. Information on the classification of genetically modified biological agents is provided within the Health and Safety Executive (HSE)'s ACGM Compendium of Guidance. Guidance from the Health and Safety Commission's Advisory Committee on Genetic Modification (HSE 2000b).

4 The Management of Health and Safety at Work Regulations (MHSWR) (1999) requires employers to ensure the health and safety at work of their employees as far as reasonably practicable. This is achieved by the production of a suitable and sufficient assessment of the risk to the health and safety of employees to which they are exposed at work, and of the risk to others arising out of their work activities.

5 The Genetically Modified Organisms (Deliberate Release and Risk Assessment – Amendment) Regulations (HSE 1997) deal with the deliberate release into the environment of genetically modified organisms to ensure adverse effects to the environment do not occur.

6 Gene Therapy Advisory Committee (GTAC) (GTAC 2000) the UK National Research Ethics Committee for Gene Therapy Clinical Research (according to the Medicines for Human Use (Clinical Trials) Regulations 2004). GTAC approve all projects that involve the deliberate introduction of genetic material into human somatic cells for therapeutic, prophylactic or diagnostic purposes, including genetically modified biological vectors such as viruses or plasmids. GTAC not only consider the scientific merits of the proposal but the potential benefits and risks (HSE 2000a). The primary concern of GTAC is whether each research proposal meets accepted ethical criteria for research on human subjects. GTAC provides advice to a wide range of agencies including local research ethics committees (HSE 2000b).

7 Other legislation that has a bearing on work with genetically modified organisms includes the Medicines for Human Use (Clinical Trials) Regulations (2004) and the Medicine Act (1971), the Personal Protection Equipment Regulations (1992), as amended 2002 (HSE 1992 amended 2002b), and part I of the Environmental Protection Act (1990).

Regulation requirements

The main requirement of The Genetically Modified Organisms (Contained Use) Regulations (HSE 2000a) is to ensure that exposure and harm to humans and the environment by GMM are reduced to the lowest level reasonably possible.

In order to do so, the regulations require organizations undertaking gene therapy to:

1 Establish a local Genetic Modification Safety Committee. All risk assessments for work with GMM must to be formally discussed and approved by the local Genetic Modification Safety Committee. It should be noted that research treatments such as gene therapy also need to be formally agreed by the health care organization's own local research ethics committee and by the Department of Health (DH)'s GTAC. The Gene Modification Safety Committee should have representation from all staff groups involved in GMM work within the organization. For health care activities this is likely to include medical, nursing, laboratory, facilities and ancillary staff representatives. The members should have sufficient depth and range of knowledge and experience to understand the risk and judge the adequacy of the risk assessment they asked to review. The conclusion of the committee should be reached by discussion and not by an individual.
2 Appoint a Biological Safety Officer (BSO) or other suitably qualified competent person to offer specialist advice on gene modification risk assessment and containment.
3 Carry out risk assessments to assess the risks to human health and to the environment.
4 Record the risk assessment and identify appropriate containment measures required.
5 Submit advanced notification to the HSE of an intention to use premises for genetic modification purposes and in certain circumstances receive HSE consent before work can start.
6 Having notified the HSE of an intention to use premises for the first time for genetic modification activity, subsequent notifications will then be dependent on the classification of activities undertaken.
7 Consideration of the recipient, the nature, activity and function of the vector, the inserted sequence, and the overall combination of host, vector and insert will need to be made before categorization can be decided. Establish the appropriate classification for the activity.
8 Implement standards of occupational and environmental safety and levels of containment appropriate to the level of risk. Whilst the contained use regulations do not include specific requirements for health surveillance for

GMM work, the MHSWR (Management of Health and Safety at Work Regulations (MHSWR) 1999) require that every employer shall ensure that his employees are provided with such health surveillance as is appropriate.
9 Identify emergency plans for dealing with adverse events involving GMM, e.g. spillage procedures.
10 Establish and implement procedures for the notification of adverse incidents associated with genetic modification activities.

The Genetically Modified Organisms (Contained Use) Regulations (HSE 2000a) and The Control of Substances Hazardous to Health (COSHH) Regulations and Approved Codes of Practice (AcoP) (HSE 2002) are enforced by the HSE. Failure to comply can lead to enforcement action and/or prosecution.

Classification

The Genetically Modified Organisms (Contained Use) Regulations (HSE 2000a) require all activities involving genetically modified organisms to be classified into one of four classes, referred to as class 1, 2, 3 or 4 (Table 19.1). Classification depends on:

■ Risk assessment factors such as the potential harmful effects of the genetically modified organisms to humans and/or the environment.
■ The characteristics of the proposed activity and the severity of any potential harmful effects.
■ The likelihood of harmful effects occurring and the level of containment required (HSE 2000a).

To assist in the determination of the appropriate classification, reference should be made to guidance contained in Schedules 3, 4, 7 and 8 of the Genetically Modified Organisms (Contained Use) Regulations (HSE 2000a). Further advice is available from the Health and Safety Commission's ACGM Compendium of Guidance, Guidance from the Health and Safety Commission's Advisory Committee on Genetic Modification (HSE 2000b).

Risk assessments

One of the most important features of The Genetically Modified Organisms (Contained Use) Regulations (HSE 2000a) is that a risk assessment must be made before any genetic modification work is undertaken. The risk assessment

Table 19.1 Classifications for genetic work as outlined in the Health and Safety Executive's ACGM Compendium of Guidance (HSE 2000b).

Class	Pathogenic to man?	Hazard to laboratory?	Transmissible in the community?	Effective prophylaxis and treatment?
1	No	No	No	Yes
2	Yes	Maybe	Unlikely	Yes
3	Yes	Yes	Maybe	Yes
4	Yes	Yes	Yes	No

process must involve the classification of the genetically modified micro-organism involved and identify the safety measures required to reduce the risk of exposure of humans and the environment to a genetically modified organism, to the lowest level reasonably practicable (HSE 2000a).

Each individual risk assessment will, therefore, vary. However, each risk assessment should identify:

- The predicted properties of the GMM to determine the hazards of the activity.
- The likelihood that in the event of exposure the activity will give rise to harm (i.e. an accident, injury, ill-health or infection).
- The appropriate containment levels required and associated safety control measures.
- The procedures for the inactivation of any waste materials produced as a result of the genetic modification activity.
- The emergency plans in place to ensure safety in the event of a foreseeable accident occurring during the activity.
- The appropriate level of training required for all personnel involved in the identified genetically modified organism activity.
- Decontamination procedures.
- Storage procedures for GMM materials.

The assessment should consider any hazards associated with the vector's pathogenicity, the inserted gene product, the area of use, and the survivability of the organism in the environment. In addition, with respect to gene therapy, the risk assessment should consider possible risks to the patients receiving the treatment, other patients and visitors in the treatment area, and to health care workers and others likely to come in contact with the genetically modified micro-organism and/or the gene therapy patient.

Once the written risk assessment has been completed (usually by the principal investigator for the study) a copy must be reviewed and approved by the local Genetic Modification Safety Committee.

Standard operating procedures

Safety operating procedures must be prepared for all areas and staff involved in the gene therapy study (HSE 2000a). This would include areas involved in preparing and administering the therapy, those involved in diagnostic investigation following the administration of the therapy, and those involved in the general care of the patient. Safety procedures for staff involved in ancillary tasks such as cleaning and waste disposal tasks should also be completed under the requirements of The Genetically Modified Organisms (Contained Use) Regulations (HSE 2000a). The safety procedure documentation must reflect the safe practices necessary for the specified gene therapy protocol and identify responsibilities for compliance in each of the work areas identified.

The structure of the safety documentation should essentially include:

- A preamble, which describes the protocol and the genetically modified organism involved and the level of risk to those potentially affected by the work activity.
- Storage and preparation procedures.
- Administration precautions for pharmacy staff.
- Safety procedures for staff involved in the care of the patient requiring gene therapy.
- Safety procedures for transportation, analysis, packaging, storage and disposal of all biological samples and specimens taken during the gene therapy treatment period.
- Waste disposal procedures.
- Action to be taken for decontamination of spills of the genetically modified organisms.
- Action to be followed for accidental exposure of staff, visitors and other patients to genetically modified organisms.
- Arrangements for staff training (HSE 2000a).

Nursing care

Potential safety issues include the immediate and long-term complications of gene therapy to the health care worker, patient, visitors and other patients. There is no current information related to the risk of health care workers to genetically modified organisms and no severe toxicity has been seen related to gene therapy (Lea 1997). However, studies are limited at this stage and, therefore, strict safety precautions must be observed at all times.

Current standards of safe practice are as follows:

1 The patient receiving gene therapy must be admitted into a single room with en-suite facilities. This room will have previously been agreed by the local Genetic Modification Safety Committee as suitable, when the protocol and risk assessment documentation was undertaken. Consideration may need to be given to the appropriateness of the ward to be used depending on the patient population and potential health issues associated with the vector used.
2 Negative pressure air conditioning is an advantage in eliminating any airborne contamination, but is not essential for Class 1 work but should be considered for higher classes.
3 Only those persons who are providing direct patient care should enter the room during the treatment period.
4 Nursing staff should observe barrier nursing principles and ensure appropriate protective clothing is worn to comply with the risk assessment, i.e. water-repellent gown, gloves, respiratory face mask, safety goggles or spectacles, plus overshoes if contamination has occurred. Risk is highest during reconstitution and administration of the therapy and less during after care (see Chapter 6).
5 Hand washing procedures should be observed before entering and when leaving the patient's room (see Chapter 5).
6 In some cases the gene therapy can be administered to patients in the outpatient setting. The therapy should be administered in a room in outpatients or a day care department that has been approved previously as suitable.

Although these patients are receiving their therapy on an outpatient basis, the restrictions and segregation that are adopted for inpatients are employed in the outpatient setting. The patient should be instructed to go directly to the designated room upon arriving at the hospital. This requirement highlights the need to protect vulnerable patients within the hospital setting.

7   While genetic modification of the vector ensures that the virulence of the vector is reduced, microbiological monitoring of blood and body fluids will be undertaken to establish when a patient is no longer excreting the vector, before barrier nursing restrictions can be reduced.

Gene therapy is still in its early stages of development (Kaneda & Tabata 2006). However, there is a need for nurses to appreciate the importance that gene therapy may play in cancer prevention and control in the future (Ghosh *et al*. 2006). Nurses must have a fundamental understanding of immunology, the administration (Loud *et al*. 2002) and the risks and potential benefits of gene therapy (Liu 2003). They must also be familiar with the gene therapy protocol to be able to provide help, support, education and advice to the patients and their families and at the same time good clinical care (Holm & Jayson 2001). Anxiety and fatigue may result from being included in a treatment trial. Patients may also experience reduced levels of concentration and therefore the nurse may need to repeat instructions and provide encouragement during the treatment period (Jenkins *et al*. 1994). Continual observations are essential to identify toxicities as soon as possible.

In a survey carried out by Jenkins *et al*. (1994), which investigated the public's perception of gene therapy, it was found that the potential benefits were thought to be cure, prevention of genetic disease, disease control, medical advance and overall benefit to humanity worldwide. However, this survey group also expressed concerns related to the risk of genetic manipulation, including the danger of error or unethical use. A more recent survey demonstrated that scientific knowledge did not appear to have an important role in determining an individual's attitude to genetic science (Sturgis *et al*. 2005). This suggests that opinion continues to be divided on the value and ethics of gene therapy (Evans *et al*. 2005).

Consent

Currently, patients in the UK enrolled in gene therapy cancer clinical trials have had advanced cancers. The GTAC, which gives approval for gene therapy research conducted on human subjects, carry out a case-by-case assessment with regard to patient group suitability. This assessment includes a review of the possible risks against the possible benefits. The GTAC needs to be convinced that the clinical management of the patient will not be impaired by the requirements of the trial (GTAC 2000).

Patients must be fully informed of the experimental nature of gene therapy treatments (Henderson *et al*. 2006). As much information as is available should be given to the patient in order for them to make an informed decision as to whether they wish to be included in the study or not (Mendell & Clark 2006). This does mean that the person obtaining consent must fully understand the trial and the control measure to prevent transmission of the genetic modification agent used for the trial (Stirling *et al*. 2004). The patient must sign a consent form (see Chapter 1).

Gene therapy options in the future

Gene therapy is a promising technique for treating disease through the modifications of genes (Byrnes 2005). Gene therapy has the potential to improve the clinical outcome of many cancers (Ohlfest *et al*. 2005). It is essential that the safety of gene therapy is a consideration by all of those people involved in the production and use of gene therapy treatments (Young *et al*. 2006). Nurses need to be familiar with current advances to provide appropriate care before, during and after gene therapy treatment (Loescher & Merkle 2005).

Procedure guidelines   Gene therapy: patient care

Preparation of patient receiving gene therapy

Action	Rationale
1 Evaluate patient's suitability for treatment.	To ensure patient's physical and psychological status is suitable for treatment and restrictions imposed by treatment (HSE 2003a: C; HSE 2005: C; Bamford *et al*. 2005: C).
2 Explain and discuss the procedure with the patient.	To ensure that the patient understands the procedure, which will enable the patient to make an informed decision regarding whether or not to participate in the study, and gives his/her valid consent (Aveyard 2002: C; Mendell & Clark 2006: R 3a; NMC 2006: C).

Procedure guidelines *(cont.)*

3 Ensure the patient is aware of the barrier nursing restrictions, and the need to remain in the room during the treatment period.	Patients who understand and have agreed the need for restrictions, are more likely to comply and be satisfied with their care (Aveyard 2004: R 1b).
4 Ensure the relatives and visitors are aware of the reasons why barrier nursing restrictions are required.	In order for relatives to be able to encourage and support the patient during the barrier nursing care (E).
5 Encourage patients to bring books and entertainment items into the room.	To prevent a feeling of loneliness and boredom (E).
6 Ensure that all personal items are washable.	In the event of contamination with genetically modified material personal items will need to be cleaned before removal from the room (E).

Preparation of room for patient receiving gene therapy

Action	Rationale
1 Place a barrier nursing sign outside the door.	To inform anyone intending to enter the room of the situation (Dhaliwal & McGeer 2005: R 1b).
2 Room should include a television and video.	To prevent the patient being bored and leaving the single room (Aveyard 2004: R 1b).
3 Room should be stocked with all necessary equipment. This will include observation equipment.	Equipment used regularly by the patient should be left within the barrier nursing area to prevent possible spread of infection (DH 2001: C).
4 Place a clinical waste bag on a bag holder in the room.	To contain all waste, including used protective clothing (DH 2006a: C).
5 Place a special waste bin with a biohazard label and a sharps disposal bin in the room.	To ensure immediate and safe disposal of special waste and sharps (DH 2006a: C).
6 Place a specimen carrying box in room.	To store and transport specimens (HSE 2003b: C).
7 Put water-repellent gowns, disposable gloves, respiratory face mask with filtering face piece protection level 3 (FFP3), safety goggles or spectacles and overshoes outside the room. Masks and goggles are only required for class 2 GMO activity or when there is the risk of airborne contamination, for example if a patient has a productive cough or a tracheostomy.	To reduce the risk of contamination to clothing, skin, eyes, nose and mouth, and to reduce the risk of inhalation or ingestion of GMO. Staff and visitors are more likely to use the protective clothing if it is readily available (HSE 1992 amended 2002b: C; DH 2005a: C).
8 Ensure hand wash basin is stocked with bactericidal detergent, paper towels and bactericidal alcoholic handrub.	To ensure hand cleaning is undertaken before and after patient contact (DH 2005a: C).

Entering the room of patient receiving gene therapy

Action	Rationale
1 Ensure staff and visitors are aware of restrictions related to entering the room.	To ensure compliance with restrictions and ensure non-essential persons do not enter the patient's room (HSE 2000b: C).

2 Visitors and staff should be restricted to essential persons only.	To restrict entry to the room to those who are aware of the need to comply to the restrictions (HSE 2000b: C; Aveyard 2002: E).
3 Pregnant staff should seek advice from occupational health staff before they enter the room.	There is no information to suggest there is a risk to the foetus, but as research is limited occupational health should undertake a risk assessment (HSE 2000b: C).
4 Young children and babies must not enter the room.	Young persons are unlikely to understand or be able to comply with restrictions (E).
5 Clean hands with bactericidal alcoholic handrub.	To reduce the risk of cross-infection (DH 2005a: C).
6 Assess the condition of the patient and the room, so that appropriate clothing can be used before entering the room. This will include: (a) Water-repellent gown. (b) Disposable gloves. (c) Respiratory face mask (FFP3) if airborne contamination is likely to occur. (d) Safety goggles or spectacles if airborne contamination is likely to occur. (e) Overshoes if contamination of the floor has occurred.	
7 Enter the room and close the door.	To reduce the risk of airborne contamination leaving the room (Kao & Yang 2006: R 3a).

Attending to patient receiving gene therapy

Action	Rationale
1 Serve meals using normal crockery and cutlery.	Nicely prepared and served food will encourage the patient to eat their food (E).
2 Dispose of any uneaten food in the clinical waste bag in the room.	Food may be contaminated by saliva (E; DH 2005b: C).
3 Wash used crockery and cutlery immediately in the ward's dishwasher.	Mechanical washing and heat will remove or kill all micro-organisms (Ayliffe *et al.* 2000: 5).
4 Place waste in yellow clinical waste bag. When half full, seal the bag with an identification tie and send for incineration.	Yellow is the recognized colour for clinical waste and this must be incinerated. To prevent contamination of the environment. To prevent overfilling of bag and potential spillage (DH 2005b: C; DH 2006a: C).
5 Label specimens and specimen request cards with a biohazard warning label, double bag in biohazard specimen carrying bag (also labelled by a biohazard warning label) and take to the appropriate laboratory in a washable, sealable box.	To warn laboratory workers of the possible risk. The box and double bag will contain spillages, if the specimen container becomes damaged (HSE 2003b: C).

Administration of gene therapy

Action	Rationale
1 Ensure only identified 'designated' staff should be involved in the administration of the gene therapy treatment.	To minimize the number of persons who could become contaminated if an accident occurs during administration of the gene therapy vaccine (E).

407

Procedure guidelines *(cont.)*

Action	Rationale
2 Staff who directly administer the gene therapy vaccine should attend the occupational health department and, if appropriate, provide a sample of blood which will be stored in a freezer.	Occupational health will ensure staff are fit to undertake this task and maintain appropriate health surveillance as required by the COSHH Regulations 2002 (HSE 2002a: C).
3 Administer the treatment using an aseptic technique. For example, intravenously, subcutaneously, directly into the tumour or via an intraperitoneal catheter (see Chapter 11).	To minimize risk of cross-infection. As far as possible the administration procedures should minimize the potential risk of airborne exposure and/or inoculation (DH 2005a: C).
4 Identify all equipment used to administer gene therapy as clinical waste and autoclave before incineration.	To comply with statutory waste disposal procedures, as there may be small amounts of gene therapy left in the administration equipment (DH 2005b: C; DH 2006a: C).

Accidental inoculation or spillage of gene therapy

Action	Rationale
1 In the event of an inoculation accident or contamination of the health care worker occurring during the administration of gene therapy, immediate action should be: (a) Make the inoculation area bleed. (b) Wash the area thoroughly. (c) Inform the occupational health department. (d) Inform the infection control officer. (e) Complete an accident/incident report form.	To ensure appropriate care is provided. An accident occurring at the time of treatment has increased significance due to the concentrated nature of the gene therapy (DH 2006b: C; HSE 2003b: C).
2 Implement the follow-up care for inoculation and contamination accidents at the time of administration, which will be included in the risk assessment documentation.	To ensure that staff are aware of appropriate emergency procedures (HSE 2000b: C).
3 In the event of a sharps accident occurring after administration of gene therapy, handle as for routine sharps accidents.	Sharps accidents that occur which are not involved with the administration of gene therapy are not as significant as those that occur when gene therapy is involved, due to the diluted nature of the gene therapy following administration (E).
4 Clear up spillages using a standard spillage kit containing chlorine releasing tablets.	To contain and remove the contamination (HSE 2003b: C).

Readmission following gene therapy

Action	Rationale
1 Barrier nursing restrictions to be reinstated, if patient is readmitted within 1 week of discharge, until the clinician can reassess the condition of the patient.	The time during which excretion of the gene therapy occurs is unknown, therefore precautions are necessary until a risk assessment shows that barrier nursing is not necessary, i.e. the patient is no longer shedding the gene therapy vector (E).

Domestic staff working with patient receiving gene therapy

Action	Rationale
1 Thoroughly prepare and clean patient's room prior to the start of the gene therapy treatment.	To provide a pleasant and safe environment for the patient (Ayliffe *et al.* 2000: E).

2 The room is only cleaned following the administration of the gene therapy, if stated in the risk assessment document.

If contamination of the environment is likely, the domestic staff should not enter the room (E).

3 The risk assessment will include information concerning the frequency with which the room is to be cleaned.

The domestic manager or supervisor needs to be informed so that the ward domestic is provided with the correct instructions (DH 2001: R1b).

4 In the event that the risk assessment states the domestic staff may enter the room, cleaning should be undertaken as for guidelines for barrier nursing (see Chapter 6).

Employing barrier nursing principles will reduce risk of contamination of staff and the environment (Lucet et al. 2005: R 1b).

5 In the event that the risk assessment states the domestic may not enter the room, the patient should be informed of this before admission and asked to undertake minor cleaning tasks. This may include flushing the toilet with disinfectant after use.

Patients expect their hospital accommodation to be kept clean by the domestic department. Prior warning that this will not occur may help prevent patient dissatisfaction and complaint. To ensure disinfection of the toilet (E).

6 Following discharge of the patient the room and bathroom should be thoroughly cleaned using a detergent/bleach solution.

To ensure any contamination is removed. Bleach is particularly useful in destroying viruses (Ayliffe et al. 2000: C).

7 Once cleaning is completed, the room can be used as normal.

Cleaning will remove any contamination, making it safe for other patients to be admitted into this area (E).

Linen used by patient receiving gene therapy
Action
1 Place used linen in a red alginate bag, then in an outer red bag.

Rationale
Red is the recognized colour for foul or infected linen. The laundry will process this type of laundry in a hot barrier wash (DH 1995: C).

Leaving the room of patient receiving gene therapy
Action
1 If wearing gloves, remove and discard them in the yellow clinical waste bag. Clean hands with bactericidal alcoholic handrub.

Rationale
To remove pathogenic organisms acquired on the gloves during contact with patient. Hands inside gloves may become contaminated following contact with the patient (DH 2001:C).

2 Remove apron, overshoes, goggles and mask, taking care not to contaminate skin or clothing. Discard in yellow clinical waste bag. Clean hands with bactericidal alcoholic handrub.

To prevent contamination of pathogenic organisms acquired during contact with patient. Hands may have become contaminated when removing protective clothing (DH 2001: C).

3 Leave room and shut the door.

To reduce the risk of airborne spread of infection (Kao & Yang 2006: R1a).

4 Clean hands with bactericidal alcoholic handrub.

Hands may have become contaminated from such items as the door handle (DH 2005a: C).

Discontinuing restrictions placed on patient receiving gene therapy
Action
1 The risk assessment documentation for the trial will state when restrictions can be discontinued. Restrictions are generally discontinued when microbiological sampling shows that the patient is no longer excreting the micro-organism.

Rationale
For some gene therapy trials it is possible to test the patient to see if they are infected. Early notification can result in a reduction in stringent barrier nursing procedures (E).

Procedure guidelines *(cont.)*

Discharge home following gene therapy

Action	Rationale
1 The patient will be discharged home when the clinician is satisfied that it is safe to do so.	Generally, restrictions are less once the patient is discharged into the community (E).
2 The patient should be asked to phone the clinician if problems occur following discharge from hospital.	It is essential that the person responsible for the research trial is available for help and advice when problems occur in the community (E).

Further advice

Health Service Executive (HSE) (2000) *A Guide to the Genetically Modified Organisms (Contained Use) Regulations.* HMSO, London. Website: www.hse.gov.uk/biosafety/gmo/index.htm.
  For advice on general policy or interpretation relating to the Contained Use Regulations 2000 refer to:
Health and Safety Executive (HSE) Health Directorate Division B, Rose Court, 2 Southwalk Bridge, London SE1 9HS. Website: www.hse.gov.uk/contact/index.htm.
  For advice on writing information leaflets for patients participating in gene therapy research, contact:
Gene Therapy Advisory Committee, Health and Safety Executive. Website: www.hse.gov.uk. Latest UK gene therapy research details available from website: www.open.gov.uk/doh/genetics/gtac.htm.

References and further reading

Anson, D.S, Smith, G.J. & Parsons, D.W. (2006) Gene therapy for cystic fibrosis airway disease – is clinical success imminent? *Curr Gene Ther*, **6**(2), 161–79.

Aveyard, H. (2002) The requirement for informed consent prior to nursing care procedures. *J Adv Nurs*, **37**(3), 243–9.

Aveyard, H. (2004) The patient who refuses nursing care. *J Med Ethics*, **30**(4), 346–50.

Ayliffe, G.A.J. *et al.* (2000) *Control of Hospital Infection. A Practical Handbook*, 4th edn. Arnold, London.

Bamford, K.B., Wood, S. & Shaw, R.J. (2005) Standards for gene therapy clinical trials based on pro-active risk assessment in a London NHS Teaching Hospital Trust. *QJM*, **98**(2), 75–86.

Bonilla, F.A. & Geha, R.S. (2006) Update on primary immunodeficiency diseases. *J Allergy Clin Immunol*, **11792**(Suppl), S435–41.

Byrnes, A.P. (2005) Challenges and future prospects in gene therapy. *Drugs*, **8**(12), 993–6.

Cantore, M. *et al.* (2003) Molecular therapy: clinical applications. Intra-arterial adenoviruses administration. *J Exp Clin Cancer Res*, **22**(4), 47–9.

DH (1995) *Hospital Laundry Arrangements for Used and Infected Linen.* Department of Health, London.

DH (2001) Standard principles for preventing hospital acquired infection. *J Hosp Infect*, **47**(Suppl), S21–37.

DH (2005a) *Saving Lives: A Delivery Programme to Reduce Healthcare Associated Infection including MRSA.* Department of Health, London.

DH (2005b) *Hazardous waste (England) regulations.* Department of Health, London.

DH (2006a) *Environment and Sustainability. Health Technical Memorandum 07-01: Safe Management of Healthcare Waste.* Department of Health, London.

DH (2006b) *Immunisation against infectious disease.* Department of Health, London.

Dhaliwal, J. & McGeer, A. (2005) Does isolation prevent the spread of methocillin-resistant *Staphylococcus aureus*? *CMAJ*, **172**(7), 875.

Edmunds, S.C. (2004) What are DNA and RNA? In: *The Biology of Cancer*, Part II, Chapter 5 (ed. J. Gabriel). Whurr Publishers, London, pp. 50–8.

Environmental Protection Act (1990) HMSO, London.

European Council Regulations (1993) No. (EEC) 2309/93. HMSO, London.

European Directive (1998) *The Contained Use of Genetically Modified Microorganisms. 98(81)EC (Amending Directive 90(219)EEC).* European Community, Brussels.

Evans, M.D., Kelley, J. & Zanjani, E.D. (2005) The ethics of gene therapy and abortion: public opinion. *Fetal Diagn Ther*, **20**(3), 223–34.

Freyta, S.O. *et al.* (2004) Gene therapy strategies to enhance the effectiveness of cancer radiotherapy. *Curr Opin Mol Ther*, **6**(5), 513–24.

Gabriel, J. (2004) What is cancer? In: *The Biology of Cancer* (ed. J. Gabriel). Whurr Publishers, London, pp. 3–10.

Gale, D.M. (2003) Molecular targets in cancer therapy. *Semin Oncol Nurs*, **19**(3), 193–205.

Gallo, P. *et al.* (2005) Adenovirus as vehicle for anticancer genetic immunotherapy. *Gene Ther Suppl*, **1**, S84–91.

Ghosh, S.S., Gopinath, P. & Ramesh, A. (2006) Adenoviral vectors: a promising tool for gene therapy. *Appl Biochem Biotechnol*, **133**(1), 9–29.

GTAC (2000) *Report of the Adenoviral Working Party.* Department of Health, London.

Health and Safety at Work Act etc. (1974) HMSO, London.

Henderson, G.E. *et al.* (2006) Therapeutic misconception in early phase gene transfer trials. *Soc Sci Med*, **62**(1), 239–53.

Holm, S. & Jayson, G. (2001) What do patients, their relatives and medical staff know about genetic therapy? *Bull Med Ethics*, **193**, 13–19.

HSE (1992) A short guide to the personal protective equipment at work regulations 1992. HSE Books, London.

HSE (1992 amended 2002b) *Personal Protection Equipment Regulations.* HSE Books, London.

HSE (1997) *Genetically Modified Organisms (Deliberate Release and Risk Assessment – Amendment) Regulations.* HMSO, London.

HSE (2000a) *The Genetically Modified Organisms (Contained Use) Regulations.* HMSO, London.

HSE (2000b) *ACGM Compendium of Guidance, Guidance from the Health and Safety Commission's Advisory Committee on Genetic Modification*, HSE Books, London.

HSE (2002a) *The Control of Substances Hazardous to Health (COSHH) Regulations and approved Codes of Practice ACoP*. HMSO, London.

HSE (2003a) *Five Steps to Risk Assessment*. HSE Books, London.

HSE (2003b) *Safe Working and the Prevention of Infection in Clinical Laboratories and Similar Facilities*. HSE Books, Norwich.

Hull, D. & Chester, M. (2002) Gene therapy trials: a patient pathway. *Nurs Stand*, 17(3), 39–42.

Jenkins J., Wheeler, V. & Albright, L. (1994) Gene therapy for cancer. *Cancer Nurs*, 17(6), 447–56.

Kaneda, Y. & Tabata, Y. (2006) Non-viral vectors for cancer therapy. *Cancer Sci*, 97(5), 348–54.

Kao, P.H. & Yang, R.J. (2006) Virus diffusion in isolation rooms. *J Hosp Infect*, 62(3), 338–45.

Kim, J. *et al.* (2002) Evaluation of E1B gene-attenuated replicating adenoviruses for cancer gene therapy. *Cancer Gene Ther*, 9(9), 725–36.

Launis, V. (2002) Human gene therapy and the slippery slope argument. *Med Health Care Philos*, 5(2), 169–79.

Lea, D.H. (1997) Gene therapy: current and future implications for oncology nursing practice. *Semin Oncol Nurs*, 13(2), 115–22.

Libermann, T.A. & Zerbini, L.F. (2006) Targeting transcription factors for cancer gene therapy. *Curr Gene Ther*, 6(1), 17–33.

Liu, K. (2003) Breakthroughs in cancer gene therapy. *Semin Oncol Nurs*, 19(3), 217–26.

Loescher, L.J. & Merkle, C.J. (2005) The interface of genomic technologies and nursing. *J Nurs Scholarsh*, 37(2), 111–19.

Loud J.T. *et al.* (2002) Applications of advances in molecular biology and genomics to clinical cancer care. *Cancer Nurs*, 25(2), 110–22.

Lucet, J.C. *et al.* (2005) Successful long term program for controlling methicillin-resistant *Staphylococcus aureus* in intensive care units. *Intensive Care Med*, 31(8), 1051–7.

Management of Health and Safety at Work Regulations (MHSWR) (1999) HMSO, London.

Medicine Act (1971) HMSO, London.

Medicines for Human Use (Clinical Trials) Regulations (2004) HMSO, London.

Mendell, J.R. & Clark, K.R. (2006) Risks, benefits, and consent in the age of gene therapy. *Neurology*, 66(7), 964–5.

NICE (2003) *Infection Control. Prevention of Healthcare-associated Infection in Primary and Community Care*. National Institute for Health and Clinical Excellence, London.

Nippert, I. (2002) The pros and cons of human therapeutic cloning in the public debate. *J Biotechnol*, 98(1), 53–60.

NMC (2006) *A–Z Advice Sheet Consent*. www.nmc.org.

O'Connor, T.P. & Crystal, R.G. (2006) Genetic medicine: treatment strategies for hereditary disorders. *Nat Rev Genet*, 7(4), 261–74.

Ohlfest, J.R., Freese, A.B. & Largaespada, D.A. (2005) Nonviral vectors for cancer gene therapy: prospects for integrating vectors and combination therapies. *Curr Gene Ther*, 5(6), 629–41.

Personal Protection Equipment Regulations (1992) HMSO, London.

Russell, S.J. & Peng, K.W. (2003) Primer on medical genomics. Part X: gene therapy. *Mayo Clin Proc*, 78(11), 1283–370.

Smith, K.R. (2003) Gene therapy: theretical and bioethical concepts. *Arch Med Res*, 34(4), 247–68.

Stirling, B., Littlejohn, P. & Willbond, M.L. (2004) Nurses and the control of infectious disease. Understanding epidemiology and disease transmission is vital to nursing care. *Can Nurse*, 100(9), 16–20.

Sturgis, P., Cooper, H. & Fife-Schaw, C. (2005) Attitudes to biotechnology: estimating the opinions of a better-informed public. *New Genet Soc*, 24(1), 31–56.

Tagawa, M. *et al.* (2006) Virology and immunology-based gene therapy for cancer. *Cancer Immunol Immunother*, 55(11), 1420–5.

Vassaux, G. & Martin-Duque, P. (2004) Use of suicide genes for cancer gene therapy: study of the different approaches. *Expert Opin Biol Ther*, 4(4), 519–30.

Wilson, J. (2006) *Infection Control in Clinical Practice*. Bailliere Tindall, London.

Woods, N.B. *et al.* (2006) Gene therapy: therapeutic gene causing lymphoma. *Nature*, 440(7088), 1123.

Young, L.S. *et al.* (2006) Viral gene therapy strategies: from basic science to clinical application. *J Pathol*, 208(2), 299–318.

Chapter 20

Haematological procedures

413 Reference material
414 Bone marrow procedures
417 Apheresis procedures (donor or therapeutic)
419 *Procedure guidelines:* Bone marrow aspiration and trephine biopsy
422 *Procedure guidelines:* Bone marrow harvest
425 *Problem solving:* Bone marrow harvest
426 References and further reading

Definition

Haematological procedures include bone marrow procedures and apheresis procedures:

- *Bone marrow procedures:* involve the removal of haematopoietic tissue from the medullary cavity of bone. The tissue is removed by either aspiration or biopsy (Perkins 2003). Needles with a range of gauges may be used and most have a removable introducer (which prevents plugging of the needle before aspiration) and a stylet that may be used to express the bone marrow biopsy sample. Some models, primarily used for sternal bone marrow aspiration procedures, have adjustable guards that limit the extent of needle penetration (Perkins 2003).
- *Apheresis:* may be described as a process by which whole blood is removed from a patient or donor, then separated into component parts to allow a desired component to be collected, while the remainder is returned to the patient or donor (Corbin *et al.* 2003). Separation of the blood components can be accomplished by filtration, centrifugation, or a combination of both. Filtration takes advantage of differences in particle size to separate blood plasma from the cellular elements. Centrifugation uses differences in specific gravity to separate and isolate blood components (Burgstaler 2003). Blood components are collected or exchanged for donor and/or therapeutic purposes.

Reference material

Bone marrow

The maturation of blood cells is termed haematopoiesis (Abboud & Lichtman 2005) and takes place in the bone marrow. At 5–9 months of foetal life, the bone marrow, liver and spleen produce the cellular components of blood. At birth the marrow of all bones is involved in haematopoiesis. During childhood there is some replacement of the haematopoietic tissue (red marrow) with fatty tissue (yellow marrow). As adults, the only sites of haematopoiesis are bones such as the pelvis and sternum (Sieff & Nathan 2000). Yellow marrow has the ability to revert to haematopoietic tissue in certain circumstances such as haemolytic anaemia (Abboud & Lichtman 2005).

Stem cells

All mature blood cells originate from one precursor cell called a stem cell. The stem cell has the ability for unlimited self-renewal (produce more stem cells) and differentiation (develop into any of the mature blood cell types) (Figure 20.1). The self-renewal and differentiation of stem cells is regulated by acidic glycoprotein molecules called haematopoietic growth factors (Traynor 2006). Some growth factors are found naturally in the plasma but others are only detectable following an inflammatory event or other stimulus (Hoffbrand *et al.* 2001). Growth factors

413

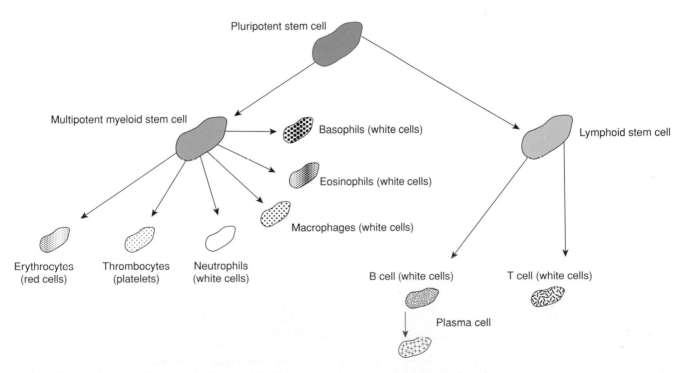

Figure 20.1 Diagrammatic representation of the stem cell and the blood cells that arise from it.

include granulocyte-colony stimulating factor (G-CSF), erythropoietin and thrombopoietin (Traynor 2006).

The first step in the differentiation process is a division of the stem cell into two main cell lineages: myeloid and lymphoid. The myeloid progenitor cell divides into red blood cells, platelets, granulocytes (neutrophils, eosinophils and basophils) and monocytes (macrophages). The lymphoid progenitor cell matures into lymphocytes (T and B). Lymphocytes, granulocytes and monocytes are all white cells (Bondurant & Koury 2003). The main function of the blood cells and the haematological values for normal adults are listed in Table 20.1.

Plasma

Plasma gives blood its liquid property to allow it to flow through the vascular system. If the cellular components of whole blood were allowed to sediment in a test tube, around 54% of the volume would be the straw-coloured plasma (Traynor 2006). Plasma consists of water, plasma proteins (e.g. fibrinogen, albumin, globulins), electrolytes (e.g. sodium, potassium, chloride) and metabolites (e.g. urea, creatinine, cholesterol). The functions of these elements include clotting, maintaining blood pressure, controlling plasma viscosity, antibody formation and regulating intra/extracellular pressure.

Bone marrow procedures

Bone marrow procedures include the following:

- Aspiration.
- Trephine biopsy.
- Harvest.

Aspiration and trephine biopsy

Bone marrow examination usually involves two separate, but interrelated, specimens. The first is a cytologic preparation of bone marrow cells obtained by aspiration of the marrow and a smear of the cells (Perkins 2003). The aspiration specimen is used to assess cell morphology (Longo 2005). The second specimen is a trephine biopsy of the bone and associated marrow, to assess overall marrow architecture, bone marrow cellularity, fibrosis, infections or infiltrative diseases (Longo 2005). Diagnosis and management of many haematologic diseases depend on examination of the bone marrow (Perkins 2003).

Common sites for bone marrow examination

Several sites may be used for bone marrow aspiration and biopsy (Figure 20.2). The site selected may reflect the normal distribution of bone marrow in relation to the age of the patient. Younger children may have marrow examinations from the anterior medial tibial area, whereas adult marrow is best sampled from the sternum at the second intercostal space or from either the anterior or posterior iliac crest area

Table 20.1 The main function of blood cells and the haematological values for normal adults (Bain 2004, Hoffbrand *et al.* 2001, Hughes-Jones *et al.* 2004, Turgeon 1999, Weatherall 2000).

Blood cell type and function	Haematological value
Red blood cells (erythrocytes): Transport oxygen from the lungs to the tissues and return carbon dioxide from the tissues to be expelled by the lungs	Men: 15 ± 2 g/dl Women: 14 ± 2 g/dl
Platelets (thrombocytes): The formation of mechanical plugs during the normal haemostatic response to vascular injury	$130–400 \times 10^9/l$
White blood cells (leucocytes): A group of diverse cells that work together to protect the body from disease and to provide immunity.	$7.0 \pm 3.0 \times 10^9/l$
White blood cell differential: **Neutrophils:** Attracted to sites of infection (chemotaxis); ingests micro-organisms (phagocytosis) and destroys them	$2.0–7.0 \times 10^9/l$
Eosinophil: Same function as the neutrophil; in addition, helps control parasitic infections; has a role in allergic responses	$0.04–0.4 \times 10^9/l$
Basophil: Has a role in immediate hypersensitivity reactions, allergic and inflammatory responses and in the control of parasitic infections.	$0.02–0.1 \times 10^9/l$
T-lymphocyte: Attacks cells bearing foreign antigens and antibody-coated cells; can help or suppress B cells (part of cell-mediated immunity)	$1.0–3.0 \times 10^9/l$
B-lymphocyte: Matures into a plasma cell, which secretes antibodies (humoral immunity).	
Natural killer lymphocyte: Attacks foreign cells and tumour cells (part of cell-mediated immunity)	
Monocyte (differentiate to macrophage in tissues): Has a role in chemotaxis, phagocytosis, killing of some microorganisms (fungi and mycobacteria), release of IL-1 and TNF which stimulate bone marrow stromal cells to produce GM-CSF, G-CSF, M-CSF and IL-6	$0.2–1.0 \times 10^9/l$

Ideal location

Posterior iliac crests   Anterior iliac crests   Sternum

Figure 20.2 Common sites for bone marrow examination, arranged in order of preference. Normally, only aspirations and not biopsies are done on the sternum because of its small size and proximity to vital organs.

(Perkins 2003). Sternal marrows do not allow a trephine biopsy to be performed, and several possible complications, including haemorrhage and pericardial tamponade, may occur if the inner table of the sternum is penetrated by the needle at areas other than the second intercostal space (Perkins 2003). In contrast, little morbidity is associated with iliac crest aspiration and biopsy, and the posterior iliac crest is the most common site for bone marrow examinations. The anterior iliac crest may be used if previous radiation, surgery, or patient discomfort does not allow a posterior approach (Perkins 2003).

Method

The specimens are collected as follows:

- *Aspiration*: an aspirate needle is inserted through the skin into the bone marrow. Once the needle is in the marrow cavity, a syringe is attached and used to aspirate liquid bone marrow. This is then spread onto slides (Hoffbrand *et al.* 2001).
- *Trephine*: a trephine needle is inserted and anchored in the bony cortex. The needle is then advanced with a twisting motion and rotated to obtain a solid piece of bone marrow. This piece is then removed along with the needle. A trephine biopsy provides a solid core of bone including marrow and is examined as a histological specimen after fixation in formalin, decalcification and sectioning (Hoffbrand *et al.* 2001).

Indications

There are a number of indications for performing a bone marrow examination (Table 20.2). These include further work-up of haematologic abnormalities observed in the

Table 20.2 Comparison of bone marrow aspiration and trephine biopsy (Hoffbrand *et al.* 2001, Perkins 2003, Longo 2005).

	Aspiration	**Trephine**
Site	Posterior/anterior iliac crest or sternum (anterior medial tibial area in children)	Posterior/anterior iliac crest
Result available	1–2 hours	1–7 days (according to decalcification method)
Main indications	Hypoproliferative or unexplained anaemia, leukopaenia, or thrombocytopaenia, suspected leukaemia or myeloma or marrow defect, evaluation of iron stores, work-up of some cases of fever of unknown origin	Performed in addition to aspiration for pancytopenia (aplastic anaemia), metastatic tumour, granulomatous infection (e.g. mycobacteria, brucellosis, histoplasmosis), myelofibrosis, lipid storage disease (e.g. Gaucher's, Niemann–Pick), any case with 'dry tap' on aspiration; evaluation of marrow cellularity
Special tests	Histochemical staining (leukaemias), cytogenetic studies (leukaemias, lymphomas), microbiology (bacterial, mycobacterial, fungal cultures), Prussian blue (iron) stain (assess iron stores, diagnosis of sideroblastic anaemias)	Histochemical staining (e.g. acid phosphatase for metastatic prostate carcinoma), immunoperoxidase staining (e.g. immunoglobulin or cell surface marker detection in multiple myeloma, leukaemia, or lymphoma; lysozyme detection in monocytic leukemia), reticulin staining (increased in myelofibrosis), microbiologic staining (e.g. acid-fast staining for mycobacteria)

peripheral blood smear, evaluation of primary bone marrow tumours, staging for bone marrow involvement by metastatic tumours, assessment of infectious disease processes including fever of unknown origin, and evaluation of metabolic storage diseases (Perkins 2003). Before a bone marrow examination is carried out, clear diagnostic goals about the information to be obtained from the procedure should be defined. Before the procedure, it should be decided whether any special studies are needed so that all the necessary specimens may be collected and handled correctly (Perkins 2003).

Special considerations

In most cases, bone marrow aspiration and biopsy may be carried out with little risk of patient discomfort, provided adequate local anaesthesia is used. Patients may describe a 'dragging sensation' during the actual aspiration procedure, even when the site is numb. Apprehensive patients may be sedated before the procedure, but this is usually not necessary (Perkins 2003).

Contraindications

The only absolute reason to avoid performing a bone marrow examination is the presence of coagulation disorders (unless correctable), which may lead to serious bleeding after the procedure. If there is a skin or soft tissue infection over the hip, a different site should be chosen (Vergidis 2004).

Complications

While mild soreness lasting 12–24 hours is common after a bone marrow examination, serious complications are rare (Vergidis 2004). Haemorrhage is the most common and most serious adverse event experienced by patients (Bain 2006). The major risk factors for haemorrhage, in order of frequency, are diagnosis of a myeloproliferative disorder, aspirin treatment, other putative platelet dysfunction, and thrombocytopenia (Bain 2005). Other complications may include:

- *Cardiac tamponade*: the actual risks associated with a sternal puncture are extremely small but penetration of the bone and damage to underlying structures is possible as the sternum is only approximately 1 cm thick in adults (Perkins 2003). The use of a guarded needle helps in preventing too deep an insertion.
- *Infection*: particularly in the neutropenic patient.
- *Bone fractures*: particularly in small children owing to the pressure exerted.

Although adverse events after trephine biopsies and bone marrow aspirates are rare, they can have considerable impact on individual patients (Bain 2005).

Post-procedural care

The following information and advice may be given to patients:

- *Wound care:* The patient should be instructed to check the site frequently and to report any bleeding (Vergidis 2004). It is routine practice to advise the patient to keep the dressing dry for 24 hours. The patient may then remove the dressing and wash as normal.
- *Pain:* The patient should be advised that minor discomfort at the biopsy site may be dealt with by simple analgesia such as paracetamol (Provan *et al.* 2004).
- *Sedation:* If the patient has had sedation, they must return to pre-procedure functional status before discharge. They should be accompanied by a responsible adult for at least 24 hours. They should receive written instructions including a contact number in the instance of an adverse event (e.g. chest pain, vomiting) and advice on not driving or making decisions or signing documents or using alcohol for 24 hours.

Bone marrow harvest

Traditionally the bone marrow was used as the primary source of stem cells for transplantation (Richardson & Atkinson 2006). One method of harvesting these stem cells is to aspirate them directly from the marrow with a bone marrow harvest needle and syringe. A volume of 800–1000 ml is aspirated from the posterior iliac crest (in order to acquire sufficient cells per kilogram of the recipient's body weight) (Outhwaite 2000). The marrow is either frozen and stored or given fresh to the recipient (Richardson & Atkinson 2006).

Indications

Every year in Britain about 24 500 people are diagnosed with a haematological malignancy such as leukaemia, lymphoma or myeloma (Leukaemia Research Fund 2005). A stem cell transplant is one possible treatment option for these diseases (Atkinson 2005). A stem cell transplant is a technique used with the aim of replacing a patient's own diseased bone marrow, with healthy stem cells. Before the patient receives the stem cells, they receive a combination of chemotherapy and radiation to destroy their own bone marrow. The healthy stem cells are either collected from a patient when in remission (autologous) or from a donor (allogeneic) (Richardson & Atkinson 2006). The stem cells are then introduced into the patient's blood stream much in the same manner as a blood transfusion. If the donated stem cells 'engraft', they begin producing normal blood cells (Atkinson 2005).

Special considerations

Bone marrow harvests are performed under general anaesthetic because:

- The procedure may last for approximately 1 hour compared with the 15–30 minutes for an aspiration and biopsy.

- Multiple puncture sites are used.
- The procedure may be painful.

Alternate sources of stem cells

With scientific advances, it is now possible to harvest stem cells from the blood stream by means of apheresis. They can be 'mobilized' into the peripheral blood following treatment with cytotoxic chemotherapy and/or the administration of the haematopoietic growth factor G-CSF. The use of peripheral blood stem cells (PBSCs) has superseded bone marrow in many transplant centres (Richardson & Atkinson 2006). Exact protocols vary according to underlying disease, treatment regimens, local practice and the type of stem cell donor.

Haematopoietic stem cells can also be obtained from the umbilical cord. Cord blood transplantation remains a specialized procedure more relevant for some areas of transplantation than others, e.g. in the paediatric setting (Richardson & Atkinson 2006).

The protocol for harvesting these alternate sources of stem cells is beyond the scope of this chapter.

Complications of the bone marrow harvest

The complications of bone marrow harvests are rare, however it remains a significant procedure and not without physical risk or psychological consequences (Blume & Amylon 2004) including:

- The general anaesthesia and associated morbidity (Rosenmayr *et al.* 2003).
- Anaemia, with resultant fatigue, due to the large amount of bone marrow that may be aspirated (Rosenmayr *et al.* 2003).
- The potential for infection at the aspiration sites (Rosenmayr *et al.* 2003).
- The potential for bone, nerve or other tissue damage at the aspiration sites (Rosenmayr *et al.* 2003).
- The possible need for allogeneic blood units and the associated transfusion risks (Rosenmayr *et al.* 2003) (see Chapter 43).

Post-procedural care

When stable, donors are transferred to the ward for further recovery, postoperative advice, medication and discharge. Guidelines to be given to donors are outlined in Table 20.3.

Donors should also be informed that it is normal to experience some pain, bruising and stiffness, feel more tired than usual and run a low-grade fever during the first week after donation. However, all donors should receive written instructions to contact the hospital if they experience any of the following symptoms (NMDP 2006):

- Temperature of 38°C or higher.
- Increased redness, bleeding, swelling, drainage or pain at the collection area.

Table 20.3 Guidelines to be given to bone marrow harvest donors post-procedure (NMDP 2006).

- The discomfort at the harvest site should resolve in about 1 week.
- Analgesia should be taken as directed.
- Aspirin should be avoided during the first week after the donation unless instructed by the medical team.
- The harvest site should be checked daily for bleeding or increasing erythema.
- The harvest site should be kept dry the night after the procedure.
- Bandages should be removed 24 hours after surgery, and replaced with an adhesive dressing.
- Some wound drainage is expected.
- Showers rather than baths should be taken for the first 2–3 days to decrease the risk of infection.
- The adhesive dressings should be changed daily after a shower until the wounds have healed.
- If bleeding occurs, firm pressure should be applied for 5 minutes, followed by an ice pack. The patient should be advised that if the bleeding does not stop after 10 minutes of constant direct pressure, they should contact the hospital.
- It is common to experience 'hard lumps' at the harvest sites where the needles were inserted. These may take a few weeks to resolve.

- Muscle weakness or severe headache within 2 weeks of donation.
- Pain more than 14 days after the donation.

Measures should be taken to alleviate and correct any adverse side-effects, e.g. more effective pain control, nerve assessment, platelet infusion or antibiotic administration. The donor should also be referred to the appropriate members of the multidisciplinary team as necessary.

Apheresis procedures (donor or therapeutic)

The basic steps in apheresis are: (i) the separation of blood components; and (ii) the removal of the desired component(s) using an on-line automated system. The ability of various techniques and equipment to carry out these basic steps determines collection efficiency and product purity (Burgstaler 2003).

Apheresis is used for a number of donor and/or therapeutic purposes. A therapeutic procedure is when a blood component is removed from a patient to decrease the amount of defective cells or deplete a disease mediator (GambroBCT 2005). A donor procedure is when a blood component is removed (e.g. stem cells, lymphocytes, platelets) to be used for therapeutic purposes (e.g. peripheral blood stem cell transplant, donor lymphocyte infusion, platelet transfusion). Some apheresis applications and indications are outlined in Table 20.4.

Table 20.4 Apheresis applications and indications (Foss 2003; Strauss 2003; GambroBCT 2005).

Applications	Indications
Therapeutic apheresis	
Plasma exchange: Removal of a patient's own plasma and replacement with appropriate fluids, e.g. albumin, fresh frozen plasma. This is in order to remove disease mediators including: <ul><li>Alloantibodies</li><li>Autoimmune antibodies</li><li>Antigen-antibody complexes</li><li>Abnormal or increased amounts of plasma protein</li><li>Very high cholesterol levels</li><li>High levels of plasma metabolic waste products</li><li>Plasma bound poisons or drugs</li></ul>	<ul><li>Thrombotic thrombocytopenia purpura</li><li>Guillain–Barré syndrome</li><li>Myasthenia gravis</li></ul>
Red blood cell exchange: Removal of large volumes of patient red blood cells and replacement with normal donor red blood cells	<ul><li>Sickle cell disease</li><li>Malaria</li><li>Babesiosis</li></ul>
Cellular depletion: Rapid removal of greatly elevated number of cells from the intravascular space. Decreases the risk associated with vascular stasis, e.g.: <ul><li>White blood cell depletion</li><li>Platelet depletion</li></ul>	<ul><li>Symptomatic leukocytosis in e.g. a patient newly diagnosed with acute myeloid leukaemia</li><li>Symptomatic thrombocytosis in a patient with thrombophilia</li></ul>
Photopheresis: Use of apheresis technology, light activated drugs, and ultraviolet light to modulate lymphocyte activity	<ul><li>Cutaneous T-cell lymphoma</li><li>Pemphigus vulgaris</li><li>Chronic graft versus host disease</li><li>Acute and chronic graft rejection</li></ul>
Immunoadsorption: Removal of a disease mediator from the patient's plasma and the subsequent return of the treated plasma to the patient	<ul><li>Immune thrombocytopenic purpura</li><li>Rheumatoid arthritis</li><li>Platelet refractoriness</li><li>Haemolytic uraemic syndrome</li></ul>
Dendritic cell collection: Removal of dendritic cells in order to manipulate them *in vitro* by providing them with tumour antigen so that they are capable of activating T-lymphocytes to fight malignancy	<ul><li>Prostate cancer</li><li>Melanoma</li><li>Multiple myeloma</li><li>Small cell lung cancer</li><li>Renal cell carcinoma</li><li>Breast cancer</li></ul>
LDL apheresis: Selective removal of LDL cholesterol from a patient's plasma through secondary processing	<ul><li>Familial hypercholesterolaemia unresponsive to drug therapy</li></ul>
Donor apheresis	
Peripheral blood stem cell collection: White cell procedure to collect haemopoietic stem cells. The collected stem cells may be used fresh or cryopreserved for both malignant and non-malignant conditions	<ul><li>Autologous stem cell collection (patient's own stem cells)</li><li>Allogeneic stem cell collection (collected from a HLA-matched related or unrelated donor)</li><li>Syngeneic stem cell collection (collected from the patient's identical twin)</li><li>Haploidentical stem cell collection (collected from either the mother or father of the patient)</li></ul>
Granulocyte collection: White cell procedure to collectic granulocytes (neutrophils) from suitable donors	<ul><li>Transfuse to neutropenic patients in order to provide adequate numbers of functional neutrophils to fight bacterial, fungal or yeast infections</li></ul>

Table 20.4   *(cont.)*

Applications	Indications
Lymphocyte collection: White cell procedure to collect lymphocytes from a related or unrelated donor for a patient following an allogeneic stem cell transplant (the donor of the graft cells is also the donor of the lymphocytes)	■ Post-allogeneic stem cell transplantation in the event of malignancy relapse ■ Non-myeloablative allogeneic stem cell transplant ■ Production of targeted cytotoxic T-lymphocytes
Platelet collection: Collection of platelets from healthy donors. Primarily the role of the blood transfusion service	■ For patients who, for a multitude of reasons, require a platelet transfusion

Method

The procedure for performing apheresis is complex and beyond the scope of this chapter. It should only be performed by specially trained operators. Further information can be gained from the respective apheresis operators' manuals.

Complications of apheresis procedures

Overall rates of adverse reactions have decreased significantly over the past two decades. Greater understanding of the physiology of apheresis has guided continued improvements in technology and the potential for untoward effects has been minimized so that most procedures are performed without adverse events. This is especially true of donation procedures, which have become very routine. Caution is in order if cell or plasma removal exceeds current guidelines or if patients have underlying instabilities that predispose them to untoward events (Crookston & Simon 2003). Issues of particular importance include:

■ *Peripheral venous access*: particular care should be taken over the peripheral venous assessment of patients and donors. Side-effects from needle insertion may include: pain, bleeding and haematoma. In addition patients and donors may suffer from needlephobia resulting in anxiety and vasovagal reactions (Dougherty 2008). When there is poor venous access, a central venous catheter needs to be placed to undertake the procedure. This has been identified as the greatest risk that patients and donors face (Stroncek *et al.* 2000). These risks are reduced by experienced personnel inserting the catheters with the assistance of ultrasound (Stroncek *et al.* 2000).

■ *Cellular loss*: as large volumes of donor or patient blood circulate through the apheresis machine, blood cells are intentionally or incidentally removed. Studies show that individual apheresis procedures produce only modest decreases in circulating blood cell counts, which are not associated with immediate toxicity (Crookston & Simon 2003). Patients with underlying instabilities may need to be supported by blood component transfusion.

■ *Anticoagulant toxicity*: during the procedure blood is prevented from clotting in the extracorporeal circuit by a citrate-based anticoagulant. This functions by binding the calcium in the blood and removing it from the clotting cascade. Donors may experience symptoms of hypocalcaemia, i.e. muscular irritability, tetany, numbness and 'pins and needles' in extremities, light-headedness, nausea and vomiting (Freshwater & Maslin-Prothero 2005). Citrate toxicity is controlled by giving the donor calcium supplements or reducing the dose of citrate administered by decreasing the blood flow rate (Stroncek *et al.* 2000).

■ *Fluid shifts*: different procedures may produce varying haemodynamic effects. Fluid overload may be a problem for patients with cardiac or renal impairment, whereas hypovolaemia may be of concern in the paediatric setting (Crookston & Simon 2003). Blood pressure should be monitored in particular, as hypotension may occur.

■ *Transfusion reaction*: with red cell and plasma exchanges, patients may experience transfusion reactions e.g. fever, chills and allergic reactions (see Chapter 43).

419

Procedure guidelines   **Bone marrow aspiration and trephine biopsy**

Equipment

1 Antiseptic skin cleaning agent (e.g. chlorhexidine gluconate 0.5% in alcohol 70%).
2 Sterile dressing pack.
3 Sterile gloves.
4 Selection of syringes and needles for administration of local anaesthetic.
5 Local anaesthetic, e.g. lidocaine 2%.
6 Marrow aspiration needle and guard.
7 Trephine biopsy needle.
8 Cytology slides and coverslips.
9 Specimen bottles (e.g. plain, formalin, EDTA and heparin).
10 Sterile dressing, e.g. mepore.
11 Scalpel.

Procedure guidelines *(cont.)*

Nurse procedure

Action	Rationale
1 Explain and provide written information about the bone marrow examination.	To ensure the patient is properly informed about the procedure (DH 2001: C; DH 2005a: C).
2 Obtain written informed consent.	To enable patients to actively participate and comply with their treatment (DH 2001: C; NMC 2006: C).
3 Check that blood parameters are within safe limits: (a) INR ≤ 1.5 (If a patient is warfarinized, they should stop their warfarin 3 days prior to procedure under the direction of a haematologist). (b) Thrombocytopenia is not a contraindication, but care should be taken to avoid trauma that is more significant than usual. (c) A platelet transfusion should be considered where applicable (Vergidis 2004).	To decrease the risk of haemorrhage, which has been identified as the most common and most serious adverse event associated with bone marrow examination (Bain 2006: C).
4 Consider oral (e.g. lorazepam) or intravenous (e.g. midazalam) sedation for very anxious patients (Giannoutsos *et al*. 2004). If intravenous sedation used, ensure appropriate resources are available as per local anaesthetic policy (cardiac monitoring, pulse oximetry, oxygen administration, reversal agent and available resuscitation equipment) (Provan *et al*. 2004).	To ensure that the procedure is performed safely and with minimal distress to the patient (E).
5 Assist the patient into the correct position, which is usually the left or right lateral position with the knees drawn up to the chest.	To access the posterior iliac crest which is the most common biopsy site in adults (E).
6 Prepare the procedure trolley and ensure that all the necessary equipment and specimen containers are readily available.	To ensure the procedure is performed efficiently and that all the necessary specimens are collected and handled correctly (Perkins 2003: C).
7 Perform the procedure aseptically. Ensure meticulous handwashing and wear sterile gloves.	To maintain asepsis throughout the procedure to minimize the risk of infection (DH 2005c: C).
8 Reassure and observe the patient throughout the procedure.	To allay anxiety and facilitate the patient's maximum co-operation (P).
9 Clean the skin thoroughly at the biopsy site with an antiseptic solution (Perkins 2003), e.g. chlorhexidine 0.5%, and alcohol solution and allow to dry (DH 2005c).	To maintain asepsis throughout the procedure to minimize the risk of infection (DH 2005c: C).
10 Administer local anaesthetic (e.g. lidocaine 2%) intradermally and subcutaneously at the site of the biopsy. Warn the patient that the drug can result in a 'stinging' sensation during administration.	To minimize pain during the procedure (P).
11 Make a small cut in the skin overlying the biopsy site with a scalpel.	To allow for better insertion of the biopsy needle through the skin and to avoid a skin 'plug' (E).

12 Insert the aspiration needle through the skin and subcutaneous tissues. Penetrate the marrow cortex 3–10 mm, with a slight rotating motion (Provan *et al.* 2004). Entrance of the needle into the bone marrow cavity may be sensed as a slight give.	To access the bone marrow for aspiration (E).
13 Remove the introducer, attach a 5 ml syringe to the needle and aspirate a volume of 0.2–2.0 ml marrow (bloody fluid) (Perkins 2003). Aspiration may cause a very brief, sharp, dragging sensation.	To aspirate liquid bone marrow in order to prepare specimens for further investigation (Hoffbrand *et al.* 2001: C).
14 If no dragging sensation is noted by the patient and no marrow is obtained, rotate the needle and apply suction again. If no marrow is obtained, another sampling site may be required (Perkins 2003).	To ensure that a sample is obtained for further investigation (E).
15 Make the smears quickly onto the cytology slides.	To avoid clotting (E).
16 Perform additional aspirations if necessary.	To provide material for flow cytometry, cytogenetics, culture, or other special studies as required (Provan *et al.* 2004: C).
17 Perform the trephine biopsy using the same skin incision if the aspirate has been performed in the iliac crest area. Use a separate biopsy needle, slightly larger than the aspirate needle (Perkins 2003).	In order to minimize the number of skin entry sites (E).
18 Advance the trephine needle to penetrate the bone cortex (Provan *et al.* 2004). The biopsy needle may require more pressure to enter the bone because of the larger bore size.	To access the bone for biopsy (E).
19 Position the trephine needle away from the area where the aspiration was performed.	To avoid collection of a specimen with extensive artifact induced by the aspiration procedure (Perkins 2003: E).
20 Remove the introducer and use firm hand pressure to advance the needle as far as possible (Provan *et al.* 2004).	To provide a solid core of bone (E).
21 Insert a stylet into the back of the needle.	To give an approximation of the size of the bone core within the needle (Perkins 2003).
22 Ensure the length of the trephine specimen is in the range of 1.6–2.0 cm (Bishop *et al.* 1992; Bain 2001; Campbell *et al.* 2003).	The analysis of the relation between length of trephine and the rate of positivity for neoplasia yielded a minimum adequate length of 1.6 cm before processing (Bishop *et al.* 1992: C).
23 Remove the needle from the bone and use the stylet to express the specimen into the appropriate container (Perkins 2003).	To collect the solid core of bone and marrow to examine as a histological specimen after fixation in formalin, decalcification and sectioning (Hoffbrand *et al.* 2001: C).
24 If no marrow can be aspirated (dry tap), make touch preparations from the biopsy (trephine roll).	To allow for cytologic examination of the bone marrow elements (Perkins 2003: C).
25 Apply manual pressure to the site for several minutes until the bleeding stops (Perkins 2003).	To achieve haemostasis (E).
26 Apply a sterile pressure dressing, e.g. gauze and mepore (Provan *et al.* 2004).	To achieve haemostasis and decrease the risk of infection at the biopsy site (E).

Procedure guidelines *(cont.)*

27 Apply pressure bandages and check the site for prolonged bleeding if a patient is thrombocytopenic (Perkins 2003).	To minimize bruising, prevent haematoma and decrease the risk of haemorrhage (Bain 2006: C).
28 Dispose of sharps as per local policy.	To ensure the safe handling and disposal of needles and other sharp instruments and to protect staff, patients and visitors from exposure to blood borne pathogens (Pratt *et al.* 2007: C).
29 Label specimens as per trust policy and send them to the appropriate laboratory department.	To prevent incorrect diagnosis and disease management through incorrectly labelled specimens (BCSH 1999: C).
30 Record the necessary information in the appropriate documents as per local policy.	To maintain accurate records (NMC 2005: C).
31 Ensure the patient has returned to pre-procedure functional status before discharge, if he/she has had sedation.	To ensure the safe management and recovery of patients receiving sedation (E).
32 Give the patient appropriate aftercare instructions (see Table 20.3).	To ensure the safe management of patients and to enable them to actively participate and comply with their treatment (DH 2001: C).

Procedure guidelines   Bone marrow harvest

There should be donor evaluation procedures in place to protect the safety of the donor and recipient. Bone marrow harvest donors (autologous or allogeneic) should be given a medical examination to confirm they are physically and emotionally fit to undergo anaesthesia and the marrow harvest (NMDP 2006). The donor's medical history, physical exam and laboratory test results should be performed according to the 'International standards for cellular therapy product collection, processing and administration' (FACT/JACIE 2006). Both the potential for disease transmission from the donor to the recipient and the risks to the donor from the collection procedure should be assessed (FACT/JACIE 2006). The allogeneic donor's suitability must be documented before the recipient's high dose therapy has begun.

The bone marrow harvest is performed under general anaesthetic in the operating room and local policy with regards to perioperative care should be followed (see Chapter 30).

Harvested bone marrow must be filtered to remove particulate matter prior to final processing and packaging for distribution or transplantation (FACT/JACIE 2006). This process must be performed under sterile conditions in the operating room at the time of harvest or in an appropriate sterile setting in the processing laboratory (FACT/JACIE 2006). Sterile in-line filters are available commercially in a collection set. The filter size may range from coarse (500 µm) to medium (300 µm) to fine (200 µm). All harvested marrow should ultimately pass through a fine filter, while other sizes may only be necessary if the marrow has a large amount of particulate matter (FACT/JACIE 2006).

Equipment

1 Skin cleaning agent.
2 A sterile collection set with transfer packs and in-line filters (e.g. 500 µm and 200 µm) containing specified anticoagulant.
3 250 ml saline with 50 ml of heparin (1000 units per ml preservative free) added in a bowl.
4 Two 11 g bone marrow harvest needles flushed with heparinized saline.
5 20 ml syringes containing 1 ml of heparinized saline.
6 Dressings.
7 Sterile gauze.
8 Sterile sheets.
9 Two receivers.
10 Face masks.
11 Sterile gowns.
12 Sterile gloves.
13 Sterile pack containing: jug, gallipot, gauze swabs, forceps, towel clips.
14 Documentation including stem cell harvest prescription.

Procedure

Action	Rationale
1 Explain and provide written information about the bone marrow harvest.	To ensure the donor is properly informed about the procedure (DH 2001: C; DH 2005a: C).
2 Obtain written informed consent.	To enable donors to actively participate and comply with their treatment (DH 2001; HTA 2006: C; NMC 2006: C).
3 Prepare the sterile procedure trolley and ensure that all the necessary equipment is available.	To ensure the procedure is performed efficiently and that the cells are collected and handled correctly (E).
4 Bring the donor into the operating room when anaesthetized and position correctly on the operating table. In adults, this is usually the prone position with hands placed above the head.	To allow marrow to be collected simultaneously from both the left and right posterior iliac crest by two practitioners (Confer 2004: C).
5 Ensure the harvest is performed as a sterile procedure: ■ Don face masks. ■ Scrub hands meticulously. ■ Don sterile gowns. ■ Don sterile gloves.	To maintain asepsis throughout the procedure to minimize the risk of infection (DH 2005c: C).
6 Clean the skin over the posterior iliac crests thoroughly with an antiseptic solution and allow to dry (DH 2005c).	To maintain asepsis throughout the procedure to minimize the risk of infection (DH 2005c: C).
7 Place four sterile drapes over the patient to maintain a sterile field: ■ One drape placed above the posterior iliac crests and spread towards the donor's head. ■ One drape placed below the posterior iliac crests and spread towards the donor's feet. ■ One drape is spread left and right of the harvest site respectively.	To maintain asepsis throughout the procedure to minimize the risk of infection (DH 2005c: C).
8 Place two receivers on the sterile towels: ■ One should contain two 11 g harvest needles (flushed with heparinized saline). ■ One should contain 20 ml syringes (flushed with heparinized saline and drawn up to 1 ml with heparinized saline).	To ensure the harvest equipment is easily accessible (E). The heparinized saline prevents the marrow from clotting in the syringe (E).
9 Locate the posterior iliac spine through palpation (Confer 2004).	To ensure the preferred site for harvest is located (E).
10 Insert the harvest needle through the skin, subcutaneous tissues, and penetrate the marrow cortex 3–10 mm, with a slight rotating motion. Entrance of the needle into the bone marrow cavity may be sensed as a slight give.	To access the marrow within the bony cortex (Confer 2004: C).
11 Remove the introducer and attach the harvest needle to a 20 ml syringe. Aspirate a volume of 10–20 ml of marrow (bloody fluid) by applying vigorous suction (Confer 2004).	To aspirate marrow from the donor. Short, vigorous aspirations are generally thought to produce a higher concentration of marrow cells relative to peripheral blood (Confer 2004: E).
12 Place filled syringes in the receiver.	To allow the nurse responsible for transferring the marrow into the sterile collection set to access them (E).

Procedure guidelines *(cont.)*

13 The nurse should: (a) Remove the filled syringe from the receiver. (b) Dispel any air from the syringe. (c) Ensure the marrow volume is recorded by a member of the theatre staff.	To ensure that the correct amount of marrow is aspirated (E).
14 The nurse should: (a) Ensure the correct volume of specified anticoagulant is added to the collection set as per local policy. (b) Gently add the marrow to the collection set. (c) Gently agitate the collection set to mix the marrow with the anticoagulant.	To prevent any clotting (E)
15 The nurse should: (a) Flush the syringe with heparinized saline (leaving 1 ml in the syringe). (b) Return it to the receiver ready for subsequent aspirations.	To ensure the practitioners performing the harvest have a supply of appropriately prepared syringes to perform the aspirations (E).
16 Advance the harvest needle several millimetres and repeat the process (Confer 2004).	To allow for several aspirations from a single bone puncture as the needle is repeatedly advanced (Confer 2004 :C).
17 After a number of aspirations from the same site, replace the introducer and move the position of the harvest needle to another place in the bone approximately 2 cm from the first entry site. *Note:* Occasionally marrow is also collected from the anterior iliac crests or the sternum. Current practice employs these supplemental sites only when the target cell dose cannot be reached by aspiration from the posterior iliac crests. This may occur if the marrow space of the crest has been compromised by e.g. trauma or radiation (Confer 2004: C).	To allow the bone to be entered multiple times through a single skin entry site. A typical collection may involve 200–300 marrow aspirations obtained through only a few skin punctures (E).
18 The nurse should: (a) Take a mid-procedure sample of aspirate from the collection set as per local policy. (b) Place the sample in a full blood count specimen container. (c) Label specimen container appropriately. (d) Send sample to the laboratory for a white cell count.	To allow the adequacy of the collection to be determined by a nucleated cell count (Confer 2004: C).
19 Continue this process until sufficient marrow has been removed. More than one skin hole may be necessary to achieve the desired volume.	To ensure the stipulated volume of marrow is harvested. The decision regarding the amount of marrow to be collected is made by the medical team (E).
20 Document the number of puncture holes made in the hospital notes.	To facilitate postoperative wound care and to maintain accurate records (NMC 2005: C).
21 The nurse should: (a) Ensure the marrow passes through the in-line filters of the collection set to the transfer pack as per manufacturer's guidelines.	To remove particulate matter (FACT/JACIE 2006: C).

22	The nurse should seal the transfer pack as per local policy.	To maintain asepsis, minimize the risk of infection and facilitate the safe transport of the cells (DH 2005c: C).
23	The nurse should record the respective volume of bone marrow on the outside of the transfer pack in millilitres.	To establish total amount of bone marrow in each bag (E).
24	Withdraw the harvest needles from the posterior iliac crest, pack sterile gauze over the left and right harvest sites respectively and maintain digital pressure until the bleeding has stopped.	To achieve haemostasis, minimize leakage and prevent the formation of a haematoma (E).
25	Dispose of sharps as per local policy.	To ensure the safe handling and disposal of needles and other sharp instruments and to protect staff, patients and visitors from exposure to blood borne pathogens (DH 2005b: C; Pratt *et al.* 2007: C).
26	Inspect the puncture sites for bleeding. Mepore and a pressure dressing may be applied over the sterile gauze.	To achieve haemostasis and decrease the risk of infection at the harvest sites (E).
27	Take the donor to the recovery room.	To ensure appropriate postoperative care (E).
28	Label each transfer pack as per local policy.	To ensure correct management of the product (FACT/JACIE 2006: C).
29	Place the transfer packs in a secondary container (e.g. a zip-type resealable bag) prior to transfer to the appropriate processing facility.	To prevent the loss of a portion of the collection, to minimize the potential of post-collection contamination of the component and to prevent potential spillage of biohazard material in areas where it may pose a risk to employees, visitors or patients (FACT/JACIE 2006: C).
30	Transport the marrow to the appropriate processing facility with the necessary forms.	To allow for cell measurement, storage and/or issue of the marrow (E).
31	Record the necessary information in the appropriate documents as per local policy.	To maintain accurate records (NMC 2005: C).
32	Ensure the donor has been given appropriate aftercare instructions (see Table 20.3).	To ensure the safe management of patients and to enable them to actively participate and comply with their treatment (DH 2001: C).

Problem solving: Bone marrow harvest

Problem	Cause	Action
Anaesthesia risks.	Reactions to the anaesthetic agents, e.g. adverse reactions, hypersensitivity reactions or idiosyncratic reactions (Confer 2004).	Instigate urgent treatment and mechanical ventilation as necessary (Confer 2004).
Infection risks.	Infections may occur at the sites of marrow collection or line insertion due to poor practitioner technique or inadequate wound care.	Ensure hand decontamination, infection control and wound care policies are followed (DH 2005c). Treat infections promptly with antibiotics if indicated (Confer 2004).

Problem solving *(cont.)*

Problem	Cause	Action
Mechanical injury risks.	The procedure of marrow collection may lead to local tissue injuries. These may include bone, nerve or vessel damage. Haemorrhage, which may be delayed can create severe pain from compression of soft tissues. Sciatic pain, lasting up to 18 months has been reported in a related marrow donor.	Refer to the medical team and physiotherapist (Confer 2004).
Transfusion risks.	Allogeneic transfusions may cause transfusion reactions, transmit viral infections and, rarely, transmit bacterial infections (Confer 2004).	Practice varies dependent on the collection physician (Confer 2004): ■ Units of autologous blood may be collected from donors a few weeks prior to the harvest for transfusion after the procedure. This practice is becoming less common. ■ Autologous red cells may be recovered from the collected bone marrow. This process has been successfully applied in children donors without compromising the quality of the marrow donation (Confer 2004). ■ Administration of erythropoietin (EPO) may also diminish the likelihood of allogeneic blood transfusion. A theoretical concern about pretreatment of donors with EPO is diminished quality of the collected marrow (Confer 2004).
Pain.	The procedure of marrow collection may lead to pain postoperatively.	Advise donors that the soreness at the collection site should ease off in around a week and to take pain medication as directed (NMDP 2006).
Fatigue.	This is related to procedure induced anaemia. The severity of anaemia is determined entirely by the donor's preoperative haemoglobin level and the net blood loss.	Transfusion of autologous blood has already been described. Other measures (NMDP 2006) include: ■ A gradual return to work (usually after 1 week). ■ Ensuring rest between periods of work. ■ Avoid strenuous activity for 3–4 weeks.

References and further reading

Abboud, C. & Lichtman, M. (2005) Structure of the marrow and the hematopoietic microenvironment. In: *Williams' Haematology* (eds M. Lichtman *et al.*), 7th edn. McGraw-Hill, London, pp. 35–72.

Atkinson, M. (2005) Communicating news of patients' deaths to unrelated stem cell donors. *Nurs Stand*, **19**(32), 41–7.

Bain, B. (2001) Bone marrow trephine biopsy. *J Clin Pathol*, **54**, 737–42.

Bain, B. (2004) *A Beginner's Guide to Blood Cells*, 2nd edn. Blackwell Publishing, Boston.

Bain, B. (2005) Bone marrow biopsy morbidity: review of 2003. *J Clin Pathol*, **58**(4), 406–8.

Bain, B. (2006) Morbidity associated with bone marrow aspiration and trephine biopsy – a review of 2004. *Haematologica*, **91**, 1293–4.

BCSH (1999) The administration of blood and blood components and the management of transfused patients. *Transfus Med*, 9, 227–38.

Bishop, B., McNally, K. & Harris, M. (1992) Audit of bone marrow trephines. *J Clin Pathol*, **45**, 1105–8.

Blume, K. & Amylon, M. (2004) The evaluation and counselling of candidates for hematopoietic cell transplantation. In: *Thomas' Hematopoietic Cell Transplantation* (eds K. Blume, S. Forman & F. Appelbaum), 3rd edn. Blackwell Publishing, Boston.

Bondurant, M. & Koury, M. (2003) Origin and development of blood cells. In: *Wintrobe's Clinical Hematology* (eds J. Greer *et al.*), 11th edn. Lippincott, Williams & Wilkins, Philadelphia, pp. 169–93.

Burgstaler, E. (2003) Current instrumentation for apheresis. In: *Apheresis: Principles and Practice* (eds B. McLeod, T. Price & R. Weinstein), 2nd edn. AABB Press, Bethesda, MD, pp. 95–130.

Campbell, J., Matthews, J. & Seymour, M. (2003) Optimum trephine length in the assessment of bone marrow involvement in patients with diffuse large cell lymphoma. *Ann Oncol*, 14, 273–6.

Confer, D. (2004) Hematopoietic cell donors. In: *Thomas' Hematopoietic Cell Transplantation* (eds K. Blume, S. Forman & F. Appelbaum), 3rd edn. Blackwell Publishing, Boston, pp. 538–49.

Corbin, F. *et al.* (2003) Development of apheresis instrumentation. In: *Apheresis: Principles and Practice* (eds B. McLeod, T. Price & R. Weinstein), 2nd edn. AABB Press, Bethesda, MD, pp. 1–27.

Crookston, K. & Simon, T. (2003) Physiology of apheresis. In: *Apheresis: Principles and Practice* (eds B. McLeod, T. Price & R. Weinstein), 2nd edn. AABB Press, Bethesda, MD, pp. 71–93.

DH (2001) *Good Practice in Consent Implementation Guide: Consent to Examination or Treatment.* HSC 2001/023. Department of Health, London.

DH (2005a) *Creating a patient-led NHS – delivering the NHS improvement plan.* Department of Health, London.

DH (2005b) *Hazardous waste (England) regulations.* Department of Health, London.

DH (2005c) *Saving Lives: a Delivery Programme to Reduce Healthcare Associated Infection including MRSA.* Department of Health, London.

Dougherty, L. (2008) Obtaining peripheral venous access. In: *Intravenous Therapy in Nursing Practice* (eds L. Dougherty & J. Lamb), 2nd edn. Blackwell Publishing, Oxford.

FACT/JACIE (2006) International standards for cellular therapy product collection, processing and administration (draft), 3rd edn. www.jacie.org/portal/jacie/about. Accessed 10/01/07.

Foss, M. (2003) Photopheresis. In: *Apheresis: Principles and Practice* (eds B. McLeod, T. Price & R. Weinstein), 2nd edn. AABB Press, Bethesda, MD, pp. 623–42.

Freshwater, D. & Maslin-Prothero, S. (eds) (2005) *Blackwell's Nursing Dictionary.* Blackwell Publishing, Oxford.

GambroBCT (2005) *Spectra™ System Therapeutics Reference Book.* GambroBCT, Denver.

Giannoutsos, I. *et al.* (2004) Performing bone marrow biopsies with or without sedation: a comparison. *Clin Lab Haematol*, 26(3), 201–4.

Hoffbrand, A.V., Pettit, J.E. & Moss, P.A.H. (2001) *Essential Haematology.* Blackwell Science, Oxford.

HTA (2006) *Human Tissue Authority Code of Practice – Consent.* Department of Health, London.

Hughes-Jones, N., Wickramasinghe, S. & Hatton, C. (2004) *Lecture Notes on Haematology*, 7th edn. Blackwell Publishing, Oxford.

Leukaemia Research Fund (2005) Facts and statistics. www.lrf.org.uk/en/1/disstahome.html. Accessed 26/9/06.

Longo, D. (2005) Examination of blood smears and bone marrow. In: *Harrison's Manual of Medicine* (eds D. Kasper, E. Braunwald & A. Fauci), 16th edn. McGraw-Hill, New York, pp. 265–7.

NMC (2005) *Guidelines for Records and Record Keeping.* Nursing and Midwifery Council, London.

NMC (2006) *A–Z Advice Sheet Consent.* www.nmc.org.

NMC (2008) *The Code: Standards of Conduct, Performance and Ethics for Nurses and Midwives.* Nursing and Midwifery Council, London.

NMDP (2006) Donor information. www.marrow.org/DONOR/index.html. Accessed 26/9/06.

Outhwaite, H. (2000) Blood and marrow transplantation. In: *Nursing in Haematological Oncology* (ed. M. Grundy). Bailliere Tindall, Edinburgh, pp. 140–55.

Perkins, S. (2003) Bone marrow examination. In: *Wintrobe's Clinical Hematology* (eds J. Greer *et al.*), 11th edn. Lippincott, Williams & Wilkins, Philadelphia, pp. 3–22.

Pratt, R. *et al.* (2007) Epic 2: National evidence-based guidelines for preventing healthcare-associated infection in NHS hospitals in England. *J Hosp Infec*, 65(1)(suppl), S2–S12.

Provan, D. *et al.* (2004) *Oxford Handbook of Clinical Haematology.* Oxford University Press, Oxford.

Richardson, C. & Atkinson, J. (2006) Blood and marrow transplantation. In: *Nursing in Haematological Oncology* (ed. M. Grundy), 2nd edn. Bailliere Tindall, Edinburgh, pp. 265–91.

Rosenmayr, A., Hartwell, L. & Egeland, T. (2003) Informed consent – suggested procedures for informed consent for unrelated haematopoietic stem cell donors at various stages of recruitment, donor evaluation, and donor workup. *Bone Marrow Transplant*, 31, 539–45.

Sieff, C. & Nathan, D. (2000) Stem cells and haemopoiesis. In: *Concise Oxford Textbook of Medicine* (eds J. Ledingham & D. Warrell). Oxford University Press, Oxford, pp. 180–3.

Strauss, R. (2003) Granulocyte (neutrophil) transfusion. In: *Apheresis: Principles and Practice* (eds B. McLeod, T. Price & R. Weinstein), 2nd edn. AABB Press, Bethesda, MD, pp. 237–52.

Stroncek, D., Confer, D. & Leitman, S. (2000) Peripheral blood progenitor cells for HPC transplants involving unrelated donors. *Transfusion*, 40, 731–41.

Traynor, B. (2006) Haematopoiesis. In: *Nursing in Haematological Oncology* (ed. M. Grundy), 2nd edn. Bailliere Tindall, Edinburgh, pp. 3–20.

Turgeon, M.L. (1999) *Clinical Haematology, Theory and Procedures*, 3rd edn. Lippincott, Williams & Wilkins, Philadelphia.

Vergidis, D. (2004) Bone aspiration and biopsy. www.emedicine.com/med/topic2971.htm#section~author_information. Accessed 29/9/06.

Weatherall, D. (2000) Haematology. In: *Concise Oxford Textbook of Medicine* (eds J. Ledingham & D. Warrell). Oxford University Press, Oxford, pp. 175–80.

Chapter 21

Intrapleural drainage

429   Reference material
434   *Procedure guidelines:* Intrapleural drain insertion
438   *Procedure guidelines:* Intrapleural drain: changing the drain bottle
439   *Procedure guidelines:* Intrapleural drain removal
441   *Problem solving:* Intrapleural drainage
442   References and further reading

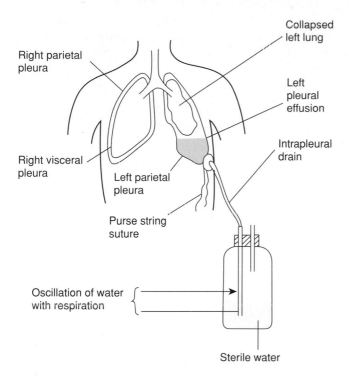

Figure 21.1 An intrapleural drain and underwater seal bottle are used to drain a left pleural effusion.

Definitions

Any abnormal collection of fluid or air in the pleural space can compress the lung, causing it to collapse either partially or fully, which can seriously compromise ventilation and the mechanics of breathing (Allibone 2003). Intrapleural drainage is a method used to remove the collection of air, fluid, pus or blood from the pleural space in order to restore normal lung expansion and function (Hyde *et al.* 1997; McMahon-Parkes 1997).

An intrapleural drain is a length of tubing, made of clear, rigid yet pliable plastic, which may have a radiopaque strip incorporated into it that enables X-ray detection. It has a proximal and distal end. The proximal end is inserted into the pleura and has a number of holes at the insertion end which facilitate drainage. The distal end is connected to the drainage system (Marieb 2001) (Figure 21.1).

Indications

Indications for chest drain insertion

- Pneumothorax:

  (a) in any ventilated patient;
  (b) tension pneumothorax after initial needle relief;
  (c) persistent or recurrent pneumothorax after simple aspiration;
  (d) large secondary spontaneous pneumothorax in patients over 50 years.

- Malignant pleural effusion.
- Empyema and complicated parapneumonic pleural effusion.
- Traumatic haemopneumothorax.
- Postoperative, e.g. thoracotomy, oesophagectomy, cardiac surgery (Laws *et al.* 2003).
- Drainage of pleural effusions.
- Drainage of chyle (digested fat drained by the lymphatic system) (Adam & Osborne 2005).

Objectives in caring for the patient with intrapleural drains

- To keep the system patent.
- To maintain sterility of the intrapleural drainage system and avoid introduction of bacteria into the intrapleural space.
- To keep the system upright and airtight (Kirkwood 2002).

Reference material

Anatomy and physiology of the pleura

Each lung is surrounded by a double membrane called the pleura. The outer membrane is the parietal pleura; this is attached to the thoracic (chest) wall and contains nerve receptors which detect pain. The inner membrane is the visceral pleura and this adheres to the lung covering the lung fissures, hilar bronchi and vessels (Figure 21.2). The pleurae are thin, serous and porous, which allows for movement of interstitial fluid across these membranes (Marieb 2001; Berne & Levy 2004; Hall &Guyton 2005; Tortora & Derrickson 2008).

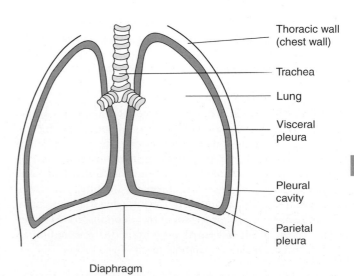

Figure 21.2 Relationship between pleural membranes, chest wall and lungs.

429

Pleural space

A space exists between the parietal and visceral pleura commonly known as the pleural space, cavity or potential space. Approximately 3–5 ml of serous fluid produced by the pleurae fills this space, enabling the pleurae to move in unison with the chest wall on inspiration. In addition, the serous fluid enables the membranes to be held closely together by surface tension forces. A careful balance is required to control the amount of fluid present in the pleural space. This balance is maintained by the oncotic pressure across the pleurae and lymphatic drainage. Approximately 1–2 litres of fluid moves across the pleural space each day (Thelan et al. 1995).

The natural recoil tendency of the lungs during breathing causes them to try and collapse, but a negative pressure is required on the outside of the lungs to keep them expanded. This is provided by the pleurae. During respiration the intrapleural pressure will vary. Before inspiration the pressure within the pleural space is equal to $-5\,\mathrm{cmH_2O}$. During inspiration there is a decrease in the intrapleural pressure due to the diaphragm being drawn down and outward with expansion of the chest. The pressure falls to $-7.5\,\mathrm{cmH_2O}$, and this results in air being drawn in for gaseous exchange (Marieb 2001). During expiration the lung returns to its preinspiratory state by elastic recoil, with collapse of the chest wall and diaphragm and the exhalation of gas, resulting in a subsequent rise in the intrapleural pressure to $-4\,\mathrm{cmH_2O}$. If there is loss of the normal negative pressure, partial or total lung collapse can occur, which can then lead to a reduction in the capacity of the lung available for effective gaseous exchange (Marieb 2001; Berne & Levy 2004; Hall & Guyton 2005; Tortora & Derrickson 2008).

Conditions that require intrapleural drainage

Pneumothorax

This can be defined as air in the pleural cavity (Kumar & Clarke 2002). When the integrity of either pleural layer is breached, air can enter the pleural cavity, causing the lung to collapse down towards the hilum (Gallon 1998).

Spontaneous pneumothorax

Spontaneous pneumothorax is a collection of air or gas in the chest that causes the lung to collapse (MedlinePlus 2006). Spontaneous pneumothorax can occur as a result of trauma, surgery, central venous catheter insertion, during positive pressure ventilation, and in those individuals with lung conditions, e.g. asthma, chronic bronchitis, tuberculosis, pneumonia or carcinoma of the lung due to the mechanical and physiological processes of these conditions (MedlinePlus 2006). If left untreated a spontaneous pneumothorax can become a tension pneumothorax.

Tension pneumothorax

A tension pneumothorax is a complete collapse of the lung. It occurs when air enters but does not leave the space around the lung (pleural space). It is a life-threatening emergency that requires immediate treatment (MedlinePlus 2006).

Pleural effusion

This is defined as an excessive amount of fluid in the pleural space (Kumar & Clarke 2002). The fluid can be composed of malignant cells, or result from an accumulation of lymph in the pleural space (chylothorax) (Kozar & Adams 2005). An effusion occurs as a result of trauma, carcinoma, heart failure, hypoproteinaemia or pneumonia. Pleural effusions occur when an imbalance in pressure allows the flow of fluid into the pleural space to exceed its absorption (Chernecky & Shelton 2001).

Care should be taken when draining pleural effusions as complications can occur, such as re-expansion of pulmonary oedema (Tang et al. 2002). No more than 1500 ml should be drained at a time, clamping the tube to interrupt drainage for 1–2 hours before recommencing or slowed to about 500 ml/h depending on haemodynamic status (Laws et al. 2003). A chest X-ray should also be performed to ascertain correct position of the drain and to detect any complications (Tang et al. 2002).

If the patient's respiratory status worsens after chest drain insertion, and proper placement of tube has been confirmed, the possibility of re-expansion pulmonary oedema should be considered; if this is present, the pleural drainage should be limited to less than 1000 ml/day and the negative pleural pressure to 5 kPa (Deshpande et al. 2003).

Haemothorax

Haemothorax is a collection of blood in the space between the chest wall and the lung (the pleural cavity), usually the result of chest injury, trauma to the heart, lungs or major vessels or in a patient who has bled on anticoagulant therapy (MedlinePlus 2006).

Haemopneumothorax

Haemothorax may also be associated with pneumothorax. Depending on the amount of blood or air in the pleural cavity, a collapsed lung can lead to respiratory and haemodynamic failure (MedlinePlus 2006).

Empyema

This is defined as pus in the pleural space. Its main causes include rupture of an abscess of the lung, following pneumonia, pulmonary tuberculosis, or an infection following thoracic surgery (Kumar & Clarke 2002).

Collective signs and symptoms

The following signs and symptoms can occur in the conditions previously mentioned, individually or together depending on the patient's condition:

- Pallor.
- Cyanosis.
- Dyspnoea.
- Increasing respiratory rate.
- Reduced breath sounds on affected side.
- Dullness of air entry, on listening to the chest with stethoscope.
- Reduced chest movement on affected side.
- Decrease in peripheral tissue oxygen saturations.
- Pleuritic chest pain.
- Cardiovascular change, i.e. increasing heart rate, decreasing blood pressure due to compression of the mediastinum and in turn the heart and surrounding vessels (Kumar & Clarke 2002).

Drain insertion site

Before insertion of an intrapleural drain the patient should have a chest X-ray reviewed by the doctor. The chest X-ray will confirm the site of the pneumothorax or effusion to be drained. Patients who are receiving anticoagulation therapy or who have platelet abnormalities should have appropriate haematological investigations (international normalized ratio [INR] or activated partial thromboplastin ratio [APTR]) to ascertain whether correction is required prior to insertion of the drain (Tang et al. 2002). If the INR or APTR is too high, bleeding could occur if left untreated.

Intrapleural drains are usually inserted in the chest, in an area which is known as the 'triangle of safety'. The mid-axillary line borders this area posteriorly, the level of the nipple inferiorly and the lateral border of the pectoralis major interiorly (Hyde et al. 1997; Peek et al. 2000; Tang et al. 2002). Once the drain has been placed in any position within the 'triangle of safety', re-expansion of the lung occurs. However, in cases of intrapleural adhesions or localized collection of pus or fluids, the doctor will need to position the tip of the drain to assist drainage (Hyde et al. 1997; Tang et al. 2002).

Drain size

The size of tube used is dependent on the reason for drainage. Whilst no large randomized trials comparing small and large bore tubes have been performed, the optimum size of drainage catheter remains controversial (Laws et al. 2003).

In the past the use of a large bore drain was recommended to prevent the blockage of chest drains, particularly by thick malignant or infected fluid (Hyde et al. 1997). However, currently the majority of physicians prefer to use smaller catheters (10–14 French [F]) and some smaller studies have shown that these are often as effective as larger bore tubes (Clementsen et al. 1998; Patz 1998). Small bore drains are more comfortable and better tolerated by the patient (Laws et al. 2003).

Securing the drain

The British Thoracic Society (Laws et al. 2003) advises that purse string stitches should not be used as they cause pain by changing a linear wound into a circular one and leave an unsightly scar. Only large and medium bore drains require suturing; small gauge chest tubes do not usually require suturing. The suture material should be strong and non-absorbable to prevent breaking, such as silk, and a mattress suture should be employed rather than a purse string suture (Laws et al. 2003).

Stripping/milking of intrapleural drains

Milking and stripping of chest tubes to keep them patent has been studied, and has shown that this increases the negative pressure in the intrathoracic cavity to -100 to -400 cmH$_2$O and subsequently it seems that milking or stripping of chest tubes on a routine basis should be avoided (Kirkwood 2002). If a chest drain becomes occluded or blocked the tubing needs to be replaced rather than milking or stripping (Avery 2000).

Clamping of intrapleural drains

The British Thoracic Society Guidelines (Miller & Harvey 1993) discourage clamping of intrapleural drains as this can prevent air leaving the pleural space. This in turn can cause a pneumothorax which could progress to a life threatening tension pneumothorax. There is also no need to clamp tubing when mobilizing or transporting patients to other departments as this may also cause a tension pneumothorax (Hyde et al. 1997; Henry et al. 2003). When changing the bottle system, it is necessary to clamp the drain for the shortest period of time possible and during this process the patient should be under close observation for any signs of deterioration in breathing (Brandt et al. 1994).

In cases of pneumothorax the chest drain should not be clamped at the time of its removal (Laws et al. 2003). The only time a non-bubbling chest drain should be momentarily clamped is in the event of disconnection, if there is damage to the drainage bottle, or to locate a leak in the drainage system (Avery 2000; Henry et al. 2003; Laws et al. 2003; Allibone 2005).

Drainage systems

Prepacked drainage systems are now available for drainage of pneumothoraces, haemothoraces or pleural effusions. The bottle has a screw top with two ports. One port has the underwater length of tubing attached. The second port has a shorter length of tubing attached which acts as the venting end and is exposed to air or could be attached to a suction unit. Venting prevents the build-up of pressure in the chest drainage system which could prevent evacuation of air or fluid (McMahon-Parkes 1997) (Figure 21.3).

431

Underwater length of tubing →

Venting port or suction port

Figure 21.3   One-bottle system.

The underwater seal occurs when there is adequate water in the bottle, usually 500 ml of water. The distal end of the intrapleural drain is then attached to the underwater seal port of the chest drain bottle and immersed 2.5 cm below the level of the water. Incoming air, bubbles through the water, which acts as a one-way valve and prevents the backflow of air into the intrapleural space (McMahon-Parkes 1997).

For more complicated pneumothoraces or haemothoraces a plastic multi-chamber system incorporates the above one-bottle system into one unit. There are three chambers: the first is for drainage, the second chamber is the underwater seal and the third chamber is the vacuum or suction control. When this system is set up, water is placed in the water seal chamber to the indicated mark, and also placed in the suction control chamber to the required level. This system is a great improvement on the previous systems and enables patient mobility (Pierce 1995) (Figure 21.4).

Maintenance of drainage systems during and after insertion

When the drain is attached to the drainage bottle bubbling or swinging should be observed; this indicates that air is being evacuated from the pleural space. As the lung re-inflates, the bubbling should decrease. If bubbling continues, a leak may be present in the patient's lung. Causes of air leaks include:

- Air in chest from a pneumothorax.
- An eyelit from chest tube outside the chest wall.
- Blocked drain may cause an air leak at puncture site.

Connection to controlled suction (A)

Clear plastic drainage tubing

Screw cap to allow easy filling of water seal

Write-on drainage record column

Mark to indicate level of water required for seal

Flood stand

Remove protective cap and connect to chest catheter

Figure 21.4   Underwater chest drainage system.

- Inadequate drain size.
- Poor tube connections.
- Poor seal around the entry site to the lung (Kirkwood 2002).

The presence of an air leak should be assessed. Bubbling can occur in the underwater seal compartment. If bubbling occurs when the patient coughs, this would usually indicate the leak is only minor. However, continuous bubbling would indicate a serious air leak in the system. The drain and tube should be inspected thoroughly down to the level of the underwater seal to eliminate any external problems such as loose tubing connections or poor seal around the drain at the insertion site. A chest X-ray should also be ordered to establish the position of the drain. Air leaks should be treated with caution and prompt action is required (such as referral to a specialist respiratory physician).

Tubing should be tailored to suit the patient's needs, allowing room to manoeuvre but preventing coiling and looping (Hyde *et al.* 1997; Avery 2000; Kirkwood 2002). Pleural effusion, impaired gas exchange and infection can also be caused by loops, coiling and kinks in the tubing as well as impeding drainage (Gorden *et al.* 1997; Kirkwood 2002) so regular inspection of tubing should be carried out.

There is debate about the most recent recommendations on taping the connection between the chest drainage bottle and drainage tubes (Godden 1998; Avery 2000), as the nurse may not be able to see if the connections have parted beneath the tape (Adam & Osborne 2005); however, without any additional method of security, such as tape, there is a risk of the drainage tubing becoming disconnected (Allibone 2005).

Dressings for insertion site

A simple dry dressing (low-linting gauze) should be applied around the drain and secured with adhesive tape during drainage and after removal of drain (Tang *et al.* 2002). Heavy strapping should be avoided as it can restrict chest movement. Dressings during the drainage procedure should be kept clean and dry and not removed until the drain is ready for removal (Tang *et al.* 1999; Avery 2000).

Pain control

On insertion of a chest drain, tissue damage occurs and this activates nerve fibres surrounding the insertion site (Gray 2000; Hilton 2004). While the drain is in place, the nerve fibres or tissue cannot heal. Therefore, the patient will experience pain throughout the insertion procedure and after the drain has been inserted (Tomlinson & Treasure 1997). Inadequate pain control can cause the patient to breathe incorrectly and the patient may try to avoid coughing, resulting in complications such as chest infections (Gray 2000). Risk can be reduced by chest physiotherapy from a physiotherapist (Gray 2000). In a study by Luketich (Luketich *et al.* 1998), 50% of patients experience pain levels of 9–10 on a scale of 0–10, with 10 being most pain imaginable. Therefore, prior to inserting an intrapleural drain unless contraindicated, pre-medication such as benzodiazepine or an opioid should be administered as prescribed (Laws *et al.* 2003). A comprehensive plan for pain control involving the patient and the health care professionals should be produced. Pain management should cover all stages of the intrapleural drainage process (Gray 2000):

- Insertion.
- Management of the intrapleural drain during the drainage process.
- Removal of the intrapleural drain.

Current protocols for the management of pain include patient-controlled analgesia, paravertebral blocks, non-steroidal anti-inflammatory drugs or transcutaneous electrical nerve stimulation (Allibone 2005).

Suction and its use

The addition of suction to the drainage system increases the negative pressure, enhancing lung re-expansion. A high-volume and low-pressure suction unit should be applied (Hyde *et al.* 1997; Tang *et al.* 2002) using pressure in the range of 5–15 kPa. The suction pressure should only be increased if the patient's pain is controlled and if the patient tolerates the increase. Once suction has been discontinued, the tubing to the underwater seal should be disconnected, otherwise this could cause positive pressure and may precipitate a tension pneumothorax (Tang *et al.* 2002) (see (A) in Figure 21.4). The suction unit should be cleaned by wiping it with a damp cloth and a mild disinfectant solution. Most suction units are fitted with a disposable air filter capsule, between the vacuum connector and the filter capsule mount. The filter prevents cross-infection and should be changed after each patient.

Chest drain removal

If a patient has had a pneumothorax, the chest drain should not be clamped at the time of its removal (Laws *et al.* 2003). The chest drain should be removed either while the patient is asked to perform a Valsalva manoeuvre or during expiration with a brisk firm movement while an assistant ties the mattress suture to close the wound (Laws *et al.* 2003). The Valsalva manoeuvre (asking the patient to hold their breath while trying to exhale out against a closed glottis, or bear down) increases the intrathoracic pressure which prevents air from entering the thoracic cavity on removal of the drain (McMahon-Parkes 1997; Avery 2000).

The decision to remove a drain is usually made by a medical practitioner based on the following criteria:

- Absence of an air leak into the chest drain bottle, usually noted when the patient exhales forcibly or coughs. When a patient is ventilated with positive pressure this will coincide with the expiration.
- Re-expansion of lung following previous discontinuation of any suction when there should be no air leak or drainage.

433

- The volume of fluid draining into the chest drain is minimal. Guidelines on what is minimal vary but less than 10 ml/h per drain has been suggested (Higgins 2006).
- There is no evidence of respiratory compromise or failure.
- There is no coagulation deficit or increased risk of bleeding (check latest coagulation results prior to removal).

- In many cases radiological evidence of the absence of air or fluid accumulation will be required before removal.

Advice should be sought from a medical practitioner if there is any doubt as to whether to remove a chest drain (Higgins 2006).

Procedure guidelines   Intrapleural drain insertion

Equipment

1 Sterile chest drain pack containing, gallipot, disposable towel, forceps, disposable scalpel and sterile low-linting gauze.
2 Suture material: silk.
3 Cleaning solution, chlorhexidine gluconate 0.5% in 70% alcohol.
4 Sterile gloves and gown.
5 Local anaesthetic, lidocaine 1%.
6 Syringes 2 × 10 ml.
7 Needles 1 × 21 gauge, 1 × 23 gauge.

8 Chest drain. Check appropriate size to be used for insertion.
9 Sterile dressing.
10 Tape.
11 Chest drain tubing.
12 Chest drain bottle.
13 Sterile water 1 litre bottle.
14 Chest drain clamps × 2.
15 Low vacuum suction pump if required.

Intrapleural drain insertion

Action	Rationale
1 Cleanse hands with alcoholic handrub. Hands to be cleansed before and after each patient contact.	To minimize the risk of infection (DH 2005a: C).
2 Explain and discuss the procedure with the patient. *Note*: the procedure might have to be performed under emergency conditions.	To ensure the patient understands why and how the procedure is to be performed and gives his/her valid consent (Laws *et al.* 2003: C; NMC 2006: C). A patient may have become acutely unwell, and so the procedure would prevent respiratory and cardiovascular collapse (Adam & Osborne 2005: E).
3 Administer analgesia prior to procedure after discussion with the doctor, about the type and route of administration. The analgesia should be given at least half an hour before the procedure.	To minimize any pain during the procedure and to ensure the patient is pain free and able to co-operate (Laws *et al.* 2003: C).
4 Administer sedation on doctor's instruction, if considered appropriate, e.g. for an anxious patient.	To relieve anxiety and allow the patient to relax and co-operate, and to enable the procedure to proceed (E).
5 Cleanse hands with alcoholic handrub.	To minimize the risk of infection (DH 2005a: C).
6 Prepare trolley, placing equipment on bottom shelf. Take to patient's bedside.	
7 Prime the underwater seal system with sufficient sterile water to cover the drainage tube. Cleanse hands with alcoholic handrub.	This prevents back flow of air or fluid into the pleural space, and marks the initial water level to allow measurement of subsequent drainage (Adam & Osborne 2005: E).
8 Assist doctor in setting up sterile procedure pack.	To minimize risk of infection and to have equipment ready (E).
9 Check the correct side of chest for drain insertion to optimize access to the triangle of safety.	To ensure drainage of correct side by checking the chest X-ray (O'Connor & Morgan 2005: E).

10 Position patient in preparation for the procedure. The patient may be positioned flat on the bed with the arm on the affected side placed behind his/her head away from the chest wall or abducted to 90°. If patient is able to sit upright, he/she can be positioned resting over a table supported by a pillow.	To facilitate insertion of the intrapleural drain. To aid patient comfort (Hyde *et al.* 1997: E).
11 Observe the patient throughout procedure, with attention to respiratory status including colour, respiratory rate, respiratory pattern, equal movement of chest and peripheral tissue oxygen saturations.	To look for any change in the patient's condition and report to the doctor, to ensure appropriate intervention, e.g. oxygen therapy (Laws *et al.* 2003: C).
Observe patient for any change to the cardiovascular system by alterations in heart rate or blood pressure.	To look for any change in the patient's condition and report to the doctor, to ensure appropriate intervention (Allibone 2003: E).
12 Communicate with the patient during the procedure and explain what is happening at each stage.	By communicating throughout the patient feels involved and informed (Laws *et al.* 2003: C).
13 Assist doctor in procedure as below:	
(a) The doctor will wash his hands with an antiseptic detergent and apply sterile gloves and a gown.	To minimize risk of infection (DH 2005a: C).
(b) The area for planned insertion of the drain will be cleaned with chlorhexidine gluconate 0.5% in alcohol and allowed to air dry.	To minimize risk of infection (DH 2005a: C).
(c) Local anaesthetic will be injected into the skin and deeper tissue (intercostal muscle and parietal pleura) along proposed insertion site.	To minimize the feeling of pain on drain insertion (Gray 2000: P).
(d) Wait 2–3 min for local anaesthetic to take.	To ensure local anaesthetic has been effective (E).
(e) An incision is then made with a scalpel to enable the intrapleural drain to be inserted.	To aid and ease the movement of the drain into the correct position (E).
(f) A finger may then be manoeuvred through to the parietal pleura to guide the drain into place, between the parietal and visceral pleurae in the pleural space for large bore chest tubes (Miller & Harvey 1993).	To aid the drain into the correct position (E). Exploration with a finger is felt to be unnecessary for the elective medical insertion of medium or small sized chest tubes (Laws *et al.* 2003: C).
(g) The drain is then clamped using two clamps until connected to the drainage system.	To prevent further lung collapse and entry of air (Laws *et al.* 2003: C).
(h) Connect the distal end of the drain to the drainage system and ensure that it is well supported and secured.	To allow for inflation of the lung or drainage of fluid, to ensure there is no movement of drain and that it remains in the correct position (Allibone 2003: E).
(i) The proximal end of the drain is secured and sutured in place with a mattress stitch. Unclamp chest drains.	To secure drain in position (Laws *et al.* 2003: C). Purse string stitches should no longer be used as they cause pain and unsightly scarring (Laws *et al.* 2003: C).
14 Clean the site and apply a dressing of gauze, then an occlusive dressing over the gauze.	To ensure site is well covered and sealed (Laws *et al.* 2003: C). To reduce risk of infection (DH 2005a: C).
15 Send patient for chest X-ray.	To ensure the correct position of the drain and to ensure that the lung has re-inflated (Laws *et al.* 2003: C).
16 Check the drain is well secured.	To prevent movement of drain or accidental disconnection of drain (Laws *et al.* 2003: C).
17 Monitor if there is bubbling/swinging of water in the bottle/tubing or drainage fluid and check there are no leaks around the site or that any loose connections exist within the drainage system.	To ensure there is no occlusion or leak which will prevent re-expansion of the lung or drainage of the fluid (Laws *et al.* 2003: C).
18 Record any bubbling, swinging and drainage on observation and fluid balance charts.	To keep acurate record of type of drainage on fluid balance chart (Laws *et al.* 2003: C; NMC 2005: C).

Procedure guidelines *(cont.)*

19 Ensure patient comfort following the procedure. Return the patient to an elevated position sitting in bed, well supported by pillows, and give further analgesia if required.	To ensure patient comfort in order to aid recovery and breathing (Allibone 2003: E).
20 Dispose of waste appropriately.	To reduce risk of cross-infection and sharps injury (DH 2005a: R Ia; DH 2005b: C).
21 Cleanse hands with alcoholic handrub.	Hands to be cleansed before and after each patient contact (DH 2005a: C).

Suction for intrapleural drainage.

Action	Rationale
1 Cleanse hands with alcoholic handrub.	To minimize the risk of infection (DH 2005a: C).
2 Communicate with the patient during the application of suction and explain what is happening at each stage.	To keep the patient fully informed. To enable the patient to feel reassured (Laws *et al.* 2003: C).
3 Discuss analgesia management with the patient. Give analgesia to the patient as prescribed.	To ensure patient comfort (Gray 2000: P).
4 Prepare the suction unit, which should be low vacuum suction (bedside suction units are high volume and therefore not suitable).	To maintain safety, ensuring the suction is set at low pressure (Laws *et al.* 2003: C).
5 Connect tube A (see Figure 21.4) to the suction unit, as directed by the medical team. Adjust the suction to required level prescribed, usually -5 cmH$_2$O (Adam & Osborne 2005), or to a level that is tolerable for the patient.	To ensure patient comfort and to ensure suction is applied (E). Higher volumes of suction may injure lung tissue (Kirkwood 2002: E).
6 Position patient to aid comfort, ensuring the patient is pain free and relaxed.	To aid breathing for lung expansion. To aid patient comfort (Gray 2000: E).
7 Monitor intrapleural drainage and record amount.	To maintain patient safety by observing level of suction and amount of fluid drained (Allibone 2003: E).
8 Check suction unit is working and suction pressure is maintained according to doctor's orders.	To maintain patient safety (Laws *et al.* 2003: C).

Post-intrapleural-drain procedure

Action	Rationale
1 Observe patient for any change in respiratory status: (a) Colour. (b) Respiratory rate and pattern. (c) Unequal chest movement. (d) Peripheral tissue oxygen saturations. (e) Blood gases.	These symptoms may indicate a change of chest drain position, occlusion of the drain or recurrence of pneumothorax or collection of fluid (Laws *et al.* 2003: C).
Observe patient for any change in cardiovascular status: (a) Heart rate. (b) Blood pressure.	May indicate pressure on the cardiovascular system (Allibone 2003: E).
Observe patient for signs of infection: (a) Temperature. (b) Exit site.	Obtain appropriate specimens (see Chapter 40) and inform medical staff (Wilson 2006: E).
2 Ensure the drain remains well secured with suture and dressing.	To prevent movement of drain and ensure safety of patient (Laws *et al.* 2003: C).

3	Ensure the drain is well positioned with no loops or kinks.	To prevent occlusion of drain (Kirkwood 2002: E).
4	Ensure drain tubing is well supported at the side of the bed using tape and clamps.	To prevent drain pulling and dragging, causing trauma to the patient or movement of or the risk of the drain falling out.
5	Ensure drain tubing and connections are secure and attached to the drainage unit.	To ensure a sealed unit exists to prevent air entry into the pleura which could lead to further lung collapse (Kirkwood 2002: E).
6	Ensure a pair of clamps is available beside the patient in case of accidental disconnection.	To clamp drain and prevent further lung collapse (Laws *et al.* 2003: C).
7	Do not clamp drains other than in the case of accidental disconnection.	To prevent a high positive pressure that can be created when the drain is clamped and which can result in a tension pneumothorax (Laws *et al.* 2003: C).
8	Ensure chest drain remains at a level below the chest at all times.	This prevents backflow of fluid into the pleural space (Laws *et al.* 2003: C).
9	Do not milk or strip tubing, rather change tubing if there is an occlusion.	Milking or stripping can cause an increase in negative pressure which could result in damage to lung tissue (Laws *et al.* 2003: C).
10	Observe volume and type of drainage; is it clear/bloodstained, etc.? Record on a fluid chart and in the nursing notes. Continue to record whether the drain is bubbling or swinging. If volumes exceed 1500 ml within the first 2 hours, clamp the tubing for 1 hour and inform doctors.	To ensure monitoring of type and volume of fluid loss. To prevent re-expansion oedema and large volume loss causing relative hypovolaemia (Laws *et al.* 2003 C).
11	Ensure that when the patient is sitting in the chair that the tubing, if coiled, is lifted periodically.	To aid drainage without letting the bottle be lifted higher than the thoracic cavity (Allibone 2003: E).
12	Position patient comfortably in bed, sitting upright, well supported by pillows.	To aid patient comfort. To aid breathing and allow for full expansion of the lungs (Laws *et al.* 2003: C).
13	Change the position of the patient while in bed.	To reduce risk of breakdown in skin integrity (E).
14	Encourage mobilization of the patient, e.g. to sit in chair and also to walk aided by physiotherapist or nurse.	To encourage patient independence and prevent complications, e.g. pulmonary embolus, deep vein thrombosis, breakdown in skin integrity (Allibone 2003: C).
15	Ensure patient maintains mobility of arm on side of drain.	To prevent complications and reduce risk of immobility of arm.
16	Ensure patient remains pain free.	To relieve pain and aid recovery (Gray 2000: P).
17	Maintain patient hygiene and mouth care. Assist patient in washing/mouth care because of restriction of movement due to drain.	To aid patient comfort and reduce the risk of infection (DH 2005a: C).
18	Maintain normal oral and dietary intake.	To aid healing process. To reduce risk of dehydration and malnutrition. To reduce risk of infection (DH 2005a: C).
19	Maintain a normal sleep pattern.	To allow patient to rest and aid recovery (E).
20	Ensure patient is kept occupied, e.g. reading, watching television, listening to the radio.	To relieve boredom and aid recovery (E).

437

Procedure guidelines Intrapleural drain: changing the bottle

Equipment

1 Cleaning solution, e.g. chlorhexidine in 70% alcohol.
2 Non-sterile gloves.
3 Tape.
4 Sterile chest drain bottle.

5 1 litre sterile water bottle.
6 Chest drain clamps × 2.
7 Procedure pack.

Changing intrapleural drain bottle

Action	Rationale
1 Cleanse hands with alcoholic handrub.	Hands to be cleansed before and after each patient contact (DH 2005a: C).
2 Explain and discuss the procedure with the patient.	To ensure the patient is well prepared, and to ensure their co-operation and consent (Laws *et al*. 2003: C; NMC 2006: C).
3 Cleanse hands with alcoholic rub and fill chest drain bottle to water fill line or until drainage tube is submerged in water.	To prevent infection and to prevent reflux of air or fluid into the lungs, and to create a water seal (Kirkwood 2002: E).
4 Undo the taping around the tubing.	
5 Clamp the tubing close to the chest wall with two clamps for the shortest time needed to change the bottles.	To prevent air entering the chest cavity causing a pneumothorax (Laws *et al*. 2003: C). Clamping the drain for long periods of time may increase the risk of pneumothorax (Laws *et al*. 2003: C).
6 Observe patient's breathing and respiratory status during the procedure.	To identify any respiratory deterioration early and report any abnormalities timely to medical team (Allibone 2005: E).
7 Clean tubing at the connection and remove full bottle and tubing and connect new bottle and tubing to clamped chest tube.	To prevent infection entering system during disconnection and connection of tubing (DH 2005a: C).
8 Ensure a secure connection, unclamp and tape.	To prevent bottle from falling over or disconnection causing air to re-enter the pleural cavity (Allibone 2005).
9 Ensure chest drain bottle is secure in metal stand on the floor.	
10 Cleanse hands with alcoholic rub.	
11 Document new bottle on fluid balance chart and in nursing documentation.	To keep accurate record of amounts drained (Allibone 2005: E; NMC 2005: C).
12 Observe patient for any changes in respiratory status as per previous instructions.	To identify any respiratory deterioration early and report any abnormalities to the medical team (Allibone 2005: E).

Procedure guidelines   Intrapleural drain removal

Equipment

1 Sterile dressing pack containing gallipot, gauze, sterile towel.
2 Cleaning solution, e.g. 0.9% sodium chloride.
3 Non-sterile gloves.
4 Stitch cutter.
5 Sterile dressing.
6 Tape.

Two nurses/assistants are required to facilitate safe removal of a chest drain. One is required to tie the suture and seal the site, and the other to remove the drain.

Intrapleural drain removal

Action	Rationale
1 Cleanse hands with alcoholic handrub.	Hands to be cleansed before and after each patient contact (DH 2005a: C).
2 Prepare patient for removal of the drain. Explain and discuss each step of the procedure with the patient.	To ensure the patient is well prepared, and to ensure their co-operation and consent (Laws *et al*. 2003: C; NMC 2006: C).
3 Encourage patient to practise breathing exercises, as these are required to help with the procedure. The patient should be instructed to take three deep breaths in and out and on the fourth breath to hold the breath in. It is on this breath that the drain will be removed, i.e. end of inspiration (Adam & Osborne 2005).	To prepare the patient and encourage co-operation (E). To allow the patient to practise the breathing exercises (E). To prevent the entry of air that can occur due to a negative intrathoracic pressure (Tomlinson & Treasure 1997; Allibone 2005: E).
4 In order to reduce the complication of recurrent pneumothorax, the Valsalva manoeuvre can be used. This requires patients to hold their breath and to bear down or try to breathe out against a closed glottis (Allibone 2005).	This increases the intrathoracic pressure, which reduces the possibility of air re-entering the pleural space through the drain site (Laws *et al*. 2003: C; Allibone 2005: E).
5 Clamping of chest drain prior to removal is not necessary.	Unnecessary clamping increases risk of pneumothorax (Laws *et al*. 2003: C; Adam & Osborne 2005).
6 Administer analgesia prior to procedure after discussion with doctor about the type and route of administration. The analgesia should be given at least half an hour before the procedure.	To minimize any pain during the procedure and to ensure the patient is pain free and able to co-operate (Gray 2000: P).
7 Administer sedation on doctor's instruction, if considered appropriate, e.g. for an anxious patient.	To relieve anxiety and allow the patient to relax and co-operate and to enable the procedure to go ahead (E).
8 Discontinue suction if in use and disconnect from venting/suction port.	To prevent a tension pneumothorax (Laws *et al*. 2003: C).
9 Cleanse hands with alcoholic handrub.	Hands need to be cleansed before and after each patient contact (DH 2005a: C).
10 Prepare trolley for procedure.	To aid the procedure (E).
11 Assist or set up the sterile procedure pack.	To minimize risk of infection and to have equipment ready (DH 2005a: C).
12 Position patient comfortably.	To aid patient comfort (E).

439

Procedure guidelines *(cont.)*

13 Place protective pad underneath the patient and drain.	To absorb any ooze from the drain. To reduce risk of contamination of the patient and bed clothing (E).
14 Cleanse hands with alcoholic handrub before touching the drain or dressing.	To reduce risk of infection (DH 2005a: C).
15 Remove dressing from around drain site, examine sutures present: (a) tube retaining suture (anchor suture) and (b) mattress suture; expose the ends of these sutures.	To prepare for drain removal and check what type of suture is present so that the suture can be used to form an airtight seal when the drain is removed (Adam & Osborne 2005: E).
16 Both assistants for the procedure must wash their hands with an antiseptic solution undertaking a full surgical scrub and apply gloves.	To reduce risk of infection (DH 2005a: C).
17 First nurse/assistant prepares mattress string suture and loosens ends ready to tie the suture when the drain is removed.	To prepare for drain removal (E).
18 Second nurse/assistant prepares and cuts the anchor suture and ensures the drain is mobile and ready to remove.	To prepare for drain removal (E).
19 Second nurse/assistant asks the patient to start deep breathing exercises: to take three deep breaths then hold his/her breath on the fourth one while the drain is pulled out steadily and smoothly. And ask the patient to perform the Valsalva manoeuvre.	To aid in drain removal. Deep breathing exercises can help to prevent a tension pneumothorax. If a drain is removed too quickly or without due care a pneumothorax can occur due to rupture of the pleura (Laws *et al.* 2003: C).
20 First nurse/assistant will then tie the mattress string suture securely to the skin.	To form an airtight seal and prevent air entry and formation of a pneumothorax (Laws *et al.* 2003: C).
21 Ask the patient to breath normally after tube is removed.	To assess if there is any air escaping from suture site (E).
22 Clean around site with 0.9% sodium chloride and apply an occlusive dressing, such as gauze soaked in flexible collodion or petroleum gauze under waterproof strapping.	To clean site, form an airtight seal and prevent air entry (E). To prevent an air leak if drain puncture site is not closed properly (Adam & Osborne 2005: E).
23 Ensure that the patient is sitting upright, and support with pillows.	To ensure patient comfort and aid respiration (Allibone 2005: E).
24 Dispose of waste appropriately.	To ensure safety and reduce risk of infection (DH 2005a: C; DH 2005b: C).
25 Document removal on fluid chart and in nursing notes.	To provide a point of reference for any queries (E).
26 A chest X-ray should be performed approximately 1 hour post-removal.	To check that a pneumothorax has not recurred (O'Connor & Morgan 2005: R 5).
27 Both the patient and the drain site should be monitored closely (Allibone 2005).	To observe for signs of respiratory distress secondary to reaccumulation of fluid/air in pleural cavity (Allibone 2005: E).
28 Cleanse hands with alcoholic handrub.	Hands need to be cleansed before and after each patient contact (DH 2005a: C).

Problem solving: Intrapleural drainage

Problem	Cause	Suggested action
Patient shows signs of respiratory distress, increased respiratory rate, uneven chest movement, decreasing peripheral tissue oxygen saturations.	Pneumothorax or tension pneumothorax.	Observe patient continually for change in vital signs. Inform doctor and administer oxygen. Prepare for reinsertion of chest drain.
Lack of drainage.	Kinking, looping or pressure on the tubing may cause reflux of fluid into the intrapleural space or may impede drainage, causing blocking of the intrapleural drain.	Check the system and straighten tubing as required. Secure the tubing to prevent a recurrence of the problem.
Fluid in drain not swinging.	Drain occluded due to position or occlusion.	Check no loops or kinks present in tubing. Lift drain, not higher than the patient's chest, to see if the obstruction will clear. Seek medical advice as the drain may need replacing.
Fluid in drain not bubbling.	Drain occluded or not correctly positioned.	Check no loops or kinks in the tubing. Lift tubing to see if it will clear.
Continual bubbling in chest drain bottle.	Air leak in system.	Check system for loose connections in tubing or around drainage unit. If no leak present in the drainage tubing the leak may be present in the lung. Inform doctor. Prepare chest drain insertion pack.
Leakage from drain site.	Bleeding or infection.	Remove the dressing and observe the site. Inform doctor, take swab. Clean and redress site. Discuss with medical team regarding prescription of antibiotic therapy.
Drainage from around drain site.	As a result of the insertion procedure. Incomplete closure with sutures. Infected insertion site.	Observe drain site, amount and type of drainage. Inform doctor. Take swab from site. Prepare suture pack to be available if required. Discuss with medical team regarding prescription of antibiotic therapy.
Accidental disconnection of the drainage tubing from the intrapleural drain.	Connections not secure.	Apply a clamp to the drain immediately in order to avoid air entering the pleural space. Re-establish the connection as soon as possible in order to re-establish drainage. If necessary, use a clean, sterile drainage tube; tubing may have been contaminated when it became disconnected. Report to the doctor, who may wish to X-ray. Record the incident in the relevant records. The patient may have been upset by the incident and will need reassurance.
Intrapleural drain falls out.	Drain not secure.	Pull the purse-string suture immediately to close the wound. Cover the wound with an occlusive sterile dressing. Check the patient's vital signs. Inform a doctor. The objective is to minimize the amount of air entering the pleural space. The drain will probably need reinserting. Prepare chest drain insertion pack. Reassure the patient with appropriate explanations.

441

Problem solving (cont.)

Problem	Cause	Suggested action
Poor arm movement.	Restriction of arm movement due to position of drain.	Encourage movement of limb to keep mobile. Adjust analgesia as required.
Pain.	Drain pulling at site.	Try repositioning tubing, so that it is not dragging or irritating skin. Give analgesia as prescribed.
Restricted mobility of patient.	Due to position of drain and attachment to the drainage unit.	Explore with the patient the movement that is possible and aid them where help is required. Encourage mobility, aid patient to sit in chair. Work in liaison with physiotherapist. Encourage patient to move in bed and change position.

References and further reading

Adam, S.K. & Osborne, S. (2005) Respiratory problems. In: *Critical Care Nursing*. 2nd edn. Oxford Medical Publications, Oxford, pp. 69–119

Allibone, L. (2003) Nursing management of chest drains. *Nurs Stand*, 17(22), 45–54.

Allibone, L. (2005) Respiratory care. Principles for inserting and managing chest drains. *Nurs Times* 101 (42), 45–9.

Avery, S. (2000) Insertion and management of chest drains. *Nurs Times*, 96, 3–6.

Berne, R.M. & Levy, M.N. (2004) Structure and function of the respiratory system. In: *Physiology*, 5th edn. Mosby, London, pp. 445–463

Brandt, M.L. *et al.* (1994) The paediatric chest tube. *Clin Intensive Care*, 5(3), 123–9.

Chernecky, C. & Shelton, B. (2001) Pulmonary complications in patients with cancer: diagnostic and treatment information for the noncritical care nurse. *Am J Nurs*, 101(5), 24A–24H.

Clementsen, P. *et al.* (1998) Treatment of malignant pleural effusion: pleurodesis using a small bore catheter. A prospective randomized study. *Respir Med*, 92, 593–6.

Deshpande, K.S., Tortolani, A.J. & Kvetan, V. (2003) Troubleshooting chest tube complications: how to prevent, or quickly correct the major problems. *J Crit Illn*, 18(6), 275–80.

DH (2005a) *Saving Lives: A Delivery Programme to Reduce Healthcare Associated Infection including MRSA*. Department of Health, London.

DH (2005b) *Hazardous waste (England) regulations*. Department of Health, London.

Gallon, A. (1998) Pneumothorax. *Nurs Stand*, 39(10), 35–9.

Godden, J. (1998) Managing the patient with a chest drain: a review. *Nurs Stand*, 12(32), 35–9.

Gorden, P.A., Norton, J.M. & Guerra, J.M. (1997) Positioning of chest drain tubes: effects on pressure and drainage. *Am J Crit Care*, 6, 33–8.

Gray, E. (2000) Pain management for patients with chest drains. *Nurs Stand*, 14(23), 40–4.

Grodzin, C.J. & Baik, R.A. (1997) Indwelling small pleural catheter needle thoracentesis in the management of large pleural effusions. *Chest*, 111(4), 981–8.

Hall, J.E. and Guyton, A.C (2005) Pulmonary ventilation. In: *A Textbook of Medical Physiology*, 11th edn. W.B. Saunders, Philadelphia, pp. 471–482.

Henry, M., Arnold, T. & Harvey, J. (2003) British Thoracic Society guidelines for the management of spontaneous pneumothorax. *Thorax*, 58, 39–52.

Higgins, D. (2006) Removal of chest drains. *Nurs Times*, 102(13), 26–7.

Hilton, P. (2004) Evaluating the treatment options for spontaneous pneumothorax. *Nurs Times*, 100(28), 32–3.

Hyde, J., Skyes, T. & Graham, T. (1997) Reducing morbidity from chest drains. *BMJ*, 314(7085), 914–15.

Kirkwood, P. (2002) Ask the experts. *Crit Care Nurse*, 22(4), 70–3.

Kozar, R. & Adams, S.D. (2005) Chylothorax. Emedicine from www.emedicine.com/med/topic381.htm. Accessed 28/08/07.

Kumar, P. & Clarke, C. (2002) *Clinical Medicine*. Mosby, St. Louis, MO.

Laws, D., Neville, E. & Duffy, J. (2003) British Thoracic Society guidelines for the insertion of a chest drain. *Thorax*, 58, 53–9.

Luketich, J.D. *et al.* (1998) Chest tube insertion: a prospective evaluation of pain management. *Clin J Pain*, 14, 152–4.

Marieb, E.N. (2001) The respiratory system. In: *Human Anatomy and Physiology*, 5th edn. John Wiley & Sons, Inc., New York. Pearson Education, San Francisco, CA. pp. 834–86.

McMahon-Parkes, K. (1997) Management of pleural drains. *Nurs Times*, 93(52), 48–52.

MedlinePlus (2006) Medical encyclopedia. www.nlm.nih.gov/medlineplus/ency/article/000100.htm. Accessed 7/08/06.

Miller, A.C. & Harvey, J.E. (1993) Guidelines for the management of spontaneous pneumothorax. *BMJ*, 307, 114–16.

NMC (2005) *Guidelines for Records and Record Keeping*. Nursing and Midwifery Council, London.

NMC (2006) *A–Z Advice Sheet Consent*. www.nmc.org.

O'Connor, A.R. & Morgan, W.E. (2005) Radiological review of pneumothorax. *BMJ*, 330, 1493–7.

Parkin, C. (2002) A retrospective audit of chest drain practice in a specialist cardiothoracic centre and concurrent review of chest drain literature. *Nurs Crit Care*, 7(1), 30–6.

Patz, E.F. (1998) Malignant pleural effusions: recent advances and ambulatory sclerotherapy. *Chest*, 113(1, Suppl 1), 74–5.

Peek, G., Morcos, S. & Cooper, G. (2000) The pleural cavity. *BMJ*, 320, 1318–21.

Pierce, L.N.B. (1995) *Guide to Mechanical Ventilation and Intensive Respiratory Care*. W.B. Saunders, London, Appendix 111, pp. 356–63.

Tang, A., Hooper, T. & Hassan, R. (1999) A regional survey of chest drains: evidence based practice? *Postgrad Med J*, 75(886), 471–4

Tang, A., Vellissaris, T. & Weeden, D. (2002) An evidence based approach to drainage of pleural cavity: evaluation of best practice. *J Eval Clin Pract*, 8(3), 333–40.

Thelan, L.A. *et al.* (1995) *Critical Care Nursing–Diagnosis and Management*, 2nd edn. Mosby, St. Louis, MO.

Tomlinson, M.A. & Treasure, T. (1997) Insertion of a chest drain: how to do it. *Br J Hosp Med*, 58(6), 248–52.

Tooley, C. (2002) The management and care of chest drains. *Nurs Times*, 98(26), 48–50.

Tortora, G.J. & Derrickson, B. (2008) The respiratory system. In: *Principles of Anatomy and Physiology*, 12th edn.

John Wiley & Sons, Inc., New York, Hoboken NJ, pp. 846–94.

Van Le, L. *et al.* (1994) Pleural effusions: outpatient management of pigtail catheter chest tubes. *Gynecol Oncol*, 54, 215–7.

Wilson, J. (2006) *Infection Control in Clinical Practice*. Bailliere Tindall, London.

Yeam, I. & Sassoon, C. (1997) Haemothorax and chylothorax. *Curr Opin Pulmon Med*, 3(4), 310–14.

Chapter 22

Last offices

445 Reference material
446 *Procedure guidelines:* Last offices
449 **Issues specific to critical care**
450 *Procedure guidelines:* Last offices: additional considerations in critical care
451 *Problem solving:* Last offices
452 *Procedure guidelines:* Last offices: requirements for people of different religious faiths
456 References
457 Further reading on religious faiths

Definition

Nursing care should not stop when the patient dies. Last offices, sometimes referred to as 'laying out', is the term for the nursing care given to a deceased patient which demonstrates continued respect for the patient as an individual (NMC 2008) and in contemporary society it is focused on attending to health, safety and legal requirements, making the body safe to handle and pleasant for others to see, whilst also respecting religious beliefs and cultural norms.

Reference material

In many societies, the care and preparation of the deceased is carried out only by close family members. In others it is undertaken by certain specialized individuals within the community (Clark 2000). For example, amongst orthodox Jews, the *chevra kadisha* or Burial Society of each community, made up of volunteers, cares for the deceased and prepares them for burial (Helman 2007). However in the UK, where of all recorded deaths, 66% of patients die in hospital (ONS 2000), it is common practice for nurses who have cared for the individual before death to care for the body after death, prior to it leaving the hospital ward or department (Berry & Griffie 2004).

There is documented evidence of nurses caring for the bodies of their deceased patients dating back to the nineteenth century (Wolf 1988). However, contemporary nursing practice is somewhat different to that of our predecessors who were required to cleanse the body of the deceased, plugging, packing and tying the patient's orifices to prevent the leakage of body fluids (Pearce 1963). Today emphasis is given to the legal issues surrounding death, the removal of invasive, defunct equipment, washing and grooming, and ensuring the correct identification of the body (Costello 2004). Such practices are being asserted by end-of-life care tools such as the Liverpool Care Pathway for the Dying (Ellershaw & Wilkinson 2003), which is fast gaining national momentum and demonstrating improvements to the care of the dying and care after death.

Whilst the procedure of last offices has its foundation in traditional cultures and has become a nursing ritual that does not have a heavy weight of research-based evidence (Cooke 2000), the administration of last offices can have symbolic meaning for nurses and can be a fulfilling experience as it is the final demonstration of respectful, sensitive care given to a patient (Nearney 1998) and also the family (Speck 1992). Last offices can mark the social transition of the person, the biological death of the patient, and begins the process of handing over care to the family and funeral director. Therefore, last offices can be considered as an important act in the rite of passage or *rite de passage* in moving the deceased into the world of the dead (Van Gennep 1972) that people in all cultures recognize. Whilst

we may not be able to locate a scientific evidence base for this clinical nursing procedure, there is a strong cultural requirement to continue with it as, 'Rituals serve to express symbolic meanings important to groups of people functioning within a subculture' (Wolf 1988, p. 59). And whilst in contemporary nursing practice and education there is a move away from ritualistic practice as it is considered as irrational and unscientific (Philpin 2002), the procedure of last offices remains a notable exception. However, this is not to say that nurses carrying out last offices do it, 'without thinking about it in a problem solving way' (Walsh & Ford 1989, p. 9) or in a way that does not recognize the individual needs of the deceased and their carers. Instead these are carried out with insight into the meanings attached to the accomplishment of this aspect of nursing care (Philpin 2002).

In administering last offices, nurses need to know the legal requirements for care of the dead and it is essential that the correct procedures are followed. Every effort should be made to accommodate the wishes of the patient's relatives (Neuberger 2004).

It is impossible to understand the laws and prohibitions about handling human bodies after death without having some idea of what that particular person's religion or philosophy has to say about the nature of human life and its value (Neuberger 1999). As the UK today is a multicultural and multifaith society, this offers a great challenge to nurses who need to be aware of the different religious and cultural rituals that may accompany the death of a patient. There are considerable cultural variations within and between people of different faiths, ethnic backgrounds and national origins and their approach to death and dying (Neuberger 1999). Whilst those who have settled in a society where there is a dominant faith or culture other than their own appear to increasingly adopt that dominant culture, in many ways they retain, almost deliberately to emphasize differences, their different practices at times of birth, marriage or death (Neuberger 1999). Approaches to death and dying also reveal as much of the attitude of society as a whole as they do about individuals within that society (Field *et al.* 1997).

Practices relating to last offices will vary depending on the patient's cultural background and religious practices (Nearney 1998). The following sections provide a guide to cultural and religious variations in attitudes to death and how individuals may wish to be treated. The information that follows is not designed to be a chapter of comparative theology. Nor is it a 'factfile' (Gunaratnam 1997; Smaje & Field 1997; Gilliat-Ray 2001) of information on culture and religion that seeks to give concrete information. Such a 'factfile' would not be appropriate as we need to be aware that whilst death and death-related beliefs, rituals and traditions can vary widely from each specific cultural group, within any given religious or cultural group there may be varying degrees of observance of these issues (Green & Green 2006) from orthodox to the agnostic and atheist. Our motivation to categorize individuals into groups with clearly defined norms can lead to a lack of understanding of the complexities of religious and cultural practice and can depersonalize individuals and their families (Smaje & Field 1997; Neuberger 1999).

Last offices for an expected death may be very different to those given to a patient who has died suddenly or unexpectedly (Docherty 2000) or in a critical care setting; therefore, these issues will be dealt with later in this chapter. In certain cases the patient's death may need to be referred to the coroner for further investigation and possible post-mortem (DH 2003). If those caring for the deceased are unsure about this, then the person in charge of the patient's care should be consulted before last offices are commenced. However, further advice on this is given in the Issues specific to critical care section, below.

Prior to the patient's death, whenever possible it is good practice to ascertain if the patient wishes to donate organs or tissue following their death. For further information on this visit: www.uktransplant.org.uk/urt.

Procedure guidelines   Last offices

. . . .

Equipment

1 Disposable plastic aprons.
2 Disposable plastic gloves.
3 Bowl of warm water, soap, the deceased's own toiletries and face cloths or disposable wash cloths and two towels.
4 Disposable razor or the patient's own electric razor, comb and equipment for nail care.
5 Equipment for mouth care including equipment for cleaning dentures.
6 Identification labels ×2.
7 Documents required by law and organization policy, e.g. notification of death cards.
8 Shroud or patient's personal clothing: night-dress, pyjamas, clothes previously requested by patient, or clothes that comply with family/cultural wishes.

9 Body bag if required (i.e. in event of actual or potential leakage of bodily fluids and/or infectious disease) and labels for the body defining the nature of the infection/disease (HSE 2003: C).
10 Gauze, waterproof tape, dressings and bandages if wounds or intravenous/arterial lines and cannulae are present.
11 Disposable or washable receptacle for collecting urine if appropriate.
12 Plastic bags for clinical and household waste.
13 Sharps bin if appropriate.
14 Laundry skip and appropriate bags for soiled linen.
15 Clean bed linen.
16 Record books for property and valuables.
17 Bags for the patient's personal possessions.

. . . .

Procedure

Action	Rationale
1 Inform the nurse in charge of the ward or unit and inform medical staff of the patient's death. Confirmation of death must be given. This is usually done by medical staff. If an expected death occurs in the event of medical staff not being available, it may be possible for the senior nurse on duty to confirm the death if an agreed local policy has been implemented (RCN 1996: C). An unexpected death must be confirmed by an attending medical officer. Confirmation of death must be recorded in a patient's medical, nursing notes and care pathway documentation if necessary.	A registered medical practitioner who has attended the deceased person during their last illness is required to give a medical certificate of the cause of death (Home Office 1971: C). The certificate requires the doctor to state on which date he/she last saw the deceased alive and whether or not he/she has seen the body after death.
2 Inform and offer support to relatives and/or next of kin. Offer support of Hospital Chaplain or other religious leader or other appropriate person, e.g. bereavement support officer. If relative(s) or next of kin are not contactable by telephone or by the GP, it may be necessary to inform the police of the death. Also inform other patients in the area of the patient's death.	To ensure relevant individuals are aware of patient's death. To provide sensitive care (Wilkinson & Mula 2003: E).

3 Ascertain if the patient had an infectious disease and whether this is notifiable or not. There are additional requirements for patients with blood-borne infections; therefore, the senior nurse on duty should be consulted and local infection control policy adhered to. Placing the deceased in a body bag is advised for all notifiable diseases and a number of non-notifiable infectious diseases (i.e. human immunodeficiency virus [HIV] and transmissible spongiform encephalopathies, e.g. Creutzfeldt–Jakob disease).

Certain extra precautions are required when handling a patient who has died from an infectious disease. However, the deceased will pose no greater threat of an infectious risk than when they were alive. It is assumed that staff will have practised universal precautions when caring for all patients, and this practice must be continued when caring for the deceased patient (HSE 2003: C).

4 Last offices should be carried out within 2–4 hours of death.

Rigor mortis can occur relatively soon after death, and this time is shortened in warmer environments (Berry & Griffie 2006: E).

5 If possible determine from the family or carers, the patient's previous wishes for care after death.

Some families and carers may wish to assist with last offices, and within certain cultures it may be unacceptable for anyone but a family member or religious leader to wash the patient (Green & Green 2006: P & C). Families and carers should be supported and encouraged to participate if possible as this may help to facilitate the grieving process (Berry & Griffie 2006: E).

6 Wash hands and put on disposable gloves and disposable plastic apron.

Personal protective equipment (PPE) must be worn when performing last offices, and is used to both protect yourself and all of your patients from the risks of cross-infection (RCN 2005: C).

7 If the patient is on a pressure-relieving mattress or device, consult the manufacturer's instructions before switching off or changing settings.

Nurses must act at all times to maintain the patient's safety when using a pressure-relieving mattress or device (RCN 2003: C & E).

8 Lay the patient on his/her back with the assistance of two nurses (adhering to your own organization's Manual Handling policy). Remove all but one pillow. Support the jaw by placing a pillow or rolled-up towel on the chest or underneath the patient's jaw. Do not bind the patient's jaw with bandages as this can leave pressure marks on the face which can be difficult to remove. Remove any mechanical aids such as syringe drivers, heel pads, etc. Apply gauze and tape to syringe driver sites and document disposal of medication (adhering to your own organization's Disposal of Medication policy). Straighten the patient's limbs.

To maintain the patient's privacy and dignity (NMC 2008: C) and for future nursing care of the body. A body with flexed limbs can be difficult to fit easily into a mortuary trolley, mortuary fridge or coffin and can cause additional distress to any carers who wish to view the body. However, if the body cannot be straightened, force should not be used as this can be corrected by the funeral director (Green & Green 2006: E).

9 Close the patient's eyes by applying light pressure to the eyelids for 30 seconds. If this is unsuccessful then a little sticky tape such as micropore can be used, and leaves no mark. Alternatively, moistened cotton wool may be used to hold the eyelids in place.

To maintain the patient's dignity (NMC 2008: C) and for aesthetic reasons. Closure of the eyelids will also provide tissue protection in case of corneal donation (Green & Green 2006: E).

10 Drain the bladder by applying firm pressure over the lower abdomen. Have a disposable or washable receptacle at the ready to collect urine. Therefore the practice of tying a bandage round a penis is not necessary and many families may find this practice unacceptable.

Because the body can continue to excrete fluids after death (Green & Green 2006: E).

Procedure guidelines *(cont.)*

11 Leakages from the oral cavity, vagina and bowel can be contained by the use of suctioning, drainage and incontinence pads respectively. Patients who do continue to have leakages from their orifices after death should be placed in a body bag following last offices. The packing of orifices can cause damage to the body and should only be done by professionals, e.g. mortuary technicians who have received specialist training.	Leaking orifices pose a health hazard to staff coming into contact with the body (HSE 2003: C; Green & Green 2006: E). Ensuring that the body is clean will demonstrate a continued respect for the patient's dignity (NMC 2008: C). The packing of orifices is considered unnecessary as it increases the rate of bacterial growth and therefore increases odour when these areas of the body are not allowed to drain naturally (Berry & Griffie 2006: E).
12 Exuding wounds or unhealed surgical scars should be covered with a clean absorbant dressing and secured with an occlusive dressing. Stitches and clips should be left intact. Stomas should be covered with a clean bag.	The dressing will absorb any leakage from the wound site (Naylor *et al.* 2001: R 2b). Open wounds and stomas pose a health hazard to staff coming into contact with the body (RCN 2005: C).
13 Remove drainage tubes, etc. unless otherwise stated, and document actions and any tubes remaining, e.g. central venous access device which should not be removed by nursing staff. Open drainage sites need to be sealed with an occlusive dressing (e.g. Tegaderm).	Open drainage sites pose a health hazard to staff coming into contact with the body (RCN 2005: C). When a death is being referred to the coroner or for post-mortem, all lines, devices and tubes should be left in place (Green & Green 2006: C).
14 Wash the patient, unless requested not to do so for religious/cultural reasons or carer's preference. Male patients should be shaved unless they chose to wear a beard in life. If shaving a man apply water-based emollient cream to the face.	For hygenic and aesthetic reasons. As a mark of respect and point of closure in the relationship between nurse and patient (Cooke 2000: C). To prevent brown streaks on the skin (Ashford and St. Peter's Hospitals NHS Trust 2005: E).
15 It may be important to family and carers to assist with washing, thereby continuing to provide the care given in the period before death.	It is an expression of respect and affection, and part of the process of adjusting to loss and expressing grief (Berry & Griffie 2006: E).
16 Clean the patient's mouth using a foam stick to remove debris and secretions. Clean dentures and replace them in the mouth if possible.	For hygenic and aesthetic reasons (Cooke 2000: C).
17 Remove all jewellery (in the presence of another nurse) unless requested by the patient's family to do otherwise. Jewellery remaining on the patient should be documented on the 'notification of death' form. Record the jewellery and other valuables in the patient's property book and store the items according to local policy. Avoid the use of the names of precious metals or gems when describing jewellery to prevent later confusion. Instead use terms such as 'yellow metal' or 'red stone'. Rings left on the body should be secured with tape, if loose.	To meet with legal requirements, cultural practices and relatives' wishes (Green & Green 2006: C).
18 Dress the patient in personal clothing or white garment, traditionally called a shroud, depending on organizational policy or relatives' wishes.	For aesthetics for family and carers viewing the body or religious or cultural reasons and to meet family's or carer's wishes (Green & Green 2006: C).

19	Ensure a correct hospital or organizational irremovable patient identification label is attached to the patient's wrist and attach a further identification label to one ankle. Complete any documents such as notification of death cards. Copies of such cards are usually required (refer to hospital policy for details). Tape one securely to clothing or shroud.	To ensure correct and easy identification of the body in the mortuary (Green & Green 2006: C).
20	Wrap the body in a sheet, ensuring that the face and feet are covered and that all limbs are held securely in position.	To avoid possible damage to the body during transfer and to prevent distress to colleagues, e.g. portering staff (Green & Green 2006: E).
21	Secure the sheet with tape.	Pins must not be used as they are a health and safety hazard to staff (Nearney 1998: E; Travis 2002: E).
22	Place the body in a sheet and then a body bag if leakage of body fluids is a problem or is anticipated, or if the patient has certain infectious diseases (see Chapter 6).	Actual or potential leakage of fluid, whether infection is present or not, poses a health hazard to all those who come into contact with the deceased patient. The sheet will absorb excess fluid (HSE 2003: C).
23	Tape the second notification of death card to the outside of the sheet (or body bag).	For ease of identification of the body in the mortuary (Green & Green 2006: E).
24	Request the portering staff to remove the body from the ward and transport to the mortuary.	Decomposition occurs rapidly, particularly in hot weather and in overheated rooms. Many pathogenic organisms survive for some time after death and so decomposition of the body may pose a health and safety hazard for those handling the body (Cooke 2000: E). Autolysis and growth of bacteria are delayed if the body is cooled.
25	Screen off area where removal of the body will occur.	To avoid causing unnecessary distress to other patients, relatives and staff (Nearney 1998: E; Travis 2002: E).
26	Remove gloves and apron. Dispose of equipment according to local policy and wash hands.	To minimize risk of cross-infection and contamination (DH 2001: R 1a).
27	Record all details and actions within the nursing documentation.	To record the time of death, names of those present, and names of those informed (NMC 2008: C).
28	Transfer property, patient records, etc. to the appropriate administrative department.	The administrative department cannot begin to process the formalities such as the death certificate or the collection of property by the next-of-kin until the required documents are in its possession (Green & Green 2006: C; NMC 2005: C).

Issues specific to critical care

Critical care, accident and emergency and other such acute settings present further issues related to last offices. These are in addition to those listed above. Issues starting with verification of death may differ; therefore, senior nursing and medical staff should be consulted before commencing last offices.

Additional practices may need to be carried out if the patient is a donor patient, particularly in the case of brain stem death (DH 1998). It is important to liaise with the transplant co-ordinator to ascertain before last offices if there are specific preparations required. In the case of a coroner-led post-mortem there may also be specific preparations required (DH 2003). Senior nursing staff or the coroner's office should be consulted to establish if this is necessary before undertaking last offices.

Procedure guidelines   Last offices: additional considerations in critical care

The following should be considered in addition to the same numbered action in the procedures listed above in Procedure guidelines: Last offices.

Procedure

Action	Rationale
3 High-risk infectious patients should be marked as such, e.g. patient with HIV, hepatitis B, on the accompanying forms, and should have hazard labels on the body bag and on the patient. Linen and waste should be treated as infected. In the case of tuberculosis, there is still a risk of expirational transmission after death. This phenomenon should be considered and communicated, especially to mortuary staff or nurses who may re-prepare the patient for a viewing at a later point in time. In certain cases (i.e. typhus, SARS [Severe Acute Respiratory Syndrome], yellow fever, anthrax, plague, rabies and smallpox) viewing should not be permitted given the high risk of transmission. In the case of highly infectious patients (e.g. notifiable) packing should be considered.	Rolling the patient in last offices may force expiration and facilitate transmission of tuberculosis. The risk of transmission remains after death in certain notifiable diseases (typhus, SARS, yellow fever, anthrax, plague, rabies and smallpox) (HSAC 2003: C). Packing may reduce the risk of transmission.
4 If the patient is not to be referred to the coroner then remove all invasive and non-invasive attachments to the patient, such as: central venous access lines, peripheral venous access lines, Swan–Ganz catheters, tracheal tubes (tracheostomy/endotracheal [ET]), drains. If a coroner's case, cap off lines and ensure no possibility of leakage. Do not remove any invasive lines.	The coroner may need to see exactly what state the patient was in at the time death and what could have contributed to cause of death (DH 2003: C). Documentation ensures that there is a record of invasive equipment in situ for the patient notes and the coroner.
11 All deceased critical care patients should be placed in a zipped plastic (body) bag. Absorbent sheets (incontinence pads) may be placed either side of the head.	There is an increased likelihood of critical care patients leaking (Travis 2002: E).
12 Consider leaving intact recent surgical dressings for wounds that could potentially leak, e.g. large amputation wounds. Reinforcement of the dressing should be sufficient.	Certain surgical wounds may have been carefully dressed in theatre and disturbing them in order to redress may precipitate leakage (Travis 2002: E).
13 Document tubes/equipment remaining, e.g. tunneled skin catheters, pacemaker, implantable cardioverter defibrillators (ICDs).	Documentation ensures that there is a record of equipment still *in situ* (Travis 2002: E).
16 Apply petroleum jelly to lips and perioral area. Suction oropharynx if patient previously intubated/had a tracheostomy.	Even if the patient is not obviously leaking from the oral cavity, secretions may accumulate in the oropharynx in previously intubated and tracheostomy patients. Petroleum jelly may prevent skin excoriation/corrosion if stomach contents aspirate (Travis 2002: E).

Problem solving: Last offices

Problem	Suggested action
Relatives not present at the time of the patient's death.	Inform the relatives as soon as possible of the death. Consider also that they may want to view the body before last offices are completed.
Relatives or next-of-kin not contactable by telephone or by the general practitioner.	If within the UK, local police will go to next-of-kin's house. If abroad, the British Embassy will assist.
Death occurring within 24 hours of an operation.	All tubes and/or drains must be left in position. Spigot any cannulae or catheters. Treat stomas as open wounds. Leave any endotracheal or tracheostomy tubes in place. Post-mortem examination will be required to establish the cause of death. Any tubes, drains etc., may have been a major contributing factor to the death.
Unexpected death.	As above. Post-mortem examination of the body will be required to establish the cause of death.
Unknown cause of death.	As above.
Patient brought into hospital who is already deceased.	As above, unless patient seen by a medical practitioner within 14 days before death. In this instance the attending medical officer may complete the death certificate if he/she is clear as to the cause of death.
Patient with leaking wounds/orifices with or without infection present. Patient with hepatitis B or who is HIV positive.	For further information see Chapter 6.
Patient who dies after receiving systemic radioactive iodine.	For further information see Chapter 36.
Patient who dies after insertion of gold grains, colloidal radioactive solution, caesium needles, caesium applicators, iridium wires or iridium hair pins.	Inform the physics department as well as appropriate medical staff. Once a doctor has verified death, the sources are removed and placed in a lead container. A Geiger counter is used to check that all sources have been removed. This reduces the radiation risk when completing the last offices procedures. Record the time and date of removal of the sources.
Patient and/or relative wishes to donate organs/tissues for transplantation.	Patients with malignancies can only donate corneas (with certain exceptions) and in some cases, heart valves and tracheas. Ultimately, this is a clinician-led decision. Contact local transplant co-ordinator as soon as decision is made to donate organs/tissue and before last offices is attempted. Obtain verbal and written consent from the next-of-kin, as per local policy. Prepare body as per transplant co-ordinator's instructions (UK Transplant, 2007).
Patient to be moved straight from ward to undertakers.	Contact senior nurse for hospital. Contact local Registry Office as release of Certificate for Burial or Cremation ('green' document) needs to be obtained. Liaise with chosen funeral directors and the deceased's family. Perform last offices as per religious/cultural/family wishes. Obtain written authority for removal of body by the funeral directors, from the next-of-kin. Document all actions and proceedings (Travis 2002: C).

Problem solving *(cont.)*

Problem

Relatives want to see the body after removal from the ward.

Suggested action

Inform the mortuary staff in order to allow time for them to prepare the body. The body will normally be placed in the hospital viewing room. Ask relatives if they wish for a chaplain or other religious leader or appropriate person to accompany them. As required, religious artefacts should be removed from or added to the viewing room. The nurse should check that the body and environment are presentable before accompanying the relatives into the viewing room. The relatives may want to be alone with the deceased but the nurse should wait outside the viewing room in order that support may be provided should the relatives become distressed. After the relatives have left, the nurse should contact the portering service who will return the body to the mortuary.

Procedure guidelines   Last offices: requirements for people of different religious faiths

The following are only guidelines: individual requirements may vary even among members of the same faith. Varying degrees of adherence and orthodoxy exist within all the world's faiths. The given religion of a patient may occasionally be offered to indicate an association with particular cultural and national roots, rather than to indicate a significant degree of adherence to the tenets of a particular faith. If in doubt, consult the family members concerned.

Bahai

1 The body of the deceased should be treated with respect. Bahai relatives may wish to say prayers for the deceased person, but normal last offices performed by nursing staff are quite acceptable.

2 Bahai adherents may not be cremated or embalmed, nor may they be buried more than an hour's journey from the place of death. A special ring will be placed on the finger of the patient and should not be removed.

3 Bahais have no objection to post-mortem examination and may leave their bodies to scientific research or donate organs if they wish.

4 Further information can be obtained from the nearest Assembly of the Bahais (see telephone directory). Alternatively, contact:
> National Spiritual Assembly of the Bahais of the United Kingdom
> 27 Rutland Gate, London SW7 1PD
> Tel: 020 7590 8792
> Email: nsa@bahai.org.uk
> Website: www.bahai.org.uk

Buddhism

1 There is no prescribed ritual for the handling of the corpse of a Buddhist person, so customary laying out is appropriate. However, a request may be made for a Buddhist monk or nun to be present.

2 As there are a number of different schools of Buddhism, relatives should be contacted for advice as some sects have strong views on how the body should be treated.

3 When the patient dies, inform the monk or nun if required (the patient's relatives often take this step). The body should not be moved for at least 1 hour if prayers are to be said.

4 There are unlikely to be objections to post-mortem examination and organ donation, although some Far Eastern Buddhists may object to this.

5 The patient's body should be wrapped in an unmarked sheet.

6 Cremation is preferred.

7 For further information contact:
> Dennis Sibley
> The Buddhist Hospice Trust
> 1 Laurel House, Trafalger Road
> Newport, Isle of Wight, PO30 1QN
> Tel: 01983 526945
> Email: dsibley@buddhisthospice.org.uk

Christianity

1 There are many denominations and degrees of adherence within the Christian faith. In most cases customary last offices are acceptable.
2 Relatives may wish staff to call the hospital chaplain, or minister or priest from their own church to either perform last rites or say prayers.
3 Some Roman Catholic families may wish to place a rosary in the deceased patient's hands and/or a crucifix at the patient's head.
4 Some orthodox families may wish to place an icon (holy picture) at either side of the patient's head.

5 For further information consult the hospital chaplain or consult the telephone directory for the local denominational minister or priest.
 Alternatively, contact:
 Hospital Chaplaincies Council
 Church House, Great Smith Street, London SW1 3NZ
 Tel: 020 7898 1894
 Useful website:
 www.nhs-chaplaincy-spiritualcare.org.uk

Humanism

1 Humanism is an approach to life based on reason and a sense of a common humanity with a recognition that moral values are founded within human nature and experience alone (BBC 2006). Therefore Humanism is not a religion but a rationalist non-religious approach to life. Humanism affirms that human beings have the right and responsibility to give meaning and shape to their own lives (BBC 2006).
2 Therefore, individuals who define themselves as Humanists should as far as possible, like all other patients, be involved in decisions relating to their care before and after death.

3 For further information contact:
 British Humanist Association
 1 Gower Street, London WC1E 6HD
 Tel: 020 70793582
 Email: info@humanism.org.uk
 Website: www.humanism.org.uk

Hinduism

1 If required by relatives, inform the family priest or one from the local temple. If unavailable, relatives may wish to read from the *Bhagavad Gita* or make a request that staff read extracts during the last offices.
2 The family may wish to carry out or assist in last offices and may request that the patient is dressed in his or her own clothes. If possible, the eldest son should be present. A Hindu may like to have leaves of the sacred Tulsi plant and Ganges water placed in his/her mouth by relatives before death. It is therefore imperative that relatives are warned that the patient's death is imminent. Relatives of the same sex as the patient may wish to wash his/her body, preferably in water mixed with water from the River Ganges. If no relatives are present, nursing staff of the same sex as the patient should wear gloves and apron and then straighten the body, close the eyes and support the jaw before wrapping in a sheet. The body should not be washed. Do not remove sacred threads or jewellery.

3 The patient's family may request that the patient be placed on the floor and they may wish to burn incense.
4 The patient is usually cremated as soon as possible after death. Post-mortems are viewed as disrespectful to the deceased person, and so are only carried out when strictly necessary. Consult the wishes of the family before touching the body.
5 For further information contact the nearest Hindu temple (see telephone directory) or:
 National Council of Hindu Temples (UK)
 40 Stoke Row, Coventry CV2 4JP
 Email: info@hinducounciluk.org
 Useful website: www.hinducounciluk.org

Jainism

1 The relatives of a Jainist patient may wish to contact their priest to recite prayers with the patient and family.
2 The family may wish to be present during the last offices and also to assist with washing. However, not all families will want to perform this task.

3 The family may ask for the patient to be clothed in a plain white gown or shroud with no pattern or ornament and then wrapped in a plain white sheet. They may provide the gown themselves.
4 Post-mortems may be seen as disrespectful, depending on the degree of orthodoxy of the patient. Organ donation is acceptable.

Procedure guidelines *(cont.)*

5 Cremation is arranged whenever possible within 24 hours of death.

6 Orthodox Jains may have chosen the path of *Sallekhana*, that is, death by ritual fasting. Sallekhana is rarely practised today although it may still have an influence on the Jain attitude to death.

7 For further information contact:
The Institute of Jainology
Unit 18, Silicon Business Centre, 26 Wandsworth Road, Greenford, Middlesex UB6 7JZ
Tel: 020 8997 2300
The Jain Centre
32 Oxford Street, Leicester LE1 5XU
Tel: 0116 254 3091
Useful website: www.jainism.org

Jehovah's Witness

1 Routine last offices are appropriate. Relatives may wish to be present during last offices, either to pray or to read from the Bible. The family will inform staff should there be any special requirements, which may vary according to the patient's country of origin.

2 Jehovah's Witnesses usually refuse post-mortems unless absolutely necessary. Organ donation may be acceptable.

3 Further information can be obtained from the nearest Kingdom Hall (see telephone directory) or:
The Medical Desk
The Watch Tower Bible and Tract Society
Watch Tower House, The Ridgeway, London NW7 1RN
Tel: 020 8906 2211
Email: his@wtbts.org.uk

Judaism

1 The family will contact their own Rabbi if they have one. If not, the hospital chaplaincy will advise. Prayers are recited by those present.

2 Traditionally the body is left for about 8 minutes before being moved while a feather is placed across the lips and nose to detect any signs of breath.

3 Usually close relatives will straighten the body, but nursing staff are permitted to perform any procedure for preserving dignity and honour. Wearing gloves, the body should be handled as little as possible but nurses may:
   (a) Close the eyes.
   (b) Tie up the jaw.
   (c) Put the arms parallel and close to the sides of the body leaving the hands open. Straighten the patient's legs.
   (d) Remove tubes unless contraindicated.
Patients must not be washed and should remain in the clothes in which they died. The body will be washed by a nominated group, the Holy Assembly, which performs a ritual purification.

4 Watchers stay with the body until burial (normally completed within 24 hours of death). In the period before burial a separate non-denominational room is appreciated, where the body can be placed with its feet towards the door.

5 It is not possible for funerals to take place on the Sabbath (between sunset on Friday and sunset on Saturday). If death occurs during the Sabbath, the body will remain with the watchers until the end of the Sabbath. Advice should be sought from the relatives. In some areas, the Registrar's office will arrange to open on Sundays and Bank Holidays to allow for the registration of death where speedy burial is required for religious reasons. The Jewish Burial Society will know whether this service is offered in the local area.

6 Post-mortems are permitted only if required by law. Organ donation is sometimes permitted.

7 Cremation is unlikely but some non-orthodox Jews are now accepting this in preference to burial.

8 For further information, contact:
The Burial Society of the United Synagogue
Tel: 020 8343 3456
The Office of the Chief Rabbi (Orthodox)
735 High Road, North Finchley, London WC1N 9HN
Tel: 020 8343 6301

Reform Synagogues of Great Britain
The Sternberg Centre for Judaism
80 East End Road, Finchley, London N3 2SY
Tel: 020 8349 4731

Union of Liberal and Progressive Synagogues
Montagu Centre, 21 Maple Street, London W1T 4BE

Mormon (Church of Jesus Christ of the Latter Day Saints)

1 There are no special requirements, but relatives may wish to be present during the last offices. Relatives will advise staff if the patient wears a one or two piece sacred undergarment. If this is the case, relatives will dress the patient in these items.

2 For further information contact the nearest Church of Jesus Christ of Latter Day Saints (see telephone directory) or:
The Church of Jesus Christ of Latter Day Saints
751 Warwick Road, Solihull, West Midlands B91 3DQ
Tel: 0121 712 1200
Useful website: www.ldschurch.org

Muslim (Islam)

1 Where possible, the patient's bed should be turned so that their body (head first) is facing Mecca. If the patient's bed cannot be moved, then the patient can be turned on to their right side so that the deceased's face is facing towards Mecca.

2 Many Muslims object to the body being touched by someone of a different faith or opposite sex. If no family members are present, wear gloves and close the patient's eyes, support the jaw and straighten the body. The head should be turned to the right shoulder and the body covered with a plain white sheet. The body should not be washed nor the nails cut.

3 The patient's body is normally either taken home or taken to a mosque as soon as possible to be washed by another Muslim of the same sex. Burial takes place preferably within 24 hours of death. Cremation is forbidden. Post-mortems are permitted only if required by law. Organ donation is not always encouraged, although in the UK a Fatwa (religious verdict) was given by the UK Muslim Law Council which now encourages Muslims to donate organs.

4 For further information contact:
IQRA Trust
3rd Floor, 16 Grosvenor Crescent, London SW1X 7EP
Tel: 020 7838 7987
Email: info@iqratrust.org
Website: www.iqratrust.org.uk

Rastafarian

1 Customary last offices are appropriate, although the patient's family may wish to be present during the preparation of the body to say prayers.

2 Permission for organ donation is unlikely and post-mortems will be refused unless absolutely necessary.

3 Useful website: www.rastafarian.net

Sikhism

1 Family members (especially the eldest son) and friends will be present if they are able.

2 Usually the family takes responsibility for the last offices, but nursing staff may be asked to close the patient's eyes, support the jaw, straighten the body and wrap it in a plain white sheet.

3 Do not remove the '5 ks', which are personal objects sacred to the Sikhs:
Kesh: do not cut hair or beard or remove turban.
Kanga: do not remove the semi-circular comb, which fixes the uncut hair.
Kara: do not remove bracelet worn on the wrist.
Kaccha: do not remove the special shorts worn as underwear.
Kirpan: do not remove the sword: usually a miniature sword is worn.

4 The family will wash and dress the deceased person's body.

5 Post-mortems are only permitted if required by law. Sikhs are always cremated.

6 Organ donation is permitted but some Sikhs refuse this as they do not wish the body to be mutilated.

7 For further information contact the nearest Sikh temple or Gurdwara (see telephone directory). Alternatively, contact:
Sikh Missionary Society UK
10 Featherstone Road, Southall, Middlesex UB2 5AA
Tel: 020 8574 1902
Sikh Educational and Cultural Association (UK)
Sat Nam Kutia, 18 Farncroft, Gravesend, Kent DA11 7LT
Tel: 01474 332356
Useful website:
www.bbc.co.uk/religion/religions/sikhism

Procedure guidelines *(cont.)*

Zoroastrian (Parsee)

1 Customary last offices are often acceptable to Zoroastrian patients.
2 The family may wish to be present during, or participate in, the preparation of the body.
3 Orthodox Parsees require a priest to be present, if possible.
4 After washing, the body is dressed in the *Sadra* (white cotton or muslin shirt symbolizing purity) and *Kusti* (girdle woven of 72 strands of lambs' wool symbolizing the 72 chapters of the *Yasna* [Liturgy]).
5 Relatives may cover the patient's head with a white cap or scarf.

6 It is important that the funeral takes place as soon as possible after death.
7 Burial and cremation are acceptable. Post-mortems are forbidden unless required by law.
8 Organ donation is forbidden by religious law.
9 For further information contact:
   The Zoroastrian Trust Funds of Europe
   440 Alexandra Avenue, Harrow, Middlesex HA2 9TL
   Tel: 020 8866 0765
   Fax: 020 8868 4572
   Email: secretary@ztfe.com
   Useful website:
   www.bbc.co.uk/religion/religions/zoroastrian

References

Ashford and St. Peter's Hospitals NHS Trust (2005) *Last Offices Nursing Procedure.* Ashford and St Peter's Hospitals NHS Trust, Kent.

Berry, P. & Griffie, J. (2006) Planning for the actual death. In: *Textbook of Palliative Nursing* (eds B. R. Ferrell & N. Coyle), 2nd edn. Oxford University Press, Oxford, pp. 561–77.

Clark, D. (2000) Death in Staithes. In: *Death, Dying and Bereavement* (eds D. Dickenson, M. Johnson & J.S. Katz). Sage Publications, London, pp. 4–9.

Cooke, H. (2000) *A Practical Guide to Holistic Care at the End of Life.* Butterworth Heinemann, Oxford.

Costello, J. (2004) *Nursing the Dying Patient: Caring in Different Contexts.* Palgrave Macmillan, Basingstoke, Hants.

DH (1998) *A Code of Practice for the Diagnosis of Brain Stem Death.* Department of Health, London. Available at: www.dh.gov.uk/assetRoot/04/03/54/62/04035462.pdf. Accessed 14/07/06.

DH (2001) Standard principles for preventing hospital acquired infections. *J Hosp Infect*, **47**(Suppl), S21–7.

DH (2003) *A Guide to the Post-mortem Examination Procedure.* Department of Health, London.

Docherty, B. (2000) Care of the dying patient. *Prof Nurse*, **15**(12), 752.

Ellershaw, J. & Wilkinson, S. (2003) *Care of the Dying. A Pathway to Excellence.* Oxford University Press, Oxford.

Field, D., Hockley, J. & Small, N. (1997) *Death, Gender and Ethnicity.* Routledge, London.

Gilliat-Ray, S. (2001) Sociological perspectives on the pastoral care of minority faiths in hospital. In: *Spirituality in Health Care Contexts* (ed. H. Orchard). Jessica Kingsley Publishers, London, pp. 135–46.

Green, J. & Green, M. (2006) *Dealing with Death: A Handbook of Practices, Procedures and Law*, 2nd edn. Jessica Kingsley Publishers, London.

Gunaratnam, Y. (1997) Culture is not enough: a critique of multiculturalism in palliative care. In: *Death, Gender and Ethnicity* (eds D. Field, J. Hockley & N. Small). Routledge, London, pp. 166–86.

HSAC (2003) *Safe Working and the Prevention of Infection in the Mortuary and Post-mortem Room.* Health and Safety Executive Books, London.

HSE (2003) *Safe Working and the Prevention of Infection in the Mortuary and Post-mortem Room.* Health and Safety Executive Books, London.

Helman, C.J. (2007) *Culture, Health and Illness*, 5th edn. Arnold, London.

Home Office (1971) *Report of the Committee on Death Certification and Coroners.* CMND 4810. HMSO, London.

Howarth, G. & Jupp. P.C. (eds) (1996) *Contemporary Issues in the Sociology of Death, Dying and Disposal.* Macmillan, Basingstoke.

Naylor, W., Laverty, D. & Mallett, J. (2001) *The Royal Marsden Hospital Handbook of Wound Management in Cancer Care.* Blackwell Science, Oxford.

Nearney, L. (1998) Last offices, part 1. *Nurs Times*, **94**(26), Insert.

Neuberger, J. (1999) Cultural issues in palliative care. In: *Oxford Textbook of Palliative Medicine* (eds D. Doyle, G. Hanks & N. MacDonald). Oxford University Press, Oxford, pp. 777–80.

Neuberger, J. (2004) *Caring for People of Different Faiths.* Radcliffe Medical Press, Abingdon, Oxon.

NMC (2005) *Guidelines for Records and Record Keeping.* Nursing and Midwifery Council, London.

NMC (2008) *The Code: Standards of Conduct, Performance and Ethics for Nurses and Midwives.* Nursing and Midwifery Council, London.

ONS (2000) NHS hospital activity by NHS Regional Office area, 2000–01. www.statistics.gov.uk. Accessed 3/5/06.

Pearce, E. (1963) *A General Textbook of Nursing.* (First published 1937.) Faber & Faber, London.

Philpin, S. (2002) Rituals and nursing: a critical commentary. *J Adv Nurs*, **38**(2), 144–51.

RCN (1996) *Verification of Death by Registered Nurses.* Issues in Nursing and Health, 38. Royal College of Nursing, London.

RCN (2003) *The Use of Pressure Relieving Devices (Beds, Mattresses and Overlays) for the Prevention of Pressure Ulcers in Primary and Secondary Care.* Royal College of Nursing, London.

RCN (2005) *Good Practice in Infection Prevention and Control. Guidance for Nursing Staff.* Royal College of Nursing, London.

Seale, C. (1998) *Constructing Death. The Sociology of Dying and Bereavement.* Cambridge University Press, Cambridge.

Smaje, C. & Field, D. (1997) Absent minorities? Ethnicity and the use of palliative care services. In: *Death, Gender and Ethnicity* (eds D. Field, J. Hockley & N. Small). Routledge, London, pp. 142–65.

Speck, P. (1992) Care after death. *Nurs Times*, 88(6), 20.

Travis, S. (2002) *Procedure for the Care of Patients Who Die in Hospital*. Royal Marsden NHS Trust, London.

UKTransplant (2007) Direct communication with UK transplant (February 2007 and August 31st 2007). See www.uktransplant.org.uk for information.

Van Gennep, A. (1972) *The Rites of Passage*. Chicago University Press, Chicago.

Walsh, M. & Ford, P. (1989) *Nursing Rituals, Research and Rational Action*. Butterworth Heinemann, Oxford.

Wilkinson, S. & Mula, C. (2003) Communication in care of the dying. In: *Care of the Dying: A Pathway to Excellence* (eds J. Ellershaw & S. Wilkinson). Oxford University Press, Oxford, pp. 74–89.

Wolf, Z. (1988) *Nurses' Work: The Sacred and the Profane*. University of Pennsylvania Press, Philadelphia.

Further reading on religious faiths

Commission for Racial Equality (1999) *CRE Factsheet: Ethnic Minorities in Britain*. CRE, London.

Eliade, M. & Couliano, I.P. (2000) *The Harper Collins Concise Guide to World Religions*. Harper, San Francisco.

Karmi, G. (1996) *The Ethnic Health Handbook. A Factfile for Health Care Professionals*. Blackwell Science, Oxford.

Keene, M. (2002) *World Religions*. Lion Publishing, Oxford.

North Kent Council for Interfaith Relations (2002) *The Spiritual and Pastoral Care of Patients in Hospital and Their Relatives*. North Kent Council for Interfaith Relations, Kent.

Rankin, J., Brown, A. & Gateshill, P. (1992) *Ethics and Religions*. Longman, London.

Sampson, C. (1982) *The Neglected Ethic: Religious and Cultural Factors in the Care of Patients*. McGraw-Hill, Maidenhead.

Bahai faith

Smith, P. (1998) *The Bahai Religion: a Short Introduction to its History and Teachings*. George Ronald, Oxford.

Smith, P. (2000) *A Concise Encyclopaedia of the Bahai Faith*. Oneworld Publications, Oxford.

Buddhism

Gyatso, G.K. (2001) *Introduction to Buddhism: An Explanation of the Buddhist Way of Life*. Tharpa Publications, Ulverston, Cumbria.

Hagan, S. (1997) *Buddhism: Plain and Simple*. Penguin, London.

Maguire, J. (2001) *Essential Buddhism: A Guide to Beliefs and Practices*. Pocket Books, New York.

Northcott, N. (2002) Nursing with dignity, part 2. Buddhism. *Nurs Times*, 98(10), 36–8.

Sibley, D. (1997) Caring for dying Buddhists. *Int J Palliat Nurs*, 3(1), 26–30.

Snelling, J. (1998) *The Buddhist Handbook: A Complete Guide to Buddhist Teaching and Practice*. Rider, London.

Stokes, G. (2000) *Buddha: A Beginner's Guide*. Hodder & Stoughton, London.

Williams, P. (1989) *Mahayana Buddhism*. Routledge, London.

Christianity

Anon (1992) *The Holy Bible*. Hodder & Stoughton, London.

Christmas, M. (2002) Nursing with dignity, part 3. Christianity I. *Nurs Times*, 98(11), 37–9.

Cross, F.L. & Livingstone, E.L. (1997) *The Oxford Dictionary of the Christian Church*. Oxford University Press, Oxford.

Edwards, D.L. (1999) *What Anglicans Believe*. Mowbray, London.

Grenz, S.J. (1998) *What Christians Believe and Why*. Paternoster Press, Carlisle.

Littleton, M. (2001) *Jesus*. John Knox Press, Westminster.

McManners, J. (ed.) (2002) *The Oxford History of Christianity*. Oxford Paperbacks, Oxford.

Papadopoulos, I. (2002) Nursing with dignity, part 4. Christianity II. *Nurs Times*, 98(12), 36–7.

Stott, J. (2002) *Basic Christianity*. Intervarsity Press, London.

Ware, T. (1997) *The Orthodox Church*. Penguin, London.

Hinduism

Cross, S. (2002) *Way of Hinduism*. Thorsons, London.

Flood, G. (2001) *An Introduction to Hinduism*. Cambridge University Press, Cambridge.

Henley, A. (1983) *Caring for Hindus and Their Families: Religious Aspects of Care*. National Extension College, Cambridge.

Jootun, D. (2002) Nursing with dignity, part 7. Hinduism. *Nurs Times*, 98(15), 38–40.

Klostermaier, K.K. (2000) *Hinduism: A Short History*. Oneworld Publications, Oxford.

Laungani, P. (1997) Death in a Hindu family. In: *Death and Bereavement Across Cultures* (eds C. Parkes, P. Laungani & B. Young). Routledge, London, pp. 52–72.

Wordsworth Classics (1997) *The Bhagavad Gita*. Wordsworth, Herts.

Humanism

BBC (2006) Religion & ethics – Humanism. www.bbc.co.uk/religion/religions/atheism/types/humanism.shtml. Accessed 16/8/06.

Jainism

Dundas, P. (2002) *The Jains*. Routledge, London.

Jehovah's Witnesses

Cumberland, W.H. (1986) The Jehovah's Witness tradition. In: *Caring and Curing: Health and Medicine in the Western Religious Traditions* (eds R. Numbers & D. Amundsen). Macmillan, New York, pp. 468–85.

Simpson, J. (2002) Nursing with dignity, part 9. Jehovah's Witnesses. *Nurs Times*, 98(17), 36–7.

The Watch Tower (2007) Medical care and blood [online] Available: www.watchtower.org/e/medical_care_and_blood.htm. Accessed 5/09/07.

Judaism

Collins, A. (2002) Nursing with dignity, part 1. Judaism. *Nurs Times*, 98(9), 33–5.

Katz, J.S. (1996) Caring for dying Jewish people in a multicultural/religious society. *Int J Palliat Nurs*, 2(1), 43–7.

Lancaster, B. (1997) *The Elements of Judaism*. Element, London.

Neuberger, J. (1999) Spiritual issues. Judaism and palliative care. *Eur J Palliat Care*, 6(5), 166–8.

Neusner, J. (2002) *Judaism*. Penguin, London.
Wigoder, N., Skolnick, F. & Himelstein, S. (2002) *The New Encyclopaedia of Judaism*. New York University Press, New York.
Wood, C. (2002) *Living Judaism*. Heinemann Library, New York.

Mormonism

Bush, L.E. (1986) The Mormon tradition. In: *Caring and Curing: Health and Medicine in the Western Religious Traditions* (eds R. Numbers & D. Amundsen). Macmillan, New York, pp. 397–420.
Eliason, E.A. (ed.) (2001) *Mormons and Mormonism*. University of Illinois Press, Illinois.

Muslim faith

Akhtar, S. (2002) Nursing with dignity, part 8. Islam. *Nurs Times*, 98(16), 40–2.
Gordon, M.S. (2002) *Islam*. Duncain Baird, London.
Henley, A. (1982) *Caring for Muslims and Their Families: Religious Aspects of Care*. National Extension College, Cambridge.
Horrie, C. & Chippindale, P. (2001) *What is Islam? A Comprehensive Introduction*. Virgin, London.
Lewis, P. (1994) *Islamic Britain*. I.B. Tauris, London.
Penguin Classics (1999) *The Koran*. Penguin, London.
Ruthven, M. (2000) *Islam: A Very Short Introduction*. Oxford University Press, Oxford.
Sarwas, G. (1998) *Islam: Beliefs and Teachings*. Muslim Educational Trust, London.
Sheikh, A. & Gatrad, A.R. (2000) *Caring for Muslim Patients*. Radcliffe Medical Press, Oxford.

Paganism

Prout, C. (1992) Paganism. *Nurs Times*, 88(33), 42–3.

Rastafarianism

Barrett, L.E. (1997) *The Rastafarians*. Beacons Press, Boston.
Baxter, C. (2002) Nursing with dignity, part 5. Rastafarianism. *Nurs Times*, 98(13), 42–3.

Sikhism

Cole, W.O. & Sambhi, P. (1995) *The Sikhs. Their Religious Beliefs and Practices*. Sussex Academic Press, London.
Gill, B.K. (2002) Nursing with dignity, part 6. Sikhism. *Nurs Times*, 98(14), 39–41.
Henley, A. (1983) *Caring for Sikhs and Their Families: Religious Aspects of Care*. National Extension College, Cambridge.
Kalsi, S.S. (1999) *The Simple Guide to Sikhism*. Global Books, New Jersey.
Mayled, J. (2002) *Living Religions. Living Sikhism*. Heinemann Library, New York.
Sambi, S.P. & Cole, W.O. (1990) Caring for Sikh patients. *Palliat Med*, 4, 229–33.
Shackle, C., Mandair, A. & Singh, G. (eds) (2000) *Sikh Religion: Culture and Ethnicity*. Routledge Curzon, New York.
Singh, D. & Smith, A. (2001) *Religions of the World*. Hodder Wayland, Hove.

Zoroastrianism

Boyce, M. (2001) *Zoroastrianism*. Routledge Curzon, New York.
Clark, P. (1998) *Zoroastranism*. Sussex Academic Press, London.
Hinnells, J.R. (1996) *Zoroastrians in Britain*. Clarendon Press, Oxford.
Kreyenbroek, P.G. (2001) *Living Zoroastrianism*. Routledge Curzon, New York.

Chapter 23

Lumbar puncture

Reference material **460**
Procedure guidelines: Lumbar puncture **463**
Problem solving: Lumbar puncture **465**
References and further reading **466**

Definition

Lumbar puncture is a medical procedure which involves withdrawing cerebrospinal fluid (CSF) by the insertion of a hollow spinal needle with a stylet into the lumbar subarachnoid space (Hickey 2003). It may be used for either therapeutic or diagnostic purposes (Barker & Chao 2002).

Indications

A lumbar puncture and withdrawal of CSF, with or without the introduction of therapeutic agents, is performed for the following purposes.

- *Diagnosis*: CSF is normally a crystal clear, colourless and sterile liquid which resembles water. Analysis of the CSF for cells not normally present may be made to determine the presence of a pathological process (Price & Madhusudan 2002). In addition, CSF pressure can be measured (Barker & Chao 2002).
- *Introduction of therapeutic agents*: for example, antibiotics or cytotoxic intrathecal chemotherapy in the presence of malignant cytology (Hickey 2003; Tervit & Phillips 2006). Since 2001 all UK trusts that undertake to administer intrathecal cytotoxic chemotherapy must ensure safe practice guidelines have been introduced and that they are fully compliant with National Guidelines on the Safe Administration of Intrathecal Chemotherapy (DH 2001).
- *Introduction of spinal anaesthesia for surgery* (Hickey 2003).
- *Introduction of radiopaque contrast medium*: used to provide radiopaque pictures (myelograms) of the spinal cord (Blows 2002). Myelograms are useful in diagnosing spinal lesions and in helping to plan surgery by isolating the level of the lesion.

Contraindications

The procedure should not be undertaken in the following circumstances.

- In patients where raised intracranial pressure (ICP) is suspected or present due to the risk of 'brain herniation' (Lindsay & Bone 2004; Belford 2005).
- In patients with papilloedema, bacterial meningitis or deteriorating neurological symptoms, where raised ICP or an intracranial mass is suspected. In this situation, neuroimaging (computed tomography [CT] or magnetic resonance imaging [MRI] scan) should be undertaken prior to lumbar puncture in order to avoid resultant potentially fatal brainstem compression, herniation or coning (Belford 2005). However, a normal CT scan does not always ensure that it is safe to perform a lumbar puncture, until better non-invasive procedures to monitor ICP become available and are routinely used, the decision to proceed must be left to clinical expertise and judgement (Hickey 2003).
- Local skin infection may result in meningitis by passage of the bacteria from the skin to the CSF during the procedure (Hickey 2003). Cutaneous or osseous infection at the site of the lumbar puncture may be considered an absolute contraindication (Hickey 2003).
- In patients who are unable to co-operate or who are too drowsy to give a history. Patient co-operation is essential to carry out a baseline neurological examination and to minimize the potential risk of trauma associated with this procedure (Barker & Chao 2002).
- In patients who have severe degenerative spinal joint disease. In such cases difficulty will be experienced both in positioning the patient and in accessing between the vertebrae (Hickey 2003).
- In those patients undergoing anticoagulant therapy or who have coagulopathies or thrombocytopenia (less than 50×10^9/litre). These patients are at increased risk of bleeding and therefore coagulopathies and thrombocytopenia must be corrected prior to undertaking lumbar puncture (Lindsay & Bone 2004).

Reference material

Anatomy and physiology

The spinal cord lies within the spinal column, beginning at the foramen magnum and terminating about the level of the first lumbar vertebra (Marieb 2004) (Figure 23.1). Like the brain, the spinal cord is enclosed and protected by the meninges, that is, the dura mater, arachnoid mater and pia mater (Barker 2002). The dura and arachnoid mater are separated by a potential space known as the subdural space. The arachnoid and pia mater are separated by the subarachnoid space which contains the CSF (Allan 2002). Below the first lumbar vertebra the subarachnoid space contains CSF, the filum terminale and the cauda equina (the anterior and posterior roots of the lumbar and sacral nerves) (Weldon 1998). So as to avoid damage to the spinal cord, it is imperative that lumbar puncture is performed below the first lumbar vertebra where the cord terminates (Figure 23.2).

The cord serves as the main pathway for the ascending and descending fibre tracts that connect the peripheral and spinal nerves with the brain (Barker 2002; Marieb 2004). The peripheral nerves are attached to the spinal cord by 31 pairs of spinal nerves.

Cerebrospinal fluid

CSF is formed primarily by filtration and secretion from networks of capillaries, called choroid plexuses, located in the ventricles of the brain. Eventually, absorption takes place through the arachnoid villi, which are finger-like projections of the arachnoid mater that push into the dural venous sinuses. CSF is clear, colourless and slightly alkaline, with a specific gravity of 1007 (Hickey 2003). In an adult, approximately 500 ml of CSF are produced and reabsorbed each day (Weldon 1998), with 120–150 ml present at one time. CSF constituents include:

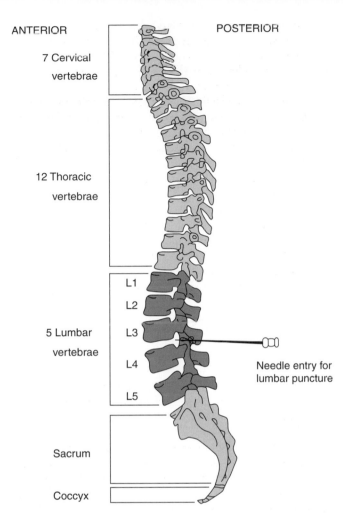

Figure 23.1 Lateral view of spinal column and vertebrae, showing needle entry site for lumbar puncture.

- Water.
- Mineral salts.
- Glucose.
- Protein (16–45 mg/dl).
- Urea and creatinine (Hickey 2003).

The functions of CSF include:

- To act as a shock absorber.
- To carry nutrients to the brain.
- To remove metabolites from the brain.
- To support and protect the brain and spinal cord.
- To keep the brain and spinal cord moist (Hickey 2003).

Sampling and CSF pressure

The amount of CSF withdrawn for sampling depends on the investigation required. In practice, approximately 5–10 ml of CSF is usually withdrawn, although investigations for cell count and Gram stain can be performed using 1 ml (Barker & Chao 2002). The pressure of CSF can be measured at the time of lumbar puncture using a manometer. Normal CSF

pressure falls within a range of 100–150 mm (Lindsay & Bone 2004). Spinal pressure may be raised in the presence of cerebrovascular accident, a space-occupying lesion or bacterial meningitis (Barker & Chao 2002).

Abnormalities of CSF

- A red discoloration of the CSF is indicative of the presence of blood, which is an abnormal finding. If the presence of blood is caused by a traumatic spinal tap, the blood will usually clot and the fluid clear as the procedure continues. If the presence of blood is due to subarachnoid haemorrhage, no clotting will occur (Lindsay & Bone 2004).
- Turbid or cloudy CSF is indicative of the presence of a large number of white cells or protein and is an abnormal finding. The causes of such turbidity include infection or the secondary infiltration of the meninges with malignant disease, e.g. leukaemia or lymphoma (Hoffbrand *et al.* 2001).
- The presence of different types of blood cells in the CSF can be diagnostic of a variety of neurological disorders, e.g.:

Figure 23.2 Lumbar puncture. Sagittal section through lumbosacral spine. The most common site for lumbar puncture is between L3 and L4 and between L4 and L5 as the spinal cord terminates at L1.

(a) Erythrocytes are indicative of haemorrhage.

(b) Polymorphonuclear leucocytes are indicative of meningitis or cerebral abcess.

(c) Monocytes are indicative of a viral or tubercular meningitis or encephalitis.

(d) Lymphocytes present in larger numbers are indicative of viral meningitis or infiltration of the meninges by malignant disease.

(e) The presence of leukaemic blast cells is indicative of infiltration of the meninges by leukaemia.

(f) Viral, bacterial or fungal cultures from the CSF sample are indicative of infection.
    (Allan 2002; Barker & Chao 2002; Hickey 2003).

Investigations

A number of tests can be performed on CSF to aid diagnosis (Lindsay & Bone 2004).

- *Culture and sensitivity*. Identifying the presence of micro-organisms would confirm the diagnosis of bacterial/fungal meningitis or a cerebral abscess. The isolation of the causative organism would enable the initiation of appropriate antibiotic or antifungal therapy.
- *Virology screening*. Isolation of a causative virus would enable appropriate therapy to be initiated promptly.
- *Serology for syphilis*. Tests include: Wasserman test (WR), venereal disease research laboratory (VDRL) and *Treponema pallidum* immobilization (TPI) test.
- *Protein*. The total amount of protein in CSF should be 15.45 mg/dl (154.5 μg/ml). Proteins are large molecules which do not readily cross the blood–brain barrier. There is normally more albumin (80%) than globulin in CSF as albumins are smaller molecules (Fischbach 2003). Raised globulin levels are indicative of multiple sclerosis, neurosyphilis, degenerative cord or brain disease. However, raised levels of total protein can be indicative of meningitis, encephalitis, myelitis or the presence of a tumour (Hickey 2003).
- *Cytology*. Central nervous system tumours or secondary meningeal disease tend to shed cells into the CSF, where they float freely. Examination of these cells morphologically after lumbar puncture will determine whether the tumour is malignant or benign (Fischbach 2003).

Instillation of chemotherapy

A number of drugs do not cross the blood–brain barrier so in the treatment and prophylaxis of some malignant diseases such as leukaemia and lymphoma, cytotoxic drugs, namely cytarabine, methotrexate and, rarely, thiopeta, may be administered intrathecally (Hoffbrand *et al.* 2006; Scurr *et al.* 2005; Coward & Cooley 2006). Hydrocortisone may also be administered intrathecally. Care must be taken when administering intrathecal cytotoxic chemotherapy so as to ensure practice is safe and fully compliant with National Guidance on the Safe Administration of Intrathecal Chemotherapy (DH 2003). This guidance was issued as a result of the 13 patients who have died or been paralysed as a result of accidental intrathecal administration of vincristine intended for intravenous administration between 1985 and 2001 (see Chapter 12).

Complications associated with lumbar puncture

- Infection (inadvertently introduced during procedure: there is a greater risk in the presence of neutropenia) (Hart 2006).
- Haemorrhage/localized bruising (may be caused by a traumatic procedure or in the presence of thrombocytopenia or a coagulopathy) (Barker & Chao 2002; Lindsay & Bone 2004).
- Transtentorial or tonsillar herniation (if Queckenstedt's test is carried out in the presence of raised ICP) (Belford 2005).
- Headache. Frequency of post-lumbar puncture headache varies among studies and between diagnostic and therapeutic procedures. The following risk factors have been identified: young age; female gender; and the presence of headache before or at the time of the lumbar puncture (Evans *et al.* 2000). Less certain risk factors include low body mass index and previous experience of post-lumbar puncture headache (Evans *et al.* 2000). Research also suggests that the size of the needle used for the lumbar puncture may contribute to headache as a large gauge needle, such as an 18 gauge, may create a larger dural opening and the tip may tear dural fibres, delaying puncture closure. To minimize the risk of headache, a 25-gauge blunt-ended needle is recommended (Connolly 1999).
- Backache.
- Leakage from puncture site (Hickey 2003).
- The combination of intrathecal methotrexate with radiotherapy may cause arachnoiditis (irritation of the meninges), cerebral atrophy and necrosing encephalopathy (Vasey & Evans 2002). Arachnoiditis has also been reported when administering intrathecal methylprednisolone (Latham *et al.* 1997).

The role of the nurse

The role of the nurse in caring for a patient undergoing a lumbar puncture procedure may include helping to explain the procedure to the patient, preparing the patient, supporting both patient and physician during the procedure and close follow-up monitoring. Education and support are essential as the patient may have concerns about this invasive procedure (Barker & Chao 2002). Preparation may include advising the patient to empty their bowels and bladder to ensure comfort, and correct and comfortable positioning during the procedure. Follow-up care will include: neurological observations; monitoring for issues such as difficulties with voiding, raised temperatures, headaches and discomfort. Analgesia and reassurance may be required (Allan 2002).

Procedure guidelines   Lumbar puncture

Equipment

1 Antiseptic skin-cleaning agents, e.g. chlorhexidine in 70% alcohol or isopropyl alcohol.
2 Selection of needles and syringes.
3 Local anaesthetic, e.g. lidocaine 1%.
4 Sterile gloves.
5 Sterile dressing pack.
6 Lumbar puncture needles of assorted sizes.
7 Disposable manometer.

8 Three sterile specimen bottles. (These should be labelled 1, 2 and 3. The first specimen, which may be bloodstained due to needle trauma, should go into bottle 1. This will assist the laboratory to differentiate between blood due to procedure trauma and that due to subarachnoid haemorrhage.)
9 Plaster dressing.

Procedure

Action	Rationale
1 Explain and discuss the procedure with the patient.	To ensure that the patient understands the procedure and gives his/her valid consent (Barker & Chao 2002: E; NMC 2006: C).
2 Patient should empty his/her bladder and bowels before procedure.	To ensure comfort (Barker & Chao 2002; Hickey 2003: E).
3 Assist patient into required position on a firm surface:	To ensure maximum widening of the intervertebral spaces and thus easier access to the subarachnoid space (Lindsay & Bone 2004: E).
(a) Lying (see Action figure 3): ■ One pillow under the patient's head. ■ On side with knees drawn up to the abdomen and clasped by the hands. ■ Support patient to maintain this position.	To avoid sudden movement by the patient which would produce trauma (Barker & Chao 2002: E).
(b) Sitting: ■ Patient straddles a straight back chair so that his/her back is facing the doctor. ■ Patient folds arms on the back of the chair and rests head on them.	This position may be used for those patients unable to maintain the lying position. It allows more accurate identification of the spinous processes and thus the intervertebral spaces (Barker & Chao 2002; Hickey 2003: E).
4 Continue to support, explain care and observe the patient throughout the procedure.	To facilitate psychological and physical well being (Barker & Chao 2002: E).
5 Assist doctor as required; doctor will proceed to: (a) Clean the skin with the antiseptic cleaning agent. (b) Identify the area to be punctured and infiltrate the skin and subcutaneous layers with local anaesthetic. (c) Introduce a spinal puncture needle between the second and third lumbar vertebrae and into the subarachnoid space. (d) Ensure that the subarachnoid space has been entered and attach the manometer to the spinal needle, if required. (e) Obtain the appropriate specimens of CSF (approx. 10 ml) for analysis. Cell count and Gram stain can be perfomed using 1 ml of fluid.	To monitor any physical or psychological changes. To ensure the removal of skin flora to minimize the risk of infection (Lindsay & Bone 2004: E). To minimize discomfort from the procedure (Barker & Chao 2002: E). This is below the level of the spinal cord but still within the subarachoid space (Lindsay & Bone 2004: E). To obtain a CSF pressure reading (normal pressure is 100–150 mmH$_2$O) (Hickey 2003; Lindsay & Bone 2004: E). To establish diagnosis (Hickey 2003: E).

Procedure guidelines *(cont.)*

(f) If intrathecal medication is to be instilled, drug and dose must be checked and administered safely acording to National Guidelines (DH 2003).	To ensure the correct drug and dosage of drug is safely administered (DH 2003: C; Coward & Cooley 2006).
(g) Withdraw the spinal needle once specimens have been obtained, appropriate pressure measurements taken and intrathecal medication administered.	To minimize the risks of the procedure (Barker & Chao 2002: E).
(h) Careful precaution should be taken when administering cytotoxic drugs and disposing of cytotoxic waste.	To protect patient and clinicians (Coward & Colley: E; DH 2005: C).
6 When the needle is withdrawn, apply pressure over the lumbar puncture site using a sterile topical swab.	To maintain asepsis and to stop blood and CSF flow (Hickey 2003: E).
7 When all leakage from the puncture site has ceased, apply a plaster dressing.	To prevent secondary infection (Allan 2002; Barker & Chao 2002: E).
8 Make the patient comfortable. He/she should lie flat or the head should be tilted slightly downwards. Time to lie flat varies from hospital to hospital, but it is usually around 4 hours if there is no headache. If the procedure has been done in an outpatient setting the patient may be discharged home after 1–2 hours but with clear instructions to lie flat in transport and at home, and to report any of the following: leakage from the site, headaches or backaches.	To avoid headache and decrease the possibility of brainstem herniation (coning) due to a reduction in CSF pressure (Barker & Chao 2002; Hickey 2003: E).
9 Remove equipment and dispose of as appropriate.	To prevent the spread of infection and reduce risk of needle stick injury (Allan 2002: E).
10 Record the procedure in the appropriate documents.	To promote continuity of care and provide an accurate record for future reference (Allan 2002: E; NMC 2005: C).
11 Ensure the specimens are labelled appropriately and sent with the correct forms to the laboratory.	To ensure that the correct results are returned to the appropriate patient's notes (Barker & Chao 2002: E).
12 Patient should be monitored for the next 24 hours with careful observation of the following:	
(a) Leakage from the puncture site.	There may be a small amount of bloodstained oozing. The presence of clear fluid should be reported immediately to the doctor, especailly if accompanied by fluctuation of other symptoms (level of consciousness, motor changes, problems voiding), as it may be a cerebrospinal leak (Barker & Chao 2002: E).
(b) Headache.	Not unusual following lumbar puncture and may be due to loss of CSF or irritation of the spinal roots. Usually relieved by lying flat and, if ordered by the doctor, a mild analgesic (Hickey 2003: E).
(c) Backache.	As above.
(d) Neurological observations/vital signs.	These may indicate signs of change in ICP (Hickey 2003: E). (For further information on neurolgical observations and vital signs, see Chapter 26.)

13 Encourage a fluid intake of 2–3 litres in 24 hours.

To replace lost fluid. Patient may have difficulty micturating due to procedure and supine position (Allan 2002; Hickey 2003: E).

Action 3 Position for lumbar puncture. Head is flexed onto chest and knees are drawn up.

Problem solving: Lumbar puncture

Problem	Cause	Suggested action
Pain down one leg during the procedure.	A dorsal nerve root may have been touched by the spinal needle.	Inform doctor, who will probably move the needle. Reassure patient.
Headache following procedure (may persist for up to a week).	Removal of the sample of CSF.	Reassure patient that it is a transient symptom. Ensure that he/she lies flat for specified period of time. Encourage a high fluid intake to replace fluid lost during procedure. Administer analgesics as ordered. If headache is severe and increasing, inform a a doctor: there is a possibility of persistent CSF leak or rising ICP (Barker & Chao 2002).
Backache following procedure.	(a) Removal of the sample of CSF. (b) Position required for puncture.	Reassure patient that it is usually a transient symptom. Ensure that he/she lies flat for appropriate period of time. Administer analgesic as ordered (Hickey 2003).
Fluctuation of neurological observations, i.e. level of consciousness, pulse, respirations, blood pressure or pupillary reaction.	Herniation (coning) of the brainstem due to the decrease of ICP. (Raised ICP is a contraindication to lumbar puncture.)	Observe patient constantly for signs of alteration in ICP. The frequency may be decreased as patient's condition allows. Report any fluctuations in these observations to a doctor immediately (Barker & Chao 2002).
Leakage from the puncture site.	(a) Resolution of bleeding. (b) Leakage of CSF.	(a) No further action required (b) Report immediately to a doctor, especially if accompanied by fluctuation in neurological observations (see Chapter 26) (Barker & Chao 2002).

References and further reading

Allan, D. (2002) Caring for the patient with a disorder of the nervous system. In: *Watson's Clinical Nursing and Related Sciences* (ed. M. Walsh), 6th edn. Balliere Tindall, Edinburgh, pp. 665–746.

Barker, E. (2002) Neuroanatomy and physiology of the nervous system. In: *Neuroscience Nursing: A Spectrum of Care* (ed. E. Barker), 2nd edn. Mosby, Phildaelphia, pp. 3–50.

Barker, E. & Chao, W.P. (2002) Neurodiagnostic and laboratory studies. In: *Neuroscience Nursing: A Spectrum of Care* (ed. E. Barker), 2nd edn. Mosby, Phildaelphia, pp. 99–130.

Belford, K. (2005) Central nervous cancers. In: *Cancer Nursing: Principles and Practice* (eds C.H. Yarbro, M.H, Frogge & M. Goodman), 6th edn. Jones & Bartlett, Boston, pp. 1089–136.

Blows, W. (2002) Diagnostic investigations, part 1: lumbar puncture. *Nurs Times*, **98**(36), 25–6.

Connolly, M.A. (1999) Clinical snapshot. Postdural puncture headache. *Am J Nurs*, **99**(11), 48–9.

Coward, M. & Cooley, H.M. (2006) Chemotherapy. In: *Nursing Patients with Cancer: Principles and Practice* (eds N. Kearney & A. Richardson). Elsevier, Edinburgh, pp. 283–302.

DH (2001) *National Guidance on the Safe Administration of Intrathecal Chemotherapy*. HSC 2001/022. Department of Health, London.

DH (2003) *Updated National Guidance on the Safe Administration of Intrathecal Chemotherapy*. HSC 2003/10. Department of Health, London.

DH (2005) *Hazardous waste (England) regulations*. Department of Health, London.

Evans, R.W. *et al.* (2000) Assessment: prevention of post-lumbar puncture headaches: report of the Therapeutics and Technology Assessment Subcommittee of the American Academy of Neurology. *Neurology*, **55**(7), 909–14.

Fischbach, F.T. (2003) *A Manual of Laboratory Diagnostic Tests*, 7th edn. Lippincott, Philadelphia.

Hart, S. (2006) Prevention of infection. In: *Nursing in Haematological Oncology* (ed. M. Grundy), 2nd edn. Balliere Tindall, Edinburgh, pp. 321–38.

Hickey, J. (ed) (2003) Cerebrospinal fluids and spinal procedures. In: *The Clinical Practice of Neurological and Neuroscience Nursing*, 5th edn. Lippincott, Philadelphia, pp. 89–91.

Hoffbrand, A.V., Moss, P.A.H. & Petit, J.E. (2006) *Haematology*, 5th edn. Blackwell Publishing, Oxford.

Latham, J.M. *et al.* (1997) The pathological effects of intrathecal betamethasone. *Spine*, **22**(14), 1558–62.

Lindsay, K.W. & Bone, I. (2004) *Neurology and Neurosurgery Illustrated*, 4th edn. Churchill Livingstone, Edinburgh.

Marieb, E.N. (2004) *Human Anatomy & Physiology*, 6th edn. Pearson, San Francisco.

NMC (2005) *Guidelines for Records and Record Keeping*. Nursing and Midwifery Council, London.

NMC (2006) *Z–Z Advice Sheet Consent*. www.nmc.org.

Price, C.G.A. & Madhusudan, S. (2002) Non Hodgkin's lymphoma. In: *Treatment of Cancer* (eds P. Price & K. Sikora), 4th edn. Arnold, London, pp. 977–95.

Richards, P. (1992) Monitoring of cerebral function. *Br J Hosp Med*, **48**(7), 390–2.

Scurr, M., Judson, I. & Root, T. (2005) Combination chemotherapy and chemotherapy principles. In: *The Royal Marsden Hospital Handbook of Cancer Chemotherapy* (eds D. Brighton & M. Wood). Elsevier, Edinburgh, pp. 17–30.

Tervit, S. & Phillips, K. (2006) Chemotherapy. In: *Nursing in Haematological Oncology* (ed. M. Grundy), 2nd edn. Balliere Tindall, Edinburgh, pp. 173–200.

Vasey, P. A. & Evans, J. (2002) Principles of Chemotherapy and Drug Development. In: *Treatment of Cancer* (eds P. Price & K. Sikora) 4th edn. Arnold, London, pp. 103–29.

Weldon, K. (1998) Anatomy and physiology of the nervous system. In: *Neuro-Oncology for Nurses* (ed. D. Guerrero). Whurr, London, pp. 1–28.

Chapter 24

Nutritional support

Reference material **468**

Procedure guidelines: Weighing the patient **479**

Procedure guidelines: Feeding an adult **481**

Procedure guidelines: Nasogastric intubation with tubes using an introducer **482**

Procedure guidelines: Nasogastric intubation with tubes without using an introducer, e.g. a Ryle's tube **484**

Procedure guidelines: Percutaneous endoscopically placed gastrostomy (PEG) tube care **486**

Procedure guidelines: Radiologically inserted gastrostomy (RIG) tube care **488**

Procedure guidelines: Jejunostomy feeding tube care **488**

Procedure guidelines: Enteral feeding tubes: administration of medication **489**

Procedure guidelines: Enteral feeding tube: unblocking **490**

Problem solving: Swallowing difficulties **491**

References and further reading **494**

Definition

Nutritional support refers to any method of giving nutrients which encourages an optimal nutritional status. It includes modifying the types of foods eaten, dietary supplementation, enteral tube feeding and parenteral nutrition (National Collaborating Centre for Acute Care 2006).

Indications

Nutritional support should be considered for anybody unable to maintain their nutritional status by taking their usual diet.

- Patients unable to eat their usual diet (e.g. because of anorexia, mucositis, taste changes or dysphagia, see Problem solving, below) should be given advice on modifying their diet.
- Patients unable to meet their nutritional requirements, despite dietary modifications, should be offered oral nutritional supplements.
- Patients unable to take sufficient food and dietary supplements to meet their nutritional requirements should be considered for an enteral tube feed.
- Patients unable to eat at all should have an enteral tube feed. Reasons for complete inability to eat include carcinoma of the head and neck area or oesophagus, surgery to the head or oesophagus, radiotherapy treatment to the head or neck, and fistulae of the oral cavity or oesophagus.
- Parenteral nutrition (PN) may be indicated in patients with a non-functioning or inaccessible gastrointestinal (GI) tract who are likely to be 'nil by mouth' for 5 days or longer. Reasons for a non-functioning or inaccessible GI tract include bowel obstruction, short bowel syndrome, gut toxicity following bone marrow transplantation or chemotherapy, major abdominal surgery, uncontrolled vomiting and enterocutaneous fistulae. Enteral nutrition should always be considered as the first option when considering nutritional support.

Patients in any group may have an increased requirement for nutrients due to an increased metabolic rate, as found in patients with burns, major sepsis, trauma or cancer cachexia (Bozzetti 2001; Thomas 2001). Patients should have nutritional requirements estimated prior to the start of nutritional support and should be monitored regularly.

Reference material

Nutrition screening

Identification of patients who are malnourished or who are at risk of malnutrition is an important first step in the patient's nutritional care. There are a number of screening tools available which consider different aspects of nutritional status. Subjective global assessment (SGA) is a comprehensive assessment but necessitates more time and expertise to

carry out than most screening. Some more simple screening tools, including the malnutrition universal screening tool (MUST) (BAPEN 2003b), based on the patient's body mass index, weight loss and illness score are less time consuming. Other tools may be specific to the patient's age or diagnosis (Kondrup *et al.* 2003). The most important feature of using any screening tool is that patients identified as requiring nutritional assessment or intervention have a nutritional care plan initiated and are referred to the dietitian for further advice if appropriate.

Assessment of nutritional status

Before the initiation of nutritional support the patient must be assessed. The purpose of assessment is to identify whether a patient is undernourished, the reasons why this may have occurred and to provide baseline data for planning and evaluating nutritional support (National Collaborating Centre for Acute Care 2006). It is useful to use more than one method of assessing nutritional status. For example, a dietary history may be used to assess the adequacy of a person's diet but does not reflect actual nutritional status, whereas percentage weight loss does give an indication of nutritional status. However, percentage weight loss taken in isolation gives no idea of dietary intake and likelihood of improvement or deterioration in nutritional status (National Collaborating Centre for Acute Care 2006).

Nutrient intake

Nutrient intake can be assessed by a diet history (Thomas & Bishop 2007). A 24-hour recall may be used to assess recent nutrient intake and a food chart may be used to monitor current dietary intake. A diet history may also be used to provide information on food frequency, food habits, preferences, meal pattern, portion sizes, the presence of any eating difficulty and changes in food intake (Reilly 1996). A food chart where all current food and fluid taken is recorded is a useful method for monitoring nutritional intake, especially in the hospital setting or when dietary recall is not reliable (Thomas & Bishop 2007).

Body weight and weight loss

Body mass index (BMI) or comparison of a patient's weight with a chart of ideal body weight gives a measure of whether the patient has a normal weight, is overweight or underweight, and may be calculated from weight and height using the following equation:

$$BMI = \frac{Weight\ (kg)}{Height\ (m)^2}$$

Tables are available to allow the rapid and easy calculation of BMI (BAPEN 2003b). These comparisons, however, are not a good indicator of whether the patient is at risk nutritionally, as an apparently normal weight can mask severe muscle wasting.

Of greater use is the comparison of current weight with the patient's usual weight. Percentage weight loss is a useful measure of the risk of malnutrition:

$$\% \text{ Weight loss} = \frac{\text{Usual Weight} - \text{Actual Weight}}{\text{Usual Weight}} \times 100$$

A patient would be identified as malnourished if they had any of the following:

- BMI less than 18.5 kg/m^2.
- Unintentional weight loss greater than 10% within the last 3–6 months.
- BMI less than 20 kg/m^2 and unintentional weight loss greater than 5% within the last 3–6 months.
  (National Collaborating Centre for Acute Care 2006.)

Sick children should have their weight and height measured frequently. It may be useful to measure on a daily basis (Shaw & Lawson 2007). These measurements must be plotted onto centile charts. A single weight or height cannot be interpreted as there is much variation of growth within each age group. It is a matter of concern if a child's weight begins to fall across the centiles or if the weight plateaus.

Obesity and oedema may make interpretation of body weight difficult; both may mask loss of lean body mass and potential malnutrition (Pennington 1997). Accurate weighing scales are necessary for measurement of body weight. Patients who are unable to stand may require sitting scales for weight to be measured.

It is often not appropriate to weigh palliative care patients who may experience inevitable weight loss as disease progresses. Psychologically it may be difficult for patients to see that they are continuing to lose weight. Measures of nutritional status such as clinical examination and current food intake may still be used in addition to measures of body weight.

Skinfold thickness

Skinfold thickness measurements can be used to assess stores of body fat. They are rarely used in routine nutritional assessment due to the insensitivity of the technique and the variation between measurements made by different observers. They are more appropriate for long-term assessments or research purposes and the technique should only be used by practitioners who are practiced in using skinfold thickness calipers because of the potential for intra-investigator variation in results (Durnin & Wolmersley 1974). Calipers are used to measure the thickness of subcutaneous fat at four sites: the triceps, biceps, subscapular and supra-iliac. The measurements can be used to determine the percentage of body fat of a person (Durnin & Wolmersley 1974). Percentage charts for skinfold thickness measurements may be used to assess nutritional status (Thomas & Bishop 2007, Appendix 6.4).

Bioelectrical impedance

Bioelectrical impedance analysis (BIA) is a simple, non-invasive and relatively inexpensive technique for measuring body composition (Janssen et al. 2000). The procedure involves the patient lying down for a period of 5–10 minutes while electrodes are connected to the hand and foot and a small undetectable electrical current is passed through the body. The speed at which this current travels through the body is influenced by the amount of water contained within the different body compartments. Tissues with a high water content (e.g. skeletal muscle) have a high electrical conductivity, whilst those with low water content (i.e. fat) act as poor conductors. BIA machines thus measure the impedance of the current as it passes through the subject. This information is then used in combination with prediction equations to calculate the volume or mass of different body compartments, which is then displayed electronically (Kyle et al. 2004a).

BIA is a technique which works well in healthy subjects but is of limited use in individuals with abnormal hydration status (e.g. severe dehydration or ascites) and is also less reliable at the extremes of BMI ranges (Kyle et al. 2004b). It is most suitable for research studies where body composition of groups of subjects is measured or for monitoring changes in nutritional status over a period of time (Buchholz et al. 2004). Importantly it is contraindicated in patients fitted with a pacemaker where the alternative skinfold thickness measurements should be used. The more expensive BIA machines also provide a measurement called 'phase angle' which has been shown to be of prognostic value in human immunodeficiency virus (HIV) (Schwenk et al. 2000) and advanced pancreatic and colorectal cancer patients (Gupta et al. 2004a, b).

Clinical examination

Observation of the patient may reveal signs and symptoms indicative of nutritional depletion.

- *Physical appearance*: emaciated, wasted appearance, loose clothing/jewellery.
- *Oedema*: will affect weight and may mask the appearance of muscle wastage. May indicate plasma protein deficiency and is often a reflection of the patient's overall condition rather than a measure of nutritional status.
- *Mobility*: weakness and impaired movement may result from loss of muscle mass.
- *Mood*: apathy, lethargy and poor concentration can be features of undernutrition.
- *Pressure sores and poor wound healing*: may reflect impaired immune function as a consequence of undernutrition and vitamin deficiencies (Thomas & Bishop 2007).

Specific nutritional deficiencies may be identifiable in some patients. For example, thiamine deficiency characterized by dementia is associated with high alcohol consumption. Rickets is seen in children with vitamin D deficiency.

Subjective global assessment

Subjective global assessment (SGA) is a clinical score, which can be obtained by a trained observer using a standardized questionnaire along with a physical examination, focused on nutritional status (Detsky *et al.* 1987). The questionnaire includes questions about food intake, physical symptoms and weight loss and therefore encompasses a number of methods of assessing nutritional status. Adaptations of the original tool have been produced including the Patient-Generated Subjective Global Assessment aimed specifically at patients with cancer (Huhmann & Cunningham 2005).

Biochemical investigations

Biochemical tests carried out on blood may give information on the patient's nutritional status. The most commonly used are:

- *Plasma proteins.* Changes in plasma albumin may arise due to physical stress, changes in circulating volume, hepatic and renal function, shock conditions and septicaemia. Plasma albumin and changes in plasma albumin are not a direct reflection of nutritional intake and nutritional status as it has been shown that these may remain unchanged despite changes in body composition (National Collaborating Centre for Acute Care 2006). In addition, albumin has a long half-life of 21 days, so it cannot reflect recent changes in nutritional intake. It may be useful to review serum albumin concentrations in conjunction with C-reactive protein (CRP), which is an acute phase protein produced by the body in response to injury or trauma. CRP greater than 10 mg/l and serum albumin less than 30 g/l suggests 'illness'. CRP less than 10 mg/l and serum albumin less than 30 g/l suggests protein depletion (Elia 2001). Prealbumin and retinol binding protein levels are more sensitive measures of nutrition support, reflecting recent changes in dietary intake rather than nutritional status. However, they may be expensive to measure (Nataloni *et al.* 1999).
- *Haemoglobin.* This is often below haematological reference values in malnourished patients (men: 13.5–17.5 g/dl; women: 11.5–15.5 g/dl). This can be due to a number of reasons, such as loss of blood from circulation, increased destruction of red blood cells or reduced production of erythrocytes and haemoglobin, e.g. due to dietary deficiency of iron or folate.
- *Serum vitamin and mineral levels.* Clinical examination of the patient may suggest a vitamin or mineral deficiency. For example, gingivitis may be due to a deficiency of vitamin C, vitamin A, niacin or riboflavin. Goitre is associated with iodine deficiency, and tremors, convulsions and behavioural disturbances may be caused by magnesium deficiency (Shenkin 2001). Serum vitamin and mineral levels are rarely measured routinely, as they are expensive and often cannot be performed by hospital laboratories.

- *Immunological competence.* Total lymphocyte count may reflect nutritional status although levels may also be depleted with malignancy, chemotherapy, zinc deficiency, age and non-specific stress (Bodger & Heatley 2001).

If a patient is considered to be malnourished by one or more of the above methods of assessment then a referral to a dietitian should be made immediately (Burnham & Barton 2001).

Calculation of nutritional requirements

Energy requirements may be calculated using equations such as those derived by Schofield (1985), which take into account weight, age, sex, activity level and clinical injury, e.g. post-surgery, sepsis or ventilator dependency. An easier and more appropriate method is to use body weight and allowances based on the patient's clinical condition (Table 24.1). Careful adjustments may be necessary in cases of oedema or obesity, in order to avoid overfeeding (Horgan & Stubbs 2003).

Fluid and nitrogen (or protein) requirements can be calculated in a similar way. If additional nitrogen is being given in situations where losses are increased, for example due to trauma, GI losses or major sepsis, then additional energy intake is required to assist in promoting a nitrogen balance. Improvement in nitrogen balance is the single nutritional parameter most consistently associated with improved outcome, and the primary goal of nutrition support should be the attainment of nitrogen balance (Gidden & Shenkin 2000). Additional fluid of 500–750 ml is necessary for every 1°C rise in temperature in pyrexial patients (Thomas 2001).

Vitamin and mineral requirements calculated as detailed in the Committee on Medical Aspects of Food Policy (COMA) Report 41 on dietary reference values (DH 1991) apply to groups of healthy people and are not necessarily appropriate for those who are ill. A patient deficient in a vitamin or mineral may benefit from additional supplements to improve a condition. For example, a malnourished patient with poor wound healing may benefit from an increase in vitamin C and zinc, although the evidence is controversial (ter Riet *et al.* 1995; Thomas 1997; Desneves *et al.* 2005). Macronutrient and micronutrient requirements

Table 24.1 Guidelines for estimation of patient's daily energy and protein requirements (per kilogram body weight).

	Normal	Pyrexia or extreme sepsis
Energy (kcal)	25	25–35
(kJ)	105	105–146
Nitrogen (g)	0.17 (0.14–0.2)	0.2–0.3
Protein (g)	1 (0.87–1.25)	1.25–1.87
Fluid (ml)	30–35	30–35 plus 2–2.5 ml per 1°C in temperature above 37°C

for children are also listed in the Committee on Medical Aspects of Food Policy (COMA) Report 41 on dietary reference values (DH 1991). Calculations are usually done with the reference nutrient intake (RNI). The child's actual body weight, not the expected body weight, is used when calculating requirements. This is to avoid excessive feeding. For a very small child, the height age instead of the chronological age is the basis of calculation (Shaw & Lawson 2007).

Planning nutritional support

Many factors, including being in hospital, need to be taken into consideration when planning nutritional support. Within the *Essence of Care* framework (DH 2001a), food and nutrition were identified by patients as a fundamental area of care that is frequently unsatisfactory within the National Health Service (NHS).

Clinical benchmarking (DH 2001a) and the *Better Hospital Food* programme) (NHS 2001) aim to address common problems that patients experience whilst in hospital. Box 24.1 outlines the benchmark for food and nutrition, identifying specific factors that need to be considered when reviewing service provision, in order to promote better practice.

Dietary supplements

These may be used to improve an inadequate diet or may be used as a sole source of nutrition if taken in sufficient quantity.

Sip feeds

These come in a range of flavours, both sweet and savoury, and are presented as a powder in a packet or ready prepared in a can, bottle or carton. Sip feeds contain whole protein, hydrolysed fat and carbohydrates. Most are called 'complete feeds' since they provide all protein, vitamins, minerals and trace elements to meet requirements if a prescribed volume is taken (Thomas & Bishop 2007). Others may be aimed at specific needs, for example high protein.

Energy supplements

Carbohydrates
Glucose polymers in powder or liquid form contain approximately 350 kcal (1442 kJ) per 100 g and 187–299 kcal (770-1232 kJ) per 100 ml respectively. Powdered glucose polymer is virtually tasteless and may be added to anything in which it will dissolve, e.g. milk and other drinks, soup, cereals and milk pudding; liquid glucose polymers may be fruit flavoured or neutral (Thomas & Bishop 2007). Such

supplements would be used to increase the energy content of the diet.

Fat
Fat may be in the form of long-chain triglycerides (LCT) or medium-chain triglycerides (MCT) and comes as a liquid which can be added to food and drinks. These oils provide 416–772 kcal (1714-3181 kJ) per 100 ml: the oils with a lower energy value are presented in the form of an emulsion and those with a higher energy value are presented as pure oil (Thomas & Bishop 2007).

Mixed fat and glucose polymer solutions and powders are available and provide 150 kcal per 100 ml or 486 kcal per 100 g, depending on the relative proportion of fat and carbohydrates in the product.

Products containing MCT are used in preference to those containing LCT where a patient suffers from GI impairment causing malabsorption. Patients require specific advice about their use to ensure that they are introduced into the diet slowly and GI tolerance is assessed (Thomas & Bishop 2007).

Always check with the manufacturer for the exact energy content of products.

Note: products containing a glucose polymer are unsuitable for patients with diabetes mellitus.

Protein supplements

These come in the form of a powder and provide 55–90 g protein per 100 g. Protein supplement powders may be added to any food or drink in which they will dissolve, e.g. milk, fruit juice, soup, milk pudding.

Energy and protein supplements are not used in isolation as these would not provide an adequate nutritional intake. They are used in conjunction with sip feeds and a modified diet. The detailed nutritional compositions of dietary supplements are available from the manufacturers.

Vitamin and mineral supplements

When dietary intake is poor a vitamin and mineral supplement may be required. This can often be given as a one-a-day tablet supplement that provides 100% of the dietary reference values. Care should be taken to avoid unbalanced supplements or those containing amounts larger than the dietary reference value (FSA 2003).

Modification of diet

Practical information on modification of diet can be found in the Royal Marsden Hospital Patient Information Series *Eating Well When You Have Cancer – A Guide for Cancer Patients* (Royal Marsden NHS Trust 2002). See also Table 24.2.

Box 24.1 Food and nutrition benchmark (*food* includes drinks) (DH 2001).

Agreed patient/client-focused outcome: patients/clients are enabled to consume food (orally) which meets their individual needs

Indicators/information that highlight concerns which may trigger the need for benchmarking activity:

- Patient satisfaction surveys
- Complaints figures and analysis
- Audit results: including catering audit, nutritional risk assessments, documentation audit, environmental audit (including dining facilities)
- Contract monitoring, e.g. wastage of food, food handling and/or food hygiene training records

- Ordering of dietary supplements/special diets
- Audit of available equipment and utensils
- Educational audits/student placement feedback
- Litigation/Clinical Negligence Scheme for Trusts
- Professional concern
- Media reports
- Sustainable Food and the NHS (Kings Fund Research Summary 2005), Food and Nutritional Care in Hospitals (Council of Europe 2003)

Factor	Benchmark of best practice
1 Screening/assessment to identify patients'/clients' nutritional needs	Nutritional screening progresses to **further assessment for all** Patients/clients identified as **'at risk' using a screening** tool that assesses body mass index and weight changes, **e.g. MUST** (National Collaborating Centre for Acute Care 2006)
2 Planning, implementation and evaluation	Plans of care based on **ongoing nutritional assessments** are of care for those patients who required advised,implemented and evaluated nutritional assessment
3 A conducive environment (acceptable sights, smells and sounds)	The environment is **conducive to** enabling the **individual** patients/clients to eat. Implementation of Protected Mealtimes
4 Assistance to eat and drink	Patients/clients **receive the care and assistance** they require with eating and drinking. Provision of eating aids where appropriate
5 Obtaining food	Patients/clients/carers, **whatever their communication needs**, have sufficient information to enable them to obtain their food. Examples include the NHS menu provision and utilizing menu translation services
6 Food provided	Food that is provided by the service **meets the needs and preferences** of individual patients/clients through audit of patient feedback and equality and diversity co-operatives
7 Food availability	Patients/clients have set meal times. Flexibility is also important, ensuring **a replacement meal is offered** if a meal is missed and patients **can access a lighter meal or snacks** at any time
8 Food presentation	Food is presented to patients/clients in a way that takes in to account portion capacity and what **appeals to them as individuals**
9 Monitoring	The amount of food patients actually eat is **monitored, recorded** and leads to **action** when cause for concern
10 Eating to promote health	**All opportunities** are used to encourage the patients/clients to eat to **promote their own health**

Other factors which may influence future food intake (e.g. surgery, chemotherapy or radiotherapy) also need to be taken into consideration when planning nutritional support, as clinical experience shows these may exert a deleterious effect on appetite and the ability to maintain an adequate nutritional intake (Newman *et al.* 1998)

Enteral tube feeding

While the majority of patients will be able to meet their nutritional requirements orally, there is a group of individuals who will require enteral tube feeding either in the short term or on a more permanent basis. Several different feeding tubes are available.

Types of enteral feed tubes

Nasogastric/nasoduodenal/nasojejunal

Nasogastric feeding is the most commonly used enteral tube feed and is suitable for short-term feeding, i.e. 2–4 weeks (National Collaborating Centre for Acute Care 2006). Fine-bore feeding tubes should be used whenever possible as

Table 24.2 Suggestions for modification of diet.

Eating difficulty	Dietary modification
Anorexia	Serve small meals and snacks, e.g. twice daily snack options Make food look attractive with garnish Fortify foods with butter, cream or cheese to increase energy content of meals Use alcohol, steroids, megestrol acetate or medroxyprogesterone as an appetite stimulant Encourage food that patient prefers Offer nourishing drinks between meals. In hospital consider a 'cocktail' drinks round.
Sore mouth	Offer foods that are soft and easy to eat Avoid dry foods that require chewing Avoid citrus fruits and drinks Avoid salt and spicy foods Allow hot food to cool before eating
Dysphagia	Offer foods that are soft and serve with additional sauce or gravy Some foods may need to be blended: make sure food is served attractively Supplement the diet with nourishing drinks between meals
Nausea and vomiting	Have cold foods in preference to hot as these emit less odour Keep away from cooking smells Sip fizzy, glucose-containing drinks Eat small frequent meals and snacks that are high in carbohydrate (e.g. biscuits and toast) Try ginger drinks and ginger biscuits
Early satiety	Eat small, frequent meals. In hospital access an 'out of hours' meal service Avoid high-fat foods which delay gastric emptying Avoid drinking large quantities when eating Use prokinetics, e.g. metoclopramide, to encourage gastric emptying

these are more comfortable for the patient than wide-bore tubes. They are less likely to cause complications such as rhinitis, oesophageal irritation and gastritis (Payne-James *et al.* 2001). Polyurethane or silicone tubes are preferable to polyvinylchloride (PVC) as they withstand gastric acid and can stay in position longer than the 10–14 day lifespan of the PVC tube (Payne-James *et al.* 2001).

A wire introducer is provided with many of the tubes to aid intubation. The position of the nasogastric tube can be checked using two methods:

- Chest X-ray.
- Testing of aspirate with pH indicator paper.

A chest X-ray must be used to confirm the position of the tube in high risk groups such as patients with oesophageal or head and neck tumours, who have impaired swallowing or who are unconscious because they are at higher risk of misplacement of the nasogastric tube. All other patients should have the position of the tube checked with syringed aspirate of gastric content. This should have a pH less than 5.5 (NPSA 2005). In accordance with National Patient Safety Agency (NPSA) guidance the following methods should **not** be used to confirm the position of a feeding tube:

- Auscultation of air insufflated through the feeding tube ('whoosh test').
- Testing the pH of the aspirate using blue litmus paper.
- Interpreting the absence of respiratory distress as an indicator of the correct positioning.
- Monitoring bubbling at the end of the tube.
- Observing the appearance of feeding tube aspirate.

In addition to the initial confirmation, the tube should be checked on a daily basis in the following situations:

- Before administering each feed.
- Before giving medication.
- Following episodes of vomiting, retching or coughing as it is likely the tube may be displaced.
- Following evidence of tube displacement (e.g. the tube appears visibly longer).

If a pH of below 5.5 is not obtained then it is highly likely that the tube has become displaced. The medical team should be contacted as the tube may need to be replaced. For further details on checking nasogastric tubes please refer to the full NPSA guidance or to local policy.

Gastrostomy

A gastrostomy may be more appropriate than a nasogastric tube where feeding is for medium- or long-term feeding. It avoids delays in feeding and discomfort associated with tube displacement (National Collaborating Centre for Acute Care 2006). Suitable patients are those undergoing radical or hyperfractionated radiotherapy to the neck or children with solid tumours. They will require long-term enteral feeding because the treatment is intensive and prolonged. A gastrostomy tube may be placed endoscopically (percutaneous endoscopically placed gastrostomy [PEG]) or radiologically (radiologically inserted gastrostomy [RIG]). They are made from polyurethane or silicone and are therefore suitable for short- or long-term feeding. A flange, flexible dome, inflated balloon or pigtail sits within the stomach and holds the tube in position. The use of conventional balloon urinary catheters is now outdated, particularly as these are at risk of allowing gastric acid to leak at the tube entry site. However, gastrostomy tubes held in place with an inflatable balloon have the benefit over urinary catheters of being less likely to leak and are also made from polyurethane or silicone rather than from PVC. Clinical trials have shown that complications with PEG tubes, such as leakage, are rare (Riera *et al.* 2002).

For long-term feeding (i.e. longer than 1 month), a gastrostomy tube may be replaced with a button which is made from silicone. The entry site for feeding is flush with the skin, making it neat and less obvious than a gastrostomy tube. This is more cosmetically acceptable, especially for teenagers, but does require a certain amount of manual dexterity from the patient (Thomas & Bishop 2007). The button is held in place by a balloon or dome inside the stomach (Griffiths 1996).

PEG tubes may be placed while the patient is sedated; thereby avoiding the risks associated with general anaesthesia.

Certain groups of patients are not suitable for endoscopy; in these cases a RIG can be used. They are indicated for oesophageal patients with bulky tumours where it would be difficult to pass an endoscope and also for head and neck patients whose airway would be obstructed by an endoscope. There is also documented risk of the endoscope seeding the tumour to the gastrostomy site when it pulls the tube past a bulky tumour although this is a rare complication (Pickhardt *et al*. 2002).

Jejunostomy

A jejunostomy is preferable to a gastrostomy if a patient has undergone upper GI surgery or has severe delayed gastric emptying; in some cases it can be used to feed a patient with pyloric obstruction (Thomas & Bishop 2007). Fine-bore feeding jejunostomy tubes may be inserted with the use of a jejunostomy kit, which consists of a needle-fine catheter. The use of needles and an introducer wire allows a fine-bore polyurethane catheter to be inserted into a loop of jejunum. Alternatively, some gastrostomy tubes allow the passage of a fine-bore tube into the jejunum.

Enteral feeding equipment

The administration of enteral feeds may be as a bolus, intermittent or continuous infusion, via gravity drip or pump-assisted (Table 24.3). There are many enteral feeding pumps available which vary in their range of flow rate from 1 ml to 300 ml per hour. The following systems may be used for feeding via a pump or gravity-drip:

- Feed is decanted into plastic bottles or PVC bags. The administration set may be an integral part of the bag. The feed is sterile until opened and decanting feed into reservoirs will increase the risk of contamination of the feed from handling (Payne-James *et al*. 2001). Malnourished and immunocompromised patients are particularly at risk from contamination and infection so this method of administration should be avoided where possible.
- The 'ready to hang system' has a glass bottle, plastic bottle or pack attached directly to the administration set. The bottles and packs are available in different types of feeds and sizes for flexibility. This is a closed sterile system. It has been shown to be successful in preventing exogenous bacterial contamination (Payne-James *et al*. 2001).

Enteral feeds

Commercially prepared feeds should be used for nasogastric, gastrostomy or jejunostomy feeding. Available in liquid or powder form, they have the advantage of being of known composition and are sterile when packaged.

1 Whole protein/polymeric feeds contain protein, hydrolysed fat and carbohydrate and so require digestion. These may provide 1.0–1.5 kcal/ml (see manufacturer's specifications). As the energy density of the feed increases so does the osmolarity. Hyperosmolar feeds tend to draw water into the lumen of the gut and can contribute to diarrhoea if given too rapidly. Fibre may be beneficial for maintaining gut ecology and function, rather than promoting bowel transit time (Thomas & Bishop 2007).
2 Feeds containing MCT. In some whole protein feeds a proportion of the fat or LCT may be replaced with MCT. The feed often has a lower osmolarity, and is therefore less likely to draw fluid from the plasma into the gut lumen. MCT is transported via the portal vein rather than the lymphatic system. These feeds are suitable for

Table 24.3 Methods of administering enteral feeds.

Feeding regimen	Advantages	Disadvantages
Continuous feeding via a pump	Easily controlled rate Reduction of GI complications	Patient connected to the feed for majority of the day May limit patient's mobility
Intermittent feeding via gravity or a pump	Periods of time free of feeding Flexible feeding routine May be easier than managing a pump for some patients	May have an increased risk of GI symptoms, e.g. early satiety Difficult if outside carers are involved with the feed
Bolus feeding	May reduce time connected to feed Very easy Minimum equipment required	May have an increased risk of GI symptoms May be time consuming

GI, gastrointestinal.

patients with fat malabsorption and maybe steatorrhoea (Cummings 2000).

3   Chemically defined/elemental feeds. These contain free amino acids, short-chain peptides or a combination of both as the nitrogen source. They are often low in fat or may contain some fat as MCT. Glucose polymers provide the main energy source. These feeds require little or no digestion and are suitable for those patients with impaired GI function (Thomas & Bishop 2007). They are hyperosmolar and low in residue.

4   Special application feeds. Low protein and mineral feeds may be used for patients with liver or renal failure. High-fat, low-carbohydrate feeds may be used for ventilated patients because less carbon dioxide is produced per calorie intake compared with a low-fat, high-carbohydrate feed.

Very high energy and protein feeds may be used where nutritional requirements are exceptionally high, e.g. burns, severe sepsis. These feeds contain approximately double the amount of energy and protein compared to standard whole protein feeds.

5   Paediatric feeds are designed for children 1–12 years old and/or 8–45 kg in weight. The protein, vitamin and mineral profile is suitable for children. Generally they are lower in osmolarity than adult feeds. The whole protein/polymeric feeds are based on cow's milk but are lactose free. Some of these feeds may contain dietary fibre. These feeds provide 1.0–1.5 kcal/ml for children who require additional energy and protein in a smaller volume. Protein hydrolysate feeds and elemental feeds are used in conditions such as food allergies or malabsorption. Some specialist centres use these feeds for enteral feeding during bone marrow transplants as children may have malabsorption caused by gut mucositis. The osmolarity of these feeds is higher than whole protein feeds. They need to be introduced carefully (Thomas & Bishop 2007).

6   Immune modulating feeds. There is evidence to show that the addition of glutamine, arginine or omega-3 fatty acids, if given preoperatively, may benefit post-surgical GI patients (Braga et al. 2002).

Up-to-date information on the exact composition of dietary supplements and enteral feeds can be obtained from the manufacturers.

Monitoring enteral tube feeding

In order to avoid complications and ensure optimal nutritional status, it is important to monitor the following in patients on enteral tube feeds:

- Oral intake.
- Body weight.
- Urea and electrolytes.
- Blood glucose.
- Full blood count.
- Fluid balance.
- Tolerance to feed, e.g. nausea, fullness and bowel activity.

- Quantity of feed taken.
- Care of tube.
- Care of stoma site.

Complications of enteral tube feeding

The type and frequency of complications related to tube feeding depend on the access route, underlying disease state, the feeding regimen and the patient's metabolic state (Payne-James et al. 2001) (Table 24.4).

Home enteral feeding

Some patients who are established on tube feeding in hospital also require enteral tube feeding at home. A multidisciplinary approach is needed for a successful discharge usually involving a dietitian, doctor, ward nurse, community nurse and general practitioner. The patient's circumstances and the ability of the patient or carers to manage the feed must be considered when the patient's discharge is being planned. Adequate time should be allowed in the hospital setting for patients to become fully accustomed to the techniques of feed administration and care of the feeding tube, prior to discharge home. Patients should also be given written information to reinforce the education they receive prior to discharge (BAPEN 1994a).

Support in the form of the general practitioner, community nurse and community dietetic services should be established before discharge. A multidisciplinary discharge meeting may be of benefit to both the patient and the professionals involved. Many of the commercial feed companies organize for the patient's feed and equipment to be delivered to the patient's home, after consultation with the local community services (BAPEN 1994a). The hospital or community dietitian can arrange this. Early notification of discharge is essential as it usually takes a minimum of 7 days to set this up.

Termination of enteral tube feeding

It is important to ensure that an individual is able to meet their nutritional requirements orally prior to termination of the feed. Ideally, the feeds should be reduced gradually, according to the dietary intake (BAPEN 1999). It may be useful to maintain an overnight feed while the patient is establishing oral intake.

Parenteral nutrition

Parenteral nutrition (PN) is the direct infusion into a vein, of solutions containing the essential nutrients in quantities to meet all the daily needs of the patient (Furst et al. 2001). While enteral feeding is the preferred route of nutritional support in terms of cost and mechanical, septic and metabolic complications (National Collaborating Centre for Acute Care 2006), PN may be indicated for patients with a

Table 24.4 Complications that may occur during enteral feeding.

Complication	Cause	Solution
Aspiration	Regurgitation of feed due to poor gastric emptying Incorrect placement of tube	Medication to improve gastric emptying, e.g. metoclopramide Check tube placement Ensure patient has head at 45° during feeding
Nausea and vomiting	Related to disease/treatment Medication such as antibiotics, analgesia, etc. Poor gastric emptying Rapid infusion of feed	Antiemetics Reduce infusion rate Change from bolus to intermittent feeding
Diarrhoea	Medication such as antibiotics, chemotherapy, laxatives Radiotherapy to pelvis Disease-related, e.g. pancreatic insufficiency Gut infection	Antidiarrhoeal agent If possible discontinue antibiotics, avoid microbiological contamination of feed or equipment Treat disease or manage symptoms Send stool sample to check for gut infection
Constipation	Inadequate fluid intake Immobility Use of opiates or other medication causing gut stasis Bowel obstruction	Check fluid balance and correct if necessary Administer laxatives/bulking agents If possible encourage mobility If in bowel obstruction, discontinue feed
Abdominal distension	Poor gastric emptying Rapid infusion of feed Constipation or diarrhoea	Gastric motility agents Reduce rate of infusion If possible encourage mobility Treat constipation or diarrhoea
Blocked tube	Inadequate flushing or failure to flush feeding tube Administration of medication via the tube	Prevent blockages by flushing with 30–50 ml water before and after feeds or medication Use liquid or finely crushed medications If blocked, try warm water, soda water, sodium bicarbonate, fizzy soft drink, enzyme preparations

prolonged ileus, uncontrolled vomiting or diarrhoea, severe radiation enteritis, short bowel syndrome or GI obstruction.

Route of administration

The traditional method of access is a central venous catheter. Central venous access is required because PN solutions are hyperosmolar and there is a risk of thrombophlebitis associated with feeding into peripheral veins (Wilson & Jordan 2001; Springhouse Corporation 2002). However, it has been shown that with care and attention, peripheral veins can be used to provide short-term peripheral PN (National Collaborating Centre for Acute Care 2006). This would be via a midline or a peripheral cannula. For the administration of PN the device should be placed in the largest vein possible, usually in the forearm away from a joint with rotation of the site every 48–72 hours (Shaw 2008) (see Chapter 45).

The major hazard associated with the delivery of PN via a central venous catheter is infection. Therefore, catheter insertion should take place using strict aseptic technique either within theatre or at the bedside (Hamilton *et al.* 1995; Fitzsimmons 1997; Benton & Marsden 2002; Weinstein

2007). A skin-tunnelled catheter is the catheter of choice for long-term nutrition but peripherally inserted central canulas (PICCs) or non-tunnelled central venous catheters can also be used in the short term. The number of lumens will depend on the patient's peripheral venous access and the number of additional therapies required. It is recommended that the minimum number of lumens is used but if additional intravenous access is required then a double or triple lumen catheter should be inserted and then one lumen should be dedicated for use with PN. If using a single lumen device, routine blood sampling and additional infusions should be carried out independently, using a separate cannula if necessary (Davidson 2005).

PN solution

The basic components of a PN regimen are provided by solutions of:

- *Amino acids* (nitrogen source). Commercially available solutions provide both essential amino acids, usually in proportions to meet requirements, and non-essential amino acids, such as alanine and glycine.

- *Glucose* (carbohydrate energy source). Glucose is the carbohydrate source of choice. It provides 3.75 kcal/g (1545 kJ/g).
- *Fat emulsion* (fat energy source). Fat generates 9 kcal/g (37 kJ/g) and its inclusion in PN is necessary to provide essential fatty acids. Fat usually provides 30–50% of non-nitrogen energy. Nitrogen: non-nitrogen energy is usually provided in the ratio of 1:150–200. An insufficient energy supply from carbohydrate and fat will encourage the use of nitrogen for energy.
- *Electrolytes*, e.g. sodium, potassium, calcium.
- *Vitamins*. Both water-soluble and fat-soluble vitamins are required.
- *Trace elements*, e.g. zinc, copper, chromium, selenium (Thomas & Bishop 2007).

Choice of a PN regimen

PN is usually administered from a single infusion container in which all the requirements for a 24-hour feed are pre-mixed. Such infusions are available as standard ready prepared bags that require the addition of vitamins, minerals and trace elements or individual bags may be made to a particular prescription and purchased from a compounding unit.

The regimen for a particular patient should be formulated according to the patient's needs for energy and nitrogen (see calculation of nutritional requirements, Table 24.1). The majority of commercial vitamin and mineral preparations aim to meet both short- and long-term requirements although appropriate monitoring is required to ensure that nutritional requirements are met.

Standard PN regimens may be suitable for some patients who require short-term nutritional support or do not appear to have excessively altered nutritional requirements.

The choice of such regimens depends on the patient's body weight and nutritional requirements. To allow for the possible need to vary the constituents of the infusion in response to changes in the patient's electrolyte or nutritional requirements, PN solutions should be ordered daily. Once compounded, most PN preparations last up to 7 days (Weinstein 2007) and need to be stored in a refrigerator. However, some triple chamber PN bags can be stored at ambient temperatures and require mixing prior to administration. These bags generally require the addition of vitamins, minerals and trace elements under aseptic conditions.

PN should be introduced slowly in the seriously ill or injured with no more than 50% of requirements given in the first 24–48 hours (National Collaborating Centre for Acute Care 2006).

Delivery of PN and recommendations for intravenous management

Administration sets should always be changed every 24 hours (Wilson & Jordan 2001; Springhouse Corporation

2002; Pratt *et al.* 2007), using an aseptic technique. Existing injection sites on the administration set should never be used for the giving of additional medications as PN is incompatible with numerous medications. Drugs may bind to the nutrients or the PN bag reducing their availability. If any additional medications, blood products or central venous pressure (CVP) readings are required then they should be given via a separate lumen or via a peripheral device.

A volumetric infusion pump must be used to ensure accurate delivery of PN. No bag should be used for longer than 24 hours (Wilson & Jordan 2001; Springhouse Corporation 2002) and rates should never be adjusted more than ±10% (Weinstein 2007).

If the infusion must be discontinued the catheter should be flushed and patency maintained. The risk of infection increases if the infusion is disconnected from the central venous device; therefore, it is not advisable to disconnect PN until the whole daily requirement has been administered (Pratt *et al.* 2007).

Monitoring of PN

During intravenous feeding monitoring is necessary to detect and minimize complications (Tables 24.5 & 24.6). Once feeding is established and the patient is biochemically stable then the frequency of monitoring may be reduced if the clinical condition of the patient permits. Additional patient monitoring such as 24-hour urine collection for urinary urea, nitrogen and serum zinc, copper or selenium may be carried out where indicated, e.g. in severe malnutrition or when PN is used for prolonged periods of time (Weinstein 2007).

Metabolic complications of PN

Metabolic complications should be detected by appropriate monitoring. Some more common complications are:

- *Fluid overload*. This may occur when other blood products and fluids are given concurrently. It may be possible to reduce the volume of a 24-hour bag of PN while maintaining the nutritional content. Pharmacy can advise on the feasibility of making such regimens.

Table 24.5 Monitoring of patients receiving parenteral nutrition. National Collaborating Centre for Acute Care (2006).

- Daily initially, reducing to twice weekly when stable
- Inspect catheter entry site daily for signs of infection or inflammation
- Inspect site of peripheral cannulae for signs of phlebitis (peripherally fed patients)
- Assess general condition daily
- Record temperature and blood pressure daily initially then as needed

Table 24.6 Biochemical monitoring of parenteral nutrition. National Collaborating Centre for Acute Care (2006).

Parameter	Frequency	Rationale	Interpretation
Sodium, potassium, urea, creatinine	Baseline Daily until stable then 1 or 2 times a week	Assessment of renal function, fluid status and Na and K status	Interpret with knowledge of fluid balance and medication
Glucose	Baseline 1 or 2 times a day (or more if needed) until stable then weekly	Glucose intolerance is common	Good glycaemic control is necessary
Magnesium, phosphate	Baseline Daily if risk of refeeding syndrome Three times a week until stable Then weekly	Depletion is common and under recognized	Low concentrations indicate poor status
Liver function tests including International Normalized Ratio	Baseline Twice weekly until stable Then weekly	Abnormalities common during parenteral nutrition	Complex, may be due to sepsis, other disease or nutritional intake
Calcium, albumin	Baseline then weekly	Hypocalcaemia or hypercalcaemia may occur	Correct measured serum calcium concentration for albumin Hypocalcaemia may be secondary to Mg deficiency Low albumin reflects disease not protein status
C-reactive protein	Baseline Then 2 or 3 times a week until stable	Assists interpretation of protein, trace elements and vitamin results	To assess the presence of an acute phase reaction The trend of results is important
Full blood count and mean cell volume	Baseline 1 or 2 times a week until stable then weekly	Anaemia due to iron or folate deficiency is common	Effects of sepsis may be important
Iron, ferritin	Baseline Then every 3–6 months	Iron deficiency common in long-term parenteral nutrition	Iron status difficult if acute phase reaction (Fe decreases and ferritin increases)
Folate, B_{12}	Baseline Then every 2–4 weeks	Iron deficiency is common	Serum folate/B_{12} sufficient, with full blood count

Monitoring of trace elements such as selenium, zinc, copper and manganese should be carried out if patients are on long-term parenteral nutrition, for example for periods longer than 1 month.

- *Hyperglycaemia*. This may occur due to stress-induced insulin resistance or carbohydrate overload. A simultaneous sliding scale insulin infusion may be required. Failure to recognize hyperglycaemia may result in osmotic diuresis.
- *Hypoglycaemia*. Abrupt cessation of PN may result in a rebound hypoglycaemia. A reduction in infusion rate to half the rate prior to stopping the infusion may help prevent this occurring.
- *Azotaemia*. Raised plasma urea may indicate renal dysfunction or dehydration. Alterations in the nitrogen and non-protein energy content of the PN may be required, or an increase in fluid input (Payne-James *et al*. 2001).
- *Hypophosphataemia*. This is associated with excessive glucose infusion and the refeeding syndrome in malnourished patients (Thorell & Nordenström 2001). It is necessary to correct phosphate levels by providing additional phosphate prior to feeding. Phosphate levels should be monitored daily at the start of feeding.

Other complications such as metabolic acidosis, electrolyte disturbances, hyperammonaemia, hypernatraemia and

Table 24.7 Criteria for determining patients at risk of refeeding problems (National Collaborating Centre for Acute Care 2006).

Patient has one or more of the following	Patient has two or more of the following
BMI < 16 kg/m²	BMI < 18.5 kg/m²
Unintentional weight loss > 15%	Weight loss > 10%
Very little nutritional intake for > 10 days	Very little nutritional intake for > 5 days
Low levels of postassium, phosphate or magnesium prior to feeding	A history of alcohol abuse or drugs including insulin, chemotherapy, antacids or diuretics

BMI, body mass index.

hypokalaemia may require a review of the PN solution, rate of administration, additional fluids, blood products and drugs.

Termination of PN

PN should not be terminated until oral or enteral tube feeding is well established (Weinstein 2007). The patient needs to be established on an adequate oral or enteral tube feed before the PN is discontinued (National Collaborating Centre for Acute Care 2006). It is important that all members of the multidisciplinary team are involved in the decision to terminate PN and that enteral intake is monitored sufficiently.

Elective removal of central venous catheter

See Chapter 45.

Home PN

There are few indications for home PN. It may be necessary in patients who have complete intestinal failure or insufficient functioning bowel to maintain an adequate nutritional status via the enteral route, e.g. short bowel syndrome due to Crohn's disease or radiation enteritis. The cost of home parenteral feeding is high and requires intensive training with an efficient and comprehensive back-up service. It is recommended that only hospitals which have the appropriate facilities to train patients and provide the necessary care in case of an emergency should be involved in home PN. There is national guidance as to the training, provision and appropriate support for such patients which should be consulted prior to any discharge of patients receiving PN (BAPEN 1994a; DH 2002).

Multidisciplinary team

It is important that all members of the multidisciplinary team, including dietitian, nurse, doctor, pharmacist, catering department and community services, are involved in the patient's nutritional care to ensure a thorough and coordinated approach to nutritional management (BAPEN 1994b; National Collaborating Centre for Acute Care 2006).

Procedure guidelines   Weighing the patient

Accurate weighing and correct documentation of the patient's weight may be necessary, for example for nutrition screening or planning of drug dosage.

Equipment

1 Scales (either sitting or standing) that are calibrated and positioned on a level surface. If electronic or battery scales are used then they must be connected to the mains or have appropriate working batteries prior to the patient getting on the scales.

Procedure

Action	Rationale
1 Position the scales for easy access and apply the brakes (if appropriate).	To ensure that the patient can get on and off the scales easily and to avoid accidents should the scales move (E).
2 Ask the patient to remove shoes and outdoor garments. The patient should be wearing light indoor clothes only (see Action figure 2).	Outdoor clothes and shoes will add additional weight and make it difficult to obtain an accurate body weight (E).
3 Ensure that the scales record zero then ask the patient to stand on scales (or sit if using sitting scales). Ask the patient to remain still and check that the patient is not supporting any weight on any object, e.g. wall, stick or feet on the floor.	To record an accurate weight (E).

Procedure guidelines *(cont.)*

4 Note the reading on the scale and record immediately taking care that it is legible. Check with the patient that the weight reflects their expected weight and that the weight is similar to previous weights recorded.

To check that the weight is correct. If the weight is not as expected then the patient should be re-weighed (E).

Action 2   Weighing a patient.

Procedure guidelines   Feeding an adult

An essential part of providing diet for a patient is to ensure that the patient is able to consume the food and fluid in a safe and pleasant environment. Some patients may require assistance with feeding or drinking and a system should be in place to ensure that these patients receive the required attention at each meal time and beverage that is provided (Nicol *et al.* 2000).

Equipment

1 Appropriate environment for eating, preferably at a dining table with chair or the patient should be positioned where the patient can sit up as much as possible in a supported midline position.
2 Clean table or tray.
3 Chair for the nurse or carer to sit with the patient.
4 Appetising meal that complies with any dietary restriction that is relevant to the patient. For example, these may include allergies, texture modifications, religious or cultural dietary requirements.

Procedure

Action	Rationale
1 Ensure the patient is comfortable, i.e. has an empty bladder, clean hands, clean mouth and if applicable clean dentures.	To make the mealtime a pleasant experience (E).
2 Wash hands thoroughly with soap and water.	Hands must be cleansed before and after patient contact to minimize cross-infection (DH 2005: C).
3 Obtain the correct food, drink, cutlery and napkin.	To prevent errors with the wrong food being served to the patient (E).
4 Protect the patient's clothing with a napkin.	To maintain dignity and cleanliness (E).
5 Assist the patient to take appropriate portions of food at the correct temperature. Tailor the size of each mouthful to the individual patient. Allow the patient to chew and swallow food before giving the next mouthful.	To make the mealtime a pleasant experience. To ensure that swallowing is not compromised if the patient feels that they must hurry with the meal (E).
6 Avoid asking questions when the patient is eating but check between mouthfuls that the food is suitable and patient is able to continue with the meal.	To reduce the risk of aspirating, which may be increased if speaking whilst eating (E).
7 Use the napkin to remove particles of food or drink from the patient's face.	To maintain dignity and cleanliness (E).
8 Ask the patient when they wish to have a drink. Tip the glass or cup gently so that the flow of liquid is controlled or use a straw if this is helpful. Take care with hot drinks to avoid offering these when too hot to drink.	To give the opportunity for the patient to swallow (E). Hot liquids may scald the patient.
9 Encourage the patient to take as much food as they feel able to eat but do not press if they have indicated that they have eaten sufficient.	To improve nutritional intake but also maintain patient dignity and choice (E).
10 After the meal assist the patient to meet hygiene needs; for example, wash hands and face and clean teeth.	To maintain patient dignity (E).

Procedure guidelines   Nasogastric intubation with tubes using an introducer

Equipment

1 Clinically clean tray.
2 Fine-bore nasogastric tube.
3 Introducer for tube.
4 Receiver.
5 Sterile water.
6 10 ml syringe.

7 Hypoallergenic tape.
8 Adhesive patch if available.
9 Glass of water.
10 Lubricating jelly.
11 Indicator strips, e.g. pH Fix, 0–6, Fisher Scientific.

Prior to performing this procedure the patient's medical and nursing notes should be consulted to check for potential complications. For example, anatomical alterations due to surgery, such as a flap repair or the presence of a cancerous tumour, can prevent a clear passage for the nasogastric tube, resulting in pain and discomfort for the patient and further complications.

Procedure

Action	Rationale
1 Explain and discuss the procedure with the patient.	To ensure that the patient understands the procedure and gives his/her valid consent (E; NMC 2006: C).
2 Arrange a signal by which the patient can communicate if he/she wants the nurse to stop, e.g. by raising his/her hand.	The patient is often less frightened if he/she feels able to have some control over the procedure (E).
3 Assist the patient to sit in a semi-upright position in the bed or chair. Support the patient's head with pillows. *Note:* The head should not be tilted backwards or forwards (Rollins 1997).	To allow for easy passage of the tube. This position enables easy swallowing and ensures that the epiglottis is not obstructing the oesophagus (E).
4 Select the appropriate distance mark on the tube by measuring the distance on the tube from the patient's ear lobe to the bridge of the nose plus the distance from the ear lobe to the bottom of the xiphisternum (see Action figures 4a & b).	To ensure that the appropriate length of tube is passed into the stomach (E).
5 Wash hands with bactericidal soap and water or bactericidal alcohol handrub, and assemble the equipment required.	Hands must be cleansed before and after patient contact to minimize cross-infection (DH 2005: R 1a).
6 Follow manufacturer's instructions to prepare the tube, e.g. injecting sterile water for injection down the tube and lubricating the proximal end of the tube with lubricating jelly.	Contact with water activates coating inside tube and on the tip. This lubricates the tube, assisting its passage through the nasopharynx and allowing easy withdrawal of the introducer (E).
7 Check that the nostrils are patent by asking the patient to sniff with one nostril closed. Repeat with the other nostril.	To identify any obstructions liable to prevent intubation (E).
8 Insert the rounded end of the tube into the clearer nostril and slide it backwards and inwards along the floor of the nose to the nasopharynx. If any obstruction is felt, withdraw the tube and try again in a slightly different direction or use the other nostril.	To facilitate the passage of the tube by following the natural anatomy of the nose (E).

9 As the tube passes down into the nasopharynx, unless swallowing is contraindicated, ask the patient to start swallowing and sipping water.

To focus the patient's attention on something other than the tube. A swallowing action closes the glottis, and crico-pharyngeal sphincter opens enabling the tube to pass into the oesophagus (Groher 1997: E).

10 Advance the tube through the pharynx, as the patient swallows until the predetermined mark has been reached. If the patient shows signs of distress, e.g. gasping or cyanosis, remove the tube immediately.

The tube may have accidentally been passed down the trachea instead of the pharynx. Distress may indicate that the tube is in the bronchus. However, absence of distress is ineffective for detecting a misplaced tube (NPSA 2005: C).

11 Remove the introducer by using gentle traction. If it is difficult to remove, then remove the tube as well.

If the introducer sticks in the tube, it may be indicative that the tube is in the bronchus (E).

12 Secure the tape to the nostril with adherent dressing tape, e.g. Elastoplast (Burns *et al.* 1995). If this is contraindicated, a hypoallergenic tape should be used. An adhesive patch (if available) will secure the tube to the cheek.

To hold the tube in place. To ensure patient comfort (E).

13 Measure the part of the visible tube from tip of nose and record in care plan. Mark the tube at the exit site (nares) (Metheny & Titler 2001).

To provide a record to assist in detecting movement of the tube (NPSA 2005: C).

14 Check the position of the tube to confirm that it is in the stomach by using the following methods:
   (a) Taking an X-ray of chest and upper abdomen.

Feeding via the tube must not begin until the correct position of the tube has been confirmed (NPSA 2005: C). To confirm placement of radiopaque nasogastric tube. X-ray of radiopaque tubes is the most accurate confirmation of position and is the method of choice in patients with altered anatomy, those who are aspirating or are unconscious with no gag reflex (NPSA 2005: C).

   (b) Aspirating 2 ml of stomach contents and testing pH indicator strips (Rollins 1997; NPSA 2005: C). When aspirated fluid for pH testing, wait at least 1 hour after a feed or medication has been administered (either orally or via the tube). Before aspirating, flush the tube with 20 ml of air to clear other substances (Metheny *et al.* 1993). A pH level of 5.5 is unlikely to be pulmonary aspirates and it is considered appropriate to proceed to feed through the tube (Metheny 2004; NPSA 2005).
   Wait at least 1 hour before aspirating to enable the feed or medication to be absorbed, otherwise an inaccurate test will be obtained (NPSA 2005: C).

Indicator strips to be used should have gradations of 0.5 or paper with a range of 0–6 or 1–11 to distinguish between gastric acid and bronchial secretions (NPSA 2005: C). To prove an accurate test result because the feed or medication may raise the pH of the stomach.

   (c) If a pH of 6.0 or above is obtained or there is doubt over the result in the range of pH 5–6 then feeding must **not** commence. The nasogastric tube may need to be repositioned or checked with an X-ray.

There is an increased risk of the nasogastric tube being incorrectly placed (NPSA 2005: C).

Procedure guidelines *(cont.)*

15 The following methods **must not** be used to test the position of a nasogastric feeding tube: auscultation (introducing air into the nasogastric tube and checking for a bubbling sound via a stethoscope), use of litmus paper or absence of respiratory distress.

These tests are not accurate or reliable as a method of checking the position of a nasogastric tube as they have been shown to give false positive results (Metheny 2004; NPSA 2005: C).

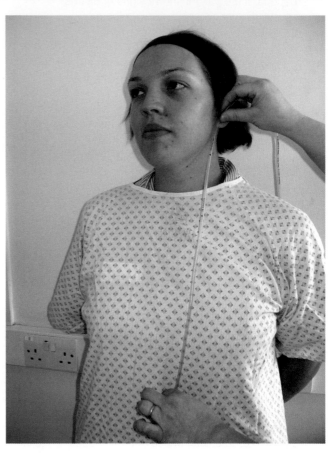

Action 4 (a & b) Measuring for a nasogastric tube.
(a) Measure from patient's ear lobe to bridge of nose.

Action 4(b) Measure from ear lobe to bottom of xiphisternum.

Procedure guidelines Nasogastric intubation with tubes without using an introducer, e.g. a Ryle's tube

It is recommended that a nasogastric tube designed for feeding purposes be used wherever possible, e.g. fine-bore feeding tube, rather than a Ryle's tube which is used for drainage of gastric contents.

Equipment

1 Clinically clean tray.
2 Nasogastric tube that has been stored in a deep freeze for at least half an hour before the procedure is to begin, to ensure a rigid tube that will allow for easy passage.
3 Topical gauze.
4 Lubricating jelly.

5 Hypoallergenic tape.
6 20 ml syringe.
7 Indicator strips, e.g. pH Fix, 0–6, Fisher Scientific.
8 Receiver.
9 Spigot.
10 Glass of water.

Procedure

Action	Rationale
1 Explain and discuss the procedure with the patient.	To ensure that the patient understands the procedure and gives his/her valid consent (E; NMC 2006: C).
2 Arrange a signal by which the patient can communicate if he/she wants the nurse to stop, e.g. by raising his/her hand.	The patient is often less frightened if he/she feels able to have some control over the procedure (E).
3 Assist the patient to sit in a semi-upright position in the bed or chair. Support the patient's head with pillows. *Note*: The head should not be tilted backwards or forwards (Rollins 1997).	To allow for easy passage of the tube. This position enables easy swallowing and ensures that the epiglottis is not obstructing the oesophagus (E).
4 Mark the distance which the tube is to be passed by measuring the distance on the tube from the patient's ear lobe to the bridge of the nose plus the distance from the ear lobe to the bottom of the xiphisternum.	To indicate the length of tube required for entry into the stomach (E).
5 Wash hands with bactericidal soap and water or bactericidal alcohol handrub, and assemble the equipment required.	Hands must be cleansed before and after patient contact to minimize cross-infection (DH 2005: R 1a).
6 Check the patient's nostrils are patent by asking him/her to sniff with one nostril closed. Repeat with the other nostril.	To identify any obstructions liable to prevent intubation (E).
7 Lubricate about 15–20 cm of the tube with a thin coat of lubricating jelly that has been placed on a topical swab.	To reduce the friction between the mucous membranes and the tube (E).
8 Insert the proximal end of the tube into the clearer nostril and slide it backwards and inwards along the floor of the nose to the nasopharynx. If an obstruction is felt, withdraw the tube and try again in a slightly different direction or use the other nostril.	To facilitate the passage of the tube by following the natural anatomy of the nose (E).
9 As the tube passes down into the nasopharynx, ask the patient to start swallowing and sipping water, enabling the tube to pass into the oesophagus (R).	To focus the patient's attention on something other than the tube. The swallowing action closes the glottis and crico-pharyngeal sphincter opens enabling the tube to pass into the oesophagus (Groher 1997: R 5).
10 Advance the tube through the pharynx as the patient swallows until the tape-marked tube reaches the point of entry into the external nares. If the patient shows signs of distress, e.g. gasping or cyanosis, remove the tube immediately.	Distress may indicate that the tube is in the bronchus. However, absence of distress is ineffective for detecting a misplaced tube (NPSA 2005: C).
11 Secure the tube to the nostril with adherent dressing tape, e.g. Elastoplast (Burns *et al.* 1995). If this is contraindicated, a hypoallergenic tape should be used. An adhesive patch (if available) will secure the tube to the cheek.	To hold the tube in place. To ensure patient comfort (E).

Procedure guidelines *(cont.)*

12 Check the position of the tube to confirm that it is in the stomach by using the following methods:

(a) Taking an X-ray of chest and upper abdomen.

To confirm placement of radiopaque nasogastric tube. X-ray of radiopaque tubes is the most accurate confirmation of position and is the method of choice in patients with altered anatomy, those who are aspirating or are unconscious with no gag reflex (NPSA 2005: C).

(b) Aspirating 2 ml of stomach contents and testing with pH indicator strips (Rollins 1997). When aspirating fluid for pH testing, wait at least 1 hour after a feed or medication has been administered (either orally or via a tube). Before aspirating, flush the tube with 20 ml of air to clear other substances (Metheny *et al.* 1993). A pH level of 5.5 is unlikely to be pulmonary aspirate and is considered appropriate to proceed to feed through the tube (Metheny 2004; NPSA 2005).

Indicator strips to be used should have gradations of 0.5 or paper with a range of 0–6 or 1–11 to distinguish between gastric acid and bronchial secretions (NPSA 2005: C). To prove an accurate test result because the feed or medication may raise the pH of the stomach. Wait at least 1 hour before aspirating to enable the feed or medication to be absorbed, otherwise an inaccurate test will be obtained (NPSA 2005: C).

(c) If a pH of 6.0 or above is obtained or there is doubt over the result in the range of pH 5–6 then feeding must **not** commence. The nasogastric tube may need to be repositioned or checked with an X-ray.

There is an increased risk of the nasogastric tube being incorrectly placed (NPSA 2005: C).

13 The following methods **must not** be used to test the position of a nasogastric feeding tube: auscultation (introducing air into the nasogastric tube and checking for a bubbling sound via a stethoscope, also known as the 'whoosh test'), use of litmus paper or absence of respiratory distress.

These tests are not accurate or reliable as a method of checking the position of a nasogastric tube as they have been shown to give false positive results (Metheny 2004; NPSA 2005: C).

Procedure guidelines   Percutaneous endoscopically placed gastrostomy (PEG) tube care

The first change of dressing should be performed 24 hours after PEG placement or earlier if indicated, e.g. the site is bleeding (Loser *et al.* 2005). Until granulation of the stoma canal has taken place the dressing should be changed daily using aseptic technique. The wound should be inspected for bleeding, erythema, secretion, induration, allergic skin reaction, etc. (Loser *et al.* 2005). This will help maintain skin integrity and detect any problems early, e.g. infection, skin breakdown.

Equipment

1 Sterile procedure pack containing gallipot, low-linting gauze.

2 0.9% sodium chloride or antiseptic solution.

Procedure

Action

1 Explain and discuss the procedure with the patient.

Rationale

To ensure that the patient understands the procedure and gives his/her valid consent (E; NMC 2006: C).

2 Perform procedure using aseptic technique.

To minimize the risk of cross-infection (DH 2005: C) (for further information see Procedure guidelines: Aseptic technique, Chapter 5).

3 Remove postprocedural dressing if in place. Observe peristomal skin and stoma site for signs of infection, irritation or excoriation.

To gain access to stoma site. To detect complications early and instigate appropriate treatment (Lynch & Fang 2004: R 5).

4 Note the number of the measuring guide on the tube closest to the end of the external fixation device. Loosen the tube from the fixation device and ease fixation device away from the abdomen. The external fixation plate should be subjected to very low traction, without tension to maintain contact of the stomach with the abdominal wall.

To ensure gastrostomy tube is reattached to the fixation device in the correct position (C & E).
To ensure stoma site is thoroughly cleaned (Lynch & Fang 2004: R 5).

5 Clean the stoma site with a sterile solution such as 0.9% sodium chloride. Using low-linting gauze dry the area thoroughly.

To remove any exudate, to prevent infection and skin excoriation (E).

6 Rotate the gastrostomy tube 360°.

To prevent the tube adhering to the sides of the stoma tract (Bumpers *et al.* 2003: R 4).

7 Gently push the external fixation device against the abdomen checking the measurement guide.

To enable the gastrostomy tube to be reattached to the fixation device (E).

8 Gently but firmly pull the gastrostomy tube and attach to the fixation device. The numbered position mark at the gastrostomy exit site will be noted in the medical and nursing notes. The fixation device should remain at the same length, so that gentle traction on the tube allows 0.5 cm give but no more for the first 14 days if the patient is not receiving chemotherapy.
If they are receiving chemotherapy it is advisable to continue with the same gentle traction for 3–4 weeks.

To ensure that the tube is correctly secured (E).

As wound healing may be impaired in chemotherapy (E).

9 Ensure the correct point on the measuring guide on the tube is placed closest to the end of the fixation device.

To ensure that the tube is correctly secured. If the patient gains weight the external fixation device should be released slightly to prevent pressure necrosis of the stoma site (Loser *et al.* 2005: C).

10 The dry dressing should be replaced daily using aseptic technique until the stoma site has no erythema or exudates or any other signs of infection. Most forms of infection can be readily treated by means of antiseptic measures and daily change of dressing using aseptic techniques (Loser *et al.* 2005). Do not replace the dressing with an occlusive type. If the patient complains of pain/discomfort administer analgesia. If this is persistent request a gastroenterology review.

To encourage wound healing.
To prevent air getting to the stoma as this may cause infection (Lynch & Fang 2004: R 5).

11 Do not use bulky dressings, particularly under the external fixation device.

This can increase the pressure on the internal retention disc or retention balloon and increase the risk of tissue necrosis and ulceration occurring in the stomach (Nutricia Clinical Care 1996: C).

12 Advise the patient not to use moisturizing creams or talcum powder around the stoma site.

To prevent infection and/or irritation to skin. The grease in creams can cause the external retention device to slip, allowing movement of the tube and increasing the risk of leakage and infection. Creams and talcs can affect the tube material, causing it to stretch or leak (Nutricia Clinical Care 1996: C). Patients should be taught how to carry out this procedure themselves. Once the stoma site has healed (approximately 10 days post-insertion), it is no longer necessary to perform an aseptic technique. A socially clean procedure using soap and water to clean the stoma site should be adopted. The tube tip should be cleaned daily using water and a small brush (Loser *et al.* 2005: R 5).

Procedure guidelines   Radiologically inserted gastrostomy (RIG) tube care

After 24 hours and during initial daily change of dressing the wound should be inspected and skin changes should be carefully noted. For the first 10 days after the gastrostomy has been inserted a nurse in hospital or suitably trained individual in the community (e.g. district or practice nurse, general practitioner) must check the tube daily. This procedure should be performed daily to maintain skin integrity and detect any problems early, e.g. infection, skin breakdown. Most forms of infection can be readily treated by means of cleaning the stoma site using aseptic technique and daily change of dressings (Loser *et al.* 2005). Antibiotics may be required in some instances.

Equipment

1 Sterile procedure pack containing gallipot, low-linting gauze.

2 Sterile 0.9% sodium chloride.

Procedure

Action	Rationale
Follow points 1, 2, 3 and 5 of care of PEG tube (see above).	
6 The dry dressing should be replaced daily using aseptic technique (Loser *et al.* 2005) until the T-Fasteners have been removed.	
Do not replace the dressing with an occlusive type.	This will prevent air getting to the stoma and may lead to infection (Lynch & Fang 2004: R 5).
7 Check that the T-fasteners are intact. These will stay in place for 10–14 days after RIG insertion.	To stablize the stomach against the abdominal wall and allow the tract to form without complications (Cook (UK) Limited 2007: C).
8 Remove the T fasteners 10–14 days after insertion and secure fixation plate 1–2 cm away from the skin. Do not rotate the tube.	To prevent the RIG tube moving into the stomach (Cook (UK) Limited 2007: C).
9 Secure the tube to the skin with hypoallergenic tape. Do not secure near the stoma site.	To prevent the weight of the tube pulling on the exit site. Tape near the stoma site will make it difficult to clean (E).
10 Advise the patient not to use moisturizing creams or talcum powder.	To prevent infection and/or irritation to the skin (E).
11 After T-fasteners have been removed do not cover the gastrostomy site with a new dressing unless there is a heavy discharge or leakage from the stoma site.	To encourage wound healing (E).

Procedure guidelines   Jejunostomy feeding tube care

This procedure should be performed daily to maintain skin integrity and detect any problems early, e.g. infection, skin breakdown.

Equipment

1 Sterile procedure pack containing gallipot, low-linting gauze.

2 Sterile 0.9% sodium chloride.

Procedure

Action	Rationale
Follow points 1, 2, 3 and 5 of care of PEG tube (see above).	
6 Check that the sutures on the retention device are intact. If not, advise medical staff and arrange for the retention device to be resutured.	To prevent accidental removal of the jejunostomy tube (E).
7 Secure the jejunostomy tube to the skin with hypoallergenic tape. The site may be covered with a dry dressing or left uncovered.	To prevent the weight of the tube pulling on the exit site (E).
8 Advise the patient not to use moisturizing creams or talcum powder.	To prevent infection and/or irritation to the skin (E).

Procedure guidelines   Enteral feeding tubes: administration of medication

Equipment

1 50 ml enteral or catheter-tipped syringe.
2 Tap water or sterile water (for jejunostomy tubes or for patients who are immunosuppressed) (NICE 2003). Water should be fresh and kept covered.
3 Mortar and pestle or tablet crusher if tablets are being administered (BAPEN 2003a: C).

Procedure

Action	Rationale
1 Check whether patient can take medication orally, whether medication is necessary or if it can be temporarily suspended.	If patient can take medication orally this reduces the risk of tube blockage (BAPEN 2003a: C).
2 Consider whether an alternative route can be used, e.g. buccal, transdermal, topical, rectal or subcutaneous.	If patient can take medication via an alternative route this reduces the risk of tube blockage (BAPEN 2003a: C).
3 Check drug is absorbed from the site of delivery.	Some drugs may not be absorbed directly from the jejunum (BAPEN 2003a: C).
4 Clean hands with bactericidal soap and water or alcoholic handgel. Put on non-sterile gloves.	To minimize cross-infection and protect the practitioner from gastric/intestinal contents (DH 2005: C).
5 Stop the enteral feed and flush the tube with at least 30 ml of water (sterile water for jejunostomy administration), using an enteral or catheter-tipped syringe.	To clear the tube of enteral feed as this may cause a blockage or interact with medications. Sterile water should be used for jejunostomy tubes as water is bypassing the protective acidic environment of the stomach (E).
6 Where there is an absolute contraindication for medicine to be taken with feed:	
(a) Stop the feed 1–2 hours before and 2 hours after administration (this will depend on the drug), e.g. for phenytoin administration, stop feed 2 hours before and 2 hours after.	To avoid interaction with enteral feed.
(b) Consult with the dietitian to prescribe a suitable feeding regimen.	To ensure that the patient's nutritional requirements are met in the time available around medicine administration (BAPEN 2003a: C).

Procedure guidelines *(cont.)*

7 Prior to preparation, check with the pharmacist which medicines should never be crushed.	Some medications are not designed to be crushed. These include: (a) Modified-release tablets: absorption will be altered by crushing, possibly causing toxic side-effects. (b) Enteric-coated tablets: the coating is designed to protect the drug against gastric acid. (c) Cytotoxic medicines: this will risk exposing the practitioner to the drug.
8 Prepare each medication to be given separately. Volumes greater than 10 ml may be drawn up in a 50 ml syringe and administered via the tube. For small volumes (less than 10 ml) follow step 11. (a) Soluble tablets: dissolve in 10–15 ml water. (b) Liquids: shake well. For thick liquids mix with an equal volume of water. (c) Tablets: crush using a mortar and pestle or tablet crusher and mix with 10–15 ml water.	To avoid interaction between different medications and to ensure solubility (BAPEN 2003a: C).
9 Never add medication directly to the enteral feed.	To avoid interaction between medicines and feed (BAPEN 2003a: C).
10 Administer the medication through the tube via a 50 ml syringe. Rinse the tablet crusher or mortar with 10 ml water, draw up in a 50 ml syringe and flush this through the tube.	To ensure the whole dose is administered (BAPEN 2003a: C).
11 If volumes of less than 10 ml are required the dose should be measured in a 10 ml oral syringe. The plunger of a 50 ml syringe should be removed and the 50 ml syringe connected with the enteral tube. The dose should then be administered into the barrel of the 50 ml syringe and the 10 ml syringe rinsed with water, which should also be administered via the barrel of the 50 ml syringe.	To ensure the whole dose is administered (BAPEN 2003a: C).
12 If more than one medicine is to be administered, flush between drugs with at least 10 ml of water to ensure that the drug is cleared from the tube.	To avoid interactions between medicines (BAPEN 2003a: C).
13 Flush the tube with at least 30 ml water following the administration of the last drug.	To avoid medicines blocking the enteral tube (BAPEN 2003a: C).
14 If the patient is on a fluid restriction or for a paediatric patient, consult the dietitian and pharmacist about the quantity of water to be given before and after medication.	To ensure that the patient does not exceed their fluid restriction or requirements (BAPEN 2003a: C).

Procedure guidelines   Enteral feeding tube: unblocking

Equipment

1 50 ml enteral or catheter-tipped syringe.

2 Tap water or sterile water (for jejunostomy tubes or for patients who are immunosuppressed) (NICE 2003). Water should be fresh and kept covered.

3 Fizzy water, e.g. soda water.

Procedure

Action	Rationale
1 Always flush the enteral tube before and after administration of feed and medication with at least 30 ml of water (sterile water for jejunostomy and for immunosuppressed patients).	To avoid the tube blocking. Sterile water should be used for jejunostomy tubes as water is bypassing the protective acidic environment of the stomach (E).
2 If the tube is blocked try to administer 50 ml warm water down the enteral tube and leave for 30 minutes. To obtain lukewarm water (40–45°C) put three-quarters of a cup (120 ml) of cold drinking tap water (sterile water for jejunostomy and for immunosuppressed patients) into a plastic cup and add a quarter of a cup (40 ml) of boiling water from the water still.	To dissolve any medication or soften any feed plugs in the tube. To prevent hot water being administered via the feeding tube (BAPEN 2003a: C).
3 Flush tube with 50 ml water.	To remove blockage (BAPEN 2003a: C).
4 If unsuccessful try to administer 50 ml fizzy water, e.g. soda water, via the enteral tube and leave for 30 minutes.	To dislodge blockage (BAPEN 2003a: C).
5 Flush tube with 50 ml water.	To remove blockage (BAPEN 2003a: C).
6 If tube is still blocked consider use of a proprietary product designed to unblock tube. Follow manufacturer's instructions (Manufacturer's recommendation: C).	To break down plug. Such products contain digestive enzymes which may break down a protein plug but they may not unblock a tube blocked with medication.
7 Do not use a syringe smaller than 50 ml.	To avoid the tube being ruptured with the high pressure of a smaller syringe.
8 If all of the above are unsuccessful then the enteral tube will need replacing.	To ensure continued enteral access for the administration of feed, fluids and medication (E).

Problem solving: Swallowing difficulties

Supervision of patients with swallowing difficulties is important, and in some cases patients may require support at meal times, or when drinking, to carry out the recommended strategies. It is important for nurses to participate in educational programmes for patients and carers in order to encourage awareness of the implications of dysphagia. Anxieties associated with dysphagia should be allayed and confidence to undertake safe eating and drinking techniques built up. Patients may experience one or a number of the following problems.

Problem	Cause	Prevention	Suggested action
Patient experiencing difficulties with drinking and/or eating (which may lead to dehydration, insufficient nutritional intake and compromised airway).	(a) *Mechanical*. Patients who have undergone surgery and/or radiotherapy to the oral cavity, pharynx, larynx, or trachea (including temporary or permanent tracheostomy) are likely to experience swallowing difficulties of a temporary or more persistent nature (Figure 24.1) (Royal College of Speech and Language Therapists 2006: C).		Refer to specialist speech and language therapist (SLT) for full assessment and management plan. Refer to dietitian for nutritional assessment and management plan.

Problem solving *(cont.)*

Problem	Cause	Prevention	Suggested action
	(b) *Neurological*. Patients who have tumours which affect the subcortical, cerebral and brainstem area (and thus the cranial nerves) may present with symptoms of dysphagia. These symptoms will continue as long as the disease and/or treatment effects are evident (Royal College of Speech and Language Therapists 2006: C).		
	(c) *Oesophageal obstruction or dysfunction*. Patients who have tumours of the upper GI tract may well experience discomfort and difficulty with the oesophageal phase of the swallow. The only way to alleviate oesophageal difficulties is through medical or surgical management. Swallowing therapy is not indicated in these circumstances, although the specialist speech and language therapist may be able to offer advice to minimize the patient's difficulties or their risk of aspiration, reflux or backflow by altering food consistencies or advising on alternative swallow strategies (E).		
Dehydration and/or difficulty in maintaining adequate hydration.	Thin liquids (e.g. water) are difficult for the patient with dysphagia to manage. Watery liquids do not retain their cohesion in the mouth and therefore pass swiftly into the pharynx. Patients may avoid liquids of this consistency and become dehydrated.	Identify patients who are at risk.	Seek medical advice on the appropriateness of intravenous hydration. A referral to a specialist SLT: to advise on other liquid consistencies; safe swallow techniques and exercises. These may help the patient to increase oral intake.
Difficulty in maintaining a clear airway (may be severe enough to block airway in tracheostomy patients).	Inability to manage secretions, indicated by drooling and/or gurgly voice. Tracheostomy patients may feel breathing is laboured (Royal College of Speech and Language Therapists 2006).	Monitor patient's progress carefully and regularly and liaise with the speech and language therapist about any changes noted.	Following assessment by specialist speech and language therapist, adjusting the patient's position may help (e.g. sitting posture and head position before and after swallowing). Oral suction may be required (see Chapter 42).

Problem	Cause	Prevention	Suggested action
Patient requires nutritional support and/or alternative feeding method.	Dysphagia and/or disease process leading to inadequate nutrition.	All patients with dysphagia should be fully assessed by a dietitian to ensure current nutritional requirements are met by nutritional support, alternative feeding method, normal diet, or a combination of these.	Nutritional support and/or alternative feeding method may be indicated following discussion with members of the multidisciplinary team. Following assessment by a specialist speech and language therapist, recommendations may be made about sitting posture, head position, and consistency of food and drink. These will be individually tailored to the patient's needs. Nursing staff should monitor progress carefully, noting changes and reporting them to the appropriate professional.
Dysphagia in oral and/or pharyngeal stages of swallowing, related to head position and/or structural or neurological deficits.	Patients with tumours of the upper GI tract may experience difficulty with the oesophageal phase of the swallow; patients with tumours affecting the brainstem/cranial nerves will experience dysphagia (Royal College of Speech and Language Therapists 2006).		Proceed as advised by the specialist speech and language therapist. Their advice may include modifications in posture. Safe swallow manoeuvres, modifying consistencies and exercises to optimize function.
Selecting suitable food and/or drink.	Not all members of the multidisciplinary team and/or catering and other staff may be aware of the extent of the patient's swallowing difficulties (E).	Liaise with specialist speech and language therapist, dietitian and catering.	Provide food and drink of a consistency which will not exacerbate the patient's problems. This might include soft foods, thickened liquids, or purées. Food and drink must be individually tailored to suit the patient.

Figure 24.1 The normal swallow. (1, tongue; 2, soft palate; 3, hyoid bone; 4, epiglottis; 5, vocal cords; 6, thyroid cartilage; 7, cricoid cartilage; 8, pharyngoesophageal sphincter; 9, trachea; 10, oesophagus.) The oral, pharyngeal and oesophageal phases are separate but highly co-ordinated (Groher 1997; Logemann 1998).

References and further reading

BAPEN (1994a) *Enteral and Parenteral Nutrition in the Community* (ed. M. Elia). British Association for Parenteral and Enteral Nutrition, Maidenhead.

BAPEN (1994b) *Organisation of Nutritional Support in Hospitals* (ed. D.B.A. Silk). British Association for Parenteral and Enteral Nutrition, Maidenhead.

BAPEN (1996) *Current Perspectives on Parenteral Nutrition in Adults* (ed. C.R. Pennington). British Association for Parenteral and Enteral Nutrition, Maidenhead.

BAPEN (1999) *Current Perspectives on Enteral Nutrition in Adults* (ed. C.A. McAtear). British Association for Parenteral and Enteral Nutrition, Maidenhead.

BAPEN (2003a) Tube feeding and your medicines: a guide for patients and carers. www.bapen.org.uk. Accessed 24/9/07

BAPEN (2003b) *Malnutrition Universal Screening Tool 'MUST' Report*. British Association for Parenteral and Enteral Nutrition, Maidenhead.

Benton, S. & Marsden, C. (2002) Training nurses to place tunnelled central venous catheters. *Prof Nurse*, **17**(9), 531–5.

Bodger, K. & Heatley, R.V. (2001) The immune system and nutrition support. In: *Artificial Nutritional Support in Clinical Practice* (eds J. Payne-James, G. Grimble & D. Silk), 2nd edn. Greenwich Medical Media, London, pp. 137–48.

Bond, S. (1997) *Eating Matters*. Centre for Health Services Research, University of Newcastle, Newcastle upon Tyne.

Bozzetti, F. (2001) Nutrition support in patients with cancer. *Artificial Nutritional Support in Clinical Practice* (eds J. Payne-James, G. Grimble & D. Silk), 2nd edn. Greenwich Medical Media, London, pp. 639–80.

Braga, M. *et al.* (2002) Preoperative oral arginine and n-3 fatty acid supplementation improves the immunometabolic host response and outcome after colorectal resection for cancer. *Surgery*, **132**, 805–14.

Buchholz, A.C., Bartok, C. & Schoeller, D.A. (2004) The validity of bioelectrical impedance models in clinical populations. *Nutr Clin Prac*, **19**, 433–46.

Bumpers, H.L. *et al.* (2003) Unusual complications of long-term percutaneous gastrostomy tubes. *J Gastrointest Surg*, **7**, 917–20.

Burke, A. (1997) *Hungry in Hospital?* Association of Community Health Councils for England and Wales, London.

Burnham, R. & Barton, S. (2001) The role of the nutrition support team. In: *Artificial Nutritional Support in Clinical Practice* (eds J. Payne-James, G. Grimble & D. Silk), 2nd edn. Greenwich Medical Media, London, pp. 241–53.

Burns, S.M. *et al.* (1995) Comparison of nasogastric tube securing methods and tube types in medical intensive care patients. *Am J Crit Care*, **4**(3), 198–203.

Cook (UK) Limited (2007) Radiologically inserted gastrostomy and gastrojejunostomy. www.cookmedical.com/esc/educationResource.do?id=Video_Tape. Accessed 24/9/07.

Council of Europe (2003) Food and nutritional care in hospitals: how to prevent undernutrition. Council of Europe www.coe.int. Accessed 24/9/07

Cummings, J.H. (2000) Nutritional management of diseases of the gut. In: *Human Nutrition and Dietetics* (eds J.S. Garrow, W.P.T. James & A. Ralph), 10th edn. Churchill Livingstone, Edinburgh, pp. 547–73.

Davidson, A. (2005) Management and effects of parenteral nutrition. *Nurs Times*, **101**(42), 28–31.

Desneves, K.J. *et al.* (2005) Treatment with supplementary arginine, vitamin C and zinc in patients with pressure ulcers: a randomized controlled trial. *Clin Nutr*, **24**(6), 979–87.

Detsky, A.S. *et al.* (1987) What is subjective global assessment of nutritional status? *J Parent Enteral Nutr*, **11**, 8–13.

DH (1991) *Dietary Reference Values for Food Energy and Nutrients for the United Kingdom*. COMA Report 41. HMSO, London.

DH (2001a) *Essence of Care – Patient Focused Benchmarking for Health Care Professionals*. Department of Health, London.

DH (2001b) Guidelines for preventing infections associated with the insertion and maintenance of central venous catheters. *J Hosp Infect*, **47**(S), S47–67.

DH (2002) *Specialised Services National Definitions Set (2nd edition) Home Parenteral Nutrition (HPN) (adult) – Definition No 12*. Department of Health, London.

DH (2005) *Saving Lives: A Delivery Programme to Reduce Healthcare Associated Infection including MRSA*. Department of Health, London.

Dorries, C.P. (2004) *Coroner's Report*. H.M. Coroner, South Yorkshire (West), 27 April 2004.

Durnin, J.B. & Wolmersley, J. (1974) Body fat assessed from total body density and its estimation from skinfold thickness: measurements on 481 men and women aged from 16 to 72 years. *Br J Nutr*, **32**, 77–9.

Elia, M. (2001) Metabolic response to starvation, injury and sepsis. In: *Artificial Nutritional Support in Clinical Practice* (eds J. Payne-James, G. Grimble & D. Silk), 2nd edn. Greenwich Medical Media, London, pp. 1–24.

Fitzsimmons, C.L. (1997) Central venous catheter placement – extending the role of the nurse. *J R Coll Phys*, **31**(5), 533–5.

FSA (2003) Safe upper levels for vitamins and minerals. Expert Group on vitamins and minerals. FSA, London.

Furst, P., Kuhn, K.S. & Stehle, P. (2001) Parenteral nutrition substrates. In: *Artificial Nutritional Support in Clinical Practice* (eds J. Payne-James, G. Grimble & D. Silk), 2nd edn. Greenwich Medical Media, London, pp. 401–34.

Gidden, F. & Shenkin, A. (2000) Laboratory support of the clinical nutrition service. *Clin Chem Lab Med*, **38**(8), 693–714.

Griffiths, M. (1996) Single-stage percutaneous gastrostomy button insertion: a leap forward. *J Parent Enteral Nutr*, **20**(3), 237–9.

Groher, M. (1997) *Dysphagia: Diagnosis and Management*, 2nd edn. Butterworth Heinemann, Boston.

Gupta, D. *et al.* (2004a) Bioelectrical impedance phase angle as a prognostic indicator in advanced pancreatic cancer. *Br J Nutr*, **92**(6), 957–62.

Gupta, D. *et al.* (2004b) Bioelectrical impedance phase angle in clinical practice: implications for prognosis in advanced colorectal cancer. *Am J Clin Nutr*, **80**(6), 1634–8.

Hamilton, H., O'Byrne, M. & Nicholai, L. (1995) Central lines inserted by clinical nurse specialists. *Nurs Times*, **91**(17), 38–9.

Heymsfield, S.B. & Matthews, D. (1994) Body composition: research and clinical advances – 1993 A.S.P.E.N. research workshop. *J Parent Enteral Nutr*, **18**(2), 91–103.

Horgan, G.W. & Stubbs, J. (2003) Predicting basal metabolic rate in the obese is difficult. *Eur J Clin Nutr*, **57**, 335–40.

Huhmann, M.B. & Cunningham, R.S. (2005) The importance of nutritional screening in cancer related weight loss. *Lancet Oncol*, **6**, 334–3.

Janssen, I. *et al.* (2000) Estimation of skeletal muscle mass by bioelectrical impedance analysis. *J Appl Physiol*, **89**, 456–71.

Kings Fund Research Summary (2005) Sustainable food and the NHS. www.kingsfund.org.uk/publications/kings_fund_publications/sustainable_food.html. Accessed 24/9/07

Kondrup, J. *et al.* (2003) ESPEN Guidelines for nutrition screening 2002. *Clin Nutr*, **22**(4), 415–21.

Kyle, U.G. *et al.* (2004a) Bioelectrical impedance analysis – part I: review of principles and methods. *Clin Nutr*, **23**, 1226–43.

Kyle, U.G. *et al.* (2004b) Bioelectrical impedance analysis – part II: utilization in clinical parctice. *Clin Nutr*, **23**, 1430–53.

Logemann, J. (1998) *The Evaluation and Treatment of Swallowing Disorders*, 2nd edn. College Hill Press, San Diego.

Loser, C.H.R. *et al.* (2005) ESPEN guidelines on artificial enteral nutrition – Percutaneous endoscopic gastrostomy (PEG). *Clin Nutr*, **24**, 848–61.

Lynch, C.R. & Fang, J.C. (2004) Prevention and management of complications of percutaneous endoscopic gastrostomy (PEG) tubes. *Practical Gastroenterology Series*, **22**, 66–76.

Metheny, N.A. (2004) Monitoring feeding tube placement – a literature review. *Nutr Clin Pract*, **19**, 487–95.

Metheny, N.A. & Titler, M.G. (2001) Assessing placement of feeding tubes. *Am J Nurs*, **101**(5), 36–45.

Metheny, N. *et al.* (1993) Effectiveness of pH measurements in predicting tube placement: an update. *Nurs Res*, **42**(6), 324–31.

Nataloni S. *et al.* (1999) Nutritional assessment in head injured patients through the study of rapid turnover visceral proteins *Clin Nutr*, **18**, 247–51.

National Collaborating Centre for Acute Care (2006) Nutrition support in adults: oral nutrition support, enteral tube feeding and parenteral nutrition. National Collaborating Centre for Acute Care, London. www.rcseng.ac.uk/publications/docs/nutrition_support_guidelines.html. Accessed 24/9/07.

Newman, L.A. *et al.* (1998) Eating and weight changes following chemoradiation therapy for advanced head and neck cancer. *Arch Otolaryngol Head Neck Surg*, **124**, 589–92.

NHS (2001) *Better Hospital Food. The NHS Recipe Book Implementation Support Pack*. HMSO, London.

NICE (2003) *Care during Enteral Feeding. Infection Control – Prevention of Health Care Associated Infection in Primary and Community Care. Clinical Guideline 2*. National Institute for Health and Clinical Excellence, London.

Nicol, M. *et al.* (2000) *Essential Nursing Skills*. Moseby, Elsevier Ltd, London.

NMC (2006) *A–Z Advice Sheet Consent*. www.nmc.org.

NPSA (2005) Reducing the harm caused by misplaced nasogastric feeding tubes. www.npsa.nhs.uk/health/display?contentId=4216. Accessed 24/9/07.

Nutricia Clinical Care (1996) *The Flocare Gastrostomy Range: a Guide to Professional Care*. Nutricia Clinical Care, Cow & Gate Nutricia, Trowbridge.

Payne-James, J., Grimble, G. & Silk, D. (2001) Enteral nutrition: tubes and techniques of delivery. In: *Artificial Nutritional Support in Clinical Practice* (eds J. Payne-James, G. Grimble & D. Silk), 2nd edn. Greenwich Medical Media, London, pp. 281–302.

Pennington, C.R. (1997) Disease and malnutrition in British hospitals. *Proc Nutr Soc*, **56**, 393–407.

Pickhardt, P.J., Rohrmann, C.A. Jr & Cossentino, M.J. (2002) Stomal metastases complicating percutaneous endoscopic gastrostomy: CT findings and the argument for radiologic tube placement. *Am J Roentgenol*, **179**(3), 735–9.

Pratt, R.J. *et al.* (2007) Epic 2: National evidence-based guidelines for preventing healthcare-associated infections in NHS hospitals in England. *J Hosp Infect*, **65**(1) (Suppl), S2–S12.

Reilly, H. (1996) Nutrition in clinical management: malnutrition in our midst. *Proc Nutr Soc*, **55**, 841–53.

Riera, L. *et al.* (2002) Percutaneous endoscopic gastrostomy in head and neck cancer patients. *J Otorhinolaryngol Relat Spec*, **64**(1), 32–4.

Rollins, H. (1997) A nose for trouble. *Nurs Times*, **93**(49), 66–7.

Royal College of Speech & Language Therapists (2006) Communicating quality 3: guidance on best practice in service organisation and provision. www.rcslt.org. Accessed 24/9/07.

Royal Marsden NHS Trust (2002) *Eating Well When You Have Cancer – A Guide for Cancer Patients*. Royal Marsden NHS Trust, London.

Schofield, W.N. (1985) Predicting basal metabolic rate. New standards and review of previous work. *Hum Nutr Clin Nutr*, **39C**(Suppl 15), 5–41.

Schwenk A. *et al.* (2000) Phase angle from bioelectrical impedance analysis remains an independent predictive marker in HIV-infected patients in the era of highly active antiretroviral treatment. *Am J Clin Nut*, **72**(2), 496–501.

Shaw, C. (2008) Parenteral nutrition. In: *Intravenous Therapy in Nursing Practice* (eds L. Dougherty & J. Lamb), 2nd edn. Blackwell Publishing, Oxford.

Shaw, V. & Lawson, M. (2007) Nutritional assessment, dietary requirements and feed supplementation. In: *Clinical Paediatric Dietetics* (eds V. Shaw & M. Lawson), 3rd edn. Blackwell Publishing, Oxford, pp. 3–20.

Shenkin, A. (2001) Adult micronutrient requirements. In: *Artificial Nutritional Support in Clinical Practice* (eds J. Payne-James, G. Grimble & D. Silk), 2nd edn. Greenwich Medical Media, London, pp. 193–212.

Springhouse (2002) Parenteral nutrition. In: *IV Therapy Made Incredibly Easy*. Springhouse Corporation, Philadelphia, pp. 269–302.

ter Reit, G., Kessels, A.G. & Knipschild, P.G. (1995) Randomised clinical trial of ascorbic acid in the treatment of pressure ulcers. *J Clin Epidemiol*, **48**(12), 1453–60.

Thomas, B. & Bishop, J. (2007) *Manual of Dietetic Practice*, 4th edn. Blackwell Publishing, Oxford.

Thomas, D.R. (1997) Specific nutritional factors in wound healing. *Adv Wound Care*, **10**(4), 40–3.

Thorell, A. & Nordenström, J. (2001) Metabolic complications of parenteral nutrition. In: *Artificial Nutritional Support in Clinical Practice* (eds J. Payne-James, G. Grimble & D. Silk), 2nd edn. Greenwich Medical Media, London, pp. 445–59.

Weinstein, S.M. (2007) Parenteral nutrition. In: *Principles and Practice of Intravenous Therapy* (ed. S.M. Weinstein), 8th edn. Lippincott, Philadelphia.

Wilson, J.M. & Jordan, N.L. (2001) Parenteral nutrition. In: *Infusion Therapy in Clinical Practice* (eds J. Hankin *et al.*). W.B. Saunders, Philadelphia, pp. 209–247.

Chapter 25

Observations

497 **Pulse**
497 Reference material
501 *Procedure guidelines:* Pulse measurement
502 **Twelve-lead electrocardiogram (ECG)**
502 *Procedure guidelines:* Electrocardiogram (ECG)
504 **Blood pressure**
504 Reference material
510 *Procedure guidelines:* Blood pressure (manual)
512 **Respiration**
513 Reference material
520 *Procedure guidelines:* Pulse oximetry
521 **Peak flow**
521 Reference material
522 *Procedure guidelines:* Peak flow reading using manual peak flow meter
522 **Temperature**
524 Reference material
528 **Urinalysis**
529 *Procedure guidelines:* Temperature measurement
530 Reference material
530 Characteristics of urine
532 *Procedure guidelines:* Urinalysis
533 **Blood glucose**
533 Reference material
536 *Procedure guidelines:* Blood glucose monitoring
538 **Central venous pressure**
538 Reference material
539 *Procedure guidelines:* Central venous pressure measurement
540 *Problem solving:* Central venous pressure (CVP)
541 References

Pulse

Definition

The pulse is a pressure wave that is transmitted through the arterial tree with each heart beat following the expansion and recoil of arteries during each cardiac cycle (Marieb & Hoehn 2007). A pulse can be palpated in any artery that lies close to the surface of the body (Figure 25.1). The radial artery at the wrist is easily accessible and therefore frequently used; there are several other clinically important areas for monitoring the pulse such as the carotid, femoral and brachial plexus (Marieb & Hoehn 2007).

Indications

The pulse is taken for the following reasons:

- To gather information on the heart rate, pattern of beats (rhythm) and amplitude (strength) of pulse.
- To determine the individual's pulse on admission as a base for comparing future measurements.
- To monitor changes in pulse.

(Marieb & Hoehn 2007).

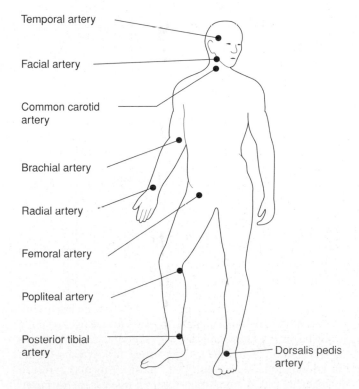

Figure 25.1 Body sites where pulse is most easily palpated. The pulse can be felt in arteries lying close to the body surface.

Reference material

In health the arterial pulse is one of the measurements used to assess the effects of activity, postural changes and emotions on the heart rate. In ill health the pulse can be used to assess the effects of disease, treatments and response to therapy. Each time the heart beats it pushes blood through the arteries. The pumping action of the heart causes the walls of the arteries to expand and distend, causing a wave-like sensation which can then be felt as the pulse (Marieb & Hoehn 2007). The pulse is measured by lightly compressing the artery against firm tissue and by counting the number of beats in a minute.

The pulse is palpated to note the following:

- Rate.
- Rhythm.
- Amplitude.

Rate

The normal pulse rate varies in different client groups as age-related changes affect the pulse rate. The approximate range is illustrated in Table 25.1 (Weber & Kelley 2003).

The pulse may vary depending on the posture of an individual. For example, the pulse of a healthy man may be around 66 beats per minute when he is lying down; this increases to 70 beats per minute when sitting up, and 80 beats per minute when he stands suddenly (Marieb & Hoehn 2007).

The rate of the pulse of an individual with a healthy heart tends to be relatively constant. However, when blood volume drops suddenly or when the heart has been weakened by disease, the stroke volume declines and cardiac output is maintained only by increasing the rate of heart beat.

Cardiac output (CO) is the amount of blood pumped out by each heart ventricle in 1 minute, while the stroke volume is the amount of blood pumped out by a ventricle with each contraction. The relationship between these and the heart rate is expressed in an equation (see below). Using normal resting values for heart rate (75 beats per minute) and stroke volume (70 ml per beat) the average adult cardiac output can be calculated (Marieb & Hoehn 2007):

$$\text{Cardiac output} = \text{Heart rate} \times \text{Stroke volume}$$

Table 25.1 Normal pulse rates per minute at various ages. From Weber & Kelley (2003).

Age	Approximate range
1 week–3 months	100–160
3 months–2 years	80–150
2–10 years	70–110
10 years–adult	55–90

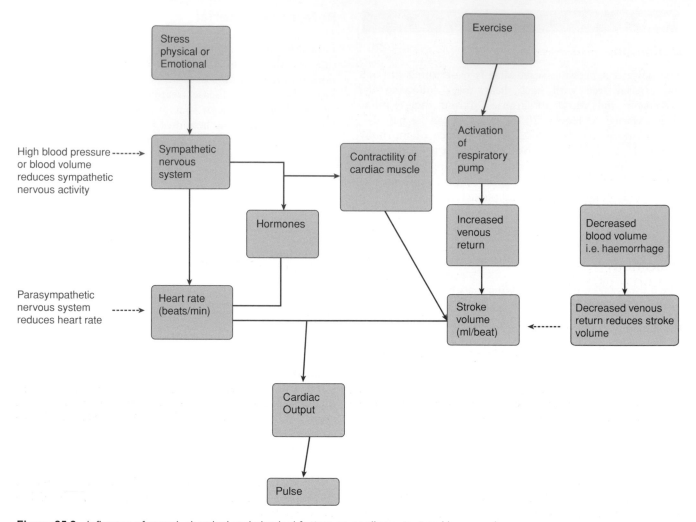

Figure 25.2   Influence of neural, chemical and physical factors on cardiac output and hence pulse.

The heart rate and hence pulse rate are influenced by various factors acting through neural, chemical and physically induced homeostatic mechanisms (Figure 25.2):

- Neural changes in heart rate are caused by the activation of the sympathetic nervous system which increases heart rate, while parasympathetic activation decreases heart rate (Thibodeau & Patton 2007).
- Chemical regulation of the heart is affected by hormones (adrenaline and thyroxine) and electrolytes (sodium, potassium and calcium) (Thibodeau & Patton 2007). High or low levels of electrolytes, particularly potassium, magnesium and calcium, can cause an alteration in the heart's rhythm and rate.
- Other factors that influence heart rate are age, sex, exercise and body temperature (Marieb & Hoehn 2007).

Tachycardia   Is defined as an abnormally fast heart rate, over 100 beats per minute in adults. This may result from a raised body temperature, increased sympathetic response due to physical/emotional stress, certain drugs or heart disease (Marieb & Hoehn 2007). Because tachycardia occasionally promotes fibrillation, persistent tachycardia is considered pathological (Marieb & Hoehn 2007).

Bradycardia (slow)   Is a heart rate slower than 60 beats per minute (Marieb & Hoehn 2007). It may be the result of a low body temperature, certain drugs or parasympathetic nervous system activation. It is also found in fit athletes when physical and cardiovascular conditioning occurs (Marieb & Hoehn 2007). This results in hypertrophy of the heart with an increase in its stroke volume. These heart changes result in a lower resting heart rate but with the same cardiac output (Marieb & Hoehn 2007). If persistent bradycardia occurs in an individual as a result of ill health, this may result in inadequate blood circulation to body tissues. A slowing of the heart rate accompanied by a rise in blood pressure is one of the indications of raised intracranial pressure (Marieb & Hoehn 2007).

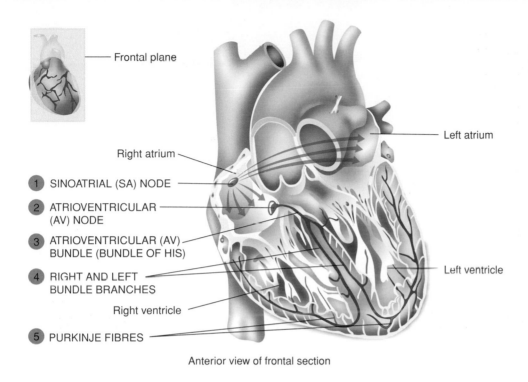

Frontal plane

Right atrium

1 SINOATRIAL (SA) NODE

2 ATRIOVENTRICULAR (AV) NODE

3 ATRIOVENTRICULAR (AV) BUNDLE (BUNDLE OF HIS)

4 RIGHT AND LEFT BUNDLE BRANCHES

Right ventricle

5 PURKINJE FIBRES

Left atrium

Left ventricle

Anterior view of frontal section

Figure 25.3 The conduction system of the heart. Autorhythmic fibres in the sinoatrial (SA) node, located in the right atrial wall, act as the heart's pacemaker, initiating cardiac action potentials that cause contraction of the heart's chambers. The conduction system ensures that the chambers of the heart contract in a co-ordinated manner. (Redrawn from Tortora & Derrickson (2007) with permission).

Rhythm   The pulse rhythm is the sequence of beats. In health, these are regular. The co-ordinated action of the muscles of the heart in producing a regular heart rhythm is due to the ability of cardiac muscle to contract inherently without nervous control (Marieb & Hoehn 2007). The co-ordinated action of the muscles in the heart results from two physiological factors:

- Gap junctions in the cardiac muscles which form interconnections between adjacent cardiac muscles and allow transmission of nervous impulses from cell to cell (Marieb & Hoehn 2007).
- Specialized nerve-like cardiac cells that form the nodal system. These initiate and distribute impulses throughout the heart, so that the heart beats as one unit (Marieb & Hoehn 2007). The nodal system is comprised of the sinoatrial node, atrioventricular node, atrioventricular bundle and the Purkinje fibres.

The sinoatrial node is the pacemaker, initiating each wave of contraction. This sets the rhythm for the heart as a whole (Figure 25.3). Its characteristic rhythm is called *sinus rhythm.*

Defects in the conduction system of the heart can cause irregular heart rhythms, or arrhythmias, resulting in unco-ordinated contraction of the heart.

Fibrillation is a condition of rapid and irregular contractions. A fibrillating heart is ineffective as a pump (Marieb & Hoehn 2007).

- *Atrial fibrillation* is a disruption of rhythm in the atrial areas of the heart occurring at extremely rapid and uncoordinated intervals. The rapid impulses result in the ventricles not being able to respond to every atrial beat and, therefore, the ventricles contract irregularly (Adam & Osborne 2005). There are many causes of this condition, but the following are the most common: (i) ischaemic heart disease; (ii) acute illness; (iii) electrolyte abnormality; and (iv) thyrotoxicosis.
- *Ventricular fibrillation* is an irregular heart rhythm characterized by chaotic contraction of the ventricles at very rapid rates (Adam & Osborne 2005). Ventricular fibrillation results in cardiac arrest and death if not reversed with defibrillation and the injection of adrenaline (epinephrine). The cause of this condition is often myocardial infarction (MI), electrical shock, acidosis, electrolyte disturbances and hypovolaemia (Resuscitation Council UK 2005).

Body fluids are good conductors of electricity so it is possible through electrocardiography to observe how the currents generated are transmitted through the heart. The electrocardiograph provides a graphic representation and record

Figure 25.4 Normal and abnormal ECG tracings. **(a)** Coarse ventricular fibrillation. **(b)** Junctional tachycardia. **(c)** ECG complexes too small; cardiac monitor did not recognize QRS complexes resulting in continuous false asystole alarms. Also difficulties may be encountered interpreting cardiac arrhythmias when the gain is set too low. **(d)** Second degree AV block Mobitz type 2.

(electrocardiogram [ECG]) of electrical activity as the heart beats (see Twelve-lead electrocardiogram (ECG) section, below). The ECG makes it possible to identify abnormalities in electrical conduction within the heart. Changes in the pattern or timing of the deflection in the ECG may indicate problems with the heart's conduction system, such as those caused by MI (Marieb & Hoehn 2007). Examples of conduction abnormalities are shown in Figure 25.4a–d.

Amplitude

Amplitude is a reflection of pulse strength and the elasticity of the arterial wall. This varies because of the alternating strong and weak ventricular contractions (Bickley & Szilagyi 2007). The flexibility of the artery of the young adult feels different from the hard artery of the patient suffering from arteriosclerosis. It takes some clinical experience to appreciate the differences in amplitude. However, it is important to be able to recognize major changes such as the faint flickering pulse of the severely hypovolaemic patient or the irregular pulse in cardiac arrhythmias.

Assessing gross pulse irregularity

Paradoxical pulse is a pulse that markedly decreases in amplitude during inspiration. On inspiration, more blood is pooled in the lungs and so decreases the return to the left side of the heart; this affects the consequent stroke volume. A paradoxical pulse is usually regarded as normal, although in conjunction with such features as hypotension and dyspnoea, it may indicate cardiac tamponade (Bickley & Szilagyi 2007).

When there is a gross pulse irregularity, it may be useful to use a stethoscope to assess the apical heart beat. This is done by placing the diaphragm of the stethoscope over the apex of the heart and counting the beats for 60 seconds. A second nurse should record the radial pulse at the same time. The deficit between the two should be noted using, for example, different colours on the patient's chart to indicate the apex and radial rates (Docherty 2002).

Conditions where a patient's pulse may need careful monitoring are described below:

- Postoperative and critically ill patients require monitoring of the pulse to assess for cardiovascular stability. The patient's pulse should be recorded preoperatively in order to establish a baseline and to make comparisons. Hypovolaemic shock post-surgery from the loss of plasma or whole blood results in a decrease in circulatory blood volume. The resulting acceleration in heart rate causes a tachycardia that can be felt in the pulse. The greater the loss in volume the more thready the pulse is likely to feel.
- Blood transfusions require the careful monitoring of the pulse as an incompatible blood transfusion may lead to a rise in pulse rate (BCSH 1999) (see Chapter 43).
- Patients with local or systemic infections or inflammatory reactions require monitoring of their pulse to detect sepsis/severe sepsis. This is characterized by a decrease in the mean arterial pressure (MAP) and a rise in pulse rate (Marieb & Hoehn 2007).
- Patients with cardiovascular conditions require regular assessment of the pulse to monitor their condition and the efficacy of medications.

Note: even where the patient has continuous ECG monitoring, such as in coronary care, Accident and Emergency (A&E) and intensive care unit (ITU), it is still essential to manually feel a pulse to determine amplitude and volume and whether the pulse is irregular.

Procedure guidelines   Pulse measurement

Equipment

1 A watch that has a second hand.

Procedure

Action	Rationale
1 Wash hands and dry hands.	To prevent cross-infection (DH 2005: C).
2 Explain and discuss the procedure with the patient.	To ensure that the patient understands the procedure and gives his/her valid consent (NMC 2006: C; NMC 2008: C).
3 Where possible, measure the pulse under the same conditions each time.	To ensure continuity and consistency in recording (E).
4 Ensure that the patient is comfortable and relaxed. *Note*: If the patient has taken any medication, this may alter the pulse rate.	To ensure that the patient is comfortable (E).
5 Place the first, second or third finger along the appropriate artery and apply light pressure until the pulse is felt (see Action figure 5).	The fingertips are sensitive to touch. Practitioners should be aware that the thumb and forefinger have pulses of their own and therefore these may be mistaken for the patient's pulse (Docherty & Coote 2006: E).
6 Press gently against the peripheral artery being used to record the pulse.	The radial artery is usually used as it is often the most readily accessible (Bickley & Szilagyi 2007: E).
7 The pulse should be counted for 60 seconds.	Sufficient time is required to detect irregularities or other defects (Bickley & Szilagyi 2007: E).
8 Record the pulse rate on appropriate documentation.	To monitor differences and detect trends; any irregularities should be brought to the attention of the appropriate senior nursing and medical teams (NMC 2008: C).

Note: In children under 2 years of age, the pulse should not be taken in this way; the rapid pulse rate and small area for palpation can lead to inaccurate data. The heart rate should be assessed by utilizing a stethoscope and listening to the apical heart beat.

Action 5 Taking a pulse.

Twelve-lead electrocardiogram (ECG)

Definition

Electrical currents generated and transmitted through the heart also spread throughout the body and can be monitored and amplified with an instrument called an electrocardiograph (Marieb & Hoehn 2007).

A 12-lead ECG is a quick non-invasive procedure of acquiring data to ascertain information about the electrophysiology of the heart (Marieb & Hoehn 2007). Electrical changes, which take place as the cardiac muscle contracts and relaxes, are recorded on the ECG trace and produces 12 different tracings from different combinations of limb and chest leads (Tortora & Derrickson 2008).

It is performed electively prior to various interventions such as surgery and anti-cancer chemotherapy. An ECG should also be considered to aid diagnosis during an acute situation, particularly in the presence of chest pain, haemodynamic disturbance or cardiac rhythm changes.

The starting point of the cardiac electrical cycle is the sinoatrial (SA) node. This is the heart's natural pacemaker, which can create impulses at 60–100 beats per minute. Its ability to spontaneously generate and discharge an electrical impulse is called automaticity (Docherty 2005).

A typical ECG consists of a series of three distinguishable waves called deflection waves (Figure 25.5). The first wave, the small P wave lasting about 0.08 seconds, results from movement of the depolarization wave from the SA node through the atria. The impulse travels from the atria to the ventricles via the atrioventricular (AV) node through internodal tracts (Lemery *et al.* 2003): this is the PR interval. From the AV node, the impulse travels down the His–Purkinje system and throughout the ventricles. The septal area con-

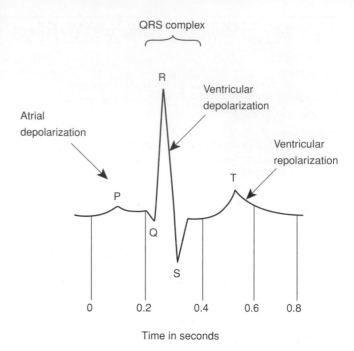

Figure 25.5   An ECG tracing illustrating normal deflection waves.

tracts before the main ventricle muscle (Tortora & Derrickson 2008) giving rise to a small negatively deflected Q wave on the ECG. The His–Purkinjie consists of His-bundle, right bundle branch, left bundle branch and Purkinjie fibres (Tortora & Derrickson 2008).

The purkinjie fibres conduct impulses through the muscle assisting depolarization almost simultaneously (Philip & Kowey 2001) giving rise to the positive R-wave deflection on the ECG, followed by an S wave as the ECG then detects the right ventricle muscle movement (Docherty 2005).

Procedure guidelines   Electrocardiogram (ECG)

Equipment

1 ECG machine with chest and limb leads labelled respectively, e.g. LA to left arm, V1 to first chest lead.
2 Disposable electrodes.
3 Swabs saturated with 70% isopropyl alcohol.
4 Abrasive strips.

Procedure

Action	Rationale
1 Wash hands using bactericidal soap and water or bactericidal alcohol handrub, and dry.	To minimize the risk of infection (DH 2005: C).

2 Explain to the patient that the ECG is to be taken, that it is not a painful procedure and that it will be useful to aid diagnosis.

To ensure that the patient understands the procedure and gives his/her valid consent (Roberts 2002: E; NMC 2006: C).

3 Ensure that the patient is comfortably positioned either lying or sitting (preferably in semi-recumbent position).

To ensure optimal recording and comfort of the patient (Roberts 2002: E).

4 Clean limb and chest electrode sites (see Action figure 4). If necessary, prepare skin by clipping hairs or use abrasive strip.

To ensure good grip and therefore good contact between skin and electrode which results in less electrical artefact (Roberts 2002: E).

5 Apply the electrodes as described in Action figure 4.

To obtain the ECG recording from vertical and horizontal planes (Roberts 2002: E).

6 Attach the leads from the ECG machine to the electrodes.

To obtain the ECG recording (Roberts 2002: E).

7 Check that the leads are connected correctly and to the relevant electrode.

To ensure the correct polarity in the ECG recording (Roberts 2002: E).

8 Ensure that the leads are not pulling on the electrodes or lying over each other.

To reduce electrical artefact and to obtain a good ECG recording (Roberts 2002: E).

9 Ask patient to relax and refrain from movement.

To obtain the optimal recording by the reduction of artefact from muscular movement (Roberts 2002: E).

10 Encourage the patient to breath normally and not to speak while ECG trace is being taken.

Speaking can alter the recording (Roberts 2002: E).

11 Check that calibration is 10 mm/mV.

To ensure standard recording to aid interpretation (E).

12 Commence the recording.

To obtain ECG.

13 In the case of artefact or poor recording, check electrodes and connections.

To ensure optimal recording (Roberts 2002: E).

14 During the procedure give reassurance to the patient.

To ensure the patient feels informed and reassured (Roberts 2002: E).

15 If necessary, record a rhythm strip utilizing leads II and V1.

To assist with interpretation if there have been any acute rhythm disturbances. Can also ensure steady baseline (Roberts 2002: E).

16 Detach ECG printout and label with patient's name, hospital number, date and time.

To ensure that the ECG is labelled with the correct patient, date and time (NMC 2005: C).

17 Inform patient that the procedure is now finished and help to remove the electrodes.

To ensure that the patient can relax and that the electrodes are removed (E).

18 Mount the ECG recording in the appropriate documentation.

To ensure that the recording does not get lost (NMC 2005: C).

19 Inform nursing and medical staff that the ECG has been completed and its location.

To enable relevant nursing and medical staff to use the ECG data in their care planning and treatment (NMC 2008: C).

Procedure guidelines (cont.)

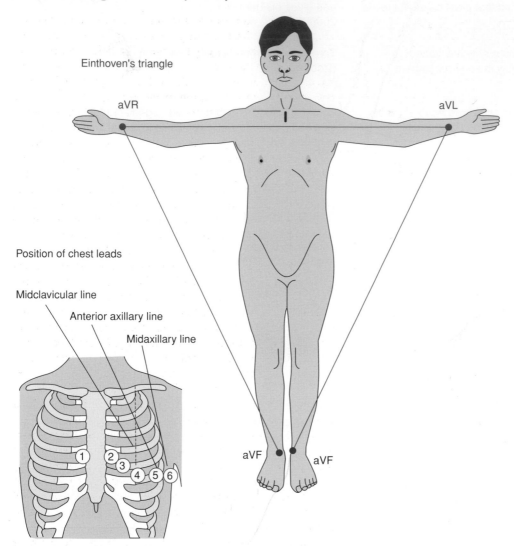

Einthoven's triangle

aVR

aVL

Position of chest leads

Midclavicular line

Anterior axillary line

Midaxillary line

1 2
3
4 5 6

aVF

aVF

Action 4   Position of electrodes for 12-lead ECG. (Redrawn from Metcalf (2000) with permission.)

Blood pressure

Definition

Blood pressure may be defined as the force exerted by blood against the walls of the vessels in which it is contained (Marieb & Hoehn 2007). Variations in blood pressure gradient provide the circulation with the force that keeps the blood moving through the body (Marieb & Hoehn 2007). Blood pressure is usually expressed in terms of millimetres of mercury (mmHg).

Indications

Blood pressure is measured for one of two reasons:

- To determine the patient's blood pressure on admission as a baseline for comparison with future measurements.

- To monitor fluctuations in blood pressure.
  (Marieb & Hoehn 2007).

Reference material

Blood flow is the volume of blood flowing through a vessel at a given time from the heart. Blood flow is equivalent to cardiac output (Marieb & Hoehn 2007). **Resistance** is the friction that occurs as the blood passes through the differently sized vessels, and impacts on the blood flow and cardiac output (Marieb & Hoehn 2007). There are three important sources of resistance: blood viscosity, vessel length and vessel diameter (Figure 25.6a, b).

Viscosity is the internal resistance to flow and may be thought of as the 'stickiness' of a fluid (Thibodeau & Patton 2007). Blood is more viscous than water due to the

(a)

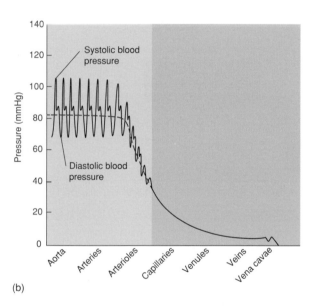

(b)

Figure 25.6 **(a)** Relationship between velocity (speed) of blood flow and total cross-sectional area in different types of blood vessels. Velocity of blood flow is slowest in the capillaries because they have the largest total cross-sectional area. **(b)** Blood pressures in various parts of the cardiovascular system. The dashed line is the mean (average) blood pressure in the aorta, arteries and arterioles. Blood pressure rises and falls with each heartbeat in blood vessels leading to capillaries. (Redrawn from Tortora & Derrickson (2007) with permission.)

elements of plasma proteins and cells that form its constituent parts, and consequently blood moves more slowly. The longer the **vessel length,** the greater the resistance encountered. The relationship between vessel length and viscosity is often constant; however, **vessel diameter** changes frequently and is an important factor in altering peripheral resistance (Thibodeau & Patton 2007). In a small blood vessel more of the fluid is in contact with the vessel walls which results in increased friction. Arterioles are the major determinants of peripheral resistance because they are small-diameter blood vessels which can expand in re-

sponse to neural and chemical controls (Thibodeau & Patton 2007).

Normal blood pressure is maintained by neural, chemical and renal controls, providing the constant blood flow around the body crucial for organ function. The neural controls operate via reflex arcs (Marieb & Hoehn 2007) derived from stretch receptors found in the wall of the proximal arterial tree, especially in the region of the aortic arch and carotid sinuses. When arterial pressure rises, there is increased stimulation of these nerve endings. The increased number of impulses along the vagus and glossopharyngeal nerves leads to reflex vagal slowing of the heart and reflex release of vasoconstrictor tone in the peripheral blood vessels. The resulting fall in cardiac output and the reduction of peripheral resistance tend to restore the blood pressure to the normal value. A fall in the arterial pressure decreases the stimulation of the arterial stretch receptors. The reflex tachycardia and vasoconstriction that ensue tend to raise the blood pressure to its normal value, forming a continuous homeostatic process (Marieb & Hoehn 2007). When the oxygen content of the blood drops sharply, chemoreceptors in the aortic arch transmit impulses to the vasomotor centre and reflex constriction occurs. The rise in blood pressure that follows helps to increase blood return to the heart and lungs (Marieb & Hoehn 2007). Renal regulation provides a major long-term mechanism of influencing blood pressure. When there is a fall in arterial pressure this results in chemical changes which lead to the release of the enzyme renin. Renin triggers a series of enzymic reactions that result in the formation of angiotensin, a powerful vasoconstrictor chemical. Angiotensin also stimulates the adrenal cortex to release aldosterone, a hormone that increases renal reabsorption of sodium. The sodium, in turn, increases the volume of water reabsorbed by the kidneys; such retention of fluid and vasoconstriction of blood vessels raises arterial pressure (Marieb & Hoehn 2007).

Blood pressure varies not only from moment to moment but also in the distribution between various organs and areas of the body. It is lowest in neonates and increases with age, weight gain, stress and anxiety (Marieb & Hoehn 2007). Shock, MI and haemorrhage are factors that cause a fall in blood pressure as they reduce cardiac output and peripheral vessel resistance or they diminish venous return after fluid loss (Figure 25.7).

Normal blood pressure

Normal blood pressure generally ranges from 100/60 to 140/90 mmHg. Blood pressure can fluctuate within a wide range and still be considered normal (Marieb & Hoehn 2007).

Systolic pressure

The systolic blood pressure is the peak pressure of blood in the arteries and is caused by the contraction of the ventricle.

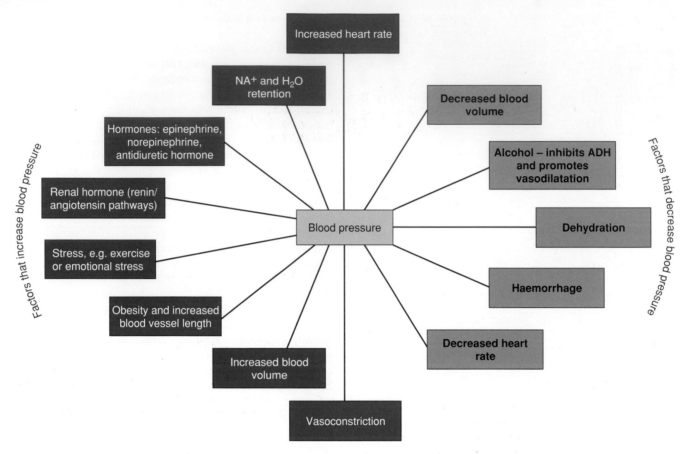

Factors that increase blood pressure

Factors that decrease blood pressure

Increased heart rate

NA+ and H₂O retention

Hormones: epinephrine, norepinephrine, antidiuretic hormone

Renal hormone (renin/angiotensin pathways)

Stress, e.g. exercise or emotional stress

Obesity and increased blood vessel length

Increased blood volume

Vasoconstriction

Blood pressure

Decreased blood volume

Alcohol – inhibits ADH and promotes vasodilatation

Dehydration

Haemorrhage

Decreased heart rate

Figure 25.7   Factors that lead to a change in blood pressure. (Redrawn from Tortora & Derrickson (2007) with permission.)

The systolic blood pressure averages around 120 mmHg in adults (Marieb & Hoehn 2007).

Diastolic pressure

The diastolic pressure is the minimum pressure of the blood against the wall of the vessel following closure of the aortic valve and is taken as a direct indication of blood vessel resistance (Marieb & Hoehn 2007).

Hypotension

Hypotension or low blood pressure is generally defined in adults as a systolic blood pressure below 100 mmHg (Marieb & Hoehn 2007). Hypotension often reflects individual variations; however, it may indicate orthostatic hypotension, i.e. postural changes that result in a lack of normal reflex response leading to a low blood pressure, or it may be the first indicator of a shock condition, e.g. septic shock, cardiogenic, hypovolaemic or toxic shock syndrome (Marieb & Hoehn 2007).

Hypertension

Hypertension is an elevation in the blood pressure and may be an acute or chronic physiological response (Marieb & Hoehn 2007). Hypertension may be a temporary response to fever, physical exertion or stress. NICE (2006) describes hypertension as persistently raised blood pressure over 140/90 mmHg. The British Hypertension Society recommends that patients who have:

- sustained blood systolic blood pressure of greater than or equal to 160 mmHg or;
- sustained diastolic blood pressure of greater than or equal to 100 mmHg,

should be commenced on antihypertensive drug treatment. Williams *et al.* (2004) further states that patients with blood pressures between 140 and 159 mmHg systolic should be offered hypertensive drug treatment if other risk factors are present, i.e. evidence of cardiovascular disease or diabetes.

Persistent hypertension is a common disease and approximately 30% of people over the age of 50 years are hypertensive (Marieb & Hoehn 2007).

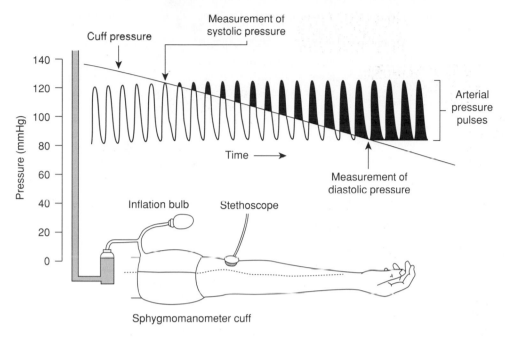

Figure 25.8 Using a sphygmomanometer, and the appearance and disappearance of Korotkoff's sounds.

Mean arterial pressure

The mean arterial pressure is the average pressure required to push blood through the circulatory system. This can be determined electronically or mathematically as well as by using an intra-arterial catheter and mercury manometer.

Mathematically, for example:

Mean arterial pressure (MAP)
= (Systolic blood pressure [SBP]
 − Diastolic blood pressure [DBP]/3) + DBP

(Adam & Osborne 2005).

A blood pressure of 130/85 mmHg gives a MAP of 100 mmHg.

Methods of recording and equipment

There are two main methods for recording the blood pressure: direct and indirect. **Direct** methods are more accurate than indirect methods. The most accurate method of measuring blood pressure involves the insertion of a minute pressure transducer unit into an artery for transmission of a waveform or digital display on a monitor. The most commonly used techniques involve placing a cannula in an artery and attaching a pressure-sensitive device to the external end (Adam & Osborne 2005).

Patients who need to be constantly monitored, e.g. in theatres, high-dependency and intensive care units, may require such devices to be used. In such patients it is essential to have an early knowledge of any change in the blood pressure, as this may indicate deterioration in the patient's condition and requires prompt treatment.

The **indirect** method is the auscultatory method. This procedure is used to measure blood pressure in the brachial artery of the arm (Evans *et al.* 2004) (Figure 25.8).

The sphygmomanometer

The sphygmomanometer consists of a compression bag enclosed in an unyielding cuff, and inflating bulb, pump or other device by which the pressure is increased, a manometer from which the applied pressure is read, and a control valve to deflate the system (Valler-Jones & Wedgbury 2005).

Manual sphygmomanometers

While mercury sphygmomanometers have been the standard method for recording blood pressure, there are concerns regarding the safety and impact on the environment of medical devices containing mercury. Following a report by the European Commission on the decommissioning of mercury (Maxon 2004), there has been no ban on the use of medical devices containing mercury in the UK. However, the Medicines and Healthcare Regulatory Agency recommends, 'the selection of mercury-free products when the ____ arises' (MHRA 2005, p. 4). If me___ are used they should be in ___ erly trained in their use and ___ or disposal, proprietary kits ___ tain the spillage and minim___ forming. While in use, the m___ ter should be kept in a vertic___ tial errors can occur (Campb___ 2001b). Local policies and the ___ tions should be followed.

The most common types of error for mercury sphygmomanometers are:

- Rapid deflation of the cuff during measurement.
- Improper placement (e.g. mercury column not vertical).
- Perished rubber tubing (McAlister & Straus 2001).
- Defective valves (Beevers *et al.* 2001b).

The other widely used type of manual sphygmomanometer is the aneroid sphygmomanometer. This is a mechanical device that measures the cuff pressure using a bellows connected to the cuff via rubber tubing. The pressure inside the bellows is transferred to a dial via a system of gears and levers (Beevers *et al.* 2001a). This type of sphygmomanometer can be calibrated properly, but is susceptible to inaccuracies or damage that would not be apparent to the user (O'Brien *et al.* 2001). The most common types of error for aneroid sphygmomanometers are:

- Non-zeroed or bent indicators.
- Cracked face plates.
- Perished rubber tubing (McAlister & Straus 2001).

In addition, there are sources of error common to all methods of manual blood pressure measuring:

- Systematic error (e.g. lack of concentration, poor hearing, inattention to audible or visual cues).
- Failure to interpret the Korotkoff sounds correctly (discussed later in this section).
- Terminal digit preference (tendency to record blood pressures ending in '5' or '0').
- Bias (e.g. recording a blood pressure corresponding to what would be expected for the patient, not the actual reading) (Beevers *et al.* 2001b).

Non-invasive automated sphygmomanometers

Automated devices to measure blood pressure have been available for some time now. Devices are manufactured for a variety of different purposes, including home use. Generally, devices intended for home use are not found to be accurate or reliable enough for clinical use (O'Brien *et al.* 2001). The British Hypertension Society and the US Association for the Advancement of Medical Instrumentation (AAMI) regularly check blood pressure measuring devices and publish recommendations for their use.

Automatic blood pressure monitors are often oscillometric devices, where the measurement of blood pressure is based on the variations of pressure in the cuff caused by the pulsing of the artery directly underneath it (Berger 2001). For this reason, placement of the cuff over the artery is essential for accurate blood pressure reading.

As with all medical devices, use should be in accordance with the procedures recommended by the manufacturer. The process of measuring an accurate blood pressure using an automated device will be similar to manual recording of blood pressure with regard to patient factors such as positioning, and placement of the cuff. All medical devices should be serviced and maintained and may need calibra-

tion at intervals. Guidance should be sought from the manufacturer.

Users of electronic sphygmomanometers should also be aware that errors in measurement (for example, if there is a weak, thready or irregular pulse) may not be readily obvious to the operator and that manual blood pressure measurement may be indicated. Those patients with muscular tremors may also experience inaccurate blood pressure readings (Beevers *et al.* 2001a).

Parts of a sphygmomanometer

Cuff

The cuff is made of washable material that encircles the arm and encloses the inflatable rubber bladder. It is secured around the arm or leg by wrapping its tapering end to the encircling material, usually by Velcro.

Inflatable bladder

A bladder that is too short and/or too narrow will give falsely high pressures. The European Society of Hypertension recommends that the centre of the bladder should cover the brachial artery and that the bladder length should be 80% of the arm circumference and the width at least 40% (O'Brien *et al.* 2003).

Control valve, pump and rubber tubing

The control valve is a common source of error. It should allow the passage of air without excessive pressure needing to be applied on the pump. When the valve is closed it should hold the mercury at a constant level and, when released, it should allow a controlled fall in the level of mercury. The rubber tubing should be long (approximately 80 cm) and with airtight connections that can easily be separated to allow rapid deflation if required.

In reviewing the methods for sphygmomanometer inaccuracies, both Campbell *et al.* (1990) and Markandu *et al.* (2000) found that errors in technique and equipment malfunction accounted for differences in readings of more than 15 mmHg. Carney *et al.* (1995) also found when evaluating 463 sphygmomanometers that only 58% were in working order.

The stethoscope

Using the stethoscope it is possible to identify a series of five phases as blood pressure falls from the systolic to the diastolic. These phases are known as Korotkoff's sounds (Figure 25.9) (Thibodeau & Patton 2007).

Korotkoff's sounds form five phases:

1 The appearance of faint, clear tapping sounds which gradually increase in intensity.
2 The softening of sounds, which may become swishing.
3 The return of sharper sounds which become crisper but never fully regain the intensity of the phase 1 sounds.
4 The distinct muffling sound which becomes soft and blowing.
5 The point at which all sound ceases.

(Evans *et al.* 2004).

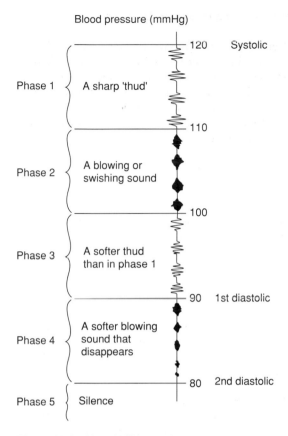

Figure 25.9   Korotkoff's sounds.

Serginson 1996; Gillespie & Curzio 1998; Beevers *et al.* 2001b). Blood pressure readings are altered by various factors that influence the patient, the techniques used and the accuracy of the sphygmomanometer. The variability of any readings can be reduced by an improved technique and by taking several readings (Campbell *et al.* 1990; Markandu *et al.* 2000). In 1981 Thompson discussed the methodology of blood pressure recording and identified poor technique and observer bias as possible sources of error. He concluded that many nurses were inadequately trained in blood pressure measurement and that more attention needed to be paid to this area. In 1996, Beevers & Beevers (1996) found that observer error could be reduced if techniques for measuring blood pressure were taught repeatedly during medical and nursing training. Furthermore, the techniques should be reinforced regularly.

Similar conclusions were found in studies by Mancia *et al.* (1987), Feher & Harris St. John (1992) and Torrance & Serginson (1996). Poor technique due to inadequate education can cause marked variation in the accuracy of measurements and can lead to inappropriate treatment decisions (Kemp *et al.* 1994; Markandu *et al.* 2000).

Regular servicing of equipment is crucial for reducing errors. Valler-Jones & Wedgbury (2005) recommend that mercury sphygmomanometers are serviced every 6–12 months, while aneroid sphygmomanometers should be serviced every 3–6 months.

Ambulatory blood pressure monitoring allows the measurement of trends in the patient's blood pressure over a longer period. For the assessment of hypertensive patients it is increasingly regarded as an important tool to assess blood pressure during normal daily activity (McAlister & Straus 2001; Williams *et al.* 2004). Ambulatory blood pressure is increasingly regarded as superior to individual blood pressure readings.

When the cuff pressure has fallen to just below the systolic pressure, a clear but often faint tapping sound suddenly appears in sequence with each cardiac contraction. The sound is produced by the transient and turbulent blood flowing through the brachial artery during the peak of each systole.

As the pressure in the cuff is reduced further, the sound becomes louder, but when the artery is no longer constricted and the blood flows freely, the sounds become muffled and then can no longer be heard. The diastolic pressure is usually defined as the cuff pressure at which the sounds disappear (Marieb & Hoehn 2007).

The stethoscope's diaphragm should be placed lightly over the point of maximal pulsation of the brachial artery (Petrie *et al.* 1997; Beevers, *et al.* 2001b; Valler-Jones & Wedgbury 2005). The diaphragm is designed to amplify low-frequency sounds such as Korotkoff's sounds (Valler-Jones & Wedgbury 2005). Excessive pressure on the stethoscope's diaphragm may partially occlude the brachial artery and delay the occurrence of Korotkoff's sounds. For this reason the diaphragm should not be tucked under the edge of the cuff (Valler-Jones & Wedgbury 2005).

Practical considerations

Much recent research has focused on the faulty techniques employed when blood pressures are taken (Campbell *et al.* 1990; Bogan *et al.* 1993; Kemp *et al.* 1994; Torrance &

Clinical considerations

Variations in the procedure and frequency of taking blood pressure may be required in different patient groups with differing conditions. With a child it is important that the correctly sized cuff is used and that the average of repeated measurements is recorded. Low diastolic pressures are common in children and thus the pressure at muffling (Korotkoff phase 4) may be difficult to determine.

Low diastolic pressures are common in elderly patients who may have atherosclerosis, and in patients with an increased cardiac output, i.e. as a result of pregnancy, exercise or hypothyroidism.

Patients with venous access devices or shunts for dialysis in their arms or superior vena cava obstruction may be unsuitable for upper arm measurements of blood pressure; however, the blood pressure may be measured in the leg or forearm. For this procedure the patient lies prone and a thigh or large cuff is used, its bladder centered over the posterior popliteal artery. The stethoscope diaphragm should be applied on the artery below the cuff. Systolic blood pressure is normally 20–30 mmHg higher in the leg than in the arm. The right sized cuff should be used for obtaining the blood pressure using the forearm, and the bladder should be centered over the radial artery below the elbow, and the cuff wrapped in a similar manner to the normal procedure. The stethoscope diaphragm should be positioned over the radial artery about 2.5 cm above the wrist. Forearm blood pressure measurements may vary significantly from an upper arm measurement, and therefore it is important to document cuff size and location (Hill & Grim 1991).

Patients who have had breast surgery with lymph node dissections and/or radiotherapy, or have lymphoedema should not have their blood pressure recorded on the affected side. This is due to the increased frailty of tissue in the area and the risk of developing lymphoedema. Patients should be told to only have their blood pressure taken on the unaffected arm or legs (Yarbro *et al.* 2005).

Conditions where a patient's blood pressure may need careful monitoring are described below:

- Patients with consistent hypotension as this could lead to renal failure.
- Hypertension is never diagnosed on a single blood pressure reading. Blood pressures are monitored to evaluate the condition of the patient and the effectiveness of medication (Williams *et al.* 2004; Marieb & Hoehn 2007).
- Postoperative and critically ill patients require monitoring of blood pressure to assess for cardiovascular stability. The patient's blood pressure should be recorded preoperatively in order to establish a baseline for comparison.
- Patients receiving intravenous infusions may require blood pressure monitoring to observe for circulatory overload. Certain chemotherapy protocols use protracted amounts of intravenous fluids. In this group of patients diuretics are frequently used to reduce the increase in blood volume which results in a rise in blood pressure. Careful monitoring of blood pressure, weight,

kidney function and electrolytes is imperative to prevent fluid overload and electrolyte imbalance (Marini & Wheeler 2006).

- Patients with local or systemic infections or neutropenia require monitoring of their blood pressure in order to detect septicaemic shock. This is characterized by a change in the capillary epithelium and vasodilatation due to circulating cell mediation (Bone 1996), which permits loss of blood and plasma through capillary walls into surrounding tissues. The decrease in the circulating volume of blood results in impaired tissue perfusion, culminating in cellular hypoxia (Thibodeau & Patton 2007).

Box 25.1   Measuring blood pressure – ten top tips (MHRA 2006)

---

1 Ensure that only clinically validated equipment is purchased and all sphygmomanometers are checked regularly: mercury devices at least 12 monthly and aneroid devices at least twice a year
2 Availability of different cuff sizes encourages cuffs being used appropriately
3 High blood pressure on the basis of anxiety should not be ruled out
4 BP should initially be measured in both arms and the arm with higher reading should be used in subsequent measurements
5 Ensure the arm is supported
6 Try to measure at the same time of day where possible
7 Be alert to 'white coat effect'
8 Remember ambulatory blood pressure measurement average day time values will be lower than hospital/surgery readings
9 Remember variability is high and blood pressure readings in patients may differ depending on time of day
10 Measurement of blood pressure by any other method is less reliable in the presence of arrhythmias

---

Procedure guidelines   **Blood pressure (manual)**

Blood pressure should be measured in both arms initially (BHS 2006; NICE 2006). A considerable number of people (particularly the elderly) can have large variations between arms. The arm with the highest reading should be the one used (Williams *et al.* 2004). Refer to Box 25.1 for recommendations from the Medicines and Healthcare Products Regulatory Agency (MHRA) 2006 for guidelines of best practice when taking patients' blood pressure.

....

Equipment

1 Sphygmomanometer.

2 Stethoscope.

....

Action

1 Explain to the patient that blood pressure is to be taken and discuss the procedure.

Rationale

To ensure that the patient understands the procedure and gives his/her consent (NMC 2006: C; NMC 2008: C).

....

2 Wash hands using bactericidal soap and water or bactericidal alcohol handrub, and dry.

To minimize the risk of infection (DH 2005: C).

....

3 Allow the patient to rest for 5 minutes either supine or seated in quiet room with comfortable temperature.	To ensure an accurate reading is obtained. Normally blood pressure readings are measured with the patient in a sitting position (BHS 2006: C).
4 Ensure that tight or restrictive clothing is removed from the arm.	To obtain a correct reading (BHS 2006: C).
5 Ensure that the upper arm is supported and positioned at heart level, with the palm of the hand facing upwards (BHS 2006).	To obtain an accurate reading. Measurements made with the arm dangling by the hip can be 11–12 mmHg higher than those made with the arm supported and the cuff at heart level. Measurements made with the arm raised can be falsely high (Beevers *et al.* 2001b: C).
6 Use a cuff that covers 80% of the circumference of the upper arm (BHS 2006).	To obtain a correct reading (BHS 2006: C).
7 Apply the cuff of the sphygmomanometer snugly around the arm, ensuring that the centre of the bladder covers the brachial artery. The lower edge of the cuff should be 2–3 cm above the arterial pulse in the antecubital fossa (Valler-Jones & Wedgbury 2005).	To obtain a correct reading (BHS 2006: C). To prevent inaccurate result due to the pressure being exerted by the cuff on the brachial artery (Valler-Jones & Wedgbury 2005: E).
8 Position the manometer within 1 m of the patient, and where it can be seen at eye level (BHS 2006).	To prevent the cuff tubing hanging down and causing a risk of being caught by objects or by the operator. The manometer should be at eye level to obtain an accurate recording (BHS 2006: C).
9 Instruct the patient to stop eating, talking, etc., during blood pressure measurement.	Activity, including eating or talking, will cause an inaccurate high blood pressure to be recorded (BHS 2006: C).
10 Inflate the cuff until the radial pulse can no longer be felt. This provides an estimation of the systolic pressure. Deflate the cuff completely and wait 15–30 seconds before continuing to measure (Hill & Grim 1991).	A low systolic pressure may be reported in patients who have an auscultatory gap. This is when Korotkoff's sounds disappear shortly after the systolic pressure is heard, and resume well above what corresponds to the diastolic pressure. About 5% of the population have an auscultatory gap and it is most common in those with hypertension (Hill & Grim 1991: E). This error can be avoided if the systolic pressure is first estimated by palpation (Hill & Grim 1991: E).
11 The cuff is then inflated to a pressure 30 mmHg higher than the estimated systolic pressure.	Pressure exerted by the inflated cuff prevents the blood from flowing through the artery (BHS 2006: C).
12 The diaphragm of the stethoscope should be placed over the pulse point of the brachial artery (see Action figure 12).	Apply just enough pressure on the stethoscope to keep it in its place over the brachial artery. Excessive pressure can distort sounds or make them persist for longer than normal (BHS 2006: C).
13 Deflate the cuff at 2 mmHg per second or per heart beat (Perloff *et al.* 1993).	At a slower rate of deflation venous congestion and arm pain can develop, resulting in a falsely low reading. At faster rates of deflation the mercury may fall too quickly, resulting in an imprecise reading (BHS 2006: C).
14 The measurement of systolic blood pressure is when a minimum of two clear repetitive tapping sounds can be heard. Diastolic pressure is measured at the point when the sound can no longer be heard.	To ensure that an accurate reading is obtained (BHS 2006: C).

Procedure guidelines *(cont.)*

15 A record should be made of the systolic and diastolic pressures and comparisons made with previous readings. It should be recorded which arm was used to take the blood pressure. Any irregularities should be brought to the attention of the medical team.

The average of two or more blood pressure readings is often taken to represent a patient's normal blood pressure.

Taking more than one measurement reduces the influence of anxiety and may provide a more accurate record (Williams *et al.* 2004: C).

Documentation should be done immediately to reduce the risk of error (Williams *et al.* 2004: C).

16 Remove the equipment and clean after use.

To reduce the risk of cross-infection (DH 2005: C).

Action 12   Manual blood pressure reading technique.

Respiration

Definition

The respiration system is a tube with many branches that end in millions of tiny hair-filled sacs called alveoli (Richardson 2006b; Tortora & Derrickson 2008). The respiratory system includes the nose, and nasal cavity, pharynx, larynx, trachea, bronchi and their smaller branches, and the lungs, which contain the terminal air sacs, or alveoli (Marieb & Hoehn 2007). The airways have three main functions (Richardson 2006b):

- To facilitate gaseous exchanges to and from the lungs.
- To protect the lungs from the entry of any foreign matter.
- To control the heat and humidity of gases.

The function of the respiratory system is to supply the body with oxygen and remove carbon dioxide. This is achieved by the diffusion of gases between the air in the alveoli of the lungs and the blood in the alveolar capillaries (Marieb & Hoehn 2007).

Indications

The respiration rate is evaluated:

- To determine a baseline respiratory rate for comparisons.
- To monitor changes in oxygenation or in respiration.
- To evaluate the patient's response to medications or treatments that affect the respiratory system.

(Tortora & Derrickson 2008).

Reference material

The body cells require a continuous supply of oxygen to carry out their vital functions and this is provided by respiration (Marieb & Hoehn 2007). To accomplish respiration, four distinct events must occur:

1 Ventilation is where air is moved into and out of the lungs so that gas in the air sacs is replenished.
2 Gaseous exchange between the blood and the alveoli.
3 Oxygen and carbon dioxide are transported to and from the lungs by the cardiovascular system. This is called respiratory transportation.
4 Internal respiration is the cellular respiration that occurs in the cell where oxygen is utilized and carbon dioxide produced.

Control of respiration

Respiratory centre

The respiratory centre generates the basic pattern of breathing. Located in the brain, it is made up of groups of nerve cells in the reticular endothelial system of the medulla oblongata. Regular impulses are sent by these cells to the motor neurones via the anterior horn of the spinal cord, which supplies the intercostal muscles and the diaphragm (Thibodeau & Patton 2007). When the motor neurones are stimulated, the muscles contract and inspiration occurs. When the neurones are inhibited, the muscles relax and expiration follows.

Although the respiratory centre generates the basic rhythm, the depth and rate of breathing can be altered in response to the body's changing needs. The most important factors are those of nervous and chemical control (Figure 25.10).

Nervous control

Lung tissue is stretched on inspiration and this stimulates afferent fibres in the vagus nerve. These impulses cause inspiration to cease and expiration occurs. Emotion, pain and anxiety also cause an increased respiratory rate (Marieb & Hoehn 2007).

Chemical control

An increase in the amount of carbon dioxide in the blood supplying the respiratory centre stimulates the respiratory centre and breathing becomes faster and deeper (Tortora & Derrickson 2008).

During exercise, carbon dioxide is produced in the muscles by the oxidation of carbohydrate. The amount of carbon dioxide in the blood increases and this stimulates the respiratory centre, producing an increase in depth and rate of respiration. More oxygen is made available in the alveoli for the blood to transport to the muscles, at the same time eliminating more carbon dioxide.

Any substance that, like carbon dioxide, lowers the pH of the blood will stimulate the respiratory centre. Figure 25.10 illustrates the factors influencing the rate and depth of breathing.

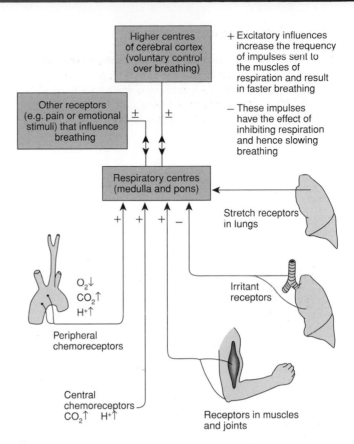

Figure 25.10 Factors influencing rate and depth of breathing.

Patients with respiratory disease, e.g. emphysema and chronic bronchitis, who maintain high levels of carbon dioxide, will have arterial oxygen levels below 9 kPa (see Chapter 38). This is termed the 'hypoxic drive'. This chronic elevation of the partial pressure of carbon dioxide results in the chemoreceptors becoming unresponsive to this chemical stimulus. The change in respiratory drive results in respiration being stimulated by decreases in oxygen levels rather than levels of carbon dioxide (Marieb & Hoehn 2007). This may be detrimental to the patient's respiration if oxygen is administered therapeutically at high levels.

Ventilation

Ventilation results from pressure changes transmitted from the thoracic cavity to the lungs (Figure 25.11). Inspiration is initiated by contraction of the diaphragm and external intercostal muscles, resulting in the rib cage rising up, and the thrusting forward of the sternum. The ribs also swing outwards, expanding the volume of the thorax (Marieb & Hoehn 2007). Because the lungs adhere tightly to the thoracic wall, attached by the layers of parietal and visceral pleura, this increases the intrapulmonary volume (Marieb & Hoehn 2007). Gases travel from an area of high pressure

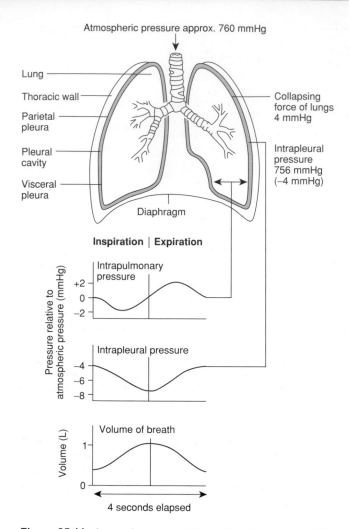

Atmospheric pressure approx. 760 mmHg

Lung

Thoracic wall

Parietal pleura

Pleural cavity

Visceral pleura

Collapsing force of lungs 4 mmHg

Intrapleural pressure 756 mmHg (−4 mmHg)

Diaphragm

Inspiration | Expiration

Intrapulmonary pressure

Intrapleural pressure

Volume of breath

Pressure relative to atmospheric pressure (mmHg)

Volume (L)

4 seconds elapsed

Figure 25.11   Intrapulmonary and intrapleural pressure relationships. Ventilation occurs due to pressure changes transmitted from the thoracic cavity to the lungs.

to areas of low pressure. The increased intrapulmonary volume results in a negative pressure of 1–3 mmHg less than the atmospheric pressure (Marieb & Hoehn 2007). The resulting pressure gradient causes air to rush into the lungs (Figure 25.12).

Expiration is largely passive, occurring as the inspiratory muscles relax and the lungs recoil as a result of their elastic properties (Marieb & Hoehn 2007). When intrapulmonary pressure exceeds atmospheric pressure this compresses the microscopic air sacs (alveoli) and an expiration of gases occurs.

A method commonly used to measure the volume of air exchanged during breathing is a **spirometer** (spiro = breathe; meter = measuring device). The record of these results is called a **spirogram** (Figure 25.13).

At rest, a healthy adult averages 12 breaths a minute, with each inhalation and exhalation moving about 500 ml of air into and out of the lungs. The volume of one breath is called the **tidal volume**. Therefore, the **minute ventilation** (**MV**) is the total volume of air inhaled and exhaled each minute which is the respiratory rate multiplied by the tidal volume which equates to 6 litres per minute (Tortora & Derrickson 2008).

Disease that affects the pleura of the individual may influence ventilation. A chest wound or rupture of the visceral pleura may allow air to enter the pleural space from the respiratory tract. The presence of air in the intrapleural space is referred to as a pneumothorax. Pleurisy, inflammation of the pleura where secretion of pleural fluid declines, causes a stabbing pain with each inspiration. Alternatively, an excessive increase in pleural secretions may hinder breathing (Marieb & Hoehn 2007). Air in the pleural space results in lung collapse (atelectasis). This affects the intrapulmonary pressure and hence ventilation.

The degree to which the lungs stretch and fill during inspiration and return to normal during expiration is due to the

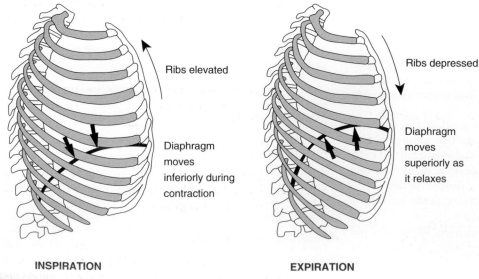

Ribs elevated

Diaphragm moves inferiorly during contraction

Ribs depressed

Diaphragm moves superiorly as it relaxes

INSPIRATION

EXPIRATION

Figure 25.12   Changes in thoracic volume during breathing.

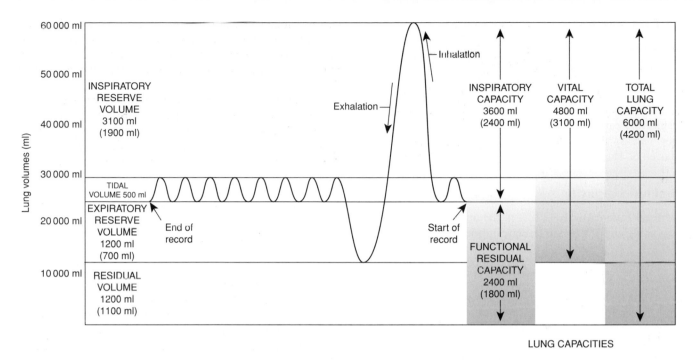

Figure 25.13 Spirogram of lung volumes and capacities. The average values for a healthy adult male and female are indicated, with values for a female in parentheses. Note that the spirogram is read from right (start of record) to left (end of record). Lung capacities are combinations of various lung volumes.

compliance and elasticity of lung tissue. Lung compliance depends on the elasticity of lung tissue and the flexibility of the thorax (Marieb & Hoehn 2007). When this is impaired, expiration becomes an active process, requiring the use of energy. The diseases that lower lung compliance are characterized by changes in the lung parenchyma. Examples include emphysema and fibrosing alveolitis, as a result of intrinsic or extrinsic means:

- **Intrinsic:**
  - severe infection;
  - rheumatoid arthritis;
  - systemic lupus erythematosus (SLE).
- **Extrinsic:**
  - pneumoconiosis;
  - psitticosis;
  - asbestosis;
  - oxygen fibrosis.

(Marieb & Hoehn 2007.)

In emphysema the lungs become progressively less elastic and more fibrous, which hinders both inspiration and expiration. The increased muscular activity results in greater energy required to breathe.

Compliance is diminished by any factor that:

- Reduces the natural resilience of the lungs.
- Blocks the bronchi or respiratory passageways.
- Impairs the flexibility of the thoracic cage.

Friction in the air passageways causes resistance and affects ventilation (Thibodeau & Patton 2007). Normally, airway resistance is reduced so that minimal opposition to airflow occurs. However, any factor that amplifies airway resistance such as the presence of mucus, tumour or infected material in the airways demands that breathing movements become more strenuous (Marieb & Hoehn 2007).

Respiratory volumes

The amount of air that is breathed varies depending on the condition of inspiration and expiration. Information about a patient's respiratory status can be gained by measuring various lung capacities, which consist of the sum of different respiratory volumes.

Tidal volume

The tidal volume (TV) is the amount of air inhaled or exhaled with each breath under resting conditions (about 500 ml) (Marieb & Hoehn 2007).

Inspiratory reserve volume

The inspiratory reserve volume (IRV) is the amount of air that can be inhaled forcibly after a normal tidal volume inhalation (about 3100 ml) (Marieb & Hoehn 2007).

Expiratory reserve volume

The expiratory reserve volume (ERV) is the maximum amount that can be exhaled forcibly after a normal tidal volume exhalation (about 1200 ml) (Marieb & Hoehn 2007).

Residual volume

The residual volume (RV) is the amount of air remaining in the lungs after a forced expiration (about 1200 ml).

Respiratory capacities

Respiratory capacities are measured for diagnostic purposes. They consist of two or more respiratory lung volumes (Marieb & Hoehn 2007).

Total lung capacity

The total lung capacity (TLC) is the amount of air in the lungs at the end of a maximum inspiration (Marieb & Hoehn 2007):

$$TLC = TV + IRV + ERV + RV \ (6000 \ ml).$$

Vital capacity

The vital capacity (VC) is the maximum amount of air that can be expired after a maximum inspiration (Marieb & Hoehn 2007):

$$VC = TV + IRV + ERV \ (4800 \ ml).$$

Inspiratory capacity

The inspiratory capacity (IC) is the maximum amount of air that can be inspired after a normal expiration (Marieb & Hoehn 2007):

$$IC = TV + IRV \ (3600 \ ml).$$

Functional residual capacity

The functional residual capacity (FRC) is the amount of air remaining in the lungs after a normal tidal volume expiration (Marieb & Hoehn 2007):

$$FRC = ERC + RV \ (2400 \ ml).$$

Dead space

A percentage of the inspired air (about 120 ml) fills the respiratory passageways and does not contribute to gaseous exchange. This is termed the anatomical dead space (Marieb & Hoehn 2007).

Gaseous exchange

Oxygen in the inspired air enters while carbon dioxide leaves the blood in the lungs in the process of ventilation. These gases move in opposite directions in the alveoli by the mechanism of diffusion (Marieb & Hoehn 2007). Adjacent to the alveoli is a dense vascular network. Oxygen moves into the alveolar capillaries and carbon dioxide moves out (Figure 25.14). This process is called gaseous exchange. Factors influencing this process include the partial pressure gradients, the width of the respiratory membrane and the surface area available (Marieb & Hoehn 2007).

The gaseous composition of the atmosphere and alveoli is demonstrated in Table 25.2. The atmosphere consists almost entirely of oxygen and nitrogen; the alveoli contain more carbon dioxide and water vapour and considerably less oxygen. These different figures reflect the following processes (Marieb & Hoehn 2007):

- Gaseous exchange in the lungs.
- Humidification of air by the respiratory passageways.
- The mixing of alveolar gas that occurs with each breath.

Respiratory transportation

Oxygen is carried in the blood in two ways, bound to the haemoglobin within the red blood cells and dissolved in plasma. Haemoglobin carries 98.5% of the oxygen from the lungs and the tissues. The amount of oxygen bound to haemoglobin depends on several factors (Marieb & Hoehn 2007):

- The partial pressure of oxygen (PaO_2) and the partial pressure of carbon dioxide ($PaCO_2$) in the blood. The gradient of partial pressure influences the rates of diffusion, the oxygen gradient being steeper than that of carbon dioxide. Carbon dioxide is transported from the tissue primarily as bicarbonate ions in the plasma (70%), whereas only small amounts are transported by haemoglobin in the red blood cells (22%) (Marieb & Hoehn 2007).
- The blood pH influences the affinity of haemoglobin for oxygen: as the pH decreases, as in acidosis, the amount of oxygen unloaded in the tissues increases (Marieb & Hoehn 2007).
- As body temperature rises above normal levels, the affinity of haemoglobin for oxygen declines, and therefore oxygen unloading is enhanced. This effect is seen in localized temperature changes such as inflammation (Marieb & Hoehn 2007).

Diseases that reduce the oxygen-carrying ability of the blood, whatever the cause, are termed anaemia. This is characterized by oxygen blood levels that are inadequate

Table 25.2   Composition of gas in the atmosphere and alveoli.

	Atmosphere inspired (%)	Alveoli (%)
Oxygen	20.9	13.7
Carbon dioxide	0.04	5.2
Nitrogen	78.6	74.9
Water	0.46	6.2

Gas exchanges occurring at the tissues

Gas exchanges occurring at the lungs

Figure 25.14   Transport and exchange of carbon dioxide and oxygen.

to support normal metabolism (Marieb & Hoehn 2007). Common causes of anaemia include:

- Insufficient number of red cells, including destruction of red cells, haemorrhage and bone marrow failure.
- Decreases in haemoglobin content, including iron deficiency anaemia and pernicious anaemia.
- Abnormal haemoglobin, including thalassaemia and sickle cell anaemia (Marieb & Hoehn 2007).

Internal respiration

Internal respiration is the exchange of gases that occurs within the tissues between the capillaries and the cells. Carbon dioxide enters the blood and oxygen moves into the cells (see Figure 25.14).

Hypoxia is the result of an inadequate amount of oxygen delivered to body tissues. The blue coloration of tissues and mucosal membranes is termed cyanosis (Marieb & Hoehn 2007).

Lung defence mechanisms

The upper airway is designed to warm, humidify and filter inspired air. The nasal passages absorb noxious gases and trap inhaled particles. Smaller particles are removed by the cough reflex.

Observation of respiration

Respirations in an individual should be observed for rate, depth and pattern of breathing (Marieb & Hoehn 2007) (Table 25.4).

Table 25.3   Respiratory rates. From Weber & Kelley (2003).

Age	Average rate/minute
Birth–6 months	30–50
6 months–2 years	20–30
3–10 years	20–28
10–18 years	12–20
Adult	15–20

Rate

Rate and depth determine the type of respiration. The normal rate at rest is approximately 14–18 breaths per minute in adults and is faster in infants and children (Table 25.3). The ratio of pulse rate to respiration rate is approximately 5 : 1 (Marieb & Hoehn 2007).

Changes in the rate of ventilation may be defined as follows. *Tachypnoea* is an increased respiratory rate, seen in fever, for example, as the body tries to rid itself of excess heat. Respirations increase by about 7 breaths per minute for every 1°C rise in temperature above normal. They also increase with pneumonia, other obstructive airway diseases, respiratory insufficiency and lesions in the pons of the brainstem (Marieb & Hoehn 2007).

Bradypnoea is a decreased but regular respiratory rate, such as that caused by the depression of the respiratory centre in the medulla by opiate narcotics, or by a brain tumour.

Depth

The depth of respiration is the volume of air moving in and out with each respiration. This tidal volume is normally about 500 ml in an adult and should be constant with each breath. A spirometer is used to measure the precise amount (see Respiratory capacities section, above). Normal, relaxed breathing is effortless, automatic, regular and almost silent (Marieb & Hoehn 2007).

Dyspnoea is undue breathlessness and an awareness of discomfort with breathing. There are several types of dyspnoea (Tortora & Derrickson 2008).

- Exertional dyspnoea is shortness of breath on exercise and is seen with heart failure.
- Orthopnoea is a shortness of breath on lying down which is relieved by the patient sitting upright. This is often caused by left ventricular failure of the heart.
- Paroxysmal nocturnal dyspnoea is a sudden breathlessness that occurs at night when the patient is lying down and is often caused by pulmonary oedema and left ventricular failure (Bickley & Szilagyi 2007).

Pattern

Changes in the pattern of respiration are often found in disorders of the respiratory control centre. Examples of changes in respiratory pattern follow.

Table 25.4   Respiratory assessment procedure.

Observation	Rationale
Rate and regularity of respiration	Very slow or rapid breathing may be a sign of oxygenation or underlying change, for example due to sepsis
Observe for signs of respiratory effort: • Nasal flaring • Pursed lips • Use of accessory muscles such as the shoulder or neck muscles (sternomastoid or scalene)	These signs may show that the patient is making extra effort in breathing and may indicate changes in the respiratory status before other observations (e.g. oxygen saturation or rate)
Listen for cough or wheezing	Dry cough may be caused by viral infection, bronchial carcinoma or congestive cardiac failure Moist cough may be due to chronic bronchitis or asthma or bacterial infection Wheezing is caused by bronchospasm or bronchial obstruction
Assess respiratory history including smoking history, history of asthma, exertional shortness of breath or other respiratory symptoms	These factors will alert the nurse to potential patient problems or concurrent conditions
Assess sputum	White or opalescent sputum may be produced by asthmatics or patients with chronic bronchitis, but does not necessarily indicate infection Thick viscous sputum that is coloured indicates infection and should be sent for microbiology culture and sensitivity Frothy sputum indicates pulmonary oedema Haemoptysis can occur with infection, pulmonary embolism, malignant disease or trauma

Hyperventilation is an increase in both the rate and depth of respiration. This follows extreme exertion, fear and anxiety, fever, hepatic coma, midbrain lesions of the brainstem, and acid–base imbalance such as diabetic ketoacidosis (Kussmaul's respiration) or salicylate overdose (in both of these situations the body compensates for the metabolic acidosis by increased respiration), as well as an alteration in blood gas concentration (either increased carbon dioxide or decreased oxygen) (Tortora & Derrickson 2008). The breathing pattern is normally regular and consists of inspiration, pause, longer expiration and another pause; this, however, may be altered by some defects and diseases. In adults, more than 20 breaths per minute is considered moderate, more than 30 is severe (Marieb & Hoehn 2007).

Apnoeustic respiration is a pattern of prolonged, gasping inspiration, followed by extremely short, inefficient expiration, seen in lesions of the pons in the midbrain.

Cheyne–Stokes respiration is periodic breathing, characterized by a gradual increase in depth of respiration followed by a decrease in respiration, resulting in apnoea.

Biot's respiration is an interrupted breathing pattern, like Cheyne–Stokes respiration, except that each breath is of the same depth. It may be seen with spinal meningitis or other central nervous system conditions.

Conditions where a patient's respirations may need careful monitoring are described below:

- Patients with conditions that affect respiration, such as those described in the text, require monitoring of respiration to evaluate their condition and the effectiveness of medication.
- Postoperative and critically ill patients require monitoring of respiration. The patient's respiration should be recorded preoperatively in order to make significant comparisons. The breathing is observed to assess for the return to normal respiratory function.
- Patients receiving oxygen inhalation therapy or receiving artificial respiration require monitoring of breathing to assess respiratory function.

Oxygen saturation

Oxygen is transported to the body's tissues in the blood. The red blood cells contain haemoglobin molecules that bind with oxygen in the lungs and transport it to the tissues where it is released. When oxygen combines with haemoglobin it forms oxyhaemoglobin. Each haemoglobin molecule has the potential to bind with four oxygen molecules. When all the binding sites for oxygen are used then the haemoglobin is saturated with oxygen.

The oxygen saturation reading is a measure of the percentage of haemoglobin molecules saturated with oxygen. The normal arterial oxygen saturation is approximately 95–98% (Woodrow 1999).

Pulse oximetry

Pulse oximetry works on the principle that blood saturated with oxygen is a different colour from blood depleted of oxygen. The probe for a pulse oximeter contains a red light source and a detector. These shine through the tissues of the body and work together to measure the colour difference between oxygenated and unoxygenated blood. The machine detects the pulse from an arterial blood source and is able to calculate the percentage of oxygen saturation by combining the detected colour changes of the blood combined with the detected pulse of the artery (Harper 2004). Because of the way the pulse oximeter works, it is susceptible to error if it is not able to accurately measure the transmission of light through the tissues or detect the pulse of the artery (Harper 2004).

Indications for pulse oximetry

- Monitoring effectiveness of oxygen therapy.
- During sedation or anaesthesia.
- During transportation of patients who are unwell and require oxygenation assessment.
- Haemodynamic instability (e.g. cardiac failure or MI) (Howell 2002).
- Respiratory illness (e.g. asthma, chronic obstructive pulmonary disease [COPD]) (Place 2000).
- Monitoring during administration of respiratory depressant drugs, e.g. opiate epidural or patient-controlled analgesia.

Possible sources of error

Light transmission:

- Barriers or obstruction, e.g. nail varnish, dirt, foreign objects, bright or fluorescent room lighting, intravenous dyes used in imaging (Harper 2004; Keenan 1995).

Pulse detection:

- Movement, rigors or shivering, poor circulation, atrial fibrillation (Woodrow 1999), vasoconstriction, arterial constriction, shock, cardiac arrest hypothermia (Howell 2002).

Limitations of pulse oximetry and oxygen saturation

Oxygen saturation is only one factor in oxygenation of the tissues. In anaemia it is possible to have high oxygen saturation readings, but inadequate amounts of oxygen reaching the tissues. Carbon monoxide (CO) exposure will lead to uptake of CO molecules in preference to oxygen (O_2). As carboxyhaemoglobin is also bright red it can lead to significant

Procedure guidelines   Pulse oximetry

Equipment

1 Pulse oximeter.

2 Alcohol swab.

Intermittent readings

Assess the patient observing correct placement of probe and for underlying problems identified above that may be influencing the reading.

Continuous readings

If the oxygen saturation monitoring is to be continuous, leaving the probe on one digit for protracted periods of time may cause pressure damage to either the skin or nail bed. There is also possibility of developing burns from the probe.

The MHRA (2001) advises to reposition the probe at least 4-hourly, or more frequently if specified by manufacturer's instructions.

Procedure

Action	Rationale
1 Explain to the patient that an oxygen saturation reading is needed and obtain consent to continue.	To ensure the patient understands the procedure and is able to provide valid consent (NMC 2006: C; NMC 2008: C).
2 Ensure that the patient is comfortable and warm enough, especially if continuous monitoring is needed.	To maintain patient comfort. Shivering will interfere with the pulse oximeter reading (Jevon 2000: E).
3 Wash and dry hands.	To minimize the risk of cross-infection (DH 2005: C).
4 Make sure the probe and equipment are clean and in good working order.	To minimize the risk of cross-infection and ensure accuracy of recording (DH 2005: C; Jevon 2000: E).
5 Select a suitable area for the probe (usually finger) and place the probe as directed by the manufacturer's instructions (see Action figure 5).	Proper function of the pulse oximeter will only be possible if the probe is placed as intended by the manufacturer (Grap 2002: E).
6 Switch the pulse oximeter machine on.	
7 Make sure that the probe sensor is detecting the pulse and that it corresponds to the patient's pulse. This will usually be indicated by a beep in time with each detected pulse or a graphical indication of the pulse on a display panel.	To ensure that the probe is detecting the pulse (Grap 2002: C).
8 Take the reading of the oxygenation saturation and document this in the patient's notes. Make a note of any oxygen administration.	To provide a written record of the patient's condition and therapy (NMC 2008: C).
9 Ensure that any abnormal reading or observation is reported to the medical team.	To ensure that any patient problems are communicated (NMC 2008: C).
10 Once oxygen saturation monitoring is completed, clean equipment and return to storage as appropriate.	Cleaning of the equipment, including the probe, will minimize the risk of cross-infection. Proper storage, including initiating battery recharging, will ensure that the equipment is ready for use when next required (DH 2005: C).

Action 5   Positioning of probe.

overestimation of oxygen saturation when using pulse oximeters (Howell 2002).

Peak flow

Definition

Peak expiratory flow rate (PEFR or peak flow) is a measurement of the highest rate at which air can be expelled from the lungs through an open mouth (Booker 2004).

Reference material

Peak flow can be used as an indication of any restriction in the airway. It is a useful aid in diagnosing and monitoring asthma and respiratory conditions (GINA 2006). PEFR is one aspect of lung function assessment and is usually used in conjunction with assessment of the lung volume and other factors to give a more complete indication of lung function (Booker 2004).

Timing of peak flow readings

For patients with asthma, the Global Initiative for Asthma (GINA) (GINA 2006) recommends measuring peak flows morning and evening before treatment is taken. In addition, a peak flow measurement should be taken 30 minutes after morning medications or nebulizers. Constriction of the airways will decrease the amount of air that can pass through and this will result in a lowered peak flow. Bronchodilators act to open the airways and allow a faster flow of air, resulting in an increase in peak flow (GINA 2006).

Factors affecting peak flow

A patient's peak flow will vary due to age, sex and ethnic origin. Respiratory problems such as asthma, COPD or emphysema will also result in a reduction in peak flow. Assessment of any impairment should be against a recognized chart of normal values (Figure 25.15) or against the patient's best recorded measurements (GINA 2006). In general, the result for a normal adult would be 400–600 litres per minute (Edmond 2002).

In patients with asthma the peak flow reading will usually vary over time and in response to medication. Any significant deterioration in peak flow may signal the onset of acute severe asthma (Box 25.2).

In the event of any life-threatening feature or pulse oximetry of less than 92%, arterial blood gases should be measured.

Blood gas markers for a severe life-threatening asthma attack are:

- Normal or high $PaCO_2$ (5–6 kPa/36–45 mmHg).
- Severe hypoxia, PaO_2 less than 8 kPa/60 mmHg regardless of oxygen therapy.
- Low pH or high H^+.

Severe and life-threatening asthma attacks can occur without patient distress. Not all features above may be evident, but

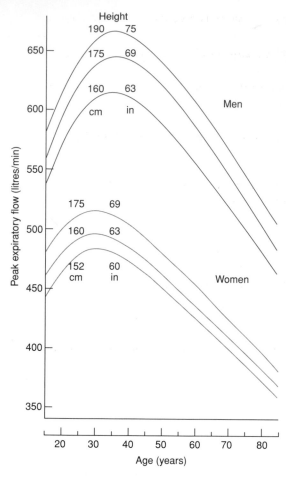

Figure 25.15 Chart of normal adult PF values. From Gregg & Nunn (1989) with permission from *BMJ*.

Box 25.2 Recognition and assessment of asthma (Edmond 2002)

Features of acute severe asthma:

- Peak flow < (less than or equal to) 50% of the predicted value (see Figure 25.14) or best readings.
- Unable to finish sentence in one breath.
- Respirations > (greater than or equal to) 25 breaths per minute.
- Pulse over 110 beats/min.

Life-threatening features:

- Peak flow < (less than) 33% of predicted or best readings.
- Cyanosis, silent chest or feeble respiratory effort.
- Bradycardia or hypotension.
- Confusion, exhaustion or coma.

if one or more symptoms are noted and there is a deterioration, the medical team should be contacted urgently (GINA 2006).

Temperature

Definition

Body temperature represents the balance between heat production and heat loss (Marieb & Hoehn 2007). All body tissues produce heat depending on how metabolically active

Procedure guidelines   Peak flow reading using manual peak flow meter

Equipment

1 Peak flow meter.

2 Observation chart.

Procedure

Action	Rationale
1 Explain the procedure to the patient and obtain consent.	To ensure the patient understands the procedure and gives valid consent (NMC 2006: C; NMC 2008: C).
2 Establish patient's current and best peak flow readings or predicted peak flow.	To allow for comparison and assessment of the patient's reading (Baillie 2001: E).
3 Wash and dry hands.	To minimize cross-infection (DH 2005: C).
4 Collect and assemble equipment. Attach mouthpiece to meter if required (see specific documentation).	

5 Move the indicator to the zero mark prior to reading.	To ensure the reading is accurate (Baillie 2001: E).
6 Sit patient in upright/usual position for readings.	To ensure consistency of readings (Baillie 2001: E).
7 Ask the patient to take a deep breath in and place their lips around the mouthpiece (see Action figure 7).	To ensure accuracy of reading (Dickinson & Martindale 2002: E).
8 Ask the patient to breathe out through the peak flow meter as hard as possible.	To ensure accuracy of reading (Baillie 2001: E).
9 Take a note of the reading. Readings may vary, so repeat process three times in total and use the best of the three readings.	To ensure accuracy of readings (Baillie 2001: C; Dickinson & Martindale 2002).
10 Return the patient to a comfortable position.	
11 Discard the used mouthpiece (if appropriate), wash your hands and store the peak flow meter ready for next use.	To minimize cross-infection (DH 2005: C).
12 Record the highest peak flow reading in the patient record, noting time of reading and any nebulized therapy. Inform medical staff of any abnormality in the reading.	To provide an accurate record of assessment (Baillie 2001: E).

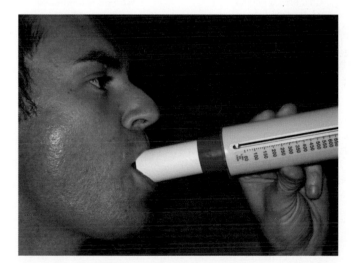

Action 7 Manual peak flow meter technique.

they are. When the body is resting, most heat is generated by the heart, liver, brain and endocrine organs (Marieb & Hoehn 2007).

Indications

Monitoring the patient's temperature is an important aspect of nursing assessment. Temperature needs to be measured accurately and monitored effectively to enable temperature changes to be detected quickly and any necessary intervention commenced (Watson 1998). Measurement of body temperature is carried out for two reasons:

- To determine the patient's temperature on admission as a baseline for comparison with future measurements.
- To monitor fluctuations in temperature.

Reference material

All tissues produce heat as a result of cell metabolism, and this is increased by exercise and activity (Marieb & Hoehn 2007). Body temperature is usually maintained between 36.0 and 37.5°C regardless of changes in the environment (Tortora & Derrickson 2008). Humans have the ability through homeostasis to ensure the core temperature that remains constant in spite of environmental changes. The body core generally has the highest temperature while the skin is the coolest (Figure 25.16). Core temperature reflects the heat of arterial blood and represents the balance between the heat generated by body tissues in metabolic activity and that lost through various mechanisms (Marieb & Hoehn 2007).

The core body temperature is set and closely regulated by the thermoregulatory centre of the hypothalamus. This comprises a group of neurones in the anterior and posterior portions, referred to as the preoptic area (Tortora & Derrickson 2008), which works as a thermostat (Figure 25.17). A relatively constant temperature is maintained by homeostasis, which is a constant process of heat gain and heat loss. The body requires stability of its temperature to produce an optimum environment for biochemical and enzymic reactions to maintain cellular function. Body temperature above or below this normal range affects total body function (Marieb & Hoehn 2007). A temperature above 41°C can cause convulsions and a temperature of 43°C renders life unsustainable.

Heat is gained through metabolic activity of the body, especially of the muscles and liver. Heat loss is achieved through the skin by the processes of radiation, convection, conduction and evaporation (Marieb & Hoehn 2007).

Various factors cause fluctuations of temperature:

- The body's circadian rhythms cause daily fluctuations. The body temperature is higher in the evening than in the morning (Marieb & Hoehn 2007). Minor & Waterhouse (1981) recorded a difference of 0.5–1.5°C between morning and evening measurements.

Figure 25.16 Body core and skin temperatures.

- Ovulation can elevate the body's temperature as it influences the basal metabolic rate (Tortora & Derrickson 2008).
- Exercise and eating cause an elevation in temperature (Marieb & Hoehn 2007).
- Extremes of age affect a person's response to environmental change. The young or elderly are unable to maintain an efficient equilibrium. Thermoregulation is inadequate in the newborn and especially in low-birth-weight babies. In older people there is an increased sensitivity to cold and the body temperature is generally lower (Nakamura *et al.* 1997).

Hypothermia Hypothermia is defined as a core temperature of 35°C that causes the metabolic rate to decrease (Trim 2005). Hypothermia may be classified as mild (32–35°C), moderate (28–32°C) and severe (less than 28°C) (Cuddy 2004). This occurs when the body loses more heat and is subsequently unable to maintain homeostasis (Neno 2005). If the temperature does fall below 35°C, the patient will start to shiver severely (Edwards 1997). However, hypothermia frequently escapes detection due to symptoms being non-specific and an oral

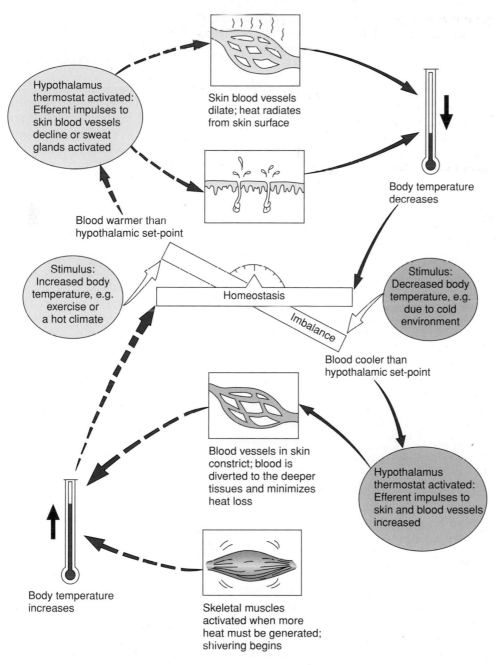

Figure 25.17 Mechanisms of body temperature regulation.

thermometer's failure to record in the appropriate range (Marini & Wheeler 2006). It can occur in all ages, but the elderly are at particular risk, and is often multifactorial in origin. It can arise as a result of:

- Environmental exposure.
- Medications that can either alter the perception of cold, increase heat loss through vasodilatation or inhibit heat generation, e.g. alcohol, paracetamol.
- Metabolic conditions, e.g. hypoglycaemia and adrenal insufficiency.

- The exposure of the body and internal organs during surgery and the use of drugs which dampen the vasoconstrictor response (Marini & Wheeler 2006).

Surgical patients having procedures greater than 1 hour have increased disruptions to normal homeostatic mechanisms resulting in a drop of temperature. Complications can include cardiovascular ischaemia, delayed wound healing and increase risk for wound infections and increase in postoperative recovery time (Wagner 2006).

Table 25.5 Non-infectious causes of hyperthermia.

Agonist drugs	Malignancy
Alcohol withdrawal	Malignant hyperthermla
Anticholinergic drugs	Neuroleptic malignant syndrome
Allergic drug or transfusion reaction	Pheochromocytoma
	Salicylate intoxication
Autonomic insufficiency	Status epilepticus
Crystalline arthritis (gout)	Stroke or central nervous system damage
Drug allergy	
Heat stroke	Vasculitis
Hyperthyroidism	

Hyperthermia   *Pyrexia* is defined as a significant rise in body temperature (Marieb & Hoehn 2007). Sudden temperature elevations usually indicate infection. However, other life-threatening non-infectious causes of fever are often overlooked (Table 25.5).

Fever caused by pyrexia is the result of the internal thermostat resetting to higher levels. This resetting of the thermostat is the result of the action of pyrogens, which are chemical substances now known to be cytokines. Cytokines are chemical mediators, which are involved in cellular immunity (Marieb & Hoehn 2007). They enhance the immune response and are released from white blood cells, injured tissues and macrophages. This causes the hypothalamus to release prostaglandins, which in turn reset the hypothalamic thermostat. The body then promotes heat-producing mechanisms such as vasoconstriction. Heat loss is reduced, the skin becomes cool and the person 'shivers'. This is often called a rigor (Marieb & Hoehn 2007). A rigor is marked by shivering and the patient complains of feeling cold. The temperature quickly rises as a result of the normal physiological response to cold. This results in the following physiological changes:

- Thermoreceptors in the skin are stimulated, resulting in vasoconstriction. This decreases heat loss through conduction and convection.
- Sweat gland activity is reduced to minimize evaporation.
- Shivering occurs, muscles contract and relax out of sequence with each other, thus generating heat.

- The body increases catecholamine and thyroxine levels, elevating the metabolic rate in an attempt to increase temperature.

(Marieb & Hoehn 2007.)

All of these changes contribute to a rise in metabolism with an increase in carbon dioxide excretion and the need for oxygen. This leads to an increased respiratory rate. When the body temperature reaches its new 'setpoint' the patient no longer complains of feeling cold, shivering ceases and sweating commences.

There are several grades of pyrexia, and these are described in Table 25.6.

There are different methods for lowering body temperature. Antipyretics, including paracetamol, can mask the function of the hypothalamus, by reducing the temperature while masking the underlying signs of disease (Cuddy 2004). It is thought that these drugs inhibit the inflammatory action of prostaglandins, affecting the hypothalamus by temporarily resetting the thermostat to normal levels. However, these drugs must be used with caution in patients with established liver disease or a history of gastric bleeding as they can cause gastric irritation and put an increased strain on a diseased liver to break down the drug.

Fanning is of benefit for moderate to high pyrexias. Fanning and tepid sponging are not recommended while the patient's temperature is still rising as this will only make the patient feel colder, cause distress (Sharber 1997) and cause the peripheral thermoreceptors to detect a decrease in temperature that leads the hypothalamus to initiate heat-gaining activities such as shivering and peripheral vasoconstriction (Krikler 1990).

Recordings of body temperature are an index of biological function and are a valuable indicator of a patient's health.

Temperature recording sites

Traditionally, the mouth, axilla or rectum have been the preferred sites for obtaining temperature readings. This is due to their accessibility. With the development of new technology the use of the tympanic membrane is increasingly popular, as it is less invasive and provides rapid results (Burke 1996). It has been suggested that tympanic membrane thermometers

Table 25.6 Grades of pyrexia.

Low-grade pyrexia	Normal to 38°C	Indicative of an inflammatory response due to a mild infection, allergy, disturbance of body tissue by trauma, surgery, malignancy or thrombosis
Moderate to high-grade pyrexia	38–40°C	May be caused by wound, respiratory or urinary tract infections
Hyperpyrexia	40°C and above	May arise because of bacteraemia, damage to the hypothalamus or high environmental temperatures

give a more accurate representation of actual body temperature, as the tympanic membrane lies close to the temperature regulation centre in the hypothalamus and shares the same artery (Van Staaij *et al.* 2003).

Oral

To most accurately measure the temperature orally, the thermometer is placed in the posterior sublingual pocket of tissue at the base of the tongue (Torrance & Semple 1998). It is important that the thermometer is placed in this region and not in the area under the front of the tongue, as there may be a temperature difference of up to 1.7°C between these areas. This temperature difference is due to the sublingual pockets being protected from the air currents, which cool the frontal areas (Neff *et al.* 1989).

This area is in close proximity to the thermoreceptors which respond rapidly to changes in the core temperature, hence changes in core temperatures are reflected quickly here (Carroll 2000; Stevenson 2004).

Oral temperatures are affected by the temperatures of ingested foods and fluids, smoking and by the muscular activity of chewing. It has been shown that oxygen therapy does not affect the oral temperature reading (Hasler & Cohen 1982; Lim-Levy 1982). A respiratory rate that exceeds 18 breaths per minute, together with a patient who smokes, will also reduce the core temperature values (Knies 2003). Oral thermometers should not be used with confused patients because of the risk of injury (Watson 1998).

Rectal

The rectal temperature is often higher than the oral temperature because this site is more sheltered from the external environment. Rectal thermometry has been demonstrated in clinical trials to be more accurate than oral or axillary thermometry; however, it is not advocated due to its invasive nature (Trim 2005). While other more precise methods can still detect fever, the rectal method offers greater precision. However, the presence of soft stool may separate the thermometer from the bowel wall and give a false reading, especially if the central temperature is changing rapidly. In infants this method is not recommended as it carries a risk of rectal ulceration or perforation (Jensen *et al.* 1994).

A rectal thermometer should be inserted at least 4 cm in an adult to obtain the most accurate reading.

Axillary

The axilla is considered less desirable than the other sites because of the difficulty in achieving accurate and reliable readings (Evans *et al.* 2004) as it is not close to major vessels, and skin surface temperatures vary more with changes in temperature of the environment (Woollens 1996).

It is usually only used for patients who are unsuitable for, or who cannot tolerate, oral thermometers, e.g. after general anaesthetic, or patients with mouth injuries (Edwards 1997).

To take an axillary temperature reading, the thermometer should be placed in the centre of the armpit, with the patient's arm firmly against the side of the chest. It is important that the same arm is used for each measurement as there is often a variation in temperature between left and right (Heindenreich & Giuffe 1990).

Whichever route is used for temperature measurement, it is important that this is then used consistently, as switching between sites can produce a record that is misleading or difficult to interpret.

Time for recording temperatures

The average person experiences circadian rhythms which make their highest body temperature occur in the late afternoon or early evening, i.e. between 4 PM and 8 PM. The most sensitive time for detecting pyrexias appears to be between 7 PM and 8 PM (Angerami 1980). Samples *et al.* (1985) found the highest temperature between 5 PM and 7 PM. These studies suggest the most useful time to measure and detect an abnormal temperature would be approximately 6 PM. This should be considered when interpreting variations in 4- or 6-hourly observations, and when taking once-daily temperatures.

Types of thermometer

A variety of thermometers are now available, from clinical glass thermometers with oral or rectal bulbs to the electronic sensor thermometer to the tympanic thermometer. Until recently, mercury in glass thermometers continued to be used, even though it has been shown they are unable to detect temperatures lower than 34.5°C (94°F) or higher than 40.5°C (105°F) (Khorshid *et al.* 2005). The MHRA (2005) advises that, for safety, equipment with mercury should be replaced where possible. They are also slow to respond to temperature changes (Marini & Wheeler 2006). O'Toole (1997) also highlights that mercury thermometers present a risk to patients of developing an infection. Therefore by using ones with disposable covers the risk of cross-infection is reduced. The use of electronic devices is therefore preferable where there are extremes of temperature or where there are temperature fluctuations. Other types of thermometer include those listed by Docherty (2000):

- Single-use plastic-coated strips with heat-sensitive recorders (dots) which change colour to indicate the temperature (record from 35.5°C to 40.4°C).
- Digital analogue probe thermometers with plastic disposable sheets (record from 32°C to 42°C).

- Invasive thermometers attached to a pulmonary artery catheter (record from 0°C to 50°C) (O'Toole 1997; Braun *et al.* 1998).

Tympanic membrane thermometer

Tympanic thermometers are small hand-held devices that have a disposable probe that is inserted into the patient's ear canal. The sensor at the end of the probe records the infrared radiation (IRR) that is emitted by the membrane, as a result of its warmth, and converts this into a temperature reading presented on a digital screen (Jevon & Jevon 2001). The probe is protected by a disposable cover, which is changed between patients to prevent cross-infection (Gallimore 2004). Van Staaij *et al* (2003) suggest that tympanic thermometers give a more accurate representation of actual body temperature because the tympanic membrane lies close to the temperature regulation centre in the hypothalamus and shares the same artery.

A common problem with using tympanic thermometers is poor technique (Gilbert *et al.* 2002), leading to inaccurate temperature measurements. The placement of the probe to fit snugly within the ear canal (see Figure 25.18) is crucial as differences between the opening of the ear canal and the tympanic membrane can be as much as 2.8°C (Hudek *et al.* 1998). Jevon and Jevon (2001) highlight other causes of false readings, which include dirty or cracked probe lens, incorrect installation of the probe cover and short time intervals between measurements (less than 2–3 minutes).

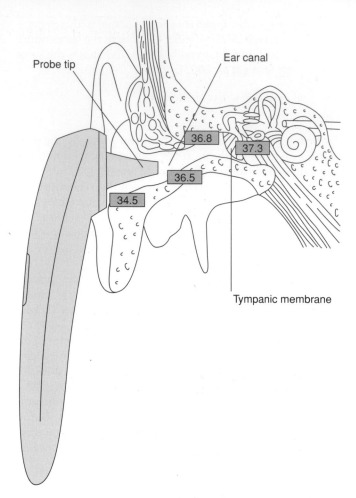

Figure 25.18 Tympanic membrane thermometer.

Conditions where a patient's temperature requires careful monitoring

1 Patients with conditions that affect basal metabolic rate, such as disorders of the thyroid gland, require monitoring of body temperature. Hypothyroidism is a condition where an inadequate secretion of hormones from the thyroid gland results in a slowing of physical and metabolic activity; thus the individual has a decrease in body temperature. Hyperthyroidism is excessive activity of the thyroid gland; a hypermetabolic condition results, with an increase in all metabolic processes. The patient complains of a low heat tolerance. Thyrotoxic crisis is a sudden increase in thyroid hormones and can cause a hyperpyrexia (Walsh 2002).

2 Postoperative and critically ill patients require monitoring of temperature. The patient's temperature should be observed preoperatively in order to make any significant comparisons. In the postoperative period the nurse should observe the patient for hyperthermia or hypothermia as a reaction to the surgical procedures (Wagner 2006).

3 Patients with a susceptibility to infection, for example those with a low white blood cell count (less than 1000 cells/mm^3), or those undergoing radiotherapy, chemotherapy or steroid treatment, will require a more frequent observation of temperature. The fluctuation in temperature is influenced by the body's response to pyrogens. Immunocompromised patients are less able to respond to infection. Bacteraemia means a bacterial invasion of the bloodstream. Septic shock is a circulatory collapse as a result of severe infection. Pyrexia may be absent in those who are immunosuppressed or in the elderly (Neno 2005).

4 Patients with a systemic or local infection require monitoring of temperature to assess development or regression of infection.

5 Pyrexia can occur when patients are receiving a blood transfusion but severe transfusion reactions usually occur within the first 15 minutes of starting (BCSH 1999).

Urinalysis

Definition

Urinalysis is the analysis of the volume and physical, chemical and microscopic properties of urine which informs the

Procedure guidelines   Temperature measurement

Equipment

1 Tympanic membrane thermometer.

2 Disposable probe covers.

Procedure

Action	Rationale
1 Explain and discuss procedure with the patient.	To ensure that the patient understands the procedure and gives his/her valid consent (NMC 2006: C; NMC 2008: C).
2 Wash and dry hands.	To minimize the risks of cross-infection and contamination (DH 2005: C).
3 Document to ensure the same ear is used for consecutive readings.	Anatomical differences between the two ears can result in a difference of up to $1°C$ (Jevon & Jevon 2001: C).
4 Remove thermometer from the base unit and ensure the lens is clean and not cracked. Use a dry wipe to clean if required.	Alcohol-based wipes should not be used as this can lead to a false low temperature measurement (Jevon & Jevon 2001: E).
5 Place disposable probe cover on the probe tip, ensuring the manufacturer's instructions are followed.	The probe cover protects the tip of the probe and is necessary for the functioning of the instrument (Jevon & Jevon 2001: E).
6 Gently place the probe tip in the ear canal to seal the opening, ensuring a snug fit.	To prevent air at the opening of the ear from entering it, causing a false low temperature measurement (Bayham *et al.* 1996: C; Jevon & Jevon 2001: E).
7 Press and release SCAN button.	To commence the instrument scanning (Bayham *et al.* 1996: C).
8 Remove probe tip from the ear as soon as the thermometer display reads DONE, usually indicated by beeps.	Measurement usually complete within 2 seconds (Bayham *et al.* 1996: C).
9 Read the temperature display.	Document in the patient's records (Jevon & Jevon 2001: C; NMC 2008: C).
10 Press RELEASE/EJECT button to discard probe cover.	Probe covers are for single use only (Jevon & Jevon 2001: E).
11 Wipe thermometer clean and replace in base unit.	To reduce the risk of cross-infection (DH 2005: C).

practitioner about the state of the body (Tortora & Derrickson 2008).

Indications

The composition of urine can change dramatically as a result of disease processes. It may contain red blood cells, glucose, proteins, white blood cells or bile (Marieb & Hoehn 2007). The presence of such abnormalities in urine is an important warning sign of illness and may be helpful in clinical assessment in the following ways:

- Screening: for systemic disease, for example, diabetes mellitus or renal conditions.
- Diagnosis: to confirm or exclude suspected conditions, for example urinary tract infection.
- Management and planning: to ascertain as a baseline, monitor progress of an existing condition and/or plan programme of care and medication (Wilson 2005).

Reference material

Urine is formed in the kidneys, which process approximately 180 litres of blood-derived fluid a day. Approximately 1% of this total actually leaves the body as urine, the rest returns to the circulation (Marieb & Hoehn 2007). Urine formation, and the simultaneous adjustment of blood composition, involves three processes (Marieb & Hoehn 2007) (Figure 25.19):

- Glomerular filtration.
- Tubular reabsorption.
- Tubular secretion.

Glomerular filtration occurs in the glomeruli of the kidney, which act as non-selective filters. Filtration occurs as a result of increased glomerular blood pressure caused by the difference in diameter between afferent and efferent arterioles. The effect is a simple mechanical filter that permits substances smaller than plasma proteins to pass from the glomeruli to the glomerular capsule (Marieb & Hoehn 2007).

Tubular reabsorption then occurs, removing necessary substances from the filtrate and returning them to the peritubular capillaries. Tubular reabsorption is an active process that requires protein carriers and energy. Substances reabsorbed include nutrients and most ions. It is also a passive process, however, driven by electrochemical gradients. Substances reabsorbed in this way include sodium ions and water. Creatinine and the metabolites of drugs are not re-absorbed either because of their size, insolubility or a lack of carriers. Most of the nutrients, 80% of the water and sodium ions, and the majority of actively transported ions are reabsorbed in the proximal convoluted tubules (Marieb & Hoehn 2007).

Reabsorption is controlled by hormones. Aldosterone increases reabsorption of sodium (and hence also water), and antidiuretic hormone (ADH) enhances reabsorption of water in the collecting tubules (Marieb & Hoehn 2007).

Tubular secretion is both an active and a passive process in which the tubules excrete drugs, urea, excess ions and other substances into the filtrate. It plays an important part in maintaining the acid–base balance of blood (Marieb & Hoehn 2007).

Regulation of urine concentration and volume occurs in the loop of Henle, where the osmolarity of the filtrate is controlled. As the filtrate flows through the tubules the permeability of the walls controls how dilute or concentrated the resulting urine will be. In the absence of ADH, dilute urine is formed because the filtrate is not reabsorbed as it passes through the kidneys. As levels of ADH increase, the collecting tubules become more permeable and water moves out of the filtrate back into the blood. Consequently, smaller amounts of more concentrated urine are produced (Marieb & Hoehn 2007).

Characteristics of urine

Urine is typically clear, pale to deep yellow in colour and slightly acidic (pH 6) (Rigby & Gray 2005), though pH can change as a result of metabolic processes or diet. Vomiting and bacterial infection of the urinary tract can cause urine to become alkaline. Urinary specific gravity ranges from 1.001 to 1.035, according to how concentrated the urine is (Fillingham & Douglas 2003; Marieb & Hoehn 2007).

The colour of urine is due to a pigment called urochrome which is derived from the body's destruction of haemoglobin. The more concentrated urine is the deeper yellow it becomes. Changes in colour may reflect diet (e.g. beetroot or rhubarb), or may be due to blood or bile in the urine (Marieb & Hoehn 2007). Often fresh urine appears turbid (cloudy), indicating there may be an infection of the urinary tract. The urinary tract is the most common site of bacterial infection. There are many predisposing factors (Figure 25.20), the most common of which is instrumentation, that is, cystoscopy and urinary catheterization (Bayer Diagnostics 1997).

Bacteriuria is defined as the presence of bacteria in the urine (Rigby & Gray 2005). Urine specimens are rarely sterile, as a result of contamination with periurethral flora during collection. Infection is distinguished by counting the number of bacteria. Significant bacteriuria is defined as a presence of more than 10^5 organisms per ml of urine in the presence of clinical symptoms. Covert bacteriuria is the presence of more than 10^5 organisms per ml of urine without clinical symptoms (Marini & Wheeler 2006) (Figure 25.21).

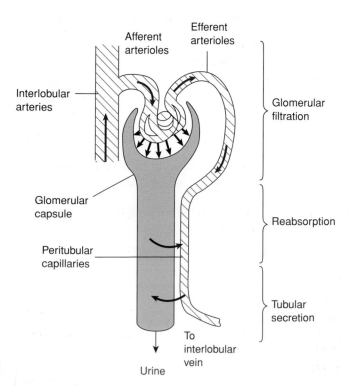

Figure 25.19 A nephron depicted diagrammatically to show the three major mechanisms by which urine is produced.

Figure 25.20 Diagramatic representation of predisposition to UTIs.

Fresh urine smells slightly aromatic. This can change as a result of disease processes such as diabetes mellitus, when acetone is present in the urine, giving it a fruity smell. The composition of urine can change dramatically as a result of disease, and abnormal substances may be present. Urinalysis can identify many of these substances, and should be part of every physical assessment (Cook 1996; Torrance & Elley 1998).

Renal clearance is the rate at which the kidneys clear a particular chemical from the plasma in a given time. Renal clearance tests are done to determine the glomerular filtration rate (GFR), which provides information about the amount of functioning renal tissue. Renal clearance tests are also done to detect glomerular damage and to follow the progress of renal disease (Marieb & Hoehn 2007).

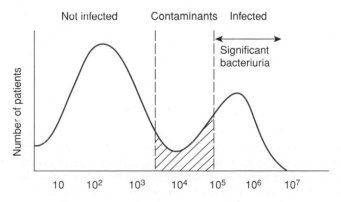

Figure 25.21 Significant bacteriuria. Specimens of urine are rarely sterile. A cut-off point is identified to distinguish true infection (significant bacteriuria) from effects of contamination from surrounding tissues.

Dipstick (reagent) tests

Strips that have been impregnated with chemicals are dipped quickly in urine and read as a means of testing urine. When dipped in urine, the chemicals react with abnormal substances and change colour. Although dipstick reagents have been primarily used as screening tools for protein or glucose in the urine, more sophisticated reagents are now available. These reagents test for nitrites and leucocyte esterase as indicators of bacterial infection. Leucocyte esterase is an enzyme from neutrophils not normally found in urine and is a marker of infection. Nitrites are produced by the bacterial breakdown of dietary nitrate, which is a waste product of protein metabolism (Rigby & Gray 2005). It is essential to use the strips according to the manufacturer's instructions and be aware of factors that may affect the results. These factors include specific drugs (Table 25.7), the quality of the urine specimen itself and the possibility that false negative results are possible.

In the microbiology laboratory, urine samples constitute about 40% of the total workload; of these, 70–80% of

Table 25.7 Routine observations of urine: possible indications and plan of action. Modified from Rigby and Gray (2005).

Observation	Possible indications	Plan of action
Colour		
Green	Pseudomonas infection, presence of bilirubin	Culture and microscopy
	Excretion of cytotoxic agents, e.g. Mitomycin or substances, e.g. Methylene Blue	Discard with care
Pink/Red	Blood	Culture and microscopy. If currently receiving chemotherapy, e.g. Ifosfamide, further mesna may need to be given.
	Excretion of cytotoxic agents, e.g. Doxorubicin	Discard with care
Orange	Excess urobiliogen, Rifampicin	Discard
Yellow	Bilirubin	Discard
Brown	Bilirubin	Discard
Odour		
Fishy	Infection	Culture and microscopy
Sweet smelling	Ketones	Culture and microscopy
Debris		
Cloudy	Infection, stale urine	Culture and microscopy
Sediment	Infection, contamination	Culture and microscopy

Table 25.8 How drugs may influence the results of reagent sticks.

Drug	Reagent test	Effect on the results
Ascorbic acid	Glucose, blood, nitrite	High concentrations may diminish colour
L-Dopa	Glucose	High concentrations may give a false negative reaction
	Ketones	Atypical colour
Nalidixic acid	Urobilinogen	Atypical colour
Probenacid		
Phenazopyridine (pyridium)	Protein	May give atypical colour
	Ketones	Coloured metabolites may mask a small reaction
	Urobilinogen, bilirubin	May mimic a positive reaction
	Nitrite	
Rifampicin	Bilirubin	Coloured metabolites may mask a small reaction
Salicylates (aspirin)	Glucose	High doses may give a false negative reaction

samples are not infected. This means that much time, energy and finances are wasted on unnecessary sample processing and investigation (Bayer Diagnostics 1997).

Further testing may be necessary, such as culture and sensitivity testing under laboratory conditions, to identify organisms responsible for infection and to determine the most effective treatment (Wilson 2005) (Table 25.8). Twenty-four hour collection is also used to measure substances such as steroids, white cells, electrolytes or to determine urine osmolarity (Tortora & Derrickson 2008).

Procedure guidelines   Urinalysis

Procedure

Action	Rationale
1 Store reagent sticks in accordance with manufacturer's instructions. This is usually a dark dry place.	Tests may depend on enzymic reaction. To ensure reliable results (Bayer Diagnostics 2006: C).
2 Explain and discuss the procedure with the patient.	To ensure that the patient understands the procedure and gives his/her valid consent (NMC 2006: C; NMC 2008: C).
3 Wash and dry hands.	To maintain infection control and prevent cross-infection (DH 2005: C).
4 Obtain clean specimen of fresh urine from patient.	Urine that has been stored deteriorates rapidly and can give false results (Bayer Diagnostics 2006: C).
5 Dip the reagent strip into the urine. The strip should be completely immersed in the urine and then removed immediately. Run edge of strip along the container. This will remove excess urine and prevent mixing of chemicals from adjacent reagent areas (Bayer Diagnostics 2006: C).	To remove any excess urine (Bayer Diagnostics 2006: C).
6 Hold the stick at an angle.	Urine reagent strips should not be held upright when reading them because urine may run from square to square, mixing various reagents (Bayer Diagnostics 2006: C).
...quired time interval before reading the strip ...olour chart (see Action figure 7).	The strips must be read at exactly the time interval specified, or the reagents will not have time to react, or may be inaccurate (Bayer Diagnostics 2006: C).

Action 7 Comparing urinalysis results.

Blood glucose

Definition

The body regulates the blood glucose levels by producing insulin. Insulin's main effect is to lower the blood glucose level, but it also influences protein and fat metabolism. If the pancreas fails to produce sufficient insulin, the level of glucose in the blood will remain high. Conversely, if too much insulin is made, or given, then the level of glucose in the blood remains low. For optimum cell function, blood glucose levels should be maintained normally at a level of 4–7 mmol/l (Ferguson 2005).

Indications

Blood glucose monitoring is used to indicate when blood glucose is not within the normal range. Conditions where a patient's blood glucose may need careful monitoring are:

- To make a diagnosis of diabetes mellitus, which is only confirmed following a glucose tolerance test (Burden 2001).
- In the acute management of unstable diabetic states: diabetic ketoacidosis, hyperosmolar non-ketotic coma and hypoglycaemia.
- To make a diagnosis of hypoglycaemia.
- To monitor and manage the treatment of both insulin-dependent diabetes mellitus (IDDM or type one) and non-insulin-dependent diabetes mellitus (NIDDM or type two).

Reference material

To maintain normal blood glucose levels, insulin and the counter-regulatory hormones, or stress hormones, must be in balance. These hormones, which include adrenaline, noradrenaline, cortisol, growth hormone and glucagon, are released in the event of stress (Sharp 1993).

During infection, major surgery or critical illness, people's regulatory hormone levels of cortisol, noradrenaline and glucagon will rise in response to the stressful event. This stimulates glycogen and fat breakdown, which causes the blood glucose levels to rise. In a healthy individual, insulin production would increase. In a person who is unable to raise his/her insulin levels, e.g. a diabetic, the result is hyperglycaemia (Curry & Weedon 1993). The majority of people who have diabetes will be known to be diabetic prior to this event, but as many as one million people in the UK have the condition and do not know it (Diabetes UK 2000). However, there may be a proportion who have had no history of such a disorder, only becoming diabetic in response to their primary illness and treatment. An example of this is steroid-induced diabetes. This diagnosis does not mean that they will remain a diabetic, but that they may need careful monitoring after their recovery.

Hypoglycaemia

Hypoglycaemia is described as a blood glucose level that is unable to meet the metabolic demands of the body (Marini & Wheeler 2006). Often young and healthy individuals can be asymptomatic during this inadequate level of glucose in the blood. Early symptoms are sweating, tremor, weakness, nervousness, tachycardia and hypertension. These symptoms depend upon not only the absolute blood glucose value but, also the rate of its decline. Severe hypoglycaemia causes mental disorientation, convulsions, unconsciousness and shock (Tortora & Derrickson 2008). The most common factors associated with hypoglycaemia include missed or delayed meals, eating less food at a meal than planned, vigorous exercise without carbohydrate compensation, taking too much diabetes medication (e.g. insulin) and drinking alcohol (Briscoe & Davis 2006).

Other causes of hypoglycaemia are:

- Infection, which can result in hepatic failure, renal insufficiency, depletion of muscle glycogen and starvation.
- Alcohol, which suppresses glyconeogenesis and nutritional intake. This induces a low insulin state, ketone production and fatty acid release.
- Hepatic failure, which can be due to tumour infiltration, cirrhosis or hepatic necrosis.
- Renal failure.
- Salicylate poisoning.
- Insulin-secreting tumours.
- Surgery.

(Marini & Wheeler 2006.)

Treatment should be by the administration of glucose. The route will depend on the conscious level of the individual and the treatment the patient has undergone. In all cases of hypoglycaemia it is vital to closely monitor the patient and recheck the serum glucose 1–2 hourly (Marini & Wheeler 2006).

Hyperglycaemia

When insulin is deficient or absent, blood glucose levels remain high after a meal. This is because insulin acts like a key, unlocking a door to allow glucose to enter the cell. If insulin is absent, the glucose is unable to enter most cells. When blood glucose levels rise, hyperglycaemic hormones are not released, but when glucose levels become excessive (hyperglycaemia) the person will feel nauseated, which precipitates the flight or fight response (Marieb & Hoehn 2007). The cells are starved of glucose and the body reacts inappropriately by producing reactions usually seen in states of fasting (hypoglycaemia). Processes such as glycogenolysis (the breakdown of glycogen to release glucose), lipolysis (the breakdown of stored fats into glycerol and fatty acids) and gluconeogenesis (the conversion of glycerol and amino acids into glucose) are instigated (Marieb & Hoehn 2007).

The blood glucose continues to rise and some of the glucose is excreted in the urine. As the level of glucose in the kidney increases, water reabsorption by the tubules becomes inhibited. This causes the body to excrete large amounts of urine (polyuria). The person will feel excessively thirsty (polydipsia) and will pass urine often and in large quantities. The person may also feel extremely hungry (polyphagia). The combination of polydipsia and polyuria will lead to dehydration, a fall in blood pressure and electrolyte imbalance. The acid–base imbalance caused by the loss of sodium (hyponatremia) and potassium (hypokalaemia) leads to the person complaining of symptoms spanning from muscle cramps, nausea, vomiting and diarrhoea to confusion, lethargy, cardiac events and coma (Marini & Wheeler 2006).

Even though there is excessive glucose in the body, the body cannot utilize it, so an alternative source of energy has to be found. To compensate, the body starts to break down its fats and protein stores for energy metabolism (Marieb & Hoehn 2007). Figure 25.22 summarizes the consequences of insulin deficiency. Fats are mobilized, which leads to high levels of fatty acids in the blood (lipidaemia). This can also cause sudden and dramatic weight loss. The fatty acid metabolites, known as ketones, accumulate in the blood more rapidly than they can be excreted or used. The blood pH will fall, resulting in ketoacidosis and ketones being excreted into the urine. If ketoacidosis is allowed to continue it can become life-threatening as it disrupts all physiological processes, including oxygen transportation and heart activity. Depression of the nervous system leads to coma and death (Marieb & Hoehn 2007).

Diabetic ketoacidosis is a common but serious condition, the mortality of which remains significant, despite aggressive treatment (Marini & Wheeler 2006). It is a result of a deficiency of insulin and a high level of stress hormones. In the diabetic patient it is usually precipitated by a poor diet and inadequate medication and can be brought on by infection. Stroke, MI, trauma, pregnancy, pancreatitis and hypothyroidism are also potential precipitants (Marini & Wheeler 2006). The most prominent metabolic changes caused by ketoacidosis are metabolic acidosis and volume depletion.

Treatment involves fluid replacement, restoration of the acid–base imbalance and careful monitoring. If patients in a ketoacidotic state do not respond to fluid replacement and correction of the pH, then other conditions such as septic shock, bleeding, adrenal insufficiency, MI and pancreatitis should be considered, and treated accordingly (Marini & Wheeler 2006).

The administration of intravenous insulin should be titrated by an infusion device, and measurements of blood glucose should be taken 1–2 hourly in order to guide the rate of insulin and fluid delivery. If the blood glucose level does not fall within the first few hours it may indicate insulin resistance and the amount of insulin may need to be increased (Marini & Wheeler 2006).

Organs/tissue involved	Organ/tissue responses to insulin deficiency	Resulting conditions:		Signs and symptoms
		In blood	In urine	
	Decreased glucose uptake and utilization	Hyperglycaemia	Glycosuria	
	Glycogenolysis		Osmotic diuresis	Polydipsia (and fatigue, weight loss)
	Protein catabolism and gluconeogenesis			Polyphagia
	Lipolysis and ketogenesis	Lipidaemia and ketoacidosis	Ketonuria	Acetone breath
				Hyperpnoea
			Loss of Na$^+$, K$^+$; electrolyte and acid–base imbalances	Nausea/vomiting/ abdominal pain
				Cardiac irregularities
				Central nervous system depression; coma

= Muscle   = Adipose tissue   = Liver

Figure 25.22 Consequences of insulin deficiency.

Note: care needs to be taken in the rapid reversal of fluid loss and electrolyte imbalance. Excessive fluids can cause sudden acid–base shifts and exacerbate hypokalaemia. Central nervous system acidosis and arrhythmias are preventable with constant monitoring. Once urine flow is re-established, potassium should be given. Magnesium and phosphate levels in the blood should also be monitored. A common complication after aggressive treatment is hypoglycaemia.

Blood glucose monitoring

Monitoring a patient's blood glucose provides an accurate indication of how the body is controlling glucose metabolism. In the short term, monitoring can prevent hypoglycaemia and ketoacidosis, and in the long term it can significantly reduce the risk of complications which affect the vascular and neural pathways by helping to maintain near-normal glucose levels (UKPDS 1998).

An advantage of blood glucose testing is that the use of blood can inform people with diabetes that their blood sugar is low or high, whereas a urine test can only indicate instances of high blood sugar (Burden 2001). The immediacy of results allows patients to receive appropriate care and advice. Blood samples can be taken from capillary, venous or arterial routes. The vessel used will depend on the accessibility of obtaining the blood sample, the frequency of testing and the condition of the patient. However, a meta-analysis questions the clinical efficiency and effectiveness of blood glucose self-monitoring (Coster *et al.* 2000).

It is essential that both the correct equipment is used and the operator is trained and proficient in its operation. Many different monitoring devices are currently available. Nursing and medical research has now been undertaken to identify the most accurate and practicable equipment (Trajanoski *et al.* 1996; Chan *et al.* 1997; Cowan 1997; Rumley 1997; Kirk & Rheney 1998; Batki *et al.* 1999).

Current methods for testing blood glucose rely on finger pricking but non-invasive blood glucose monitoring devices are being developed which would enable automatic detection of hypoglycaemia or hyperglycaemia (American Diabetes Association 2001). Non-invasive monitoring means checking blood glucose levels without puncturing the skin for a blood sample. One device approved is worn like a wristwatch and measures blood glucose via interstitial fluid (Pickup 2000).

Point-of-care testing (POCT), sometimes referred to as near-patient testing, is any test performed for a patient by a health care professional outside the laboratory setting (MDA 2002a). There is a significant risk for errors to occur when using POCT. The Department of Health (DH) issued a hazard warning in 1987 and again in a 1996 safety notice. These warnings highlighted the need for formal training and strict quality control (DH 1996). Quality assurance in relation to POCT is defined as the measures taken to ensure the test results are reliable (MDA 2002a); this also aims to maintain the competency of all users. These hazard notices drew attention to the fact that a management or therapeutic decision based on an unreliable blood glucose result can prove fatal. Inaccurate results are often due to incorrect timing of the test, insufficient amount of blood taken and smearing of the sample (Heenan 1990). Staff undertaking POCT should be aware that certain patient conditions may lead to false and misleading results. The testing of blood glucose in the blood may be affected by the following:

- Hyperlipaemia (containing abnormal fat concentrations, for example cholesterol above 56.5 mmol/l). May elevate readings.
- Haematocrit values. If extremely high, i.e. above 55%, and blood glucose values are above 11 mmol/l, the value may be up to 15% too low. If the haematocrit level is low, i.e. less than 35%, the value may be up to 10% too high.
- Dialysis treatment. May elevate readings.
- Bilirubin values above 0.43 mmol/l, e.g. in jaundice. May elevate readings.
- Intravenous infusion of ascorbic acid (vitamin C). May depress readings.
- When there has been peripheral circulatory failure, e.g. following severe dehydration caused by hyperglycaemic–hyperosmolar state with or without ketoacidosis, hypotension, shock or peripheral vascular disease. In these cases the results of the blood sample taken from the peripheral blood, e.g. from a finger prick, may be much lower than laboratory measurements taken from venous or arterial sources. In these cases treatment should be based on laboratory measurements only (Sandler et al. 1990).

The DH report (1996) highlights that there must be standardization in training, reliability and quality control. In order to achieve this, the following aspects need to be considered when selecting POCT blood glucose monitoring equipment:

1 Equipment is designed for use by non-laboratory staff and is suitable for use in the clinical environment.
2 All the equipment used is compatible and will give reliable results.
3 The biochemistry laboratory is involved in the purchase and maintenance of the equipment. This may involve the purchase of one type of device from one company for the whole hospital, to reduce costs and provide standardization (Lowes 1995).
4 The product should be easy to use and the staff should be involved in the choice of the device (Kirk & Rheney 1998).
5 The ongoing cost and maintenance of the device need to be considered; this should include buying strips, control solutions and the replacement of devices (Kirk & Rheney 1998).
6 There are written standard operating procedures available and kept with the device.
7 Training is given to the operators and records are kept of this. After training the following learning outcomes should be demonstrated by the operator (MDA 2002a):

(a) *Knowledge of the basic principle of measurement and normal ranges.*
(b) *The proper use of the equipment as laid down by the operating instructions and specifications (Bayne 1997).*
(c) *The consequences of improper use.*
(d) *Health and safety procedures for the collection of blood samples, i.e. to prevent spillage and needlestick injuries.*
(e) *The importance of complete documentation.*
(f) *Use of appropriate calibration and quality control techniques.*
(g) *An understanding that blood sugar analysis should only be used as a guide and a tool, with diagnosis and treatment decisions being based on confirmed laboratory results (DH 1996).*

There is a requirement to monitor the quality of the results of the device and the person operating it. This is both a hospital and a government directive (MDA 2002a). Independent quality control should be carried out with the collaboration of the biochemistry laboratory. External auditing of quality control should be undertaken and this may be provided in the package offered by the company.

Procedure guidelines   Blood glucose monitoring

Only nursing staff who have obtained a certificate of training for the equipment should undertake this task.

Equipment

1 Blood glucose monitor.
2 Test strips.
3 Control solution.
4 Single-use safety lancets.
5 Gloves.

Procedure

Action	Rationale
1 Before taking the device to the patient the monitor needs to be checked for the following: (a) That one pack of test strips is open and has not been left exposed to the air and that they are in date.	To ensure accuracy of the result. The quality control and checks have been carried out in order to ensure the safety of the patient (Roche Diagnostics 2004: C).

(b) That the monitor and the test strips have been calibrated together.

(c) That if a new pack of strips is required, the monitor is recalibrated.

(d) That a high and low internal quality control test is carried out prior to any patient sample being measured.

(e) That the result of the internal quality control is recorded in the equipment log book and signed.

2 Explain the procedure to the patient. Some patients may want to look away at the sight of a needle.	The patient should be aware of the procedure in order to allay some of his/her anxieties, and to be able to co-operate in the procedure (NMC 2008: C).
3 Patients should be advised to wash their hands prior to blood sampling. The use of alcohol rub should be avoided. Encourage patients to keep their hands warm until sampling has been performed.	To ensure a non-contaminated result. To encourage good blood flow (Cowan 1997: E).
4 Ask the patient to sit or lie down.	To ensure the patient's safety as some patients may feel faint when blood is taken (Roche Diagnostics 2004: C).
5 Wash your hands, and put on gloves.	To minimize the risk of cross-infection. To minimize the risk of contamination (DH 2005: C).
6 Use a single-use lancet (DH 1996) and if the lancet has depth settings ensure correct setting (most commonly the middle setting (Roche Diagnostics 2004).	To minimize the risk of cross-infection and accidental needlestick injury. Disposable lancets are advised following an outbreak of hepatitis B in French and US hospitals (DH 1996; Roche Diagnositcs 2004: C).
7 Take a blood sample from the side of the finger using the lancet, ensuring that the site of piercing is rotated. Avoid frequent use of the index finger and thumb. The finger may bleed without assistance, or may need assistance by 'milking' to form a droplet of blood which is large enough to cover the test pad.	The side of the finger is used as it is less painful and easier to obtain a hanging droplet of blood. The site is rotated to reduce the risk of infection from multiple stabbing, the areas becoming toughened and to reduce pain (Roche Diagnostics 2004: C).
8 Apply the blood to the testing strip. Some test strips are hydrophilic and are dosed/filled from the side and are not dropped directly onto the strip.	The window on the test strip allows verification of a correctly dosed strip (Roche Diagnostics 2004: C).
9 Dispose of lancet in a container designed for sharps.	To reduce the risk of needlestick injury (Roche Diagnostics 2004: C).
10 Depending on the type of monitor, the procedure will differ. See individual manuals and hospital policies.	To ensure the accuracy of the result (Roche Diagnostics 2004: C).
11 Once the result is obtained, record immediately.	To ensure the accuracy of the result (Roche Diagnostics 2004: C).
12 Dispose of waste appropriately. Remove gloves and dispose.	To reduce the risk of cross-infection (DH 2005: C).
13 Make the patient comfortable and observe site of test for bleeding.	To ensure the patient's comfort (E).
14 Wash and dry hands.	To prevent cross-infection (DH 2005: C).

Central venous pressure

Definition

Central venous pressure (CVP) is the pressure of blood returning to or filling the right atrium. It indicates blood volume, vascular tone and cardiac function (Hudek *et al.* 1998).

CVP is usually used to assess blood volume and to guide fluid management, particularly in patients with hypovolaemia following trauma, shock, burns or sepsis (Kumar & Clark 2005). It is important to remember that CVP can be affected by:

- Intrathoracic pressure.
- Vascular tone.
- Obstruction.

(Woodrow 2002.)

Reference material

CVP monitoring is often misleading if interpreted as an isolated reading. In order to obtain maximum benefits, trend measurements over a period of time should be studied and correlated with the patient's clinical status (Udwadia 2005), as a reflection of level of hydration and cardiac function. Clinical observations such as auscultation of breath sounds, heart and respiratory rate, ECG, neck vein distension and urine output are all paramount when interpreting the meaning of the CVP recording (Morton *et al.* 2005).

The CVP should be measured at the right atrial level, as it is a measure of the pressure of blood returning to the right atrium (Woodrow 2002). CVP is usually recorded at the mid-axilla (Figure 25.23).

Ideally, the patient should lie flat in a supine position to reflect the right atrial pressure. However, many breathless patients cannot tolerate lying supine, therefore the measurement can also be taken in a semi-recumbent or recumbent position (Hatchett 2000). If the patient is supine an alternative position is via the sternal angle. It is important to use just one method, to promote consistency, as readings from the sternal angle are about 5 cm lower than those taken from the mid-axilla (Hatchett 2000; Woodrow 2002). It is vital that the site from which the measurement is being recorded is marked and documented to maintain the continuity and accuracy of the trend of the CVP (Mooney 2003). It is essential that the patient is fully informed before a CVP measurement is carried out, ensuring that any anxieties are relieved and the patient is aware of the procedure to be undertaken.

CVP measurements can be recorded either manually, using a water manometer set, or electronically, using a transducer. Electronic measurement is most commonly used in the critical care environment.

Zeroing a CVP

Zeroing a CVP is an essential part of measurement. This is a technique used to ensure the atmospheric pressure at the point of measurement is read as zero. In critical care areas CVPs are usually measured by monitors that can be set to zero electronically once the transducer is placed at right atrial level, with flow from the transducer open to air, but closed to the patient (Woodrow 2002). When measuring with water manometers, which are used on the wards, the zero should align with the right atrial level. This is usually checked by a spirit level.

Reading CVP

After zeroing, the chamber should be filled with fluid nearly to the top. This is done by turning the flow tap to allow fluid, such as saline to flow into the measuring chamber, while closing the flow to the patient. Care should be taken not to get the air filter at the top wet, as a wet filter will resist air entry and give a false raised reading. The tap should then be turned so the fluid flow is stopped and the chamber opened to the patient. Gravity will cause the water level to fall until resistance from the patient's CVP matches the pressure

Figure 25.23 Measuring a CVP using a water manometer. Adapted from Edwards and Manley (1998).

of gravity. However, slight changes in pressure caused by the patient's respiration, usually 1 cm, will make the fluid fall in a swinging pattern, until it oscillates between two figures. The intrathoracic pressure represented by the fluid level in the chamber falls on inspiration so the higher figure should be recorded. CVP can be measured in either millimetres of mercury (mmHg) or centimetres of water (cmH$_2$O) (Woodrow 2002).

Normal pressures

A normal CVP value should be 5–10 mmHg mid-axilla or 0–5 mmHg sternal angle (Henderson 1997), which is 7–14 cmH$_2$O mid-axilla or 0–7 cmH$_2$O sternal angle. A low CVP usually indicates fluid loss through haemorrhage or excessive diuresis; poor venous return and peripheral vasodilatation can also lower the CVP. In some patients there can be a discrepancy between CVP and left-side heart filling pressures. False high CVP can be seen in patients with the following conditions:

- Tricuspid valve regurgitation.
- Congestive cardiac failure.
- Pulmonary valve stenosis.
- Pulmonary artery hypertension.
- Severe pulmonary embolism.
- COPD.

(O'Neill & Le Grove 2003.)

These patients can have a high CVP measurement yet be hypovolaemic. For this reason, comparing changes in a CVP measurement with a baseline measurement is more beneficial than noting the initial recording (O'Neill & Le Grove 2003). Various other factors like lumen occlusion/obstruction and user error can also give high CVP readings (Woodrow 2002).

Procedure guidelines   Central venous pressure measurement

Equipment

1 Spirit level.
2 Manometer.
3 Drip stand.
4 Central venous pressure (CVP) monitoring intravenous administration set.
5 Intravenous fluid.

Procedure

Action	Rationale
1 Explain and discuss the procedure with the patient.	To ensure that the patient understands the procedure and gives his/her valid consent (NMC 2006: C; NMC 2008: C).
2 Wash and dry hands.	To maintain infection control and minimize the risk of cross-infection (DH 2005: C).
3 Ascertain the point of CVP reading, i.e. sternal angle or mid-axilla. If the patient agrees, this point should be marked on the patient and noted in the care plan chart for future reference.	CVP must always be read from the same point because the sternal angle reading is about 5 cmH$_2$O higher than the mid-axilla reading (Edwards 2000: E).
4 Assist the patient to get into a supine, recumbent or semi-recumbent position to a maximum angle of 45°.	The position of the patient must allow the baseline of the manometer to be level with the patient's right atrium. If the patient is upright or is lying on his/her side, the right atrium will not be in line with the sternal angle or the mid-axilla. However, if it is impossible for the patient to be in any other position, the CVP reading may be recorded with the patient sitting up at a 90° angle, but this must be recorded on the observation chart (Edwards 2000: E).
5 Position the manometer so that the baseline is level with the right atrium.	To obtain an accurate CVP reading, the baseline and the right atrium must be level (Edwards 2000: R; E).
6 Loosen the securing screw and slide the scale up or down until the baseline zero is lined up with the zero on the arm of the spirit level (see Figure 25.23).	To remove the effect of extraneous pressure and to ensure the baseline is always the same in order to have a single point of reference (Edwards 2000: R; E).

Procedure guidelines *(cont.)*

7 Check that the baseline and right atrium are level by extending the arm of the spirit level to the sternal angle or to the mid-axilla. Move the manometer until the bubble is between the parallel lines of the spirit level (see Figure 25.23).	To ensure a more accurate reading (Edwards 2000: E).
8 Care should be taken when flushing the catheter regarding the volume and type of fluid.	To ensure the patency of the catheter and to check for leaks, kinks, blockages, etc. To ensure that correct solution is used to flush, e.g. 0.9% sodium chloride or dextrose, and not a solution containing drugs (Edwards 2000: E).
9 Turn off the three-way tap to the patient (see Figure 25.23). Allow the manometer to fill slowly.	To allow the intravenous fluid to run into the manometer. To avoid: (a) Bubbles, which cause inaccurate readings. (b) Overfilling of, and spillage from, the manometer that would put the patient at risk from infection (Edwards 2000: E).
10 Turn off the three-way tap to the intravenous fluid (see Figure 25.23).	To allow fluid from the manometer to enter the patient's right atrium (Edwards 2000: E).
11 The column of water should fall rapidly.	Indicating patency of the catheter, resulting in an accurate CVP reading (Edwards 2000: E).
12 When the level of fluid in the manometer ceases to drop, and oscillates with the patient's respirations, the reading can be taken.	The pressure of the column of water in the manometer now equals the pressure in the right atrium (Edwards 2000: E).
13 Turn off the three-way tap to the manometer.	To restore infusion via the intravenous catheter (Edwards 2000: E).
14 Readjust the infusion rate.	To ensure correct rate setting (E).
15 Wash and dry hands.	To maintain infection control and minimize the risk of cross-infection (DH 2005: C).
16 Record the CVP measurement on the appropriate chart. Compare this measurement with the patient's acceptable CVP limits as stated by the medical team.	Acceptable CVP values vary with the patient observations and his/her overall condition. Deviations from these limits may require urgent medical intervention (E).

Problem solving: Central venous pressure (CVP)

Problem	Cause	Suggested action
Inaccurate central venous pressure (CVP) readings.	Patient in a position different from that in which the initial reading was taken. Reference point on the patient not observed.	Position should be documented in the patient's records. Zero of the manometer must be level with the patient's right atrium at the point marked on the patient, i.e. mid-axilla or sternal angle.
	Faulty pressure reading technique.	If the CVP reading is outside the limits deemed acceptable for that patient and it is considered to be an accurate reading, recheck it after 15 or 30 minutes and inform a doctor if unchanged.

Problem	Cause	Suggested action
Elevated CVP.	Increased intrathoracic pressure caused by coughing, increased movement or pain.	Encourage coughing before taking the reading. Ensure that the patient is comfortable and pain free.
	Lower extremities elevated.	Position the patient so that he/she is lying in a supine position.
	Patient having intermittent positive-pressure ventilation.	Read the CVP at the end expiratory level (lowest point of fluctuation). This will always be higher than the 'normal' reading.
	Anxiety and/or restlessness.	Verify the cause of the anxiety or restlessness and take action to reassure patient.
	Blood in progress via the CVP catheter.	Flush the catheter with 0.9% sodium chloride and read again.
	Shivering and/or muscular spasm, e.g. post-anaesthetic reaction (see Chapter 30).	Assess the patient's condition, e.g. pulse, blood pressure, temperature. Check that the patient is warm enough. Inform a doctor.
Low CVP reading.	Leak in the system or equipment adjusted inaccurately.	Check and readjust the system.
	Changing of the patient's position from recumbent to semi-recumbent.	Reread with the patient in the recumbent position.

References

Adam, S. & Osborne, S. (2005) *Critical Care Nursing: Science and Practice*. Oxford University Press, Oxford.

American Diabetes Association (2001) Clinical practice recommendations. *Diabetes Care*, **24**, 580–2.

Angerami, E.L.S. (1980) Epidemiological study of body temperature in patients in a teaching hospital. *Int J Nurs Stud*, **17**, 91–9.

Armstrong, R.S. (2002) Nurse's knowledge of error in blood pressure measurement technique. *Int J Nurs Prac*, **8**(3), 118–26.

Baillie, L. (2001) *Developing Practical Nursing Skills*. Arnold, London.

Batki, A. *et al* (1999) Selecting blood glucose monitoring systems. *Prof Nurse*, **14**(10), 715–23.

Bayer Diagnostics (1997) *Urinary Tract Infection*. Technical Information Bulletin No. 8. Bayer Diagnostics, Newbury.

Bayer Diagnostics (2006) *Your Practical Guide to Urine Analysis*. Bayer Diagnostics, Newbury.

Bayham, E. *et al.* (1996) *First Temp Genius. Clinical Considerations for Use of First Temp & First Temp Genius Infrared Tympanic Thermometers*. Sherwood Medical Company, USA.

Bayne, C. (1997) How sweet it is: glucose monitoring equipment and interpretation. *Nurs Manage*, **28**(9), 52–4.

BCSH (1999) The administration of blood and blood components and the management of transfused patients. *Transfus Med*, **9**, 227–38.

Beevers, M. & Beevers, G.B. (1996) Blood pressure measurement in the next century, a plea for stability. *Blood Press Monit*, **1**(2), 117–20.

Beevers, G., Lip, G.Y.H. & O'Brien, E. (2001a) Blood pressure measurement, part 1. Sphygmomanometry: factors common to all techniques. *BMJ*, **322**(7292), 981–5.

Beevers, G., Lip, G.Y.H. & O'Brien, E. (2001b) Blood pressure measurement, part 2. Conventional spyygmomanometry: technique of auscultatory blood pressure measurement. *BMJ*, **322**(7292), 1043–7.

Berger, A. (2001) How does it work? Oscillatory blood pressure monitoring devices. *BMJ*, **323**(7318), 9–19.

Bickley, L. & Szilagyi, P. (2007) *Bates' Guide to Physical Examination and History Taking*, 9th edn. Lippincott Williams & Wilkins, Philadelphia.

Bogan, B., Kritzer, S. & Deane, D. (1993) Nursing student compliance to standards for blood pressure measurement. *J Nurse Educ*, **32**(2), 90–2.

Bone, R.C. (1996) The pathogenesis of sepsis and rationale for new treatments. Proceedings of the International Intensive Care Conference, Barcelona.

Booker, R. (2004) Best practice in the use of spirometry. *Nurs Stand*, **19**(48), 149–54.

Braun, S.K., Preston, P. & Smith, R.N. (1998) Getting a better read on thermometry. *Reg Nur*, **61**(3), 57–60.

Briscoe, V.J & Davis, S.N. (2006) Hypoglycemia in type 1 and 2 diabetes: physiology, pathophysiology and management. *Clinical Diabetes*, **24**(3), 115–21.

British Hypertension Society (BHS) (2006) FACT FILE 01/2006. www.bhsoc.org/bhf-factfiles/bhf-factfile-Jan2006.doc. Accessed 21/11/07.

British Thoracic Society (2004) British guidelines on the management of asthma, revised edition. www.brit-thoracic.org.uk/guidelines%201997_asthma_html. Accessed 01/07.

British Thoracic Society Standards of Care Committee (1997) Current best practice for nebuliser treatment. *Thorax*, **52**(Suppl 2), S1-S3.

Burden, M. (2001) Diabetes blood glucose monitoring. *Nurs Times*, **97**(8), 36–9.

Burke, K. (1996) The tympanic membrane thermometer in paediatrics: a review of the literature. *Accid Emerg Nurs*, **4**(4), 190–3.

Campbell, N.R. *et al.* (1990) Accurate, reproducible measurement of blood pressure. *Can Med Assoc J*, **143**(1), 19–24.

Carney, S.L. *et al.* (1995) Hospital sphygmomanometer use; an audit. *J Qual Clin Pract*, **15**(1), 17–22.

Carroll, M. (2000) An evaluation of temperature measurement. *Nurs Stand*, **14**(44), 39–43.

Chan, J. *et al.* (1997) Accuracy, precision and user-acceptability of self blood glucose monitoring machines. *Diabetes Res Clin Pract*, **36**(2), 91–104.

Cook, R. (1996) Urinalysis: ensuring accurate urine testing. *Nurs Stand*, **10**(46), 49–55.

Coster, S. *et al.* (2000) Self monitoring in type 2 diabetes mellitus: a meta-analysis. *Diabet Med*, **17**(11), 755–61.

Cowan, T. (1997) Blood glucose monitoring devices. *Prof Nurse*, **12**(8), 593–7.

Cuddy, M. (2004) The effects of drugs on thermoregulation. *Advanced Practice in Acute Critical Care*, **15**(2), 238–53.

Curry, M. & Weedon, L. (1993) Balancing act. *Nurs Times*, **89**(23), 50–2.

DH (1996) *Extra-Laboratory Use of Blood Glucose Meters and Test Strips: Contraindications, Training and Advice to Users.* Medical Devices Agency Adverse Incident Centre Safety Notice 9616, June. Department of Health, London.

DH (2005) *Saving Lives: a Delivery Programme to Reduce Healthcare Associated Infection Including MRSA: Skills for Implementation.* Department of Health, London. See www.dh.gov.uk/publications. Accessed 01/07.

Diabetes UK (2000) *Diabetes in the UK – The Missing Millions.* Diabetes UK, London.

Dickinson, A. & Martindale, G. (2002) Caring for the patient with a respiratory disorder. In: *Watson's Clinical Nursing and Related Sciences* (ed. M. Walsh), 6th edn. Bailliere Tindal, Edinburgh, pp. 333–370.

Dobbin, K. (2002) Noninvasive blood pressure monitoring protocols for practice: applying research at the bedside. *Crit Care Nurse*, **22**(2), 123–4.

Docherty, B. (2000) Temperature recording. *Prof Nurse*, **16**(3), 943.

Docherty, B. (2002) Cardiorespiratory physical assessment for the acutely ill. *Br J Nurs*, **11**(11), 750–8.

Docherty, B. (2005) The arteriovenous system: part one, the anatomy. *Nurs Times*, **101**(34), 28–9.

Docherty, B. & Coote, S. (2006) Monitoring the pulse as part of the track and trigger. *Nurs Times*, **102**(43), 28–9. See www.nursingtimes.net/nursingtimes/pages/monitoringthepulseaspartof-trackandtrigger. Accessed 18/12/06.

Edmonds, C. *et al.* (2006) Disorders of the respiratory system. In: *Nursing Practice, Hospital & Home, the Adult* (eds M. Alexander, J. Fawcett & P. Runciman). Churchill Livingstone, London, pp. 73–103.

Edwards, S. (1997) Measuring temperature. *Prof Nurse*, **13**(2), 55–7.

Edwards, S.L. (2000) Maintaining an adequate circulation. In: *Surgical Nursing Advanced Practice* (eds K. Manley & L. Bellman). Churchill Livingstone, London, pp. 507–37.

Edwards, L. & Manley, K.L. (1998) *Care of Adults in Hospital.* Edward Arnold, London.

Evans, D. *et al.* (2004) *Vital Signs.* The Joanna Briggs Institute, Australia.

Feher, M. & Harris St. John, K. (1992) Blood pressure measurement by junior hospital doctors: a gap in medical education? *Health Trends*, **24**(2), 59–61.

Ferguson, A. (2005) Blood glucose monitoring. *Nurs Times*, **101**(38), 28–9.

Fillingham, S. & Douglas, J. (2003) *Urological Nursing*, 3rd edn. Bailliere Tindal, London.

Gallimore, D. (2004) Reviewing the effectiveness of tympanic thermometers. *Nurs Times*, **100**(32), 32–5.

Gilbert, M., Barton, A.J. & Counsell, C.M. (2002) Comparison of oral and tympanic temperatures in adult surgical patients. *Appl Nurs Res*, **15**(1), 42–7.

Gillespie, A. & Curzio, J. (1998) Blood pressure measurement: assessing staff knowledge. *Nurs Stand*, **12**(23), 35–7.

GINA (2006) Global strategy for asthma management and prevention. www.ginasthma.org. Accessed 4/12/06.

Grap, M. (2002) Protocols for practice, applying research at the bedside. *Crit Care Nurse*, **22**(3), 69–74.

Gregg, I. & Nunn, A.J. (1989) New regression equations for predicting peak flow expiratory flow in adults. *BMJ*, **298**, 1068–70.

Harper, J. (2004) Post-anaesthesia care unit nurses' knowledge of pulse oximetry. *J Nurs Staff Dev*, **20**(4), 177–80.

Hasler, M. & Cohen, J. (1982) The effect of oxygen administration on oral temperature assessment. *Nurs Res*, **31**, 265–8.

Hatchett, R. (2000) Central venous pressure measurement. *Nurs Times*, **96**(15), 49–50.

Heenan, A. (1990) Blood glucose measurement. *Nurs Times*, **86**(4), 65–8.

Heindenreich, T. & Giuffe, M. (1990) Postoperative temperature measurement. *Nurs Res*, **39**(3), 153–5.

Henderson, N. (1997) Central venous lines. *Nurs Stand*, **11**(42), 49–56.

Hill, M.N. & Grim, C.M. (1991) How to take a precise blood pressure. *Am J Nurs*, **91**(2), 38–42.

Howell, M. (2002) The correct use of pulse oximetry in measuring oxygen status. *Prof Nurse*, **17**(7), 416–18.

Hudek, C.M., Gallo, B.M. & Morton, P.G. (1998). *Critical Care Nursing: a Holistic Approach*, 7th edn. Lippincott, New York.

Jensen, B.N. *et al.* (1994) The superiority of rectal thermometry to oral thermometry with regard to accuracy. *J Adv Nurs*, **20**, 660–5.

Jevon, P. (2000) Pulse oximetry – 2. *Nurs Times*, **96**(27), 43–4.

Jevon, P. & Jevon, M. (2001) Using a tympanic thermometer. *Nurs Times*, **97**(9), 43–4.

Keenan, J. (1995) Pulse oximetry (cardiology update). *Nurs Stand*, **9**, 35–55.

Kemp, F., Foster, C. & McKinlay, S. (1994) How effective is training for blood pressure measurement? *Prof Nurs*, **9**(8), 521–4.

Khorshid, L. *et al.* (2005) Comparing mercury-in-glass, tympanic and disposable thermometers in measuring body temperature in healthy young people. *J Clin Nurs*, **14**(4), 496–500.

Kirk, J. & Rheney, C. (1998) Important factors of blood glucose meters. *J Am Pharm Assoc*, **8**(2), 210–19.

Knies, R. (2003) Temperature measurement in acute care: the who, what, where, when, why, and how? www.enw.org/Research-Thermometry.htm. Accessed 30/1/07.

Krikler, S. (1990) Pyrexia: what to do about temperatures. *Nurs Stand*, **4**(25), 37–8.

Kumar, P. & Clark, M. (2005) *Clinical Medicine*, 6th edn. Elsevier Saunders, Edinburgh.

Lemery, R. *et al.* (2003) Anatomic description of Bachmann's bundle and its relation to the atria septum. *Am J Cardiol*, **91**(12), 1482–5.

Lim-Levy, F. (1982) The effect of oxygen inhalation on oral temperature. *Nurs Res*, **31**, 150–2.

Lowes, L. (1995) Accuracy in ward-based blood glucose monitoring. *Nurs Times*, **91**(13), 44–5.

Mancia, G. *et al.* (1987) Alerting reaction and rise in blood pressure during measurement by physician and nurse. *Hypertension*, **9**, 209–15.

Marieb, E.M. & Hoehn, K. (2007) *Human Anatomy and Physiology.* Pearson Benjamin Cummings, San Francisco.

Marini, J.J. & Wheeler, A.P. (2006) *Critical Care Medicine: the Essentials.* Lippincott Williams & Wilkins, Philadelphia.

Markandu, N.D. *et al.* (2000) The mercury sphygmomanometer should be abandoned before it is prescribed. *J Hum Hypertens*, 14(3136), 31–6.

Maxon, P. (2004) Mercury flows in Europe and the World: the impact of decommissioned Chlor-Alkali plants. European Commission, Brussels.

McAlister, F.A. & Straus, S. (2001) Evidence based treatment for hypertension – measurement of blood pressure an evidence based review. *BMJ*, 322, 908–11.

MDA (2002a) Self monitoring in type 2 diabetes mellitus: a meta-analysis. *Diabet Med*, 17(11), 755–61.

MDA (2002b) *Management and Use of IVD Point-of-Care Test Devices*. Medical Devices Agency, London.

Metcalfe, H. (2000) Recording a 12-lead electrocardiogram – 1. *Nurs Times*, 96(19), 43–4.

MHRA (2001) Tissue necrosis caused by pulse oximeter probes. SN2001(08). www.mhra.gov.uk/home. Go to publications and safety notices. Accessed 7/12/2006.

MHRA (2005) Report of the independent advisory group on blood pressure monitoring in clinical practice. www.mhra.gov.uk/home. Go to medical advice alerts. Accessed 7/12/06.

MHRA (2006) Medical device alert ref. MDA/2006/037. Blood pressure monitors and sphygmomanometers.www.mhra.gov.uk/home. Accessed 7/12/2006.

Minor, D.G. & Waterhouse, J.M. (1981) *Circadian Rhythms and the Human*. Wright, Bristol.

Mooney, G. (2003) What you need to know about central venous lines. *Nurs Times*, 99(10), 28–29.

Morton, P.G., Tucker, T. & Van Rueden, R. (2005) *Critical Care Nursing: a Holistic Approach*, 8th edn. Lippincott Williams & Wilkins, Philadelphia.

Nakamura, K. *et al.* (1997) Oral temperatures in the elderly in nursing homes in summer and winter in relation to activities of daily living. *Int J Biometerol*, 40(2), 103–6.

Neff, J. *et al.* (1989) Effect of respiratory rate, respiratory depth, and open versus closed mouth breathing on sublingual temperature. *Res Nurse Health*, 12, 195–202.

Neno, R. (2005) Hypothermia: assessment, treatment and prevention. *Nurs Stand*, 19(20), 47–52.

NICE (2006) CG 34. *Hypertension: Management of Hypertension in Adults in Primary Care*. National Institute of Health and Clinical Excellence, London.

NMC (2005) *Guidelines for Records and Record Keeping*. Nursing and Midwifery Council, London.

NMC (2006) *A–Z Advice Sheet Consent*. www.nmc.org.

NMC (2008) *The Code: Standards of Conduct, Performance and Ethics for Nurses and Midwives*. Nursing and Midwifery Council, London.

O'Brien, E. *et al.* (2001) Blood pressure measuring devices: recommendations of the European Society of Hypertension. *BMJ*, 322(7285), 531–6.

O'Brien, E. *et al.* (2003) European Society of Hypertension recommendations for conventional, ambulatory and home blood pressure measurement. *J Hypertens*, 21, 821–48.

O'Neill, D. & Le Grove, A. (2003) Monitoring critically ill patients in accident and emergency. *Nurs Times*, 99(45), 32–5.

O'Toole, S. (1997) Alternatives to mercury thermometers. *Prof Nurse*, 12(11), 783–6.

Perloff, D. *et al.* (1993) Human blood pressure determined by sphygmomanometry. *Circulation*, 88(5), 2460–70.

Petrie, J.C. *et al.* (1997) *British Hypertension Society: Recommendations on Blood Pressure Measurement*, 2nd edn. British Hypertension Society, London.

Philip, J.P. & Kowery, P.R. (2001) *Cardiac Arrhythmia: Mechanisms, Diagnosis and Management*, 2nd edn. Lippincott Williams & Wilkins, Philadelphia.

Pickup, J. (2000) Sensitive glucose sensing in diabetes. *Lancet*, 355(9202), 426–7.

Place, B. (2000) Pulse oximetry: benefits and limitations. *Nurs Times*, 96(26), 42.

Resuscitation Council UK (2005) *Resuscitation Guidelines*. RCUK Publications, London.

Richardson, M. (2006a) The respiratory system. Part 1: nose, pharynx and larynx. *Nurs Times*, 102 (21), 24–5.

Richardson, M. (2006b) The respiratory system. Part 2: trachea to alveoli. *Nurs Times*, 102 (22), 24–5.

Rigby, D. & Gray, K. (2005) Understanding urine testing. *Nurs Times*, 101(12), 60–1.

Roberts, A. (2002) The role of anatomy and physiology in interpreting ECGs. *Nurs Times*, 98(20), 34–36.

Roche Diagnostics (2004) Accu-Chem Safe T-Pro Plus: Information Leaflet. Roche, East Sussex.

Rumley, A. (1997) Improving the quality of new patient blood glucose measurement. *Ann Clin Biochem*, 34(Part 2), 281–6.

Samples, F. *et al.* (1985) Circadian rhythms: basis for screening for fever. *Nurs Res*, 34(6), 377–9.

Sandler, M. *et al.* (1990) Misleading capillary glucose measurements. *Pract Diab Int*, 7, 210.

Sharber, J. (1997) The efficacy of tepid sponge bathing to reduce fever in young children. *Am J Emerg Med*, 15(2), 188–92.

Sharp, S. (1993) Blood glucose monitoring in the intensive care unit. *Br J Nurs*, 2(4), 209–14.

Sims, J. (1996) Making sense of pulse oximetry and oxygen dissociation curve. *Nurs Times*, 92(1), 34–5.

Stevenson, T. (2004) Achieving best practice in routine observation of hospital patients. *Nurs Times*, 100(30), 34–5.

Thibodeau, G. & Patton, K.T. (2007) *Anatomy and Physiology*, 6th edn. Mosby Elsevier, St. Louis MO.

Thompson, D.R. (1981) Recording patients' blood pressure: a review. *J Adv Nurs*, 6(4), 283–90.

Torrance, C. & Elley, K. (1998) Urine testing 2 – urinalysis. *Nurs Times*, 94(5), Supp 1–2.

Torrance, C. & Semple, M. (1998) Recording temperature. *Nurs Times*, 94(2), Supp 1–2.

Torrance, C. & Serginson, E. (1996) Student nurses' knowledge in relation to blood pressure measurement by sphygmomanometry and auscultation. *Nurse Educ Today*, 16(6), 397–402.

Tortora, G.J. & Derrickson, B. (2008) *Principles of Anatomy and Physiology*, 12th edn. John Wiley & Sons, Inc., New York.

Trajanoski, Z. *et al.* (1996) Accuracy of home blood glucose meters during hypoglycaemia. *Diabetes Care*, 19(12), 1412–15.

Trim, J. (2005) Monitoring temperature. *Nurs Times*, 101(20), 30–31.

Udwadia, F.E. (2005) *Principles of Critical Care*, 2nd edn. Oxford University Press, Oxford.

UKPDS (1998) Tight blood pressure control and risk of macrovascular and microvascular complications in type 2 diabetes. *BMJ*, 317(7160), 703–13.

Valler-Jones, T. & Wedgbury, K. (2005) Measuring blood pressure using the mercury sphygmomanometer. *Br J Nurs*, 14(3), 145–50.

Van Staaij, B.K. *et al.* (2003) Accuracy and feasibility of daily infrared tympanic membrane temperature measurements in identification of fever in children. *Int J Pediatr Otorhinolaryngol*, 67, 1091–7.

Wagner, D. (2006) Unplanned perioperative hypothermia. *AORN J*, 83(2), 470–6.

Walsh, M. (2002) *Watson's Clinical Nursing and Related Sciences*, 6th edn. Bailliere Tindall, London.

Watson, R. (1998) Controlling body temperature in adults. *Nurs Stand*, 12(20), 49–55.

Weber, J. & Kelley, J. (2003) *Health Assessment in Nursing*, 2nd edn. Lippincott Williams & Wilkins, Philadelphia.

Williams, B. *et al.* (2004) Guidelines for management of hypertension: report of the fourth working party of the British Hypertension Society, BHS IV. *J Hum Hypertens*, 18, 139–85.

Wilson, L.A. (2005) Urinalysis. *Nurs Stand*, 19(35), 51–4.

Woodrow, P. (1999) Pulse oximetry. *Nurs Stand*, 13(42), 42–6.

Woodrow, P. (2002) Central venous catheters and central venous pressure. *Nurs Stand*, 16(26), 45–51.

Woollens, S. (1996) Temperature measurement devices. *Prof Nurse*, 11(8), 541–7.

Yarbro, C.H., Frogge, M.H.M. & Goodman, M. (2005) *Cancer Nursing: Principles and Practice*, 6th edn. Jones and Barlett, Sudbury.

Chapter 26

Observations: neurological

Reference material 546
Procedure guidelines: Neurological observations and assessment 553
References and further reading 556

546

Definition

Neurological observation relates to the assessment and evaluation of the integrity and function of an individual's nervous system (Rowley & Fielding 1991).

Indications

An accurate neurological assessment is essential in planning patient care. Neurological observations are required to monitor and evaluate changes in the nervous system by indicating trends, thus aiding diagnosis and treatment, which in turn may affect prognosis and rehabilitation (Carlson 2002a; Kaye 2005).

Reference material

Changes in neurological status can be rapid and dramatic or subtle, developing over minutes, hours, days, weeks or even months depending on the insult (Aucken & Crawford 1998). Therefore the frequency of neurological observations will depend upon the patient's condition and the rapidity with which changes are occurring or expected to occur.

Neurological function is assessed by observing five critical areas:

- Level of consciousness.
- Pupillary activity.
- Motor function.
- Sensory function.
- Vital signs.

Consciousness

Consciousness is a state of awareness of self and the environment and is dependent upon two components:

- Arousability.
- Awareness.

(Carlson 2002a.)

Arousability

This depends on the integrity of the reticular activating system (RAS). The core of nuclei which make up the RAS extends from the brainstem to the thalamic nuclei in the cerebral hemispheres (Figure 26.1). Thus cognitive ability depends on the ability of the cerebral cortex to permit reciprocal stimulation and conscious behaviour. Consciousness therefore depends on the intactness of the cerebral cortex and the RAS and their ability to communicate effectively (Carlson 2002b; Fairley & McLernon 2005).

Awareness

This requires an intact cerebral cortex to interpret sensory input and respond accordingly. This is the content of the consciousness (Scherer 1986; Bateman 2001).

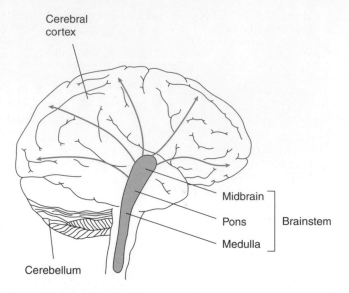

Figure 26.1 Reticular activating system.

Levels of consciousness may vary and are dependent on the location and extent of any neurological damage (Aucken & Crawford 1998). Previous and/or co-existing problems should be heeded when noting levels of consciousness, for example deafness, hemiparesis/hemiplegia.

Level of consciousness

Alterations in level of consciousness can vary from slight to severe changes, indicating the degree of brain dysfunction (Aucken & Crawford 1998). Consciousness ranges on a continuum from alert wakefulness to deep coma with no apparent responsiveness. Therefore, nurses must ensure that families and friends are involved at initial history taking and throughout care so as to chronicle accurately any change in neurological symptoms.

Terms such as 'fully conscious', 'semiconscious', 'lethargic' or 'stuporous' to describe levels of consciousness are subjective and open to misinterpretation. Thus, level of consciousness is often measured using the Glasgow Coma Scale (GCS), which was developed in 1974 at the University of Glasgow by Teasdale and Jennett (1974) (Table 26.1; Figure 26.2). The GCS was designed to grade the severity of impaired consciousness in patients with traumatic head injuries or intracranial surgery (Aucken & Crawford 1998). The GCS is now used worldwide; it is objective and provides a reliable and easy-to-use measure of conscious level. For example, a GCS score less than 8 is equated with a state of coma (NICE 2003). When used consistently, the GCS provides a graphical representation that shows improvement or deterioration of the patient's conscious level at a glance (see Figure 26.2). The National Institute for Health and Clinical Excellence (NICE) (2003) advocates the use of the GCS for assessment and classification of all head injury patients.

Table 26.1 Scoring activities of the Glasgow Coma Scale. Scores are added, with the highest score 15 indicating full consciousness. From Aucken and Crawford (1998) and Carlson (2002a).

Category	Score	Response
Eye opening:		
Spontaneous	4	Eyes open spontaneously without stimulation
To speech	3	Eyes open to verbal stimulation (normal, raised or repeated)
To pain	2	Eyes open with painful/noxious stimuli
None	1	No eye opening regardless of level of stimulation
Verbal response:		
Orientated	5	Able to give accurate information regarding time, person and place
Confused	4	Able to answer in sentences using correct language but cannot answer orientation questions appropriately
Inappropriate words	3	Uses incomprehensible words in a random or disorganized fashion
Incomprehensible sounds	2	Makes unintelligible sounds, e.g. moans and groans
None	1	No verbal response despite verbal or other stimuli
Best motor response:		
Obeys commands	6	Obeys and can repeat simple commands, e.g. arm raise
Localizes to pain	5	Purposeful movement to remove painful stimuli
Normal flexion	4	Withdraws extremity from source of pain, e.g. flexes arm at elbow without wrist rotation in response to painful stimuli
Abnormal flexion	3	Decorticate posturing (flexion of arms, hyperextension of legs) spontaneously or in response to noxious stimuli
Extension	2	Decerebrate posturing (limbs extended and internally rotated) spontaneously or in response to noxious stimuli
None	1	No response to noxious stimuli. Flaccid limbs

Assessment of level of consciousness

Assessment using the GCS involves three phases (Teasdale & Jennett 1974):

1 Eye opening.
2 Evaluation of verbal response.
3 Evaluation of motor response.

Evaluation of eye opening

Eye opening indicates that the arousal mechanism in the brain is active. Eye opening may be: spontaneous; to speech, e.g. spoken name; to painful stimulus; or not at all. Arousal (eye opening) is always the first measurement undertaken when performing the GCS, as without arousal, cognition cannot occur (Aucken & Crawford 1998). It must, however, be remembered that swollen or permanently closed eyes (e.g. after tarsorrhaphy surgery in which the upper and lower eyelids are partially or wholly joined to protect the cornea; Martin 2003) will not open and do not necessarily indicate a falling conscious level.

Evaluation of verbal response

Verbal response may be:

- *Orientated*: the patient is aware of self and environment.
- *Confused*: the patient's responses to questions are incorrect and patient is unaware of self or environment.
- *Inappropriate words:* the patient responds using intelligible words which are unsuitable as responses.

- *Incomprehensible*: the patient may moan and groan without recognizable words.
- *Absent*: the patient does not speak or make sounds at all.

The absence of speech may not always indicate a falling level of consciousness. The patient may not speak English (though he/she can still speak), may have a tracheostomy or may be dysphasic. The patient may have a motor (expressive) dysphasia, and therefore be able to understand but unable to find the right word, or a sensory (receptive) dysphasia, being unable to comprehend what is being told to them (Aucken & Crawford 1998; Shah 1999). At times patients with expressive dysphasia may also have receptive problems; therefore it is important to make an early referral to a speech and language therapist. The nurse should also bear in mind that some patients may need a lot of stimulation to maintain their concentration to answer questions, even though they can answer them correctly. It is, therefore, important to note the amount of stimulation that the patient required as part of the baseline assessment (Aucken & Crawford 1998).

Evaluation of motor response

To obtain an accurate picture of brain function, motor response is tested by using the upper limbs because responses in the lower limbs reflect spinal function (Aucken & Crawford 1998). The patient should be asked to obey commands;

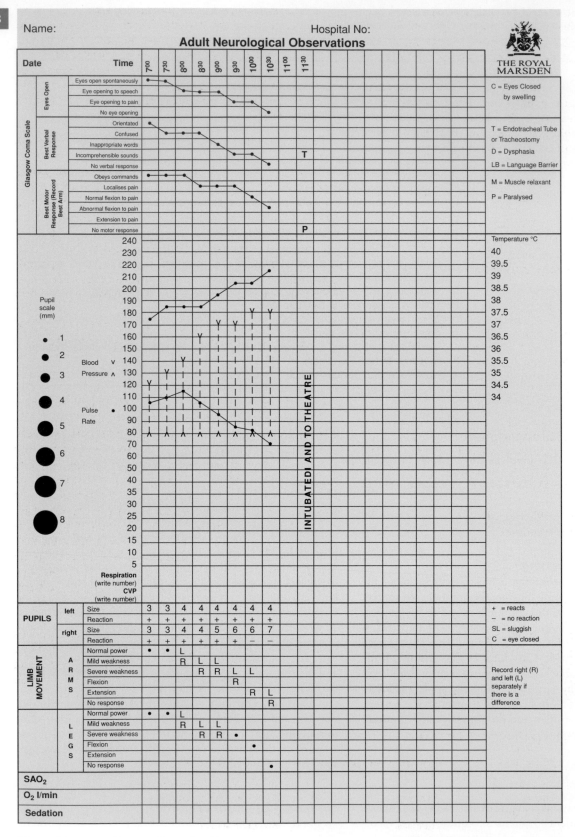

Figure 26.2 The Glasgow Coma Scale.

for example, the patient should be asked to squeeze the examiner's hands (both sides) with the best motor response recorded. The nurse should note power in the hands and the patient's ability to release the grip. This is because some patients with cerebral dysfunction, for example those with diffuse brain disease, may show an involuntary grasp reflex where stimulation of the palm of their hand causes them to grip (Aucken & Crawford 1998). If movement is spontaneous, the nurse should note which limbs move, and how, for example whether the movement is purposeful.

Response to painful stimulus may be:

- *Localized*: the patient moves the other hand to the site of the stimulus.
- *Flexor*: the patient's limb flexes away from pain.
- *Extensor*: the patient's limb extends from pain.
- *Flaccid*: no motor response at all.

(Aucken & Crawford 1998; Shah 1999.)

Application of painful stimuli

Painful stimuli should be employed only if the patient does not respond to firm and clear commands. It is always important that the least amount of pressure to elicit a response is applied so as to avoid bruising or paining the patient. As such, it should only be undertaken by experienced professionals (for suggested methods, see below).

As the ability to localize pain is lost, various responses may be observed when painful stimuli are applied (Carlson 2002a). It is important to note, when applying a painful stimulus, that the brain responds to central stimulation and the spine responds first to peripheral stimulation (Aucken & Crawford 1998).

Central stimulation can be applied in the following ways (Aucken & Crawford 1998; Carlson 2002a; Price 2002):

- *Trapezium squeeze*: using the thumb and two fingers, hold 5 cm of the trapezius muscle where the neck meets the shoulder and twist the muscle.
- *Supraorbital pressure*: running a finger along the supraorbital margin, a notch is felt. Applying pressure to the notch causes an ipsilateral (on that side) sinus headache. This method is not to be used if the facial or cranial bones are unstable, facial fractures are suspected, after facial surgery or if the assessor has sharp fingernails.

- *Sternal rub*: using the knuckles of a clenched fist to grind on the centre of the sternum. When applied adequately, marks are left on the skin as sternal tissue is tender and bruises easily. Please note that because of the danger of bruising, this method should not be used for repeated assessment but may be indicated if a decision as to whether to re-scan or alter management, e.g. proceed to surgery, is necessary.

Peripheral stimulation can be applied in the following way:

Place the patient's finger between assessor's thumb and a pencil or pen. Pressure is gradually increased over a few seconds until the slightest response is seen. Any finger can be used, although the third and fourth fingers are often most sensitive (Frawley 1990). Please note that because of the risk of bruising, pressure should not be applied to the nail bed. It must be remembered that nail bed pressure is a peripheral stimulus and should only be used to assess limbs that have not moved in response to a central stimulus (Aucken & Crawford 1998).

It cannot be overemphasized that the above methods of patient assessment should only be undertaken by appropriately qualified and trained nurses.

Evaluation of pupillary activity

Careful examination of the reactions of the pupils to light is an important part of neurological assessment (Table 26.2). The size, shape, equality, reaction to light (both direct and consensual responses, that is, the response from the eye that is not directly exposed to light) and position of the eyes should be noted. Are the eyes deviated upwards or downwards? Are both eyes conjugate (moving together) or dysconjugate (not moving together)? Impaired pupillary accommodation (adjustment of the eye resulting in pupil constriction or dilation) signifies that the midbrain itself may be suffering from pressure exerted by a swelling mass in the brain. Pupillary constriction and dilation are controlled by cranial nerve III (oculomotor) and any changes may indicate pressure on this nerve or brainstem damage (Figure 26.3) (Fuller 2004).

It should be noted that 'normal' visual function depends on a full and conjugate range of eye movements (involving cranial nerves III, IV, VI) in addition to normally functioning optic and oculomotor nerves and an intact visual centre in the occipital cortex (Aucken & Crawford 1998).

Table 26.2 Examination of pupils. From Fuller (2004).

Observation	Pupil size	Pupil reactiveness	Possible indication
Pupils equal	Pinpoint	—	Opiates or pontine lesion
	Small	Reactive	Metabolic encephalopathy
	Mid-sized	Fixed	Midbrain lesion
		Reactive	Metabolic lesion
Pupils unequal	Dilated	Unreactive	IIIrd nerve palsy
	Small	Reactive	Horner's syndrome

Figure 26.3 Diagrammatic representation of pressure from expanding mass and/or cerebral oedema.

Evaluation of motor function

Damage to any part of the motor nervous system can affect the ability to move. After assessing motor function on one side of the body the contralateral muscle group should also be evaluated to detect asymmetry. Motor function assessment involves an evaluation of the following:

- Muscle strength.
- Muscle tone.
- Muscle co-ordination.
- Reflexes.
- Abnormal movements.

(Aucken & Crawford 1998; Fuller 2004.)

Muscle strength

This involves testing the patient's muscle strength against the pull of gravity and then against one's own resistance. Changes in motor strength especially between right and left sides may indicate imminent neurological failure (Carlson 2002a).

Muscle tone

This involves flexing and extending the patient's limbs on both sides and noting how well such movements are resisted. Increased resistance would denote increased muscle tone and vice versa.

Muscle co-ordination

Any disease or injury that involves the cerebellum or basal ganglia will affect co-ordination. Assessment of hand and leg co-ordination can be achieved by testing the rapidity and rhythm of alternating movements and of point-to-point movements.

Reflexes

Among the most important reflexes are: blink, gag and swallow, oculocephalic and plantar:

- *Blink*: this is a protective reflex and can be affected by damage to the Vth cranial nerve (trigeminal) and the VIIth cranial nerve (facial). Absence of the corneal reflex (Vth and VIIth cranial nerves) may result in corneal damage. Facial weakness (VIIth cranial nerve) will affect eye closure.

- *Gag and swallow*: damage to the IXth cranial nerve (glossopharyngeal) and Xth cranial nerve (vagus) may impair protective reflexes. These two cranial nerves are always assessed together as their functions overlap. Muscle innervation of the palate is from the vagus, while sensation is supplied by the glossopharyngeal nerves (Aucken & Crawford 1998; Fuller 2004).
- *Oculocephalic*: this reflex is an eye movement that occurs only in patients with a severely decreased level of consciousness. In conscious patients this reflex is not present. When the reflex is present, the patient's eyes will move in the opposite direction from the side to which the head is turned. However, in patients with absent brainstem reflexes, the eyes will appear to remain stationary in the centre. Assessing this reflex should not be carried out if there is suspected instability of the cervical spine as this reflex can involve head movement which could exacerbate any spinal injury (Aucken & Crawford 1998).
- *Plantar*: Abnormalities of plantar reflex will help to locate the anatomical site of the lesion. Upgoing plantar (extension) reflex is termed 'positive Babinski' and indicates an upper motor neurone lesion. It should be noted that in babies under 1 year of age upgoing plantar is normal (Aucken & Crawford 1998).

Abnormal movements

When carrying out neurological observations, any abnormal movements such as seizures, tics and tremors must be noted.

Sensory functions

Constant sensory input enables an individual to alter responses and behaviour to suit the environment. When disease or injury damages the sensory pathways, the sensory responses are always affected. Any assessment of sensory function should include an evaluation of the following:

- Central and peripheral vision.
- Hearing and ability to understand verbal communication.
- Superficial sensations (light touch, pain) and deep sensations (muscle and joint pain, muscle and joint position).
  (Carlson 2002a; Fuller 2004.)

Vital signs

It is recommended that assessments of vital signs should be made in the following order:

1 Respirations.
2 Temperature.
3 Blood pressure.
4 Pulse.

(See also Chapter 25.)

Respirations

Of these four vital signs, respiratory patterns give the clearest indication of how the brain is functioning because the complex process of respiration is controlled by more than one area of the brain. Any disease or injury that affects these areas may produce respiratory changes. The rate, character and pattern of a patient's respiration must be noted. Abnormal respiratory patterns are listed in Table 26.3.

Constant re-evaluation of the patient's ability to maintain and protect their airway is a concern when there is evidence of reduced consciousness or coma (GCS score is less than 8). At this stage, muscles often become flaccid and the use

Table 26.3 Abnormal respiratory patterns.

Type	Pattern	Significance
Cheyne–Stokes	Rhythmic waxing and waning of both rate and depth of respirations, alternating regularly with briefer periods of apnoea. Greater than normal respiration, i.e. 16–24 breaths per minute	May indicate deep cerebral or cerebellar lesions, usually bilateral; may occur with upper brainstem involvement
Central neurogenic hyperventilation	Sustained, regular, rapid respirations, with forced inspiration and expiration	May indicate a lesion of the low midbrain or upper pons areas of the brainstem
Apnoeustic	Prolonged inspiration with a pause at full inspiration; there may also be expiratory pauses	May indicate a lesion of the lower pons or upper medulla, hypoglycaemia or drug-induced respiratory depression
Cluster breathing	Clusters of irregular respirations alternating with longer periods of apnoea	May indicate a lesion of lower pons or upper medulla
Ataxic breathing	A completely irregular pattern with random deep and shallow respirations; irregular pauses may also appear	May indicate a lesion of the medulla

Table 26.4 Frequency of observations.

Category	Frequency	Rationale
All patients diagnosed as suffering from neurological or neurosurgical conditions. Unconscious patients (including ventilated and anaesthetized)	At least 4-hourly, affected by the patient's condition. Frequency indicated by patient's condition	To monitor the condition of the patient so that any necessary action can be instigated. To monitor the condition closely and to detect trends so that appropriate action may be taken

of the recovery position may need to be considered. Patients who have deteriorated may require adjuncts to protect the airway and possibly artificial ventilation (Resuscitation Council (UK) 2006). Close working liaison with physiotherapists and speech and language therapists is important to minimize the danger of chest infections.

Temperature

Damage to the hypothalamus, the temperature-regulating centre, may result in grossly fluctuating temperatures (Fairley & McLernon 2005).

Blood pressure, pulse and respirations

Observations of blood pressure, pulse and respirations will provide evidence of increased intracranial pressure. When intracranial pressure is greater than 33 mmHg for even a short time, cerebral blood flow is significantly reduced. The resulting ischaemia stimulates the vasomotor centre, causing systemic blood pressure to rise. The patient becomes bradycardic and the respiratory rate falls. Abnormalities of blood pressure and pulse usually occur late, after the patient's level of consciousness has begun to deteriorate. This change in the blood pressure was first described by Cushing and is known as the Cushing reflex (Carlson 2002b).

Frequency of observations

The frequency and type of neurological observation are matters of much debate (Price 2002). It is therefore not possible to be prescriptive, as the frequency will depend on the underlying pathology and possible consequences. For example, in a patient with a head injury and a skull fracture there may be bruising to the brain (contusion), cerebral oedema and an extradural haemorrhage which may increase in size. The bruising and oedema may develop over a couple of days and gradually give rise to subtle neurological changes, whilst the extradural haemorrhage can develop very quickly and cause profound neurological changes over a matter of a few hours. Therefore such a patient may require frequent 30-minute GCS observations for the first 6 hours followed by 1–2-hourly observations for a further 48 hours. The nurse must be competent and take appropriate action if changes in

the patient's neurological status occur, as well as reporting any subtle signs that may indicate deterioration, e.g. if the patient is incontinent, reluctant to eat, drink or initiate interaction. It should never be assumed that difficulty to rouse a patient is due to night-time sleep as even a deeply asleep patient with no focal deficit should respond to pain. Therefore if the patient requires an increased amount of stimulus to achieve the same GCS score, this may also be a pointer to subtle deterioration (Table 26.4) (Aucken & Crawford 1998; Waterhouse 2005).

General points

The initial assessment of a patient should include a history (taken from relatives or friends if appropriate), including noting changes in mood, intellect, memory and personality, since these may be indicators of a long-standing problem, e.g. brain tumour (Belford 2005).

Visual acuity

The clarity or clearness of vision may be tested using Snellen's chart, which uses decreasing letter size, or newspaper prints, with and without glasses if worn.

Visual fields

Lesions at different points in the visual pathways affect vision (Table 26.5). It should be noted that loss of vision is always described with reference to the visual fields rather than the retinal fields (Weldon 1998).

Table 26.5 Visual pathways. From Fuller (2004).

Defect	Implication
Monocular field defects	Lesion anterior to optic chiasm
Bitemporal field defects	Lesion at the optic chiasm
Homonymous field defects	Lesion behind the optic chiasm
Congruous homonymous field defects	Lesion behind lateral geniculate bodies

Procedure guidelines   Neurological observations and assessment

Note. the following describes a full neurological assessment. It may be inappropriate, unnecessary or impossible for the nurse to carry out all of the procedures every time the patient is observed.

Equipment

1 Pen torch.
2 Thermometer.
3 Sphygmomanometer.
4 Tongue depressor.

5 Low-linting swabs.
6 Patella hammer.
7 Neurotips™ (refer to action 27).
8 Two test tubes (refer to action 28).

Procedure

Action	Rationale
1 Inform the patient of the procedure, whether conscious or not, and explain and discuss the observations.	Sense of hearing is frequently unimpaired even in unconscious patients. It is important, as far as is possible, that the patient understands the procedure and gives his/her valid consent (DH 2001: C; NMC 2006: C).
2 Talk to the patient. Note whether he/she is alert and is giving full attention or whether he/she is restless or lethargic and drowsy. Ask the patient who he/she is, the correct day, month and year, where he/she is, and to give details about family.	To establish whether the patient's level of consciousness is deteriorating. If the patient is becoming disorientated, changes will occur in this order: (a) Disorientation as to time. (b) Disorientation as to place. (c) Disorientation as to person (Aucken & Crawford 1998: R 5).
3 Ask the patient to squeeze and release your fingers (include both sides of the body) and then to stick out their tongue.	To evaluate motor responses and to ensure that the responses are equal and are not reflexive (Carlson 2002a: R 5).
4 If the patient does not respond, apply painful stimuli. Suggested methods have been discussed earlier.	Responses grow less purposeful as the patient's level of consciousness deteriorates. As the condition worsens, the patient may no longer localize pain and respond to it in a purposeful way (Aucken & Crawford 1998: R 5).
5 Record, precisely, the findings, recording the patient's best response. Write exactly what stimulus was used, where it was applied, how much pressure was needed to elicit the response, and how the patient responded.	Vague terms can be easily misinterpreted. Accurate recording will enable continuity of assessment and comply with NMC guidelines (NMC 2005: C).
6 Extend both hands and ask the patient to squeeze your fingers as hard as possible. Compare grip and strength.	To test grip and ascertain strength. Record best arm in GCS chart to reflect best outcome (Carlson 2002a: R 5).
7 Darken the room, if necessary, or shield the patient's eyes with your hands.	To enable a better view of the eye (E).
8 Ask the patient to open their eyes. If the patient cannot do so, hold the eyelids open and note the size, shape and equality of the pupils.	To assess the size, shape and equality of the pupils as an indication of brain damage. Normal pupils are spherical, usually at mid-position and have a diameter ranging from 2 to 5 mm (Shah 1999: R 5).
9 Hold each eyelid open in turn. Move torch towards the patient from the side. Shine it directly into the eye. This should cause the pupil to constrict promptly.	To assess the reaction of the pupils to light. A normal reaction indicates no lesions in the area of the brainstem regulating pupil constriction (Aucken & Crawford 1998: R 5).

Procedure guidelines *(cont.)*

10 Hold both eyelids open but shine the light into one eye only. The pupil into which the light is not shone should also constrict.	To assess consensual light reflex. Prompt constriction indicates intact connections between the brainstem areas regulating pupil constriction (Scherer 1986: R 5).
11 Record unusual eye movements.	To assess cranial nerve damage (Aucken & Crawford 1998: R 5).
12 Note the rate, character and pattern of the patient's respirations.	Respirations are controlled by different areas of the brain. When disease or injury affects these areas, respiratory changes may occur (Carlson 2002a: R 5).
13 Take and record the patient's temperature at specified intervals.	Damage to the hypothalamus, the temperature-regulating centre in the brain, will be reflected in grossly abnormal temperatures (Fairley & McLernon 2005: R 5).
14 Take and record the patient's blood pressure and pulse at specified intervals.	To monitor signs of increased intracranial pressure. Hypertension and bradycardia usually occur late, after the patient's level of consciousness has begun to deteriorate. Call for medical assistance as soon as it is evident that there is a deterioration in the patient's level of consciousness (Scherer 1986: R 5; Tortora & Derrickson 2008: R 5).
15 Ask the patient to close the eyes and hold the arms straight out in front, with palms upwards, for 20–30 seconds. The weaker limb will 'fall away'.	To show weakness and difference in limbs (Carlson 2002a: R 5).
16 Stand in front of the patient and extend your hands. Ask the patient to push and pull against your hands. Ask the patient to lie on his/her back in bed. Place the patient's leg with knee flexed and foot resting on the bed. Instruct the patient to keep the foot down as you attempt to extend the leg. Then instruct the patient to straighten the leg while you offer resistance. *Note*: if a patient cannot follow the instruction due to a language barrier or unconsciousness, observe spontaneous movements and note how strong they appear. Then, if necessary, apply painful stimuli.	To test arm strength. If one arm drifts downwards or turns inwards, it may indicate hemiparesis. To test flexion and extension strength in the patient's extremities by having patient push and pull against your resistance (Carlson 2002a: R 5).
17 Flex and extend all the patient's limbs. Note how well the movements are resisted.	To test muscle tone (Carlson 2002a: R 5).
18 Ask the patient to pat the thigh as fast as possible. Note whether the movements seem slow or clumsy. Ask the patient to turn the hand over and back several times in succession. Evaluate co-ordination. Ask the patient to touch the back of the fingers with the thumb in sequence rapidly.	To assess hand and arm co-ordination. The dominant hand should perform better (Carlson 2002a: R 5).
19 Extend one of your hands towards the patient. Ask the patient to touch your index finger, then his/her nose, several times in succession. Repeat the test with the patient's eyes closed.	To assess hand and arm co-ordination/cerebellar function (Carlson 2002a: R 5).
20 Ask the patient to place a heel on the opposite knee and slide it down the shin to the foot. Check each leg separately.	To assess leg co-ordination (Fuller 2004: R 5).

21 Ask the patient to look up or hold the eyelid open. With your hand, approach the eye unexpectedly or touch the eyelashes.

To test the corneal (blink) reflex (Fuller 2004: R 5).

22 Ask the patient to open the mouth, and hold down the tongue with a tongue depressor. Touch the back of the pharynx, on each side, with a low-linting swab.

To test the gag reflex (Fuller 2004: R 5).

23 Ask the patient to lie on his/her back in bed. Place your hand under the knee, raise and flex it. Tap the patellar tendon. Note whether the leg responds.

To assess the deep tendon knee-jerk reflex (Fuller 2004: R 5).

24 Stroke the lateral aspect of the sole of the patient's foot. If the response is abnormal (Babinski's response), the big toe will dorsiflex and the remaining toes will fan out.

To assess for upper motor neurone lesion (Fuller 2004: R 5).

25 Ask the patient to read something aloud. Check each eye separately. If vision is so poor that the patient is unable to read, ask the patient to count your upraised fingers or distinguish light from dark.

To test for visual acuity (Fuller 2004: R 5).

26 Occlude the ear with a low-linting swab. Stand a short way from the patient. Whisper numbers into the open ear. Ask for feedback. Repeat for both ears.

To test hearing and comprehension (Fuller 2004: R 5).

27 Ask the patient to close the eyes. Using the point of a Neurotip™ (sharp instrument for applying pressure) stroke the skin. Use the blunt end occasionally. Ask patient to tell you what is felt. See if the patient can distinguish between sharp and dull sensations.

To test superficial sensations to pain (Fuller 2004: R 5).

28 Ask the patient to close the eyes. Fill two test tubes with water: one warm, one cold. Touch the patient's skin with each test tube and ask patient to distinguish between them.

To test superficial sensations to temperature (Fuller 2004: R 5).

29 Stroke a low-linting swab lightly over the patient's skin. Ask the patient to say what he/she feels.

To test superficial sensations to touch (Fuller 2004: R 5).

30 Ask the patient to close the eyes. Hold the tip of one of the patient's fingers between your thumb and index finger. Move it up and down and ask the patient to say in which direction it is moving. Repeat with the other hand. For the legs, hold the big toe.

To test proprioception. *Definition of proprioception*: the receipt of information from muscles and tendons to the labyrinth that enables the brain to determine movements and the position of the body (Tortora & Derrickson 2008).

31 Should seizures (epilepsy/fits) occur, maintain airway if possible by placing the patient in the recovery position.
    Do not insert artificial airway into patient's mouth during the tonic/clonic phase.
    Record type of seizure, duration, any warning (aura) or incontinence the patient may have, as well as any postictal (after the fit) weakness (Todd's paralysis) or increase in drowsiness.
    Ensure the patient is closely observed until back to previous conscious level prior to ictus (fit).
    Anticonvulsants may be required as prescribed.

To maintain patient's safety and to assist in the diagnosis of any underlying pathology (E).

References and further reading

556

Aucken, S. & Crawford, B. (1998) Neurological observations. In: *Neuro-Oncology for Nurses* (ed. D. Guerrero). Whurr, London, pp. 29–65.

Bateman, D. (2001) Neurological assessment of coma. *J Neurol Neurosurg Psychiatry*, **71**(Suppl 1), i13–17.

Belford, K. (2005) Central nervous system cancers. In: *Cancer Nursing: Principles and Practice* (eds C. Henke- Yarbro, M. Frogge & M. Goodman), 6th edn. Jones and Bartlett, Sudbury MA, pp. 1089–136.

Carlson, B.A. (2002a) Neurologic clinical assessment. In: *Critical Care Nursing: Diagnosis and Management* (eds L. Urden, K. Stacy & M. Lough), 4th edn. Mosby, St. Louis, pp. 645–57.

Carlson, B.A. (2002b) Neurologic anatomy and physiology. In: *Critical Care Nursing: Diagnosis and Management* (eds L. Urden, K. Stacy & M. Lough), 4th edn. Mosby, St. Louis, pp. 617–44.

DH (2001) Good practice in consent implemation guide: consent to examination or treatment. www.dh.gov.uk. Accessed 24/9/07.

Fairley, S. & McLernon S. (2005) Neurological problems. In: *Critical Care Nursing: Science and Practice* (eds Adam S. Osborne S.), 2nd edn. Oxford University Press, Oxford, pp. 285–327.

Frawley, P. (1990) Neurological observations. *Nurs Times*, **86**(35), 29–34.

Fuller, G. (2004) *Neurological Examinations Made Easy*, 3rd edn. Churchill Livingstone, Edinburgh.

Jennett, B. & Teasdale G. (1984) *An Introduction to Neurosurgery*, 4th edn. William Heinemann Medical Books, London, pp. 23–9.

Kaye, A.H. (2005) Neurological assessment and examination. *Essential Neurosurgery*, 3rd edn. Blackwell Publishing, Oxford, pp. 1–14.

Lower, J. (2003) Using pain to assess neurological response. *Nursing*, **33**(6), 56–7.

Martin, E.A. (2003) *Oxford Concise Colour Medical Dictionary*, 3rd edn. Oxford University Press, Oxford.

NICE (2003) *Head Injury: Triage, Assessment, Investigation and Early Management of Head Injury in Infants, Children and Adults*. National Institute for Clinical Excellence, London.

NMC (2005) *Guidelines for Records and Record Keeping*. Nursing and Midwifery Council, London.

NMC (2006) *A–Z Advice Sheet Consent*. www.nmc.org.

Price, T. (2002) Painful stimuli and the Glasgow Coma Scale. *Nurs Crit Care*, **7**(1), 17–23.

Resuscitation Council (UK) (2006) Airway management and ventilation. In: *Advanced Life Support*, 5th edn. Resuscitation Council (UK), London, pp. 41–57.

Rowley, G. & Fielding, K. (1991) Reliability and accuracy of the Glasgow Coma Scale with experienced and inexperienced users. *Lancet*, **337**(8740), 535–8.

Scherer, P. (1986) The logic of coma. *Am J Nurs*, **86**, 542–9.

Shah, S. (1999) Neurological assessment. *Nurs Times*, **13**, 49–56.

Teasdale, G. & Jennett, B. (1974) Assessment of coma and impaired consciousness: a practical scale. *Lancet*, **2**, 81–4.

Tortora, G.J. & Derrickson B. (2008) *Principles of Anatomy and Physiology*, 12th edn. John Wiley & Sons Ltd, Chichester.

Waterhouse, C. (2005) The Glasgow Coma Scale and other neurological observations. *Nurs Stand* **19**(33), 56–64.

Weldon, K. (1998) Neurological observations. In: *Neuro-Oncology for Nurses* (ed. D. Guerrero). Whurr, London, pp. 1–28.

Chapter 27

Pain management and assessment

Reference material **558**
Procedure guidelines: Pain control: assessment and education **572**
of patient prior to surgery
Procedure guidelines: Pain assessment chart: chronic **573**
References and further reading **573**

Definition

Pain is not a simple sensation but a complex phenomenon having both a physical and an affective (emotional) component. To reflect this, the International Association for the Study of Pain (IASP) (1994) published the following definition of pain: 'An unpleasant sensory and emotional experience associated with actual or potential tissue damage, or described in terms of such damage'. Pain is subjective and another favoured definition for use in clinical practice, proposed originally by McCaffery (1968) and cited in McCaffery (2000, p. 2), is: 'Pain is whatever the experiencing person says it is, existing whenever the experiencing person says it does'.

Many factors influence the expression of pain and may be associated with the patient, the nurse or the clinical environment (organizational aspects) (Carr & Mann 2000a).

Reference material

There are several ways to categorize the types of pain that occur; for example, acute or chronic, nociceptive (somatic or visceral) or neuropathic. It is increasingly recognized that acute and chronic pain may represent a continuum rather than distinct separate entities, combine different pain mechanisms and vary in duration (ANZCA and Faculty of Pain Medicine 2005).

Acute pain

The IASP has defined acute pain as: 'Pain of recent onset and probable limited duration. It usually has an identifiable temporal and causal relationship to injury or disease' (Ready & Edwards 1992, p. 1). Acute pain is produced by a wide range of physiological processes, and includes inflammatory, neuropathic, sympathetically maintained, visceral and cancer pain (Walker *et al.* 2006).

Chronic pain

Chronic pain is usually prolonged and defined as pain that exists for more than 3 months (IASP 1996). It is often associated with major changes in personality, lifestyle and functional ability (Foley 2004). Chronic pain occurs as a result of both cancer and non-malignant chronic conditions such as neuropathic, musculoskeletal, and chronic postoperative pain syndromes.

The term breakthrough pain is widely used. Within the medical literature other terms are referred to in the description of breakthrough pain including episodic pain, exacerbation of pain, pain flare, transient pain and transitory pain (Colleau 1999). This is further discussed below.

Assessment of pain

Assessment is a key step in the process of managing pain. The aim of assessment is to identify all the factors, physi-

cal and non-physical, that affect the patient's perception of pain. A comprehensive clinical assessment is essential to gain a thorough understanding of the patient's pain, select an appropriate analgesic therapy, evaluate the effectiveness of interventions and modify therapy according to the patient's response.

Acute pain assessment for surgical patients

For surgical pain to be controlled effectively, pain must be assessed regularly and systematically. The process of pain assessment begins before surgery and continues through to discharge.

Assessment of the psychosocial aspects of acute pain

A number of psychosocial factors can influence pain. Pain is an individual, multifactorial experience influenced by previous pain events, beliefs about pain and pain management, anxiety, mood and culture (ANZCA and Faculty of Pain Medicine 2005). Patients may be anxious about the outcome of the surgery or how pain will be controlled, particularly if they have bad memories of previous pain experiences (Audit Commission 1997; Carr & Mann 2000b). Anxiety in turn exacerbates pain by increasing muscle tension. Providing patients with appropriate support and information to address these concerns can reduce both anxiety and postoperative pain (Audit Commission 1997; Kalkman *et al.* 2003).

Assessment of pre-existing pain

Patients who have been taking regular opioid analgesics for a pre-existing chronic pain problem may require higher doses of analgesia to manage an acute pain episode (Macintyre 2001; Lewis & Williams 2005; Mehta & Langford 2006). It is therefore important to take a history of pre-existing pain and analgesic use so that appropriate analgesic measures can be planned in advance of surgery.

Assessment of location and intensity of pain

Location

Many complex surgical procedures involve more than one incision site and the nature and extent of pain at each site may vary. A careful assessment of the location and type of pain is required, because each pain problem may respond to different pain management techniques. Pain location may also help to determine why pain is exacerbated by certain movements or positions (Anderson & Cleeland 2003).

Intensity

As part of the assessment process it is important to assess the intensity of pain. Only then can the effects of any intervention be evaluated and care modified as appropriate. The simplest techniques for pain measurement involve the use of a verbal rating scale, numerical rating scale or visual analogue scale. Using one of these scales, patients are asked to match pain intensity to the scale.

Three principles apply to the use of these scales:

- The patient must be involved in scoring his/her own pain intensity. It provides the patient with an opportunity to express their pain intensity and also what it means to them and the effect it has on their lives. This is important because health care professionals frequently underestimate the intensity of a patient's pain and effectiveness of pain relief (Drayer *et al.* 1999; Loveman & Gale 2000; Idvall *et al.* 2002).
- Pain intensity assessment should incorporate different components of pain. This should include assessment of static (rest) pain and dynamic pain (on sitting, coughing or moving the affected part). For example, in a postoperative patient this is important to prevent complications of delayed recovery such as chest infections and emboli (deep vein thrombosis, pulmonary embolism) and to determine if analgesia is adequate for return of normal function (Macintyre & Ready 2001; Hobbs & Hodgkinson 2003).
- It is important to remember that a complete picture of a patient's pain cannot be derived solely from the use of a pain scale (Lawler 1997). Ongoing communication with the patient is required to uncover and manage any psychosocial factors that may be affecting the patient's pain experience.

Chronic pain assessment

The prevalence of chronic pain is approximated at being between 30–50% among patients with cancer who are undergoing active treatment for a solid tumour and between 70 and 90% among those patients with advanced disease (Portenoy & Lessage 1999). For example, approximately two-thirds of advanced cancer patients will also complain of anorexia, one-half will have a symptomatic dry mouth and constipation, and one-third will suffer nausea, vomiting, insomnia, dyspnoea, cough or oedema (Donnelly & Walsh 1995). It is clear from these figures that chronic pain assessment cannot be seen in isolation; identification of all related symptoms is of equal importance as they will contribute to a lowered pain threshold (the lowest stimulus intensity at which a person perceives pain) and impaired pain tolerance (the greatest stimulus intensity causing pain that a person is prepared to tolerate) (Grond *et al.* 1996). Furthermore, chronic cancer pain is often multifactorial. Adequate pain assessment requires a comprehensive evaluation of all factors that play a significant role in the cancer pain experience (Zaza 2002).

A diagnosis of cancer does not necessarily mean that the malignant process is the cause of the pain. Pain in chronic cancer may be:

- Caused by the cancer itself.
- Caused by treatment.

- Associated with debilitating disease, such as a pressure ulcer.
- Unrelated to either the disease or the treatment, such as headache.

(Twycross & Wilcock 2001.)

It is imperative to ascertain the patients' current level of anxiety and depression and to understand each patient's own understanding of the meaning of pain (Foley 2004). The cause of *each* pain should therefore be identified carefully; many pains unrelated to the cancer will respond to specific treatment. If the pain is due to the cancer, then it is important to determine the precise mechanism of pain because treatment will vary accordingly. Patients with cancer may experience a range of psychological and spiritual problems that extend far beyond the experience of physical pain (Paz & Seymour 2004). The concept of total pain reminds practitioners that pain is a deeply personal experience and that one of the greatest challenges is for nurses to be able to facilitate the expression for each individual of that particular pain (Krishnasamy 2001). Pain assessment needs to acknowledge these facts and particular attention must be paid to factors that will modulate pain sensitivity (Table 27.1).

Assessment tools for acute and chronic pain

Accurate pain assessment is a prerequisite of effective control and is an essential component of nursing care. In the assessment process, the nurse gathers information from the patient that allows an understanding of the patient's experience and its effect on the patient's life. The information obtained guides the nurse in planning and evaluating strategies for care. Pain is rarely static; therefore, its assessment is not a one-time process but is ongoing.

Pain assessment is difficult to achieve. For example, the tendency suggested by both research and clinical practice is for the patient not to report any pain or to do so inadequately or inaccurately, minimizing the pain experience (McCaffery & Beebe 1989). Nurses are influenced by a number of variables when assessing the amount of pain a patient is suffering (Kitson 1994). Pargeon and Hailey (1999) demonstrated that health care providers usually over- or underestimate a patient's pain. It has also been suggested that nurses do not

Table 27.1 Factors affecting pain sensitivity.

Sensitivity increased	Sensitivity lowered
Discomfort	Relief of symptoms
Insomnia	Sleep
Fatigue	Rest
Anxiety	Sympathy
Fear	Understanding
Anger	Companionship
Sadness	Diversional activity
Depression	Reduction in anxiety
Boredom	Elevation of mood

possess sufficient knowledge to care for patients in pain (Mc-Caffery & Ferrell 1997; Drayer *et al.* 1999). A survey of over 3000 nurses (McCaffery & Robinson 2002) demonstrated that nurse education has improved confidence in the pain assessment process but that further education continues to be required in the pharmacology of pain medications and addressing nurses' fears of opioid addiction and respiratory depression, which continue to contribute to the under-treatment of pain.

A variety of pain assessment tools exist which can be used to assist nurses to assess pain and plan nursing care. They enable pain to be successfully assessed and monitored (Walker *et al.* 1987; McCaffery & Beebe 1989; Twycross *et al.* 1996) and improve communication between staff and patients (Raiman 1986). Higginson (1998, p. 150) notes that: 'Taking assessments directly from the patient is the most valid way of collecting information on their quality of life'. Encouraging patients to take an active role in their pain assessment by using pain tools helps to increase their confidence and makes them feel part of the pain management process.

Some degree of caution, however, must be exercised with the use of pain assessment tools. The nurse must be careful to select the tool that is most appropriate for a particular type of pain experience. For example, it would not be appropriate to use a pain assessment tool that had been designed for use with patients with chronic pain, to assess postoperative pain. Furthermore, pain tools should not be used totally indiscriminately. Walker *et al.* (1987) found that pain tools appeared to have little value in cases of unresolved or intractable pain.

The most commonly used pain assessment tools meet the following criteria (Fitzpatrick *et al.* 1998):

- Simplicity: ease of understanding for all the patient groups.
- Reliability: reliability of the tool when used in similar patient groups; results are reproducible and consistent.
- Valid: the tool measures the patient's perception of pain.
- Sensitivity: sensitivity of the tool to the patient's pain.
- Accuracy: accurate and precise recording of data.
- Interpretable: meaningful pain scores or data are produced.
- Feasiblity/practicality: the degree of effort involved in using the tool is acceptable; a practical tool is more likely to be used by patients and nursing staff.

The use of pain assessment tools for acute pain has been shown both to increase the effectiveness of nursing interventions and to improve the management of pain (Scott 1994; Harmer & Davies 1998). Several pain assessment tools are available. Verbal Descriptor Scales (VDS) are based on numerically ranked words such as 'none', 'mild', 'moderate', 'severe' and 'very severe' for assessing both pain intensity and response to analgesia. Numerical Rating Scales (NRS) have both written and verbal forms. The written forms are described as either a vertical or a horizontal line with '0' indicating no pain located on one extremity of the line and '10' indicating severe pain at the other extremity. This type of scale is easily used as a verbal scale of 0–10 if patients are unable to see or focus on a written scale. Although originally published as a line with a scale of 0–10 there are many versions of it (Flaherty 1996). Since many of these scales focus on assessing the intensity of pain, it is important that nurses do not neglect to combine their use of these tools with an assessment of the patient's psychosocial needs.

For practical purposes, a combined pain assessment and observation chart is frequently used in the postoperative period. The Royal Marsden Hospital Postoperative Observation and Pain Assessment Chart is an example of one of these (Figure 27.1). The patient's assessment of their pain is recorded on the numerical rating pain scale at the bottom of the chart at the same time that other observations are carried out (usually 2–4 hourly but more frequently if pain is not controlled).

Other pain assessment tools have been developed to capture the multidimensional nature of pain. These specifically measure several features of the pain experience. This includes the location and intensity of pain, pattern of pain over time, the effect of pain on the patient's daily function and activities, the effect on the patient's mood and the ability to interact and socialize with others. Examples of these include the McGill Pain Questionnaire (MPQ) (Melzack 1975) and the Brief Pain Inventory (BPI) (Cleeland 1991). These are more commonly used in chronic pain assessment.

Neuropathic pain is defined as pain due to a disturbance of function or pathological change in a nerve (Merskey & Bogduk 1994). Patients may describe spontaneous pain (those that arise without detectable stimulation) and evoked pain (abnormal responses to stimuli) (Bennett 2001). The Leeds Assessment of Neuropathic Symptoms and Signs (LANSS) pain scale (Bennett 2001) was developed to more accurately assess this type of pain.

The Royal Marsden NHS Foundation Trust currently uses a patient held pain tool for patients with chronic cancer pain (Figure 27.2).

The need for effective acute pain control

There are several reasons why pain needs to be well-controlled following surgery, not least that patients have a right to expect adequate treatment of pain and that all members of the health care team have an ethical obligation to provide it (Audit Commission 1997). It is now known that under-treatment of acute pain coupled with the physiological response to surgery, known as the stress response, can have a number of adverse consequences (Macintyre & Ready 2001). Uncontrolled pain can lead to increased anxiety, fear, sleeplessness and muscle tension which further exacerbate pain. It can delay the recovery process by hindering mobilization and deep breathing, which increases the risk of a patient developing a deep vein thrombosis, chest infection or pressure ulcer. Pain can also lead to significant delays in gastric emptying and a reduction in intestinal motility (Macintyre & Ready 2001). With severe pain, activity of the sympathetic nervous system and the neuroendocrine

Patient Name:_____   Hosp. No.: _____   C.U./Consultant:_____

POST OPERATIVE OBSERVATION AND PAIN ASSESSMENT CHART

The Royal Marsden NHS Trust

Date	
Time	
Temp	40°C, 39°C, 38°C, 37°C, 36°C, 35°C

BLOOD PRESSURE / PULSE

220-, 210-, 200-, 190-, 180-, 170-, 160-, 150-, 140-, 130-, 120-, 110-, 100-, 95-, 90-, 85-, 80-, 75-, 70-, 65-, 60-, 55-, 50-, 45-, 40-, 35-, 30-, 25-, 20-

Oxygen Saturation If on oxygen add amount

Respiratory rate

Sedation Score

Hourly Rate of Epidural/IV Infusion

S/C Analgesia Continuous (C), Intermittent (I)

PCA Accumulative Total

Height of Epidural Block

Nausea and Vomiting

Bowels

CVP

Drain 1, 2, 3

Pain Score (0–10): At Rest, On Movement

Figure 27.1   The Royal Marsden Hospital Postoperative Observation And Pain Assessment Chart.

The Royal Marsden NHS Trust
Patient Held Pain Chart

Surname:

Who completed the assessment:
(specify if nurse or family member helped)

First name:

Date of this assessment:

Instructions for use:

1. This chart is for you to complete (you may want your family or a nurse to help you)

2. Work through the questions in section 1 and 2 of the chart. Do ask for help if you are not clear about any of the questions.

3. When you get to section 3 use the instructions at the top of the sheet to help you keep an ongoing record of your pain and the effect of any pain treatments.

Please keep this chart with you because the nurses and doctors who are looking after you will use it to help manage your pain(s)

Section 1: Where is your pain?

Please draw on the body outlines below to show where you feel pain. Label each site A, B, C, etc. or use a different colour

Section 2: Questions about your pain

How would you describe your pain(s) at the site(s) you drew on the body diagram? (e.g. aching, tender, sharp, shooting, burning).

What helps reduce your pain(s) at each site? (e.g. specific drugs, activities or treatments such as massage).

What makes your pain worse at each site? (e.g. specific activity or heat/cold).

How often do you get pain at each site? (e.g. all the time or at different times during the day).

How do you feel when you are in pain and how has it changed your daily activities? (e.g. moving, sleeping).

Section 3: Scoring and recording your pain scores

Pain Scores

0	= No pain
1–4	= Mild pain
5–6	= Moderate pain
7–9	= Severe pain
10	= Worst pain imaginable

Instructions for scoring and recording pain scores

1) In the column marked Pain scores use the scoring system shown here to record your pain score(s) at each site (see columns A, B, C, etc.) where you feel pain.
2) Score your pain at regular intervals. Do this before your pain treatments (e.g. analgesics/pain medicines, massage) and 30–45 minutes afterwards so that you can see if they have helped.

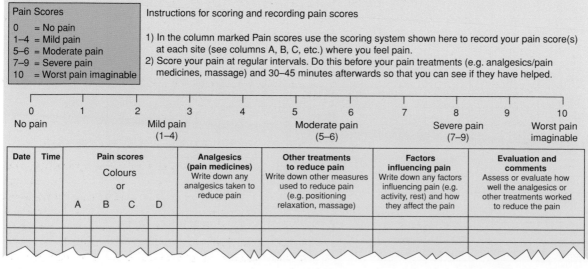

Date	Time	Pain scores Colours or A B C D	Analgesics (pain medicines) Write down any analgesics taken to reduce pain	Other treatments to reduce pain Write down other measures used to reduce pain (e.g. positioning relaxation, massage)	Factors influencing pain Write down any factors influencing pain (e.g. activity, rest) and how they affect the pain	Evaluation and comments Assess or evaluate how well the analgesics or other treatments worked to reduce the pain

Figure 27.2   The Royal Marsden Hospital Patient Held Pain Chart.

'stress response' cause platelet activation, changes in regional blood flow and stress on the heart. These can lead to impaired wound healing and myocardial ischaemia (Macintyre & Ready 2001). There is evidence to suggest that in the long term, poorly controlled acute pain may lead to the development of chronic pain. Perkins and Kehlet (2000) established that moderate to severe acute postoperative pain was a predictor for developing chronic pain after breast surgery, thoracic surgery and hernia repair.

Management of chronic pain

The control of pain is directed by the 'Analgesic Ladder', which was presented by the World Health Organization (WHO) in 1996 (Figure 27.3). The simple principles are such that pharmacological intervention begins on the first step of the ladder and proceeds upwards as and when the pain reaches a higher level and the current analgesia is no longer effective. Analgesia should be administered 'around the clock' (ATC) to enable chronic persistent pain to be controlled. It is important to remember that the patient will experience different types of pain due to different aetiological and physiological changes, manifested through the cancer trajectory (e.g. bone pain, neuropathic pain). It is important to make an assessment of each pain separately, since the pain may need to be managed in a different manner and one analgesic intervention will rarely be sufficient. Often the best practice is to combine the baseline analgesia with an appro-

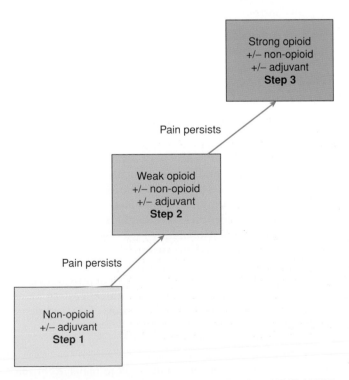

Figure 27.3 The Analgesic Ladder. Modified from WHO (1996).

Table 27.2 The use of adjuvant drugs (co-analgesics).

Type	Use	Examples
Non-steroidal anti-inflammatory drugs (NSAIDs)	Bone pain Muscular pain Inflammation Visceral pain	Diclofenac Naproxen Ibuprofen
Steroids	Pressure Bone pain Inflammation Raised intracranial pressure	Dexamethasone Prednisolone
Tricyclic antidepressants	Neuropathic pain	Amitriptyline
Anticonvulsants		Sodium valproate Carbamazepine Gabapentin Pre Gabalin
Antibiotics	Infection	Flucloxacillin Trimethoprim
Benzodiazepines	Anxiety	Diazepam Clonazepam
Antispasmodics	Spasms	Baclofen
Bisphosphonates	Bone pain	Sodium clodronate Disodium pamidronate Zoledronic acid

priate adjuvant treatment in order to achieve maximum pain control (Table 27.2).

Oral administration of therapeutic interventions may not always be appropriate. In chronic pain the European Association of Palliative Care (EAPC) recommends that if patients can no longer manage the oral route, the preferred alternative route is subcutaneous, which is simple and less painful than the intramuscular route (Hanks et al. 2001). In rare circumstances when rapid titration of analgesia is required the intravenous route may also be used if patients have established intravenous access.

Accurate ongoing assessment is imperative for efficient and effective pain control.

The management of pain following surgery

Since nurses, surgeons, anaesthetists, pain specialists, pharmacists and physiotherapists are all involved in the management of surgical pain, teamwork is essential. Professionals must reach clear agreement as to their individual roles so that patients receive the best possible care from preadmission through to discharge (Audit Commission 1997).

A wide variety of pharmacological and non-pharmacological techniques are available for the management of surgical pain. The following basic principles apply to their use:

1 Tailor the treatments to:
   (a) Meet individual needs.
   (b) Prevent pain, rather than allowing it to become established.
2 Whenever possible, choose the simplest and safest techniques to achieve the desired level of pain relief (McQuay *et al*. 1997).
3 Use the WHO Analgesic Ladder (see Figure 27.3) to select the most appropriate analgesics for mild, moderate and severe acute pain.
4 Choose the most appropriate route for giving analgesia.
5 Combine techniques to provide balanced analgesia and enhance overall pain control (Kehlet 1997).
6 Ensure patients receive regular antiemetics to control postoperative nausea and vomiting. Vomiting increases muscle tension and exacerbates pain.

Acute pain

Pharmacological techniques

Opioid analgesics

Opioids are the first-line treatment for pain that follows major surgery. Interpatient opioid requirements vary greatly (Macintyre & Jarvis 1996) and opioid doses need to be titrated carefully to achieve pain relief to suit each individual patient while minimizing any unwanted side-effects (McQuay *et al*. 1997; see Chronic pain section for further details on side-effects).

A number of opioids are used for controlling pain following surgery. These include morphine, diamorphine, fentanyl and oxycodone. The most common routes of opioid administration are intravenous, epidural, subcutaneous, intramuscular or oral.

Evidence for the concept of opioid rotation when patients have intolerable opioid related side-effects originates from cancer pain studies (Quigley 2004) but it may be a useful strategy to consider in the management of acute pain as well.

Intravenous analgesia

Continuous intravenous infusions of opioids such as morphine, diamorphine and fentanyl are effective for controlling pain in the immediate postoperative period. Their use is often restricted to critical care units where patients can be closely monitored because of the potential risk of respiratory depression (Macintyre & Ready 2001). Compared with patient-controlled analgesia (PCA; see next paragraph) continuous infusions of opoids for acute pain management in a general ward setting resulted in a fivefold increase in the incidence of respiratory depression (Schug & Torrie 1993).

Patient-controlled analgesia (PCA) is an alternative and safer technique for giving intravenous opioids (usually morphine, diamorphine or fentanyl) in the ward environment (Sidebotham *et al*. 1997). With PCA, patients self-administer intermittent doses of opioids, by using an infusion pump and timing device. When in pain, the patient presses a button con-

nected to the pump and a set dose of opioid is delivered (usually intravenously but it may also be given subcutaneously) to the patient (Macintyre & Ready 2001).

There are a number of advantages of using PCA:

- PCA is more likely to maintain reasonably constant blood concentrations of the opioid within the analgesic corridor. This is the blood level where analgesia is achieved without significant side-effects. The flexibility of PCA helps to overcome the wide interpatient variation in opioid requirements (Macintyre & Ready 2001).
- PCA allows patients to titrate analgesia against daily variations in the pain stimulus (Tye & Gell-Walker 2000). By using a PCA pump, patients can administer analgesia as soon as pain occurs and titrate the dose of analgesia according to increases and decreases in the pain stimulus. This is particularly helpful for controlling more intense pain during movement.
- PCA prevents delays in patients receiving analgesics (Chumbley *et al*. 2002).

Whilst PCA may be very effective for controlling pain for a number of patients undergoing surgery (Macintyre 2001), it is not suitable for the following groups (Tye & Gell-Walker 2000):

- Patients who are unable to activate the PCA device due to problems with dexterity or visual impairment.
- Patients who are unable to understand the concept of PCA, particularly the very young or patients who are confused.
- Patients who do not wish to take responsibility for their pain control.

(For further details about the use of PCA pumps see Chapter 13.)

Epidural analgesia

Epidural analgesia refers to the provision of pain relief by continuous administration of analgesic pharmacological agents (usually low concentrations of local anaesthetics and opioids) into the epidural space via an indwelling catheter (ANZCA and Faculty of Pain Medicine 2005). Giving analgesia epidurally is a particularly valuable technique for the prevention of postoperative pain in patients undergoing major thoracic, abdominal and lower limb surgery, and can sometimes be used to manage the pain associated with trauma. Commonly used opioids for epidural analgesia include fentanyl and diamorphine (Wheatley *et al*. 2001). Combinations of low concentrations of local anaesthetic agents and opioids have been shown to provide consistently superior pain relief compared with either drug alone (Macintyre & Ready 2001). Further details of this technique are given in Chapter 29.

Subcutaneous analgesia

Opioids are often given subcutaneously to manage chronic cancer pain. More recently, there has been an increase in the use of subcutaneous opioids for postoperative pain control. Both PCA- and nurse-administered opioid injections of morphine, diamorphine or oxycodone via an indwelling subcutaneous cannula have been used successfully to manage postoperative pain (Vijayan 1997). An advantage of giving analgesia subcutaneously is that it avoids the problems associated with maintaining intravenous access.

Intramuscular analgesia

Until the early 1990s regular 3–4-hourly intramuscular injections of opioids such as pethidine, morphine or preparations containing morphine (Omnopon) were routinely used for the management of postoperative pain. Because alternative techniques such as PCA and epidural analgesia are available, intramuscular analgesia is now used less frequently. Some useful algorithms have been developed to give guidance on titrating intramuscular analgesia (Harmer & Davies 1998; Macintyre & Ready 2001). Absorption via this route may be impaired in conditions of poor perfusion (e.g. in hypovolaemia, shock, hypothermia or immobility). This may lead to inadequate early analgesia (the drug cannot be absorbed properly and reach systemic circulation and forms a drug depot) and late absorption of the drug depot (where the drug has remained in the muscular tissue and is absorbed only once perfusion is restored) (ANZCA and Faculty of Pain Medicine 2005).

Oral analgesia

Oral opioids are used less frequently in the immediate postoperative period because many patients may be nil by mouth or on restricted oral intake for a period of time. Often this route is used if patients require strong analgesics following discontinuation of epidural or intravenous analgesia. Morphine is an ideal oral preparation because it is available as a tablet (Sevredol) or an elixir (Oramorph). Oxycodone can be given as second line opioid treatment if patients are allergic/sensitive to or fail to respond to morphine.

Opioids for mild to moderate pain and non-opioid analgesics

Paracetamol and paracetamol combinations

The use of non-opioid analgesics such as paracetamol or paracetamol combined with a weak opioid such as codeine is recommended for managing pain following minor surgical procedures or when the pain following major surgery begins to subside (McQuay et al. 1997). Paracetamol can also be given rectally if the oral route is contraindicated. An intravenous preparation of paracetamol is now available and can provide effective analgesia after surgical procedures (Romsing et al. 2002). It is more effective and of faster onset than the same dose given enterally. The use of the intravenous form should be limited to patients where the enteral route cannot be used.

Paracetamol taken in the correct dose of not more than 4 g per day is relatively free of side-effects. When used in combination with codeine preparations, the most frequent side-effect is constipation.

Tramadol

Another opioid for mild to moderate pain, which has been shown to be an effective analgesic for postoperative pain, is tramadol (McQuay & Moore 1998; Reicin et al. 2001). Although tramadol does have some side-effects, which include nausea and dizziness, it is free of non-steroidal anti-inflammatory drug (NSAID) side-effects and causes less constipation than codeine preparations and opioids (Bamigbade & Langford 1998). The combination of tramadol with paracetamol is more effective than either of the two components administered alone (McQuay & Edwards 2003).

Non-steroidal anti-inflammatory drugs

Non-steroidal anti-inflammatory drugs (NSAIDs) have been shown to provide better pain relief than paracetamol combinations for acute pain (McQuay et al. 1997). These drugs can be used alone or in combination with both opioid and non-opioid analgesics. Two commonly used NSAIDs are diclofenac, which can be administered orally, enterally or rectally, and ibuprofen, which is available only as an oral or enteral preparation. The disadvantage of both of these is that often side-effects such as coagulation problems, renal impairment and gastrointestinal disturbances limit their use. Newer COX 2-specific NSAIDs have the advantage that they are associated with similar analgesia and anti-inflammatory effects (Reicin et al. 2001) but have no effect on platelets or the gastric mucosa (Rowbotham 2000). As a result coagulation problems and gastrointestinal irritation are likely to be significantly reduced. However, recently several of these drugs have been withdrawn from the market due to long-term cardiovascular side-effects and it will take time for newer products with an improved safety profile to re-establish themselves in practice (ANZCA and Faculty of Pain Medicine 2005).

Nitrous oxide (Entonox)

Inhaled nitrous oxide provides analgesia that is short acting and works quickly. It has a special role in managing pain associated with wound dressings and drain removal (see Chapter 28 on the use of Entonox).

Local anaesthetics

In addition to epidural analgesia, local anaesthetics may be used to block individual or groups of peripheral nerves during surgical procedures and to infiltrate surgical wounds at the end of an operation (Carroll & Bowsher 1993). Occasionally these techniques may be used to extend the duration of postoperative analgesia beyond the finite period that a single injection technique provides (ANZCA and Faculty of Pain Medicine 2005). Techniques include regular intermittent bolus doses or continuous infusions of local anaesthetic.

Non-pharmacological techniques for acute and chronic pain

Optimal pain control is more likely to be achieved by combining non-pharmacological techniques with pharmacological techniques. Despite the lack of research evidence to support the effectiveness of many non-pharmacological techniques, their benefits to patients and families should not be underestimated.

Psychological interventions

A number of simple psychological interventions can improve a patient's pain control by:

- Reducing anxiety, stress and muscle tension.
- Distraction (distraction plays a role in pain management by pushing awareness of pain out of central cognition).
- Increasing control and pain-coping mechanisms.
- Improving general well-being (Zarnegar & Daniel 2005).

Some simple interventions include the following.

Creating trusting therapeutic relationships

By creating trusting relationships with patients, nurses are instrumental in reducing anxiety and helping patients to cope with pain (Carr & Mann 2000b). Nurses can help to create a trusting relationship by:

- Listening to the patient.
- Believing the patient's pain experience (Seers 1996).
- Acting as a patient advocate.
- Providing patients with appropriate physical and emotional support.

The use of gentle humour

Pasero (1998) suggests that many patients find gentle humour an effective way of coping with pain. Humour may be particularly helpful prior to a painful procedure as it can have a lasting effect. In the clinical setting, humorous tapes, books and videos can be made available for patient use.

Information/education

Patient information/education can make all the difference between effective and ineffective pain relief. Information/education helps to reduce anxiety (Hayward 1975; Taylor 2001) and enables patients to make informed decisions about their care. Patients should be given specific information about why pain control is important, what to expect in terms of pain relief, how they can participate in their management and what to do if pain is not controlled. Some caution is required, however, because not all patients respond positively to the same level of information. Patients with

high levels of anxiety may find that detailed information can increase their anxiety and influence their pain control. To avoid this, patients can be given a choice of whether or not they receive simple or detailed information (Mitchell 1997).

Relaxation

Whilst scientific evidence for the effectiveness of relaxation techniques is limited (Carroll & Seers 1998; Seers & Carroll 1998), a number of studies have shown benefits for patients experiencing pain (Sloman et al. 1994; Good et al. 1999; Lang et al. 2000). Payne (1995) describes several relaxation techniques ranging from simple breathing techniques to progressive muscle relaxation and more complex techniques. One simple relaxation technique script that has been adapted for use at The Royal Marsden Hospital is outlined in Box 27.1. This technique can be taught to patients and used during painful procedures or at times when the patient feels anxious or stressed. Patients should be encouraged to practise the technique to gain mastery.

Music

The use of taped music in the health care setting can also provide relaxation and distraction from pain (Beck 1991; Good 1996; Heiser et al. 1997; Good et al. 1999). Setting up a library of taped music (e.g. easy listening, classical) and having personal stereos available for patient use is a simple way to provide patients with relaxing music.

Art

Art therapies have also been used to assist the patient in moving the focus of attention away from the physical sensation of pain to other aspects of the person (Trauger-Querry & Haghighi 1999). The skills of an art therapist are required to ensure the successful use of this intervention.

Physical interventions

In addition to psychological interventions, a number of physical interventions can be helpful in reducing pain.

Comfort measures

Simple comfort measures such as careful body positioning (for example, supporting a painful arm on a pillow) and the use of soft and therapeutic mattresses (Ballard 1997) can help to improve patient comfort and pain control.

Exercise

Both passive and active physical exercises may benefit patients by increasing range of motion (Feine & Lund 1997), preventing joint stiffness and muscle wasting which may further compound pain problems. Exercise should always be tailored to the patient's tolerance and stamina. A simple exercise regimen which is practised regularly and supervised by

---

Box 27.1   Simple relaxation technique script

Please note that breathing during this technique should be normal for the patient in their present condition.

1   Loosen any tight clothing and position yourself comfortably, either lying or sitting. Have your arms and legs uncrossed. Ensure your back and head are well supported.
2   Allow both your hands to rest on your abdomen, one on top of the other. It may be helpful to place a pillow on your lap for your hands to rest on.
3   Gently allow your eyes to close. Breathe normally in and out through your nose if you find this comfortable.
4   As you breathe in, be aware of your abdomen rising gently under your hands (do not force this movement).
5   As you breathe out, be aware of your abdomen relaxing under your hands.
6   Let your shoulders relax and drop down.
7   Let your jaw relax.
8   Now keep your attention softly focused on the rise and fall of your abdomen as this movement follows each breath.
9   Repeat steps 4–8 for between 3 and 5 minutes or longer if appropriate.

During the exercise

As you become aware of any thoughts that arise, let them go and just bring your attention back to the rise and fall of the abdomen. If you are still having difficulty focusing on the technique try saying the following phrases: 'I am relaxed' or 'I feel calm'.

To finish the exercise

Now slowly become aware of your surroundings, stretch out your fingers and toes, gently open your eyes and come back to the room.

---

a therapist can help patients feel better and more in control as well as having benefits in terms of pain relief.

Rest

In addition to exercise, teaching patients to rest comfortably in any position when in pain is a meaningful action and the base from which a person can learn to move more easily (O'Connor & Webb 2002). A person with a terminal illness may experience restriction of movement and neuromuscular pain with increased tension. For these patients, learning to rest and letting go of any tension can be helpful. O'Connor and Webb (2002) describe a specific method for resting known as the Feldenkrais method. Using this, a person can be taught how to rest comfortably in any position: this may be lying down, sitting or standing.

Transcutaneous electrical nerve stimulation

Transcutaneous electrical nerve stimulation (TENS) is thought to work by sending a weak electrical current through the skin to stimulate the sensory nerve endings. Depending on the stimulation parameters used, TENS is thought to modulate pain impulses by closing the gate to pain transmission within the spinal cord by stimulating the release of natural pain-relieving chemicals in the brain and spinal cord (King 1999).

To date there is limited scientific evidence for the effectiveness of TENS. Despite this, many health care professionals use TENS for a variety of chronic pain conditions and support the view that this is a useful form of analgesia (Walsh 1997). In contrast, TENS has not been found to improve the control of acute pain following surgery (McQuay *et al.* 1997).

Acupuncture

This involves placing fine solid needles into the skin at acupoints or trigger points. Although the exact mechanism of action is unknown, acupuncture is believed to work in part by stimulating release of the body's own natural opioids. Although there is also limited scientific evidence for the pain-relieving effects of acupuncture, largely due to the poorly controlled studies (Ezzo *et al.* 2000), it is used widely and has an important role in pain management.

Heat therapies

For decades superficial heat therapy has been used to relieve a variety of muscular and joint pains, including arthritis, back pain and period pain. There is much anecdotal and some scientific evidence to support the usefulness of heat as an adjunct to other pain treatments (Akin *et al.* 2001; Nadler *et al.* 2002; Robinson *et al.* 2002).

Heat works by:

- Stimulating thermoreceptors in the skin and deeper tissues, thereby reducing the sensitivity to pain by closing the gating system in the spinal cord.
- Reducing muscle spasm.
- Reducing the viscosity of synovial fluid which alleviates painful stiffness during movement and increases joint range (Carr & Mann 2000b).

In the home environment people use a variety of different methods for applying heat therapies, such as warm baths, hot water bottles, wheat-based heat packs and electrical heating pads. In the hospital setting caution is required with this equipment as it does not reach health and safety standards (no even and regular temperature distribution) and there have been incidences of serious burns (Barillo *et al.* 2000). Carr and Mann (2000b) note that heat therapy should not be used immediately following tissue damage as it will increase swelling. The Medicines and Healthcare Products Regulatory Agency (MHRA 2005) has documented evidence of burns caused by using heat patches or packs and therefore urge caution in their use and also recommend regular checking of skin throughout therapy.

Cold therapies

Cold therapies can also be used to stimulate nerves and modulate pain (Carr & Mann 2000b). Cold may be particularly valuable following an acute bruising injury where it can help to reduce inflammation and limit further damage. Cold can be applied in the form of crushed ice or gel-filled cold packs which should be wrapped in a towel to protect the skin from an ice burn.

Chronic pain

Pharmacological techniques

Using the WHO Analgesic Ladder (1996)

The Analgesic Ladder was designed as a framework for the management of chronic pain (see Figure 27.3). There are several drugs available to manage chronic pain and the Analgesic Ladder allows the flexibility to choose from the range according to the patient's requirements and tolerance (Hanks *et al.* 2001).

Step 1: non-opioid drugs

Examples of non-opioid drugs include paracetamol, aspirin and NSAIDs that are effective for mild to moderate pain. These drugs are especially effective for musculoskeletal and visceral pain (Twycross & Wilcock 2001).

Step 2: opioids for mild to moderate pain

Examples of opioids for mild to moderate pain include codeine, dihydrocodeine, tramadol and oxycodone (steps 2 and 3). These drugs are used when adequate pain management is not achieved with the use of non-opioids and are usually used in combination formulations. It is not recommended to administer another analgesic from the same group if the drug being used is not controlling the pain. Uncontrolled pain needs to be assessed and managed with the titration of an opioid by moving up the Analgesic Ladder. The exception to this would be if the patient was experiencing intolerable side-effects on the weak opioid and an alternative drug may be beneficial.

In recent studies tramadol has been recognized as being efficacious in the management of chronic cancer pain of moderate severity (Davis *et al.* 2005). It is uncertain whether tramadol is more effective in neuropathic pain than other opioids for mild to moderate pain; one report suggests a reduction in allodynia (pain from stimuli which is not normally painful) (Sindrup & Jensen 1999; Twycross & Wilcock 2001). Nurses should be aware that there are circumstantial reports that suggest tramadol lowers seizure threshold, and therefore care needs to be taken in those patients who have a history of epilepsy, as well as any other medications that may contribute to the lowering of the seizure threshold for example tricyclic antidepressants and selective serotonin reuptake inhibitors (SSRIs) (Twycross & Wilcock 2001). Few patients with severe pain will achieve a satisfactory level of pain control with tramadol. It is available in immediate and modified release preparations.

Step 3: opioids for moderate to severe pain

Morphine   A large amount of information and research is available concerning morphine and therefore it tends to be the drug of choice within this category (Hanks *et al.* 2001, 2004). It is available in oral, rectal, parenteral and intraspinal preparations. A recent study of 43 European Palliative Care Units showed that morphine was the most frequently used opioid for moderate to severe pain, with over 50% of patients taking oral or parenteral preparations (Klepstad *et al.* 2005). All strong opioids require careful titration from an expert practitioner. It is better to begin with a small dose, usually one that is equivalent to the previous medication, and increase gradually in conjunction with careful assessment of its effectiveness (Hanks *et al.* 2001). Titration begins with the immediate-release form which is available in tablet (Sevredol) or elixir (Oramorph) preparations, and once pain control is achieved the patient can be converted to a modified release preparation that acts over a 12- or 24-hour period (Zomorph or MXL respectively).

Breakthrough analgesia is administered using the equivalent 4-hourly dose of the immediate-release form. This dose can be given as required (hourly) and subsequent adjustments can be made to the modified form if the patient is requiring more than three breakthrough doses in a 24-hour period (Hanks *et al.* 2001).

Patients should be informed of potential side-effects such as constipation, nausea and increased sleepiness, in order to allay any fear. The patient should also be told that nausea and drowsiness are transitory and normally improve within 48 hours, but that constipation can be an ongoing problem and it is recommended that a laxative should be prescribed at the same time as the opioid is started. It is recommended that the most effective laxative for this group of patients is a combination of both a softening and a stimulating laxative (Davis *et al.* 2005).

Patients often have many concerns about commencing strong drugs such as morphine. Frequent fears centre around addiction and believing that its use signifies the terminal phase of the illness (McQuay 1999). Time should be taken to reassure patients and their families and provide verbal and written information. Although morphine is still considered to be the opioid drug of choice for moderate to severe pain (Hanks *et al.* 2001), alternative opioids allows the practitioner to carefully assess the patient on an individual basis and select the most appropriate opioid to use.

Durogesic (fentanyl) Fentanyl is a strong opioid, available in a patch, which is recommended in patients who have stable pain requirements. Transdermal patches are available in 12 (new size), 25, 50, 75 or 100 μg. It is reported to have an improved side-effect profile in comparison to morphine (Ahmedzai & Brooks 1997), although some patients experience nausea and mild drowsiness (BMA/Royal Pharmaceutical Society of Great Britain 2008) and occasionally patients may develop a reaction to the adhesive in the patch (Ling 1997). Use of the patch has increased because it allows the patient freedom from taking tablets.

Changing of the patch is recommended every 3 days, and steady plasma levels are reported to be reached after 8–16 hours (Zech *et al.* 1994), although in some patients it may be necessary to change it more frequently. The patch should be applied to skin that is free from excess hair and any form of irritation and should not be applied to irradiated areas. It is advisable to change the location on the body to avoid an adverse skin reaction. Occasionally difficulties arise relating to the titration of the patch as each patch is equivalent to a range of morphine (Table 27.3). For breakthrough pain, if patients are able to take oral medications then an immediate release preparation, for example immediate release morphine sulphate (oramorph/sevredol), at the appropriate dose can be used. An immediate-release fentanyl lozenge is available for use in breakthrough or incident pain. The advantage of oral transmucosal fentanyl citrate (OTFC) is its fast onset via the buccal mucosa (5–15 minutes) and its short duration (up to 2 hours). It is available in a range of doses (200–1600 μg) but there is no direct relation between the baseline analgesia and the breakthrough dose. Titration can be difficult and lengthy as the recommended starting dose is 200 μg with titration upwards (Portenoy *et al.* 1999).

Fentanyl is also available in parenteral preparations. There are potential problems with fentanyl due to dose limitations. The ampoules are available in 50 μg/1 ml. If the dose required is too large a volume to use in the syringe driver, then alfentanil may be a useful alternative (Dickman *et al.* 2002).

Palladone (hydromorphone) Palladone (hydromorphone) is mostly used when patients experience unacceptable drowsiness with morphine. It is similar to morphine in its pharmacokinetic profile and it is approximately 5.0–7.5 times more potent than morphine. It is available in immediate-release and sustained-release preparations and titration occurs in the same manner as morphine (Hays *et al.* 1994).

The side-effects are similar to those of morphine (Ellershaw 1998).

Methadone Methadone is a synthetic opioid developed more than 40 years ago (Riley *et al.* 2006). It is available in oral, rectal and parenteral preparations. There has been some reluctance amongst professionals to use methadone, which arose from the difficulties experienced in titrating the drug due to its long half-life (15 hours) that caused accumulation to occur, especially in the elderly (Gannon 1997). There are different methods of achieving effective titration (Gannon 1997); for example, one regimen is to calculate one-tenth of the total daily dose of morphine (maximum starting dose must not exceed 30 mg). Administer the methadone to the patient on an as-required basis but not within 3 hours of the last fixed dose. The total dose required over a 24-hour period is calculated after 5–6 days, divided and given as a two or three times daily regimen and this avoids the build-up of methadone within the body (Morley & Makin 1998). Titration is recommended within a hospital setting to ensure accurate administration. This can be difficult for patients because they have to experience pain before they are administered a dose of methadone in the titration period.

Methadone can be a cheap, effective alternative to morphine if titration is supervised by the specialist pain or palliative care team (Gardner-Nix 1996).

Methadone is particularly useful in patients with renal failure. Morphine is excreted via the kidneys and if renal failure occurs this may lead to the patient experiencing severe drowsiness as a result of culmination of morphine metabolites (Gannon 1997). Methadone is lipid soluble and is metabolized mainly in the liver. About half of the drug and its metabolites are excreted by the intestines and half by the kidneys.

Table 27.3 Oral morphine conversion to Durogesic (fentanyl) patch.

4-hourly oral morphine dose (mg)	Durogesic patch strength (μg/hour)	24-hour morphine dose (mg)
20	25	135
25–35	50	135–224
40–50	75	225–314
55–65	100	315–404
70–80	125	405–494
85–95	150	495–584
100–110	175	585–674
115–125	200	675–764

A 12 μg/hour Durogesic DTrans (fentanyl transdermal system with matrix technology) patch has been introduced to aid dose titration between 25 and 75 μg/hour.

Oxycodone Oxycodone is available as an immediate or modified release tablet and titration should occur in the same way as morphine. Oxycodone is a useful opioid as an alternative to morphine (Riley *et al.* 2006). It has similar properties to morphine and can be administered orally, rectally, intraspinally and parenterally. Oxycodone has similar side-effects and it is usually given 4–6 hourly. Oxycodone has an analgesic potency of 1.5–2.0 times higher than morphine. It has similar side-effects to morphine, although oxycodone has been found to cause less nausea (Heiskanen and Kalso 1997) and significantly less itchiness (Mucci-LoRusso *et al.* 1998).

Diamorphine Diamorphine is used parenterally in a syringe driver for the control of moderate to severe pain when patients are unable to take the oral form of morphine. It is calculated by dividing the total daily dose of oral morphine by three. Breakthrough doses are calculated by dividing the 24-hour dose of diamorphine by six and administering on an as-required basis (Hanks *et al.* 2004). A recent problem with the supply of Diamorphine nationally has resulted in centres using morphine sulphate or an alternative opioid as a substitute.

Nasal analgesia It is suggested that the nasal route may be effective for a number of opioids (Hanks *et al.* 2004). Nasal diamorphine spray has been shown to provide effective pain relief in Accident and Emergency Departments in children and teenagers who are experiencing acute pain. This approach is being investigated in adult cancer patients with acute, episodic pain (Hanks *et al.* 2004).

Alfentanil Alfentanil is also a useful alternative to diamorphine and is used as an alternative opioid for those patients who have renal impairment. The onset of action is rapid owing to a more rapid blood–brain equilibration. It is 10 times more potent than diamorphine (i.e. diamorphine 10 mg = alfentanil 1 mg). The breakthrough dose can be calculated as one-tenth of the 24-hour dose as opposed to the usual one-sixth. For example 1 mg of alfentanil over 24 hours will require a breakthrough dose of alfentanil 0.1 mg. It is beneficial when high doses are required as it comes in ampoules of 1 mg/2 ml and 5 mg/1 ml and smaller volumes can be used (Hill 1992).

Buprenorphine Buprenorphine is an alternative strong opioid available in a patch form. The patch has similar advantages to fentanyl but does not contain a reservoir of the drug. Instead it is contained in a matrix form with effective levels of the drug being reached within 24 hours. Titration is recommended with an alternative opioid initially and then transfer to the patch when stable requirements have been reached. The patches are available in strengths of 5, 10 and 20 µg/hour at a lower dose patch (Butrans) that

should be worn continuously by the patient for 7 days. The higher dose patch (Transtec) of 35, 52.5 and 70 µg/hour is now licensed to be used up to 96 hours or twice weekly for patient convenience. Conversion is based on the chart supplied by the pharmaceutical company which demonstrates equivalent doses. Buprenorphine is also available as a sublingual tablet, which is titrated from 200 to 800 µg 6-hourly. Conversion is based on multiplying the total daily dose of buprenorphine by 100 to give the total daily dose of morphine (i.e. 200 µg buprenorphine/8-hourly = 600 µg buprenorphine/24 hours = 60 mg morphine/24 hours) (Budd 2002).

Cannabis Studies are currently taking place to examine the potential benefits of using cannabis for the management of chronic conditions, e.g. multiple sclerosis and cancer. Good-quality research is sparse (Wall *et al.* 2001) but there are a number of studies that allude to its benefits in managing chronic pain, spasticity and muscle spasms (Martyn 1995; Consroe 1997).

Breakthrough analgesia

Breakthrough pain refers to a transitory exacerbation of pain experienced by the patient who has relatively stable and adequately controlled background pain (Portenoy *et al.* 2004). There should not be a time limit on this type of prescription because it would need to be given when and if the patient demonstrated any signs of discomfort or pain (with the exception of renal failure where dosages would need to be limited).

Breakthrough doses are calculated on a 4-hour equivalence; for example, if a patient was prescribed 60 mg MXL (a modified form of morphine given once a day), the equivalent breakthrough dose would be 10 mg of the immediate-release formulation. If several breakthrough doses are required within a 24-hour period, then the background analgesia (long-acting form) would have to be increased (McMillan 2001). However, it is important to recognize the classifications of breakthrough pain, as increasing the background dose will not always be indicated.

Breakthrough pain can be classified as follows:

(a) Spontaneous pain: this type of pain occurs unexpectedly.

(b) Incident pain: this pain is related to specific events and can be classified into four categories (Davies 2006):

1 Volitional pain is precipitated by a voluntary act, for example walking.

2 Non-volitional pain is precipitated by an involuntary act, for example coughing.

3 Procedural is a type of pain related to a therapeutic intervention, for example wound dressing.

4 End-of-dose failure is related to analgesic dosing (declining analgesic levels).

The use of opioids in renal failure

Renal failure can cause significant and dangerous side-effects due to the accumulation of the drug. Basic guidelines for pain management in renal failure include:

- Reduce analgesia dose and/or dose frequency (6-hourly instead of 4-hourly).
- Select a more appropriate drug (non-renally excreted).
- Avoid modified release preparations.
- Seek advice from a specialist pain/palliative care team and/or pharmacist (Farrell & Rich 2000).

Adjuvant drugs (co-analgesics)

Adjuvant drugs are a miscellaneous group of drugs whose primary indication is for conditions other than pain which may however relieve pain in specific circumstances (Twycross & Wilcock 2001). Examples of this category of drugs include NSAIDs, steroids, antibiotics, antidepressants, anti-epileptics, N-methyl-D-aspartate (NMDA) receptor channel blockers, antispasmodics and muscle relaxants (Twycross & Wilcock 2001).

The WHO Analgesic Ladder recommends the use of these drugs in combination with non-opioids, opioids for mild to moderate pain and opioids for moderate to severe pain (see Table 27.2).

Cancer treatment interventions

In addition to pharmacological and non-pharmacological strategies, treatment of cancer pain may be managed most effectively with radiotherapy, surgery, chemotherapy, hormonal manipulation and bisphosphonates. Many palliative care units/hospices may not have access to these interventions and, indeed, careful consideration must be given to ensure that the advantages achieved from any proposed treatment are not outweighed by the potential side-effects and consequent poor quality of life. The aim of these treatments would be to reduce the overall size of the tumour(s), and therefore to improve symptom control; and this must be clearly indicated to the patient (Twycross & Wilcock 2001).

Opioids and driving

In 2004 a publication in *Palliative Medicine* offered guidance for professionals on the advice they should offer to patients who were taking opioids and driving. One of the contributors to the guidance was the medical advisor to the Driver and Vehicle Licensing Agency (DVLA) (Pease *et al.* 2004). Advice to patients should include:

(a) A patient should not drive:
  - For 5 days after starting or changing the dose of the recommended opioid.
  - If they feel sleepy

- After drinking alcohol or taking strong opioids which have not been recommended by the doctor or non-medical prescriber, e.g. cannabis.
- On days when additional breakthrough medication of an opioid has been taken.

(b) Patients can restart driving:
  - After 5 days starting or changing the dose of the recommended opioid and if the patient does not feel sleepy. But the patient:
    - should make the first trip short;
    - on roads that the patient is familiar with;
    - at a time when the traffic is not too busy, and
    - have an experienced driver accompany the patient as this may be helpful.

(c) Patients do not need to inform the DVLA about starting an opioid but may need to inform them of other aspects relating to their illness. The patient should be encouraged to inform their insurance company about their current state of health and current medications.

Anaesthetic interventions

Sometimes it is difficult to attain and maintain adequate pain control without significant side-effects and it is in situations such as this that anaesthetic interventions may be of benefit.

Effective control can be achieved by epidural or intrathecal (spinal) infusions:

- as single injections for simple nerve blocks or;
- regional nerve blocks which target individual nerves, plexuses or ganglia (Hicks & Simpson 2004).

Examples include managing pelvic pain and post-radiation brachial plexopathy. These interventions can be useful, but careful consideration and assessment must take place to ensure that any potential side-effects are discussed with the patient (anaesthetic interventions may severely limit the patient's activities) and that future planning is addressed with the patient and family as an epidural/intrathecal infusion may limit discharge options for the patient who is dying.

Conclusion

The management of acute and chronic pain is a constant challenge to the health care professional. Accurate assessment of the type and site of each pain, accompanied by careful monitoring and reviewing of any intervention, are essential in order to provide care that benefits the patient and does not impinge on his or her quality of life.

Nurses are in an ideal situation to promote a trusting relationship with the patient by encouraging the patient to express any concerns, thus allowing the patient adequate opportunities to work in partnership and be an active participant in his or her pain management programme.

Procedure guidelines   Pain control: assessment and education of patient prior to surgery

Procedure

Action	Rationale

1 If patient has had previous surgery, ask for details of:
  (a) Previous and current pain control methods (pharmacological and non-pharmacological).
  (b) Effectiveness of these methods.
  (c) Experience of side-effects, such as nausea and vomiting.
	To ensure previous experiences are taken into consideration when planning pain control. To allay any fears based on previous experience. To ensure care is planned to minimize side-effects such as nausea and vomiting (Audit Commission 1997: C).

2 Assess patient for pre-existing long-term pain problems. Obtain information on:
  (a) Pain type, location and intensity.
  (b) Use of analgesics.
	To plan in advance of surgery the pain control methods that will be used to manage both the patient's long-term and anticipated postoperative pain (Lewis & Williams 2005: R 5).

3 Check patient suitability for various pain control methods, e.g. renal function, clotting abnormalities, dexterity, visual impairment.	To avoid the use of inappropriate pain control methods, e.g.:
	  (a) Diclofenac in renal impairment.
	  (b) Epidural analgesia with clotting abnormalities.
	  (c) PCAs, if lack of dexterity or visual impairment makes the patient incapable of pressing the demand button which is connected to the pump (Mehta & Langford: R 4).

4 Liaise with multidisciplinary team and patient to select most appropriate pain control method(s).	To ensure effective collaboration between the patient and team in order to optimize postoperative pain control (Halaszynski *et al.* 2004: R 4).

5 Explain and discuss with patient:
  (a) How pain will be assessed and the use of a pain Scale.
 	
  (b) How pain will be controlled.
 	
  (c) Goals for pain control at rest and on movement.
	To allay anxiety and promote patient well-being and control.
	To encourage active involvement in pain control. To give the patient a chance to ask questions (E).
	To ensure the patient understands the rationale for pain control during deep breathing and movement. This will help prevent postoperative complications, e.g. chest infections (Knoerl *et al.* 1999: R 3).

6 Provide patient with written information about pain control.	To support verbal information (Chumbley *et al.* 2002: R 4).
7 Where appropriate, demonstrate the use of pain control methods before surgery.	To ensure the patient has the skill and knowledge to effectively use the pain control methods chosen, e.g. PCAs (Chumbley *et al.* 2002: R 4).

Procedure guidelines   Pain assessment chart: chronic

Procedure

Action	Rationale
1 Explain the purpose of using the chart to the patient.	To ensure that the patient understands the procedure and gives his/her valid consent and co-operation (Witt-Sherman *et al.* 2004: R 4; NMC 2006: C).
2 Encourage the patient, where appropriate, to identify pain him/herself.	The body outline (see Figure 27.2) is a vehicle for the patient to describe his/her own pain experience (Witt-Sherman *et al.* 2004: R 4).
3 When it is necessary for the nurse to complete the chart, ensure that the patient's own description of his/her pain is recorded.	To reduce the risk of misinterpretation (E).
4 (a) Record any factors that influence the intensity of the pain, e.g. activities or interventions that reduce or increase the pain such as distractions or a heat pad.	Ascertaining how and when the patient experiences pain enables the nurse to plan realistic goals. For example, relieving the patient's pain during the night and while he/she is at rest is usually easier to achieve before relief from pain on movement (Davis & McVicker 2000: E).
(b) Record whether or not the patient is pain free at night, at rest or on movement.	To ascertain an understanding of the experience of pain for the patient (Twycross & Wilcock 2001: R 5).
(c) Record frequency of pain, what helps to relieve the pain, what makes the pain worse and how the patient feels when they are in pain.	
5 Index each site (A–D; see Figure 27.2) in whatever way seems most appropriate, e.g. shading or colouring of areas or arrows to indicate shooting pains.	This enables individual pain sites to be located (Witt-Sherman *et al.* 2004: R 4).
6 Give each pain site a numerical value according to the key to pain intensity or the pain scale and note time recorded.	To indicate the intensity of the pain at each site (Turk & Okifuji 1999: E).
7 Record any analgesia given and note route and dose.	To monitor efficacy of prescribed analgesia. (Twycross & Wilcock 2001: R 5)
8 Record any significant activities that are likely to influence the patient's pain.	Extra pharmacological or non-pharmacological interventions might be indicated (Turk & Okifuji 1999: E; RCN 2005: C).

Note: fixed times for reviewing the pain have been omitted intentionally to allow for flexibility. It is suggested that, initially, the patient's pain is reviewed by the patient and nurse every 4 hours. When a patient's level of pain has stabilized, recordings may be made less frequently, e.g. 12-hourly or daily. The chart should be discontinued if a patient's pain becomes totally controlled.

References and further reading

Ahmedzai, F. & Brooks, D. (1997) Transdermal Fentanyl versus Oral Morphine in Cancer Pain: Preference, Efficacy and Quality of Life. *J Pain Symptom Management* 13, 254–61.

Akin, M. *et al.* (2001) Continuous low-level topical heat in the treatment of dysmenorrhea. *Obstet Gynecol*, 97(3), 343–9.

Anderson, K.O. & Cleeland, C.S. (2003) The assessment of cancer pain. In: *Cancer Pain: Assessment and Management* (eds E.D. Bruera & R.K. Portenoy). Cambridge University Press, Cambridge, pp. 51–66.

ANZCA and Faculty of Pain Medicine (2005) *Acute Pain Management: Scientific Evidence*, 2nd edn. Australian and New Zealand College of Anaesthetists, Melbourne, Victoria, Australia.

Audit Commission (1997) *Anaesthesia under Examination*. Audit Commission, Oxford.

Ballard, K. (1997) Pressure-relief mattresses and patient comfort. *Prof Nurse*, 13(1), 27–32.

Bamigbade, T. & Langford, R. (1998) Tramadol hydrochloride: an overview of current use. *Hosp Med*, **59**(5), 373–6.

Barillo, D. *et al.* (2000) Burns caused by medical therapy. *J Burn Care Rehabil*, **21**(3), 269–73.

Beck, S. (1991) The therapeutic use of music for cancer-related pain. *Oncol Nurse Forum*, **18**(8), 1327–37.

Bennett, M. (2001) The LANSS pain scale: the Leeds assessment of neuropathic symptoms and signs. *Pain*, **92**, 147–57.

BMA/Royal Pharmaceutical Society of Great Britain (2008) *British National Formulary*. Pharmaceutical Press, Oxford.

Budd, K. (2002) *Evidence-based Medicine in Practice. Buprenorphine: a Review*. Haywood Medical, London.

Carr, E. (1990) Post-operative pain: patient expectations and experiences. *J Adv Nurs*, **15**(1), 89–100.

Carr, E. & Mann, E. (2000a) Recognising the barriers to effective pain relief. In: *Pain: Creative Approaches to Effective Management*. Macmillan Press/Bournemouth University, London, pp. 109–29.

Carr, E. & Mann, E. (2000b) Managing chronic pain. In: *Pain: Creative Approaches to Effective Management*. Macmillan Press/Bournemouth University, London, pp. 81–108.

Carroll, D. & Bowsher, D. (1993) *Pain Management and Nursing Care*. Butterworth Heinemann, Oxford.

Carroll, D. & Seers, K. (1998) Relaxation for the relief of chronic pain: a systematic review. *J Adv Nurs*, **27**(3), 476–87.

Caunt, H. (1992) Reducing the psychological impact of postoperative pain. *J Nurs*, **1**(1), 13–19.

Chumbley, G.M., Hall, G.M. & Salmon, P. (2002) Patient-controlled analgesia: what information does the patient want? *J Adv Nurs*, **39**(5), 459–71.

Cleeland, C.S. (1991) The brief pain inventory. www.mdanderson.org/pdf/bpilong. Accessed 24/9/07.

Coda, B. *et al.* (1997) Comparative efficacy of patient-controlled administration of morphine, hydromorphone, or sufentil for the treatment of oral mucositis following bone marrow transplantation. *Pain*, **72**(3), 333–46.

Colleau, S.M. (1999) The significance of breakthrough pain in cancer. *Cancer Pain Release*, **12**, 1–4.

Consroe, P. (1997) The perceived effects of smoked cannabis on patients with multiple sclerosis. *Eur Neurol*, **38**(1), 44–8.

Davies, A. (2006) *Cancer-related Breakthrough Pain*. Oxford Pain Mnagement Library, Oxford.

Davis, B.D. & McVicker, A. (2000) Issues in effective pain control: from assessment to management. *Int J Palliat Nurs*, **6**(4), 162–9.

Davis, M., Glare, P. & Hardy, J. (2005) *Opioids in Cancer Pain*. Oxford University Press, Oxford.

Dickman, A., Littlewood, C. & Varga, J. (eds) (2002) Drug information. In: *The Syringe Driver. Continuous Subcutaneous Infusions in Palliative Care*. Oxford University Press, Oxford, pp. 11–58.

Donaldson, G. *et al.* (1997) Comparative efficacy of patient controlled administration of morphine, hydromorphone or sufentil for the treatment of oral mucositis following bone marrow transplantation. *Pain*, **72**(3), 333–46.

Donnelly, S. & Walsh, D. (1995) The symptoms of advanced cancer. *Semin Oncol*, **22**(2 Suppl 3), 67–72.

Drayer, R.A., Henderson, B.S. & Reidenberg, M. (1999) Barriers to better pain control in hospitalised patients. *J Pain Symptom Control*, **17**(6), 434–40.

Ellershaw, J. (1998) Hydromorphone: a new alternative to morphine. *Prescriber*, **9**(4), 21–7.

Ezzo, J. *et al.* (2000) Is acupuncture effective for the treatment of chronic pain? A systematic review. *Pain*, **86**(3), 217–25.

Farrell, A. & Rich, A. (2000) Analgesic use in patients with renal failure. *Eur J Palliat Care*, **7**(6), 201–5.

Field, L. (1996) Are nurses still underestimating patients' pain post-operatively? *Br J Nurs*, **15**(13), 778–84.

Feine, J. & Lund, J. (1997) An assessment of the efficacy of physical therapy and physical modalities for the control of chronic musculoskeletal pain. *Pain*, **71**(1), 5–23.

Fine, P.G. *et al.* (1991) An open label study of oral transdermal fentanyl citrate (OTFC) for the treatment of breakthrough cancer pain. *Pain*, **45**, 149–53.

Fitzpatrick R. *et al.* (1998) Evaluating a patient based outcome measure for use in clinical trials. *Health Technol Assess*, **21**, 95–102.

Flaherty, S.A. (1996) Pain measurement tools for clinical practice and research. *J Am Assoc Nurse Anesth*, **64**, 133–40.

Foley, K. (2004) Pain assessment and cancer pain syndromes. In: *Oxford Textbook of Palliative Medicine* (eds D. Doyle *et al.*), 3rd edn. Oxford Medical Publications, Oxford, pp. 298–316.

Gannon, C. (1997) The use of methadone in the care of the dying. *Eur J Palliat Care*, **4**(5), 152–8.

Gardner-Nix, J. (1996) Oral methadone for managing chronic non malignant pain. *J Pain Symptom Control*, **11**(5), 321–2.

Good, M. (1996) Effects of relaxation and music on postoperative pain: a review. *J Adv Nurs*, **24**, 905–14.

Good, M. *et al.* (1999) Relief of postoperative pain with jaw relaxation, music and their combination. *Pain*, **81**(1–2), 163–72.

Good, M. *et al.* (2005) Relaxation and music reduce pain following intestinal surgery. *Res Nurs Health*, **28**, 240–51.

Gould, T. *et al.* (1992) Policy for controlling pain after surgery: effect of sequential changes in management. *Br Med J*, **305**(6863), 1187–93.

Grond, S. *et al.* (1996) Assessment of cancer pain: a prospective evaluation. *Pain*, **64**(1), 107–14.

Halaszynski, T.M., Juda, R. & Silverman, D.G. (2004) Optimizing postoperative outcomes with efficient preoperative assessment and management. *Crit Care Med*, **32**(4), S76–86.

Hamrin, E., Sjostrom, B. & Unosson, M. (2002) Patient and nurse assessment of quality of care in postoperative pain management. *Qual Saf Health Care*, **11**, 327–34.

Hanks, G., Cherny, N. & Fallon, M. (2004) Opioid analgesic therapy. In: *Oxford Textbook of Palliative Medicine* (eds D. Doyle *et al.*), 3rd edn. Oxford Medical Publications, Oxford, pp. 316–342.

Hanks, G. & Expert Working Group of the European Association for Palliative Care (1996) Morphine in cancer pain: modes of administration. *Br Med J*, **3**(12), 823–6.

Hanks, G.W. (1991) Opioid-responsive and opioid non-responsive pain in cancer. *Br Med Bull*, **47**, 718–31.

Hanks, G.W. *et al.* (2001) Morphine and alternative opioids in cancer pain: the EAPC recommendations. *Br J Cancer*, **84**(5), 587–93.

Harmer, M. & Davies, K. (1998) The effect of education, assessment and a standardised prescription on postoperative pain management. *Anaesthesia*, **53**(5), 424–30.

Hays, H. *et al.* (1994) Comparative clinical efficacy and safety of immediate release and controlled release hydromorphone for chronic severe pain. *Cancer*, **74**(6), 1808–16.

Hayward, J. (1975) *Information, a Prescription against Pain, the Study of Nursing Care*. Research Project, Series 2(5). Royal College of Nursing, London.

Heiser, R. *et al.* (1997) The use of music during the immediate postoperative recovery period. *AORN J*, **65**(4), 777.

Heiskanen, T. & Kalso, E. (1997) Controlled-release oxycodone and morphine in cancer related pain. *Science Direct* **73**(1), 37–45.

Hicks, F. & Simpson, K.H. (eds) (2004) Regional nerve blocks. In: *Nerve Blocks in Palliative Care.* Oxford University Press, Oxford, pp. 53–55.

Higginson, I. (1998) Can professionals improve their assessments? *J Pain Symp Manage,* **15**(3), 149–50.

Hill, H.F. (1992) Patient controlled analgesic infusions: alfentanil versus morphine. *Pain,* **49**(3), 301–10.

Hobbs, G.J. & Hodgkinson, V. (2003) Assessment, measurement, history and examination. In: *Clinical Pain Management: Acute Pain* (eds D.J. Rowbotham & P.E. Macintyre). Arnold Publishers, London pp. 93–112.

IASP (1994) IASP pain terminology. www.iasp-pain.org/terms. Accessed 17/7/06.

IASP (1996) Classification of chronic pain. *Pain,* **3**(Suppl), 51–226.

Idvall, E. *et al.* (2002) Patient and nurse assessment of quality of care in postoperative pain management. *Qual Saf Health Care,* **11,** pp. 327–34.

Kalkman, C.J. *et al.* (2003) Preoperative prediction of severe postoperative pain. *Pain,* **105,** 415–23.

Kehlet, H. (1997) Multimodal approach to control of postoperative pathophysiology and rehabilitation. *Br J Anaesth,* **78**(5), 606–17.

King, A. (1999) *King's Guide to TENS for Health Professionals.* King's Medical Physio-Med Services, Glossop, Derbyshire.

Kitson, A. (1994) Post-operative pain management: a literature review. *J Clin Nurs,* **3**(1), 7–18.

Klepstad, P. *et al.* (2005) Pain and pain treatments in European palliative care units. A cross sectional survey from the European Association for Palliative Care Research Network. *Palliat Med,* **19**(6), 477–84.

Knoerl, D.V., Faut-Callohan, M. & Paice, J. (1999) Preoperative PCA teaching program to manage postoperative pain. *Medsurg Nurs,* **8,** 25–33 & 36.

Krishnasamy, M. (2001) Pain. In: *Cancer Nursing Care in Context* (eds J. Corner & C. Bailey). Blackwell Science, Oxford, pp. 339-350.

Lang, E. *et al.* (2000) Adjunctive non-pharmacological analgesia for invasive medical procedures: a randomised trial. *Lancet,* **355**(9214), 1486–90.

Lawler, K. (1997) Pain assessment. *Prof Nurs Study,* **13**(1, Suppl), S5–8.

Lewis, N.L. & Williams, J. (2005) Acute pain management in patients receiving opioids for chronic cancer pain. *Continuing Education in Anaesthesia, Critical Care and Pain,* **5**(4), 127–9.

Ling, J. (1997) The use of transdermal fentanyl in palliative care. *Int J Palliat Nurs,* **3**(2), 65–8.

Loveman, E. & Gale, A. (2000) Factors influencing nurses inferences about patient pain. *Br J Nurs,* **9**(6), 334–7.

Macintyre, P.E. & Jarvis, D.A. (1996) Age is the best predictor of postoperative morphine requirements. *Pain,* **64,** 357–64.

Macintyre, P.E. (2001) Safety and efficacy of patient-controlled analgesia. *Br J Anaesth,* **87**(1), 36–46.

Macintyre, P.E. & Ready, L. (2001) *Acute Pain Management. A Practical Guide.* W.B. Saunders, London.

Martyn, C. (1995) 'N = 1' cross-over trial using nabilone in a patient with multiple sclerosis. *Lancet,* **345**(8949), 579.

McCaffery M. (1968) *Nursing practice theories related to cognition, bodily pain and man environment.* Student store, UCLA, Los Angeles.

McCaffery, M. (1990) Nursing approaches to non-pharmacological pain control. *Int J Nurs Stud,* **27**(1), 1–5,

McCaffery, M. (2000) *Nursing Management of the Patient with Pain,* 3rd edn. Lippincott, Philadelphia.

McCaffery, M. & Beebe, A. (1989) Perspectives on pain. In: *Clinical Manual for Nursing Practice,* pp. 1–5. Mosby, St Louis.

McCaffery, M. & Ferrell, B.R. (1997) Nurses' knowledge of pain assessment and management: how much progress have we made? *J Pain Symp Manage,* **14**(3), 175–88.

MaCaffery, M. & Pasero, C. (2003) Breakthrough pain: it's common in patients with chronic pain. *Am J Nurs,* **103**(4), 83–6.

McCaffery, M. & Robinson, E.S. (2002) Your patient is in pain—here's how you respond. *Nursing,* **32**(10), 36–47.

McMillan, C. (2001) Breakthrough pain: assessment and management in cancer patients. *Br J Nurs,* **10**(13), 860–6.

McQuay, H. (1990) The logic of alternative routes. *J Pain Symp Manage,* **5**(2), 75–7.

McQuay, H. (1999) Opioids in pain management. *Lancet,* **353,** 2229–32.

McQuay, H. & Edwards, J. (2003) Meta-analysis of single dose oral tramadol plus acetaminophen in acute postoperative pain. *Eur J Anaesthesiol,* **28**(Suppl), 19–22.

McQuay, H. & Moore, A. (1998) Oral tramadol versus placebo, codeine and combination analgesics. In: *An Evidence Based Resource for Pain.* Oxford University Press, Oxford, pp. 138–46.

McQuay, H., Moore, A. & Justins, D. (1997) Treating acute pain in hospital. *Br Med J,* **314**(7093), 1531–5.

Mehta, V. & Langford, R.M. (2006) Acute pain management for opioid dependent patients. *Anaesthesia,* **61,** 269–76.

Melzack, R. (1975) The McGill Pain Questionnaire: major properties and scoring methods. *Pain,* **1,** 277–99.

Merskey, H. & Bogduk, N. (1994) *Classification of Chronic Pain.* 2nd edn. IASP Press, Seattle.

MHRA (2005) *Medical Device Alert.* Ref. MDA/2005/027. MHRA, London.

Mitchell, M. (1997) Patients' perceptions of pre-operative preparation for day surgery. *J Adv Nurs,* **26**(2), 356–63.

Morley, J.S. & Makin, M.K. (1998) The use of methadone in cancer pain poorly responsive to other opioids. *Pain Rev,* **5,** 51–8.

Mucci-LoRusso, P. *et al.* (1998) Controlled release oxycodone compared with controlled release morphine in the treatment of cancer pain: a randomised, double-blind, parallel group study. *Eur J Pain,* **2,** 239–49.

Nadler, S. *et al.* (2002) Continuous low-level heat wrap therapy provides more efficacy than ibuprofen and acetaminophen for acute low back pain. *Spine,* **27**(10), 1012–17.

NMC (2006) *A–Z Advice Sheet Consent.* www.nmc.org.

O'Connor, M. & Webb, R. (2002) Learning to rest when in pain. *Eur J Palliat Care,* **9**(2), 68–71.

Pargeon, K.L. & Hailey, B.J. (1999) Barriers to effective cancer pain management: a review. *J Pain Symp Manage,* **5,** 358–68.

Pasero, C. (1998) Pain control – is laughter the best medicine? *Am J Nurs,* **98**(12), 12–14.

Payne, R. (1995) *Relaxation Techniques: a Practical Handbook for Health Care Professionals.* Churchill Livingstone, Edinburgh.

Paz, S. & Seymour, J.E. (2004) Pain theories, evaluation and management. In: *Palliative Care Nursing* (eds S. Payne *et al.*). Open University Press, Berkshire, pp. 260–298.

Pease, N., Taylor, H. & Major, H. (2004) Strong painkillers and driving. *Palliat Med,* **18,** 663–8.

Perkins, F.M. & Kehlet, H. (2000) Chronic pain as an outcome of surgery. *Anasthesiology,* **93,** 1123–33.

Portenoy, R.K. & Lesage, P. (1999) Management of cancer pain. *Lancet,* **353,** 1695–1700.

Portenoy, R.K., Payne, R. & Coluzzi, P. (1999) Oral transmucosal fentanyl citrate (OTFC) for the treatment of breakthrough pain in cancer patients: a controlled dose titration study. *Pain,* **79,** 303–12.

Portenoy, R.K. *et al.* (2004) Difficult pain problems: an integrated approach. In: *Oxford Textbook of Palliative Medicine* (eds D. Doyle *et al.*). Oxford University Press, Oxford, pp. 316–36.

576

Poyhia, R. *et al.* (1993) Oxycodone an alternative to morphine for cancer pain. A review. *J Pain Symp Manage*, 8, 63–7.

Quigley, C. (2004) Opioid switching to improve pain relief and drug tolerability. *Cochrane Database Syst Rev*, 3 CD004847.

Raiman J. (1986) Pain relief-a two way process. *Nursing Times*, 82(15), 24–28.

Ready, L. & Edwards, W. (1992) *Management of Acute Pain: a Practical Guide*. IASP Publications, Seattle.

Reicin, A. *et al.* (2001) Efficacy of single-dose and multidose rofecoxib in the treatment of post orthopedic surgery pain. *Am J Orthoped*, 30(1), 40–8.

Riley, J. *et al.* (2006) Opioids in palliative care. *Eur J Palliat Care*, 13(6), 230–3.

Robinson, V.A. *et al.* (2002) Thermotherapy for treating rheumatoid arthritis. Cochrane Database of Systematic Review 2002, Issue 2, Article No. CD002826. Doi: 10: 1002/14651858.

Romsing, J., Moiniche, S. & Dahl, J.B. (2002) Rectal and parenteral paracetemol, and paracetemol in combination with NSAIDs for postoperative analgesia. *Br J Anaesth*, 88, 215–26.

Rowbotham, D. (2000) Non-steroidal anti-inflammatory drugs and paracetamol. In: *Chronic Pain*. Martin Dunitz, London, pp. 19–26.

Saunders, C. & Sykes, N. (1993) *The Management of Terminal Malignant Disease*, 3rd edn. Hodder & Stoughton, Boston.

Schug, S.A. & Torrie, J.J. (1993) Safety assessment of postoperative pain management by an acute pain service. *Pain*, 55, 387–91.

Scott, I. (1994) Effectiveness of documented assessment of post operative pain. *Br J Nurs*, 3(10), 494–501.

Seers, K. (1996) The patients' experiences of their chronic nonmalignant pain. *J Adv Nurs*, 24(6), 1160–8.

Seers, K. & Carroll, D. (1998) Relaxation techniques for acute pain management: a systematic review. *J Adv Nurs*, 27(3), 466–75.

Sidebotham, D. *et al.* (1997) The safety and utilization of patient controlled analgesia. *J Pain Symp Manage*, 14(4), 202–9.

Sindrup, S. & Jensen, T. (1999) Efficacy of pharmacological treatments of neuropathic pain: an update and effect related to mechanism of drug action. *Pain*, 83, 389–400.

Sloman, R. *et al.* (1994) The use of relaxation for the promotion of comfort and pain relief in persons with advanced cancer. *Contemp Nurse*, 3(1), 6–12.

Tasmuth, T., Estlandberg, A. & Kalso, E. (1996) Effect of present pain and memory of past post-operative pain in women treated with surgery for breast cancer. *Pain*, 68(2–3), 343–7.

Taylor, H. (2001) Pain management supplement. The importance of providing good patient information. *Prof Nurse*, 17(1), 34–6.

Trauger-Querry, B. & Haghighi, K. (1999) Balancing the focus: art and music therapy for pain and symptom management in hospice care. *Hospice J*, 14(1), 25–37.

Turk, D.C. & Okifuji, A. (1999) Assessment of patients' reporting of pain: an integrated perspective. *Lancet*, 353, 1784–9.

Twycross, R. & Wilcock, A. (2001) *Symptom Management in Advanced Cancer*, 3rd edn. Radcliffe Medical Press, Oxford.

Twycross, R., Harcourt, J. & Bergl, S. (1996) A survey of pain in patients with advanced cancer. *J Pain Symp Manage*, 12(5), 273–82.

Tye, T. & Gell-Walker, V. (2000) Patient-controlled analgesia. *Nurs Times*, 96(25), 38–9.

Vijayan, R. (1997) Subcutaneous morphine – a simple technique for postoperative analgesia. *Int J Acute Pain*, 1(1), 21–6.

Walker, S.M., MacIntyre, P.E. & Visser, E. (2006) Acute pain management: current best practice evidence provides guide for improved practice. *Pain Med*, 7(1), 3–5.

Walker, V.S. *et al.* (1987) Pain assessment charts in the management of chronic cancer pain. *Palliat Med*, 1, 111–16.

Wall, J., Davis, S. & Ridgway, S. (2001) Cannabis: its therapeutic use. *Nurs Stand*, 16(10), 39–44.

Walsh, D. (ed) (1997) Review of clinical studies on TENS. In: *TENS: Clinical Applications and Related Theory*. Churchill Livingstone, London, pp. 83–101.

Wheatley, R., Schug, S. & Watson, D. (2001) Safety and efficacy of postoperative epidural analgesia. *Br J Anaesth*, 87(1), 47–61.

WHO (1996) *Cancer Pain Relief*. World Health Organization, Geneva.

Witt-Sherman, D. *et al.* (2004) Learning pain assessment and management. A goal of the end-of-life nursing education consortium. *J Contin Edu Nursing* 35(3), 107–20.

Zarnegar, R. & Daniel, C. (2005) Pain management programmes. Continuing education in anaesthesia. *Crit Care Pain J*, 5(3), 80–3.

Zaza, C. (2002) Cancer pain and psychosocial factors: a critical review of the literature. *J Pain Symptom Manage*, 24(5), 526–40.

Zech, D., Lehmann, A. & Grond, S. (1994) A new treatment option for chronic cancer pain. *Eur J Palliat Care*, 1(1), 26–30.

Chapter 28

Pain management: Entonox administration

Reference material 579
Procedure guidelines: Entonox administration 581
Problem solving: Entonox administration 582
References and further reading 583

Definition

Entonox (BOC 1995), a gaseous mixture of 50% nitrous oxide (N$_2$O) and 50% oxygen (O$_2$), is a patient-controlled, inhaled analgesic which is used for the short-term relief of acute pain (Stannard & Booth 1998). Nitrous oxide is a colourless, sweet smelling gas with powerful analgesic properties and it is supplied in premixed cylinders (Bruce & Franck 2000). The gas is inhaled and self-administered by the patient using a demand unit attached to a face mask or a mouthpiece. The nitrous oxide component of the gas acts as a powerful analgesic producing similar physiological effects to opioids (Gillman & Lightigfeld 1994), whilst the oxygen component has an antihypoxic effect (Faddy & Garlick 2005), ensures good cerebral perfusion and enhanced recovery (Peate & Lancaster 2000).

Mode of action

Although the exact mechanism of nitrous oxide is unknown, its effects take place within the pain centres of the brain and spinal cord and are related to the release of endogenous neurotransmitters such as opioid peptides and serotonin and the activation of certain opioid receptors (Fang *et al.* 1997; Gillman & Lightigfeld 1998). N-methyl-D-aspartate (NMDA) receptor currents were inhibited by nitrous oxide and it is known that these receptors are involved with many central nervous system pathways (Jevtovic-Todorovic *et al.* 1998). The release of these neurotransmitters is thought to activate descending pain pathways which modulate pain transmission in the spinal cord (Maze & Fujinaga 2000). Pulmonary transfer of nitrous oxide is rapid, with onset of effect in seconds and full analgesic effect within 1–2 minutes. It is also rapidly eliminated from the blood, via the lungs, when inhalation ceases (Trojan *et al.* 1997).

Indications

There are several advantages to using Entonox:

- As the gas is inhaled it is painless when compared to systemic methods of administering analgesia (such as injections).
- It has a rapid onset of effect.
- The side-effects are few and are self limiting as the gas is self administered.
- It does not depress respiratory or cardiovascular function.
- Effects wear off rapidly; usually within 5 minutes.
- The patient is in full control, which can reduce anxiety (BOC 2001).

Because of these properties Entonox is an ideal agent for short-term pain relief following injury or trauma and during therapeutic and investigative procedures. It is used in a variety of settings including Accident and Emergency (O'Sullivan & Benger 2003), obstetrics (Rosen 2002), paediatrics (Bruce & Franck 2000; Pickup & Pagdin 2001), endoscopy /biopsy procedures (Forbes & Collins 2000; Manikandan *et al.* 2003) and the ambulance service.

Indications for Entonox use include:

- Wound and burn dressing, wound debridement and suturing.
- Normal labour.
- Changing or removing of packs and drains.
- Removal of sutures from sensitive areas, e.g. the vulva.
- Invasive procedures such as catheterization and sigmoidoscopy.
- Removal of radioactive intracavity gynaecological applicators.
- Altering the position of a patient who experiences incident pain.
- Manual evacuation of the bowel in severe constipation.
- Acute trauma, e.g. applying orthopaedic traction following pathological fracture, reduction of joint dislocation.
- Physiotherapy procedures, particularly postoperatively.

Contraindications

Entonox should not be used with any of the following conditions:

- Maxillofacial injuries (BOC 2000), as the patient may not be able to hold the mask tightly to the face or use the mouthpiece adequately. There is a risk of causing further damage to facial wounds and there may also be a significant risk of blood inhalation.
- Head injuries with impairment of consciousness.
- Heavily sedated patients, as they would be unable to breathe in the Entonox on demand and to potentiate sedation further may be hazardous.
- Intoxicated patients, as drowsiness and aspiration would be a hazard in the event of vomiting.
- Pneumothorax, air embolism, bowel obstruction or abdominal distension (BOC 2000). The nitrous oxide constituent of Entonox passes into any air-filled cavity within the body faster than nitrogen passes out. As the gas expands this is likely to result in a build-up of tension, which will increase the patient's symptoms.
- Decompression illness or a recent dive (the 'bends'), as nitrous oxide escapes into the bloodstream and increases the size of the nitrogen bubbles in the tissues.
- Laryngectomy patients, as they will be unable to use the apparatus.
- Temperatures of below −6°C as the gases separate (BOC 1995). If this occurs the cylinders will initially deliver a high concentration of oxygen but will eventually deliver nearly pure nitrous oxide.

Cautions

Prior to Entonox use consideration should be given to the following:

- The high level of oxygen (50%) in Entonox may depress respiration in patients who have chronic obstructive pulmonary disease and are carbon dioxide (CO_2) retainers.
- Entonox should not be used as a replacement for procedures requiring increased levels of medical intervention where intravenous analgesia or general anaesthesia is required.
- As a precaution the British Oxygen Company (BOC) (1995) data sheet recommends that patients should avoid driving or operating machinery for 12 hours after Entonox administration.

Reference material

Patient assessment prior to use

The patient's ability to administer Entonox safely and effectively (particularly the very young or old) must be assessed prior to use. Patients should be able to:

- Understand the instructions for Entonox use.
- Hold the demand valve to self-administer the gas.
- Inhale the gas through the mask or mouthpiece whilst breathing normally (patients who have impaired lung function may not be able to inhale the gas sufficiently to provide adequate analgesia).

Equipment

Cylinders

Two types of Entonox cylinder are available from the BOC: the light-weight cylinders (available from 2001: size HX [10 litres] or CD [2 litres]) and the older style F size cylinders (10 litres). All cylinders have blue and white markings on their shoulder (Figure 28.1).

The light-weight cylinders have the following advantages:

- They are easier to carry.
- They have a live contents gauge.
- Changing an empty cylinder is simple because it is not necessary to fit a regulator or use a cylinder key.

The smaller CD-size cylinders tend to be used in ambulances and by midwives for their portability in home births. Some clinical areas may have piped Entonox, such as Accident and Emergency departments, High Dependency Units and Critical Care Units. The larger HX cylinders would require a trolley to move them around so are more suitable for ward areas.

Figure 28.1   Entonox CD-size cylinder (courtesy of BOC Medical Gases).

Demand apparatus

There are a number of different companies that supply the demand apparatus for self-administered Entonox use. Examples of these include the Ease demand valve (Sabre Medical) and the Carnet single-patient-use demand valve (Figure 28.2).

Use of bacterial filters

Because Entonox equipment is a potential source of cross-infection, bacterial filters (single-use only) should be fitted between the face mask mouthpiece and demand valve if the demand valve is not for single use (Chilvers & Weisz 2000). Face masks and mouthpieces must also be single-use only and disposable once therapy ceases. Local policies must also be followed for the cleaning/sterilization of equipment between patient use.

Principle of administration

Entonox is designed for self-administration by the patient. This method of administration makes use of a demand unit which safeguards the patient from excess inhalation

580

cause prolonged exposure to Entonox causes inactivation of vitamin B_{12}, impaired folate metabolism and pernicious anaemia (BOC 2000), it is recommended that:

- Entonox is used on a short-term rather than a long-term basis.
- Exposure to Entonox should not be for more than 6 hours continuously (BOC 1995).
- If daily use is required for more than 4 days, this should be accompanied by twice-weekly blood tests to check for changes in red and white blood cells (BOC 1995). Consideration should also be given to the administration of B_{12} and folate supplements.

Prescribing of Entonox

In a number of health care settings, nurses, midwives and physiotherapists may be able to administer Entonox without a written prescription from a doctor providing there is a local patient group direction to allow this (see Chapter 11). Where this is the case, Entonox can be used more readily and time is not wasted waiting for a medical prescription. Non-medical

Figure 28.2 Example of a demand valve apparatus (courtesy of BOC Medical Gases).

of Entonox. The demand unit ensures that gas can be obtained only by the patient inhaling from the mouthpiece or mask and producing a negative pressure (Figure 28.3). The gas flow stops when the patient removes the mouthpiece or mask from their face. Thus patients are able to self-regulate the dose of Entonox (a method of patient-controlled analgesia). Therefore, the patient must hold the mask firmly over the face or mouthpiece to the lips to produce an airtight fit and breathe in before the gas will flow. Expired gases escape by the expiratory valve on the handpiece. It is essential to adhere to this method of self-administration as it is then impossible for patients to overdose themselves because if they become drowsy they will relax their grip on the handset and the gas flow will cease when no negative pressure is applied. However, should inhalation continue, light anaesthesia supervenes and the mask drops away as the patient relaxes. Entonox may be self-regulated, but additionally may be administered by attendant medical personnel trained in its use, e.g. within obstetric/Accident and Emergency units, and accident ambulances.

Entonox has an oxygen content two-and-a-half times that of air and is, therefore, a good way of giving extra oxygen as well as providing analgesia.

Duration and frequency of administration

The duration and frequency of Entonox administration should always be tailored to individual patient needs. Be-

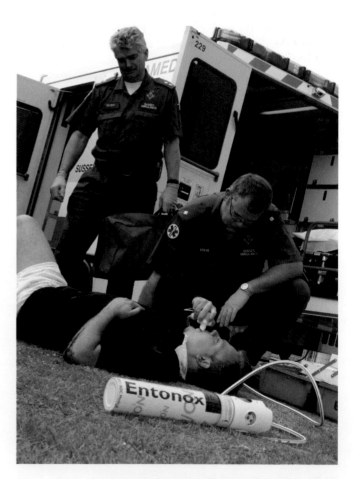

Figure 28.3 A patient administering Entonox through a mouthpiece (courtesy of BOC Medical Gases).

prescribers who have completed the relevent training as an independent prescriber may also prescribe Entonox if this is within their area of competence.

Staff training

Where Entonox is available for patient use it is important that staff are given appropriate theoretical and practical training (BOC 1998; Peate & Lancaster 2000). This can be supplied by BOC Medical and certificated.

Use during pregnancy and lactation

It has been suggested that prolonged exposure to high levels of nitrous oxide may affect a woman's ability to become pregnant (Ahlborg *et al.* 1996). Mild skeletal teratogenic changes have been observed in pregnant rat embryos when

the dam (pregnant mother) has been exposed to high levels of nitrous oxide during the period of organogenesis. However, no increased incidence of foetal malformation has been discovered in eight epidemiological studies and case reports in humans (BOC 1995). No published material shows that nitrous oxide is toxic to the human foetus. Therefore, there is no absolute contraindication to its use in the first 15 weeks of pregnancy.

Complications

Inappropriate inhalation of Entonox will ultimately result in unconsciousness, passing through stages of increasing light-headedness and intoxication. The treatment is removal to fresh air, mouth-to-mouth resuscitation and, if necessary, the use of an oxygen resuscitator (BOC 1995).

Procedure guidelines   Entonox administration

Equipment

1 Entonox cylinder and head.
2 Face mask and/or mouthpiece.
3 Sterile bacterial filter.

Procedure

Action	Rationale
1 Explain and discuss the procedure with the patient.	To ensure that the patient understands the procedure and gives his/her valid consent (NMC 2006: C). To reduce patient anxiety (Royal College of Anaesthetists 2006: C).
2 Turn on the Entonox supply from the cylinder. (If using the older type cylinder the tap should be turned in an anticlockwise direction.)	To ascertain whether there is any Entonox in the cylinder (BOC 1999: C).
3 Examine the gauge to determine how much gas is in the cylinder.	To ensure an adequate supply of gas throughout the procedure (BOC 1999: C).
4 Ensure that the patient is in as comfortable a position as possible.	To promote patient comfort (BOC 1999: C).
5 Demonstrate how to use the apparatus by holding the mask tightly to your face, replacing the mask/mouthpiece that you have used. Explain to the patient that when he/she breathes in and out regularly and deeply a hissing sound will be heard, indicating that the gas is being inhaled.	To ensure that the patient understands what to do and what to expect before any painful procedure commences (BOC 1999: C).
6 Allow the patient to practise using the apparatus.	To enable the patient to adopt the correct technique and for the nurse to observe the analgesic effect of the gas before the procedure commences (BOC 1999: C).

Procedure guidelines *(cont.)*

7 Encourage the patient to breathe gas in and out for at least 2 minutes before commencing any painful procedure.	To allow sufficient time for an adequate circulatory level of nitrous oxide to provide analgesia. (When the patient inhales, gas enters first the lungs then the pulmonary and systemic circulations. It takes 1–2 minutes to build up reasonable concentrations of nitrous oxide in the brain) (BOC 1999: C).
8 During the procedure encourage the patient to breathe in and out regularly and deeply.	To maintain adequate circulatory levels, thus providing adequate analgesia (BOC 1999: C).
9 At the end of the procedure observe the patient until the effects of the gas have worn off.	Some patients may feel a transient drowsiness or giddiness and should be discouraged from getting out of bed until these effects have worn off. It is rare for the patient to experience transient amnesia (BOC 1999: C).
10 Evaluate the effectiveness of Entonox with the patient throughout, and following procedures, by verbal questioning and encouraging the patient to self-assess the analgesic effect.	To establish whether the Entonox has been a useful analgesic for the procedure. This should then be documented to assist any subsequent procedures, e.g. dressing changes (BOC 1999: C).
11 Turn off the Entonox supply from the cylinder. (If using the older type cylinder the tap should be turned in a clockwise direction. The gauge should read 'Empty' when turned off.)	To avoid potential seepage of gas from the apparatus (BOC 1999: C).
12 Depress the diaphragm under the demand valve.	To remove residual gas from tubing (BOC 1999: C).
13 Follow local policies/guidelines for the cleaning and sterilization of expiratory valve and tubing, and face mask (or disposal if single use). Filters and mouthpieces should be discarded after use.	To reduce the risk of cross-infection (BOC 1999: C).
14 Record the administration on appropriate documentation.	To promote continuity of care, maintain accurate records and provide a point of reference in the event of any queries (BOC 1999: C; NMC 2005: C).

Problem solving: Entonox administration

Problem	Cause	Suggested action
Patient not experiencing adequate analgesic effect.	Entonox cylinder empty. Apparatus not properly connected.	Check before procedure commences.
	Patient not inhaling deeply enough (BOC 2000).	Encourage the patient to breathe in until a hissing noise can be heard from the cylinder. Reassess suitability of patient for Entonox use. The patient may not be strong enough to inhale deeply or may have reduced lung capacity.

Problem	Cause	Suggested action
	Patient inhaling pure oxygen, i.e. cylinder has been stored below −6°C and nitrous oxide has liquified and settled at the bottom of the cylinder (All cylinders should be stored horizontally at a temperature of 10°C or above for 24 hours before use.) (BOC 1995).	Initially safe, but later the patient may inhale pure nitrous oxide and be asphyxiated. Discontinue the procedure. Ensure adequate warming of the cylinder and inversion of the cylinder to remix the gases adequately.
	Not enough time has been allowed for nitrous oxide to exert its analgesic effect.	Allow at least 2 minutes of Entonox use before commencing the procedure.
Patient experiences generalized muscle rigidity.	Hyperventilation during inhalation (BOC 2000).	Discontinue Entonox and allow the patient to recover. Explain the procedure again, stressing deep and regular inspiration. Use a mouthpiece in place of a mask.
Patient unable to tolerate a mask.	Smell of rubber, feeling of claustrophobia.	Use a mouthpiece in place of a mask.
Patient feels nauseated, drowsy or giddy.	Effect of nitrous oxide accumulation (BOC 2000).	Discontinue Entonox administration: the effect will then rapidly disappear.
Patient afraid to use Entonox.	Associates gases with previous hospital procedures, e.g. anaesthesia before surgery (BOC 2000).	Reassure patient and reiterate instructions for use and short-term effects.

References and further reading

Ahlborg, G. Jr, Axelsson, G. & Bodin, L. (1996) Shift work, nitrous oxide exposure and spontaneous abortion among Swedish midwives. *Occup Environ Med*, **53**, 374–8.

BOC (1995) *BOC Gases Data Sheet: Entonox*. BOC Group, Manchester.

BOC (1998) *Entonox: the Non-invasive Patient Controlled Analgesic. Suggested Protocol Document*. BOC Group, Manchester.

BOC (1999) Inhalation Pain Control (video). BOC Group, Manchester.

BOC (2000) *Entonox: Controlled Pain Relief Reference Guide*. BOC Medical, Manchester.

BOC (2001) *Entonox: Controlled Pain Relief*. BOC Medical, Manchester.

Bruce, E. & Franck, L. (2000) Self-administered nitrous oxide (Entonox) for the management of procedural pain. *Paediatr Nurs*, **12**(7), 15–19.

Chilvers, R. & Weisz, M. (2000) Entonox equipment as a potential source of cross-infection. *Anaesthesia*, **55**(2), 176–9.

Faddy, S.C. & Garlick, S.R. (2005) A systematic review of the safety of analgesia with 50% nitrous oxide: can lay responders use analgesic gases in the prehospital setting. *Emerg Med J*, **22**, 901–6.

Fang, F., Guo, T.Z. & Davies, M.F. (1997) Opiate receptors in the periaqueductal grey mediate analgesic effect of nitrous oxide in rats. *Eur J Pharmacol*, **336**(2–3), 137–41.

Forbes, G.M. & Collins, B.J. (2000) Nitrous oxide for colonoscopy: a randomised controlled study. *Gastrointest Endosc*, **51**, 271–7.

Gillman, M. & Lightigfeld, F. (1994) Pharmacology of psychotropic analgesic nitrous oxide as a multipotent opioid agonist. *Int J Neurosci*, **76**, 5–12.

Gillman, M. & Lightigfeld, F. (1998) Clinical role and mechanisms of action of analgesic nitrous oxide. *Int J Neurosci*, **93**(1–2), 55–62.

Jevtovic-Todorovic, V., Todorovic, S.M. & Mennerick, S. (1998) Nitrous oxide (laughing gas) is an NMDA antagonist, neuroprotectant and neurotoxin. *Nat Med*, **4**, 460–3.

Manikandan, R. *et al.* (2003) Nitrous oxide vs periprostatic nerve block with 1% lidocaine during transrectal ultrasound guided biopsy of the prostate: a propective, randomised, controlled trial. *J Urol*, **170**, 1881–3.

Maze, M. & Fujinaga, M. (2000) Recent advances in understanding the actions and toxicity of nitrous oxide. *Anaesthesia*, **55**(4), 311–4.

NMC (2005) *Guidelines for Records and Record Keeping*. Nursing and Midwifery Council, London.

NMC (2006) *A–Z Advice Sheet Consent*. www.nmc.org.

O'Sullivan, I. & Benger, J. (2003) Nitrous oxide in emergency medicine. *Emerg Med J*, **20**, 214–7.

Peate, I. & Lancaster, J. (2000) Safe use of medical gases in the clinical setting: practical tips. *Br J Nurs*, **9**(4), 231–6.

Pickup, S. & Pagdin, J. (2001) Procedural pain: Entonox can help. *Paediatr Nurs*, **12**(10), 33–6.

Rosen, M.A. (2002) Nitrous oxide for relief of labour pain: a systematic review. *Am J Obstet Gynecol*, **186**, S110–26.

Royal College of Anaesthetists (2006) *Raising the Standard: Information for Patients* (ed. J.R. Colvin), 2nd edn. Section 1 Key issues in developing new materials. Royal College of Anaesthetists, London, pp. 14–29.

Stannard, C.F. & Booth, S. (1998) Management of pain following trauma. In: *Churchills Pocket Book of Pain*. Churchill Livingstone, Edinburgh, p. 178.

Trojan, J., Saunders, B.P. & Woloshynowych, M. (1997) Immediate recovery of psychomotor function after patient administered nitrous oxide/oxygen inhalation for colonoscopy. *Endoscopy*, **29**(1), 17–22.

Pain management: epidural and intrathecal analgesia

Reference material 586
Epidural/intrathecal analgesia for patients with intractable chronic and cancer pain 591
Procedure guidelines: Epidural/intrathecal catheter for chronic pain: 592
preinsertion management
Procedure guidelines: Epidural/intrathecal catheter insertion 593
Procedure guidelines: Epidural/intrathecal infusion: setting up utilizing an 594
ambulatory pump
Procedure guidelines: Epidural/intrathecal catheter for chronic pain management: 595
post-insertion management
Procedure guidelines: Epidural/intrathecal exit site dressing change 596
Procedure guidelines: Epidural/intrathecal analgesia top up (bolus) 597
Procedure guidelines: Discharge planning for patients with epidural/intrathecal 597
catheter in situ
Procedure guidelines: Epidural/intrathecal catheter removal 599
Problem solving: Epidural/intrathecal infusions of local anaesthetic agents and 599
opioids: management of side-effects
Problem solving: Epidural/intrathecal insertion: complications 601
Problem solving: Epidural/intrathecal catheter: issues with pump and site 602
References and further reading 603

Definition

The spinal cord rests in a medium of cerebrospinal fluid (CSF), which is contained by the protective membrane of the dura mater. Analgesics applied outside the dura mater are termed epidural analgesia, and medications given into the CSF are termed intrathecal analgesia (Sloan 2004). The term 'spinal analgesia' refers to both the epidural and intrathecal route (Day 2001; Sloan 2004).

Epidural analgesia is the administration of analgesics (local anaesthetics and opioids with or without adjuvants such as corticosteroids and clonidine) into the epidural space via an indwelling catheter (ANZCA 2005). This technique enables analgesics to be injected close to the spinal cord and spinal nerves where they exert a powerful analgesic effect. It is one of the most effective techniques available for the management of acute pain (Macintyre & Ready 2001; Wheatley et al. 2001).

Intrathecal analgesia is the administration of analgesic drugs (as listed above) directly into the CSF in the intrathecal space (Urdan et al. 2006). Analgesic drugs given via this route are 10 times as potent as those given into the epidural space so doses given are much smaller. This method can use either an external infusion pump or can be part of a fully implantable reservoir system (Dickson 2004).

For cancer patients who do not obtain pain relief from treatment with opioids administered orally, rectally, by injection or continuous infusion, there is evidence that both epidural and intrathecal analgesia can be effective (Ballantyne & Carwood 2005).

Advantages

There are three main advantages in using epidural or intrathecal analgesia:

- It has the potential to provide effective dynamic pain relief for many patients (Wheatley et al. 2001).
- The combination of local anaesthetic agents with opioids has a synergistic action that allows the concentration of each drug to be reduced. This limits the unwanted side-effects of each drug (Fotiadis et al. 2004).
- There is also evidence that the use of epidural analgesia may reduce the stress response to surgery or trauma, thereby reducing morbidity, recovery time and hospital stay (Kehlet 1997).

Indications

- Provision of analgesia during labour.
- As an alternative to general anaesthesia, e.g. in severe respiratory disease or for patients with malignant hyperthermia.
- Provision of postoperative analgesia. Epidural analgesia has been used since the late 1940s as a method of controlling postoperative pain (Chapman & Day 2001).

- Provision of analgesia for pain resulting from trauma, e.g. fractured ribs, which may result in respiratory impairment due to pain on breathing.
- Management of chronic intractable pain in patients who experience the following:
  - Unacceptable side-effects with systemic opioids.
  - Unsuccessful treatment with opioids via other routes despite escalating doses.
  - Severe neuropathic pain due to tumour invasion or compression of nerves.
        (Smitt et al. 1998; Mercadante 1999; Day 2001).
- To relieve muscle spasm and pain resulting from lumbar cord pressure due to disc protrusion or local oedema and inflammation.

Contraindications

These may be absolute or relative.

Absolute

- Patients with coagulation defects, which may result in haematoma formation and spinal cord compression, e.g. iatrogenic (anticoagulated patient) or congenital (haemophiliacs), or thrombocytopenia due to disease or as the result of anticancer treatment (Horlocker & Wedel 1998).
- Local sepsis at the site of proposed epidural or intrathecal injection; the result might be meningitis or epidural abscess formation.
- Proven allergy to the intended drug.
- Unstable spinal fracture.
- Patient refusal to consent to the procedure.

Relative

- Unstable cardiovascular system.
- Spinal deformity.
- Raised intracranial pressure (a risk of herniation if a dural tap occurs).
- Certain neurological conditions, for example multiple sclerosis, where an epidural may result in an exacerbation of the disease (Hall 2000).
- Unavailability of staff trained in the management of epidural or intrathecal analgesia (Macintyre & Ready 2001). Hall (2000) notes that staff managing patients with epidural or intrathecal analgesia should have undertaken a period of formal training to care for patients safely and competently.

Reference material

Anatomy of the epidural and intrathecal space
(Figure 29.1)

The spinal cord is covered by the meninges; the *pia mater* is closely applied to the cord, and the *arachnoid mater* lies closely with the outer, tough covering of the *dura mater* (Day 2001).

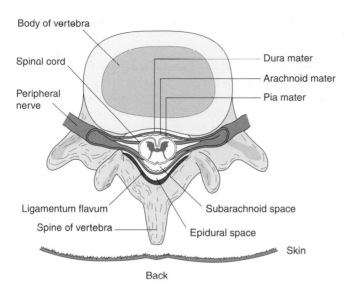

Figure 29.1 Diagram of the spinal spaces. (Courtesy of Day 2001.)

The epidural space lies between the spinal dura and ligamentum flavum. The contents of the epidural space include a rich venous plexus, spinal arterioles, lymphatics and extradural fat.

The intrathecal space (often also termed the subarachnoid space) lies between the arachnoid mater and pia mater and contains the CSF (Chapman & Day 2001).

There are 31 pairs of spinal nerves of varying size. These nerves pass out through the intervertebral foramina between each vertebra (Chapman & Day 2001). The two main groups of nerve fibres are:

- *Myelinated*. Myelin is a thin, fatty sheath which protects and insulates the nerve fibres and prevents impulses from being transmitted to adjacent fibres.
- *Unmyelinated*. Delicate fibres, more susceptible to hypoxia and toxins than myelinated fibres.

The spinal nerves are composed of a posterior and anterior root, which join to form a spinal nerve:

- *Posterior root*. Transmits ascending sensory impulses from the periphery to the spinal cord.
- *Anterior root*. Transmits descending motor impulses from the spinal cord to the periphery by means of its corresponding spinal nerve.
  (Day 2001; Chapman & Day 2001; Urdan *et al.* 2006).

Specific skin surface areas are supplied/innervated by each of the spinal nerves. These skin areas are known as dermatomes (McCaffery & Pasero 1999) (Figure 29.2).

Classes of epidural and intrathecal drugs and mechanism of action

Three classes of drugs are commonly used to provide epidural or intrathecal analgesia: opioids, local anaesthetic

agents and adjuvant drugs such as corticosteroids and clonidine.

Opioids

Whilst a number of different opioids have been used for epidural and intrathecal analgesia, two of the most commonly used are diamorphine and fentanyl (Cook *et al.* 1997; Romer & Russell 1998; Bannon *et al.* 2001). When either of these opioids is injected into the *epidural* space, part of the opioid dose:

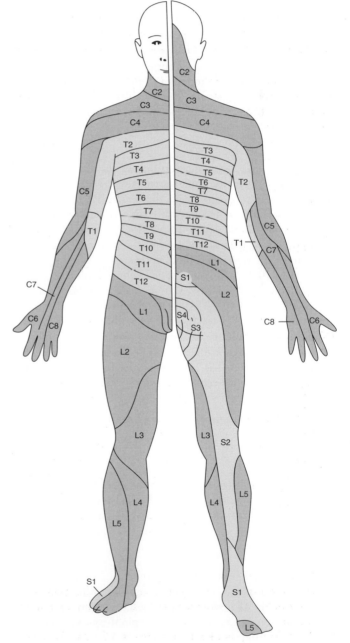

Figure 29.2 Dermatomes. (Redrawn with permission from Walsh 1997.)

- Crosses the dura and arachnoid membrane and enters the CSF. From the CSF a proportion of the drug is taken up into the spinal cord and reaches the opioid receptors in the spinal cord. Once bound to the opioid receptors, this results in blocking of pain impulses.
- Enters the systemic circulation and contributes to analgesia.
- Binds to the epidural fat and does not contribute to analgesia.

When opioids are placed directly into the CSF in the *intrathecal* space they attach directly to the opioid spinal cord receptor sites (Urdan *et al.* 2006).

Fentanyl differs from diamorphine in that it is more lipid soluble. This means that it passes more easily into the CSF, gaining faster access to the opioid receptors and having a more rapid onset of action. Fentanyl also has a shorter duration of action (1–4 hours) as opposed to diamorphine (6–12 hours) (Macintyre & Ready 2001).

Local anaesthetic drugs

Commonly used local anaesthetic agents include bupivacaine, levobupivacaine and ropivacaine. These drugs gain access to the nerve roots and the spinal cord by crossing the dura and subarachnoid membranes (Macintyre & Ready 2001). They inhibit pain transmission by blocking sodium ion channels which are involved in the propagation of electrical impulses along the spinal nerves.

The dose of a local anaesthetic agent will also determine which nerves are blocked. Low concentrations of bupivacaine (e.g. 0.100–0.125%) preferentially block nerve impulses in the smallest diameter nerve fibres, which include the pain and temperature sensory fibres. As the larger diameter motor fibres are less likely to be blocked with concentrations of 0.100–0.125% bupivacaine, the incidence of leg weakness is reduced and the patient is able to mobilize.

Adjuvant drugs

Corticosteroids

Although not licensed for epidural or intrathecal use, corticosteroid injections are often used to relieve pain caused by inflammatory irritation of nerve roots (Papagelopoulos *et al.* 2001).

Clonidine

Clonidine is a mixed α-adrenergic agonist. Although its exact mechanism of action is unknown, clonidine is believed to enhance analgesia provided by spinal opioids and local anaesthetic drugs (Smith & Elliott 2001). Clonidine has a specific role in the management of neuropathic pain in patients with advanced cancer (Mercadante 1999).

Methods of administration

Continuous infusion

Continuous infusions of epidural drugs are the most effective way of providing dynamic pain relief after major surgical procedures (Kehlet & Holte 2001). Continuous infusions of intrathecal analgesic drugs have been shown to be effective in the management of chronic intractable pain (Ballantyne & Carwood 2005). Continuous infusions can be given by either a syringe pump or a designated infusion pump system. The effectiveness of this method of administering drugs is dependent on a number of factors including the combination of drugs used, the position of the spinal catheter at a level appropriate to the site of surgery or pain (Weetman & Allison 2006) and the volume of the local anaesthetic agent infused (Hall 2000; Chapman & Day 2001).

Combination of drugs used

Epidural or intrathecal infusions of local anaesthetic and opioid combinations are commonly used in the UK (Wheatley *et al.* 2001; Baker *et al.* 2004). The rationale behind their combined use is based on the observation that better analgesia is achieved with lower doses of each drug, therefore minimizing drug-related side-effects produced by higher concentrations (Curatolo *et al.* 1998; Fotiadis *et al.* 2004). Although the solutions used will vary with the clinical situation, common solutions are bupivacaine 0.1–0.125% with 2–4 μg/ml of fentanyl.

Position of epidural or intrathecal catheter

Local anaesthetic drugs block nerve fibres at spinal segments adjacent to their site of administration. To ensure the local anaesthetic agent spreads to the dermatomes or nerves supplying the area of pain (e.g. the surgical site, or the pain location caused by a tumour), the tip of the spinal catheter should be placed within the mid-dermatomal distribution of the pain site (Table 29.1). This achieves optimal analgesia using the least amount of drugs. If the catheter is placed below the dermatomes supplying the pain site then analgesia is likely to be inadequate (Macintyre & Ready 2001).

Volume of infusion

As the volume of local anaesthetic agent influences the number of spinal nerves that are blocked, it is important to maintain the hourly infusion rate at a volume which keeps the appropriate nerves blocked (Hall 2000; Chapman & Day 2001).

Table 29.1   Optimal catheter location for different surgical sites.

Surgical site	Catheter location
Thoracic	T6–T9
Upper abdominal	T7–T10
Lower abdominal	T9–L1
Hip/knee	L1–L4

588

Bolus injections

Bolus injections of opioids and local anaesthetic agents are used infrequently to manage postoperative pain but are more commonly used for managing labour pain (Grond *et al.* 2000).

Patient-controlled epidural analgesia

The use of patient-controlled epidural analgesia (PCEA) has gained popularity in recent years because it enables patients to control their analgesia. For patients with postoperative or chronic pain, PCEA is used more effectively in combination with a low-dose background infusion (Wheatley *et al.* 2001). This ensures a baseline level of analgesia which can then be supplemented by the patient when required.

Monitoring

When caring for a patient receiving epidural or intrathecal analgesia, it is important to monitor the patient for the following:

- Signs of drug-related side-effects.
- Pain intensity.
- Signs of complications due to the epidural or intrathecal procedure.

Drug-related side-effects

There are a number of drug-related side-effects associated with epidural/intrathecal opioids and local anaesthetic agents.

Opioids

- *Respiratory depression*: this is due to the action of opioids on the respiratory centre. Respiratory depression may occur at two different time intervals.
  - Early: usually within 2 hours of the opioid injection. This may occur if high blood levels of the opioid follow absorption from the epidural space into the systemic circulation (Macintyre & Ready 2001).
  - Late: this may not be seen for 6–12 hours after an opioid is given. It results from rostral migration of the drug in the CSF to the brainstem and respiratory centre (Macintyre & Ready 2001). This is less likely to occur with lipid-soluble opioids such as fentanyl.
- *Sedation*: although there may be many different causes of sedation, epidural/intrathecal opioids can cause sedation owing to their effect on the central nervous system. Opioid-induced sedation is often an early warning sign of respiratory depression.
- *Nausea and vomiting*: nausea and vomiting is caused by the action of opioids on the vomiting centre in the brainstem and stimulation of the chemoreceptor trigger zone in the fourth ventricle of the brain.

- *Pruritus*: although the exact mechanism is unknown, pruritus is presumed to be centrally mediated and a consequence of activation of opioid receptors in the spinal cord (Sands *et al.* 1998).
- *Urinary retention*: this is due to opioid inhibition of the micturition reflex which is evoked by increases in bladder volume.

Local anaesthetic agents

- *Hypotension*: this can be caused by two mechanisms. Firstly, local anaesthetic agents can spread outside the epidural/intrathecal space, blocking the sympathetic nerves. This results in peripheral vasodilatation and hypotension. It is most likely to occur if a bolus dose of local anaesthetic agent (e.g. 10 ml of 0.25% bupivacaine) is given to improve pain control (Macintyre & Ready 2001). Secondly, if the local anaesthetic agent spreads above the T4 dermatome (nipple line) the cardio-accelerator nerves may become blocked, leading to bradycardia and hypotension (Macintyre & Ready 2001).
- *Motor blockade*: this will depend on the concentration and total dose of local anaesthetic agent used and the position of the epidural/intrathecal catheter (Hall 2000). Motor blockade occurs when the local anaesthetic agent blocks the larger diameter motor nerves. Leg weakness will occur if the motor nerves supplying the legs are blocked.
- *Urinary retention*: as with epidural/intrathecal opioids, blockade of the nerves supplying the bladder sphincter can cause urinary retention.

Routine monitoring of the patient for these side-effects must be carried out to facilitate early management. The patient's blood pressure, respiratory rate and peripheral tissue oxygenation should be monitored continuously initially and then according to local policy and as the patient's condition dictates.

For guidance on managing the side-effects associated with epidural/intrathecal opioids and local anaesthetic agents, see Problem solving: management of side-effects, p. 599.

Pain assessment

Pain should be assessed (at rest and on movement) at the same time that the patient's routine observations are carried out. Simple numerical (e.g. 0–10 where 0 is no pain and 10 is the worst pain imaginable) or verbal rating scales (e.g. none, mild, moderate, severe, or very severe) can be used.

Inadequate postoperative pain management can lead to physiological complications (respiratory, cardiovascular, gastrointestinal and endocrine systems) and adverse effects (behavioural, such as reduced mobility, and psychological, such as increased anxiety and reduced mood) (Macintyre & Ready 2001). Thus, when patients are assessed the practitioner should ensure the patient can take a deep breath and cough and mobilize with a minimal level of pain to reduce the impact of the physiological, behavioural and psychological effects of undertreated acute pain.

When used for chronic pain management the aim of epidural/intrathecal analgesia is to improve the overall quality of life of the patient. Although it is acceptable to use the above pain assessment rating scales, a more in-depth pain assessment scale may be used such as the Brief Pain Inventory (BPI) (Cleeland 1991).

If pain is not controlled and the infusion has already been titrated according to hospital guidelines, the pain/anaesthetic team should be contacted for advice after checking the following:

- The catheter is still in situ.
- The catheter is still connected to the bacterial filter.
- There are no leaks within the system.
- The height of the epidural/intrathecal block. This will indicate whether the block has fallen below the upper limit of the incision or pain site. To check the height of the block use a small piece of ice or cold solution (ethyl alcohol): start at the top of the chest above the patient's incision or pain site. Gently dab the ice (or apply the cold solution) down each side of the patient's body (one side and then the other). Use a dermatome map to assess the upper and lower limit where the sensation changes (see Figure 29.2).

If the height of the block has fallen below the upper limit of the incision or pain site, the pain/anaesthetic team may undertake the following: give the patient a bolus dose of local anaesthetic agent to re-establish the block; reposition the epidural catheter. If either of these fail, other methods of analgesia need to be considered.

Complications of epidural and intrathecal analgesia

As with any invasive technique, epidural/intrathecal analgesia results in potential complications, many of which are rare. They include the following.

Haematoma

An epidural haematoma can arise from trauma to an epidural blood vessel during catheter insertion or removal. Although the incidence of a haematoma occurring is extremely rare, particular care must be taken in patients receiving thromboprophylaxis (see Procedure guidelines: Epidural intrathecal catheter removal, below). Initial symptoms include back pain and tenderness. As the haematoma expands to compress the nerve roots or the spinal cord, this proceeds to sensory/motor weakness (Chapman & Day 2001).

Abscess formation

Wheatley et al. (2001) note that infection can be introduced into the epidural space from an exogenous source via contaminated equipment or drugs or from an endogenous source, leading to bacteraemia which seeds to the insertion site or catheter tip. Alternatively the catheter can act as a wick through which the infection tracks down from the entry site on the skin to the epidural/intrathecal space. Symptoms include back pain and tenderness accompanied by redness with a purulent discharge from the catheter exit site (Day 2001).

Complications specific to epidural analgesia

Dural puncture

This usually occurs when the dura mater is inadvertently punctured during the placement of the epidural catheter. The incidence of a dural puncture arising during placement of the catheter is approximately 0.32–1.23% (Wheatley et al. 2001). The main symptom is a headache, which arises from leakage of CSF through the dura.

Catheter migration

Catheter migration is extremely rare, occurring in less than 0.2% of patients (Wheatley et al. 2001). The catheter may migrate into either a blood vessel or the CSF. If the catheter migrates into a blood vessel, opioid or local anaesthetic toxicity will occur. Opioid toxicity results in sedation and respiratory depression. Local anaesthetic toxicity results in circumoral tingling, numbness, twitching, convulsions and apnoea (Pasero & McCaffery 1999). If the catheter migrates into the CSF the epidural opioids and local anaesthetic agents may reach as high as the cranial subarachnoid space. If this occurs the respiratory muscles are paralysed together with the cranial nerves, resulting in apnoea, profound hypotension and unconsciousness (Macintyre & Ready 2001).

Complications specific to intrathecal analgesia

Meningitis is a rare complication of intrathecal analgesia. The epidural route is often considered safer as the intact dura serves as an effective barrier to the spread of infection to the subarachnoid space. In fact similar infection rates are reported with both intrathecal and epidural administration (Mercadante 1999). The incidence of major infections varies widely but is reported by Ballantyne and Carwood (2005) as zero and as approximately 5% by Sloan (2004) for epidural and intrathecal therapy with external pump systems.

If the patient presents with headaches, fever, neck stiffness or photophobia they must be reviewed as a matter of urgency by the medical/anaesthetic team, as if meningitis is suspected CSF samples can be obtained and sent to microbiology for analysis, and antibiotic therapy initiated promptly (Day 2001; Baker et al. 2004).

Equipment and prescription safety checks

When a patient is receiving a continuous infusion of epidural/intrathecal analgesia it is advisable to carry out the safety checks given in Table 29.2 at least once per shift.

Table 29.2 Epidural/intrathecal analgesia: safety checklist.

Checklist	Rationale
Check the prescription and rate of the epidural/intrathecal infusion	To ensure epidural/intrathecal drugs are being administered correctly
Check the epidural/intrathecal infusion/syringe pump extension set is connected to the epidural catheter and not to any other access device	To ensure drugs are administered via the correct route
Check the bacterial filter is securely attached to the epidural/intrathecal catheter	To prevent accidental disconnection of the catheter from the filter
Check that the dressing over the epidural/intrathecal catheter exit site is secure	To prevent catheter dislodgement and minimize the risk of contamination of the catheter site

Epidural/intrathecal analgesia for patients with intractable chronic and cancer pain

Epidural and intrathecal analgesia are well-established techniques for managing intractable cancer pain (Mercadante 1999). A number of special considerations apply to the use of epidural/intrathecal analgesia in the chronic pain setting.

Indications

There are three main indications for using epidural/intrathecal analgesia in patients with intractable cancer pain (Mercadante 1999):

- Patients treated with systemic opioids but who suffer from unacceptable side-effects.
- Unsuccessful treatment with strong opioids despite escalating doses.
- Severe neuropathic pain due to tumour invasion or compression (Smitt *et al.* 1998).

Factors to consider before using epidural/intrathecal analgesia

Prior to using epidural/intrathecal analgesia for intractable chronic or cancer pain, the following issues should be addressed with the patient, family and primary health care team.

Patient/family

The concentration of analgesics needed to provide sufficient analgesia for patients with chronic cancer pain is often higher than the concentrations used postoperatively. As a result, drug-related side-effects such as motor weakness and urinary retention can occur. Some patients find these side-effects un-

acceptable and may prefer to avoid epidural/intrathecal analgesia altogether. Therefore, it is recommended that patients are thoroughly evaluated before they are selected as candidates for chronic intraspinal drug therapy (Wallace 2002). A discussion must therefore take place with the patient and family to ensure that they are aware of these potential side-effects and are willing to continue with epidural/intrathecal analgesia. The patient should also be informed that they will need to spend a period of time in hospital following insertion of the catheter, to allow for dose adjustment and ensure that side-effects are minimized and optimum pain management achieved.

Primary health care team

If it is anticipated that the patient will go home with a continuous epidural or intrathecal infusion, the patient's general practitioner and district nursing team should be consulted at the outset to determine whether they are willing to be involved and/or trained in the management of epidural/intrathecal analgesia care.

Arrangements should also be made with the primary health care team for the provision of a suitable epidural/intrathecal pump and the supply of reconstituted syringes/infusion bags.

Drugs and doses

Epidural/intrathecal infusions of local anaesthetic–opioid combinations are frequently used for the management of intractable chronic and cancer pain.

Opioids

The most commonly used opioids are morphine, diamorphine and fentanyl. Although there is a lack of consensus over the method of converting from a systemic to an epidural/intrathecal opioid, Mercadante (1999) recommends that if converting from oral morphine, a starting dose of roughly 10% of the oral opioid should be given epidurally and then titrated to effect. For example, if a patient was receiving a total daily dose of 180 mg morphine sulphate orally, this would convert to total daily dose of 18 mg of morphine via the epidural route. Stevens and Ghazi (2000) recommend that the intrathecal dose will be 10% of the calculated epidural dose. Thus, in the above example the intrathecal dose would be the epidural dose (18 mg) divided by 10 which would covert to a total daily dose of 1.8 mg of morphine via the intrathecal route.

Local anaesthetic drugs

Bupivacaine is the local anaesthetic agent of choice owing to its long duration of action and predominant action on sensory rather than motor fibres (Mercadante 1999). The starting concentration of bupivacaine can range from 0.125% to 0.25% but concentrations of 0.5% may be required to block resistant pain. Concentrations above 0.25% are associated

591

with motor block (weakness) and autonomic block (urinary retention requiring catheterization).

Monitoring after insertion of epidural/intrathecal for chronic pain

For the first 24 hours after epidural/intrathecal insertion, the patient should be monitored for signs of drug-related side-effects or uncontrolled pain. Intravenous access should be maintained for at least 24 hours so that emergency drugs and fluids can be given if necessary.

After 24 hours, providing the patient's condition is stable, routine monitoring of respiratory rate and cardiac function is not usually required unless indicated clinically by the patient's condition or by local policy guidelines. This allows monitoring for patient safety immediately post-insertion whilst minimizing invasive procedures in patients with chronic pain problems. Ongoing assessment of pain and observation for any signs of infection (temperature monitoring and observation of the catheter exit site) should be continued for the duration of epidural/intrathecal analgesia.

Discharge planning

If the patient is to go home with an epidural/intrathecal infusion, discharge planning should begin prior to insertion of the spinal catheter. Primary care teams, patients and their families will need to be trained and supplied with the appropriate equipment, drugs, catheter filters, information about the infusion pump, how to identify a catheter-related or systemic infection and what to do if pain occurs or complications arise. Contact numbers must be available in case specialist advice is needed.

Minimizing infection

Infection is a complication with long-term epidural or intrathecal analgesia.

Tunnelling the epidural intrathecal catheter

To minimize the risk of a serious infection (e.g. epidural abscess, meningitis), it is common to tunnel the epidural/intrathecal catheter during insertion. This reduces the speed at which a local infection can spread along the catheter before reaching the epidural/intrathecal space (Baker *et al.* 2004). Once a local infection is suspected at the tunnelled site, treatment with antibiotics should be prompt to prevent a systemic infection. See the Intrathecal analgesia section in the Complications of epidural and intrathecal analgesia section for management of suspected meningitis.

Epidural intrathecal filter changes

De Cicco *et al.* (1995) found that the use of bacterial filters during prolonged epidural catheterization maintained an unmodified antimicrobial function for more than 60 days when perfused with reduced volumes of drugs. It is recommended that bacterial filters should only be changed every 4–6 weeks unless blocked (De Cicco *et al.* 1995; Mercadente 1999). More frequent filter changes have been associated with an increased risk of microbial colonization as a direct result of the manipulations (De Cicco *et al.* 1995). Therefore it is recommended that epidural/intrathecal filters should only be changed every 4–6 weeks unless blocked (De Cicco *et al.* 1995; Mercadante 1999).

Procedure guidelines   Epidural/intrathecal catheter for chronic pain: preinsertion management

If the patient is taking a slow-release preparation of morphine, e.g. MST or MXL, they should be converted to immediate-release morphine, either orally, intravenously or as a subcutaneous infusion for 24 hours before the insertion of the catheter. This is in order to minimize the risk of opioid overdose and the risk of respiratory depression. Once it has been decided that the patient is to have an epidural or intrathecal infusion for pain management, a decision will need to be made regarding its fixation. As the catheter may need to stay in situ for several weeks/months it will either be tunnelled subcutaneously or anchored in place with medical glue and sutures.

....

Procedure

Action	Rationale
1 Explain and discuss the procedure with the patient and relatives/carers. Ensure the patient understands the potential side-effects of epidural/intrathecal analgesia for chronic pain management as discussed earlier in the chapter. Ensure the patient and family are also aware of the need for complex discharge planning, which may delay discharge if it is proposed that the patient returns home with the epidural or intrathecal analgesia. Obtain written consent.	To ensure that the patient understands the procedure and gives his/her valid consent (DH 2001: C; Wallace 2002: R 5; NMC 2006b: C).

Procedure guidelines   Epidural/intrathecal catheter insertion

Note: patients undergoing epidural/intrathecal analgesia should always have a venous access device in situ before the procedure. This is because, although rare, a reaction to the opioid or local anaesthetic solution (e.g. respiratory depression or sympathetic blockade) may require immediate access to the venous system. The procedure should be performed in a clinical area with access to full resuscitation equipment.

Equipment

1 Chlorhexidine in 70% alcohol.
2 Local anaesthetic.
3 Selection of needles and syringes.
4 Sterile dressing pack.
5 Face mask.
6 Tuohy needle or assorted gauge lumbar puncture needles.

7 Epidural/intrathecal catheter.
8 Bacterial filter.
9 Moisture responsive transparent dressing and dressing tape to secure catheter (Cousins *et al.* 2003: E).

Procedure

Action	Rationale
1 Explain and discuss the procedure with the patient. If the intention is to provide postoperative analgesia then explanation and consent should have been discussed the day before surgery.	To ensure that the patient understands the procedure and gives his/her valid consent (NMC 2006b: C) and to ensure patient has time to assess information and ask questions (DH 2001: C).
2 Assist the patient into the required position: (a) Lying: Patient should be lying comfortably on a firm surface. Position pillow under patient's head. On side with knee drawn up to the abdomen and clasped by the hands. Support the patient in this position.	To allow identification of the spinal processes and intervertebral discs (Brown 1999: E).
(b) Sitting: Patient sits on firm surface with arms resting on a table, and with the head resting on the arms.	To ensure maximal widening of the intervertebral spaces which will provide easy access to the epidural/intrathecal space (Brown 1999: E).
3 Support, encourage and observe the patient throughout the procedure.	As the procedure takes place behind the patient, reassurance is very important (Chapman & Day 2001: E).
4 Assist the doctor as required. The doctor will proceed as follows: (a) Clean the skin with alcohol-based solution (e.g. chlorhexidine in 70% isopropyl alcohol).	To clean skin and minimize risk of contamination (Kinirons *et al.* 2001: R 1b; Hebl 2006: R 5).
(b) Identify the area to be punctured and inject the skin and subcutaneous layers with local anaesthetic.	To ensure the spinal catheter is inserted at the correct level to provide analgesia and numb the skin prior to insertion of the Tuohy needle (Brown 1999: E).
(c) Introduce Tuohy or spinal needles usually between the identified vertebrae.	To access the epidural or intrathecal space (Brown 1999: E).
(d) Ensure epidural/intrathecal space has been entered.	To prevent anaesthesia being given directly into spinal cord or intravenously by means of the dural veins (Brown 1999: E).
(e) Inject test dose of drug (may be performed).	To ensure the position of the needle (Brown 1999: E).
(f) Thread spinal catheter through barrel of Tuohy needle.	To facilitate intermittent topping-up of anaesthesia and to allow greater control (Brown 1999: E).
(g) Attach the bacterial filter.	To prevent injection of contaminants into spinal space (Brown 1999: E).
(h) Apply transparent occlusive dressing and tape to the catheter insertion site.	To prevent the catheter being dislodged, to aid visibility and minimize contamination of the site (Baker *et al.* 2004: E).
(i) Inject solution into epidural/intrathecal space via catheter.	To provide anaesthesia (Brown 1999: E).

Procedure guidelines (*cont.*)

5	Position the patient according to the doctor's instructions, tilting if appropriate.	To ensure spread of solution to provide optimum effect (Brown 1999: E).
6	Take vital signs observations of blood pressure, pulse, respiratory rate and sedation score as dictated by the anaesthetist in the immediate post-insertion period. After this refer to local guidelines for frequency of observations required.	To monitor for signs of hypotension and respiratory depression (Weetman & Allison 2006: E).
7	Make the patient comfortable. Usually the patient is nursed flat for the first 3–6 hours, then slowly elevated into a sitting position. Bedclothes should not constrict the feet.	To ensure that any CSF leak is minimized and to prevent the patient developing a headache. To prevent the development of footdrop due to motor and sensory alterations caused by local anaesthetics (E).
8	Assess pain regularly using a visual analogue scale or pain chart if appropriate. Observe the patient's movements and facial expressions. Discuss insufficient or ineffective analgesia with the anaesthetist.	To ensure optimal pain management and that the patient is involved in his/her pain management (Macintyre & Ready 2001: E).

Procedure guidelines   Epidural/intrathecal infusion: setting up utilizing an ambulatory pump

This is a clean aseptic technique.

Procedure

Action	Rationale
1 Check the prescribed drugs and dilutent against the prescription. If not dispensed in infusion bags prepared aseptically in a special unit, specific local arrangements should be agreed between anaesthetists, pharmacists and ward/theatre/recovery staff for the preparation of the solution.	To ensure correct infusion is ready to connect. Except in special circumstances, the solutions should be prepared aseptically in a special unit (Royal College of Anaesthetists 2004: C).
Attach relevant extension set; apply drug information label. Recheck against prescription.	Clear labelling must be used to distinguish solutions for epidural/intrathecal infusion from all other infusions (Royal College of Anaesthetists 2004: C).
2 Check patency of epidural/intrathecal catheter as described in local policy or guidelines.	To ensure the catheter is in the correct position (E).
3 Insert the extension set into the pump and prime the extension set following the manufacturer's instructions for use of the pump.	To ensure the set is free from air when the infusion is commenced, thus minimizing the risk of air entering the catheter (E).
4 Open the sterile bacterial filter using a non-touch technique.	To minimize the risk of introducing any contaminants and micro-organisms into the epidural/intrathecal space via the filter (E).
5 Attach the extension set to the bacterial filter and start the pump.	To ensure the pump is working and the drugs are being delivered (E).
6 Place pump and infusion bag into the lock box or 'carry bag/pouch', ensuring that the tubing is not kinked.	To ensure comfort for the patient and to avoid obstruction to the infusion (E).

Procedure guidelines   Epidural/intrathecal catheter for chronic pain management: post-insertion management

It should be noted that the monitoring required in this patient group is different from that required in the postoperative setting. In the chronic setting, patients have already been taking opioids and have not received a general anaesthetic and are therefore less likely to suffer respiratory depression or alterations to their blood pressure (De Leon-Casasola *et al.* 1993).

Respiratory and cardiac function assessment

Action	Rationale
1 Monitor the patient's respiratory and cardiovascular function whilst in a recovery or high dependency area for 1 hour post-insertion.	To monitor for signs of respiratory depression and hypotension and to allow for immediate intervention where indicated (E).
2 On return to the ward for a minimum of 4 hours perform hourly assessment of: respiratory rate and SaO_2, blood pressure and pulse.	To monitor for signs of respiratory depression and hypotension and to allow for intervention if indicated (E).
3 If patient is stable, 4-hourly observations of the above for 24 hours. After 24 hours if patient is stable, respiratory and cardiac monitoring should only be reintroduced if deemed necessary by the multidisciplinary team for the individual patient or as dictated by local policy. Monitoring will continue for temperature measurements and observation for signs of localized or systemic infection for the duration of the epidural or intrathecal analgesia therapy.	To monitor patient safety whilst minimizing invasive procedures in patients with chronic pain problems (E).

Pain assessment

Action	Rationale
1 Assess the patient for their comfort/freedom from pain at rest and on movement, utilizing the same tool as used preinsertion.	This allows the practitioner and the patient to make a valid comparison (JCAHO & NPC 2001: C).
2 Pain assessment should be performed by the practitioner and patient/family together.	To gain the patient's trust and to give the patient some control over their quality of life (Higginson 1998: E).
3 Pain assessment should be performed initially at least hourly and then a minimum of 4-hourly until the patient and clinician feel that an optimum target has been achieved.	To aid patient comfort and the adjustment of drug dosages (JCAHO & NPC 2001: C).
4 Document pain assessment.	To provide the patient/family with a visual record of achievement and to allow continuity of information for different clinicians (Higginson 1998: E).
5 Assess sensory and mobility quality.	Monitor for any loss of sensation, bladder function and motor function (E).

Procedure guidelines   Epidural/intrathecal exit site dressing change

The dressing over the epidural/intrathecal exit site needs to fulfil the following three functions:

1 To help secure the epidural/intrathecal catheter.
2 To minimize the risk of infection.
3 To allow observation of the site without disturbing the dressing.

A transparent moisture responsive occlusive dressing (e.g. Tegaderm™ or Opsite IV 3000™) fulfils these functions. Opsite IV 3000™ has been found to perform well as an epidural catheter fixation product (Lawler & Anderson 2002). The epidural/intrathecal site should be inspected daily and the dressing changed at least once weekly or more frequently if there is any serous discharge from the site.

Equipment

1 Sterile dressing pack.
2 Skin cleaning agent, e.g. chlorhexidine in 70% alcohol.

3 Transparent occlusive dressing.

Procedure

Action	Rationale
1 Explain and discuss the procedure with the patient.	To ensure that the patient understands the procedure and gives his/her valid consent (DH 2001: C; NMC 2006b: C).
2 Wash hands with soap and water. Clean trolley (or plastic tray in the community) with chlorhexidine in 70% alcohol with a paper towel.	To minimize cross-infection (Preston 2005: C). To provide a clean working surface (Parker 2004: E).
3 Position the patient comfortably on their side or sitting forward so that the site is easily accessible without undue exposure of the patient.	To maintain the patient's dignity and comfort. This is especially important when carers are attending to an area that is not visible to the patient (Chapman & Day 2001: E).
4 Prepare trolley or tray with sterile field and cleaning solution.	To minimize risk of infection and ensure equipment available (Preston 2005: C).
5 Remove old dressing and place in disposable bag.	To prevent cross-infection (E).
6 Wash hands with bactericidal handrub.	To minimize the risk of microbial contamination (E).
7 Observe site for any signs of infection such as redness, swelling or purulent discharge. If any of these are present contact the hospital anaesthetic/pain team for advice.	To ensure careful monitoring of site to minimize the chance of any infection (Royal College of Anaesthetists 2004: C).
8 Clean site with skin-cleaning agent (chlorhexidine in 70% alcohol)	To minimize the risk of infection (Mimoz et al 1999: R 1b; Kinirons et al. 2001: R 1b; Hebl 2006: R 5).
9 Apply transparent occlusive dressing over the whole area.	To anchor the epidural/intrathecal catheter, minimize the risk of infection and allow observation of the epidural/intrathecal site (Burns et al. 2001: R 1b; Royce et al. 2006: E).
10 Ensure that the patient is comfortable.	
11 Dispose of all material in the clinical waste bag.	To prevent environmental contamination (Preston 2005: C).
12 Wash hands with soap and water.	To reduce the risk of cross-infection (Preston 2005: C).

Procedure guidelines   Epidural/intrathecal analgesia top up (bolus)

This procedure is usually performed by the doctor. Local anaesthetics or opioids may be given by nursing or midwifery staff as part of an extended role, according to local policy. This should follow an agreed period of education and supervised practice, which must be documented. This is a clean aseptic procedure. Most epidural/intrathecal infusion pumps allow a bolus dose to be programmed and delivered from the pump. This prevents the administration line and bacterial filter from being accessed and thus minimizes the risk of introducing infection. Intrathecal bolus doses are usually only given by the doctor.

Equipment

1 Antiseptic cleaning agent.
2 Syringes and needles.
3 Drug prescribed.
4 Water or 0.9% sodium chloride for injection as necessary.
5 Patient's prescription chart.
6 Sterile hub or bung.

Procedure

Action	Rationale
1 Wash hands with soap and water or bactericidal handrub.	To reduce the risk of cross-infection (Preston 2005: C).
2 Check the drug to be administered and diluents, according to policy.	To ensure the correct drug, amount and concentration is administered to the correct patient (NMC 2006a: C).
3 Draw up the drug as per local policy.	To maintain safe practice in medicines management (NMC 2006a: C).
4 Check patient's nameband against prescription.	To ensure the correct drug, amount and concentration is administered to the correct patient (NMC 2006a: C).
5 Clean the access portal of the bacterial filter.	To prevent the introduction of contaminants and micro-organisms into the epidural space (E).
6 Inject drug as prescribed.	To give the drug to the patient (E).
7 Monitor blood pressure, pulse and respirations at least every 5 minutes for 30–45 minutes.	To monitor for signs of hypotension and respiratory depression (side-effects of local anaesthetic and opioid drugs) (Coniam & Mendham 2005a: C).
8 Dispose of the equipment appropriately.	To prevent injury to patients, staff and to comply with medicines management policy (NMC 2006a: C).
9 Document the bolus dose administration in the medical and nursing records.	To aid communication and dissemination of information between members of the multidisciplinary team (NMC 2005: C).

Procedure guidelines   Discharge planning for patients with epidural/intrathecal catheter in situ

An epidural/intrathecal infusion should not be seen as a barrier to the patient leaving hospital. Patients can be safely managed in the community provided the following areas are addressed.

Procedure

Action	Rationale
1 Convert patient's infusion to one that requires the minimum of changing, i.e. an infusion bag and ambulatory pump rather than a 20 ml syringe and syringe driver.	This will reduce the workload of the patient/family or district nurse and also minimizes the number of interruptions to the patient circuit, thus minimizing the chance of microbial contamination (E).

Procedure guidelines (*cont.*)

2 Ensure that the patient will not be alone at home.

Epidural/intrathecal catheters can obstruct, become dislodged and the battery can fail on the device: most patients need immediate reassurance and practical help in these situations (Day 2001: E).

3 Arrange preparation of epidural/intrathecal drug infusion bags, usually in batches to provide enough delivery for 1 week. This can be arranged at the cancer centre or the referring hospital if they have the appropriate pharmaceutical arrangements.

Pharmacy reconstitution ensures aseptic preparation, thus minimizing the chance of microbial contamination, and reduces the workload and anxiety for family/district nurse. It should also be noted that epidural/intrathecal infusions may contain a combination of drugs and pharmacy reconstitution may help to reduce preparation error (E).

4 Discuss how the infusion bags will be collected each week; they cannot be posted because they contain drugs that are categorized as controlled drugs.

The method of collection needs to be discussed at an early stage with the family/district nurse to ensure continuity of infusion bag delivery and avoid any anxiety or delay to discharge (E).

5 The patient/family should be provided with the following equipment to take home:
   (a) Spare battery.
   (b) Bottle of bactericidal handrub.
   (c) Bottle of chlorhexidine in 70% alcohol.
   (d) Sterile gauze.
   (e) Syringes and needles.
   (f) 0.9% Sodium chloride for injection.
   (g) One spare bacterial filter and screw connector.
   (h) One week's supply of reconstituted epidural/intrathecal infusion bags.
   (i) Written advice re contact numbers/troubleshooting and prescription.

To ensure that the first week of therapy continues smoothly.

6 Patient/family and district nurse/general practitioner should be taught and trained in the following areas:
   (a) Setting up the infusion.
   (b) The functions of the ambulatory device, including alarms and visual displays.
   (c) Loading the administration set into the pump and priming the set.
   (d) Observation of the epidural/intrathecal site for signs and symptoms which would indicate an infection, e.g. redness, tenderness, swelling, leakage or pus.
   (e) The prescribed therapy for breakthrough pain.
   (f) Troubleshooting (as described below).
   (g) The procedure for obtaining medical/nursing help locally or at the cancer centre 24 hourly and every day of the week.
   (h) Dressing of the epidural/intrathecal site.

To reduce anxiety and increase patient comfort and trust (E).
To ensure that the patient/family and community team feel confident: (i) in using the infusion pump; (ii) in troubleshooting pump problems; (iii) where to seek help if they experience any problems (E).

7 Arrange any appropriate follow-up. This will be determined by the clinical status of the patient.

Patient may not return to the hospital for follow-up unless there are any problems if the intent is to move the patient's care to the community team, for example, in the terminal phase of illness when the patient may wish to be at home. However, contact with the community team should be maintained to ensure any problems with the epidural/intrathecal system are dealt with swiftly (E).

Procedure guidelines   Epidural/intrathecal catheter removal

Note: before an epidural/intrathecal catheter is removed it is essential to consider the clotting status of the patient's blood. If the patient is fully anticoagulated a clotting profile must be performed and advice sought from the medical staff as to when the catheter can be removed. If the patient is receiving a prophylactic anticoagulant the following guidelines are recommended (Vandermeulen *et al.* 1994; Horlocker & Wedel 1998; Rowlingson & Hanson 2005).

- Low-dose low molecular weight heparin. If this is given once daily the epidural/intrathecal catheter should be removed at least 12 hours after the last injection and several hours prior to the next dose (the timing will depend on the manufacturer's recommended guidelines, e.g. Tinzaparin [Leo Laboratories Ltd] recommend epidural or spinal catheters are removed a minimum of 4 hours before the subsequent dose).
- Unfractionated heparin. The epidural/intrathecal catheter should be removed following local guidelines and the advice of the anaesthetic/pain management team.

Equipment

1 Dressing pack.
2 Skin cleaning agent, e.g. chlorhexidine in 70% alcohol.

3 Occlusive dressing.

Procedure

Action	Rationale
1 Explain and discuss the procedure with the patient.	To ensure the patient understands the procedure and gives his/her valid consent (DH 2001: C; NMC 2006b: C).
2 Wash hands with bactericidal soap and water or bactericidal alcohol handrub.	To minimize cross-infection (Preston 2005: C).
3 Open dressing pack.	
4 Wash hands and remove tape and dressing from catheter insertion site.	To minimize risk of cross-infection (Preston 2005: C).
5 Gently, in one swift movement, remove the catheter. Check that the catheter is intact. This can be done by observing that the tip of the catheter is marked blue and that the 1 cm marks along the length of the catheter are all intact. Add to document that catheter removed intact.	To ensure the catheter is removed intact with the minimum of discomfort to the patient (E).
6 Clean around the catheter exit site using skin cleaning agent.	To minimize contamination of site by micro-organisms (E).
7 Apply an occlusive dressing and leave in situ for 24 hours. The epidural/intrathecal tip may be sent for culture and sensitivity if infection is suspected, or according to local policy.	To prevent inadvertent access of micro-organisms along the tract (E).

Problem solving: Epidural/intrathecal infusions of local anaesthetic agents and opioids: management of side-effects

Problem	Cause	Suggested action
Respiratory depression.	*Increasing age.* Elderly patients are more susceptible to the side-effects of opioids due to age-related alterations in the distribution, metabolism and excretion of drugs.	If respiratory rate falls to 8 breaths a minute or below: (a) Stop the epidural/intrathecal infusion. (b) Summon emergency assistance. (c) Commence oxygen via face mask and encourage the patient to take deep breaths.

Problem solving *(cont.)*

Problem	Cause	Suggested action
		(d) Review current analgesic prescription and consider reducing opioid and local anaesthetic doses before resuming the infusion (Macintyre *et al.* 2003).
	Concurrent use of systemic opioids or sedatives. Patients receiving opioids by epidural/intrathecal infusion should not be given opioids by any other route unless given in the palliative care setting for breakthrough pain.	1 Stop the epidural/intrathecal infusion. 2 Stay with the patient and monitor respiratory rate, sedation score and peripheral tissue oxygenation (using a pulse oximeter) continuously. 3 Commence oxygen therapy. 4 Consider giving naloxone if prescribed by anaesthetist or patient unrousable and naloxone already prescribed (when utilized for acute pain management). 5 Review analgesia: stop any other opioids prescribed and consider changing parameters of epidural/intrathecal infusion. (Pasero & McCaffery 1999: E.)
Sedation: 1 *Mild:* patient drowsy but easy to rouse. 2 *Severe:* patient difficult to rouse.	See under Respiratory depression, above	1 If patient has mild sedation, consider reducing the rate of the infusion or the dose of opioid or taking the opioid out of the infusion. 2 If patient is difficult to rouse and opioid toxicity/overdose is suspected, follow management for respiratory depression.
Hypotension.	Patients with hypovolaemia. Patients with a high thoracic epidural in whom the concentration of local anaesthetic agent and volume of infusion cause blockade of the cardio-accelerator nerves.	If blood pressure falls suddenly: (a) Stop the epidural/intrathecal infusion. (b) Summon emergency assistance. (c) Administer oxygen via face mask or nasal cannula. (d) Stay with the patient and monitor blood pressure at 5 minute intervals. (e) Ensure polyfusor of Haemacel or Gelofusine is readily available and use if prescribed by the anaesthetist. (f) Vasoconstrictor agents such as ephedrine or metaraminol may need to be given by the anaesthetic team if hypotension does not respond to a fluid challenge of Haemacel or Gelofusine. (Macintyre & Ready 2001.)
Motor blockade.	More likely to occur when higher concentrations of local anaesthetic agents are given by continuous infusion. If a high concentration of a local anaesthetic agent is administered via a low lumbar epidural/intrathecal catheter then the lumbar motor nerves are likely to be blocked, causing leg weakness.	Do not attempt to mobilize patient if leg weakness is evident. Contact pain or anaesthetic team for advice: reducing the concentration of the local anaesthetic agent or the rate of the epidural/intrathecal infusion may help to resolve this problem (Pasero & McCaffery 1999).

Problem	Cause	Suggested action
Nausea and vomiting.	Previous episodes of nausea and vomiting with opioids. Exacerbated by low blood pressure.	Regular administration of antiemetics. Treat other causes, e.g. low blood pressure. Consider use of non-pharmacological methods (e.g. stimulation of the P6 acupressure point) (Lee & Done 2004).
Pruritus (usually more marked over the face, chest and abdomen).	Previous pruritus with opioids.	Administer an antihistamine such as chlorpheniramine (may be contraindicated in patients who are becoming increasingly sedated) or a small dose of naloxone (administer with caution as this can easily reverse analgesia). If pruritus does not resolve consider switching to another opioid or removing the opioid from the infusion (Pasero & McCaffery 1999).
Urinary retention.	More likely to occur if opioids and local anaesthetic agents are infused in combination.	Catheterize patient.

Problem solving: Epidural/intrathecal insertion: complications

Problem	Signs and symptoms	Suggested action
Dural puncture.	Headache.	Bedrest: headache will be less severe if patient lies flat. Replacement fluids either intravenously or orally to encourage formation of CSF. Administer analgesics for headache. If headache does not settle, contact the anaesthetic team who may consider an epidural blood patch to seal the puncture (Gaiser 2006).
Catheter migration into an epidural blood vessel.	If catheter migrates into a blood vessel signs of opioid or local anaesthetic toxicity can occur: *opioid*: sedation and respiratory depression; *local anaesthetic*: circumoral tingling and numbness, twitching, convulsions and apnoea.	Stop epidural infusion. Contact pain/anaesthetic team or summon emergency assistance. Treat the patient for complications of opioid or local anaesthetic overdose. If necessary support ventilation (Chapman & Day 2001).
Catheter migration across the dura into the CSF (from the epidural space into the intrathecal space).	If an epidural catheter migrates into the CSF the analgesic solution may reach as high as the cranial subarachnoid space. If this occurs the respiratory muscles are paralysed together with the cranial nerves, resulting in apnoea, profound hypotension and unconsciousness. This is because intrathecal doses are calculated as one-tenth of the epidural dose and migration from the epidural space to the intrathecal space leads to a drug overdose.	Stop epidural infusion. Summon emergency assistance. Prepare emergency equipment to support respiration and ventilate lungs. Prepare emergency drugs and intravenous fluids and administer as directed. Prepare equipment for intubation.

601

Problem solving *(cont.)*

Problem	Signs and symptoms	Suggested action
Epidural haematoma.	Back pain and tenderness and nerve root pain with sensory and motor weakness.	Urgent neurological assessment. Computed tomography (CT) or magnetic resonance imaging (MRI) scan to accurately diagnose if there is nerve or spinal cord compression. If a haematoma is diagnosed prepare patient for urgent surgery. (Chapman & Day 2001). To avoid haematoma on removal of epidural in patients treated with prophylactic anticoagulants, see guidelines for timing of removal.
Epidural abscess.	Back pain and tenderness. May have redness and purulent discharge from catheter exit site. May also develop nerve root signs with neuropathic pain and sensory/motor weakness.	If the epidural catheter is still in situ, remove and send tip off for culture and sensitivity. Treat with antibiotics. Carry out CT or MRI scan and refer for urgent neurosurgery to prevent paraplegia (Chapman & Day 2001: E).
Meningitis.	Headaches, fever, neck stiffness, photophobia.	Assist anaesthetist/doctor to obtain CSF sample for microbiology analysis. Initiate antibiotic therapy as per hospital policy. Non pharmacological measures for symptom management, e.g. dim lights. If the infection does not respond to antibiotics it may be necessary to remove the catheter and convert back to systemic analgesia until meningitis has resolved (Mercadante 1999).
Intrathecal catheter granulona (an inflammatory mass that forms around the catheter tip).	Pain, parasthesia, numbness in lower extremeties that may progress to paresis.	MRI scan to diagnose the problem. Stop infusion (granulomas may resolve on their own once the infusion is stopped Du Pen (2005)).

Problem solving: Epidural/intrathecal catheter: issues with pump and site

The following can be used by nursing staff and then adapted for use by the patient/family.

Problem	Cause	Suggested action
Ambulatory pump auditory alarm.	Battery failure is most likely.	Stop pump, remove old and replace with new battery; ensure battery is fitted up snugly to connections. Turn on pump and ensure light indicator is flashing.
	Catheter occlusion.	Stop pump, draw up 0.9% sodium chloride and flush catheter. If catheter clears reattach pump, press start and ensure light indicator is flashing. If catheter is still obstructed and will not flush, phone cancer centre/general practioner.

Problem	Cause	Suggested action
Sudden acute pain.	Catheter obstruction; catheter movement; change in pathology.	Check the catheter for any obvious problems which can be quickly resolved such as catheter disconnection. If the catheter has blocked or migrated outwards, stop the infusion pump and give the patient a breakthrough dose of analgesia orally or subcutaneously. Inform general practitioner and/or hospital anaesthetic/pain team as soon as possible. If the patient has had an exacerbation of pain due to disease progression, follow advice from hospital team (the infusion rate may require titrating or the concentration of drugs may need to be changed).
Disconnection of epidural/intrathecal catheter from filter.	Patient movement: typically turning in bed at night.	Stop the pump. Wrap the disconnected end of the catheter in a piece of sterile gauze and contact the district nursing/hospital team for advice. Suggested procedure for district nursing/hospital team (Langevin *et al.* 1996): ▪ Clean approximately 15 cm of the disconnected catheter with chlorhexidine in 70% alcohol. Allow to air dry completely. ▪ Using sterile scissors, cut the cleaned catheter 10 cm away from the contaminated end. ▪ Insert the cleaned end of catheter into a sterile screw connector and catheter filter. ▪ Change the epidural/intrathecal infusion extension set and recommence infusion.
Redness, swelling or leakage of discoloured fluid from site.	Infection *or* local irritation at site from skin interaction with the plastic catheter.	Contact general practitioner and hospital anaesthetic/pain team. If infection is suspected, the patient should be started on antibiotics to prevent spread of any infection into the epidural space. It may be necessary to remove the catheter if the patient has a temperature, there is pus at the exit site or if the patient has back pain.

References and further reading

ANZCA (2005) Epidural analgesia. In: *Acute Pain Management: Scientific Evidence*, 2nd edn. Australia and New Zealand College of Anaesthetics, Melbourne, Australia.

Baker, L. *et al.* (2004) Evolving spinal analgesia practice in palliative care. *Palliat Med*, **18**, 507–15.

Ballantyne, J.C. & Carwood, C.M. (2005) Comparative efficacy of epidural, subarachnoid and intracerebroventricular opioids in patients with pain due to cancer. *Cochrane Database Syst Rev*, **2**, CD005178.DOI:10.1002/14651858.

Bannon, L., Alexander-Williams, M. & Lutman, D. (2001) A national survey of epidural practice. *Anaesthesia*, **56**(10), 1021–2.

Brown, D.L. (1999) *Atlas of Regional Anaesthesia*, 2nd edn. W.B. Saunders Company, Philadelphia.

Burns, S.M. *et al.* (2001) Intrapartum epidural catheter migration: a comparative study of three dressing applications. *Br J Anaesth*, **86**(4), 565–7.

Chapman, S. & Day, R. (2001) Spinal anatomy and the use of epidurals. *Prof Nurs*, **16**(6), 1174–7.

Cleeland, C.S. (1991) The brief pain inventory. www.mdanderson.org/topics/paincontrol. Accessed 24/9/07.

Coniam, S. & Mendham, J. (2005) Management of acute pain: principles and practice. In: *Principles of Pain Management for Anaesthetists*. Hodder Arnold, London, pp. 74–5.

Cook, T., Eaton, J. & Goodwin, A. (1997) Epidural analgesia following upper abdominal surgery: United Kingdom practice. *Acta Anaesthesiol Scand*, **41**(1), 18–24.

Cousins, K. *et al.* (2003) Intrathecal catheters: developing consistency in filter use and dressings in Perth, Australia. *Int J Palliat Nurs*, **7**(9), 308–14.

604

Curatolo, M., Peterson-Felix, S., & Scaramozzino, P. (1998) Epidural fentanyl, adrenaline and clonidine as adjuvants to local anaesthetics for surgical anaesthesia: meta analysis of analgesia and side effects. *Acta Anaesthesiol Scand*, **42**, 910–20.

Day, R. (2001) The use of epidural and intrathecal analgesia in palliative care. *Int J Palliat Care*, 7(8), 369–74.

De Cicco, M. *et al.* (1995) Time-dependent efficacy of bacterial filters and infection risk in long-term epidural catheterisation. *Anesthesiology*, **82**, 765–71.

De Leon-Casasola, O.A. *et al.* (1993) A comparison of postoperative epidural analgesia between patients with chronic cancer taking high doses of oral opioids versus opioid-naïve patients. *Anesth Analg*, 76, 302–7.

Du Pen, A. (2005) Care and management of intrathecal and epidural catheters. *J Infusion Nursing*, **28**(6), 377–81.

DH (2001) Good practice in consent implementation guide: consent to examination or treatment. www.dh.gov.uk/en/Publicationsandstatistics/Publications/PublicationsPolicyAndGuidance/DH_4005762. Accessed 24/9/07.

Dickson, D. (2004) Risks and benefits of long term intrathecal analgesia. *Anaesthesia*, **59**, 633–5.

Fotiadis, R.J. *et al.* (2004) Epidural analgesia in gastrointestinal surgery. *Br J Surg*, **91**, 828–41.

Gaiser, R. (2006) Postdural puncture headache. *Curr Opin Anaesthesiol*, **19**, 249–53.

Grond, S. *et al.* (2000) Epidural analgesia for labour pain: a review of availability, current practices and influence on labour. *Int J Acute Pain Manage*, 3(1), 31–43.

Hall, J. (2000) Epidural analgesia management. *Nurs Times*, 96(28), 38–9.

Hebl, J.R. (2006) The importance and implications of aseptic techniques during regional anaesthesia. *Reg Anesth Pain Med*, **31**, 311–23.

Higginson, I. (1998) Can professionals improve their assessments? *J Pain Symptom Manage*, **15**(3), 149–50.

Horlocker, T. & Wedel, D. (1998) Spinal and epidural blockade and perioperative low molecular weight heparin: smooth sailing on the Titanic. *Anaesth Analg*, 8, 1153–6.

JCAHO & NPC (2001) Pain: current understanding of assessment, management and treatments. www.jcaho.org. Accessed 8/06.

Kehlet, H. (1997) Multimodal approach to control postoperative pathophysiology and rehabilitation. *Br J Anaesth*, 78(5), 606–17.

Kehlet, H. & Holte, K. (2001) Effect of postoperative analgesia on surgical outcome. *Br J Anaesth*, **87**(1), 62–72.

Kinirons, B. *et al.* (2001) Chlorhexadine versus povidine iodine in preventing colonisation of continuous epidural catheters in children. *Anaesthesiology*, **94**, 239–44.

Langevin, P. *et al.* (1996) Epidural catheter reconnection: safe and unsafe practice. *Anesthesiology*, 85(4), 883–8.

Lawler, K. & Anderson, T. (2002) Regional trial of five epidural fixation products and a commonly used control. *Pain Network Newsletter*, Spring, pp. 6–8.

Lee, A. & Done, M.L. (2004) Stimulation of the wrist acupuncture point P6 for preventing post-operative nausea and vomiting. *Cochrane Database Syst Rev*, 3, CD003281.DOI: 10.1002/14651858.

Leo Laboratories Ltd (2004) Tinzaparin sodium 10 000 IU/ml. Product information leaflet. www.emc.medicines.org.uk. Accessed 02/06.

Macintyre, P. & Ready, L. (2001) Epidural and intrathecal analgesia. In: *Acute Pain Management. A Practical Guide*, (eds P. Macintyre & L. Ready) 2nd edn. W.B. Saunders, London.

Macintyre, P., Upton, R. & Ludbrook, G.L. (2003) Pain in the elderly. In: *Clinical Pain Management: Acute Pain* (eds D.J. Rowbotham & P.E. Macintyre), pp. 157–58. Arnold, London.

Mackenzie, A.R. *et al.* (1998) Spinal epidural abscess: the importance of early diagnosis and treatment. *J Neurosurg Psychiatry*, 65(2), 209–12.

McCaffery, M. & Pasero, C. (1999) *Pain: Clinical Manual*. Mosby, St. Louis, MO.

Mercadante, S. (1999) Problems of long-term spinal opioid treatment in advanced cancer patients. *Pain*, 79(1), 1–13.

Mimoz, O., Karim, A. & Cosseron, M. (1999) Chlorhexidine compared with povidone-iodine as skin preparation before blood culture. A randomised controlled trial. *Ann Intern Med*, 131(11), 834–7.

NMC (2005) *Guidelines for Records and Record Keeping*. Nursing and Midwifery Council, London.

NMC (2006a) *Medicines Management Advice Sheet*. Nursing and Midwifery Council, London.

NMC (2006b) *A–Z Advice Sheet Consent*. www.nmc.org.

Papagelopoulos, P. *et al.* (2001) Treatment of lumbosacral radicular pain with epidural steroid injections. *Orthopedics*, **24**(2), 145–9.

Parker, L.J. (2004) Decontamination of medical devices: legislation and compliance to practice. *Br J Nurs*, **13**(17), 1028–32.

Pasero, C. & McCaffery, M. (1999) Providing epidural analgesia. *Nursing*, 29(8), 34–42.

Preston, R.M. (2005) Aseptic technique: evidence-based approach to patient safety. *Br J Nurs*, **14**(10), 540–5.

Richardson, J. (2001) Post-operative epidural analgesia: introducing evidence-based guidelines through an education and assessment process. *J Clin Nurs*, **10**(2), 238–45.

Romer, H. & Russell, G. (1998) A survey of the practice of thoracic epidural analgesia in the United Kingdom. *Anaesthesia*, 53(10), 1016–22.

Rowlingson, J.C. & Hanson, P.B. (2005) Neuraxial anesthesia and low-molecular-weight heparin prophylaxis in major orthopedic surgery in the wake of the latest American Society of Regional Analgesia Guidelines. *Anesth Analg*, **100**, 1482–8.

Royal College of Anaesthetists (2004) *Good Practice in the Management of Continuous Epidural Analgesia in the Hospital Setting*. Royal College of Anaesthetists, London.

Royce, C.F., Hall, J. & Royce, A.G. (2006) The 'mesentery' dressing for epidural fixation. *Anaesthesia*, **61**, 713.

Sands, R., Yarussi, A. & de Leon-Casasola, D. (1998) Complications and side-effects associated with epidural bupivacaine/morphine analgesia. *Acute Pain*, 1(2), 43–50.

Sloan, P.A. (2004) The evolving role of interventional pain management in oncology. *J Support Oncol*, 2(6), 491–503.

Smith, H. & Elliott, J. (2001) Alpha2 receptors and agonists in pain management. *Curr Opin Anaesthesiol*, **14**, 513–18.

Smitt, P. *et al.* (1998) Outcome and complications of epidural analgesia in patients with chronic cancer pain. *Cancer*, 83(9), 2015–22.

Stevens, R.A. & Ghazi, S.M. (2000) Routes of opioid analgesic therapy in the management of cancer pain. *Cancer Control*, 7(2), 132–41.

Urdan, L.D., Stacy, K.M. & Lough, M.E. (2006) Pain and pain management. In: *Thelan's Critical Care Nursing Diagnosis and Management*. Mosby Elsevier, St Louis, MO.

Vandermeulen, E., Van Aken, H. & Vermylen, J. (1994) Anticoagulants and spinal-epidural anaesthesia. *Anaesth Analg*, 79(6), 1165–77.

Wallace, M.S. (2002) Treatment options for refractory pain: the role of intrathecal therapy. *Neurology*, 59(Suppl 2), S18–24.

Walsh, D. (1997) *TENS: Clinical Applications and Related Theory*. Churchill Livingstone, Edinburgh.

Weetman, C. & Allison W. (2006) Use of epidural analgesia in post-operative pain management. *Nursing Standard* Jul 12–18; 20(44):54–64.

Wheatley, R., Schug, S. & Watson, D. (2001) Safety and efficacy of postoperative epidural analgesia. *Br J Anaesth*, 87(1), 47–61.

Chapter 30

Perioperative care

Preoperative care 606
Reference material 606
Procedure guidelines: Antiembolic stockings: fitting and wearing 608
Procedure guidelines: Preoperative care 611
Intraoperative care 613
Reference material 613
Procedure guidelines: Intraoperative care 616
Postanaesthetic recovery 617
Reference material 617
Procedure guidelines: Postanaesthetic recovery 620
Problem solving: Postanaesthetic recovery 623
Procedure guidelines: Postoperative recovery 625
References and further reading 627

Definition

Perioperative care refers to the nursing care delivered to a patient before (pre), during (intra) and after (post) surgery.

Preoperative care

Definition

Preoperative care is the assessment and preparation, physical and psychological, of a patient before surgery.

Objectives

Physical

- To assess the physical condition of the patient so that potential problems can be anticipated and prevented.
- To ensure that the patient understands the need to be in an optimum physical condition before surgery.
- To minimize postoperative complications, e.g. by teaching the patient deep breathing exercises, leg exercises and their importance to the individual's well-being postoperatively.

Psychological

- To ensure that the patient is fully informed and understands the nature of anaesthetic, surgery and possible complications.
- To minimize anxiety for the patient and help them to identify and implement useful coping mechanisms.
- To inform and ensure the patient understands what to expect postoperatively, e.g. presence of possible drains, catheters, pumps and monitors that may be necessary.

Reference material

Patient education and postoperative pain

Research has shown that preoperative patient education not only meets patients' information needs but also assists patients in reducing anxiety levels and promotes the patients' well being (Walker 2002). Patient information booklets can also help patients to have a greater understanding of surgery and what is expected of them.

Preoperative education can address some of the patients' concerns and fears. As pain and anaesthesia are patients' greatest worries, they need to be discussed in the preoperative period so that anxiety can be reduced (Mitchell 2000), which may result in patients requiring less analgesia (Beddows 1997). Preoperative visiting by recovery staff allows patients to ask questions, which could help them to manage their anxiety and provide baseline information about patients, which is important for effective management postoperatively, for example, of pain management. It also gives

information to the surgical team to allow them to maintain continuity of care in the operating department (Beddows 1997).

The control of pain whilst the patient is still in the operating theatre and whilst recovering from his/her surgery is vital to further reduce anxiety and general well being. Use of patient-controlled analgesia (PCA) gives the patient a sense of autonomy, which may decrease anxiety and which will in turn influence the patient's pain perception (Field & Adams 2001). For further information see Chapter 27, Pain management and assessment.

Skin preparation

Traditionally patients had their operation site and surrounding area shaved the night before surgery in the belief that hair removal reduces the incidence of wound infection postoperatively. However, this method of hair removal can injure the skin and may increase the risk of infection by producing microscopic infected lacerations, so hair needs to be removed only from the area immediately around the site of incision. This should be done with depilatory cream the day before the operation. If this is not possible then shaving should take place in the anaesthetic room prior to surgery, using electric clippers. It should not be done in the operating room as this is a source of infection (Kjonniksen *et al.* 2002).

Preoperative fasting

General anaesthesia carries the risk of the patient inhaling gastric contents during induction, which could lead to serious complications and can even be fatal (Dean & Fawcett 2002). Ensuring that the patient understands the rationale for fasting is important in order to reduce anxiety. For elective surgery patients are kept 'nil by mouth' long enough to allow the stomach to empty. This means that patients can have water or clear fluids up to 3 hours before surgery and solid foods up to 6 hours provided this is light food (RCN 2005). However, gastric emptying can be delayed by anxiety or the action of some opiates, for example morphine (O'Callaghan 2002), so it is important to be aware of this when deciding when to commence patients 'nil by mouth'. Most patients prefer not to eat but would like to have a drink to keep their mouth moist before surgery and so are happy to comply with the 3 hours fasting for water and clear fluids.

Antiembolic stockings (graduated elastic compression stockings)

Patients should be assessed for the individual risk factors for venous thromboembolism (VTE), i.e. deep vein thrombosis (DVT) and pulmonary embolism (PE) when hospitalized in order to determine the most appropriate thromboprophylaxis (House of Commons Health Committee 2005; NICE 2007). Patients at higher risk include those with major illness e.g. acute cardiac or respiratory failure, major surgery, older patients, patients who are obese or with a previous history of DVT or PE (SIGN 2002; NICE 2007). All patients requiring an inpatient stay for surgery should have prophylactic treatment to reduce the risk of DVT, which may include anticoagulation and mechanical compression methods, for example antiembolic stockings and intermittent pneumatic compression methods (SIGN 2002; Roderick *et al.* 2005; NICE 2007). Patients should be given verbal and written information before surgery about the risks of VTE and the effectiveness of prophylaxis (NICE 2007). It is estimated that 20% of patients undergoing major surgery will develop a DVT with the risk increasing to 40% of patients undergoing major orthopaedic surgery (SIGN 2002). Mechanical compression methods reduce the risk of DVT by about two-thirds when used as monotherapy and by about half when added to pharmacological methods (Roderick *et al.* 2005). Graduated compression stockings (antiembolic) promote venous flow and reduce venous stasis not only in the legs but also in the pelvic veins and inferior vena cava (Hayes *et al.* 2002; Rashid *et al.* 2005; Roderick *et al.* 2005).

Thigh-length graduated compression/antiembolic stockings should be fitted from the time of admission to hospital unless contraindicated, for example peripheral arterial disease or diabetic neuropathy (NICE 2007, p. 121), and until the patient has returned to their usual level of mobility. Thigh-length stockings are difficult to put on and can roll down creating a tourniquet just above the knee restricting blood supply, so patient monitoring and/or assistance should take place to ensure that stockings are fitted smoothly, are not rolled down or the top band not folded down. If thigh-length stockings are inappropriate for a particular patient for reasons of compliance or fit, knee-length stockings may be used as a suitable alternative. It has been suggested that 15–20% of patients cannot effectively wear antiembolic stockings because of unusual limb size or shape (SIGN 2002). In reality, knee-high stockings have the advantage of simplicity, with greater patient compliance and economy (Byrne 2002; Barker & Hollingsworth 2004; Parnaby 2004). When applying the stockings, it is important that correct measurements are taken so that the appropriate stocking size is fitted for optimum effectiveness. The stocking compression profile should be equivalent to the Sigel profile, and approximately 18 mmHg at the ankle, 14 mmHg at the mid-calf and 8 mmHg at the upper thigh (NICE 2007, p. 52).

During surgery the use of heel supports which reduce the pressure on the calves on the operating table will also encourage venous return. The use of intermittent calf compression air boots that promote venous flow during surgery have also been reported to be effective (Davis & O'Neill 2002; NICE 2007). The intermittent calf compression boots can be used in conjunction with antiembolic stockings providing double protection. The only time this needs to be reviewed is when the patient is placed in Lloyd Davis position as there is a risk of developing compartment syndrome (see Positioning section, below). In this instance either the antiembolic stockings or the intermittent calf compression boots should

be used: this decision will be made by the surgeon and the anaesthetist.

Assessment of latex allergy

Natural rubber latex is a durable flexible material composed of natural proteins and added chemicals. In the health care setting, natural rubber latex is present in gloves and other medical devices such as catheters and wound drains. Latex allergy results in a reaction to one or more of the components of natural rubber latex (AORN 2004).

As part of the patient's preoperative assessment, allergy status must be established. This information must be communicated to all members of the health care team and departments that the patient may visit including theatre, recovery, pathology and radiology. The assessment should cover the following known risk factors for latex allergy (AORN 2004):

- History of multiple surgeries beginning at an early age (e.g. spina bifida, urinary malformation).
- Known food allergies (avocado, chestnut or banana).
- History of an allergic reaction to latex.
- History of an allergic reaction during an operation.
- Past experience of itchy skin, skin rash or redness when in contact with rubber products.
- Past skin irritation from an examination by a doctor or dentist wearing rubber gloves.
- Past sneezing, wheezing or chest tightness when exposed to rubber.

Assessment and monitoring for symptoms of latex allergy in both the conscious and unconscious patient is required at all stages of perioperative care (Table 30.1).

Table 30.1 Symptoms of latex exposure and possible anaphylaxis.

The conscious patient	The unconscious patient
Itchy eyes	Facial oedema
Generalized pruritis	Urticaria/rash
Shortness of breath	Skin flushing
Sneezing/wheezing	Bronchospasm
Nausea	Laryngeal oedema
Oedema	Hypotension
Vomiting	Tachycardia
Abdominal cramp	Cardiac arrest
Diarrhoea	
Feeling faint	

Management of the patient with known latex allergy

Patients identified as having an allergy to natural latex rubber need to be treated in a latex-free environment following these recommendations:

- The theatre must be cleaned with latex-free gloves and equipment.
- All latex products removed or covered with plastics so that the rubber elements are not exposed.
- All health care staff must be made aware of the adverse reactions that could occur following the patient's exposure to natural rubber latex.
- All health care staff in direct contact with the patient must wear vinyl gloves during procedures and in the vicinity of the patient.
- The patient should be first on the operating list.
- Where a type I (immediate hypersensitivity reaction) allergy is suspected, suitable clinical management procedures must be ready for use in the event of the patient having a hypersensitivity reaction.
- A latex-free contents box or trolley (this holds stock of all latex-free products that will be required during surgery and anaesthetic) should be ready in every theatre department and in recovery room. There should be a list of all latex-free equipment with the manufacturers listed available in the box or trolley.

Further guidance may be sought from the Association of Perioperative Registered Nurses (AORN) proposed latex guideline at www.aorn.org/proposed/latex.htm (accessed 16/2/06).

Procedure guidelines   Antiembolic stockings: fitting and wearing

Note: antiembolic stockings are also known as graduated elastic compression stockings or thromboembolic deterrent stockings (TEDS).

Equipment

1 Tape measure.
2 Antiembolic stockings (calf or thigh length).
3 Apron.
4 Patient records/documentation.

Procedure

Action

Patient assessment for antiembolic stockings

1 Assess and record in the patient's documentation the patient's risk factors for venous thromboembolism (VTE), i.e. deep vein thrombosis (DVT) and pulmonary embolism (PE).
Examples of risk factors:
 (a) patient undergoing major surgery or abdominal/pelvic surgery;
 (b) immobility, e.g. prolonged bedrest;
 (c) active cancer;
 (d) severe cardiac failure or recent myocardial infarction;
 (e) acute respiratory failure;
 (f) elderly;
 (g) previous history of DVT or PE;
 (h) acute infection/inflammation;
 (i) diabetes;
 (j) smoker;
 (k) obesity;
 (l) gross varicose veins;
 (m) paralysis of lower limbs;
 (n) clotting disorders;
 (o) hormone replacement therapy;
 (p) oral contraceptives;
 (q) pregnancy;
 (r) puerperium;
 (s) anaesthesia.
(SIGN 2002; House of Commons Health Committee 2005; Rashid *et al.* 2005; NICE 2007)

Rationale

All patients admitted to hospital should undergo a risk assessment for venous thrombosis to determine the most appropriate preventative measures, i.e. thromboprophylaxis (SIGN 2002: C; House of Commons Health Committee 2005: C; Roderick *et al.* 2005: C; NICE 2007: C).
The higher the number of risk factors the greater the risk for VTE (SIGN 2002: C; NICE 2007: C).

2 Assess and record in the patient's documentation the patient's suitability for antiembolic stockings, identifying whether the patient has any contraindications for wearing antiembolic stockings.

To comply with national guidelines and hospital policy/guidelines.
To ensure that antiembolic stockings are fitted correctly and to reduce the complications associated with antiembolic stockings (SIGN 2002; NICE 2007: C).

Contraindications:
(a) Severe peripheral arterial disease (SIGN 2002).
(b) Severe peripheral neuropathy (SIGN 2002).
(c) Vascular disease resulting from congestive heart conditions (House of Commons Health Committee 2005).
(d) Gangrene.
(e) Pulmonary oedema or massive oedema of the legs (House of Commons Health Committee 2005).
(f) Major leg deformity (SIGN 2002).
(g) Certain types of skin disease, e.g. weeping skin lesions/dermatitis (SIGN 2002).

The stockings would hinder healing of local leg conditions, e.g. dermatitis (C).

(h) Recent skin graft (Rashid *et al.* 2005).
(i) Cellulitis (Rashid *et al.* 2005).
(j) Pressure sores to heels (NICE 2005; Rashid *et al.* 2005).

Pressure sores are a complication of antiembolic stockings and stockings should not be applied (NICE 2005: C).

3 Explain and discuss the procedure with the patient and provide written information as follows:

To ensure that the patient understands the procedure and gives his/her valid consent (NMC 2005: C; NMC 2006: C).
To ensure that the patient understands how to fit and wear stockings including self-care measures and what to report to the nurse so as to detect complications early, e.g. pressure sores, circulation difficulties of wearing antiembolic stockings (SIGN 2002: C; NICE 2007: C).

(a) Reasons for wearing antiembolic stockings.
(b) How to fit and wear stockings.
(c) What to report to the nurse, e.g. any feelings of pain or numbness or skin problems.
(d) Skin care, i.e. wash and dry legs daily.
(e) Reasons for early mobilization and adequate hydration.
(f) Reasons against crossing of legs or ankles.
(g) Length of time that the stockings should be worn, e.g. until they return to their usual level of mobility.

Measuring for and fitting of antiembolic stockings

4 Perform hand hygiene and put on apron prior to the procedure.

To prevent cross-infection (Pratt *et al.* 2007).

5 Place the tape measure around the calf at the greatest point and measure the calf circumference (and leg measurements) according to the manuafacturer's instructions, recording the measurements in the patient's documentation.

To comply with the manufacturer's instructions (C). Incorrect sizing causes swelling and bruising to ankles and can constrict blood supply leading to long term complications (C).

6 Check pedal pulses are intact.

To ensure the patient has good circulation to the feet and antiembolic stockings are not contraindicated (SIGN 2002: C; NICE 2007: C).

Apply the antiembolic stocking to the legs according to the manufacturer's instructions. Refer to the Procedure guidelines: Compression garments (elastic): application of, Chapter 9.

To ensure correct size of stocking is fitted correctly (C).

Procedure guidelines *(cont.)*

Daily care of patient wearing antiembolic stockings

7 Remove stockings daily, observing for pain, skin damage, circulation difficulties which may arise as a result of wrinkling, etc. of stocking, but for no more than 30 minutes: confirm size is applicable (SIGN 2002).

To review calf and/or leg measurements to ensure stockings fit correctly (SIGN 2002: C; NICE 2005:C). Reported complications of wearing antiembolic stockings include pressure sores (NICE 2005:C) and circulation difficulties, e.g. arterial occlusion, thrombosis, gangrene (SIGN 2002: C). The circulation complications can be linked to the tourniquet effect of bunched-up stockings combined with swelling of the leg (SIGN 2002; House of Commons Health Committee 2005).

8 Where worn, ensure that antiembolic stockings are of the correct size and fit smoothly. Check the colour and tips of the toes. *Note*: top band of stockings must not be turned down.

To prevent a tourniquet effect if the stocking rolls down (C). To ensure the blood supply is not compromised (C).

9 Encourage early mobilization. For patients on bedrest, encourage deep breathing and exercises of the leg hourly; flexion/extension and rotation of the ankles.

To improve venous circulation (SIGN 2002: C; NICE 2007: C).

10 Encourage patient to sit with legs up when resting.

It is recognized that this will reduce limb swelling and promote venous return by its gravitational effect; however, there is little scientific data to clarify that this does reduce the risk of VTE. *Note*: care should be taken with patients with ischaemic legs (NICE 2007: C).

11 Monitor for signs of DVT or PE and report to medical staff immediately:
  (a) Complaints of calf or thigh pain.
  (b) Erythema, warmth, tenderness and abnormal swelling of the calf or thigh in the affected limb.
  (c) Numbness or tingling of the feet.
  (d) Dyspnoea, chest pain or signs of shock.
  (e) Pain in the chest, back or ribs which gets worse when the patient breathes in deeply.
  (f) Coughing up blood.

To monitor for signs of DVT and PE (Rashid *et al.* 2005: C; NICE 2007: C).

12 Monitor whether the patient has adequate hydration.

To ensure the patient is adequately hydrated (SIGN 2002: C; NICE 2007: C).

13 Record temperature daily.

To detect infection early and signs of inflammation associated with venous thrombosis (C).

14 Launder according to the manufacturer's instructions.

To reduce the risk of cross-infection and patient comfort (C).

Discharge care of patient with antiembolic stockings

15 On discharge from hosptial, check the patient understands the following:
  (a) Signs and symptoms of DVT.
  (b) Correct use of prophylaxis at home, e.g. how to wear antiemoblic stocking correctly.
  (c) Implications of not using prophylaxis correctly.
  (d) To continue to undertake leg exercises if immobile.
  (e) To avoid long periods of travel for 4 weeks after an operation.

To reduce the risks of developing a DVT or PE after an operation and to ensure that the patient reports any symptoms promptly to enable the early detection and management of DVT and/or PE (NICE 2007: C).

Procedure guidelines   Preoperative care

Equipment

1 Identification bracelets.
2 Allergy bands if necessary.
3 Theatre gown.
4 Cotton-based underwear or disposable pants can be worn if they do not interfere with surgery.
5 Antiembolic stockings if appropriate.
6 Labelled containers for dentures, glasses and/or hearing aid if necessary.

7 Hypoallergenic tape.
8 Patient records/documentation including medical records, consent form, X-ray films, blood test results, anaesthetic assessment, record and preoperative checklist.

Procedure

Action	Rationale
1 Assess the preoperative education received by the patient and ensure that it is complete and understood.	To ensure that the patient understands the nature and outcome of the surgery to reduce anxiety and possible postoperative complications (Walker 2002: R).
2 Check that the patient has undergone relevant investigative procedures, e.g. X-ray, electrocardiogram (ECG), blood test and that these are included with the patient's notes.	To ensure all relevant information is available to the nurses, anaesthetists and surgeons (AORN 2000: C).
3 (a) Check and confirm pregnancy status on all women of childbearing age. If a pregnancy test is required, ensure the result is known to all health care professionals involved in the operation.	To eliminate the possibility of unknown pregnancy prior to the planned surgical procedure.
(b) If appropriate, ask the patient if they are menstruating and ensure that they have a sanitary towel in place and not a tampon.	This is to prevent infection if the tampon is left in place for longer than 2 hours (www.tamponalert.org.uk: C).
4 Check the consent form is correctly completed, signed and dated.	To comply with legal requirements and hospital policy and to ensure that the patient has understood the surgical procedure (NMC 2006: C).
5 Check the operation site is marked correctly.	To ensure the patient undergoes the correct surgery for which he/she has consented (AORN 2000: C).
6 Check that the patient has undergone preanaesthetic assessment by the anaesthetist.	To ensure that the patient can be given the most suitable anaesthetic and any special requirements for anaesthetic have been highlighted (AORN 2000: C).
7 Record the patient's pulse, blood pressure, respirations, temperature and weight.	To provide baseline data for comparison intra and postoperatively. The weight is recorded so that the anaesthetist can calculate the correct dose of drugs to be administered (AORN 2000: C).
8 Instruct the patient to shower or bath as close to the planned time of the operation as possible and before a premedication is administered, if appropriate.	To minimize risk of postoperative wound infection and prevent patient accidents (Pratt et al. 2007: R).
9 Assist the patient to change into a theatre gown after having a shower/bath.	To reduce the risk of cross-infection, ease of access to operation site and soiling of patient's own clothes (Pratt et al. 2007: R).

Procedure guidelines *(cont.)*

10 Long hair should be held back with, for example, a non-metallic tie.	For safety to prevent hair getting caught in equipment and to reduce the risk of infection (E).
11 All jewellery, cosmetics, nail varnish and clothing, other than the theatre gown, are to be removed. Wedding rings may be left in situ, but must be covered and secured with hypoallergenic tape.	Metal jewellery may be accidentally lost or may cause harm to the patient, e.g. diathermy burns. Facial cosmetics make the patient's colour difficult to assess. Nail varnish makes the use of the pulse oximeter, used to monitor the patient's pulse and oxygen saturation levels, impossible and masks peripheral cyanosis (Vendovato et al. 2004: C).
12 Disposable or cotton underwear could be worn unless the patient is undergoing major urology or gynaecology procedure.	To maintain patient's dignity (NMC 2008: C).
13 Valuables should be placed in the hospital's custody and recorded according to the hospital policy.	To prevent loss of valuables (E).
14 Check whether patient micturated before premedication.	To prevent urinary incontinence when sedated and/or unconscious and possible contamination of sterile area (E).
15 Apply antiembolic stockings correctly.	To reduce the risk of postoperative deep vein thrombosis or pulmonary emboli (NICE 2007: C).
16 Ensure the patient is wearing an identification bracelet with the correct information.	To ensure correct identification and prevent possible patient misidentification (AORN 2000: C).
17 Ensure the patient is wearing an allergy alert band if appropriate.	To reduce allergic reactions to known causative agents and to alert all involved in the care of the patient in the operating theatre (AORN 2004: C).
18 Check when patient last had food or drink and ensure that it was at least 6 hours before planned operation time.	To reduce the risk of regurgitation and inhalation of stomach contents on induction of anaesthesia (Dean & Fawcett 2002: C).
19 Note whether the patient has dental crowns, bridge work or loose teeth.	The anaesthetist needs to be informed to prevent accidental damage. Loose teeth or a dental prosthesis could be inhaled by the patient when an endotracheal tube is inserted.
20 Ensure prosthesis, dentures and contact lenses are removed. Make a note of unremovable prosthesis (e.g. knee replacement) on the preoperative checklist.	To promote patient safety during surgery, e.g. dentures may obstruct airway, contact lenses can cause cornea abrasions.
21 Spectacles may be retained until the patient is in the anaesthetic room. Hearing aids may be retained until the patient has been anaesthetized. (These may be left in position if a local anaesthetic is being used.) Any prosthesis should then be labelled clearly and retained in the recovery room.	To allow the patient to communicate fully, thus reducing anxiety and enabling the patient to understand any procedures carried out (P).
22 Complete the preoperative checklist by asking the patient and checking records and notes before giving any premedication.	Questioning premedicated patients is not a reliable source of checking information as the patient may be drowsy and/or disorientated (AORN 2000: C).

23 Give the premedication, if prescribed, in accordance with the anaesthetist's instructions.	Different drugs may be prescribed to complement the anaesthetic to be given, e.g. Temazepam to reduce patient anxiety by inducing sleep and relaxation (C).
24 Advise the patient to remain in bed once the premedication has been given and to use the nurse call systems if assistance is needed.	To reduce the risk of accidental patient injury as the premedication may make the patient drowsy and disorientated (E).
25 Ensure the patient is supported fully on the canvas, especially the head, when transferred from the ward bed to the trolley.	To reduce the risk of injury to the neck, etc. during transfer from the ward to the operating theatre (AORN 2001: C).
26 Ensure that all relevant information, e.g. X-rays, notes, blood results, accompany the patient to the operating theatre.	To prevent delays which can increase the patient's anxiety and to ensure that the anaesthetist and surgeon have all the information they require for the safe treatment of the patient (C).
27 The patient should be accompanied to the theatre by a ward nurse who remains present until the patient has been checked by the anaesthetic assistant/nurse and/or anaesthetized.	To reduce patient anxiety and ensuring a safe environment during induction (C).
28 The ward nurse should give a full handover to the anaesthetic nurse or operating department practitioner on arrival in the anaesthetic room, using patient records and the preoperative checklist.	To ensure the patient has the correct operation. To ensure continuity of care and to maintain the safety of the patient by exchanging all relevant information (AORN 2000: C).

613

Intraoperative care

Definition

Intraoperative care is the physical and psychological care given to the patient in the anaesthetic room and theatre until transfer to the recovery room.

Objectives

- To ensure that the patient understands what is happening at all times in order to minimize anxiety.
- To ensure that the patient has the correct surgery for which the consent form was signed.
- To ensure patient safety at all times and minimize postoperative complications by:

  (a) Giving the required care for the unconscious patient.
  (b) Ensuring injury is not sustained from hazards associated with the use of swabs, needles, instruments, diathermy and power tools.
  (c) Minimizing postoperative problems associated with patient positioning, such as nerve or tissue damage.
  (d) Maintaining asepsis during surgical procedures to reduce the risk of postoperative wound infection in accordance with hospital policies on infection control.

Reference material

Diathermy

Diathermy is used routinely during operations to control haemorrhage by cauterizing blood vessels or cutting body tissues. Diathermy is potentially hazardous to the patient if used incorrectly. It is important that all theatre nurses know how to test and use all diathermy equipment in their department to prevent patient injury (Aigner et al. 1997; Wicker 2000; Molyneux 2001).

The main risk when using diathermy is of thermoelectrical burns. The most common cause is incorrect application of the patient plate or a break in the connecting lead (Vendovato et al. 2004) or if the patient is in contact with metal. The machine will automatically switch off if the neutral electrodes become loose from the patient or will alarm, but if the patient is in contact with metal this is a little harder to identify. To prevent these injuries only equipment fitted with adaptive neutral electrodes should be used.

Other causes of burns include skin preparation solutions or other liquids pooling around the plate site (Fong et al. 2000). With alcohol-based skin preparations especially, the skin should be allowed to dry before diathermy is used, as the alcohol can ignite (Fong et al. 2000). If the patient's position is changed during the operation the patient plate should be rechecked to ensure that it is still in contact and that the connecting clamp or lead is not causing pressure in the new position.

Use of diathermy and the plate position should be noted on the nursing care plan, and the patient's skin condition (plate site, pressure areas, and other areas where exposure to metal could have occurred) should be checked before the patient is transferred to the recovery unit.

The use of electrosurgical diathermy unit during surgical procedures results in a smoke by-product from the coagulation or cutting of tissue. This smoke plume can be harmful to the perioperative personnel because it can contain (Allen 2004):

- Toxic gases and vapors such as benzene, hydrogen cyanide and formaldehyde.
- Bioaerosols.
- Dead and live cellular material, including blood fragments.
- Viruses.

To reduce the risk for staff and patients, an efficient filtered evacuation system should be used, such as a smoke evacuation machine; piped hospital suction must not be used (Scott *et al.* 2004).

Patient positioning

The position of the patient on the operating table must be such as to facilitate access to the operation site(s) by the surgeon, and the patient's airway for the anaesthetist. It will also be dependent upon the type of surgery being performed, position of monitoring equipment and intravenous devices in situ. It should not compromise the patient's circulation, respiratory system or nerves. Preoperative assessment will identify patients with particular needs such as weight, nutritional state, age, skin condition and pre-existing disease which may necessitate extra precautions during positioning. Pre-existing conditions such as backache or sciatica can be exacerbated, particularly if the patient is in the lithotomy position as the sciatic nerve can be compressed against the poles (AORN 2001). Most postoperative palsies are due to improper positioning of the patient on the operating table (Ulrich *et al.* 1997). Consideration by and the co-operation of all theatre personnel can help prevent many of the postoperative complications related to intraoperative positioning and remains a team responsibility (McEwen 1996; AORN 2001).

All movements of the limbs of the unconscious patient should take into account the anatomy and natural planes of movement of that limb to avoid stretching and pressure on the related nerve planes (AORN 2001). Hyperabduction of the arm when placed on a board, for example, could stretch the brachial plexus, causing some postoperative loss of sensation and reduced movement of the forearm, wrist

and fingers. The ulnar and radial nerves may be affected by direct pressure as a result of insufficient padding on arm supports.

Compartment syndrome is a life-threatening complication of the Lloyd Davies position and occurs when perfusion falls below tissue pressure in a closed anatomical space or compartment such as hand, forearm, buttocks, legs, upper arms and feet. It develops through a combination of prolonged ischaemia and reperfusion of muscle within a tight osseofascial compartment (Turnbull *et al.* 2002). Untreated it can lead to necrosis, functional impairment, possible renal failure and death (Callum & Bradbury 2000; Paula 2002).

If patients are placed in Lloyd Davies position and Trendelenburg tilt for longer than 4 hours, the legs should be removed from the support every 2 hours, or as close to 2 hours as possible, for a short period of time to prevent reperfusion injury (Raza *et al.* 2004).

The use of compression stockings and intermittent compression devices in the Lloyd Davies position need to be reviewed as this may contribute to compartment syndrome (Turnbull & Mills 2001). There is insufficient evidence to suggest use of one device over another will reduce the risk of compartment syndrome, nor is there enough evidence to recommend use of both devices at the same time because this will place pressure on the calf in the Lloyd Davies position. The use of devices will depend very much on the surgeon and anaesthetist and the patient's comorbidity.

All equipment that may be needed to support the patient during surgery, e.g. the table, arm supports, Lloyd Davies poles, lithotomy poles and securing straps, should be checked to ensure that they are in working order, clean and free from sharp edges. Metal parts that may come into contact with the patient should be covered as there is an increased risk of burns if diathermy is used (Vendovato *et al.* 2004). Pressure-relieving devices should be placed at the patient's elbows and heels, and pillows positioned between the legs if the patient is lying in a lateral position. Special consideration should also be given to vulnerable points or areas such as heels, elbows, ears, the head, back and sacrum where pressure-relieving devices, such as gel pads, should be used (AORN 2001).

When a patient is transferred between the trolley or bed and operating table, adequate personnel should be present to ensure patient and staff safety (AORN 2001). It is recommended that an approved rolling or sliding device is used to transfer patients from the trolley to operating table, in compliance with legislation on manual handling. Safe manual handling and the safety of the patient depend on the participation of the correct number of staff in the specified handling manoeuvre. There should be a minimum of four staff: one at either end of the patient to support the head and the feet and one on either side.

Additional staff may be required if weight of the patient is over 90 kilos.

Control of infection and asepsis in operating theatres

The term asepsis means the absence of any infectious agents. The aseptic technique is the foundation on which contemporary surgery is built (Gruendemann & Meeker 1983). The aim of operating theatres is to provide an area free from infectious agents. Large quantities of bacteria are present in the nose, mouth, on the skin, hair and on the attire of personnel; therefore, people entering the operating theatres wear clean scrub suits and lint-free surgical hats to eliminate the possibility of these bacteria, hair or dandruff being shed into the environment (Tammelin *et al.* 2000). Sterile gowns and gloves are worn to prevent cross-infection. Well-fitting shoes with impervious soles should be worn and regularly cleaned to remove splashes of blood and body fluids (Woodhead *et al.* 2002). Face masks are worn to prevent droplets falling from the mouth into the operating field. The extent to which face masks are capable of preventing droplet spread is disputed (Lipp & Edwards 2002). It is, however, accepted that masks offer protection to the wearer from blood splashes and for safety reasons should be worn by the scrub team.

Presurgical hand washing is essential to the maintenance of asepsis in the operating theatre. New research has recommended a 1-minute hand wash with a non-antiseptic soap followed by hand rubbing with liquid aqueous alcoholic solution, prior to each surgeon's first procedure of the day. Before subsequent procedures the process should be repeated. This has been shown to be as effective as traditional hand scrubbing with antiseptic soap in preventing surgical site infections (Parienti *et al.* 2002). However, the traditional 3-minute first scrub of the day is recommended for all intermediate, major and complex cases.

Surgical gloves have a dual role, acting as a barrier for personal protection from the patient's blood and other exudate and preventing the bacterial transfer from the surgeon's hand to the operating site. It has been suggested that double gloving significantly reduces the number of perforations to the innermost glove in high-risk surgical patients, thus reducing infection rates during surgical procedures (Tanner & Parkinson 2002).

Universal precautions should be taken in theatres to minimize the risk of infection from blood and body fluids. These include the wearing of gloves, masks, barrier gowns and aprons. Protective eyewear or face shields should be worn during procedures likely to cause splashes or droplets of blood or generate bone chips (Tokars *et al.* 1995). Instruments must be handled carefully, and needle holders and forceps used to manipulate sutures to minimize the risk of needlestick or sharps injury.

The female patients of menstruating age also need to be made aware of the dangers of using tampons which can cause infection leading to toxic shock syndrome. At the time of admission it is important to ask the patients if they are menstruating and to highlight the dangers of using tampons during surgery. If these are left in situ for longer than 6 hours infection may develop (see www.tamponalert.org.uk/akta/tss, leaflet 2000 pdf, accessed 26/3/07).

Laparoscopic surgery

Laparoscopy has evolved from a diagnostic modality into a widespread surgical technique. Advantages for the patient include: a shorter stay in hospital, reduced postoperative pain and a shorter recovery period. However, this technique is not without its complications (O'Malley & Cunningham 2001). Laparoscopic surgery is now common in operating departments, and it is important that potential complications are identified and steps taken to minimize risk to the patient, both during surgery and in the recovery period. Patients should be prepared psychologically and physically for an open procedure, which may be undertaken under certain circumstances. Instruments and supplies for an open procedure must be readily available in the operating theatre.

Laparoscopy involves insufflation of the abdomen with carbon dioxide (CO_2). Prolonged insufflation can cause hypothermia since although the gas temperature in the hose equals room temperature, the temperature in the abdomen can decrease to $27.7°C$ due to high gas flow and the large amounts of gas used (Jacobs *et al.* 2000). Sharma *et al.* (1997) refer to the increased risk of hypercarbia and surgical emphysema during insufflation with CO_2. Careful monitoring and recording of the patient's vital signs, including oxygen saturation and expiratory gas levels, are therefore essential during laparoscopy.

Haemorrhage can occur during the procedure and may be difficult to detect because surgeons have a limited view of the area being operated upon. Electrosurgical injuries to organs may occur as a result of capacitive coupling (Wu *et al.* 2000) (capacitive coupling is the transfer of electrical currents from the active electrode through coupling of stray currents into other conductive surgical equipment). Theatre staff must be aware of potential complications and ensure that equipment is used safely and according to the manufacturer's instructions.

The equipment used for laparoscopic surgery is very specialized and can be daunting for theatre staff. AORN recommends that all equipment is regularly and competently maintained and a maintenance record kept in a log (AORN 2000; Wicker & O'Neill 2006). Policies and procedures should be developed for the checking procedure, and all staff thoroughly instructed in the operation of laparoscopic equipment.

615

Procedure guidelines   Intraoperative care

Procedure

Action

Rationale

In the anaesthetic room

1 Ensure all the equipment to be used is checked and in working order before the operating list commences, including suction, the anaesthetic machine, medical gases, monitoring equipment, diathermy and operating table.

To ensure all necessary equipment is present and to prevent accidental injury due to faulty equipment (C).

2 Greet the patient by name. Confirm with the ward nurse that it is the correct patient for the scheduled operation.

To reduce patient anxiety (P).

3 Identify the patient by checking the identification band (name and patient number) against the patient's notes and the operating list.

To safeguard against patient misidentification. Questioning the premedicated patient can be unreliable (AORN 2000: C).

4 Check and confirm the correct completion of the preoperative checklist.

To ensure that all of the listed measures have been completed and that any additional information has been recorded (E).

5 Check that the results of the investigative procedures, e.g. blood results, X-rays, etc., are included with the patient's notes.

To ensure that all of the required results are available for the theatre team's use (E).

6 Maintain a calm, quiet environment and explain all the procedures to the patient including the monitoring of blood pressure, pulse and oxygen saturation.

To reduce anxiety and enhance the smooth induction of anaesthesia (C).

7 When the patient is anaesthetized ensure that the eyes are closed and secured with hypoallergenic tape.

To prevent corneal damage due to eyes drying out or accidental abrasion.

In the operating room

8 Prior to transferring the patient from the trolley to the operating table check with the anaesthetist that the patient's airway is protected, patent and safe.

To prevent complications with breathing (E).

9 Ensure that there are adequate staff to transfer the patient onto the operating table. Ensure the brakes on the trolley and operating table have been applied. Ensure the patient's head and limbs are supported when transferring to the operating table.

To prevent patient injury during the transfer between trolley and operating table (AORN 2001: C).

10 When transferring the patient ensure all limbs are supported and secure on the table. Ensure adequate padding and cushioning of bony prominences. The patient's position will be dictated by the nature of the surgery but must take into account the requirements of the anaesthetist and the physical needs of the patient.

If the patient is unconscious and unable to maintain a safe environment, support is necessary to prevent injury. Nerve damage due to compression or stretching must be prevented.
The patient is especially at risk from damage due to pressure and stretching, so measures to maintain the skin's integrity are vital (AORN 2001: C).

11 Ensure the patient is covered by the gown or blanket. These items should only be removed immediately before surgery.	To maintain the patient's dignity. To help prevent a reduction in body temperature or accidental hypothermia (E).
12 Use a warm air mattress on the operating table. Ensure all fluids used are warmed if possible.	To help maintain the patient's body temperature and prevent postoperative complications due to hypothermia (E).
13 Ensure diathermy patient plate is attached securely in accordance with the manufacturer's instructions and hospital policy.	To ensure that no injury is sustained from the use of diathermy during surgery (Molyneux 2001: C).
14 Follow hospital policy for the checking of swabs, needles and instruments.	To ensure that swabs, needles and instruments are accounted for at the end of the operation (C).
15 Follow hospital policy for the disposal of sharps and clinical waste.	To reduce the risk of injury to the patient and staff (Pratt *et al.* 2007: C).

In the recovery room

16 The scrub nurse accompanies the patient with the anaesthetist to the recovery area. A handover is given that includes:	To ensure continuity and effective communication of care for the patient. To ensure that the recovery nurse has all the information required to assess the patient's recovery needs (C).
(a) The surgical procedure performed.	The actual procedure performed may be different from the proposed procedure (E).
(b) Information including allergies or pre-existing medical conditions, e.g. diabetes mellitus.	To highlight specific potential postoperative complications to be assessed and monitored (E).
(c) The patient's cardiovascular state and pattern of anaesthesia used.	To maintain the patient's immediate postoperative safety with cardiovascular system and airway (E).
(d) The presence, position and nature of any drains, infusions or intravenous or arterial devices.	To ensure care and management of these drains is continued and the positioning of the patient is assessed to prevent any occlusion of drains or infusions (F).
(e) Information about any anxieties of the patient expressed before surgery, such as a fear of not waking after anaesthesia or fear about coping with pain.	To ensure appropriate action can be taken as the patient regains consciousness and to enable an assessment of the efficacy of nursing interventions used (E).
(f) Specific instructions from the anaesthetist for postoperative care.	To facilitate effective communication of the patient's care and treatment (C).
(g) All information is to be recorded in the perioperative nursing care plan.	

Postanaesthetic recovery

Definition

Postanaesthetic recovery involves the short-term critical care required by patients during their immediate postoperative period within the recovery room, until they are stable, conscious, orientated and safe to transfer back to the ward environment.

Indication

All patients having undergone surgery and anaesthesia but not those who are transferred directly to the Critical Care Unit.

Reference material

The postanaesthetic recovery room is an area within the operating department specifically designed, equipped and staffed for the support, monitoring and assessment of patients through the reversing stages of anaesthesia.

The recovery period is potentially hazardous. Therefore, when the patient arrives in the postanaesthetic recovery room, individual nursing care is required until patients are able to maintain their own airway (AAGBI 2002). While the majority of patients can be expected to achieve uneventful recovery, 24% of all patients have complications (Hines *et al.* 1992). Although nausea and vomiting are high on the list of complications (Jolley 2001), the most notable are respiratory and circulatory complications. Obstruction of the upper airway is the most common respiratory complication in the immediate postoperative period (Dhara 2006). Close observation and appropriate action can prevent the sequence of respiratory obstruction resulting in hypoxia leading to cardiac arrest (Peskett 1999).

Layout of equipment

The need for speed, efficiency and economy of movement is essential when time becomes a critical factor in the ultimate safety of the patient in the recovery room. Thus, the basic equipment for monitoring airway maintenance, pulse oxymetry and non-invasive blood pressure monitoring and piped gases and suction must be available at the patient's head in each recovery bay. Equipment should be compatible between operating theatre and recovery room. This must be arranged for ease of access and always be clean and in full working order. Further support equipment, such as nerve stimulator, should be available centrally, whenever possible being stored on trolleys for ease of transportation (AAGBI 2002).

Assessment for discharge

The length of patient's stay in the recovery room is dependent on the patient's cardiovascular and respiratory condition and the rate at which that patient recovers physically and emotionally from the anaesthetic. A prior knowledge of the patient's cardiovascular and respiratory parameters as well as past medical history obtained through preoperative contact is of great value when assessing their return to normal state. It also has the advantage of helping the patient to orientate to time and place, as familiarity generates a degree of security and confidence. The patients must meet the following criteria before they can be discharged from recovery room to the ward:

- The patient is fully conscious, able to maintain own airway, exhibits protective airway reflexes and is orientated.
- Respiratory function and good oxygenation is being maintained.
- The cardiovascular system is stable with no unexplained cardiac irregularity. The specific values of pulse and blood pressure are within normal preoperative limits on consecutive observation.
- There is no persistent or excessive bleeding from wound or drainage sites.

- Patients with urinary catheters have passed adequate amounts of urine (more than 0.5 ml/kg/hour) (Eltringham et al. 1989).
- Pain and emesis should be controlled and suitable analgesia and antiemetic regimes should be prescribed by the anaesthetist (AAGBI 2002).
- Body temperature is at least 36°C (Kean 2000).

Discharge from the recovery room is the responsibilty of the anaesthetist but the recovery staff are responsible for keeping the anaesthetist informed about any changes in the patient's condition that may arise during the recovery phase. This could be cardiovascular, respiratory or the level of consciousness. The recovery staff use the discharge criteria (Figure 30.1) as an assessment tool to determine whether the patient has achieved optimum recovery to enable them to return back to the ward safely. However, if there any changes in the patient's condition this needs to be discussed with the anaesthetist who should come and assess the patient before their return to the ward.

Local and regional anaesthesia

Patients having surgical procedures performed under local or spinal anaesthesia, whether intra- or extra- (epi) dural, will require a period of postoperative observation, although the priorities of their care will be geared towards different considerations, such as hypotension, headaches and dizziness (AAGBI 2002).

Summary

Postanaesthetic care can best be described and understood as a series of many nursing procedures performed in sequence and simultaneously on patients who are in an artificially induced and traumatized condition. These patients will display varying degrees of responsiveness and physical and emotional states. It is important to establish a rapport with each individual to gain the patient's confidence and co-operation and to aid assessment. It is also necessary to understand that when emerging from the final stage of anaesthesia, some patients can behave in an emotional and disinhibited fashion, at variance with their normal behaviour (Eckenhoff et al. 1961). These displays are always transient and fortunately patients seldom have any recollection of them. Most patients will have an uneventful recovery following surgery. However, recovery can be adversely affected by the extent and length of both surgery and anaesthesia.

		Yes	No
Respiratory Function			
1.	Is the patient able to maintain their airway without assistance?		
2.	Does the patient have a regular respiratory pattern and show no signs of cyanosis?		
3.	Is the patient's respiratory rate > 10 and < 24 breaths per minute?		
4.	Are oxygen saturation readings > 95% or the same as the patient's pre-operative oxygen saturation readings on air / prescribed oxygen?		
Cardiovascular Function			
5.	Is the patient's pulse and blood pressure within pre-operative range? If not – is the anaesthetist satisfied with the patient's observations?		
6.	Is the patient's temperature between 36°C and 37.5°C?		
7.	Are drains(s) and wound(s) free from excessive bleeding i.e. < 50 ml blood / hour in drain or wound dressing requiring reinforcement/pressure?		
8.	Are the drain(s) unclamped and vacuumed if appropriate? *State if not applicable*		
9.	Is the patient free from neurovascular compromise? For example: check limb/flap observations, i.e. colour, warmth, blanching, sensation and movement, which are performed following limb reconstructive surgery. *State if not applicable*		
Level of Consciousness			
10.	Is the patient conscious, orientated, able to lift head off pillow, can cough and take deep breath? (*Patient must have a minimum score of 8 on the SALIM score on discharge*) *If patient is confused – was the patient confused pre-operatively?*		
Fluid Administration & Management			
11.	Is the patient's fluid balance satisfactory? For example: no signs of fluid overload – breathlessness, tachycardia, generalized oedema or dehydration – dry skin, poor urine output, bradycardia (refer to fluid balance chart if appropriate).		
12.	Are the infusion sites satisfactory, i.e. patent and secured?		
13.	Are all infusions and infusion administration sets appropriately labelled, e.g. Patient Controlled Analgesia, Epidural, Blood, Platelets, Insulin etc. and three-way taps removed?		
14.	If catheterized, is the patient passing acceptable volumes of urine, i.e. 1–1.5 ml/kilogram/hour?		
Nausea & Vomiting			
15.	Has the patient stated their nausea or vomiting is controlled (**see nausea & vomiting score**)? If not, state actions taken.		
16.	Is the nasogastric tube correctly positioned, secured, patent and the drainage satisfactory, i.e. < 100 ml immediate post operation? *State if not applicable*		
Pain			
17.	Has the patient stated their pain is controlled? (**Is the pain score < 5 on movement, whilst coughing or taking a deep breath?**)		
18.	If nerve block or epidural analgesia – is the height of the nerve/epidural block recorded and the rate of the epidural analgesia recorded? *State if not applicable & delete as appropriate*		
Follow up care			
19.	Are IV fluids, analgesia and anti-emetics prescribed for the next 24 hours if appropriate?		
20.	Are the surgeon's post-operative written instructions clear and available?		
21.	**Has the anaesthetist agreed the patient is fit for discharge from recovery?** *NB If patient has had an adverse event or been in recovery > 2 hrs has the anaesthetist reviewed their condition?*		
FOR INFORMATION ONLY			
22.	Has the patient passed urine post-operatively? *State if not applicable*		
23.	Is the patient's property accompanying them back to the ward area? *State if not applicable*		

	Signature	Full Name (PRINT)	Date	Time
Recovery Room Nurse / Operating Department Practitioner (ODP)				
Ward/Unit Nurse				

Time of Patient's Discharge from Recovery: ....(24 hr clock)

Figure 30.1   Recovery discharge criteria. Used with permission from The Royal Marsden NHS Foundation Trust (2007).

619

Procedure guidelines   Postanaesthetic recovery

Equipment in the recovery room

1 Theatre trolley bed, which must incorporate the following features:
   (a) Oxygen supply.
   (b) Trendelenburg tilt mechanism.
   (c) Adjustable cot sides.
   (d) Adjustable back rest.
   (e) Brakes.
   (f) Radio translucency.

2 Basic equipment required for each patient:
   (a) Oxygen supply, preferably wall-mounted with tubing, face masks (with both fixed and variable settings), a T-piece system and full range of oropharyngeal and nasopharyngeal airways.
   (b) Suction: regulatable with tubing, and a range of nozzles and catheters.
   Note: spare oxygen cylinders with flowmeters and an electrically powered portable suction machine should always be available in case of pipeline failure.
   (c) Sphygmomanometer and stethoscope. Automatic blood pressure recorders are a valuable means of saving time and of minimizing disturbance to patients, especially those in pain or disorientated, and leaving the nurse's hands free to attend to other needs. However, such equipment can be non-functioning in certain cases, e.g. shivering or profoundly bradycardic patients, and is subject to electrical and mechanical failure. Therefore, manual equipment must always be available.
   (d) Pulse oximeter, whenever possible.
   (e) Miscellaneous items: receivers, tissues, disposable gloves, sharps container and waste receptacle.

3 Essential equipment centrally available for respiratory and cardiovascular support:
   (a) Self-inflating resuscitator bag, e.g. Ambu bag and/or Mapleson C circuit with face mask.
   (b) Full intubation equipment: laryngoscopes with spare bulbs and batteries, range of endotracheal tubes, bougies and Magill's forceps, syringe and catheter mount.
   (c) Anaesthetic machine and ventilator.
   (d) Wright respirometer.
   (e) Cricothyroid puncture set.
   (f) Range of tracheostomy tubes and tracheal dilator.
   (g) Intravenous infusion sets and cannulae, range of intravenous fluids.
   (h) Central venous cannulae and manometer.
   (i) Emergency drug box/trolley: contents in accordance with current hospital policy.
   (j) Defibrillator.

4 Standard equipment for routine nursing procedures such as dressing trolley.

Procedure

The following recommended actions are not necessarily listed in order of priority. Many will be carried out simultaneously and much will depend on the patient's condition, surgery and level of consciousness. All actions must be accompanied by commentary and explanation regardless of the apparent responsiveness, as the sense of hearing returns before the patient's ability to respond (Levinson 1965).

Action	Rationale
1 Assess the patency of the airway by feeling for movement of expired air.	To determine the presence of any respiratory depression or neuromuscular blockade. Observe chest and abdominal movement, respiratory rate, depth and pattern (Drummond 1991: C).

(a) Listen for inspiration and expiration. Apply suction if indicated. Observe any use of accessory muscles of respiration and check for tracheal tug.

To ensure airway is clear and laryngeal spasm is not present.

(b) If indicated, support the chin with the neck extended.

In the unconscious patient the tongue is liable to fall back and obstruct the airway, and protective reflexes are absent (E).
Foreign matter can obstruct the airway or cause laryngeal spasm in light planes of anaesthesia. It can also be inhaled when protective laryngeal reflexes are absent (Dhara 2006: C).

(c) Suction of the upper airway is indicated if gurgling sounds are present on respiration and if blood secretions or vomitus are evident or suspected, and the patient is unable to swallow or cough either at all or adequately. Suction must be applied with care to avoid damage to mucosal surfaces and further irritation or initiation of a gag reflex or laryngeal spasm.

(d) Endotracheal suction is performed following the same procedure as that for suction of tracheostomy tubes. (For further information see the procedure section in Chapter 42.)

To maintain the patency of the tube and remove secretions (Dhara 2006: C).

(e) Apply a face mask and administer oxygen at the rate prescribed by the anaesthetist. If an endotracheal tube or laryngeal mask is in position, check whether the cuff or mask is inflated and administer oxygen by means of a T-piece system.

To maintain adequate oxygenation. Oxygen should be administered to all patients in the recovery room (Nimmo et al. 1994: C).

(f) Observe skin colour and temperature. Check the colour of lips and conjunctiva, then peripheral colour and perfusion.

Central cyanosis indicates impaired gaseous exchange between the alveoli and pulmonary capillaries. Peripheral cyanosis indicates low cardiac output (Nimmo et al. 1994: C).

2 Feel and assess the pulse. The patient's position will probably mean that the head, carotid, facial or temporal arteries will offer the easiest access. Note the rate, rhythm and volume, and record.

To assess cardiovascular function and establish a postoperative baseline for future comparisons (Peskett 1999: C).

3 Obtain full information about:
- Anaesthetic technique, potential problems and the patient's general medical condition.
- Surgical procedure performed.
- The presence of drains and packs.
- Amount of blood loss.
- Specific postoperative instructions.

To ensure effective communication of the patient's care and treatment and to aid the planning of subsequent care.

Note: the information gained from point 3 will be recorded within the patient's records, but an initial verbal handover will ensure that there is no delay in providing immediate care.

4 Perform and record blood pressure, pulse and respiratory rate measurements on reception and at a minimum of 5-minute intervals unless the patient's condition dictates otherwise.

To enable any fluctuations or gross abnormalities in cardiovascular and respiratory functions to be detected immediately (Peskett 1999: C).

Procedure guidelines *(cont.)*

5 Check the temperature of the patient, especially those who are at high risk of hypothermia, e.g. the elderly, children, those who have undergone long surgery or where large amounts of blood or fluid replacement therapy have been used. Temperature must be measured hourly or half hourly if hypothermic. Use Bairhugger blankets and extra blankets to warm the patient.

More than 70% of patients undergoing surgery experience some degree of postoperative hypothermia (Wagner 2003: C). The symptoms of hypothermia can mimic those of other postoperative complications, which may result in inappropriate treatment. Hypothermia interferes with the effective reversal of muscle relaxants, so monitor patients who are shivering, restless, confused or with respiratory depression (Bowers Feldman 1988: C). Shivering puts an increased demand on cardiopulmonary systems as oxygen consumption is increased (Bowers Feldman 1988: C; Frank *et al.* 1993: C). Other complications such as arrhythmias or myocardial infarct can result and the longer the duration of the postoperative hypothermia, the greater the patient mortality (Crayne *et al.* 1988: C; Frank *et al.* 1993: C).

6 Check and observe wound site(s),dressings and drains. Note and record leakage/drainage on the postoperative chart and also on the drain bottle/bag.

To assess and monitor for signs of haemorrhage (Eltringham *et al.* 1989: C).

7 Check intravenous infusions are running at the correct prescribed rate and the site of the venous device is satisfactory.

Care of venous devices/sites prevents complications and ensures fluid replacement and balance is achieved safely (E).

8 Check the prescription chart for medications to be administered during the immediate postoperative period, e.g. analgesia, antiemetic.

To treat symptoms swiftly and appropriately and to monitor their effectiveness (E).

9 Remain with the patient at all times. Assess level of consciousness during reversing stages of anaesthesia, observing for returning reflexes, i.e. swallowing, tear secretion and eyelash and lid reflexes and response to stimuli: both physical (*not* painful) and verbal (do not shout).

To monitor progress from unconscious state to rousable and orientated (AAGBI 2002: C).

10 Orientate the patient to time and place as frequently as is necessary.

To alleviate anxiety, provide reassurance, and gain the patient's confidence and co-operation. Premedication and anaesthesia can induce a degree of amnesia and disorientation (C).

11 Give mouth care. (For further information, see Procedure guidelines, Chapter 32.)

Preoperative fasting, drying gases and manipulation of lips, etc., leave mucosa vulnerable, sore and foul tasting (E).

12 After regional and/or spinal anaesthesia, assess the return of sensation and mobility of limbs. Check that the limbs are anatomically aligned.

To prevent inadvertent injury following sensory loss (AAGBI 2002: C).

Problem solving: Postanaesthetic recovery

Note: any concern/abnormality regarding the patient's condition requires a thorough holistic, individual assessment prior to any interventions. Liaise with appropriate medical colleagues accordingly.

Problem	Cause	Suggested action
Airway obstruction.	Tongue occluding the airway.	Support chin forward from the angle of the jaw. If necessary insert a Guedel airway. Use a nasopharyngeal airway if the teeth are clenched or crowned.
	Foreign material, blood, secretions, vomitus.	Apply suction. Always check for the presence of a throat pack.
	Laryngeal spasm.	Increase the rate of oxygen. Assist ventilation with an Ambu bag and face mask. If there is no improvement, inform anaesthetist and have intubation equipment ready. Offer the patient reassurance by talking to them and telling them what you are doing.
Hypoventilation.	Respiratory depression from medications, e.g. opiates, inhalations, barbiturates.	Inform the anaesthetist, keeping oxygen on and administer antagonist on instruction, e.g. naloxone (opiate antagonist), doxapram (respiratory stimulant). *Note*: if naloxone is given it can reverse the analgesic effects of opiates and has a duration of action of only 20–30 minutes. The patient must be observed for signs of returning hyperventilation (Nimmo *et al.* 1994).
	Decreased respiratory drive from a low partial pressure of carbon dioxide ($PaCO_2$), loss of hypoxic drive in patients with chronic pulmonary disease.	Administer oxygen using a Venturi mask with graded low concentrations (Atkinson *et al.* 1982).
	Neuromuscular blockade from continued action of non-depolarizing muscle relaxants, potentiation of relaxants caused by electrolyte imbalance, impaired excretion with renal or liver disease.	Inform the anaesthetist, have available neostigmine and glycopyrolate, or atropine potassium chloride and 10% calcium chloride. Often the degree of blockade is mild and will wear off in minutes without treatment, but it is extremely frightening and patients will need continuous reassurance that their condition is not unnoticed and is resolving and that they will not be left alone.
Hypotension.	Hypovolaemia.	Take manual reading of the blood pressure. Take central venous pressure (CVP) readings if catheter is in place. Give oxygen. Lower the head of the trolley unless contraindicated, e.g. hiatus hernia, gross obesity. Check the record of anaesthetic agents used which might cause hypotension, e.g. enflurane, beta-blockers, nitroprusside, opiates, droperidol, sympathetic blockade following spinal anaesthesia. Check the peripheral perfusion. If the CVP is low, increase intravenous infusion unless contraindicated, e.g. congestive cardiac failure. Check drains and dressings for visible bleeding and haematoma. Inform the anaesthetist or surgeon.
Hypertension.	Pain, carbon dioxide retention. This may be due to retention during laparoscopic procedures.	Treat pain with prescribed analgesia and provide a quiet environment to enable them to rest/sleep. Pain from certain operation sites can also be alleviated by changing the patient's position.
	Fluid overload.	Check fluid balance sheet and the rate of intravenous infusion.

623

Problem solving *(cont.)*

Problem	Cause	Suggested action
	Distended bladder.	Offer a bedpan or urinal and if necessary catheterize the patient.
	Some anaesthetic drugs given during reversal of anaesthetic.	Check the prescription chart for those patients on regular antihypertensive therapy. If the situation is not resolved inform the anaesthetist. Also check patient's past medical history.
Bradycardia.	Very fit patient, opiates, reversal agents, beta-blockers, pain, vagal stimulation, hypoxaemia from respiratory depression.	Connect the patient to the ECG monitor to exclude heart block and monitor cardiac activity. Ascertain pre-operative cardiac function. Check the prescription chart and anaesthetic sheet for medication administered that may cause bradycardia. Inform and liaise with the anaesthetist.
Tachycardia.	Pain, hypovolaemia, some anaesthetic drugs, e.g. ephedrine, septicaemia, fear, fluid overload.	Assess patient's pain and provide analgesia. Check the anaesthetic chart to ascertain which anaesthetic drugs were used. Connect the patient to the ECG monitor to exclude ventricular tachycardia. Provide reassurance for the patient. Assess fluid balance.
Pain.	Surgical trauma, worsened by fear, anxiety and restlessness.	Provide prescribed analgesia and assess its efficacy. Reassure and orientate the patients, who can be unaware that surgery has been performed, in which case their pain is more frightening. Try positional changes where feasible, e.g. experience has shown that after breast surgery some relief can be obtained from raising the back support by 20–40°; patients with abdominal or gynaecological surgery can be more comfortable lying on their side; elevate limbs to reduce swelling where appropriate. Unless significant relief is obtained, inform the anaesthetist and the pain control specialist nurse.
Nausea and vomiting.	Anaesthetic agents, opiates, hypotension, abdominal surgery, pain; high-risk patients who have a history of postoperative nausea and vomiting.	Administer intravenous antiemetics and monitor effectiveness. Encourage slow, regular breathing. If the patient is unconscious, turn onto the side, tip the head down and suck out pharynx, give oxygen. *Note*: have wire-cutters available if the jaws are wired.
Hypothermia.	Depression of the heat-regulating centre, vasodilatation, following abdominal surgery, large infusions of unwarmed blood and fluids.	Use extra blankets or a Bairhugger (Kumar *et al.* 2005). Monitor the patient's temperature. Administer warm intravenous fluids. In the event of bladder irrigation this should also be warmed but care has to be taken that the temperature of the warming cabinet is not too hot as this could burn the patient. The temperature should be the same as normal body temperature.
Shivering.	Some inhalational anaesthetics, hypothermia.	Give oxygen, reassure the patient and take patient's temperature. Provide a Bairhugger and warm blankets.
Hyperthermia.	Infection, blood transfusion reaction.	Give oxygen, use a fan or tepid sponging if this is warranted. Medical assessment of antibiotic therapy and obtaining blood cultures. Administer intravenous paracetamol if prescribed.

624

Problem	Cause	Suggested action
	Malignant hyperpyrexia (above 40°).	Malignant hyperpyrexia is a medical emergency and a malignant hyperpyrexia pack with the necessary drugs should be readily available at a central point in theatre. All personnel must know its location.
Oliguria.	Mechanical obstruction of catheter, e.g. clots, kinking.	Check the patency of the catheter. Consider bladder irrigation. If clots present, inform surgeon.
	Inadequate renal perfusion, e.g. hypotension, systolic pressures under 60 mmHg, hypovolaemia, dehydration.	Take blood pressure and CVP if available. Increase intravenous fluids. Inform the anaesthetist.
	Renal damage, e.g. from blood transfusion, infection, drugs, surgical damage to the ureters.	Refer to the anaesthetist or surgeon.

Procedure guidelines   Postoperative recovery

Equipment

After discharge from the recovery room to the ward, the nursing care given during the postoperative period is directed towards the prevention of those potential complications resulting from surgery and anaesthesia which might be anticipated to develop over a longer period of time.

Consideration of the psychological and emotional aspects of recovery will of necessity be altered by the changed state of consciousness, awareness and knowledge of patients and their differing responses to surgery, diagnosis and treatment.

Potential respiratory complications

Action	Rationale
1 Observe respirations, noting rate and depth and any presence of dyspnoea or orthopnoea: (a) Observe chest movement for equal, bilateral expansion. (b) Observe colour and perfusion. (c) Position the patient to facilitate optimum lung expansion and reinforce preoperative teaching of deep breathing exercises and coughing.	Respiratory function postoperatively can be influenced by a number of factors: increased bronchial secretions from inhalation anaesthesia; decreased respiratory effort from opiate medication; pain or anticipation of pain from surgical wounds; surgical trauma to the phrenic nerve; pneumothorax as a result of surgical or anaesthetic procedures. All factors limiting the adequate expansion of the lung and the ejection of bronchial secretions will encourage the development of atelectasis and consolidation of the affected lung tissue (AAGBI 2002: C).
2 Change position of patients on bedrest every 2–3 hours.	To prevent and monitor formation of pressure sores and tissue viability (NICE 2007: R).
3 Provide adequate prescribed analgesia.	Patients in pain are more likely to be disorientated and show signs of high blood pressure and tachycardia (Nimmo et al. 1994: C).
4 Record temperature and pulse. If sputum produced, observe nature and quantity for culture.	If infection follows there may be a rise in temperature, pulse and respiratory rate (C).

Procedure guidelines (cont.)

Potential circulatory complications

Deep venous thrombosis and pulmonary embolus

Action	Rationale
1 Encourage early mobilization where patient's condition allows. For patients on bedrest, encourage deep breathing and exercises of the leg: flexion/extension and rotation of the ankles.	Patients are at increased risk of developing deep venous thrombosis as a result of muscular inactivity, postoperative respiratory and circulatory depression, abdominal and pelvic surgery, prolonged pressure on calves from lithotomy poles, etc., increased production of thromboplastin as a result of surgical trauma, pre-existing coronary artery disease (Rashid *et al.* 2005: C).
2 Where worn, ensure that antiembolic stockings are of the correct size and fit smoothly.	Incorrect sizing causes swelling and bruising to ankles and can constrict blood supply leading to long-term complications (NICE 2007: R).
3 Advise against crossing of legs or ankles.	To prevent constriction of blood supply and swelling.
4 Record temperature.	
5 Report any complaints of calf or thigh pain to medical staff.	To monitor for signs of DVT.
6 Observe for any dyspnoea, chest pain or signs of shock.	To monitor for signs of PE.

Haemorrhage

Action	Rationale
1 Observe dressings, drains and wound sites, and quantity and nature of drainage. Observe pulse, blood pressure, respirations and colour.	Early haemorrhage may occur as the patient's blood pressure rises. Record postoperatively re-establishing blood flow or blood as a result of the slipping of a ligature or the dislodging of a clot (Peskett 1999: C).
2 Observe wound for redness, tenderness and increased temperature.	Secondary haemorrhage may occur after a period of days as a result of infection (E).

Potential fluid and electrolyte imbalance and malnutrition

Action	Rationale
1 Maintain accurate records of intravenous infusions, oral fluids, wound and stoma drainage, nasogastric drainage, vomitus, urine and urological irrigation.	Preoperative fasting and dehydration, increased secretion of antidiuretic hormone, blood loss and paralytic ileus all contribute to potential fluid and electrolyte imbalance. Vomiting and stasis of intestinal fluid may lead to potassium depletion (Jolley 2001: C).
2 Observe nature and quantity of all drainage, aspirate, faeces, etc.	To monitor and replace fluid loss and to detect any abnormality as a result of surgery, e.g. a breakdown in anastomosis (E).
3 Give prescribed antiemetics if nausea or vomiting occur.	To make the patient comfortable (Jolley 2001: C).
4 Observe state of mouth for coating, furring and dryness.	To maintain oral hygiene and to assess for thrush and hydration (Jolley 2001: C).

5 Encourage oral fluids as soon as the patient is able to take them unless the nature of the surgery contraindicates this.	To encourage hydration, and promote diuresis and digestion. Also to maintain oral hygiene (Jolley 2001: C).
6 Encourage early resumption of diet.	Return to an adequate nutritional state is necessary for wound healing (see Chapter 48); it is particularly important that diabetic patients should return to their preoperative insulin/diet regime to avoid increased risk of metabolic disturbance (E).

Potential pain

Action	Rationale
1 Observe the patient, noting physiological signs indicative of pain, e.g. sweating, tachycardia, hypotension, pallor or flushed appearance.	These are the first indications of pain related to intraoperative trauma and postoperative complications (E).
2 Note restlessness, immobility and facial expressions.	Continuous severe pain can cause restlessness, anxiety, insomnia and anorexia, and may thus interfere with recovery by impeding deep breathing, mobilization and nutrition (E).
3 Listen to the patient and ascertain the location and nature of the pain. If necessary, use a pain scale chart (see Chapter 27).	Communication skills are necessary for the effective assessment and alleviation of pain as there may be multiple contributory factors, both physical and emotional in origin (C).
4 Administer prescribed analgesia and observe effect.	To relieve and control pain and if necessary to review pain relief available (E).
5 Try changing position of patient. Give attention, information and reassurance; assist with relaxation exercises.	To promote comfort and reduce anxiety due to pain (E).

References and further reading

AAGBI (2002) *Immediate Postanaesthetic Recovery*. Association of Anaesthetists of Great Britain and Ireland, London.

Aigner, N. *et al.* (1997) Complications in the use of diathermy. *Burns*, **23**, 256–64.

Allen, G. (2004) Smoke plume evacuation. *AORN J*, **79**(4), 866–70.

AORN (2000) Recommended practices for safety through identification of potential hazards in the perioperative environment. *AORN J*, **72**(4), 690–8.

AORN (2001) Recommended practices for positioning the patient in the perioperative practice setting. *AORN J*, **73**(1), 231–8.

AORN (2004) Latex guidelines, *AORN J*, **70**(3), 653–8, 660–4, 666, 668–72.

Atkinson, R.S. *et al.* (1982) *A Synopsis of Anaesthesia*, 9th edn. John Wright, Bristol.

Barker, S.G.E. & Hollingsworth S.J. (2004) Wearing graduated compression stockings: the reality of everyday deep vein thrombosis prophylaxis. *Phlebology*, **19**(1), 52–3.

Beddows, J. (1997) Alleviating pre-operative anxiety in patients: a study. *Nurs Stand*, **11**(37), 35–8.

Bowers Feldman, M.E. (1988) Inadvertent hypothermia, a threat to homeostasis in the postanaesthetic patient. *J Postanaesth Nurs*, **3**(2), 82–7.

Bryne, B. (2002) Deep vein thrombosis prophylaxis: the effectiveness and implications of using below knee or thigh length graduated compression stockings. *J Vasc Nurs*, **20**(2), 53–9.

Callum, K. & Bradbury, A (2000) ABC of arterial and venous disease: acute limb ischaemia. *BMJ*, **320**(7237), 764–7.

Crayne, H.E. *et al.* (1988) Thermoresuscitation for postoperative hypothermia using reflective blankets. *AORN J*, **47**(1), 222–3, 226–7.

Davis, P. & O'Neill, C. (2002) The potential benefits of intermittent pneumatic compression in the prevention of deep venous thrombosis. *J Orthopaed Nurs*, **6**(2), 95–100.

Dean, A. & Fawcett, T. (2002) Nurse's use of evidence in preoperative fasting. *Nurs Stand*, **17**(12), 33–37.

Dhara, S. (2006) Complications in the recovery room. *Singapore Med J*, **38**(5), 190–1.

Drummond, G.B. (1991) Keep a clear airway. *Br J Anaesth*, **66**, 153–66.

Eckenhoff, J.E., Kneale, D.H. & Dripps, R.D. (1961) The incidence and aetiology of postanaesthetic excitement. *Anaesthesiology*, **22**, 667–73.

Eltringham, R. *et al.* (1989) *Post Anaesthetic Recovery. A Practical Approach*, 2nd edn. Springer, Berlin.

Field, L. & Adams, N. (2001) Pain management 2: the use of psychological approaches to pain. *Br J Nurs*, **10**(15), 971–4.

Fong, E.P., Tan, W.T. & Chye, L.T. (2000) Diathermy and alcohol skin preparations – a potential disastrous mix. *Burns*, 26(7), 673–5.

Frank, S.M., Beattie, C. & Christopher, R. (1993) Unintentional hypothermia is associated with postoperative myocardial ischaemia *Anaesthesiology*, 78, 468–76.

Gruendemann, B. & Meeker, H.M. (1983) *Alexander's Care of the Patient in Surgery*, 7th edn. Mosby, St. Louis, MO.

Hayes, C.A., Lehman, J.M. & Castonguay, P. (2002) Graduated compression stocking: updating practice, improving compliance. *Med Surg Nurs*, 11(4), 163–7.

Hines, R. *et al.* (1992) Complications occurring in the postanaesthesia care unit: a survey. *Anaesth Analg*, 74, 503–9.

House of Commons Health Committee (2005) *The Prevention of Venous Thromboembolism in Hospitalised Patients*. House of Commons Health Committee Second Report 2004–2005. The Stationary Office, London.

Hukushi, G. *et al.* (2007) Deep vein thrombosis prophylaxis methods. *AORN J*, 85(2), 265–6.

Jacobs, V.R. *et al.* (2000) Intraoperative evaluation of laparoscopic insufflation technique for quality control in the OR. *J Soc Laparoendoscopic Surg*, 4(3), 189–95.

Jolley, S. (2001) Managing post-operative nausea and vomiting. *Nurs Stand*, 15(40), 47–52.

Juzo (2006) *Application of Compression Stockings*. Juzo UK Ltd, Dundee, Scotland.

Kean, M. (2000) Adult/elderly care nursing. A patient temperature audit within a theatre recovery unit. *Br J Nurs*, 9(3), 150–6.

Kjonniksen, I. *et al.* (2002) Preoperative hair removal – a systematic literature review. *AORN J*, 75(5), 928–34, 936, 938.

Kumar, S. *et al.* (2005) Effects of perioeprative hypothermia and warming in surgical practice. *Int Wound J*, 2(3), 193–201.

Levinson, B.W. (1965) States of awareness during general anaesthesia. Preliminary communication. *Br J Anaesth*, 37(7), 544–6.

Lipp, A. & Edwards, P. (2002) Disposable surgical face masks for preventing surgical wound infection in clean surgery. *Cochrane Database Syst Rev*, 1: CD002929.

McEwen, D.R. (1996) Intra-operative positioning of surgical patients. *AORN J*, 63(6), 1059–63, 1066–79, 1080–6.

Mitchell, M. (2000) Nursing interventions for pre-operative anxiety. *Nurs Stand*, 14(37), 40–3.

Molyneux, C. (2001) Open forum. Electrosurgery policy, 'Electrosurgery in perioperative practice'. *Br J Periop Nurs*, 11(10), 424.

NICE (2005) *The Prevention and Treatment of Pressure Ulcers*. National Institute for Health and Clinical Excellence, London.

NICE (2007) Venous thromboembolism: reducing the risk of venous thromboembolism (deep vein thrombosis and pulmonary embolism) in inpatients undergoing surgery. Full guidance. National Collaborating Centre for Acute Care, Royal College of Surgeons for England, London. www.guidance.nice.org.uk/CG/published/CG46. Accessed 30/4/07.

Nimmo, W.S. *et al.* (eds) (1994) *Anaesthesia*, 2nd edn. Blackwell Science, Oxford.

NMC (2005) *Records and Record Keeping*. Nursing and Midwifery Council, London.

NMC (2006) *A–Z Advice Sheet Consent*. www.nmc.org.

NMC (2008) *The Code: Standards of Conduct, Performance and Ethics for Nurses and Midwives*. Nursing and Midwifery Council, London.

O'Callaghan, N. (2002) Pre-operative fasting. *Nurs Stand*, 16(36), 33–7.

O'Malley, C. & Cunningham, A.J. (2001) Physiologic changes during laparoscopy. *Anesthesiol Clin North Am*, 19(1), 1–19.

Parienti, J.J. *et al.* (2002) Hand-rubbing with an aqueous alcoholic solution vs. traditional surgical hand-scrubbing and 30-day surgical site infection rates: a randomised equivalence study. *JAMA*, 288(6), 722–7.

Parnaby, C. (2004) The new antiembolism stocking. *Br J Perioper Nurs*, 14(7), 302–7.

Paula, R. (2002) Richard Paula Compartment Syndrome Extremity. www.emedicie.com/emerg/topic739.htm. Accessed 11/4/07.

Peskett, M.J. (1999) Clinical indicators and other complications in the recovery room or postanaesthetic care unit. *Anaesthesia*, 54(12), 1143–9.

Pratt, R.J. *et al.* (2007) Epic 2: national evidence-based guidelines for preventing healthcare-associated infections in NHS hospitals in England. *J Hosp Infect*, 65, S1–64.

Rashid, S.T. *et al.* (2005) Venous thromboprophylaxis in UK medical patients. *J R Soc Med*, 98, 507–12.

Raza, A., Byrne, D. & Townell, N. (2004) Lower limb (well leg) compartment syndrome after urological pelvic surgery. *J Urol*, 171(1), 5–11.

RCN (2005) *Perioperative Fasting in Adults and Children. A RCN Guideline for the Multidisciplinary Team*. Royal College of Nursing, London.

Roderick, P. *et al.* (2005) Towards evidence-based guidelines for the preventions of venous thromboembolism: systematic reviews of mechanical methods, oral anticoagulation, dextran and regional anaesthesia as thromboprophylaxis. *Health Technol Assess*, 9(49), 1–78.

Scott, E., Beswick, A. & Wakefield, K. (2004) The hazards of diathermy plume. *Br J Perioper Nurs*, 14(10), 453–6.

Sharma, K.C. *et al.* (1997) Laparoscopic surgery and its potential for medical complications. *Heart Lung: J Acute Crit Care*, 26(1), 52–67.

SIGN (2002) *Prophylaxis of Venous Thromboembolism Guidelines*. Scottish Intercollegiate Guidelines Network, Edinburgh.

Tammelin, A., Domicel, P. & Hambraeus, A. (2000) Dispersal of methicillin-resistant *Staphylococcus epidermidis* by staff in an operating suite for thoracic and cardiovascular surgery: relation to skin carriage and clothing. *Hosp Infect*, 44(2), 119–26.

Tanner, J. & Parkinson, H. (2002) Double gloving to reduce surgical cross-infection. *Cochrane Database Syst Rev*, 1(3): CD003087.

Tokars, J.I. *et al.* (1995) Skin and mucous membrane contacts with blood during surgical procedures: risk and prevention. *Epidemiology*, 16(12), 703–11.

Turnbull, D. & Mills, G. (2001) Compartment syndrome associated with the Lloyd Davies position. *Anaesthesia*, 56(10), 980–7.

Turnbull, D. *et al.* (2002) Calf compartment pressures in the Lloyd Davies position, a cause for concern? *Anaesthesia*, 57(9), 905–8.

Ulrich, W. *et al.* (1997) Damage due to patient positioning in anaesthesia and surgical medicine. *Anaesthesiol Intens Med Notfallmed Schmerzther*, 32(1), 4–20.

Vendovato, J.W., Polvora, P. & Leonardi, D.F. (2004) *Burns as a Complication of the Use of Diathermy*. American Burn Association no. 0273 8481/2004. *J Burn Care Rehab*, 25(1), 120–123.

Wagner, D.V. (2003) Impact of perioperative temperature management on patient safety. *SSM*, 9(4), 38–43.

Walker, J.A. (2002) Emotional and psychological preoperative preparation in adults. *Br J Nurs*, 11(8), 567–75.

Wicker, P. (2000) Back to basics. Electrosurgery in perioperative practice. *Br J Periop Nurs*, 10(4), 221–6.

Wicker, P. & O'Neill, J. (2006) *Caring for the Perioperative Patient*. Blackwell Publishing, Oxford.

Woodhead, K., Taylor, E. & Bannister, G. (2002) Behaviours and rituals in the operating theatre: a report from the Hospital Infection Society Working Party on Infection Control in Operating Theatres. *Hosp Infect*, 51(4), 241–55.

Wu, M.P. *et al.* (2000) Complications and recommended practices for electrosurgery in laparoscopy. *Am J Surg*, 179(1), 67–73.

Chapter 31

Personal hygiene: eye care

Reference material **630**
Procedure guidelines: Eye swabbing **637**
Procedure guidelines: Artificial eye care **638**
Procedure guidelines: Contact lens care **639**
Procedure guidelines: Eye drop instillation **641**
Procedure guidelines: Eye ointment instillation **642**
Procedure guidelines: Eye irrigation **643**
Procedure guidelines: Eyelid closure for comatose patients **645**
References and further reading **646**

Definition

Eye care is the practice of assessing, cleaning or irrigating the eye and/or the instillation of prescribed ocular preparations (Stollery *et al.* 2005).

Indications

Eye care may be necessary under the following circumstances:

- To relieve pain and discomfort.
- To prevent or treat infection.
- To prevent or treat injury to the eye.
- To detect disease at an early stage.
- To detect drug-induced toxicity at an early stage.
- To prevent damage to the cornea in sedated or unconscious patients.
- To maintain contact lenses and care for false eye prostheses.
- Eye care may also include patient education and health and safety advice.

(Cunningham & Gould 1998; Boyd-Monk 2005; Stollery *et al.* 2005)

Reference material

If able, and after appropriate instruction, patients should be encouraged to carry out many of the procedures involved

in eye care themselves. However, in the case of postoperative, physically limited or unconscious patients, it is often the nurse who is responsible for eye care. A poor eye care technique may lead to the transmission of infection from one eye to the other or the development of irreversible damage to the eye (Ashurst 1997; Cunningham & Gould 1998). In some cases this can lead to loss of sight.

Anatomy and physiology

The eye consists of three main areas: the orbit, the globe (eyeball) and the extrinsic structures. The orbit, or socket, is formed by seven bones of the skull and is lined with fat; it supports and protects the globe and its accessory structures (blood vessels and nerves) and provides attachments for the ocular muscles (Stollery *et al.* 2005).

The globe is approximately 2.5 cm in diameter and can be divided into three layers (Figure 31.1):

- The outer layer or fibrous tunic, composed of the cornea and sclera.
- The middle layer or vascular tunic, composed of the choroid, ciliary body and iris.
- The inner layer or nervous tunic, composed of the retina.

The function of the outer layer is protective and gives shape to the eyeball. The middle layer contains the globe's vascular supply and is darkly pigmented. The inner layer, or retina,

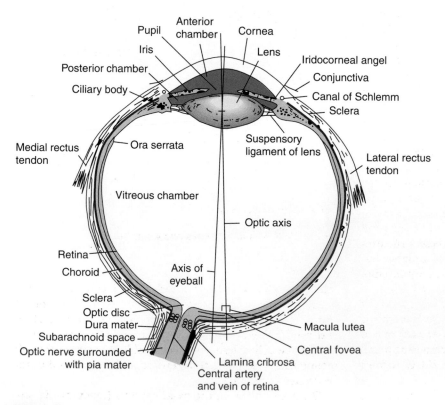

Figure 31.1 Horizontal section through eyeball at level of optic nerve. Optic axis and axis of eyeball are included.

contains the light-sensitive cells known as the rods and cones and is also the site of the macula lutea (yellow spot), which contains the central fovea (the area of highest visual acuity). Extrinsic structures of the eye include the eyelids, eyelashes, eyebrows and lacrimal (tear) apparatus. These structures protect the globe from external injury (Stollery *et al.* 2005). The blood vessels inside the eye may be readily viewed with an ophthalmoscope and examined for changes due to systemic diseases, such as diabetes or hypertension, or local disease processes, such as senile macular degeneration (Tortora & Derrickson 2008).

The optic nerve which is responsible for vision (cranial nerve II) exits the eye to the side of the macula lutea at an area called the optic disc, sometimes called the anatomical blind spot. The optic nerve passes from the orbit, through the optic foramen and into the brain. The two separate optic nerves meet at the optic chiasma and some optic nerve fibres cross over here to the opposite side of the brain. The nerves then continue along the optic tracts and terminate in the thalamus. From there projections extend to the visual areas in the occipital lobe of the cerebral cortex (Tortora & Derrickson 2008) (Figure 31.2). An additional blind spot, or area of depressed vision called a scotoma, may be indicative of a brain tumour. For example, in pituitary gland tumours it is common to develop bilateral defects in the field of vision due to invasion of the optic chiasm (Goodman & Wickham 2005).

The inside of the globe is divided into two chambers by the lens: the anterior cavity, anterior to the lens, and the vitreous chamber, posterior to the lens. The anterior cavity is divided into the anterior chamber and the posterior chamber by the iris. It contains a clear, watery fluid called the aqueous humour. The vitreous chamber is filled with a jelly-like substance called the vitreous body or vitreous humour. Together these two fluid-filled cavities help maintain the shape of the eyeball and the intraocular pressure (Marieb 2001; Tortora & Derrickson 2008) (Figure 31.3).

The aqueous humour is continuously secreted by the ciliary process (a part of the ciliary body) located behind the iris. This fluid then permeates the posterior chamber, passing between the lens and the iris, and flows through the pupil into the anterior chamber. From the anterior chamber the aqueous humour drains into the scleral venous sinus (canal of Schlemm) and is absorbed back into the blood stream. The aqueous humour is the principal source of nutrients and waste removal for the lens and cornea, as these structures have no direct blood supply. If the outflow of aqueous humour is blocked, excessive intraocular pressure may develop, leading to the disease process known as glaucoma. This excess pressure can cause degeneration of the retina, which may result in blindness (Lee 2006). The vitreous humour is a clear gelatinous substance which fills the vitreous chamber, which unlike the aqueous humour, is produced during foetal development and is never replaced (Marieb 2001; Tortora & Derrickson 2008).

Tears are produced in the lacrimal glands located at the upper, outer edge of the eye (Figure 31.4). They are excreted

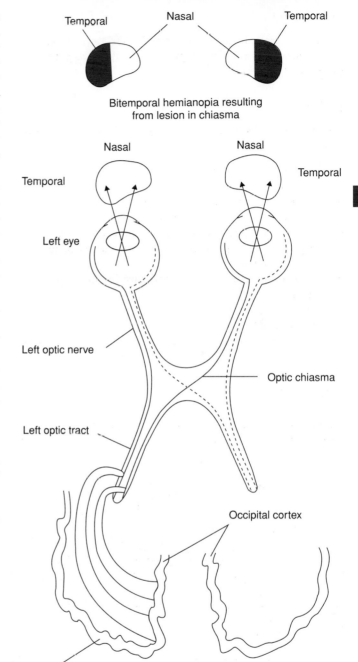

Figure 31.2 Visual pathways and visual fields.

onto the upper surface of the globe and washed over the ocular surface by the action of blinking. The function of tears is to clean, moisten and lubricate the ocular surface and eyelids. Tears also provide antisepsis as they contain an enzyme called lysozyme that is able to rupture the cell membranes of some bacteria leading to their lysis and death (Forrester *et al.* 2002).

The tears collect in the nasal canthus (inner, medial aspect of the eye) where they drain into the upper and lower

Figure 31.3 Anterior cavity in front of lens is incompletely divided into anterior chamber (anterior to iris) and posterior chamber (behind iris), which are continuous through pupil. Aqueous humour, which fills the cavity, is formed by ciliary processes and reabsorbed into venous blood by the canal of Schlemm.

lacrimal puncti which drain into the lacrimal sac. From here the tears pass into the nasolacrimal duct and empty into the nasal cavity (Marieb 2001; Tortora & Derrickson 2008).

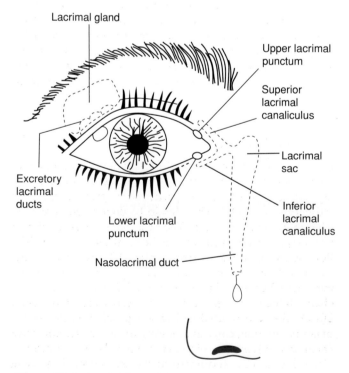

Figure 31.4 Lacrimal apparatus.

General principles of eye care

Aseptic technique is necessary only in certain circumstances, for example, when the eye is damaged or following ophthalmic surgery.

Position of patient

The patient should be sitting or lying with his or her head tilted backwards and chin pointing upwards. This allows for easy access to the eyes and is usually a good position for patient comfort and compliance (Stollery *et al.* 2005).

Position of light source

A good light source is necessary prior to commencing eye care procedures to enable careful assessment of the eyes and to avoid damage to their delicate structures. The light source should be positioned above and behind the nurse. It should never be allowed to shine directly into the patient's eyes, as this will be extremely uncomfortable for the patient.

Instillation of drops

Most types of drops are instilled into the inferior fornix, the pocket formed by gently pulling on the lower eyelid (see Action figure 7 in Procedure guidelines: Eye drops instillation, below), as the conjunctiva in this area is less sensitive than that overlying the cornea. Administering medications into this area prevents immediate loss of the drops into the nasolacrimal drainage system. Exceptions to this instillation technique are as follows:

- *Drugs used to lubricate the cornea*: oil-based drops produce less corneal reaction than aqueous ones as they do not feel as cold to the cornea when administered. They may therefore be instilled directly into the inferior fornix.
- *Anaesthetic drops*: the first drop should be instilled into the inferior fornix for absorption and then directly onto the cornea one drop at a time until the patient is no longer able to feel the drops.
- *Drops used to treat the nasal passages*: these should be instilled at the nasal canthus end of the eye.
- The number of drops instilled depends on the type of solution used and its purpose. Usually, one drop only is ordered and will be sufficient if it is instilled in the correct manner. The exceptions to the 'one-drop' rule are:
- *Oil-based solutions*: these are used for lubricating the eyeball. Usually one drop is instilled and repeated as required.
- *Anaesthetic drops*: Used to anesthetize the eye, one drop should be instilled at a time. This is repeated until the drop cannot be felt on the eye.

If two different preparations are required at the same time an interval of 5 minutes should lapse before the second preparation is instilled to prevent dilution or overflow (BNF 2006).

The dropper should be held as close to the eye as possible without touching either the lids or the cornea (see Action figure 7 in Procedure guidelines: Eye drop instillation, below). This will avoid corneal damage and reduce the risk of cross-infection. If the drop falls from too great a height it is difficult to control and will also be uncomfortable for the patient. The eye should be closed for as long as possible after application, preferably for 1–2 minutes.

A variety of droppers and bottles are available for the instillation of eye preparations. These include pipettes, bottles incorporating pipettes, plastic bottles with a dropper attachment and single dose packs. Pipettes are easy to use but need to be dried and sterilized between doses. Plastic bottles can be squeezed and so avoid the need for a pipette and they are also cheaper than glass bottles with a dropper. Each patient should have their own individual eye drop container for each eye and single dose containers should be used for all patients in eye clinics or in accident and emergency departments (BNF 2006).

Instillation of ointments

Ointments are also applied to the upper rim of the inferior fornix using a similar technique to eye drops (see Action figure 7 in Procedure guidelines: Eye ointment instillation, below). A 2 cm line of ointment should be applied from the nasal canthus outwards. Similarly to the instillation of eye drops, the nozzle should be held approximately 2.5 cm above the eye to avoid contact with the cornea and eyelids.

Contact lenses and eye preparations

Contact lenses may affect the distribution and absorption of eye preparations. Some drugs and preservatives in eye preparations may accumulate in soft hydrogel lenses and induce a toxic reaction. For these reasons contact lenses should be removed prior to instillation of eye drops or ointments and not worn for the period of treatment (BNF 2006). Eye drops can be instilled over rigid contact lenses (BNF 2006).

Care of contact lenses

Contact lenses are thin, curved discs made of hard or soft plastic or a combination of both. Hard contact lenses are made of a rigid plastic that does not absorb water or saline solutions and can be worn for a maximum of 12–14 hours continuously. Soft contact lenses are more pliable, retain more water and so can be worn for up to 30 days and cleaned once weekly. Ill-fitting lenses may reduce the tear film between lens and cornea which may result in oxygen deprivation of the cornea leading to corneal oedema and blurred vision. Further damage to the corneal epithelial cells may lead to corneal abrasion and pain (Marsden & Spence 2006). Gas-permeable lenses are a combination of both hard and soft and permit oxygen to reach the cornea, providing greater comfort, and can be left in for several days (Olver & Cassidy 2005).

Most people look after their own contact lenses. Cleaning and storage solutions depend on the type of lenses used: manufacturers provide specific instructions for the care of their products. They should be stored in a container with slots for right (R) and left (L) eye, so they can be worn in the correct eye. Seriously ill patients should have their lenses removed and stored correctly until they can reinsert their own lenses. Contact lenses are stored in a sterile solution, usually sodium chloride, when they are not in the eye. This helps to lubricate the lens and enable the lens to glide over the cornea, reducing the risk of injury (Kozier *et al.* 1998).

Eye irrigation

Eye irrigation is most often perfomed to remove foreign bodies or caustic substances from the eye, e.g. domestic cleaning agents or medications, particularly cytotoxic material (Stollery *et al.* 2005). This should be done as soon as possible to minimize damage. The procedure is also used as a preoperative preparation or to remove infected material. The fluids most commonly used are sterile 0.9% sodium chloride, 'for irrigation', or sterile water, 'for irrigation'. However, using water may result in deeper corneal damage by corrosive chemicals due to water's hypotonic nature (Kuckelkorn *et al.* 2002). The volume used will vary depending on the degree of contamination; copious amounts are needed for corrosive chemicals and smaller volumes for removal of eye secretions. The solution may be directed to the area affected by using intravenous tubing. To avoid physical damage, the tubing

633

should be held approximately 2.5 cm from the eye (Stollery *et al.* 2005).

Care of the insensitive eye

If the eye-blink reflex is absent the eye's surface will dry out, causing irreversible corneal damage. The cornea may become ulcerated or infected, leading to scarring and possibly loss of vision (Carlson 2002: E). This is a particular problem in the sedated, ventilated or unconscious patient. When the patient has lost this protective reflex, the nurse must initiate interventions to maintain eye moisture and corneal integrity. The surface of the eye and surrounding structures should be kept clean and moist by gentle cleaning with sterile 0.9% sodium chloride and, when necessary, the instillation of lubricating preparations. If there is no eye-blink reflex the eyelids should be kept closed by the use of hypoallergenic tape (Suresh *et al.* 2000). If the eyes become infected the relevant medication should be prescribed and administered.

With each of these measures care must be taken not to spread infection between the eyes. Any alteration to the appearance of the eye must be reported to the doctor.

Artificial eyes

These are made of glass or plastic; some are permanently implanted. Most people who have artificial eyes care for them themselves. If the patient is unconscious it is not necessary to remove the eye regularly for cleaning.

For all procedures which involve removal or insertion of contact lenses or prosthetic eyes the patient should be encouraged to remove/insert the lens/prosthetic themselves as they will have developed their own particular methods. However, the nurse must observe as the patient may still need education to improve upon their technique.

Eye medications

Drugs may be given either systemically or topically to exert an effect on the eye (BNF 2006). However, if given systemically the prescribing doctor needs to take account of the blood–aqueous barrier which exists within the eye. This barrier is selective in allowing drugs to pass into the intraocular fluids. The permeability of this barrier may increase during inflammatory conditions or following paracentesis, the removal of excess fluid with a needle or cannula (Andrew 2006).

Medications applied topically meet some resistance at the barrier presented by the lacrimal system (tear film barrier). A further barrier is the cornea which is selectively permeable and only allows the passage of water and not drugs. However, corneal resistance may alter if there is damage to the corneal epithelium (Kirkwood 2006). Many drugs will produce a similar effect on both the healthy and diseased eye. Drugs for use in the eye are usually classified according to their action.

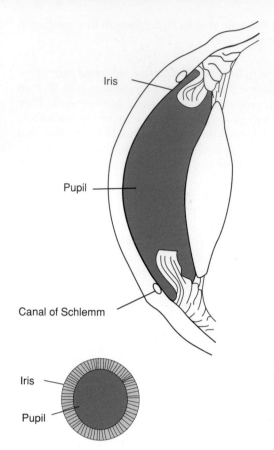

Figure 31.5 Effects of mydriatics.

Mydriatics and cycloplegics

These drugs cause pupil dilation and produce their effects by paralysing the ciliary muscle, stimulating the dilator muscle of the pupil (Figure 31.5) or by a combination of both (see Action figure 7 in Procedure guidelines: Eye drop instillation, below). They are used mainly for diagnostic purposes and most have an anticholinergic action. The most commonly used preparations are cyclopentolate hydrochloride, tropicamide and atropine (BNF 2006).

Miotics

These drugs produce their effects by contracting the ciliary muscle and constricting the pupil (Figure 31.6). Miotics help in the drainage of aqueous humour and are used primarily in the treatment of glaucoma. Examples are pilocarpine and carbachol (BNF 2006).

Local anaesthetics

These render the eye and the inner surfaces of the lids insensitive. They are used before minor surgery, removal of foreign bodies and tonometry (measurement of intraocular pressure). The most widely used eye anaesthetics are oxybuprocaine and amethocaine (BNF 2006).

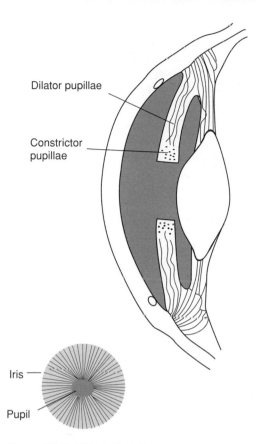

Iris

Pupil

Figure 31.6 Effect of miotics.

Anti-inflammatories

Anti-inflammatory drugs include steroids, antihistamines, lodoxamide and sodium cromoglycate. The most commonly used steroid preparations are dexamethasone, prednisolone and betamethasone (BNF 2006).

Corticosteroid eye drops should be used with caution as they can cause cataract formation or a gradual rise in intraocular pressure in a small percentage of people, particularly if they have a history of glaucoma (Forrester *et al.* 2002).

Antibacterials/antivirals/antifungals

Antibacterials and antivirals can be used for the active treatment of infections or as prophylactic treatment for eye surgery, after removal of a foreign body or following an eye injury. Antibiotic preparations in common use are chloramphenicol, neomycin and framycetin. Aciclovir is the only commonly used antiviral available as an eye preparation although Ganciclovir is licensed for the treatment of acute herpetic keratitis (BNF 2006). Antifungal preparations are not available so the patient needs to be referred to a specialist centre.

Artificial tears

Artificial tears are used when there is a deficiency in natural tear production. This can be due to a disease process,

postradiotherapy treatment, as a side-effect of certain drugs or when the eye-blink reflex is absent. These artificial lubricants commonly contain hypromellose or hydroxyethylcellulose (BNF 2006). Additionally, pilocarpine can be given orally. The severity of the problem and the patient's choice will determine the treatment.

Toxic effects of some systemic drugs on the eye

As the eye may be the first place to show signs of systemic disease, so some systemic drugs may show their toxic effects in the eye; this is in part due to the small mass and the relatively high vasculature of the eye. The integrity, thus permeability of the blood–aqueous barrier may be a determining factor. These effects range from pruritis, irritation, redness, epiphora (excess tear production with overflow), photophobia and blepharoconjunctivitis (inflammation of the eyelids and conjunctiva), to disturbance of vision (Andrew 2006).

Particular effects of specific drugs are listed below:

- *Methotrexate and related antimetabolites*: these drugs may cause blepharoconjunctivitis. They may also induce photophobia, epiphora, periorbital oedema and conjunctival hyperaemia.
- *5-Fluorouracil (5-FU)*: 5-FU can cause canalicular fibrosis and oculomotor disturbances (probably secondary to a local neurotoxicity affecting the brain-stem).
- *Antihistamines*: these drugs decrease tear production and may lead to 'dry eye', especially in patients with Sjögren's syndrome (a wasting disease of the salivary glands), ocular pemphigus (rare, autoimmune disease of the skin), those who wear contact lenses and in the elderly.
- *Tamoxifen*: this drug can cause subepithelial whirl-like deposits in the cornea, and retinal lesions.
- *Indomethacin*: this can cause: blurred vision, corneal deposits and retinal pigmentary toxicity.
- *Oral contraceptives*: these can stimulate corneal steeping and intolerance to contact lenses.
- *Atropine, scopolamine and belladonna-like substances*: such drugs cause mydriasis (widening of the pupil) and cycloplegia (paralysis of the ciliary muscle that moves the iris).
- *Corticosteroids*: prolonged use of corticosteroids produces posterior subcapsular cataracts and can increase intraocular pressure.
- *Chloramphenicol*: chloramphenicol treatment can lead to optic neuritis.
- *Ethambutol*: this drug can cause damage to the optic nerve.
- *Rifampicin*: stains soft contact lenses and alters tear coloration.
- *Digoxin*: in overdose results in blurred vision and yellow/green vision.
- *Antidepressants*: may cause a rise in intraocular pressure causing acute glaucoma.
- *Amiodarone*: may increase corneal opacity.
- *Ciprofloxacin*: may deposit in the corneal epithelium.

635

- *Beta-blockers*: may affect lacrimation causing reduced tear secretion and dry eye.
- *Oxygen*: in neonates, high concentrations for a long period can cause retrolental fibroplasia (abnormal proliferation of fibrous tissue behind the lens causing blindness).

(Forrester *et al.* 2002; Abdollahi *et al.* 2004; Andrew 2006; BNF 2006)

Tumours of the eye

There are a number of benign lumps associated with the anatomical structures of the eye. Meibomian cysts (or chalazion) may present as painful eyelid swelling due to a blocked meibomian duct of which there are 20–30 in each eyelid (Stollery *et al.* 2005). Other benign conditions include papilloma (warts in epithelial calls caused by the papilloma virus), retention cysts (blockage of excretory duct) and sebaceous cysts (Olver & Cassidy 2005).

Primary tumours of the eye

Tumours of the eye may exhibit a range of signs and symptoms depending on which structures are affected. Within the globe retinoblastoma (malignant tumour of the retina) and malignant melanoma are most common. They may go undiagnosed for some time unless they cause a disturbance in the visual field, for example if they are situated in the macula lutea or cause retinal detachment (Ward *et al.* 2006).

Because of the highly vascular nature of the globe, metastases may be more common.

Tumours of the orbit are rare: the most common are rhabdomyosarcomas in children and lymphomas in adults (Char 1993). Orbital tumours may push the eye away from its normal visual axis in a sagittal or vertical plane. In almost all cases the direction of displacement is opposite to the growing tumour (Moeloek 1993). Lack of room for growth may cause proptosis (protrusion of the eye). The average volume of the eye is 24 ml and an increase of only 4 ml will cause a 6 mm proptosis. This proptosis and accompanying diplopia (double vision) can be disfiguring and distressing symptoms for the patient (Char 1993; Souhami & Tobias 2005). Proptosis may also be a sign of thyroid eye disease or Graves' ophthalmopathy especially if the proptosis is bilateral (Ryder 2006).

Basal cell carcinoma (BCC) or rodent ulcer and squamous cell carcinoma (SCC) are fairly common tumours of the extrinsic structures such as the eyelids particularly in the elderly (Lindgren *et al.* 1998; Finger 2000). BCC grow slowly and rarely metastasize but can spread by direct growth into adjacent structures such as the orbit and ultimately even the brain. SCC is less common than BCC but it grows more rapidly and may metastasize to regional lymph nodes, particularly in the neck (McQueen 2006).

Investigations

Comprehensive clinical examination by a specialist consultant is imperative. Additional investigations may include:

- Histology.
- Computed tomography (CT).
- Magnetic resonance imaging (MRI).
- Orbital venography: radiographic visualization of ophthalmic veins using radio-opaque dye.
- Carotid angiography: to assess blood supply to the ophthalmic artery.
- Ultrasound.

The last three techniques have become less popular with the advent of CT and MRI (Lund 1987). Histological confirmation of the tumour type should be performed if possible, by either biopsy or cytology. Care needs to be taken during these procedures as tumour spillage, haemorrhage and blindness are potential risks with either method of sampling. If the tumour is encapsulated it is suggested that it be excised in entirety (Souhami & Tobias 2005).

Treatment

The treatment of any eye malignancy is always based on the principle of curing the disease and preserving sight. In the instance of large or invasive tumours this is not always possible so the aim then is to maintain a suitable cosmetic appearance. The treatment will depend on the size, histology of the tumour, anatomical location of the structures affected and current evidence of the efficacy of treatments available.

Small tumours may be controlled with surgical excision, ablative therapies (cryotherapy or photocoagulation, for example), brachytherapy ('short distance' therapy, see Chapter 35) external beam radiotherapy or chemotherapy. When the tumour is very extensive and/or the eye is beyond the point of useful recovery then enucleation (removal of the globe) is considered the treatment of choice (Souhami & Tobias 2005). If there is local spread of the tumour then adjuvant chemotherapy may be indicated (Goddard *et al.* 1999).

Summary

Like most disfigurements of the head and neck, orbital tumours are also difficult to camouflage. Commonly patients will wear tinted glasses, or wear an eye pad/protector so that it looks more like protection from an eye injury rather than camouflage of a tumour. Eye patches are occasionally worn, but most patients feel that this is indicative of eye loss.

Patients with orbital disease need skilled emotional support. This is particularly true if the disease is inoperable and/or end stage. The tumour may be exophytic (growing outwards), proptosed (abnormal protuberance/bulging out) or causing splaying of the nasal and ethmoid bones. Such disfiguring complications may lead to social isolation, avoidance and despair. These patients not only live with disfigurement and dysfunction, but also the threat to their survival from the disease process. Nursing and medical staff in specialist centres are more likely to have the experience and knowledge required in dealing with these relatively rare and demanding disease processes and their consequences.

In addition, they may be more aware of community support networks and can ensure that, when necessary, patients are referred to an appropriate specialist prosthetic department.

Primarily, the nurse will be involved in helping the patient cope with the diagnosis and treatment of their disease, care of the eye (or cavity if enucleation has been performed) and any prostheses the patient has had fitted. Reintegration into the community and workplace must be followed up closely through outpatient clinics or via telephone contact to help reduce any feelings of isolation and abandonment once discharged from hospital. Further nursing interventions include observation and early detection of any eye irregularities and clinical management of symptoms. This will involve assessment and management of pain (see Chapter 27), maintaining the eye in a clean and comfortable state and administering eye preparations as prescribed. The eye may need to be covered for protection, patient comfort or as a means of camouflage.

Eye care of the comatose patient

The comatose patient may be unconscious due to injury or deliberate sedation in a critical care environment. The hygiene needs of these patients need to be addressed by nursing staff involved in their care (see Chapter 44). The loss of the physical and biological protective functions may result in damage to the eye. Muscle relaxants administered to sedated patients can reduce the contraction of the orbicularis oculi muscle thus inhibiting full eyelid closure, reduce the blink reflex and random eye movement resulting in diminished tear film coverage of the eye. This desiccation (drying) of the eye may result in exposure keratopathy or superficial corneal abrasions (Ashurst 1997; Cunningham & Gould 1998; Joyce & Evans 2006). To prevent drying of the eye regular interventions such as hygiene and/or administration of products are recommended. Paraffin preparations such as Lacri-Lube® have been shown to offer eye protection in the compromised eye (Ezra *et al.* 2005).

Procedure guidelines   Eye swabbing

Equipment

1 Sterile dressing pack.
2 Sterile low linting swab.

3 Sterile 0.9% sodium chloride for irrigation or sterile water for irrigation.

Procedure

Action	Rationale
1 Explain and discuss the procedure with the patient.	To ensure that the patient understands the procedure and gives his/her valid consent (NMC 2006: C).
2 Assist the patient into the correct position: (a) Head well supported and tilted back. (b) Preferably the patient should be in bed or lying on a couch.	The patient needs to be discouraged from flinching or making unexpected movements and so should be in the most comfortable, pain free position possible at the start of the procedure (Shaw 2006: R 5).
3 Ensure an adequate light source, taking care not to dazzle the patient.	To enable maximum observation of the eyes without causing the patient harm or discomfort (Shaw 2006: R 5).
4 Wash hands thoroughly using bactericidal soap and water or bactericidal alcohol handrub, then dry hands.	To reduce the risk of cross-infection (DH 2005: C).
5 Always treat the uninfected or uninflamed eye first.	To reduce the risk of cross-infection (NT 2003: R 5).
6 Always bathe lids with the eyes closed first.	To reduce the risk of damaging the cornea and to remove any crusted discharge (E).
7 Using a slightly moistened low-linting swab, ask the patient to look up and gently swab the lower lid from the inner canthus outwards. Use an aseptic technique for the damaged or postoperative eye.	If the swab is too wet the solution will run down the patient's cheek. This increases the risk of cross-infection and causes the patient discomfort. Swabbing from the nasal corner outwards avoids the risk of swabbing discharge into the lacrimal punctum, or even across the bridge of the nose into the other eye. Aseptic technique reduces the risk of cross-infection (DH 2005: C).

Procedure guidelines (*cont.*)

8 Ensure that the edge of the swab is not above the lid margin.	To avoid touching the sensitive cornea (E).
9 Using a new swab each time, repeat the procedure until all the discharge has been removed.	To reduce risk of cross-infection (DH 2005: C).
10 Gently swab the upper lid by slightly everting the lid margin and asking the patient to look down. Swab from the nasal corner outwards and use a new swab each time until all discharge has been removed.	To effectively remove any foreign material from the eye (E). To reduce the risk of cross-infection (DH 2005: C).
11 Once both eyelids have been cleaned and dried, make the patient comfortable.	To ensure patient comfort (E).
12 Remove and dispose of equipment.	To keep area clean and reduce risk of cross-infection (DH 2005: C).
13 Wash hands.	To reduce the risk of cross-infection (DH 2005: C).
14 Record the procedure in the appropriate documents.	To monitor trends and fluctuations (NMC 2005: C).

Note: for information about obtaining an eye swab for pathological investigations, see Chapter 40.

Procedure guidelines   **Artificial eye care**

Equipment

1 Sterile dressing pack.
2 Sterile 0.9% sodium chloride for irrigation.

3 Low-linting gauze.

Procedure
Removal of artificial eye

Action	**Rationale**
1 Explain and discuss the procedure with the patient.	To ensure that the patient understands the procedure and gives his/her consent (NMC 2006: C).
2 Wash hands thoroughly using bactericidal soap and water or bactericidal alcohol handrub.	To reduce the risk of cross-infection (DH 2005: C).
3 Wearing gloves and with the dominant hand, gently pull the eyelid downwards and exert slight pressure below the eyelid to overcome the suction, enabling the prosthesis to be removed (see Action figure 3).	To minimize patient discomfort (E).
4 Rinse and drain the eye socket with sterile 0.9% sodium chloride.	To remove any loose debris and to minimize damage caused by touch (E).
5 Clean the eye with sterile 0.9% sodium chloride.	To prevent the build up of debris and to reduce the risk of infection (DH 2005: C).

Insertion of artificial eye

Action	**Rationale**
1 Explain and discuss the procedure with the patient.	To ensure that the patient understands the procedure and gives his/her consent (NMC 2006: C).

638

2 Wash hands thoroughly using bactericidal soap and water or bactericidal alcohol handrub.	To reduce the risk of cross-infection (DH 2005: C).
3 Wearing gloves and with the dominant hand, gently lift up the upper eyelid and pull down the lower eyelid. With the other hand, hold the prosthesis between the thumb and index finger and gently insert it.	To minimize patient discomfort and ensure correct insertion (E).

639

(a)   (b)

Action 3   Removing an artificial eye.

Procedure guidelines   Contact lens care

Procedure
Removal of hard contact lenses

Action	Rationale
1 Explain and discuss the procedure with the patient.	To ensure that the patient understands the procedure and gives his/her consent (NMC 2006: C).
2 Wash hands thoroughly using bactericidal soap.	To reduce the risk of cross-infection (DH 2005: C).
3 Using thumb and forefinger separate the eyelids. Keeping the eyelid stationary, place the index finger on the lens. Gently move the lens to one side of the cornea and pull away (see Action figure 3).	To minimize corneal trauma (Stollery *et al.* 2005: R 5).
4 Store lenses in the appropriate solution as recommended by the manufacturers and ensure lenses are placed in the correct left and right storage pots.	To prevent deterioration and contamination (Stollery *et al.* 2005: R 5).
5 Refer to manufacturer's instructions for further storage information, particularly if patient will not be using the lenses for a lengthy period of time.	To prevent deterioration of lens and growth of organisms (C).

Procedure guidelines (*cont.*)

Removal of soft contact lenses

Action

1 Explain and discuss the procedure with the patient.

2 Wash hands thoroughly using bactericidal soap.

3 Wearing gloves, gently pinch the lens between the thumb and index finger (see Action figure 3).

4 Store lenses in the appropriate solution as recommended by the manufacturers and ensure lenses are placed in the correct left and right storage pots.

5 Refer to manufacturer's instructions for further storage information, particularly if patient will not be using the lenses for a lengthy period of time.

Rationale

To ensure that the patient understands the procedure and gives his/her consent (NMC 2006: C).

To reduce the risk of cross-infection (DH 2005: C).

To encourage the lens to fold together, allowing air to enter underneath the lens for easy removal (C).

To prevent deterioration and contamination (Stollery *et al.* 2005: E).

To prevent deterioration and growth of organisms (C).

(a)　　　(b)　　　(c)

Action 3(a)   Removing hard contact lenses.

(a)　　　(b)

Action 3(b)   (a) Moving a soft lens down the interior part of the sclera. (b) Removing a soft lens by pinching it between the pads of the thumb and index finger.

Procedure guidelines   Eye drop instillation

Equipment

1 Sterile dressing pack.
2 Sterile 0.9% sodium chloride for irrigation or sterile water for irrigation.
3 Appropriate eye drops.
4 Low-linting swab.

Procedure

Action	Rationale
1 Explain and discuss the procedure with the patient.	To ensure that the patient understands the procedure and gives his/her valid consent (NMC 2006: C).
2 If there is any discharge, proceed as for eye swabbing.	To remove any infected material and thus ensure adequate absorption of the drops (C).
3 Consult the patient's prescription sheet, and ascertain the following. (a) Patient identification. (b) Drug. (c) Dose. (d) Date and time of administration. (e) Route and method of administration, including which eye the drops are prescribed for. (f) Expiry date on bottle. (g) Validity of prescription. (h) Signature of prescriber.	To ensure that the patient is given the correct drug in the prescribed dose in the correct eye, and that the drug has not expired (NMC 2008: C).
4 Assist the patient into the correct position, i.e. head well supported and tilted back.	To ensure that drops are instilled into the pocket of the inferior fornix and to avoid excess solution running down the patient's cheek (Stollery et al. 2005: E).
5 Wash hands thoroughly using bactericidal soap and water or bactericidal alcohol handrub, and dry them.	Asepsis is essential when the patient has a damaged eye or has just had an operation on the eye. Infection can lead to loss of an eye (DH 2005: C).
6 Place a wet low-linting swab on the lower lid against the lid margin and gently pull down to evert the lower eyelid.	To absorb any excess solution which may be irritating to the surrounding skin and open the inferior fornix (E).
7 Ask the patient to look up immediately before instilling the drop (see Action figure 7).	This opens the eye and allows the drop to be instilled into the upper rim of the inferior fornix. If drop instilled too soon, the patient may blink as the drop is instilled (E).
8 Ask the patient to close the eye for approximately 1 minute. Keep the wet low-linting swab on the lower lid.	To ensure adequate absorption of the fluid and to avoid excess running down the cheek (Stollery et al. 2005: E).
9 Make the patient comfortable.	
10 Remove and dispose of equipment.	To keep area clean and reduce risk of cross infection (DH 2005: C).
11 Wash hands with bactericidal soap and water.	To reduce the risk of cross-infection (DH 2005: C).
12 Complete the patient's recording chart and other hospital and/or legally required documents.	To maintain accurate records. To provide a point of reference in the event of any queries. To prevent any duplication of treatment (NMC 2005: C).

641

Procedure guidelines (*cont.*)

Action 7   How to instil eye drops.

Procedure guidelines   Eye ointment instillation

Equipment

1 Sterile dressing pack.
2 Sterile 0.9% sodium chloride for irrigation or sterile water for irrigation.

3 Appropriate eye ointment.
4 Low-linting swab.

Procedure

Action	Rationale
1 Explain and discuss the procedure with the patient.	To ensure that the patient understands the procedure and gives his/her valid consent (NMC 2006: C).
2 If there is any discharge, and to remove any previous application of ointment, proceed as for eye swabbing.	To remove any infected material and previous ointment to allow for absorption of ointment (C).
3 Consult the patient's prescription sheet, and ascertain the following: (a) Patient identification. (b) Drug. (c) Dose. (d) Date and time of administration. (e) Route and method of administration, including which eye the ointment is prescribed for. (f) Expiry date on bottle. (g) Validity of prescription. (h) Signature of prescriber.	To ensure that the patient is given the correct drug in the prescribed dose in the correct eye, and that the drug has not expired (NMC 2008: C).
4 Wash hands thoroughly using bactericidal soap and water or bactericidal alcohol handrub.	To reduce the risk of cross-infection (DH 2005: C).
5 Place a wet low-linting swab on the lower lid against the lid margin.	To absorb excess ointment which may be irritating to the surrounding skin (E).
6 Gently pull on the low-linting swab. Ask the patient to look up immediately before applying the ointment.	To allow the application to be made inside the lower lid into the lower fornix (E).

7 Apply the ointment by gently squeezing the tube and, with the nozzle 2.5 cm above the eye, drawing a line along the inner edge of the lower lid from the nasal corner outwards (see Action figure 7).	To reduce the risk of cross-infection, contamination of the tube and trauma to the eye (Stollery *et al.* 2005: E).
8 Ask the patient to close the eye and remove excess ointment with a new wet low-linting swab.	To avoid excess ointment irritating the surrounding skin (E).
9 Warn the patient that, when the eye is opened, vision will be a little blurred for a few minutes.	To prepare patient and to avoid anxiety (Stollery *et al.* 2005: E).
10 Make the patient comfortable.	
11 Remove and dispose of equipment.	To keep area clean and reduce risk of cross infection (DH 2005: C).
12 Wash hands with bactericidal soap and water.	To reduce the risk of cross-infection (DH 2005: C).
13 Complete the patient's recording chart and other hospital and/or legally required documents.	To maintain accurate records. To provide a point of reference in the event of any queries. To prevent any duplication of treatment (NMC 2005: C).

Action 7 How to instil eye ointment.

Procedure guidelines Eye irrigation

Equipment

1 Sterile dressing pack.
2 Sterile 0.9% sodium chloride for irrigation or sterile water for irrigation (in an emergency tap water may be used).
3 Receiver.
4 Towel.
5 Plastic cape.
6 Irrigating flask.
7 Warm water in a bowl to warm irrigating fluid to tepid temperature.
8 Anaesthetic drops.

Procedure

Action	Rationale
1 Explain and discuss the procedure with the patient.	To ensure that the patient understands the procedure and gives his/her valid consent (NMC 2006: C).
2 Instil anaesthetic drops if required (proceed as for instillation of eye drops).	To avoid any discomfort (Marsden 2006: R 5).

Procedure guidelines (*cont.*)

3 Prepare the irrigation fluid to the appropriate temperature by placing in bowl of water until warmed.	Tepid fluid will be more comfortable for the patient. The solution should be poured across the inner aspect of the nurse's wrist to test the temperature (E).
4 Assist the patient into the appropriate position: (a) Head comfortably supported with chin almost horizontal. (b) Head inclined to the side of the eye to be treated.	To avoid the solution running either over the nose into the other eye to avoid cross-infection or out of the affected eye and down the side of the cheek (DH 2005: C). To reduce risk of cross-infection (DH 2005: C).
5 Wash hands using bactericidal soap and water or bactericidal alcohol handrub, and dry.	To prevent washing the discharge down the lacrimal duct or across the cheek (E).
6 If there is any discharge proceed as for eye swabbing.	
7 If possible remove any contact lens, proceed as for contact lens removal.	To ensure no reservoir of chemical remains in the eye (Marsden 2006: E).
8 Ask the patient to hold the receiver against the cheek below the eye being irrigated.	To collect irrigation fluid as it runs away from the eye (E).
9 Position the towel and plastic cape.	To protect the patient's clothing (E).
10 Hold the patient's eyelids apart, using your first and second fingers, against the orbital ridge.	The patient will be unable to hold the eye open once irrigation commences (E).
11 Do not press on the eyeball.	To avoid causing the patient discomfort or pain (E).
12 Warn the patient that the flow of solution is going to start and pour a little onto the cheek first.	To allow time to adjust to the feeling of water flow (E).
13 Direct the flow of the fluid from the nasal corner outwards (see Action figure 13).	To wash away from the lacrimal punctum and prevent contaminating other eye (E).
14 Ask the patient to look up, down and to either side while irrigating.	To ensure that the whole area including fornices are irrigated (Stollery *et al.* 2005: E).
15 Evert upper and lower lids whilst irrigating.	To ensure complete removal of any foreign body (E).
16 Keep the flow of irrigation fluid constant.	To ensure swift removal of any foreign body (Marsden 2006: E).
17 When the eye has been thoroughly irrigated, ask the patient to close the eyes and use a new swab to dry the lids.	For patient comfort (E).
18 Take the receiver from the patient and dry the cheek.	To prevent spillage of receiver contents and promote patient comfort (E).
19 Make the patient comfortable.	
20 Remove and dispose of equipment.	To keep area clean and reduce risk of cross-infection (DH 2005: C).
21 Wash hands with bactericidal soap and water.	To reduce the risk of cross-infection (DH 2005: C).
22 Complete the patient's recording chart and other hospital and/or legally required documents.	To maintain accurate records. To provide a point of reference in the event of any queries. To prevent any duplication of treatment (NMC 2005: C).

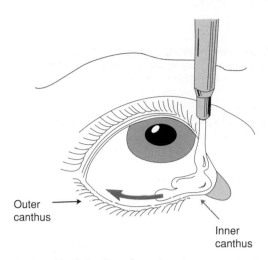

Outer
canthus

Inner
canthus

Action 13   Irrigation of eye from inner to outer canthus.

Procedure guidelines   Eyelid closure for comatose patients

If necessary clean and apply medication as outlined above.

Equipment

1 Sterile dressing pack.
2 Sterile 0.9% sodium chloride for irrigation or sterile water.

3 Hypoallergenic tape.

Procedure

Action	Rationale
1 Explain the procedure to the patient.	Hearing is often still present in unconscious patients so it is good practice to explain the procedure.
2 Wash hands thoroughly using bacterial soap and water or bactericidal alcohol handrub, then dry hands.	To reduce the risk of cross-infection (DH 2005: C).
3 Always treat and clean the uninfected or uninflamed eye first.	To reduce the risk of cross-infection (DH 2005: C).
4 Lubricate the eyelids (following procedure as outlined above for instillation of ointment).	To prevent corneal surface drying (Cunningham & Gould 1998: R 3a).
5 Gently hold down upper eyelid until it meets the lower lid.	To ensure there is no gap between eyelids (Joyce & Evans 2006: R 3a).
6 Place hypoallergenic tape across upper eyelid ensuring that there are no eyelashes caught underneath the tape.	To keep eyes closed and ensure patient does not feel pain when tape is removed (P).
7 Remove and dispose of equipment.	To keep area clean and reduce risk of cross-infection (DH 2005: C).
8 Wash hands.	To reduce the risk of cross-infection (DH 2005: C).
9 Record the procedure in the appropriate documents.	To monitor trends and fluctuation (NMC 2005: C).

References and further reading

Abdollahi, M. *et al.* (2004) Drug-induced toxic reactions in the eye. *J Infus Nurs*, **27**(6), 386–98.

Andrew, S. (2006) Pharmacology. In: *Ophthalmic Care* (ed. J. Marsden). Whurr, Chichester, pp. 42–65.

Ashurst, S. (1997) Nursing care of the mechanically ventilated patient in ITU: 1. *Br J Nurs*, **6**(8), 447–54.

BNF (2006) *British National Formulary No. 51*. British Medical Association, London.

Boyd-Monk, H. (2005). Bringing common eye emergencies into focus. *Nursing*, **35**(12), 46–51.

Carlson, B.A. (2002) Neurologic disorders. In: *Critical Care Nursing: Diagnosis and Management* (eds L. Urden, K. Stacy & M. Lough), 4th edn. Mosby, St. Louis, MO, pp. 671–700.

Char, D.H. (1993) Management of orbital tumours. *Mayo Clin Pract*, **68**, 1081–96.

Cunningham, C. & Gould, D. (1998) Eyecare for the sedated patient undergoing mechanical ventilation: the use of evidence-based care. *Int J Nurs Stud*, **35**, 32–40.

DH (2005) *Saving Lives: A Delivery Programme to Reduce Healthcare Associated Infection Including MRSA*. Department of Health, London.

Ezra, D. *et al.* (2005) Preventing exposure keratopathy in the critically ill: a prospective study comparing eye care regimes. *Br J Ophthalmol*, **89**, 1068–9.

Finger, P.T. (2000) Tumour location affects the incidence of cataract and retinopathy after ophthalmic plaque radiation therapy. *Br J Ophthalmol*, **84**(9), 1068–70.

Forrester, J. *et al.* (2002). *The Eye: Basic Science in Practice*, 2nd edn. Saunders, Edinburgh.

Foss, A.J.E. *et al.* (1999) Modelling uveal melanoma. *Br J Ophthalmol*, **83**, 588–94.

Goddard, A.G., Kingston, J.E. & Hungerford, J.L. (1999) Delay in diagnosis of retinoblastoma: risk factors and treatment outcome. *Br J Ophthalmol*, **83**(12), 1320–3.

Goodman, M. & Wickham, R. (2005) Endocrine malignancies. In: *Cancer Nursing: Principles and Practice* (eds C. Yarbo, M. Hansen Frogge & M. Goodman), 6th edn. Jones and Bartlett, Sudbury, MA, pp. 1215–43.

Joyce, N. & Evans, D. (2006) Eye care for patients in the ICU. *Am J Nurs*, **106**(1), 72AA–DD.

Kirkwood, B. (2006) The cornea. In: *Ophthalmic Care* (ed. J. Marsden). Whurr, Chichester, pp. 339–69.

Kozier, B. *et al.* (1998) Assisting with hygiene. In: *Fundamentals of Nursing: Concepts, Process, Practice*. Addison-Wesley, Menlo Park, CA, pp. 729–84.

Kuckelkorn, R. *et al.* (2002) Emergency treatment of chemical and thermal eye burns. *Acta Ophthalmol Scand*, **80**(1), 4–10.

Lee, A. (2006) The angle and aqueous. In: *Ophthalmic Care* (ed. J. Marsden). Whurr, Chichester, pp. 420–60.

Lindgren, G., Diffey, B.L. & Larko, O. (1998) Basal cell carcinoma of the eyelids and solar ultraviolet radiation exposure. *Br J Ophthalmol*, **82**(12), 1412–5.

Lund, V.J. (1987) The orbit. In: *Otolaryngology* (ed. A.G. Kerr), 5th edn. Butterworth, London.

Marieb, E.N. (2001) *Human Anatomy and Physiology*, 5th edn. Benjamin Cummings, San Francisco.

Marsden, J. (2006) The care of patients presenting with acute problems. In: *Ophthalmic Care* (ed. J. Marsden). Whurr, Chichester, pp. 209–52.

Marsden, J. & Spence, D. (2006) Optics. In: *Ophthalmic Care* (ed. J. Marsden). Whurr, Chichester, pp. 20–41.

McQueen, L. (2006) Eyelids and lacrimal drainage system. In: *Ophthalmic Care* (ed. J. Marsden). Whurr, Chichester, pp. 276–306.

Moeloek, N.F. (1993) Updates in orbital tumours. *Eye Sci*, **9**(1), 40–4.

NMC (2005) *Guidelines for Records and Record Keeping*. Nursing and Midwifery Council, London.

NMC (2006) *A–Z Advice Sheet Consent*. www.nmc.org.

NMC (2008) *Standards for Medicines Management*. Nursing and Midwifery Council, London.

NT (2003) NT skills update – eye care. *Nurs Times*, **99**(8), 28.

Olver, J. & Cassidy, L. (2005) *Ophthamology at a Glance*. Blackwell Science, Malden, MA.

Ryder, A. (2006) The orbit and extraocular muscles. In: *Ophthalmic Care* (ed. J. Marsden). Whurr, Chichester, pp. 510–53.

Shaw, M.E. (2006) Examination of the eye. In: *Ophthalmic Care* (ed. J. Marsden). Whurr, Chichester, pp. 66–84.

Souhami, R. & Tobias, J. (2005) *Cancer and its Management*, 5th edn. Blackwell Publishing, Oxford.

Stollery, R., Shaw, M. & Lee, A. (2005) *Ophthalmic Nursing*, 3rd edn. Blackwell Publishing, Oxford.

Suresh, P. *et al.* (2000) Eye care for the critically ill. *Intensive Care Med*, **26**, 162–6.

Tortora, G.J. & Derrickson, B. (2008) *Principles of Anatomy and Physiology*, 12th edn. John Wiley & Sons, Ltd, Chichester.

Ward, B., Raynel, S. & Catt, G. (2006) The uveal tract. In: *Ophthalmic Care* (ed. J. Marsden). Whurr, Chichester, pp. 396–420.

Chapter 32

Personal hygiene: mouth care

Reference material **648**
Procedure guidelines: Mouth care **654**
Problem solving: Mouth care **656**
References and further reading **657**

Definition

Good mouth care (oral hygiene) is a vital part of nursing care and includes the careful assessment, correct care and the appropriate treatment of the oral cavity including the teeth and mouth (Roberts 2004). White (2004) states that while this is an essential part of nursing care it is an often overlooked aspect of patient care both in the community and hospital setting.

Oral hygiene has been given a much greater profile since its inclusion as one of the clinical benchmarks proposed in *The Essence of Care* (DH 2001). There is still a danger that with the increasing demands made on nursing time and lack of knowledge that oral care may be one of the first things to be set aside (Fitzpatrick 2000; Miller & Kearney 2001; Southern 2007). Damage to the oral cavity secondary to lack of care, disease or treatment may cause multiple problems to the patient and reduce their quality of life (White 2000; Miller & Kearney 2001; Borbasi *et al.* 2002; Sonis *et al.* 2004). The main aims of oral care are to (Cooley 2002):

- Keep the mucosa clean, soft, moist and intact and to prevent infection.
- Keep the lips clean, soft, moist and intact.
- Remove food debris as well as dental plaque without damaging the gingiva.
- Alleviate pain and discomfort and enhance oral intake.
- Prevent halitosis and freshen the mouth.

Reference material

Anatomy and physiology

The mouth is the oval cavity at the anterior end of the digestive tract (Marieb 2004). It consists of the mouth cavity (cavum oris proprium) and the vestibule (vestibulum oris), which is bounded by the lips containing the cheeks, gums, teeth, tongue, hard and soft palate (Thiobodeau & Patton 2007).

The oral cavity is lined with a mucous membrane consisting of three layers: top layer, sub-mucosa and basement layer, consisting of multiple layers of cells, including epithelial and connective tissue (Martini 2007). It is worth noting that damage to the oral mucosa may take place on any or on all of these layers, and while the oral cavity may look normal, damage may still be occurring (Sonis 2004). The oral mucosa is an area of rapid replication designed to meet the constant demands of activities such as chewing and talking, and it is thought that the epithelial layer of the oral mucosa is replaced every 7–14 days (Sonis 2004). The tongue forms the greater part of the floor of the oral cavity.

The mouth has three main functions: (i) to enable ingestion of food and fluids; (ii) to aid communication; and (iii) to support breathing (along with the nasal cavity) (Thiobodeau & Patton 2007).

The mouth is lubricated by secretions from the salivary glands: parotid, submandibular and sublingual. It is believed that as much as 1.5 litres of saliva are produced each day (Dickinson & Porter 2006). The functions of saliva are both protective (preventing infection) and digestive (supporting chewing and swallowing of food) in nature (Sreebny 2000).

Predisposing factors to poor oral health may include:

- Inability to take adequate fluids leading to dehydration and dryness of mucosa.
- Poor nutritional status leading to poor cellular repair and vitamin deficiencies.
- Insufficient saliva production leading to infection and dryness of the mucosa.
- Major intervention altering oral status; surgery, radiotherapy or chemotherapy causing structural changes.
- Lack of knowledge, ability or motivation towards maintaining oral hygiene.
- Other factors: pre-existing dental problems, co-morbidities, drug/oxygen therapy causing dryness, age (children and older adults), genetic factors, alcohol and tobacco use (Barasch & Peterson 2003; Beck 2004).

Oral complications

Oral complications may manifest as taste changes, pain, ulcers, infection, bone and dentition changes, bleeding and functional disorders affecting verbal and non-verbal communication, chewing and swallowing, and respiration (Porter 1994). Stomatitis (inflammation of the oral cavity) results from damage to the mucous membrane and may be induced by trauma, infection or by factors that decrease the proliferation rate of the cells (e.g. chemotherapy and radiotherapy). Oral mucositis is the term usually used to describe the inflammation and ulceration of the oral mucosa associated with chemotherapy and radiation (Dodds 2004). Although not fully understood, it is now clear that the mucosal damage related to cytotoxic treatment is a complex process and thought to consist of five simultaneous phases of mucosal damage consisting of: initiation, up-regulation, signalling and amplification, ulceration and healing (Sonis 2004). Many of the new and developing treatments for oral mucositis in the cancer care setting are aimed at preventing damage in these identified phases (Sonis 2004).

Xerostomia (oral dryness) is often but not always linked to salivary gland dysfunction; oral dryness can be caused by other factors including the continued use of oxygen therapy and inadequate hydration. Salivary gland dysfunction, which may be permanent or temporary, is an alteration in the production and composition of saliva and can be extremely distressing to patients (preventing sleep, causing difficulty in talking, eating and swallowing, and allowing oral pathogens to develop) (Torres *et al.* 2002; Davies 2005). While many patients may experience xerostomia and/or salivary dysfunction, some studies have shown that over 80% of dying patients may suffer from this condition (Chaushu *et al.* 2000; Davies *et al.* 2002). In the cancer setting salivary function can be affected by chemotherapy, radiotherapy and other drugs, including cyclizine and hyoscine (Cheng 2006). The production of saliva may be completely destroyed by radiation to the oral region as the salivary glands are highly sensitive to radiation (Shih *et al.* 2003). While a complex problem, good oral care can provide relief from this distressing symptom (Cheng 2006).

The oral cavity harbours a variety of endogenous bacteria which do not normally pose problems and serve to prevent other forms of pathogens from developing in the cavity (Sonis 2004). However, an inadequate functioning immune system secondary to disease and/or systemic treatments such as cytotoxic therapy (cancer setting), immunosuppression drugs (organ transplant setting) and antifungal therapies may increase the pathogenicity of these organisms leading to local infection. Common organisms include *Pseudomonas*, *Klebsiella*, *Escherichia coli* and *Candida* species (Porter 1994). Local infection may lead to a secondary infection or systemic infection (septicaemia), particularly when the mucosa barrier is damaged (Blijlevens *et al.* 2000).

Halitosis (oral offensive odour) may be very distressing for the patient and for family members (Shorthose & Davies 2005). It is thought that many people in the general population suffer from this condition (Loesche & Kazor 2002). The cause can be either physiological (food debris, epithelial cells, blood cells, saliva), or due to an underlying disease (infection, inflammation, malignancy) (Shorthose & Davies 2005). Careful brushing of the tongue to remove debris, advice on diet, smoking cessation, the use of mouthwashes and where possible treating the underlining cause can relieve this distressing symptom (Shorthose & Davies 2005).

Mouth care

Mouth care involves; patient education and support, regular oral assessment, appropriate frequency of care and the use of oral care equipment and agents. It is clear that nurses do not always feel they have the correct skills and knowledge to support patients with mouth care (Fitzpatrick 2000; Ohrn *et al.* 2000; Southern 2007). Cheng (2006) suggests that in order to achieve compliance, oral care should be realistic, simple and acceptable to patient and family members in hospital, hospice, nursing homes and home care settings.

Oral assessment

Thorough and correct oral assessment is required in planning effective care (Eilers 2004; Sonis *et al.* 2004; Jaroneski 2006; Quinn *et al.* 2007). Assessment of the oral cavity is required to: (i) provide baseline data; (ii) monitor and evaluate response to care and treatment; and (iii) identify new problems as they arise (Holmes & Mountain 1993).

A number of oral assessment tools have been developed including: World Health Organization (WHO) Mucositis Scale (WHO 1979), National Cancer Institute Common Toxicity Criteria (NCI-CTC) (National Institutes of Health 1987), Oral Mucositis Index (OMI) (Schubert *et al.* 1992) and Oral Assessment Guide (OAG; Eilers *et al.* 1988). While some of

these assessment tools have been designed specifically for use in the oncology setting, their relevance and applicability to other settings is clear. The tools share much in common in that all include subjective and objective measures, and include the assessment of: the oral cavity, the presence or absence of erythema, ulcers, pain, saliva, and the ability to eat or drink. In most clinical situations it is essential that the patient is involved in the oral assessment process. In order to fully assess the oral cavity in the cancer setting, the eight areas most susceptible to cytotoxic damage must be inspected (Box 32.1).

> **Box 32.1** Areas of oral cavity most susceptible to cytotoxic damage
>
> - Upper lip (labial mucosa)
> - Lower lip (labial mucosa)
> - Right buccal mucosa
> - Left buccal mucosa
> - Right lateral and ventral tongue
> - Left lateral and ventral tongue
> - Floor of mouth
> - Soft palate
> (Sonis 2004)

Holmes and Mountain (1993) evaluated three oral assessment tools for reliability, validity and clinical usefulness. In their conclusion they showed a preference for that developed by Eilers *et al.* (1988), but stressed that further work is required to develop a tool that is entirely satisfactory for use in clinical practice and future research. Andersson *et al.* (1999) found that Eilers' oral assessment guide with minor amendments for patients undergoing high-dose chemotherapy treatment was a reliable and clinically useful tool for assessing the oral cavity status and determining changes. Other studies have shown a preference for the NCI-CTC and WHO assessments because these simple scales enable the clinical team to consistently correctly assess the oral cavity (Sonis *et al.* 2004; Stone *et al.* 2007). The choice of assessment tool to be used should be decided on, after careful consideration of the clinical environment; however, the WHO scale is simple and easy to use in all clinical settings. Recognizing the need for guidance, a European group of nurses, physicians and dentists have developed recommendations that should be considered when assessing the oral cavity (Quinn *et al.* 2007).

Frequency of care

Dodd *et al.* (2000) concluded that the incidence of oral complications was reduced by the frequency of care rather than the agents employed. However, there has been little research to indicate the most effective frequency. Various suggested time intervals including 2-hourly, 4-hourly, after meals and before bed have been proposed (Beck 2004).

649

Following a review of earlier studies Krishnasamy (1995) recommends the following:

- Four-hourly care will reduce the potential for infection from micro-organisms.
- Two-hourly care will reduce mouth care problems and ensure patient comfort.
- One-hourly care is recommended for patients requiring oxygen therapy, those who are mouth breathing, who have an infected mouth or are unconscious (intubated and dying patients).

There is however a need for further research and frequency of care should be carefully considered in each particular clinical situation (McNeill 2000). Basic oral care should always include the removal of any debris to prevent infection and steps to keep the mucosa moist in order to provide comfort (Sonis 2004).

Oral care equipment

A variety of equipment that may be used in caring for the mouth has been reported in the literature, including toothbrush, foam-stick, dental floss and gauze. The most appropriate piece of equipment should be determined by its efficacy together with its potential to damage the gingiva. The use of the toothbrush is well supported by the literature and is the most effective tool at removing debris from the teeth and gums, including plaque (Clay 2000; Xavier 2000; Pearson & Hutton 2002). The foamstick, however, can cause less trauma, particularly when oral care includes free surgical flaps and skin grafts (Hahn & Jones 2000) or oral bleeding occurs as a result of thrombocytopenia (Walton et al. 2002). Care must be taken to ensure that the toothbrush is kept free from infection as toothbrushes have been shown to harbour organisms such as group A beta-haemolytic streptococci, staphylococci, Candida and Pseudomonas (Brook & Gober 1998). These organisms have been found to contribute to persistent oropharyngeal infections (Brook & Gober 1998; Taji & Rogers 1998). Borowski et al. (1994) demonstrated that good oral hygiene, such as brushing the gingiva and teeth, can help to decrease the incidence of septicaemia.

Maintaining good oral hygiene

In most clinical situations oral care should include tooth brushing and rinsing of the mouth to remove debris and reduce oral complications (Beck 2004). Nurses should:

- Encourage/support patient to clean teeth with toothpaste and toothbrush (removing debris) after meals. Toothpaste must be removed from the oral cavity through thorough rinsing as prolonged contact with teeth and mucosa of some agents (glycerine) can cause damage.
- Encourage/support the patient to keep mucosa and lips moist (sipping fluids/application of oral lubricant, such as petroleum gel, KY gel, Vaseline).

- Consider use of sodium chloride 0.9%, to be swilled in the mouth and discarded to help cleanse the mouth and remove any debris.
- Possible use of chlorhexidine gluconate 0.2% 5 ml, four times a day, which should be retained in the mouth for at least 1 minute before discarding.
- Consider use of other oral care agents and analgesia; glycerin, nystatin, paracetamol, aspirin, opiates.
- Care should be delivered in a dignified and gentle manner (Sweeney 2005).

Oral care agents

The choice of an oral care agent will be dependent on the aim of care. The agent may be used to remove debris and plaque, prevent superimposed infection, alleviate pain, provide comfort, stop bleeding, provide lubrication or treat specific problems (Dickinson & Porter 2006). A wide variety of agents are available and should be determined by the individual needs of the patient and the particular clinical situation together with a detailed nursing assessment. There is ongoing debate on the efficacy of the agents presently available and there remains insufficient evidence to clearly state the best agents to use in the clinical setting. Most of the agents described below are included in *The Royal Marsden Hospital Prescribing Guidelines for Mouth Care* (Royal Marsden Hospital 2002).

Normal saline (sodium chloride 0.9%)
The use of normal saline is supported by a number of authors as part of a patient's oral care. This relatively cheap and generally well-tolerated solution can be rinsed in the mouth and then discarded. It helps to loosen and remove debris, moistens the mucosa, helps alleviate discomfort and promote healing (Madeya 1996; Cheng et al. 2001).

Chlorhexidine gluconate
Chlorhexidine is a compound with broad-spectrum antimicrobial activity that results in binding to and sustained release from mucosal surfaces (Ferretti et al. 1990). While chlorhexidine continues to be widely used in clinical settings its efficacy has been widely debated in certain clinical situations. Ferretti et al. (1990) in their study found that it had protected patients in their study group from infection and helped to resolve existing infections, reducing soft tissue disease and oral microbial burden. Likewise, Rawlins and Trueman (2001) believe that chlorhexidine can greatly reduce bacteria in seriously ill patients. However, some studies have shown that it is not effective as a prophylatic treatment in the cancer setting (Worthington et al. 2003). In one study of 222 outpatients, Dodd et al. (1996) found that chlorhexidine as a mouthwash was no more effective than water in preventing chemotherapy-induced mucositis. While Foote et al. (1994) showed that patients receiving chlorhexidine mouthwash while undergoing radiation therapy showed a trend to develop more mucositis than those receiving a placebo mouthwash, leading to the hypothesis that chlorhexidine

may be detrimental in this clinical setting. Having reviewed the existing evidence, Barasch *et al.* (2006) advise against the use of chlorhexidine for chemotherapy-induced mucositis. It is clear that chlorhexidine should be used with caution and further research needs to be done within this area.

Antifungal treatment

Nystatin is the best known and most commonly used antifungal agent (Campbell 1995). It is an antifungal antibiotic that is used as an oral suspension (Finlay & Davies 2005). Barkvoll *et al.* (1989) showed in their in vitro study that combinations of nystatin and chlorhexidine gluconate were not effective against *Candida albicans* and recommended that the most efficient treatment plan must be restricted to the use of one of these drugs alone.

Fluconazole is an antifungal that has been demonstrated to be effective in the treatment of candidiasis of the oropharynx, oesophagus and a variety of deep tissue sites (Brammer 1990). Fluconazole can be administered as a capsule, suspension or as an intravenous infusion. Although most patients will not require fluconazole as a prophylactic measure, it may be given prophylactically in certain clinical settings when patients are severely immunocompromised (haemato-oncology/stem cell transplant setting). It is often the treatment of choice for suspected fungal infection (Finlay & Davies 2005). Other antifungal drugs may include: amphotericin, ketoconazole, miconazole and itraconazole (Finlay & Davies 2005).

Sucralfate

Sucralfate is a complex of aluminium hydroxide and sulphated sucrose which may be used to protect the oral mucosa. In one study, Barker *et al.* (1991) showed that consistent daily oral hygiene and use of a mouth-coating agent such as sucralfate in patients receiving radiotherapy results in less pain, may reduce weight loss and interruption of radiation therapy because of severe mucositis. However, Barasch *et al.* (2006) having reviewed the literature do not recommend the use of sucralfate for radiotherapy-induced mucositis. Some reduction in pain and increase in oral intake have been shown in patients with chemotherapy-induced ulcerating or erythematous mucositis taking oral sucralfate (Rattan *et al.* 1994). However, Chiara *et al.* (2001) performed a pilot study to assess the efficacy of sucralfate gel for the treatment of chemotherapy-induced mucositis and found that the suspension did not demonstrate any significant advantage over the placebo used. Further research is therefore needed. The administration of sucralfate and enteral feeds should be separated by 1 hour to avoid interactions and used with extreme caution in patients with renal impairment (Royal Pharmaceutical Society of Great Britain 2006).

Fluoride

Fluoride helps to prevent and arrest tooth decay, especially radiation caries, demineralization and decalcification. Following its use, no food or fluids should be taken for at least 30 minutes in order for it to work (Cooke 1996).

Artificial saliva

Saliva substitutes duplicate the properties of normal saliva (Kusler & Rambur 1992). They buffer the acidity of the mouth and lubricate the mucous membranes (Heals 1993).

Over-the-counter oral mouthwashes should be used with caution and the ingredients should be critically assessed before use as some ingredients, including alcohol, can cause further discomfort to an already damaged mucosa (Sonis 2004).

Problems

Fungal

Oral candidiasis is known to be the cause of most oral fungal infections. It usually occurs as a result of both host factors (immunosuppression, nutritional problems) and mucosal damage secondary to treatment (Finlay & Davies 2005).

Prophylaxis

Nystatin mouthwash 1 ml used four times a day. This should be rinsed around the mouth and retained for at least 1 minute before swallowing. Dentures must be removed prior to rinsing. One millimetre of nystatin oral suspension can be added to the water to soak acrylic dentures (Walton *et al.* 2002). If using chlorhexidine, a time interval of 15–30 minutes should be allowed between administration of chlorhexidine and nystatin to ensure efficacy.

Treatment

Surgical patients:

- First-line: nystatin 5 ml four times a day.
- Second-line: fluconazole 50 mg tablet or sugar-free suspension, daily for 7 days.

Radiotherapy/chemotherapy patients:

- First-line: fluconazole 50 mg orally, daily for 7 days. Use 100 mg intravenously daily if patients cannot tolerate oral therapy.
- Second-line: fluconazole 200–400 mg intravenously daily until able to tolerate oral therapy.

Viral infections

Many viral infections may not require any specific treatment. However, infections such as herpes simplex virus will require treatment with topical 5% aciclovir, while severely immunocompromised patients may require systemic treatment with aciclovir or other antiviral agents to prevent and treat infection (Bagg 2005b). Other viral infections will require careful treatment consideration.

Bacterial infections

Bacterial infections of the oral cavity may require treatment with antibiotics. Clinicians should liaise with the microbiology department about the most appropriate use of drug. Bacterial abscesses within the mouth may require drainage

651

DH (2005) *Saving Lives: a Delivery Programme to Reduce Health-care Associated Infections including MRSA: Skills for Implementation*. Department of Health, London.

Dickinson, L. & Porter, H. (2006) Oral care. In: *Nursing in Haematological Nursing* (ed. M. Grundy), 2nd edn. Balliere Tindall, Edinburgh, pp. 371–86.

Dodds, M.J. (2004) The pathogenesis and characterisation of oral mucositis associated with cancer therapy. *Oncol Nurs Forum*, **31**(4), 5–11.

Dodd, M.J. *et al.* (1996) Randomized clinical trial of chlorhexidine versus placebo for prevention of oral mucositis in patients receiving chemotherapy. *Oncol Nurs Forum*, **23**(6), 921–7.

Dodd, M.J. *et al.* (2000) Randomised clinical trial of the effectiveness of three commonly used mouthwashes to treat chemotherapy-induced mucositis. *Oral Surg Oral Med Oral Path*, **90**(1), 39–47.

Dose, A.M. (1992) Cryotherapy for prevention of 5-fluorouracil-induced mucositis. Cancer nursing, changing frontiers. Proceedings of the 7th International Conference of Cancer Nursing. *Eur J Cancer Care*, **2**(1), 95–7.

Dudjak, L. (1987) Mouth care for mucositis due to radiation therapy. *Cancer Nurs*, **10**, 131–40.

Eilers, J. (2004) Nursing interventions and supportive care for the prevention and treatment of oral mucositis associated with cancer treatment. *Oncol Nurs Forum*, **31**(4), 13–23.

Eilers, J. *et al.* (1988) Development, testing and application of the oral assessment guide. *Oncol Nurs Forum*, **15**(3), 325–30.

Feber, T. (1996) Management of oral mucositis in oral irradiation. *Clin Oncol*, **8**, 106–11.

Ferretti, G.A. *et al.* (1990) Chlorhexidine prophylaxis for chemotherapy- and radiotherapy-induced stomatitis: a randomised double-blind trial. *Oral Surg Oral Med Oral Pathol*, **69**(3), 331–7.

Finlay, I. & Davies, A. (2005) Fungal infections. In: *Oral Care in Advanced Disease* (eds A. Davies & I. Finlay). Oxford University Press, Oxford, pp. 55–72.

Fitzpatrick, J. (2000) Oral health care needs of dependent older people: responsibilities of nurses and care staff. *J Adv Nurs*, **32**(6), 1325–32.

Foote, R.L. *et al.* (1994) Randomized trial of a chlorhexidine mouthwash for alleviation of radiation-induced mucositis. *J Clin Oncol*, **12**(12), 2630–3.

Grealy, L. (1994) *Autobiography of a Face*. Harperennial, New York.

Hahn, M.J. & Jones, A. (2000) Mouth care. In: *Head and Neck Nursing*. Churchill Livingstone, London, pp. 35–57.

Heals, D. (1993) A key to well being: oral hygiene in patients with advanced cancer. *Prof Nurse*, **8**(6), 391–8.

Holmes, S. (1990) *Cancer Chemotherapy*. Lisa Sainsbury Foundation. Austen Cornish, London, pp. 180–1.

Holmes, S. & Mountain, E. (1993) Assessment of oral status: evaluation of three oral assessment guides. *J Clin Nurs*, **2**, 35–40.

Howarth, H. (1977) Mouth care procedures for the very ill. *Nurs Times*, **73**, 354–5.

Jaroneski, L.A. (2006) The importance of assessment rating scales for chemotherapy-induced oral mucositis. *Oncol Nurs Forum*, **33**(6), 1085–93.

Johnson, J.T. *et al.* (1993) Oral pilocarpine for post irradiation xerostomia in patients with head and neck cancer. *N Engl J Med*, **329**(6), 390–5.

Jones, A.L. & Gore, M.E. (1995) Medical treatment of malignant tumours of the mouth, jaw and salivary glands. In: *Malignant Tumours of the Mouth, Jaws and Salivary Glands* (eds J.D. Langdon & J.M. Henk), 2nd edn. Edward Arnold, London, pp. 123–35.

Kannan, V. *et al.* (1997) Efficacy and safety of granulocyte macrophage-colony stimulating factor (GM-CSF) on the frequency and severity of radiation mucositis in patients with head and neck carcinoma. *Int J Radiat Oncol Biol Phys*, **37**(5), 1005–10.

Keefe, D.M. *et al.* (2007) Mucositis Study Section of the Multinational Association of Supportive Care in Cancer and the International Society for Oral Oncology. *Cancer*, **109**(5), 820–31.

Killoy, W.J. (1998) Chemical treatment of periodontitis: local delivery of antimicrobials. *Int Dent J*, **3**(Suppl), 305–15.

Kozier, B. *et al.* (2003) Hygiene. In: *Fundamentals of Nursing: Concepts, Process & Practice*. Pearson Education, New Jersy, pp. 695–755.

Krishnasamy, M. (1995) Oral problems in advanced cancer. *Eur J Cancer Care*, **4**, 173–7.

Kusler, D.L. & Rambur, B.A. (1992) Treatment for radiation-induced xerostomia: an innovative remedy. *Cancer Nurs*, **15**(3), 191–5.

Larson, P.J. *et al.* (1998) The PRO-SELF mouth aware programme: an effective approach for reducing chemotherapy-induced mucositis. *Cancer Nurs*, **21**(4), 263–8.

Lippold, A.J.C. & Winton, F.R. (1972) *Hearing and Speech Human Physiology*. Churchill Livingstone, Edinburgh, pp. 443–64.

Loesche, W.J. & Kazor, C. (2002) Microbiology and treatment of halitosis. *Periodontol 2000*, **28**, 256–79.

Madeya, M.L. (1996) Oral complications from cancer therapy. Part 2: nursing implications for assessment and treatment. *Oncol Nurs Forum*, **23**(5), 808–19.

Mahood, D.J. *et al.* (1991) Inhibition of fluorouracil-induced stomatitis by oral cryotherapy. *J Clin Oncol*, **9**(3), 449–52.

Makkonen, T.A. *et al.* (2000) Granulocyte macrophage-colony stimulating factor (GM-CSF) and sucralfate in prevention of radiation-induced mucositis: a prospective randomised study. *Int J Radiat Oncol Biol Phys*, **46**(3), 525–34.

Marieb, E.N. (2004) *Human Anatomy & Physiology*, 6th edn. Pearson, San Francisco.

Martini, F. (2007) *Fundamentals of Anatomy and Physiology*, 7th edn. Benjamin Cummings, San Francisco, CA.

Mascarin, M. *et al.* (1999) The effect of granulocyte colony-stimulating factor on oral mucositis in head and neck cancer patients treated with hyperfractionated radiotherapy. *Oral Oncol*, **35**, 203–8.

McGuire, D.B. *et al.* (2006) The role of basic oral care and good clinical practice principles in the management of oral mucositis. *Support Care Cancer*, **14**, 541–5.

McNeill, H.E. (2000) Biting back at poor oral hygiene. *Inten Crit Care Nurs*, **16**, 367–72.

Miller, M. & Kearney, N. (2001) Oral care for patients with cancer: a review of the literature. *Cancer Nurs*, **24**(4), 241–54.

National Institutes of Health (1987) *Consensus Development Conference Statement on Oral Complications of Cancer Therapies: Diagnosis, Prevention, and Treatment*. National Cancer Institute, **7**(17), 1–11.

Nicolatou, O. *et al.* (1998) A pilot study of the effect of granulocyte-macrophage colony-stimulating factor on oral mucositis in head and neck cancer patients during X-radiation therapy. *Int J Radiat Oncol Biol Phys*, **42**(3), 551–6.

NMC (2006) *A–Z Advice Sheet Consent*. www.nmc.org.

Ohrn, K.E.O., Wahlin, Y.B. & Sjoden, P.O. (2000) Oral care in cancer nursing. *Eur J Cancer Care*, **9**, 22–9.

Pearson, L.S. (1996) A comparison of the ability of foam swabs and toothbrushes to remove dental plaque: implications for nursing practice. *J Adv Nurs*, **23**(1), 62–9.

Pearson, L.S. & Hutton, J.L. (2002) A controlled trial to compare the ability of foam swabs and toothbrushes to remove dental plaque. *J Adv Nurs*, **39**(5), 480–9.

Porter, H.J. (1994) Mouth care in cancer. *Nurs Times*, **90**(14), 27–9.

Porter, H.J. (2000) Oral care. In: *Nursing in Haematological Oncology* (ed. M. Grundy). Harcourt, London, pp. 371–85.

Quinn, B. *et al.* (2007) Ensuring accurate oral mucositis assessment in the European Group for Blood and Marrow Transplantation Prospective Oral Mucositis Audit. *Eur J Oncol Nurs*, **11**(Supp 1), 10–18.

Rattan, J. *et al.* (1994) Sucralfate suspension as a treatment of recurrent aphthous stomatitis. *J Intern Med*, **236**, 341–3.

Rawlins, C.A. & Trueman, J.W. (2001) Effective mouth care for seriously ill patients. *Prof Nurs*, **16**(14), 1025–8.

Ripamonti, C. & Fulfaro, F. (2005) Taste disturbance. In: *Oral Care in Advanced Disease* (eds A. Davies & I. Finlay). Oxford University Press, Oxford, pp. 115–24.

Roberts, J. (2004) Developing an oral assessment and intervention tool for older people. In: *Trends in Oral Health Care* (ed. R. White). Quay Books, Wiltshire, pp. 11–35.

Rovirosa, A., Ferre, J. & Biete, A. (1998) Granulocyte macrophage-colony stimulating factor mouthwashes heal oral ulcers during head and neck radiotherapy. *Int J Radiat Oncol Biol Phys*, **41**(4), 747–54.

Royal Marsden Hospital (2002) *The Royal Marsden Hospital Prescribing Guidelines for Mouth Care*. Drugs and Therapeutic Advisory Committee, September. The Royal Marsden Hospital, London.

Royal Pharmaceutical Society of Great Britain (2006) *British National Formulary*. RFS Publishing, Bedfordshire.

Rubenstein, E.B. *et al.* (2004) Clinical practice guidelines for the prevention and treatment of cancer therapy-induced oral and gastrointestinal mucositis. *Cancer*, **100**(9 Suppl), 2026–46.

Schubert, M.M. *et al.* (1992) Clinical assessment scale for rating of oral mucosal changes associated with bone marrow transplantation. *Cancer*, **69**, 2469–77.

Shih, A. *et al.* (2003) Mechanisms for radiation-induced oral mucositis and the consequences. *Cancer Nurs*, **26**(3), 222–9.

Shorthose, K. & Davies, A. (2005) Halitosis. In: *Oral Care in Advanced Disease* (eds A. Davies & I. Finlay). Oxford University Press, Oxford, pp. 125–32.

Smith, A.J. *et al.* (1996) The efficacy of an anti-gingivitis chewing gum. *J Clin Periodontol*, **23**(1), 19–23.

Sonis, S. (2004) The pathobiology of mucositis. *Nat Rev Cancer*, **4**(4), 277–84.

Sonis, S. *et al.* (2004) Perspectives on cancer therapy-induced mucosal injury: pathogenesis, measurement, epidemiology, and consequences for patients. *Cancer Suppl*, **100**(9), 1995–2025.

Southern, H. (2007) Oral care in cancer nursing: nurses' knowledge and education. *J Adv Nurs*, **57**(6), 631–8.

Spijkervet, F.K. & Sonis, S.T. (1998) New frontiers in the management of chemotherapy-induced mucositis. *Curr Opin Oncol*, **10**(Suppl 1), S23–7.

Sprinzl, G.M. *et al.* (2001) Local application of granulocyte-macrophage colony stimulating factor (GM-CSF) for the treatment of oral mucositis. *Eur J Cancer*, **37**, 2003–9.

Sreebny, L.M. (2000) Saliva in health and disease: an appraisal and update. *Int Dent J*, **50**, 140–61.

Sreebny, L.M., Zhu, W.X. & Meek, A.G. (1995) The preparation of an autologous saliva for use with patients undergoing therapeutic radiation for head and neck cancer. *J Oral Maxillofac Surg*, **53**(2), 131–9.

Stiff, P. (2001) Mucositis associated with stem cell transplantation: current status and innovative approaches to management. *Bone Marrow Transplant*, **27**, S3–11.

Stone, B. *et al.* (2005) Improving oral care: quality control of oral mucositis assessment in the EBMT prospective oral mucositis audit. *Bone Marrow Transplant*, **37**(1), S273–274.

Stone, R. *et al.* (2007) Management of oral mucositis at European transplantation centres. *Eur J Oncol Nurs*, **11**(Suppl 1), 3–9.

Sweeney, M.P. *et al.* (1995) Oral health in elderly patients. *Br J Nurs*, **4**(20), 1204–8.

Sweeney, P. (2005) Oral hygiene. In: *Oral Care in Advanced Disease* (eds A. Davies & I. Finlay). Oxford University Press, Oxford, pp. 21–36.

Taji, S.S. & Rogers, A.H. (1998) ADRF Trebitsch Scholarship. The microbial contamination of toothbrushes. A pilot study. *Aust Dent J*, **43**(2), 128–30.

Thiobodeau, G.A. & Patton, K.T. (2007) *Anatomy & Physiology*, 6th edn. Elsevier, St Louis, MO.

Torres, S.R. *et al.* (2002) Relationship between salivary flow rates and *Candida* counts in subjects with xerostomia. *Oral Surg Oral Med Oral Path*, **93**(2), 149–54.

Toth, B.B. & Frame, R.T. (1983) Dental oncology. *Curr Probl Cancer*, **10**, 7–35.

Toth, B.B., Chambers, M.S. & Fleming, T.C. (1996) Prevention and management of oral complications associated with cancer therapies: radiotherapy/chemotherapy. *Texas Dent J*, **113**(6), 23–9.

Walton, J.C., Miller, J. & Tordecilla, L. (2002) Elder oral assessment and care. *ORL Head Neck Nurs*, **20**(2), 12–19.

Waly, N.G. (1995) Local antifibrinolytic treatment with tranexamic acid in hemophiliac children undergoing dental extractions. *Egypt Dent J*, **41**(1), 961–8.

White, R. (2004) Oral health assessment: a review of current practice. In: *Trends in Oral Health Care* (ed. R. White). Quay Books, Wiltshire, pp. 1–10.

White, R.J. (2000) Nurse assessment of oral health: a review of practice and education. *Br J Nursing*, **9**(5), 260–6.

WHO (1979) *Handbook for Reporting Results of Cancer Treatment*. Offset Publications, Geneva, **48**, pp. 15–22.

Worthington, H.V., Clarkson, J.E. & Eden, O.B. (2003) Interventions for the prevention of oral mucositis for patients with cancer receiving treatments. *Cochrane Database Syst Rev*, **2**.

Xavier, G. (2000) The importance of mouth care in prevention. *Nurs Stand*, **14**(18), 47–51.

Yusef, Z.W. & Bakri, M.M. (1993) Severe progressive periodontal destruction due to radiation tissue injury. *J Periodontol*, **64**(12), 1253–8.

Chapter 33

Personal hygiene: skin care

661 Reference material
664 *Procedure guidelines:* Bed bathing a patient
666 References and further reading

Definition

Personal hygiene is the physical act of cleaning the body to ensure that the skin, hair and nails are maintained in an optimum condition (DH 2001a). The prevention of infection is also pertinent and will be referred to within the text (see also Chapter 6).

Reference material

'Cleanliness is not a luxury in a highly developed country, it is...a basic human right' (Young 1991, p. 54). When an individual becomes ill, he or she may depend on others to perform this elementary intervention. If this occurs, it is important that the nurse is able to appropriately observe and assess the patient.

Hygiene is a personal entity and everyone will have their own individual requirements and standards of cleanliness. In this way, 'nurses must take care not to impose their own norms on patients and clients and should respect their autonomy in decisions concerning care' (Spiller 1992, p. 431). When assessing personal considerations, the patient's religious and cultural beliefs should be taken into account. Personal hygiene is individual to that person and is also based on family influences, peer groups, economic and social factors (Cooper 1994). Various examples of this will be discussed in this chapter.

In Western culture, privacy is of the utmost importance and considered to be a basic human right. In some cultures, modesty is crucial, e.g. for Muslims, and can cause problems in the hospital setting (Neuberger 1987). Patients will feel a great deal of embarrassment having to depend on another person to help/assist them with this extremely private act and consideration should be given to their personal needs (Wagnild & Manning 1985; Spiller 1992). It is therefore surprising to find that such little reference is made to these elements in the literature. The nurse's role is continued provision of appropriate levels of cleanliness (Young 1991), which promotes 'comfort, safety and well-being' for the patient, and should be carried out with skill and knowledge (Whiting 1999, p. 339). Frequently, the time taken to attend to personal hygiene will provide ample opportunity for communication. Wilson states:

> ...a bedbath facilitates listening and enables the nurse to pick up cues to a patient's anxieties and fears. It provides the time and opportunity for the nurse to offer support and encouragement when difficult situations have to be confronted, solutions sought and decisions made.
>
> (Wilson 1986, p. 81)

This also focuses on the nurse's ability to be with the patient as well as provide for the patient (Campbell 1984) and is part of the essence of nursing care (Kitson 1999). This derives from theorists such as Henderson (1966) and Nightingale (1969) focusing on the aspect of patient-centred care or holistic care. This is as essential when thinking of the personal hygiene of patients as it is about the uniqueness of patients, their needs and how they wish to be treated.

It is during the delivery of personal hygiene that the nurse is able to demonstrate a wide range of skills such as assessment, communication, observation and caring for the patient. This can be the most significant social interaction of the day for the patient, as the nurse develops a deeper understanding of the patient's personality and needs, providing a personal bond between the nurse and patient (Hector & Touhy 1997). Health care assistants with a recognized qualification such as a National Vocational Qualification (NVQ) can complement the role of the qualified nurse in the implementation of planned care. It is vital that health professionals share their knowledge and any changes identified during procedures; personal feedback and documentation are good vehicles for this.

Nursing models, which provide a conceptual framework for practice, all make some reference to meeting the patient's hygiene needs. Roper *et al.* (1981) adapted Henderson's original concept of nursing (Henderson 1966) to develop a model reflecting the activities of daily living. Another example was given by Orem (1980) who focused on the ability of the patient to self-care and refers to the universal self-care requisites of the skin, nail and hair condition and the patterns of standard hygiene. Gordon (1994) discusses formulation of nursing diagnosis. Following assessment, clusters of actual or potential health problems are established; specific diagnosis are used to describe these. Clinical knowledge is then applied, to provide problem solving activities to achieve a set outcome.

Benchmarking is a valid framework by which nurses can establish and share best practice throughout the work environment. Three benchmarks, hygiene, self-care and privacy and dignity cited in the *Essence of Care* (CH 2001a), are important to consider when reviewing patient hygiene, and the needs should be carried out to an uncompromising standard (Geraghty 2005):

- All patients are assessed to identify the advice and/or assistance required in maintaining and promoting their individual personal hygiene.
- Planned care is negotiated with patients and/or their carers and is based on assessment of their individual needs.
- Patients have access to an environment that is safe and acceptable to the individual.
- Patients are expected to supply their own toiletries but single-use toiletries are provided until they can supply their own.
- Patients have access to the level of assistance that they require to meet their individual personal hygiene (DH 2001a).

Areas of care

Skin care

A definition of healthy skin is that it is fulfilling all of its functions, so an individual's quality of life is not adversely affected (Penzer & Finch 2001). Being the largest organ of the body, maintaining its integrity is essential to the prevention of infection and the promotion of both physical and psychological health. The skin has several functions (Burr & Penzer 2005):

- Regulation of temperature.
- Physical protection and immunological protection.
- Excretion and preservation of water balance.
- Sensory perception.
- Psycho-social: how the individual is perceived.

It is made up of three layers: the epidermis, dermis and the deep subcutaneous layer.

The *epidermis* is the outer coating of the skin and contains no blood vessels or nerve endings. The cells on the surface are gradually shed from the surface and replaced by new cells which have developed from the deeper layers; this process takes approximately 28 days. The epidermis has hairs, sweat glands and the ducts of sebaceous glands passing through it. It provides an efficient natural barrier (Burr & Penzer 2005).

The *dermis* is the thicker layer which contains blood vessels, nerve fibres, sweat and sebaceous glands and lymph vessels. It is made up of white fibrous tissue and yellow elastic fibres which give the skin its toughness and elasticity. It provides the epidermis with structural and nutritional support (Holloway & Jones 2005).

The *subcutaneous layer* contains the deep fat cells (areolar and adipose tissue) and provides the heat regulation factor for the body. It is also the support structure for the outer layers of the skin (Ross & Wilson 2001). Maintaining the skin integrity, through good personal hygiene, will allow this complex process to provide the efficient natural barrier.

It is important to remember the skin is a changing organ, affected by internal and external factors, temperature, air humidity and age (Burr & Penzer 2005). It has a great ability to adapt to changes in the environment and stimuli; however, it will be affected by ill health and immobility (McLoughlin 2005). Its integrity, continuity and cleanliness are essential to maintain its physiological functions.

The ageing process can adversely affect the skin structure. Skin tissue becomes thin, less elastic and resistant to trauma and shearing forces. The blood supply is reduced as cells replace more slowly; affecting healing. Transmission from sensory receptors on stimuli slows and can lead to damage. The natural oils produced decline and can lead to dry skin which increases the risk of infection and tissue breakdown (Penzer & Finch 2001) (see Chapter 48). Hence extra care and vigilance should be taken when washing and drying elderly patients; nursing interventions can protect and restore the skin's natural barrier (Ersser *et al.* 2005).

An initial assessment using observational skills is essential to ascertain the skin's general condition, colour, texture, smell and temperature (Penzer & Finch 2001). To accurately observe and assess changes in the skin, an understanding of the structure and function and factors that cause disruption is essential, so as to identify those at increased risk (Ersser *et al.* 2005).

Several factors may influence the appearance of the tissue:

- Nutritional and hydration state: imbalances will cause loss of elasticity and drying of the skin. Oedema will cause stretching and thinning of the skin (Potter & Perry 1995).
- Incontinence: the presence of urine and faeces on the skin increase the normal pH of 4.0–5.5 and makes the skin wet. This rise of pH and excess moisture increase the risks of tissue breakdown and infection (Ersser *et al.* 2005).
- The individual's age, health and mobility status (Smoker 1999), e.g. presence of pressure ulcers (see Chapter 48).
- Treatment therapies, e.g. radiotherapy (skin may become moist and cracked), chemotherapy (some cytotoxic agents such as methotrexate can cause erythematous rashes) and continuous infusions of 5-fluorouracil (5-FU) can cause a condition called palmar–plantar erythrodysesthesia syndrome, which presents with cracking and epidermal sloughing of the palms and soles (Lokich & Moore 1984). A low platelet count can lead to an increased risk of bruising and a decrease in the white blood cells can influence the rate of healing. Steroids may cause the skin to become papery and fragile (see Chapters 35 & 48).
- Any concurrent conditions, e.g. eczema, psoriasis, diabetes, or stress can affect the ability of skin to maintain its integrity (Holloway & Jones 2005).

Frailty and the presence of pressure ulcers, redness, abrasions, cuts, papery skin and open wounds should prompt the nurse to take extra care in the bathing procedure. Involving patients in their care plans ensures that correct and/or preferred lotions are used. Persistent use of some soaps can alter the pH of the skin and remove the natural oils, leading to drying and cracking (Smoker 1999), and provide an ideal environment for bacteria to multiply (Holloway & Jones 2005). According to Ersser *et al.* (2005), patients with dry skin have a 2.5-fold likelihood of skin break down. In addition, patients may like to use moisturizers and this should be respected and applied accordingly. Care should be taken with skin folds and crevices, paying particular attention to thorough drying of the areas and observing for any breaks in the skin. It is recommended that the skin is patted and not rubbed, to reduce damage caused by friction (Ersser *et al.* 2005).

A growing body of evidence is recommending a move away from traditional washing using soap and water, for some of the reasons mentioned previously. Penzer and Finch (2001) and Burr and Penzer (2005) recommend a soap substitute using emollient therapy, for washing and moisturizing to seal the skin. In a literature review of hygiene practices, the use of soap and water remains common practice; however several studies suggest skin cleansers, for example emollient creams, followed by moisturizing, may be less likely to disrupt the skin barrier and have a therapeutic benefit (Ersser *et al.* 2005). A different range of products are allowing the patient to play a more active role (Collins & Hampton 2003). Prepackaged clothes impregnated with cleanser and moisturizer are a cost-effective, evidence-based alternative (Sheppard & Brenner 2000). They require no rinsing and are as effective at cleansing and more skin preserving than soap and water (Byers *et al.* 1995).

Frequently, patients may have intravenous devices and wound drains inserted as part of their therapy and these should be handled with caution to prevent the hazards of introducing infection or of 'pulling' the tubes.

Patients who require assistance may be able to have a bath or shower depending on their level of dependence. Alternatively, assistance with care may occur by the bedside or in bed as 'bed bathing'. When practising bed bathing the nurse informs the patient of his/her plan of care, seeking consent from the patient or patient's family/carer, especially if hoists, slides or transfer sheets are to be used. The nurse must also respect cultural and religious factors, privacy and dignity at all times, e.g. some people prefer to sit under running water as opposed to sitting in a bath (Sampson 1982).

- Those following Islam must do ablution (Wudhu, to use the Islamic term) before the daily prayer, which is the formal washing of the face, hands and forearms, etc. One of the criteria for cleanliness is washing after the use of the lavatories. Any traces of urine or faeces must be eliminated by washing with water, at least. The use of toilet tissues for cleaning is not sufficient. With such emphasis on washing and personal hygiene, adhering to the practical teaching of Islam on washing would enhance personal hygiene for the individual and therefore reduce the chance of disease and sickness individually and subsequently for the whole society.
- Hindus also place importance on washing before prayer; they believe the left hand should dominate in this process and therefore do not eat with the left hand as it is deemed unclean.
- Sikhs place great importance on not shaving or cutting hair, choosing to comb their hair twice a day, wash regularly, and wear their hair underneath a turban in a sign of respect for God.

Perineal/perianal care

When the nurse is performing care for the perineal/ perianal area, the patient may be embarrassed or humiliated. Care should be taken to maintain privacy at all times. It is important that informed consent is sought. This requires the nurse and patient to engage in a two-way process: where agreement is given for the nurse to provide care (DH 2001b).

It is important to be meticulous with this area, especially for those people who may be prone to infection (see Chapter 18).

Problems arising from treatment therapy, for example radiotherapy, fistulae, diarrhoea, constipation and urinary tract infections, require additional vigilance with cleanliness and patients should be encouraged at every opportunity to perform this themselves (see Chapter 35) (Haisfield Wolfe 1998).

Ideally, perineal hygiene should be attended to after the general bath or, at the very least, the water and wipes should be changed and cleaned once utilized (Gooch 1989; Gould 1994) due to the large colonies of bacteria that tend to live in or around this area (Gould 1994). It is generally acknowledged that soap and lotions administered improperly to the perineum/perianal area can cause irritation and infection (Ersser *et al.* 2005; Holloway & Jones 2005). Many nurses will use soap or a similar chemical derivative in order to promote and ensure thorough cleaning, but frequently lack of knowledge can lead to further problems and discomfort for the patients (Lindell & Olsson 1989). It is suggested that warm water alone be used to avoid irritating the mucous membranes which become sensitive during the ageing process.

Hair care

The way a person feels is often related to their appearance. Hair care can be complex: consideration should be given to the patient's personal preferences.

Washing of the hair can be difficult if a patient is bedbound, but there are several ways to manage this. To wash a patient's hair, move the patient to the top of the bed and hang their head over the end. The patient's condition must be assessed before performing this task; for example, it would not be appropriate for patients with head and neck or spinal injuries. Shampooing frequency depends on the patient's wellbeing and his/her hair condition. Referral to a hairdresser may also be appropriate.

Grooming the hair provides an ideal opportunity to observe for dandruff, psoriasis, flaky skin and head lice. Head lice are extremely infectious so it is imperative to treat the hair with a medicated shampoo from the pharmacy as soon as possible. Hospital policy/protocol should be followed regarding the disposal of infected linen. Towel drying of hair should occur. Hairdryers can be used with the consent of the patient: use of a hairdryer may not be appropriate if patient has had recent alopecia due to chemotherapy. Hairdryers should be checked for safety by the hospital electrician.

A patient's cultural and religious beliefs should always be taken into consideration when attending to his/her hair. Some religions do not allow hair washing or brushing, while others may require the hair to be covered by a turban. Similarly, in some countries facial hair is significant and should never be removed without the patient's/relatives' consent. Always establish any preferences before beginning care.

In the oncology setting, chemotherapy is an established treatment and some cytotoxic drugs can cause alopecia (loss of hair). The patient's physical, psychological and social needs are affected by the loss of hair. Special care and skilled advice are required regarding the adjustment to hair loss. Referral to the hospital surgical appliance officer is appropriate to discuss the choice and fitting of a wig. A shampoo with a neutral pH is recommended for patients who are at risk of alopecia. Prevention of alopecia is discussed further in Chapter 39.

663

Care of the beard and moustache is also important. Excess food can often become lodged here so regular grooming is essential for hygiene and comfort purposes. Beard trimmers can be used as appropriate.

Care of the nails and feet

The feet and nails require special care in order to avoid pain and infection occurring. Nails should be trimmed correctly. Specialist advice from a chiropodist can be useful. Chronic diseases such as diabetes and the long-term use of steroids can result in problems such as pressure ulcers, breakdown of the skin integrity and delays in the healing process. Special attention should be paid to cleaning the feet and in between the toes to avoid any fungal infection (Geraghty 2005). Powders and creams are available that help with the treatment of infections and odour management, e.g. miconazole nitrate 2% for fungal infections.

Care of the ears and nose

Lack of attention to cleaning the ears and nose can lead to impairment of the senses. Usually these small organs require minimal care, but observation for a buildup of wax in the ears and deposits in the nose is essential to maintain patency.

Special care should be taken to avoid damage to the aural cavity or ear drum. Clean area with cotton wool or gauze and warm water.

Patients undergoing enteral feeding and oxygen therapy should have regular nasal care to avoid excessive drying and excoriating of the delicate air passages. Gentle cleaning of the nasal mucosa with wool/gauze and water is recommended and application of a thin coating of a water-based lubricant to prevent discomfort can be beneficial; this will remove debris and maintain a moist environment (Geraghty 2005).

Patients who have had piercing of the ears or nose will require cleaning of the holes to avoid the risk of infection. Gently cleaning around the piercing area, cotton wool/gauze and warm water should be used and the area towel dried. Observe for inflammation or oozing. If this occurs, inform the patient and doctor. Remove device on consent of the patient if inflammation or oozing occurs.

Eye care

Specific aspects of eye care, e.g. irrigation, are referred to in Chapter 31.

In general, the eye structure and delicate surface are protected by the tears that maintain the eye's moistness, but in a patient who is unconscious, drying of the eye may occur (Ross & Wilson 2001). Gentle cleaning with low-linting gauze and 0.9% sodium chloride will be sufficient to prevent infection and will keep the eyes moist. The eye is an important organ of communication and consideration should always be given to a patient's sight aids, e.g. glasses, contact lenses. Assistance may be required to help clean these aids and advice regarding the most appropriate method should be sought, preferably from the patient.

Some patients may have an artificial eye and care should be taken to ensure this remains clean. Advice regarding the ideal method of removal and insertion should be sought, from the local ophthalmology service or nursing team in ophthalmology unit.

Mouth care

Mouth care, e.g. cleaning and infection control, is referred to in Chapter 32.

Summary

Personal hygiene of patients is an integral part of the role of the nurse, creating a bond with the patient. In doing this, the nurse is able to spend time with his/her patient listening to issues, concerns or fears the patient may have regarding admission, treatment, discharge planning or prognosis. This may help to build a therapeutic relationship.

The nurse must recognize the uniqueness of the patient who may depend on others to assist them in times of ill health; respect and thought should be given to individual preferences (Whiting 1999). Comfort, cleanliness, availability of washing facilities, privacy and assistance from nurses were expressed as being important in providing hygiene care by patients in a recent ward audit (unpublished) at The Royal Marsden Hospital.

The world of nursing is ever changing, and there is a risk that activities such as attending to the personal hygiene of patients may become devalued or just another routine. The literature supports the enhanced quality of care to patients, when hygiene needs are attended to by qualified/experienced practitioners (Carr-Hill *et al.* 1992). Personal hygiene is considered part of the essence of care that nurses should never treat as ritualistic.

Procedure guidelines   **Bed bathing a patient**

Procedure

Prior to each part of the procedure, explain and obtain agreement from the patient. The procedure can provide the opportunity to build the nurse/patient relationship, during this time patients can discuss the issues troubling them. Planned care is negotiated with the patient and is based on assessment of their individual needs. Planned care should be documented and changed according to the patient's/carer's needs on a daily basis. Before commencing this procedure, read the patient's care plan, manual handling documentation and risk assessment to gain knowledge of safe practice.

Action	**Rationale**
1 Assess and plan care with the patient and family/friend if desired. Note personal preferences, addressing religious and cultural beliefs.	To plan care and encourage participation and independence (NMC 2008: E, C).
2 Clear area of any obstacles, ensure environment warm and draw curtains/close doors to guarantee privacy and dignity.	To maintain comfort, a safe environment and promote privacy and dignity (NMC 2008: C, E).
3 Offer patient urinal, bedpan or commode.	To reduce any disruption to procedure and prevent any discomfort (NMC 2008: C, E).
4 Collect all equipment by bedside: ■ Clean bed linen. ■ Bath towels. ■ Laundry skip, applying local guidelines for soiled and/or infected linen. ■ Flannels, preferably disposable. ■ Toiletries, as preferred by patient. ■ Clean clothes as desired. ■ Wash bowl and warm water; ensure bowl is cleaned with hot soapy water before use. ■ Comb/brush/razor/scissors/nail clippers. ■ Equipment for oral hygiene. ■ Any manual handling equipment.	To minimize time away from patient during procedure. Disposable flannels are preferable as this reduces the risk of infection. To meet patient preference during procedure (NMC 2008: E, P, R).
5 Wash hands; use disposable gloves and aprons according to local guidelines.	To minimize risk of cross-infection (DH 2005: R).
6 Assist patient with removal of clothing, cover patient with bath towel or fleece and fold back bedclothes.	To maintain privacy and dignity and body temperature (NMC 2008: C, E).
7 Ask patient whether they use soap on the face, wash, rinse and dry face, neck and ears.	To promote cleanliness and independence (NMC 2008: C, E).
8 Assist male patients with facial shaving, apply chosen shaving foam/soap. Ensure skin is taut, begin shaving from cheeks down to neck in short strokes. Rinse razor as required. Change water and rinse face with clean water. Utilize electric shaver as desired.	To promote positive body image (C).
9 Wash, rinse and pat dry top half of body, starting with the side furthest away from you. Care needs to be taken not to wet drains/dressings and IV devices. Apply toiletries as required.	To promote patient well-being and cleanliness and reduce the risk of cross-infection (NMC 2008: C, E, R).
10 Change the water, and your disposable gloves. Inform the patient that you are going to wash around the genitalia, gain verbal consent from the patient or ask the patient if they wish to wash this area themselves. Using a separate flannel or wipe, wash around the area, then dry the area. Remove gloves, dispose as per hospital policy. If there is an indwelling catheter, put on your gloves and wash the tubing away from the genitalia area, dry tubing and remove gloves as per hospital policy. (Patients may prefer to do this themselves.) When washing this area, remember female patients wash from the front to back. Male patients should draw back the foreskin if uncircumcised when washing the penis.	To reduce risk of infection and to maintain a safe environment (NMC 2008: C, E, R).

665

Procedure guidelines (*cont.*)

11 Change water and gloves, ensuring patient has nurse call bell, and is covered.	To maintain cleanliness, preserving dignity and privacy (NMC 2008: C, E).
12 Wash, rinse and pat dry legs, starting with the side furthest away from you. Assess the need for possible chiropody referral. Roll patient, wash back, then using disposable flannel wash sacral area, observing pressure areas. Cover areas that are not being washed. Return patient onto their back, ensure they are covered. Apply toiletries as required.	To prevent and treat pressure ulcers, ensuring appropriate referrals are made (E).
13 Inspect finger and toenails, clean under nails using nail file. Cut or clip finger nails to top level of finger, edges can be shaped using an emery board. Toenails should be cut/clipped straight across. Note any areas of skin dryness, inflammation, callouses.	To enhance positive body image and patient comfort and reduce risk of infection (NMC 2008: C, E, R).
14 Replace clothes and change bottom sheet whilst patient is being turned, if they are to remain in bed. Ensure a minimum of two nurses are present during this procdure.	To reduce unnecessary activity for patient and nurse. To maintain safety of patient and safe manual handling, following risk assessment (NMC 2008: C, E).
15 Provide appropriate equipment and assist patient, if required, to brush teeth and/or rinse mouth.	To maintain good oral hygiene (E).
16 Dry and comb patient's hair as desired.	To enhance patient comfort, and to promote positive body image (NMC 2008: C, E).
17 Remake top bedclothes.	
18 Help patient to sit or lie in desired position.	To enhance patient comfort and reduce risk of pressure ulcers (NMC 2008: C, E).
19 Remove equipment from bedside; replace patient's possessions in their appropriate place. Place locker, bedside table and call bell within reach.	To maintain a safe environment and promote patient independence (NMC 2008: C, E).
20 Remove apron and gloves and dispose of them according to local rules.	To prevent cross-infection (Pratt *et al.* 2001: R).
21 Wash hands, use alcohol based hand wash.	
22 Document any changes in planned care.	To provide recorded documentation of care and aid in communication to the multiprofessional team (C, E, R).

References and further reading

Armstrong-Esther, C.A. (1981) Skin introduction. *Nursing*, **1** (26), 1115.

Burr, S. & Penzer, R. (2005) Promoting skin health. *Nurs Stand*, **19**(36), 57–65.

Byers, P.H. *et al.* (1995) Effects of incontinence care cleansing regimens on skin integrity. *J Wound Ostomy Continence Nurs*, **22**(4), 187–92.

Campbell, A. (1984) Nursing, nurturing and sexism. In: *Moderated Love: A Theology of Professional Care*. Society for Promoting Christian Knowledge, London.

Carr-Hill, R., Dixon, P. & Gibbs, I. (1992) *Skill Mix and the Effectiveness of Nursing Care*. Centre for Health Economics, York.

Clinical Skills (2003) Bed baths. *Nurs Times*, **99**(5), 29.

Collins, F. & Hampton S. (2003) The cost effective use of Bagbath: a new concept in patient hygiene. *Br J Nurs*, **12**(16), 985–90.

Cooper, C. (1994) Hygiene and the client. In: *Knowledge to Care* (eds C.A. McMahon & J. Harding). Blackwell Scientific, Oxford.

DH (2001a) *Essence of Care*. HMSO, London.

DH (2001b) *Reference Guide to Consent for Examination or Treatment*. Department of Health, London.

DH (2005) *Saving Lives: A Delivery Programme to Reduce Healthcare Associated Infection including MRSA*. Department of Health, London.

Ersser, S.J. *et al.* (2005) A critical review of the inter-relationship between skin vunerability and urinary incontinence and related nursing intervention. *Int J Nurs Stud*, **42**, 823–35.

Geraghty, M. (2005) Nursing the unconcious patient. *Nurs Stand*, **20**(1), 54–64.

Gooch, J. (1989) Skin hygiene. *Prof Nurse*, **5**(1), 13–17.

Gordon, M. (1994) *Nursing Diagnosis: Process and Application*, 3rd edn. Mosby, St Louis.

Gould, D. (1994) Helping the patient with personal hygiene. *Nurs Stand*, **8**(34), 30–2.

Haisfield Wolfe, M.E. (1998) Providing effective perineal–rectal skin care to patients with cancer. *Oncol Nurs Forum*, **25**(3), 472.

Hector, L.M. & Touhy, T.A. (1997) The history of the bath: from art to task? Reflections for the future. *J Gerontol Nurs*, **23**(5), 7–15.

Henderson, V. (1966) *The Nature of Nursing*. Collier Macmillan, London.

Holloway, S. & Jones, V. (2005) The importance of skin care and assessment. *Br J Nurs*, **14**(22), 1172–6.

Kitson, A. (1999) The essence of nursing. *Nurs Stand*, **13**(23), 42–6.

Lindell, M. & Olsson, H. (1989) Lack of care givers' knowledge causes unnecessary suffering in elderly patients. *J Adv Nurs*, **14**, 976–9.

Lokich, J.J. & Moore, C. (1984) Chemotherapy associated palmar plantar erythrodysesthesia syndrome. *Ann Intern Med*, **101**, 798–800.

McLoughlin, C. (2005) A guide to wash creams. *Prof Nurse*, **20**(6), 46–7.

Neuberger, J. (1987) *Caring for Dying People of Different Faiths*, 2nd edn. Mosby, London.

Nightingale, F. (1969) *Notes on Nursing*. Dover Publications, New York.

NMC (2008) *The Code: Standards of Conduct, Performance and Ethics for Nurses and Midwives*. Nursing and Midwifery Council, London.

Orem, D. (1980) *Nursing – Concepts of Practice*, 2nd edn. McGraw Hill, New York.

Penzer, R. & Finch, M. (2001) Promoting healthy skin in older people. *Nurs Stand*, **15**(34), 46–52.

Potter, P.A. & Perry, G. (1995) *Basic Nursing Theory and Practice*. Mosby, London.

Pratt, R.J. *et al.* (2001) Guidelines for preventing infections associated with the insertion and maintenance of short-term indwelling urethral catheters in acute care. *J Hosp Infect*, **47**(Suppl), S39–46.

Roper, N. *et al.* (1981) *Learning to Use the Process of Nursing*. Churchill Livingstone, Edinburgh.

Ross, J. & Wilson, K. (2001) *Anatomy and Physiology in Health and Illness*. Churchill Livingstone, Edinburgh.

Sampson, C. (1982) *The Neglected Ethic; Religious and Cultural Factors in the Care of Patients*. McGraw-Hill, London, p. 36.

Sheppard, C.M. & Brenner, P.S. (2000) The effects of bathing and skin care practices on skin quality and satisfaction with an innovative product. *J Gerontol Nurs*, **26**(10), 36–45.

Smoker, A. (1999) Skin care in old age. *Nurs Stand*, **13**(48), 47–53.

Spiller, J. (1992) For whose sake – patient or nurse? *Prof Nurse*, **7**(7), 431–4.

Wagnild, G. & Manning, R.W. (1985) Convey respect during bathing procedures. *J Gerontol Nurse*, **11**(12), 6–10.

Whiting, L.S. (1999) Maintaining patient's personal hygiene. *Prof Nurse*, **14**(5), 338–40.

Wilson, M. (1986) Personal cleanliness. *Nursing*, **3**(2), 80–2.

Young, L. (1991) The clean fight. *Nurs Stand*, **5**(35), 54–5.

Chapter 34

Positioning

669 Reference material
669 Principles of positioning
669 Medical considerations
670 Positioning in bed
670 *Procedure guidelines:* Positioning the patient supine
671 *Procedure guidelines:* Positioning the patient sitting in bed
672 *Procedure guidelines:* Positioning the patient side lying
673 Guidance for assisting patients to move
674 *Procedure guidelines:* Moving from lying to sitting: assisting the patient
675 *Procedure guidelines:* Positioning the patient in a chair
675 *Procedure guidelines:* Moving from sitting to standing: assisting the patient
681 *Procedure guidelines:* Walking: assisting the patient
682 *Procedure guidelines:* Positioning to minimize the work of breathing
683 *Procedure guidelines:* Positioning to maximize ventilation/perfusion (*V/Q*) matching and oxygenation
684 Positioning of patients with cardiorespiratory compromise
684 Positioning to maximize the drainage of respiratory secretions
684 Positioning the patient with neurological impairment
686 *Procedure guidelines:* Positioning the neurological patient with tonal problems
688 *Procedure guidelines:* Positioning the preoperative and postoperative amputee patient
688 Positioning and amputee management
689 References and further reading

Definition

The verb positioning is defined as 'a way in which someone or something is placed or arranged' (Pearsall 2001, p. 1116). In medical terms the word position relates to body position or posture. Positioning lies within the broader context of manual handling, which incorporates 'transporting or supporting a load (including lifting, putting down, pushing, pulling, carrying or moving) by hand or bodily force' (HSE 1992). In this chapter the principles of positioning will relate to the patient, but the practitioner needs to ensure that they consider their own position regarding the safety aspects of manual handling as advised by government and local policy and the manual handling advisor or the physiotherapist.

This chapter aims to provide guidance on various aspects of positioning patients acknowledging the need to be clinically effective and, where possible, evidence based.

The main objectives of the chapter are to:

1 Outline the general considerations of positioning.
2 Provide guidance on the principles of positioning whether the patient is in bed, sitting or mobilizing.
3 Review optimal positioning and modifications for patients requiring different clinical needs.
4 Provide suggestions for further reading.

Reference material

This chapter relates to conscious adults (for positioning of the unconscious patient see Chapter 44) and does not cover positioning in children or neonates.

· Positioning is an important aspect in patient care because of its effect on the patient physically, physiologically and psychologically. It can have a major influence on patient recuperation and well being, addressing patients' impairments in order to optimize their function and participation in society. Although important, positioning must not be seen in isolation and is just one aspect of patient management within the context of preventative, rehabilitative, supportive and palliative rehabilitation models (Dietz 1981). Positioning is often used to provide a starting point to maximize the benefit of other interventions such as bed and breathing exercises, optimal rest, and rehabilitation to facilitate recovery.

It is essential to frequently evaluate the effect that positioning has on the individual and/or different pathologies to ensure that the intervention is helping to achieve the desired result or goal. This relates to considering whether the positioning procedure is being clinically effective and, where possible, is evidence based.

Points to consider regarding the clinical effectiveness of positioning are:

- Is the timing right to consider positioning? For example, is the pain relief adequate?
- Is it being carried out in the correct way? This relates to manual handling with regard to preventing trauma either to the patient or the practitioner.

- Is the required position taking into account all the pertinent needs of the patient? This emphasizes the need to consider the patient in a holistic manner.
- Is it achieving the desired or detrimental result?

Principles of positioning

Positioning is indicated for patients who are acutely ill or require bed rest when normal functioning is impaired. The aim of positioning is to reduce impairment, facilitate function, and alleviate symptomatic discomfort and to assist future rehabilitation where appropriate. The main principles underpinning all interventions regarding patient positioning focus on the short- and long-term goals of rehabilitation and management for each specific patient. It is imperative that a thorough assessment is carried out prior to any intervention in order to plan goals of treatment. Regular reassessment is required to allow for modification of plans to allow for changes in status. It may be necessary to compromise on one principle depending on the overall goal. For example, for the palliative patient, it may be that the primary aim of any intervention is to facilitate comfort at the cost of reducing function.

The principles of positioning are based on patterns of posture which maximize function with minimal amount of effort (Gardiner 1973) without causing damage to the body system (Pope 1996). These basic principles of positioning can be applied regardless of a patient's pathology.

To achieve a good position of the patient in bed the following points should be considered:

- wounds;
- pain;
- weakness;
- tonal changes;
- sensory changes;
- limitations of joint range;
- oedema;
- skin blistering;
- medical devices associated with treatment, e.g. catheter, intravenous infusion, venous access devices, drains;
- cardiovascular and respiratory status;
- cognitive state.

Medical considerations

Skin integrity should be assessed prior to positioning and vulnerable areas protected and placed so as to minimize harmful contact with other surfaces (see Chapter 48).

Patients may have complex symptoms that require control prior to moving or positioning. It is important to time the intervention to allow adequate time for medication to take effect or to ensure the patient is given a breakthrough dose before moving (see Chapter 27).

It is important to establish spinal stability before positioning or moving the patient. Suspected or confirmed spinal instability should be managed in accordance to local policy (see Chapter 41).

669

Caution should be taken in patients with known, possible pathological fracture(s) or pain. Before a lesion becomes apparent radiologically at least 50% of bone mass must be lost; so that pain may precede radiological changes (McGarvey 1990).

Fatigue can be a distressing symptom, so advice and help should be given to the patient to pace their everyday activities. Barsevick *et al.* (2002, p. 71) describe energy conservation as 'the deliberate planned management of one's personal energy resources in order to prevent their depletion'. Prioritizing activities may help to avoid engaging in tasks that are unnecessary or of little value (Cooper 2006). Sometimes it may be appropriate to assist with activities such as washing and dressing to help conserve energy for more meaningful or pleasurable activities.

Medical considerations for patient on bed rest

Patients with acute medical conditions and decreased mobility are at risk of secondary complications of bed rest such as pulmonary embolus (PE) (Reidel 2001), deep vein thrombosis (DVT) or respiratory infection (Convertino *et al.* 1995).

The severity of an illness may leave no choice except bed rest, but the rest itself is rarely beneficial. Historically patients complaining of pain, dyspnoea, neurological dysfunction and fatigue were advised to rest. However, inactivity may cause (Creditor 1993; Doyle *et al.* 2004):

- Deconditioning of many of the body's systems (particularly in cardiorespiratory and musculoskeletal systems).
- A worsening of symptoms.
- Fear of movement.
- Loss of independence.
- Social isolation.

Therefore, patients should be encouraged or assisted, to mobilize or change position, at frequent intervals. This so that deconditioning is minimized, unless their medical condition or fatigue makes this inappropriate. Early referral to therapy services is advantageous. If bed rest is unavoidable then the following factors should be taken into account:

- Patient comfort and adequate support.
- Avoidance of the complications of prolonged bed rest (see Chapter 33).
- Consideration regarding the optimal frequency of position change.

Patients on bed rest should be encouraged to practice regular deep breathing to maximize their respiratory function.

They should also be encouraged to practice active or passive movements, as advised by the physiotherapist, in order to (Adam & Forrest 1999):

- Maintain full joint range.
- Maintain full muscle length and extensibility.
- Assist venous return.
- Maintain sensation of normal movement.

Active ankle movements are to be encouraged to assist the circulation, as failure to exercise the calf muscle for prolonged periods may result in limited or poor blood circulation in the lower leg and increase the risk of DVT (O'Donovan *et al.* 2006).

Positioning in the bed

The body should be supported to maintain its natural contours, symmetry and alignment (Carter & Edwards 1996).

Procedure guidelines   Positioning the patient supine

......

Equipment

1 Pillows.
2 Towels.
3 Bed extension for tall patients.

......

Procedure

Action	Rationale
1 (a) Place one pillow squarely under the patient's head according to patient comfort.	To support the head in a neutral position and to compensate for the natural lordosis of the cervical spine (E).
For patients with a tracheostomy, endotracheal tube, soft tissue structural involvement or head and neck surgery take care not to occlude or displace tubes or increase pressure to vulnerable areas. Or:	To ensure the airway is patent (E). To increase patient support and comfort (E).
(b) Use two pillows in a 'butterfly' position so that two layers of pillow support the head and one layer of pillow under each shoulder. Or:	This may be necessary for the patient with pain, breathlessness (see Respiratory section, below) or an existing kyphosis (E).
(c) Use a folded towel if this provides natural spinal alignment (E).	To prevent excess neck flexion (E).

......

2 Ensure the patient lies centrally in the bed.	To ensure spinal and limb alignment (E).
3 Place pillows and/or towels under individual limbs to provide maximum support for patient with painful, weak or oedematous limbs.	To ensure patient comfort (E, P)
4 Ensure patient's feet are fully supported by the mattress. For taller patients use a bed extension if required.	To ensure patient comfort (E, P).
5 Place pillow at the end of the hospital bed to support ankle at 90° of flexion if the patient has weakness or is immobile. Refer to the occupational therapist or physiotherapist for orthosis/splinting if the patient is unable to actively flex their foot. Refer to the physiotherapist if the patient has a neurological pathology for advice regarding positioning to reduce altered tonal influences (R) (E).	To ensure patient comfort (E, P). To prevent loss of ankle movement (E).

671

Procedure guidelines   Positioning the patient sitting in bed

Patients should be encouraged to sit up in bed periodically if their medical condition prevents them from sitting out in the chair (Figure 34.1). If the patient is unable to participate fully in the procedure, manual handling equipment should be used to help achieve the desired position.

Attention should also be given to sitting posture. One of the most common causes of low back pain is poor posture and may frequently be brought on by sitting for a long time in a poor position (McKenzie 1985) as it causes an increase in pressure in the disc (Norris 1995).

Patients who have suspected or confirmed spinal instability should be nursed flat unless medical staff instruct otherwise. Patients should lie flat to prevent dural headache following lumbar puncture unless local policy states otherwise.

Equipment

1 Pillows.
2 Manual handling equipment may be required, e.g. sliding sheets or a hoist depending on local policy.

Procedure

Action	Rationale
1 Ask the patient to sit up in bed. The angle at which the patient sits may be influenced by pain, fatigue, abdominal distension or level of confusion/agitation.	To encourage haemodynamic stability (E). To enable effective breathing pattern: maximizing basal expansion (Pryor & Webber 2002: R 4).
2 Ask the patient to position their hips in line with the hinge of the automatic mattress elevator or backrest of the bed.	To ensure good postural alignment, i.e. flexing at the hip when sitting up in bed (E). To prevent strain on the spine (E, R).
3 Place a pillow under the patient's knees or use the electrical control of the bed to slightly bend the patient's knees. Extra care should be taken if the patient has a femoral line or is on haemofiltration.	To reduce strain on the lumbar spine (E). To maintain the position (E).
4 Place a pillow under individual or both upper limbs for patients with a chest drain, upper limb weakness, trunk weakness, surgery involving shoulder/upper limb/breast/thorax, fungating wounds involving axilla, breast and shoulder, upper limb /truncal lymphoedema or fractures involving ribs or upper limbs.	To provide upper limb support (E). To maintain trunk alignment (E). To encourage basal expansion (Pryor & Webber 2002: E, R 4).

Procedure guidelines *(cont.)*

Figure 34.1   Sitting up in bed.

Procedure guidelines   Positioning the patient side lying

This can be a useful position for patients with:
1 Compromised venous return, e.g. pelvic/abdominal mass, pregnancy.
2 Global motor weakness.
3 Risk of developing pressure sores.
4 Unilateral pelvic or lower limb pain.
5 Altered tone (see Positioning the patient with neurological impairment section, below).
6 Fatigue.
7 Chest infection, for gravity-assisted drainage of secretions.
8 Lung pathology, to optimize ventilation and perfusion matching.
9 Abdominal distension, e.g. ascites, bulky disease, to optimize lung volume (for more information on the above three points (7, 8, 9) see Positioning of patients with cardiorespiratory compromise section, below).
See Figure 34.2

Equipment

1 Pillows.
2 Manual handling equipment may be required, e.g. sliding sheets or a hoist depending on local policy.

Procedure

Action	Rationale
1 Place one or two pillows in 'butterfly' position under the patient's head ensuring the airway remains patent. Extra care should be taken for those patients with a tracheostomy, central lines or recent head and neck surgery.	To support the head in mid-position (E). To support shoulder contours (E).
2 Ask/assist the patient to semiflex the underneath leg at the hip and the knee. Extra care should be taken with the degree of flexion for those patients who have hip or knee pain or loss of movement, fracture involving the femur or pelvis, leg oedema, femoral lines or other venous access devices.	To support the patient in a stable position and prevent rolling (E).

3 (a)	Ask/assist the patient to semi-flex the uppermost leg at the hip and knee. Use a pillow to support under the leg placed on the bed. Or:	To prevent lumbar spine rotation (E). To support the pelvic girdle (E).
(b)	Place a pillow between the patient's knees.	To aid pressure care (E).

| 4 | Place the underneath arm in front with scapula protracted (this would not be appropriate for patients with shoulder pathology). Extra care should be taken with patients with low tone in the affected arm, lymphoedema or who have access lines in that arm. | To promote patient comfort (E, P).
To promote shoulder alignment (E).
To provide additional support and comfort (E, P). |

Note: care should be taken in lying the patient directly over the greater trochanter as this increases pressure at this interface and the risk of developing pressure sores (Hawkins *et al.* 1999).

Figure 34.2 Side lying.

Guidance for assisting patients to move

This section covers general principles of assisting patients to move, enhancing their rehabilitation process by avoiding unnecessary debilitation. It serves as a guide only, is not prescriptive and does not attempt to cover mandatory local manual handling issues. Each situation should be risk assessed on an individual basis as part of standard nursing assessment.

Particular thought should be given to the patient's:

- Previous functional status.
- Consent and compliance to treatment or activity.
- Medical stability.
- Environmental safety.
- Level of consciousness.
- Symptom control.
- Muscle strength.
- Sensation.

- Co-ordination and balance.
- Cognitive function.
- Level of fatigue.
- Cardiovascular/respiratory status.

In order to assist recovery, postural alignment is essential to improve motor control. The term motor control is broadly defined as: 'the control of both movement and posture' (Shumway-Cook & Woollacott 1995, p. 3).

Postural alignment helps the patient develop an initial position that is (Shumway-Cook & Woollacott 1995, p. 224):

(a) appropriate for the task;
(b) efficient with respect to gravity, i.e. minimal muscle activity required to maintain the position; and
(c) maximizes stability, allowing postural control.

Procedure guidelines   Moving from lying to sitting: assisting the patient

See Figures 34.3, 34.4 and 34.5.

Equipment

1 Manual handling equipment may be required, e.g. sliding sheets or a hoist depending on local policy.

Action	Rationale
1 Ask the patient to bend both knees and turn their head towards the direction they are moving. Abdominal wounds should be supported by the patient's hands. Extra care should be taken with patients who have joint pathology, oedema, ascites or positional vertigo.	To assist the patient to roll using their body weight (E).
2 Ask patient to reach toward the side of the bed with the uppermost arm and roll on to their side.	
3 Ask the patient to bend their knees and lower their feet over the edge of the bed.	
4 Ask the patient to push through the underneath elbow and the upper arm on the bed to push up into sitting. As the patient sits up monitor changes in pain or dizziness which could indicate postural hypotension or vertigo. Be aware that the patient with neurological symptoms or weakness may not have safe sitting balance.	To help to lever the patient into a sitting position using the weight of their legs (E).
5 Achieve upright sitting position with appropriate alignment of body parts.	To ensure safe sitting position achieved.

Figure 34.3   Lying to sitting (stage 1).

Figure 34.4   Lying to sitting (stage 2).

Figure 34.5   Lying to sitting (stage 3).

Procedure guidelines   Positioning the patient in a chair

. . . .

Equipment

1 Upright chair with arms.
2 Manual handling equipment may be required, e.g. a hoist depending on local policy.
3 Pillows/rolled up towel.
4 Footstool if the patient has lower limb oedema.

. . . .

Procedure

Action	Rationale
1 Ask the patient to sit well back in the chair. They should have a maximum 90° angle at their hips and knee joints. The patient may not be able to achieve this position if they have pain, abdominal distension or hip/back pain. It may be necessary to refer the patient to the occupational therapist for chair raises, a cushion or appropriate seating if a comfortable or safe position cannot be achieved.	To provide a stable base of support for balance (E). To ensure good body alignment (E). To achieve a safe sitting position (E).
2 Place a pillow or rolled up towel in the small of the patient's back as is comfortable for the patient.	To allow the patient's back to be supported in a good position (E).
3 Ensure the patient's feet are resting on the floor or supported surface. Use pillows or a rolled up towel to support under the feet if necessary.	To provide postural alignment and support the lumbar spine (E).
4 If the patient has a lower leg oedema use a foot stool placed under the patient's limb ensuring the whole leg and foot is supported and avoiding hyperextension at the knees.	To improve venous drainage.
5 Discourage the patient from crossing their legs.	To reduce risk of developing a DVT (O'Donovan *et al.* 2006: R 4).

675

Procedure guidelines   Moving from sitting to standing: assisting the patient

If the patient stands from the side of a hospital bed, it is helpful to raise the bed slightly to reduce the work of standing for the patient to ensure that hips are level or higher than the knees with the feet in contact with the floor. A physiotherapy referral may be appropriate. See Figures 34.6 and 34.7.

. . . .

Equipment

1 Walking aid if required (if previously issued by physiotherapist).
2 Suitable non-slip, well-fitting, supportive and flat footwear (if not available then bare feet are preferable to socks or stockings which may slip).

. . . .

Procedure

Action	Rationale
1 Ask the patient to lean forward and move their bottom closer to the front of the chair or edge of the bed.	To bring the patient's weight over their feet (E).

. . . .

2 Ask the patient to move their feet back so they are slightly tucked under them with their feet hip width apart.	To provide a stable base prior to moving (E).
3 Instruct the patient to lean forward from their trunk.	To help initiate movement (E). To facilitate a normal pattern of movement (E).
4 Instruct the patient to push through their hands on the arms of the chair or surface on which they are sitting as they stand. Encourage a forward and up motion whilst extending their hips and knees.	To minimize energy expenditure (E).
5 As the patient stands observe changes in pain or dizziness.	To be aware of postural hypotension (E).
6 Once standing, ask the patient to stand still for a moment to ensure balance is achieved before the patient attempts to walk.	To ensure safe static standing (E).

676

Figure 34.6 Sitting to standing (stage 1).

Figure 34.7 Sitting to standing (stage 2).

Walking

'Walking requires alternating support on one leg and then the other' (Gillis 1989, p.671). Successful walking is dependent on three specific functional tasks (Gillis 1989):

1 Weight acceptance.
2 Single limb support.
3 Limb advancement.

Patients may use a variety of different walking aids to help them mobilize. All aids are designed to improve balance and therefore reduce the risk of falls.

It is assumed that patients will take equal amounts of body weight through both legs, defined as being fully weight bearing (FWB). If a patient has to be non-weight bearing (NWB) or partially weight bearing (PWB) this will be due to bone or joint pathology, e.g. fracture, joint instability, inflammation or infection. Restrictions in weight bearing should always be clearly documented and communicated by the medical staff. Weight bearing will also be affected by pain, weakness, sensory changes and confidence. If the patient has difficulty mobilizing, appears unsafe or is at risk of falling for any reason refer for physiotherapy assessment.

A physiotherapist will assess and issue the patient with an appropriate walking aid. All patients should be given verbal and written instructions on their use. If they are unsure, please refer to the patient information sheets for instructions (Boxes 34.1, 34.2 and 34.3).

Box 34.1   Using your walking sticks

Your physiotherapist has suggested that you would benefit from using a walking stick. This fact sheet is to remind you of the most important points that your physiotherapist has shown you. Your walking stick will help to give you more support when standing and walking. It can help you take weight off one leg if you have pain or weakness. It can also help with improving your balance.

Standing
- Use your arms to push up from the surface you are sitting on.
- Hold the stick in your stronger hand or the opposite hand to the painful or weak leg.

Walking

- Place the stick in front of you.
- Step forwards with your weaker leg so it is level with the stick.
- Lean on the stick and take a normal step with the other leg.
- Repeat this sequence always moving the stick forwards before or at the same time as the weaker leg as advised by your physiotherapist.
- It may take a bit of practice for you to get into a rhythm.

Sitting
- Always turn so you are backing towards the bed or chair.
- When you can feel the bed or chair on the backs of your legs, reach back with your hand to feel the arm of the chair or bed surface.
- Slowly sit down.

Continued on p. 678

Box 34.1 *(cont.)*

Stairs

Going up:

- Hold on to the banister with the stick in the other hand.
- Pushing down on the stick and banister, step up with the stronger leg.
- Bring the stick and weaker leg up to join the stronger leg on the same step.
- Repeat this sequence.

Going down:

- Hold on to the banister with the stick in the other hand.
- Place the stick on to the step below.
- Step down with the weaker leg.
- Lean on the stick and banister as you step down with the stronger leg on to the same stair.
- Repeat this sequence.

Take extra care using your stick where:

- There are loose rugs or carpet edges: try to remove or tape down.
- The floor is wet.
- The floor is rough or uneven.

Care and maintenance of your stick

You should wipe the stick down with warm soapy water and dry thoroughly with a soft cloth once a week or more frequently if necessary. Check the stick weekly for signs of wear and tear:

- Is the rubber tip worn or showing poor tread?
- Is the wood cracked or splintered?

©The Royal Marsden NHS Foundation Trust

Box 34.2   Using your elbow crutches

Your physiotherapist has suggested you use elbow crutches to help you walk. This fact sheet is to remind you of the most important points that your physiotherapist has shown you.

   Your crutches will help to give you more support when standing and walking. They can help you take weight off one leg if you have pain or weakness. They can also help with improving your balance.

Standing
- Hold both crutches in one hand making an 'H' shape.
- Push up with the other hand from the surface you are sitting on. Don't put your arms through the rings until you are standing up.
- When you are standing, pass one crutch over to the other hand and put hands through the rings one at a time.
- Get your balance before beginning to walk.

Walking

- Place the crutches in front of you.
- Step forwards with your weaker leg level with the crutches.
- Lean on the crutches and take a normal step with the other leg.
- Repeat this sequence always moving the crutches forwards before or at the same time as the weaker leg as advised by your physiotherapist.
- It may take a bit of practice for you to get into a rhythm.
- If your physiotherapist has shown you a different way to walk with crutches then follow the advice given to you.

Sitting

- When sitting down always turn so you are backing towards the bed or chair.
- When you can feel the bed or chair on the backs of your legs, pass one crutch over in to the other hand so you are holding both crutches in one hand.
- Take your hands out of the rings and make an 'H' shape with the crutches.
- Reach back with your free hand to feel the arm of the chair or bed surface.
- Slowly sit down.

Stairs

Going up:

- Hold on to the banister with both crutches in the other hand as demonstrated by your physiotherapist. The second crutch should be held horizontally as demonstrated by your physiotherapist.
- Pushing down on the crutches and banister, step up with stronger leg.
- Bring the crutches and weaker leg up to join the strong leg on the same step.
- Repeat this sequence.

Continued on p. 680

Box 34.2 (*cont.*)

Going down:

- Hold on to the banister with both crutches in the other hand as demonstrated by your physiotherapist.
- Place the crutches on to the step below.
- Step down with the weaker leg.
- Lean on the crutch and banister as you step down with the strong leg on to the same stair.
- Repeat this sequence.
- Always remember to keep the crutches with the weak leg on the lower level.

Take extra care using your crutches where:

- There are loose rugs or carpet edges: try to remove or tape down.
- The floor is wet.
- The floor is rough or uneven.

Care and maintenance of your crutches

You should wipe the crutches down with warm soapy water and dry thoroughly with a soft cloth once a week or more frequently if necessary.
Check the crutches weekly for signs of wear and tear:

- Are the rubber tips worn and showing poor tread?
- Are the hand grips loose or cracked?
- Is the metal tubing cracked or damaged?

©The Royal Marsden NHS Foundation Trust

Box 34.3 Using your walking frame

Your physiotherapist has suggested that you would benefit from using a walking frame. This fact sheet is to remind you of the most important points that your physiotherapist has shown you. Your walking frame should help to give you more support when standing and walking. It can also help you take weight off one or both of your legs if you have pain or weakness. The walking frame can also help with improving your balance.
Your physiotherapist will have assessed the height of the frame when it was given to you.
There should be no need to adjust the height again.

Standing

- Always push up with your arms from the surface you are sitting on or from the arms of the chair.
- Shuffle to the edge of the chair or bed.
- Lean forwards and stand up pushing with your arms.
- Never put your hands on the frame until you are standing.
- Do not pull on the frame as it may tip back.

Walking

- Move the frame in front of you and lean on it.
- Step forwards into the middle of the frame. If you walk too far into the frame it may become unbalanced and tip backwards.
- If you have one leg that is weaker or painful step forward with that leg first.
- Always have both hands on the frame and do not try and carry anything while you are walking.

Sitting

- Always turn the frame using small steps, so you are backing towards the bed or chair.
- When you feel the bed or chair on the back of your legs, reach back with your hands one at a time, to hold the arms of the chair or surface of the bed.
- Slowly sit down.

Box 34.3 *(cont.)*

Do not use your frame:

- Where there are loose rugs or carpet edges: always remove or tape down.
- Where the floor is wet.
- Where there is not enough space to turn the frame.
- Where there are stairs or steps.
- Where the floor is rough or uneven.
- Outside.

Care and maintenance of the frame

You should wash the frame down with warm soapy water and dry thoroughly with a soft cloth once a week or more frequently if necessary. Check the frame regularly for signs of wear and tear:

- Are the rubber tips worn and showing poor tread?
- Has the frame become wobbly or unstable?
- Are the hand grips loose or cracked?
- Is the metal tubing cracked or damaged?

©The Royal Marsden NHS Foundation Trust

Procedure guidelines Walking: assisting the patient

Equipment

1 Walking aid (see later).
2 Suitable non-slip, well-fitting, supportive and flat footwear (if not available then bare feet is preferable to socks or stockings which may slip).

Action	Rationale
1 Stand next to and slightly behind the patient. If patient requires support place your arm nearest the patient lightly around their pelvis. Your other hand should hold the patient's hand closest to you. Observe changes in pain as the patient walks.	To give appropriate support (E). To increase patient's confidence (E, P).
2 Give verbal supervision/cueing as required to achieve safe walking.	To provide encouragement (E). To ensure patient safety (E).

Procedure guidelines   Positioning to minimize the work of breathing

The aim of any position is to restore a normal frequency (rate) and depth (tidal volume) of breathing in order to achieve efficient, adequate ventilation.

The positions will usually be used in conjunction with other interventions, e.g. breathing control and specific muscle relaxation, to achieve reduced work of breathing. These may include attention to symptom control (e.g. pain), environmental control (e.g. reducing unnecessary noise stressors).

Repositioning can cause a temporary fall in SaO_2 or a raised respiratory rate due to the work undertaken. If the fall is greater than 4% points or recovery time is protracted supplemental oxygen delivery may be required. If the clinical signs remain altered from normal then an alternative position may be indicated.

Procedure

Action

1 As shown in Action figure 1, the resting positions include:
- High side lying (see Action figure 1a).
- Forward lean sitting (see Action figure 1b).
- Relaxed sitting (see Action figure 1c).
- Forward lean standing (see Action figure 1d).
- Relaxed standing (see Action figure 1e).

Rationale

These positions all serve to:
- Support the body reducing the overall use of postural muscle and oxygen requirements.
- Improve lung volumes.
- Optimize the functional positions of the respiratory (thoracic and abdominal) muscles (Dean 1985: R 4, E, P).

(a)

(d)

(b)

(c)

(e)

Action 1   (a–e) Positions to support breathing.

Procedure guidelines   Positioning to maximize ventilation/perfusion (*V*/*Q*) matching and oxygenation

For optimal gaseous exchange to take place it is necessary to have an adequate perfusion of blood and a regular supply of inspired air (ventilation) in the same area of the lung. Ventilation and perfusion are not exactly matched even in the normal lung but can be changed by positional alteration to improve oxygenation and reduce the requirements for supplemental oxygenation (see Figures 34.8 and 34.9 and Chapter 38). In the presence of respiratory pathology, *V*/*Q* matching is better in the non-affected areas (Jones & Moffatt 2002). Where there is cardiac compromise, if there is an increase in heart rate or alteration in blood pressure, the head of the bed may need to be gradually raised until signs normalize.

The ideal positioning for *V*/*Q* matching will be determined by a number of factors:

- The cardiorespiratory pathophysiology.
- Co-existence of other pathophysiology.
- Auscultatory findings.
- X-ray or computed tomography (CT) findings.

In the spontaneously breathing patient

Action	Rationale
1 Supported side lying on the unaffected side for unilateral lung disease.	Maximizes *V*/*Q* in the unaffected lung as the ventilation and perfusion are both preferentially distributed to the dependent areas of the lungs (West *et al.* 1964: R 4; Zach *et al.* 1974: R 4, E, P).
2 High supported sitting for bilateral lower lobe pathology or multi-lobe pathology.	Due to the effects of shunting in multi-lobe lung pathology perfusion may best match ventilation in supported high sitting (Dean 1985: R 4, E, P).

In patients receiving positive pressure ventilation

Each individual patient should be positioned according to their pathology and responses to the principles outlined below. Where positive pressure ventilation is delivered maximum ventilation will occur in the non-dependent regions, whilst the perfusion is still preferentially delivered to the dependent areas. This may vary again where there is respiratory pathology causing ventilatory shunt, whereby pulmonary venous blood re-enters the arterial circulation without being ventilated and hence not oxygenated (Wagner & West 2005).

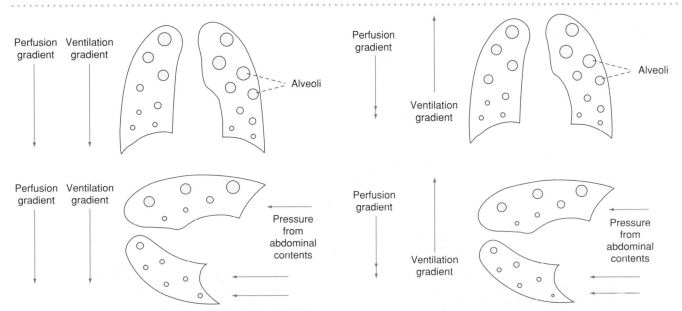

Figure 34.8 Effect of gravity on the distribution of ventilation and perfusion in the lung in the upright and lateral positions. From Hough (2001) with permission.

Figure 34.9 Effect of controlled mandatory ventilation on ventilation and perfusion gradients. In contrast to spontaneous respiration, the perfusion gradient increases downwards and the ventilation gradient is reversed. From Hough (2001) with permission.

Positioning of patients with cardiorespiratory compromise

The causes of cardiorespiratory compromise may be multifactorial and should be established before undertaking positioning interventions. Compromise may be due to medical intervention (e.g. surgery, side-effects of medication), metabolic, surgical or primary cardiorespiratory pathologies.

The guidelines regarding assisting patients to move are applicable to this group. However, particular observation is required regarding their response to the interventions and specific modifications may be required (e.g. increased assistance, paced activity or provision of supplemental oxygen) for the duration and recovery period following the procedure.

The main aim of positioning management of the patient with respiratory symptoms is to use gravity to:

- Minimize the work of breathing.
- Maximize the drainage of respiratory secretions.
- Maximize ventilation/perfusion (V/Q) matching and oxygenation.

In many instances positioning may combine the above aims to enhance medical management by the use of the effects of gravity upon the cardiovascular and respiratory systems. This may reduce the need for more invasive intervention (Jones & Moffatt 2002), i.e. assisted ventilation. As such, the most advantageous positioning should be integrated into the overall 24-hour plan, and positions that may have an adverse effect should be avoided (Brown *et al.* 1996).

It should be remembered that thoracic and abdominal muscles contribute to normal breathing patterns and that any compromise of the abdominal muscle activity (e.g. due to abdominal surgery, ascites or deconditioning) may lead to an alteration in the normal cardiorespiratory function and the ability to generate an effective cough (Hodges & Gandevia 2000).

Positioning to maximize the drainage of respiratory secretions

Sputum retention may lead to an increased bacterial load for the patient and may compromise respiratory functioning by causing airway obstruction leading to segmental atelectasis or lobar collapse increasing the mortality.

Optimal positioning for the gravity assisted positions to facilitate the drainage of respiratory secretions will be determined by a number of factors:

- The cardiorespiratory pathophysiology.
- Co-existence of other pathophysiology.
- Auscultatory findings.
- X-ray or CT findings.

Where secretions are found in a specific segment, the patient should be specifically positioned to place the bronchus of each bronchopulmonary segment perpendicular to gravity

in order to be drained. Advice may be given by the physiotherapist on these positions.

The positions will usually be used in conjunction with other techniques to facilitate the clearing of respiratory secretions. These may be specific breathing and clearance techniques and/or other manual techniques.

If the respiratory muscles are ineffective the patient may not be able to clear secretions independently. Positions to reduce the work of breathing and optimize respiratory muscle function (see the above section) may enhance this. If clearance is still not effective then the physiotherapist may use or will advise the use of other techniques (Hough 2001; Jones & Moffatt 2002; Pryor & Webber 2002).

Positioning the patient with neurological impairment

For those with acute and long-standing neurological issues principles of positioning can be applied at any time along their treatment trajectory; those with rehabilitation potential; deteriorating function and those requiring palliative management for each of these clinical presentations. This relates to problems associated with abnormal tone, abnormal movement patterns, sensory and perceptual problems. The general principles of positioning discussed earlier can be applied for this group of patients. However, the complexity of these patients highlights the difficulty of a uniform approach to overall management. Therefore, this section will look at some of the variations in treatment of this patient group and suggest some principles to be considered when positioning these patients.

Disease or damage to the central or peripheral nervous system can lead to temporary or permanent complex physical, cognitive, psychological and psychosocial problems (Brada 1995; Lindsay & Bone 1997; Guererro 1998; Ellison & Love 2000; Kirschblum *et al.* 2001; Tookman *et al.* 2004). Their problems may include:

- Weakness: unilateral, bilateral or global.
- Sensory changes.
- Balance problems.
- Perceptual problems.
- Visual problems.
- Cognitive problems.
- Dysphagia.
- Dysphasia.
- Behavioural changes.

If a person with a neurological presentation is unable to move, they are deprived of the physical benefits of movement including:

- Sensory–motor appreciation.
- Posture and balance control.
- Maintenance of joint and soft tissue range of movement.
- Maximization of functional independence.
- Minimization of tonal changes such as spasticity (Hawkins *et al.* 1999).
- Cardiorespiratory fitness (Convertino *et al.* 1995).

This section will cover recommendations for assisting patients presenting with physical neurological symptoms affecting their central nervous systems (CNS) and peripheral nervous systems (PNS) as a consequence of their disease or treatment itself. These may include:

- Hemiparesis or monoparesis.
- Hemiaesthesia.
- Peripheral motor/sensory neuropathies.

Spinal cord compression will not be covered in this section (see Chapter 41).

Positioning can additionally offer control of positional influences of unwanted reflex activity for patients with altered tone (Davies 1985; Edwards 1996b; Jackson 1998). Many positions advocated relate to the desire to avoid the development of abnormal patterns of movement associated with altered tone through minimizing the influence of primitive developmental reflexes (Bobath 1990). The three reflexes identified whose 'release' can be influenced are: (i) the tonic labyrinth reflex; (ii) the symmetrical tonic neck reflex; and (iii) the asymmetrical tonic neck reflex (Davies 1985; Jackson 1998 citing Carr & Kenney 1992; Davies 2000). Davies (2000) describes these primitive reflexes:

The tonic labyrinthine reflex is evoked by changes in the position of the head in space; originating at otolithic organs of the labyrinths and believed to be integrated at brainstem levels. In supine, extensor tone increases throughout the body with resultant extension of head, spine and limb extension and shoulder retraction. In prone lying, flexor tone increases throughout the body. This may only be seen as a reduction in extensor tone in a patient with severe spasticity. The influence of relative head position to body will also be noticed in sitting or standing and may affect functional movement or position.

The symmetrical tonic neck reflex is a proprioceptive reflex, elicited by stretching of the muscles and joints of the neck. When the head extends, extensor tone in the arms and flexor tone in the legs increases. When the head is flexed, the extensor tone in the lower limbs increases, with more flexor tone in arms. This position can be seen where the patient sits unsupported or is half lying in bed with their head flexed; their affected leg extends and affected arm flexes more. This can also be seen when a patient is sitting unsupported in a chair or wheelchair.

The asymmetrical tonic neck reflex is elicited as a proprioceptive response from the muscles of the joints and neck. Extensor tone increases in the limbs on the same side to which the head is turned. The limbs on the occipital side show an increase in flexor tone. Patients who have poor mobility requiring wheelchair dependence may have an increase in lower limb flexor tone on their weak side as well as affecting their arm. Here, a flexion contracture of the knee may develop requiring effective management strategies recommended by therapists following individual patient assessment.

Davies (1985, 2000) describes positioning for stroke patients and urges the avoidance of flat supine positioning due to its influence on the tonic neck and labyrinthine reflexes potentially resulting in an increase in inappropriate extensor activity throughout the body.

However, today there appears an overall lack of consensus in clinicians' actual practice regarding the key components of the positions necessary to limit the onset of spasticity and unwanted patterns of movement developing (Jackson 1998; Chatterton *et al.* 2001). A survey of physiotherapists specializing in treatment of stroke patients identified the most common aims of positioning for patients with neurological problems were: modulation of muscle tone (93%); prevention of damage to affected limbs (92%); and supporting and stabilizing body segments (91%) (Chatterton *et al.* 2001). These factors promote recovery in patients with neurological presentations where recovery is likely (Pope 1996; Edwards 1998; Hawkins *et al.* 1999; Barnes 2001b). The evidence for positioning neurological patients is drawn from parallel literature for patients presenting with similar neurological symptoms and impairments affecting their function as a consequence of illness such as stroke and head injury (Davies 1985; Bobath 1990; Lynch & Grisogono 1991; Carter & Edwards 1996; Hawkins *et al.* 1999).

Joint protection

Positioning is suggested as a strategy to prevent hemiplegic shoulder pain and to prevent loss of range of movement (Kaplan 1995; Dean *et al.* 2000; Ada *et al.* 2005). This is a goal of rehabilitation to prevent the patient's functional deterioration (Gloag 1985). Dean *et al.* (2000) identified that these complications often prevent a patient's full participation in rehabilitation; contributing to poor upper limb functional outcome. Several factors were described for this:

- Glenohumeral subluxation due to lack of muscular activity around the shoulder.
- Trauma to the shoulder complex through unsuitable exercise.
- Trauma through inappropriate handling of the patient by staff during transfers.

Although their study failed to demonstrate significantly altered outcomes in pain and range through positioning the shoulder, Dean *et al.* (2000) acknowledged that consistency in education was essential for these common problems. Ada *et al.* (2005) recommended that patients with little upper limb function in the early stages post-stroke undergo a programme of positioning of the affected shoulder. This incorporated 45° shoulder abduction and comfortable external rotation for at least 30 minutes a day in addition to standard therapy. Their study showed statistical significance in maintaining shoulder range when compared with patients who received standard upper limb care of arm support and exercise only. Such specific joint positioning requires assessment by the physiotherapist for each individual patient.

Altered tone and abnormal patterns of movement

Tone is defined clinically as, 'the resistance that is encountered when the joint of a relaxed patient is moved passively' (Britton 1998, p. 57). Alterations in tone will affect functional recovery in patients with neurological problems and require careful management. This can be through positioning, splinting if required and oral and focal pharmacological intervention (Barnes 2001a).

Increased tone and spasticity are disorders of spinal proprioceptive reflexes. Spasticity is defined as:

a motor disorder characterised by a velocity dependent increase in tonic stretch reflexes (muscle tone) with exaggerated tendon jerks, resulting from hyper excitability of the stretch reflex, as

one component on the upper motor neurone syndrome (Barnes 2001a, p.1).

Abnormal movement patterns exist where there is interruption of the key components for normal movement. Normal movement is dependent on a neuromuscular system that can receive, integrate and respond appropriately to multiple intrinsic and extrinsic stimuli. Where this is altered through CNS or PNS disease, abnormal movement patterns will exist. Key components include:

- Normal postural tone.
- Reciprocal innervation of muscles.
- Sensory: motor feedback and feedforward.
- Balance reactions (Edwards 1996a).
- Biomechanical properties of muscle (Edwards 1998).

Procedure guidelines   Positioning the neurological patient with tonal problems

Positional influences in the patient with neurological impairment may affect spinal, pelvic and shoulder girdle alignment with risk of soft tissue shortening due to potential:
- Flattened lumbar spine.
- Extended thoracic spine.
- Pelvis tilted backwards.
- Retracted hip.
- Elevated shoulder, retracted scapula.
- Feet tend toward plantar flexion.

Therefore, additional considerations should be applied for the neurological patient with severe tonal management issues. These should always be discussed with the physiotherapist. Appropriate seating is also advocated as an adjunct to management (Pope 1996; Kirkwood & Bardslay 2001). Referral to the occupational therapist and physiotherapist is essential for assessment where this is required. See Figures 34.10 and 34.11.

Equipment
1 Pillows or towels (as guidance or basic positioning).
2 Foot resting splint if required.

Procedure

Action	Rationale
1 Follow basic positioning advice for positioning the patient in supine, side lying and sitting in bed as described in the above procedure guidelines for positioning patients.	To promote alignment of body segments for patients with high or low tone due to abnormal influences of primitive developmental reflexes resulting in asymmetrical posture in these patients (Davies 1985; Bobath 1990; Lynch & Grisogono 1991; Carter & Edwards 1996: R 4, E).

2 Consider and apply possible modifications as specified below:
(a) *Supine* (see Action figure 2a):
  ■ Place pillow under hemiplegic hip for alignment.
  ■ Place additional pillows or wedge under knees and/or head.
  ■ Place pillow to support feet in neutral/plantargrade position.
  ■ Apply foot resting splint (ankle foot orthosis [AFO]) to weak foot and ankle if recommended. NB. Ensure the splint is fitting correctly.
  ■ Place pillow under weak arm.
	To control pelvic and spinal alignment (E).
	To optimize patient comfort (E, P).
	
	To maintain joint and soft tissue range (ACPIN 1998: C, E; Edwards 1998; Barnes 2001a: R 4).

(b) *Side lying* (see Action figure 2b):
- Place pillow under head and in front of trunk.

To support the patient's affected shoulder and upper limb due to a risk of trauma, pain, muscle and soft tissue shortening (Dean *et al.* 2000; Ada *et al.* 2005: R 2b, E).
To reduce the influence of primitive developmental reflexes and asymmetrical posturing of head and trunk in patients with high or low tone (E).
May be effective in maintaining opposing trunk muscles (E).

Action 2   Positioning the patient with neurological weakness. **(a)** Side lying: affected arm supported on pillow. **(b)** Supine: affected arm supported on pillow.

The influence of altered tone and abnormal patterns of movement are key to therapeutic theories supporting treatment of recovery of motor control associated with patients with neurological problems. Patients attempt to perform functional skills as prerequisites of activities of daily living, but without appropriate background postural tone and normal properties of muscle, these movements will be performed in an abnormal way.

Soft tissue changes and contractures

Soft tissue changes and contractures occur through disuse in normal muscle (Jones & Moffatt 2002). With increased tone joint range and subsequent function is at risk. Restriction in the range of movement is not always simply through increased tone of the relevant muscles. The surrounding soft tissues, tendons, ligaments and the joints themselves can develop changes resulting in decreased compliance leading to an increased likelihood of them being maintained in a shortened position (Barnes 2001a). This creates a secondary biomechanical component of spasticity and is often seen in patients with functional mobility problems. Adaptation of the mechanical properties of muscle also contribute to increased tone in patients with hypertonia (O'Dwyer *et al.* 1996). It is possible, but not proven, that maintaining a joint through a full range of movement may prevent the longer term development of soft tissue contractures (Barnes 2001a).

Environment and positioning

Problems of perception are considered to be one of the main factors limiting functional motor recovery following stroke (Baer & Durward 2004). These can be applied to patients with disease or illness affecting their CNS. Here, the patient fails to respond appropriately to stimuli presented on their hemiplegic side, the contralateral side to the brain lesion; the left is more commonly affected following right parietal lesions (Lindsay & Bone 1997; Baer & Durward 2004). Environmental factors such as correct positioning are essential for ensuring optimal level of function for each individual (Edwards 1996b). Clinical management strategies include:

- Addressing the patient from the affected side.
- Deliberate placement of items such as drinks on that side.
- Advice to carers to position themselves on the patient's affected side whilst talking to them in order to orientate them to their affected side.
- Positioning the patient on their 'affected side' enabling function with their 'sound side'.
- Positioning the patient on their 'unaffected side', orientating the patient to their affected side.

Limited evidence exists to suggest the benefit of this (Baer & Durward 2004). However, it is recognized as a useful treatment adjunct for these patients by experienced occupational therapists and physiotherapists, through promotion of sensory awareness/appreciation, including perception and body image and enabling function (Davies 1985; Bobath 1990; Lynch & Grisogono 1991; Greive 1993; Carter & Edwards 1996).

Rehabilitation opportunity

Patients with neurological illness or disease present with an assortment of clinical symptoms. Positioning can assist in their holistic management and allow future opportunity for rehabilitation where their disease allows. Additional considerations for this patient group include the patient's:

- Respiratory function (see earlier section).
- Swallowing function; a referral to a speech and language therapist is recommended for any patient at risk.

- Cognitive function; a referral to occupational therapy or clinical psychology is recommended.

Appropriate management of these factors will influence the patient's future rehabilitation opportunity and will contribute to their recovery and/or management from an early stage. The latter are not covered in this book.

Procedure guidelines   Positioning the preoperative and postoperative amputee patient

Equipment

1 Stump board (for below knee amputees sitting out in wheelchair).
2 Pillows.

Action	Rationale
Upper limb amputee	
1 Ensure patient is maintaining full range of motion of all joints of the upper limb.	To prevent contractures in case of possible prosthetic rehabilitation and functional use (E, P).
Positioning the below knee amputee	
1 Maintain knee extension:	
(a) **In bed**: do not place towel or pillow under knee unless supporting whole of stump, i.e. do not encourage the knee to be maintained in a flexed position.	To prevent knee flexion contracture (E). To aid stump oedema management (E). To promote healing (E).
(b) **In chair**: use stump board on wheelchair if one has been issued.	To support knee joint (E, P). To prevent excessive knee flexion (E). To aid stump oedema management (White 1992: R 4, E, P). To protect the residual limb (E, P).
Positioning the above knee amputee	
1 Maintain hip in a neutral position:	To maintain hip extension (E).
(a) **In bed**: ensure patient is periodically lying supine. Or:	To prevent hip flexion contracture (E).
(b) Consider prone lying or side lying with hip in neutral position.	To avoid shortening of hip flexors and abductors (E).
(c) **In sitting**: ensure that patient does not place towel or pillow under stump.	To prevent excessive hip flexion (E).

Note: Following lower limb amputation patients should be mobilized with caution, particularly if a prosthetic assessment is planned. This is because standing for long periods or hopping can:
- Negatively influence stump oedema and wound healing.
- Overtire a patient particularly elderly patients or those who are physically de-conditioned prior to the amputation.
- Encourage the patient to adopt poor gait patterns due to excessive weight bearing on the remaining limb leading to difficulty with prosthetic rehabilitation.

Positioning and amputee management

The main goal of positioning with regard to amputee management is the prevention of contractures (particularly if the patient's goal is prosthetic rehabilitation) and help controlling stump oedema in order to assist wound healing.

Patients will need to be comprehensively assessed by the key professionals to identify realistic goals and ensure adequate pain management (BACPAR 2006). Where possible the process of positioning starts at the preoperative stage when the affected limb is often painful and therefore the patient may adopt positions of comfort that can lead to contractures.

These positions are often maintained post-amputation due to comfort and habit but are also due to changes in muscle balance. For example, above knee amputees may adopt a flexed position of their stump due to an alteration in muscle balance and pain but this can lead to contracture over time if not corrected (Engstrom & Van de Ven 1999). Contractures can profoundly affect the potential for prosthetic rehabilitation so early correct positioning is paramount in this cohort of patients (Munin *et al.* 2001).

Amputation affecting either an upper or lower limb will alter the patient's centre of gravity resulting in decreased balance and likelihood to adopt poor postures. Although the guidelines regarding sitting or walking a patient outlined above are applicable to this client group, particular care needs to be taken with regard to body symmetry and posture when the patient is lying, sitting or mobilizing.

Conclusion

This chapter has discussed the aims and general principles of positioning in order to help optimize function for patients. These principles of positioning can apply to all patients regardless of their diagnosis. However, attention has been drawn to specific patient groups where additional considerations and/or modifications are required.

It is essential that maximum function and quality of life are achieved through early assessment and treatment including positioning, timely rehabilitation and provision of equipment. It highlights the need for early identification of problems and early referral to appropriate key health professionals for individual patient assessment. This helps to provide effective, patient-focused holistic management and care.

References and further reading

ACPIN (1998) *Clinical Practice Guidelines on splinting adults with neurological dysfunction.* Association of Physiotherapists Interested in Neurology, Chartered Society of Physiotherapy, London.

ACPOPC (1993) *Physiotherapy in Oncology and Palliative Care: Guidelines for Good Practice.* Association of Physiotherapists in Oncology and Palliative Care, Chartered Society of Physiotherapy, London.

Ada, L. *et al.* (2005) Thirty minutes of positioning reduces the development of shoulder external rotation contracture after stroke: a randomised controlled study. *Arch Phys Med Rehabil*, **86**, 230–4.

Adam, S. & Forrest, S. (1999) ABC of intensive care: other supportive care. *BMJ*, **319**, 175–8.

Anderson, F.A. & Spencer, F.A. (2003) Risk factors for venous thromboembolism. *Circulation*, **107**, 9–16.

BACPAR (2006) *Clinical Guidelines for the Pre and Post Operative Management of Adults with Lower Limb Amputation.* The Chartered Society of Physiotherapy, London.

Baer, G. & Durward, B. (2004) Stroke. In: *Physical Management in Neurological Rehabilitation* (ed M. Stokes), 2nd edn. Elsevier Mosby, Edinburgh, pp. 75–101.

Barnes, M.P. (2001a) An overview of the clinical management of spasticity. In: *Upper Motor Neurone Syndrome and Spasticity: Clinical Management and Neurophysiology* (eds M.P. Barnes & G.R. Johnson). Cambridge, Cambridge University Press, pp. 1–11.

Barnes, M.P. (2001b) Spasticity: a rehabilitation challenge in the elderly. *Gerontology*, **47**(6), 295–9.

Barsevick, A.M. *et al.* (2002) A pilot study examining energy conservation for cancer treatment-related fatigue. *Cancer Nurs*, **25**(5), 333–41.

Bausewein, C., Borasio, G.D. & Voltz, R. (2004) Brain tumours. In: *Oxford Textbook of Palliative Medicine* (eds D. Doyle *et al.*). Oxford University Press, Oxford, pp. 727–30.

Beck, L.A. (2003) Cancer rehabilitation: can it make a difference? *Rehab Nurs*, **28**(2), 42–7.

Bobath, B. (1990) *Adult Hemiplegia: Evaluation and Treatment.* Heinemann, Oxford.

Brada, M. (1995) Central nervous system tumours. In: *Oncology: A Multidisciplinary Textbook* (ed. A. Horwich). Chapman & Hall, London, pp. 395–416.

Britton, T.C. (1998) Abnormalities of muscle tone and movement. In: *Neurological Physiotherapy* (ed. M. Stokes). Mosby, London, pp. 57–65.

Brown, A. *et al.* (1996) *Physiotherapy Management of the Spontaneously Breathing, Acutely Breathless, Adult Patient – A Problem Solving Approach.* Association of Chartered Physiotherapists in Respiratory Care, London.

Carr, E.K. & Kenney, F.D. (1992) Positioning the stroke patient: a review of the literature. *Int J Nur Stud*, **29**, 335–6.

Carter, P. & Edwards, S. (1996) General principles of treatment. In: *Neurological Physiotherapy: A Problem Solving Approach* (ed S. Edwards). Churchill Livingstone, London, pp. 87–113.

Chatterton, H.J., Pomeroy, V.M. & Gratton J. (2001) Positioning for stroke patients: a survey of physiotherapists' aims and practices. *Disabil Rehabil*, **23**(10), 413–21.

Convertino, V.A., Bloomfield, S.A. & Greenleaf, J.E. (1995) An overview of the issues: physiological effects of bed rest and restricted physical activity. *Med Sci Sport Ex*, **29**(2), 187–90.

Cooper, J. (2006) *Occupational Therapy in Oncology and Palliative Care.* John Wiley & Sons, Ltd, Chichester.

Corcoran, P.J. (1991) Use it or lose it – the hazards of bed rest and immobility. *West J Med*, **154**(5), 536–8.

Creditor, M.C. (1993) Hazards of hospitalization of the elderly. *Ann Intern Med*, **118**(3), 219–23.

CSP (2002) Guidance on the manual handling for physiotherapists. www.csp.org.uk. Accessed 21/07/2003.

CSP (2003) CSP position statement: the role of physiotherapy for people with cancer. Chartered Society of Physiotherapy. www.csp.org.uk. Accessed 21/07/2003.

Davies, P.M. (1985) *Steps to Follow: a Guide to the Treatment of Adult Hemiplegia.* Springer-Verlag, Berlin.

Davies, P.M. (2000) *Steps to Follow: the Comprehensive Treatment of Adult Hemiplegia*, 2nd edn. Springer-Verlag, Berlin.

Dean, C.M., Makey, F.H. & Katrak, P. (2000) Examination of shoulder positioning after stroke: a randomised controlled pilot trial. *Aust J Physiother*, **46**, 35–40.

Dean, E. (1985) Effect of body positioning on pulmonary function. *Phys Ther*, **65**, 613–18.

DH (2000) The NHS cancer plan: a plan for investment, a plan for reform. www.doh.gov.org. Accessed 18/5/06.

Dietz, J.H. (1981) *Rehabilitation Oncology.* John Wiley & Sons, Inc., New York.

Doyle, D. *et al.* (2004) *Oxford Textbook of Palliative Medicine*, 3rd edn. Oxford University Press, Oxford.

Doyle, L., McClure, J. & Fisher, S. (2004) The contribution of physiotherapy to palliative medicine. In: *Oxford Textbook of Palliative Medicine* (eds D. Doyle *et al.*), 3rd edn. Oxford University Press, Oxford, pp. 1050–56.

Edwards, S. (1996a) An analysis of normal movement as the basis for development of treatment techniques. In: *Neurological Physiotherapy: a Problem Solving Approach.* Churchill Livingstone, London, pp. 15–40.

Edwards, S. (1996b) Abnormal tone and movement as a result of neurological impairment. In: *Neurological Physiotherapy: a Problem Solving Approach*. Churchill Livingstone, London, pp. 63–86.

Edwards, S. (1998) Physiotherapy management of established spasticity in spasticity rehabilitation. In: *Spasticity Management* (ed. G. Sheean). Churchill Communications Europe Ltd, London, pp. 71–90.

Ellison, D. & Love, S. (2000) Classification and general concepts of CNS neoplasms and astrocytic neoplasms. In: *Neuropathology: a Reference Text of CNS Pathology* (eds D. Ellison & S. Love). Mosby, London.

Engstrom, B. & Van de Ven, C. (1999) *Therapy for Amputees*, 3rd edn. Churchill, Harcourt Brace & Co, Edinburgh.

Fulton, C. (1994) Physiotherapy in cancer care: a framework for rehabilitation. *Physiotherapy*, 80(12), 830–4.

Fyfe, N. *et al.* (1993) Orthoses, mobility and environmental control systems. In: *Neurological Rehabilitation* (eds R. Greenwood *et al.*). Churchill Livingstone, London, pp. 229–44.

Gardiner, M.D. (1973) *The Principles of Exercise Therapy*. Bell & Sons, London.

Gillis, M.K. (1989) Observational gait analysis. In: *Physical Therapy* (eds R.M. Scully & M.R. Barnes). Lippincott, Philadelphia, pp. 670–95.

Gloag, D. (1985) Rehabilitation after stroke: what's the potential? *Br Med J*, 290, 699–701.

Greive, J. (1993) *Neuropsychology for Occupational Therapists: Assessment of Perception and Cognition*. Blackwell Publishing, London.

Guererro, D. (1998) *Neuro-oncology for Nurses*. Whurr, London.

Hawkins, S., Stone, K. & Plummer, L. (1999) An holistic approach to turning adults. *Nurs Stand*, 6(14), 51–6.

Hodges, P.W. & Gandevia, S.C. (2000) Changes in intra-abdominal pressure during postural and respiratory activation of the human diaphragm. *J Appl Physiol*, 89(3), 967–76.

Hough, A. (2001) *Physiotherapy in Respiratory Care: an Evidence-Based Approach to Respiratory and Cardiac Management*, 3rd edn. Nelson Thornes Ltd., Cheltenham.

HSE (1992) *Manual Handling Operations Regulations*. HMSO, London.

Jackson, J. (1998) Specific treatment techniques. In: *Neurological Physiotherapy* (ed. M. Stokes). Mosby, London, pp. 299–311.

Jones, M. & Moffatt, F. (2002) Deconditioning. In: *Cardiopulmonary Physiotherapy* (ed. A. Watts). BIOS Scientific Publishers Ltd, Oxford, pp. 129–38.

Kaplan, M.C. (1995) Hemiplegic shoulder pain – early prevention and rehabilitation. *Am J Phys Med Rehabil*, 162(2), 151–152.

Kirkwood, C.A. & Bardslay, G.I. (2001) Seating and positioning in spasticity. In: *Upper Motor Neurone Syndrome and Spasticity: Clinical Management and Neurophysiology* (eds M.P. Barnes & G.R. Johnson). Cambridge University Press, Cambridge, pp. 122–141.

Kirschblum, S. *et al.* (2001) Rehabilitation of persons with central nervous system tumours. *Cancer*, 92(54), 1029–38.

Lindsay, K.W. & Bone, I. (1997) *Neurology and Neurosurgery Illustrated*, 3rd edn. Churchill Livingstone, London.

Lynch, M. & Grisogono, V. (1991) *Strokes and Head Injuries: a Guide for Patients, Families, Friends and Carers*. John Murray, London.

McGarvey III, C.L. (1990) *Physical Therapy for the Cancer Patient*. Churchill Livingstone, New York.

McKenzie, R. (1985) *Treat Your Own Back*. Spinal Publications, New Zealand.

Munin, C. *et al.* (2001) Predictive factors for successful early prosthetic ambulation among lower limb amputees. *J Rehabil Res Dev*, 38(4), 379–84.

National Council for Hospice and Specialist Palliative Care Services (NCHSPCS) (2000) *Fulfilling Lives: Rehabilitation in Palliative Care*. Land and Unwin, Northamptonshire.

NHSE (1995) A policy framework for commissioning cancer services: a report by the Expert Advisory Group on Cancer to the Chief Medical Officers of England and Wales (Calman–Hine Report). National Health and Safety Executive, Department of Health, London. Available from www.doh.gov.org. Accessed 21/03/2007.

NICE (2002) *Guidance on Cancer Services: Improving Outcomes in Breast Cancer*. National Institute for Health and Clinical Excellence, London.

NICE (2004) *Guidance on Cancer Services: Improving Supportive and Palliative Care for Patients with Cancer*. National Institute for Health and Clinical Excellence, London, pp. 134–147.

NICE (2005) *Guidance on Cancer Services: Improving Outcomes for People with Tumours of the Brain and Central Nervous System*. National Institute for Health and Clinical Excellence, London.

Norris, C.M. (1995) Spinal stabilisation 2. Limiting factors to end stage motion in the lumbar spine. *Physiotherapy*, 81(2), 64–72.

O'Donovan K. *et al.* (2006) An investigation of recommended lower leg exercises for induced calf muscle activity. International Association of Science and Technology for Development. Proceedings of the 24th IASTED International Conference on Biomedical Engineering, Innsbrook.

O'Dwyer, N.J., Ada, L. & Neilson, P.D. (1996) Spasticity and muscle contracture following stroke. *Brain*, 119, 1737–49.

Pearsall, J. (ed.) (2001) *The Concise English Dictionary*, 10th edn. Oxford University Press, Oxford.

Pope, P. (1996) Postural management and seating. In: *Neurological Physiotherapy: a Problem Solving Approach* (ed S. Edwards). Churchill Livingstone, London, pp. 135–60.

Pryor, J.A. & Webber, B.A. (2002) Physiotherapy techniques. In: *Physiotherapy for Respiratory and Cardiac Problems: Adults and Paediatrics* (eds J.A. Pryor & S.A. Prasad). Churchill Livingstone, Edinburgh, pp. 189–230.

Reidel, M. (2001) Acute pulmonary embolism 1: pathophysiology, clinical presentation, and diagnosis. *Heart*, 85(2), 229–40.

Russell, L. (2004) Patient repositioning revisited. *J Wound Care*, 13(8), 328–9.

Shumway-Cook, A. & Woollacott, M. (1995) *Motor Control: Theory and Practical Applications*. Williams and Wilkins, Baltimore.

Stokes, M. (2004) *Physical Management in Neurological Rehabilitation*, 2nd edn. Elsevier Mosby, Edinburgh.

Tookman, A.J., Hopkins, K. & Scharpen-von-Heusson, K. (2004) Rehabilitation in palliative medicine. In: *Oxford Textbook of Palliative Medicine* (ed. D. Doyle), 3rd edn. Oxford University Press, Oxford, pp. 1019–32.

Wagner, P.D. & West, J.B. (2005) Ventilation, blood flow and gas exchange. In: *Textbook of Respiratory Medicine* (eds R.J. Mason *et al.*), 4th edn. Elsevier Saunders, Philadelphia, pp. 51–85.

West, J.B., Dollery, C.T. & Naimark, A. (1964) Distribution of blood flow in isolated lung; relation to vascular and alveolar pressures. *J Appl Physiol*, 19, 713–24.

White, E. (1992) Wheelchair stump boards and their use in lower limb amputees. *Br J Occupat Ther*, 55(5), 174–8.

WHO (2001) International classification for functioning and health. World Health Organization. www3.who.int/icf/icftemplate.cfm. Accessed 9/2/07.

Zach, M.B., Pontoppidan, H. & Kazemi, H. (1974) The effect of lateral positions on gas exchange in pulmonary disease. *Am Rev Respir Dis*, 110, 49–55.

Chapter 35

Radioactive source therapy: sealed sources

Sealed radioactive source therapy **692**
Reference material **692**
Remote afterloading **698**
Reference material **698**
Procedure guidelines: Sealed radioactive sources insertion: patient care **702**
Procedure guidelines: Intraoral sealed radioactive sources: patient care **704**
Procedure guidelines: Iridium and caesium gynaecological sources **705**
(manual and afterloaded): patient care
Procedure guidelines: Gynaecological caesium and iridium wires removal **706**
Problem solving: Gynaecological caesium and iridium wires **708**
Procedure guidelines: Selectron treatment: patient care **708**
Procedure guidelines: Selectron applicator removal **709**
Problem solving: Selectron treatment **710**
Procedure guidelines: Radioactive seeds (e.g. iodine-125): patient care **711**
Procedure guidelines: Breast sealed radioactive sources: patient care **712**
Procedure guidelines: Interstitial perineal template (Hammersmith hedgehog) **712**
Useful websites **714**
References and further reading **714**

Sealed radioactive source therapy

Definition

Sealed radioactive sources are usually powders or solids enclosed in a casing which is inserted into the patient (Hart 2006). Generally, there is little risk of spreading radioactive contamination from these sources, unless the casing is cracked during sterilization. Radioactive iridium-198 is a solid metal, which may be made into alloy wires and used for direct insertion into tissues or cavities. Although not sealed in a metal casing, the methods applied to the use of sealed sources are also applied to this substance. Sealed source therapy is also referred to as brachytherapy. The word brachytherapy comes from the Greek 'brachy', which means close by, and from 'therapia', meaning therapy. This implies that brachytherapy refers to a radioactive source that is inserted in or placed near the tumour (Hoskin & Coyle 2005). The principles of radiation protection, distance, time and shielding (which minimize personal exposure to radiation), must be applied when working with sealed sources to ensure that all unnecessary exposure is avoided (Hart 2006).

Indications

Permanent or temporary insertions of small, sealed sources are used to deliver very high doses of radiation into tumours or tumour-bearing tissue while giving rapidly diminishing doses to adjacent structures. This will limit the damage caused to normal tissue (Nag 2004). A specific dose of radiation will be received by the cancer. This is delivered continuously over a period of minutes, hours or days.

Reference material

Measures of radiation

Ionizing radiation is the term used to describe energetic particles (e.g. alpha, beta) or electromagnetic waves with a wavelength of no more than 100 nanometres because they are capable of producing ions by ejecting electrons from their atoms (DH 2000).

Radiation kills by causing ionization within living cells. The activity of radioisotopes was at one time measured in millicuries (mc), but the standard unit is now the becquerel (Bq). A becquerel is the Système International (SI) unit of activity and is 1 disintegration per second:

$$k \text{ (kilo)} = 1 \times 10^3$$
$$M \text{ (mega)} = 1 \times 10^6, \text{ e.g. megabecquerel (MBq)}$$
$$G \text{ (giga)} = 1 \times 10^9$$

The half-life of a radioactive substance is the time taken for it to decay to half its original number of radioactive atoms (Bomford 2002a). The sensitive target appears to be deoxyribonucleic acid (DNA) in the nucleus of the cell. The ionizing radiation thus passes through the cells and tissues, and the dose of radiation received is measured in terms of energy absorbed. The unit of absorbed dose is the gray:

$$100 \text{ centigray (cGy)} = 1 \text{ gray (Gy)}$$

For the purposes of radiation protection of staff and patients, the dose to the whole body must be known. Whereas the absorbed dose is measured in gray, the dose to the whole body is measured in sieverts. For instance, for staff over 18 years of age who are not pregnant, wearing a monitoring badge to monitor exposure to radiation, the annual dose limit is 20 millisieverts (mSv), but doses allowed to staff should be kept below 6 mSv where practicable (DH 1999).

Ionizing radiation regulations

The use of ionizing radiation is governed by strict regulations. In 1995 the Advisory Group on ionizing radiation was formed whose responsibilities included to review work related to radiation relevant to human health. This included occupational, public health, environment and research. In April 2005, The National Radiological Protection Board merged with the Health Protection Agency (HPA) to form the new Radiation Protection Division. The HPA has a statutory responsibility for advising UK government departments and those with responsibility for using ionizing and non-ionizing radiation, on the risk to human beings from radiation exposure. The importance of these groups cannot be underestimated. Research evaluating the cancer risk following radiation exposure that occurred following the Japanese atomic bomb, along with the knowledge that has been gained from patients who have received radiotherapy treatment for a primary cancer and who later developed a second primary cancer, highlights the risk that exposure to radiation may cause cancers. This knowledge has enabled the therapeutic benefit of treatment to be evaluated against the risk of developing a second cancer (Advisory Group on Ionising Radiation 2003).

The Ionising Radiations Regulations 1999 place duties on employers and employees to ensure the safe use of ionizing radiations in the workplace (DH 1999). The Ionising Radiation (Medical Exposure) Regulations 2000 lay down basic measures for the health protection of individuals undergoing medical exposures. These regulations require medical exposures to ionizing radiations to be justified and authorized and the doses received by the individuals must be kept as low as reasonably practicable (ALARP) and within recommended limits (DH 2000). The Medicines (Administration of Radioactive Substances) Regulations 1978 impose duties on those responsible for administering radioactive substances. A patient may receive a radioactive substance provided the patient's medical consultant has obtained a certificate from the Department of Health (DH) to enable them to administer that substance (DH 1978).

To help ensure compliance with the regulations the following must be in place:

- The area in which work with ionizing radiation is undertaken must be designated as a controlled area if special procedures are required to restrict significant exposures (i.e. 6 mSv per year) or to reduce the probability and magnitude of radiation accidents occurring. The area may otherwise need to be designated as a supervised area if a person may be exposed to more than 1 mSv per year.
- Local rules must be written for each controlled or supervised area.
- Staff monitoring must be performed in controlled areas.
- A Radiation Protection Adviser must be appointed to provide advice on all aspects of radiation protection.
- Radiation Protection Supervisors must be appointed for all controlled areas to ensure that the local rules for their area are being followed.
- Protocols and procedures must be written for all medical exposures to ionizing radiation.
- Practitioners (persons who justify and authorize the medical exposure) and operators (persons who undertake any practical aspect of the medical exposure) must be appointed and they must comply with the written protocols and procedures.
- Referrers (persons who refer patients for examination or treatment) must be identified.
- Staff training must be provided. This must include adequate theoretical knowledge and practical experience to ensure both their own and the patient's safety.
- Patients must be given adequate information so that they may give informed consent for therapy exposures to ionizing radiation.
- Patients must receive adequate instructions to ensure they fully understand the restrictions associated with their treatment.
- Visitors must receive adequate information to ensure they understand the restrictions and the risks associated with their potential exposure to ionizing radiation from the radioactive substances administered to patients.
- A quality assurance programme must be established to ensure that the policies, procedures and protocols are being performed satisfactorily and comply with agreed standards.
- A quality control clinical audit must be undertaken to ensure the quality assurance programme is followed. (DH 1978, 1999, 2000.)

Patient assessment

All patients who have been referred for treatment with radioactive sources must be assessed by the interdisciplinary staff associated with their treatment to ensure the treatment being planned will be successful (DH 2000) (see Preparation of the patient section, below). This assessment should establish that the patient can understand and is able to follow the restrictions imposed by the treatment. Difficulties understanding the spoken word, being deaf or hard of hearing,

being partial or totally sightless, having problems feeding or walking, being incontinent or being in need or in receipt of psychological or psychiatric support, will all require extra time being spent with the patient. Patients with these difficulties will need to be assessed to ensure they are suitable for sealed radioactive source therapy, as it is essential that the radiation restrictions necessary for these treatments will not cause the patients any additional problems (Hoskin & Coyle 2005). The assessment would normally be initially undertaken in the outpatient department and then on admission to the ward. If potential problems are indicated during the assessment, the doctor responsible for the patient should be informed and the nursing and physics staff involved with the treatment should be asked for help and advice.

Use of contamination monitor

Waste and equipment must be monitored before being removed from controlled areas where patients have received or are receiving therapy using interstitial or intracavitary sealed sources. This monitoring will establish that sources, which might have been dislodged from the patient, are not present amongst the items being removed (Hart 2006). Before using a contamination monitor it is important to check that the monitor's batteries are fully charged. The background reading on the monitor must then be noted before undertaking the monitoring. The background must be reasonably low (normally less than 10 counts per second), otherwise it will be difficult to detect small levels of radioactivity present on the item being monitored. If the background reading immediately outside the treatment room is found to be high it will be necessary to monitor the items further away where the background is lower. Items should be monitored by passing the monitor's probe over each item, while watching for fluctuations in the count rate. If an item is found to be contaminated (indicated by a sustained increase in count rate), it should either be returned to a safe location in the treatment room or set aside in a designated area while help is sought from the patient's doctor and from the physics department (Bomford 2002a).

Incident procedure

If an accident or incident has occurred or if one is suspected, the immediate priority is to ensure the safety of patients, staff and visitors and take whatever action is practicable to prevent further damage or injury (see Procedure guidelines: Sealed radioactive sources insertion: patient care, below). As soon as immediate care has been provided, all accidents, untoward incidents and near misses, irrespective of severity, must be reported on an incident report form. Proactive and reactive risk management processes are important. These processes should identify areas of potentially higher risk or allow lessons to be learnt from past incidents and accidents. This will allow the implementation of appropriate action plans to reduce the probability and/or severity of an incident occurring or recurring.

Radioactive isotopes used as sealed sources

Most radioactive isotopes used as sealed sources for brachytherapy emit both beta (β) and gamma (γ) radiation. Brachytherapy is either intracavitary, where radioisotope sources are placed in pre-existing body cavities (such as the uterine cavity or vagina), or interstitial, where radioisotope sources are inserted directly into the tissues in tubes or needles (Hoskin & Coyle 2005).

The radiation useful in treating malignant disease includes X-rays, produced artificially by electron bombardment of a metal target, and gamma rays, a natural emission in the nuclear decay of radioisotopes. They are sometimes referred to as 'photon' radiation. Beta particles are also capable of ionization; these are distinguishable from electromagnetic radiation by their characteristic of carrying a negative electrical charge. Beta particles result when a neutron within the nucleus disintegrates to form a proton and an electron. The electron is ejected from the nucleus, producing beta radiation (IPEM/RCN 2002).

Caesium-137

Caesium-137 is a radioisotope that can be used in the form of interstitial implants or in intracavitary applicators. This treatment allows a highly conformal dose of radioactivity to be delivered directly to the site of the cancer (Karakoyun-Celik *et al.* 2005). It has a half-life of 30 years and has largely replaced radium as a source of brachytherapy.

Oral implants

Caesium-137 can be used in a needle-like implant that is inserted directly into the tissue surrounding the tumour. This is a fairly common treatment for early lesions of the cheek, lip and anterior two-thirds of the tongue (Leborgne *et al.* 2002; Nutting *et al.* 2006). Oral implants have the advantage of allowing preservation of the structure and function of the tongue whilst avoiding the toxicity of external beam radiotherapy to the oral mucosa (Wadsley *et al.* 2003). If bone involvement is suspected, e.g. in the mandible, alternative external treatment will be given.

The sources (Figure 35.1) are inserted in theatre under a general anaesthetic. They are inserted individually in a predetermined pattern so that the implant covers the whole growth, with a safety margin of at least 1 cm. Each needle

Figure 35.1   Caesium-137 needles.

is positioned by pushers so that its eye, through which silk is threaded, is just visible beneath the mucosal surface. Each silk is then stitched to the tongue with a single suture. When all the needles have been inserted, the silks are counted and gathered together. They are threaded through a piece of rubber to prevent friction and trauma to the mouth. The silks are strapped to the cheek to prevent any needle being swallowed should it work loose. Small beads are attached to the ends of the threads to facilitate counting the needles. X-rays are always taken to check the positions of the needles and to enable estimation of the dose distribution (Takacsi-Nagy *et al.* 2001).

Gynaecological applicators

Caesium-137 can be used in applicators. The most common malignancies treated by the use of radioactive applicators are tumours of the female genital tract (Kucera *et al.* 2001). Intracavitary applicators are used which deliver a high dose to the region of the cervix, the paracervical tissue, the upper part of the vagina and the uterine body.

Iridium-192

Iridium-192 is a radioisotope which can be used in the form of pins or wires in interstitial therapy (Fung 2002). Its half-life is 74.2 days. Iridium-192 is used because of the low energy of its gamma emission compared to caesium, which simplifies radiation protection, and because in the form of a platinum–iridium alloy it can be drawn into thin flexible wires. The wires consist of an active platinum–iridium alloy core encased in a sheath of platinum 10 μm thick, which screens out the beta radiation from the iridium-192.

Iridium-192 can now be made with a very high specific activity, that is, in a very radioactive form. High activity sources of iridium are used in high dose-rate remote afterloading systems, which reduce the amount of radiation to which clinical oncologists and other staff are exposed.

Iridium-192 implants are used under the following circumstances:

- As a treatment for small primary lesions, for example, tongue or breast lesions (Lapeyre *et al.* 2004).
- As a 'boost' dose after external radiotherapy for larger primary tumours or where nodes are also involved (Grabenbauer *et al.* 2001).
- To treat recurrence (Nutting *et al.* 2006).

Iridium-192 hair pin and single pin types of implants are usually used intraorally (Figure 35.2). They are slotted into tissue using steel guides to obtain accurate alignment. Radiological examination is used to check the position of the guides before the iridium is inserted. The pins are held in place by sutures.

The staff of the physics department are normally responsible for calculating how long a radioactive implant is to stay in place. This is usually about 6 days, depending on the

Figure 35.2   Iridium-192 pins. (a) Iridium single pin. (b) Iridium hair pin.

size of the tumour. Removal is carried out in theatre by the clinical oncologist.

Iridium-192 wires are usually used for head and neck, breast or lesions of vulva or perineum (Figure 35.3). Polythene or metal cannulae are inserted under a general anaesthetic. In the case of breast lesions, both ends of each tube protrude through the skin. Correct alignment is established often with the aid of a Perspex template which fits over the breast and holds the metal cannulae in the correct alignment. In the case of vulval or perineal insertions, only one end of the tube protrudes. For these, alignment of the sources may be achieved by using a Perspex template and vaginal obturator.

The iridium wire source is afterloaded, usually on the ward, and the wires are held in the cannulae with crimped lead washers (see Figure 35.3). The tiny size of the high activity iridium-198 source in high dose rate machines may allow some interstitial brachytherapy to be given as a few

Figure 35.3   Iridium-192 wire in polythene cannula. Typical assembly in tissue.

treatments of several minutes each, in contrast to the single treatment of many hours' duration which is necessary with low-activity iridium wire (Hart 2006).

The clinical oncologist is responsible for calculating how long a radioactive implant should stay in place. This is usually for 3–6 days, depending on the size of the tumour. Removal of the implant is usually carried out on the ward.

The above procedures are safe and deliver a dose that is higher that can be achieved by eternal beam radiation alone, and leads to improved organ preservation rates (Karakoyun-Celik et al. 2005).

Interstitial perineal template

Iridium-192 interstitial brachytherapy can be used to treat locally advanced or recurrent tumours. Interstitial brachytherapy is a suitable alternative to standard intracavitary brachytherapy where the patient is considered unsuitable because the dose distribution may be suboptimal (Agrawal et al. 2005). Side-effects expected are similar to those from afterloading techniques and are considered to be acceptable (Syed et al. 2002). Late side-effects, such as fistulae and bowel complications requiring surgery in some patients, have been documented (Nag et al. 2002).

In a study to evaluate the long-term efficacy and safety of transperineal interstitial implant for advanced pelvic malignancy, it was found that this treatment offered a 5- and 10-year disease-free survival of 48% for patients aged 45 years and less, and an 80% disease-free survival in patients aged over 45 years (Budrukkar et al. 2001).

The device itself consists of two acrylic cylinders and an acrylic template with an array of holes that serve as guides for trocars and a cover plate (Figure 35.4). The cylinders are usually placed in the vagina but can also be used in the rectum for rectal tumours. They are then fastened to the template, so that a fixed geometric relationship among the tumour volume and normal structures, i.e. bladder and rectum, is produced. This ensures that the source placement is preserved throughout the course of the implantation. The iridium wire is then manually afterloaded and held in place with a crimped washer to prevent movement of the source during treatment (see Figure 35.3).

Nursing care is similar to the care that patients receive for intracavitary brachytherapy (see Procedure guidelines,

Figure 35.4   Interstitial perineal template device.

Iridium and caesium gynaecological sources (manual and afterloaded): patient care, below).

Iodine-125

Seeds of iodine-125 have replaced those of gold-198. The half-life of iodine-125 is 60 days. Some therapists believe that there is a radiobiological advantage to this long half-life in treating slowly growing tumours such as carcinoma of the prostate (Blank *et al.* 2000).

Seeds are inserted into the tissue that is to be irradiated, under ultrasound or image intensifier control. The patient requires a general anaesthetic for the insertion.

Because the energy of the gamma-ray emission from iodine-125 is very low compared with that of gold-198, large numbers of seeds are required, which means that more precautions must be taken in order to achieve a regular geometrical arrangement to ensure satisfactory distribution of the dose (Stock *et al.* 2000).

Implanted iodine-125 source is a well-established procedure and an increasing number of patients throughout the world are treated in this manner (Anglesio *et al.* 2005). Current evidence on the safety and efficacy of this treatment supports its use (NICE 2005). Complications include incontinence, obstructive urinary symptoms, rectal symptoms and sexual dysfunction. The impotence rate was 10–15% compared with 45% of those patients undergoing radical prostatectomy (NICE 2005). One quality-of-life study found that quality of life was worse during the first 4 weeks following treatment but returned to baseline values 1 year after implant (Zelefsky 2006).

It is important that the patient understands the uncertainties of iodine-125 seed therapy and the alternative treatment options. Included in the informed consent should be that:

- The patient understands that it's not clear how the procedure affects general health and the chance of the cancer returning in the long term (Wust *et al.* 2004).
- The patient understands what is involved and the alternative options.
- The results of the treatment are monitored: the length of time depending on the type of cancer and how advanced it is (NICE 2005).

Application of sources

Small sealed sources inserted into the body may take the form of:

- *Intracavitary applicators*, i.e. sources that are placed in natural cavities and usually held in place by packing.
- *Interstitial implants*, i.e. sources that are inserted directly into the tumour-bearing tissue (Hoskin & Coyle 2005).

(*Note*: sources held in plastic surface applicators or moulds are applied directly to superficial cancers.)

Intracavitary applicators and interstitial implants can be used in three forms:

- The source is preloaded in the applicator before it is placed in the patient for a fixed length of time, e.g. caesium-137 needles and iridium-192 hair pins.
- Permanent insertion in the case of iodine-125 seeds, which, once inserted, would be difficult to remove. The available data shows that, except in the case where the patient's partner is pregnant at the time of implantation, no restrictions are required once the patient is discharged home. Written information must be given to the patient on discharge, this must include the following:

  1   There is the possibility of triggering certain types of security radiation monitors.
  2   In most cases brachytherapy does not make the patient infertile, therefore the patient needs to be aware of the limited risk of genetic effects for a child.
  3   The implant should be discussed if future surgery is planned.
  4   Specific instruction should be available if the patient dies and cremation is required (The International Commission on Radiological Protection 2005).

- Whilst the patient is an inpatient all urine should be checked to ensure no seed has become dislodged. If it has become dislodged, the loose seed should be placed in a lead pot with long-handled forceps; any seed in a catheter bag should be saved to be collected by the Trust radiation protection service, which is generally the Physics department.
- Afterloading systems: where the applicator is placed in position and the radioactive source is inserted when the position of the applicator and the condition of the patient are satisfactory. Insertion of the sealed source can be undertaken manually in the case of iridium-192 wires or by remote control, as in the case of the low dose rate Selectron machine and the high dose rate microSelectron machine.

Afterloading techniques have the advantage of allowing the source carrier to be accurately positioned (Teruya *et al.* 2002), and for the sources to be withdrawn to a radiation-proof safe during patient care, sparing staff from radiation exposure.

The proportions of radioisotope (initially radium and latterly caesium) within the intrauterine tube and the vaginal ovoids (oval-shaped applicators) are calculated to give a constant dose rate to a geometrical point A when using different lengths of intrauterine tube and different sizes of vaginal ovoids. This constancy of dose rate when using applicators of different sizes is an important aspect of the Manchester system.

Afterloading brachytherapy

The basis of afterloading brachytherapy is that applicators are placed within the cervix and vaginal fornices, and that the radioisotope is only introduced into these when the applicators are correctly positioned, check radiographs have been taken and the patient is comfortable and in a protected environment (Hoskin & Coyle 2005). The sources may then be inserted either manually or by remote control. Manual methods are common and have the advantage of being cheap, but do not entirely protect staff as the sources have to be inserted by staff and cannot be removed for short periods while a patient's needs are attended to. Remote systems have the advantage of complete protection of staff, but have the disadvantage of high cost and the need for interlocking mechanisms (Bomford 2002b). These ensure that the correct source has been inserted into the correct applicator for the programmed length of time.

Remote afterloading systems allow the dose rate of brachytherapy to be increased. Classically, the dose rate with the Manchester system was approximately 50 cGy per hour to point A. With modern engineering methods, caesium pellets can be produced which will allow a dose rate of between 150 and 200 cGy per hour to point A. Many systems now use sources that allow a higher than standard dose rate to be delivered. This has the advantage of reducing treatment time (Kuipers *et al.* 2001).

If the concept of increasing dose rate is taken further, high dose rate brachytherapy, delivering doses at rates in excess of 1 Gy per minute to point A, offers the possibility of very short treatment times. This allows complete geometrical stability of the applicator during the treatment and makes a higher patient throughput possible. However, there is considerably less time for repair of radiation damage to normal tissues in a high dose rate treatment and, therefore, such treatments have to be fractionated over several days, in contrast to the continuous treatment given by a low dose rate brachytherapy implant. High-dose brachytherapy produces survival rates comparable to low-dose brachytherapy although complications can occur. Treatment regimens for patients with gynaecological cancers generally involve surgery, external beam radiotherapy and brachytherapy and this has proved to be both effective and tolerable (Chen *et al.* 2004).

Intracavitary applicators

Intracavitary applicators are inserted under a general anaesthetic, and the position of the applicator is checked by X-ray before the patient returns to the ward. A urinary catheter is also inserted in theatre to reduce the risk of the sources becoming dislodged by the patient when micturating.

Several different types of applicator are available and choice is usually determined by the site of the tumour, the anatomy of the patient and the preference of the treatment centre. The most commonly used types of applicator are described below (also see Figure 35.5).

Manchester applicator
Manchester applicators in their original form were live sources enclosed in intrauterine tubes of varying lengths and vaginal applicators (ovoids) of varying sizes. The applicators

Figure 35.5 Gynaecological caesium applicators. Arrangement of brachytherapy sources in the uterus and vagina for treatment of cervical carcinoma. Sources may be active or, more usually these days, afterloaded into applicators along catheters protruding from the vagina. (a) Manchester applicator. (b) Modified Stockholm applicator. (c) Fletcher applicator. (d) Dobbie applicator.

were inserted under general anaesthetic and held in place by a gauze pack. More recently, the applicators have been modified for either manual or remote afterloading at either low or high dose rate, but the principle of the three applicator system remains. Removal of the applicators or, if still used, the live sources is carried out on the ward and may require administration of Entonox as analgesia.

Stockholm applicator
This is used for carcinoma of the body of the uterus or cervix. Usually a uterine tube and two vaginal packets are inserted. Occasionally, if the vaginal vault is small, one packet is

697

omitted or replaced by a vaginal tube. The radioactive material is held in place with a proflavine-soaked gauze pack. It is usually left in place for 22 hours. Tubes and packets have strings attached for removal and colour-coded beads indicate which should be removed first (Bomford 2002b).

Modified Stockholm applicator

This is used for carcinoma of the body of the uterus and cervix. It consists of a uterine tube and a square box which connect together by a point and a hole. The vagina is then packed with gauze saturated with proflavine. They are usually left in place for 20 hours. The box should be removed first (Bomford 2002b).

Fletcher applicator

This is used for carcinoma of the corpus or cervix, but the patient needs to have a fairly capacious vaginal vault. Hollow applicators, a uterine tube and two vaginal ovoids are inserted in theatre and loaded with the radioactive sources later, on the ward, by the radiotherapist. The apparatus is held in place with a proflavine pack. Long ends project through the vulva so that after loading can be carried out. These insertions are usually left in place for 60–72 hours. No strings are needed as the apparatus itself projects from the vulva (Bomford 2002b).

Dobbie applicator

This is used to irradiate the whole vagina. A Perspex cylindrical applicator, with radioactive sources in the centre, is inserted into the vagina and sutured in place to the vulva. It may be used with low or high dose rate sources. Strings are attached to the applicator for removal (Bomford 2002b).

Manual afterloading systems

Manual afterloading systems are largely being replaced by remote systems, but they are still used in a few centres and are widely used in developing countries.

The plastic applicator tubes follow the pattern of the Manchester system with an intrauterine tube and two vaginal ovoids (oval intracavity applicators inserted into the vagina). The plastic tubes are designed to be disposed of after a single use. Insertion of the tubes takes place under general anaesthetic, after which confirmatory X-rays are taken with dummy sources in place. As with the classical Manchester system there are varying lengths of intrauterine tube and sizes of ovoids.

If the X-rays are satisfactory and once the dosimetry has been calculated, the radioactive caesium sources are introduced on their carrying rods using long-handled forceps. Once in place a silver metal cap is screwed over the end of the plastic tube to hold the sources securely.

Manual afterloading does not permit, for reasons of staff safety, the use of high activity sources and treatment may last many hours or even several days. When treatment is complete the caps are removed from the tubes and the sources are

withdrawn and placed immediately in a lead storage vessel. The plastic applicator tubes are then removed.

It is particularly important to observe for displacement or extrusion of the applicator tubes over the long treatment times. It is customary to mark the thigh level with the end of the applicator tubes and to compare this alignment at regular intervals as the treatment progresses. In addition, the silver metal caps should be monitored regularly for any loosening or displacement (Bomford 2002b).

Remote afterloading

Definition

Remote-controlled afterloading machines transfer active sources from a radiation-proof safe to the patient only when it is safe to do so (Hoskin & Coyle 2005).

Indications

Remote-controlled afterloading machines are gradually replacing conventional intracavitary caesium applicators as well as other manual and mechanical afterloading techniques (Bomford 2002b).

The low dose rate Selectron is used predominantly for the treatment of gynaecological cancers. While the high dose rate microSelectron is also regularly used in the treatment of gynaecological cancers, in some cases it may also be useful in the treatment of bronchial or oesophageal or other intraluminal carcinomas (Tessa et al. 2005; Ung et al. 2006).

Reference material

The low dose rate Selectron

The Selectron unit comprises a lead-shielded safe containing caesium-137 sources in the form of small spherical pellets, a microprocessor, keyboard, display unit and printer (Figure 35.6). Leading from the Selectron unit are either three or six flexible plastic transfer tubes corresponding to numbered treatment channels. Each tube ends in a fragile plastic catheter which is inserted into the appropriately numbered applicator and secured by a coupling device. The unit has a supply of compressed air and it is air pressure that the system uses to transfer the sources from the safe within the unit to the applicators along the connecting tubes. Operation of the unit is initiated from a remote-control unit situated outside the protected treatment area (Hoskin & Coyle 2005).

The Selectron provides an accurate and safe method of radiotherapy treatment for cancers of the cervix, uterus and upper part of the vagina.

The advantages of the Selectron system are threefold:

- Remote afterloading eliminates contact with radioactive material and protects personnel. The Selectron unit is switched off each time someone enters the patient's room, and only once all staff leave the room will the selectron

Figure 35.6   Selectron unit.

unit be switched back on. This will automatically re-turn the radioactive pellets into the applicators, and the treatment that was temporarily discontinued, will recommence (Hart 2006).

- It allows highly accurate dosimetry.
- The activity of the caesium-137 sources is such (up to 1.5 GBq) that treatment times for patients are considerably shorter than with conventional techniques.

Patients have hollow, lightweight stainless steel applicators positioned in the operating theatre under a general anaesthetic. These are usually modified Manchester or Fletcher type applicators consisting of a uterine tube and two vaginal ovoids held in place with a proflavine-soaked vaginal packing. However, several other applicators are available. Accurate positioning of the applicators is confirmed by taking X-rays with dummy sources in situ and the optimum source configuration is selected, taking account of individual anatomical variations.

The Selectron is programmed by the physicist. For each treatment channel being used, active source pellets are interspersed with inactive stainless steel spacer pellets to achieve the desired dose distribution (Hoskin & Coyle 2005). The treatment time required to reach the prescribed dose is also entered. With a six-channel Selectron unit it is possible to treat two patients with three applicators each simultaneously. The radiotherapist is responsible for connecting the transfer tubes to the applicators. The transfer tubes are led over a bed bracket which supports the weight of the tubes

and prevents traction being applied to the applicators in the patient. If the wrong catheter is connected to the applicator, the system will fail to operate.

Operating the Selectron

Treatment is commenced by activation of the remote control unit when all staff have left the treatment area. While treatment is in progress it can be interrupted and restarted from the remote control unit by pressing the stop and start buttons. The display panel indicates which channels are being used for treatment and which are unused with red and green lights respectively. The time of the longest treatment is displayed on the panel and a telephone intercom system, for example, allows for communication with the patient without the need to interrupt treatment (Hoskin & Coyle 2005).

Interrupting the treatment by pressing the green stop button results in the sources being withdrawn into the Selectron unit and stops the timer. This allows nursing staff to enter the treatment area in safety and give routine or specific care to the patient. Pressing the red start button transfers the sources back into the applicators and restarts the timer. The red lights demonstrate that the channels are operating again satisfactorily.

The system has built-in safety features. In the event of a failure in the system, treatment stops automatically. An audible and visual alarm at the remote control unit alerts staff to a problem and indicates whether this is a fault related to the air or power supply, the pellets or the timer. There is an optional nurse station display unit with a similar alarm indicator which also emits an audible signal when treatment has been interrupted. This helps to prevent treatment being inadvertently left interrupted for long periods.

A record of any break in treatment is shown on the printout from the unit itself, together with any programming or system fault. These appear as an error code and can be identified by reference to the Selectron user's manual.

At the end of the treatment time, all sources will be withdrawn automatically from the applicators back into the Selectron unit. When two patients are being treated simultaneously termination of the treatment of one patient may be some time before that of the other. This means the timer will register the longer treatment time, but the indicator lights for the channels used for the first patient will have changed from red to green.

Additional safety features include a door switch facility to retract sources immediately if the door to the treatment area is opened when treatment is in progress, and/or Geiger dose meters visible when entering the treatment area and approaching the patient, which indicate when there are radioactive sources either in the patient or in the connecting tubes.

The high dose rate microSelectron

The operating principles of the high dose rate (HDR) microSelectron are similar to those of the low dose rate (LDR)

Selectron. LDR Selectron applicators are afterloaded with active sources interspersed with inactive spacers to produce the correct isodose pattern. HDR microSelectron machines, on the other hand, achieve the desired isodose pattern with a single iridium-192 source which moves within the applicators and stops at preset positions for predetermined dwell times.

The HDR microSelectron delivers radiation at approximately 100 times the rate of the LDR Selectron and treatment times are therefore much shorter. It has the added advantage of applicators with a smaller diameter which can be put in place under local anaesthetic in the outpatients' department and is a suitable alternative for patients who may not be able to tolerate the demands of LDR (Hoskin & Coyle 2005).

Once in position, HDR microSelectron intracavitary applicators are fixed to the treatment couch by means of an adjustable clamp. Movement of the applicators is therefore minimal and dosimetry calculations accurately represent actual treatment. In addition, more constant and reproducible geometry of source positioning is possible (Jones *et al.* 1999).

Treatment protocols generally consist of two treatments but can involve as many as five. Following explanation and support for the patient (Faithfull & Wells 2003), the procedure is carried out under local anaesthetic. For the first treatment a urinary catheter is passed and the balloon inflated with dilute contrast medium. Check X-rays are taken once the applicator tubes are in place to collect information, which is fed into the Selectron planning computer and used to calculate the treatment time (Hoskin & Coyle 2005).

The HDR microSelectron follows the same principles for programming and treatment as the LDR Selectron. When treatment is complete the applicators and catheter are removed and the patient is free to go home. A case report found that patients undergoing treatment with HDR microSelectron for gynaecological cancer found the experience acceptable (Tan *et al.* 2004). Adequate preparation of the patient about treatment options is essential. The time spent preparing the patient for radiotherapy makes them better equipped to make informed decisions related to their care (Wallace *et al.* 2006). A poorly prepared patient may be more anxious and less able to follow instructions, less tolerant of the implant procedure (Montgomery *et al.* 1997). An assessment of patients' physical and emotional needs must be made prior to each treatment to identify whether any aspect of the treatment is problematic (Faithfull & Wells 2003).

The advantages of the HDR microSelectron are:

- The shorter treatment time reduces variations in the patient's position and allows more accurate dosimetry (Jones *et al.* 1999).
- Treatment lasts only minutes, minimizing the need for immobilization and reducing discomfort and the risk of complications associated with bed-rest.

- Treatment can be offered on an outpatient basis with a consequent reduction in cost.
- As an alternative to LDR, which may be more suitable for some patients.
- Complication rates are comparable with low dose brachytherapy (Wong *et al.* 2003).

Complications of intracavitary radiotherapy for gynaecological cancers

Radiation-induced early complications of intracavitary treatment are generally mild. They include, during treatment, pain and nausea and, following treatment, radiation-induced fatigue, diarrhoea, urinary frequency, dysuria, vaginal discharge and perineal irritation (Faithfull & Wells 2003). Severe reactions are rare, but may include severe or prolonged proctitis in patients with pre-existing bowel disease, and urgency and frequency of micturition, nocturia and dysuria. Late complications may include bowel and bladder complications (Shang-Wen *et al.* 2003).

Preparation of patient

Information about radiation therapy should be given to patients and carers when therapy is first discussed to allay fears and misconceptions about radiotherapy. Verbal information should be reinforced with written material to prepare the patient, reduce anxiety and promote coping (Faithfull & Wells 2003). A contact name and telephone number are useful for patients who wish to obtain further information at a later date.

Information for gynaecological patients receiving radiotherapy can be divided into three categories: (i) disease and treatment; (ii) short- and long-term side-effects; and (iv) sexuality.

All patients should have a thorough nursing assessment undertaken to assess their suitability for the treatment, both in the outpatients department and on admission to the ward. This will ensure that they are able to comply with the demands of the treatment. Any doubt due to the patient's physical or psychological problems and concerns can then be discussed with the patient and their medical team. This will allow for action to be taken, either to improve the patient's general condition so they are suitable for treatment or to postpone or cancel the radioactive sealed source therapy in favour of a more suitable treatment option (Velji & Fitch 2001).

LDR often follows 5 weeks of external beam radiotherapy of the pelvis (Petereit *et al.* 1998). This may mean that patients are already experiencing a number of symptoms at the time of the planned sealed source therapy. These may include radiation-induced enteritis, nausea, fatigue and skin reactions. Management of these symptoms may be required before LDR can be considered.

Prior to the procedure, it should be explained to patients that they will require an indwelling catheter and will be connected to the Selectron unit with flexible plastic tubes. Patients should be prepared for the noises made by the Selectron system, especially when sources are being transferred in and out of the applicators. Some patients may find the prospect of treatment alarming (Gosselin & Waring 2001) and may prefer to receive regular sedation for the duration of treatment. Patients' movements will need to be restricted during their treatment and they will be required to lie flat to maintain the pelvis in roughly the same position. This is to ensure that there is no significant movement of the applicators. The patient may be allowed to have a maximum of two pillows to support their head if this improves their comfort during treatment. Where practicable, the patient should be closely monitored during treatment. This can be achieved by the use of CCTV, telephone or intercom access for the patient and nurse, and a nurse call system, all of which provides further reassurance for patients.

Vaginal care following intracavitary treatment

Because the vaginal canal is included in the radiation field, vaginal stenosis, fibrosis, loss of elasticity and lubrication, and a decrease in sensation may develop after treatment if prophylactic measures are not taken (Muscari Lin et al. 1999).

To help prevent changes due to radiation, women who are sexually active should continue to have regular intercourse after any discomfort caused by an acute radiation reaction has resolved. Alternatively, a dilator can be used to keep the vagina open and stretched. Water-soluble lubricants may alleviate the dry mucosa, and hormone therapy, if appropriate, may be given orally or vaginally to increase natural lubrication (Blake et al. 1998).

Women can consider using a dilator once treatment has been completed for 2–6 weeks. Initially, the dilator should be inserted into the vagina daily for 5–10 minutes (removing and reinserting three or four times). A water-soluble lubricant should be used to ensure ease of insertion (Robinson et al. 1999). Following advice from a doctor or nurse specialist, frequency of dilatation can be reduced to between three times and once per week.

In addition some clinical oncologists recommend douching during radiotherapy and following brachytherapy, continuing for up to 8 weeks, to avoid infections and the formation of adhesions. Douching can be seen as controversial due to a theoretical risk of causing tumour cells to be transported and lodged further away from the site of the original tumour (Blake et al. 1998). The decision to use douching should therefore be made in discussion with the patient, her consultant and clinical nurse specialist. Douching should not be carried out, however, if there is a risk of haemorrhage from a persistent tumour (Blake et al. 1998).

Patients are encouraged to douche once a day using a disposable douche and tap water. Douching should continue until symptoms have resolved and advice has been given by a doctor or nurse specialist.

A review of 107 patients who had received radiotherapy found that advice from doctors and alternative practitioners such as nurses and dietitians was valuable in managing complications (Gami et al. 2003). A further study found that many of the patients' symptoms were not directly related to radiotherapy as patients often had other clinical problems which were readily treatable (Andreyev et al. 2005).

Follow-up care

Remote-controlled afterloading brachytherapy is a safe and effective treatment for cervical cancer, and has the added advantage of eliminating radiation exposure to staff, visitors and other patients. However, side-effects can occur including signs and symptoms associated with menopause in premenopausal women (Muscari Lin et al. 1999). A 20-year evaluation of the long-term survival and safety of interstitial and intracavitary brachytherapy in the treatment of carcinoma of the cervix found a reasonable chance of cure with acceptable morbidity (Syed et al. 2002).

Teruya et al. (2002) found that all patients included in a retrospective review of HDR microSelectron therapy had vaginal mucosal changes, but had no complaints regarding sexual functioning. Cancer treatment can cause persistent changes to the vagina which results in considerable distress by compromising sexual activity (Bergmark et al. 1999); patients need to be reassured that many women regain their capacity for sexual activity and enjoyment. Sexual counselling may improve outcome. Counselling should focus on self-esteem, body image and sexuality (Farrell 2002). Male partners of women with cancer reported difficulty in knowing how to behave and how to communicate with their partners (Lalos et al. 1995). Almost all male partners were given the news of the diagnosis exclusively by their ill partner, which provoked feelings of anger and bitterness (Lalos 1997). Coping improved if the men were integrated in the patient's care from the time the diagnosis of cancer was made (Lalos et al. 1995).

Discharge of the patient

Patients are usually discharged on the day of completion of brachytherapy. They must void urine normally following removal of the urinary catheter. Patients are sometimes unsteady on their feet after prolonged bed rest and may require assistance. They should be informed that normal bowel actions may not return for a day or so; advice on managing diarrhoea or constipation should be given. Light spotting or discharge from the vagina is normal. If patients experience pain or any more marked bleeding, hospital staff should be contacted immediately. Symptoms of urinary tract infection such as dysuria and/or elevated temperature should also be reported.

Procedure guidelines   Sealed radioactive sources insertion: patient care

Procedure

Action	Rationale
1 Before treatment begins, ensure the room is set up appropriately. This includes placing a lead pot and long-handled forceps in the room to hold any dislodged sources.	To reduce unnecessary time spent in the room once patient returns from theatre (Hart 2006: E).
2 Switch on controlled area radiation warning light outside the room and check it is working correctly.	To warn staff, visitors and other patients of the radiation risk and to ensure only trained personnel enter the room (Hart 2006: E).
3 Place radiation warning notice outside patient's room.	To ensure only authorized personnel enter the room (E).
4 Place lead shields in position at the door. All staff entering the room should work behind the lead shield when in close contact with the patient.	To reduce radiation exposure of staff in close contact with the patient (Hart 2006: E).
5 When transferring patients from theatre to ward, the nurse and porter should remain at the head and foot of the bed and at least 120 cm from the centre of the bed in the event of any delay in the transfer. If the source is intraoral, the nurse should stand at the foot of the bed.	To minimize the risk of exposure to radiation (E).
6 A yellow radiation hazard board should accompany the patient back from theatre. This must remain at the bottom of the bed or outside the cubicle until the source is removed.	To alert everybody that the patient has a radioactive source (E).
7 Nursing staff must calculate the time allowed with the patient in any 24-hour period. This time should be written on the yellow warning notice on the bed or cubicle door.	To minimize exposure to radiation (Hart 2006: E).
8 A contamination monitor should be available on the ward.	To monitor radioactivity if a dislodged source is suspected, e.g. in the bed linen (Hart 2006: E).
9 Whilst one nurse should be responsible for planning the nursing care of the patient, the time spent with the patient should be shared between all suitably trained nurses and all time spent in performing nursing procedures must be kept to a minimum. Only those staff whose presence is necessary should spend time with the patient.	To minimize the risk of overexposure to radiation (Hart 2006: E).
10 Every nurse must wear a radiation badge above the level of the lead shield.	To record the extent of exposure to radiation (DH 1999: C).
11 All bed linen and waste materials removed from the patient area should be monitored before being removed from the ward.	To prevent loss of an accidentally dislodged source (Hart 2006: C).
12 If a source becomes dislodged, use the long-handled forceps to put the source into a lead pot. Care should be taken not to damage the source. It must never be handled directly with the fingers.	To minimize the dose of radiation received (Hart 2006: E).

13 Visitors must seek permission each time they wish to enter the room. Visitors must remain at least 120 cm away from the patient. Visitors must always sit behind one of the bed shields. The visit should not last longer than the time shown on the warning notice. No children or pregnant women are allowed to visit.

To minimize the risk of overexposure to radiation (Ionising Radiation (Medical Exposure) Regulations, DH 2000: C).

14 When the patient needs to visit another department, for example to X-ray, the following must be ensured:

In order that medical care can continue to be provided while the patient is receiving radioactive sealed source therapy (E).

(a) That the receiving department is aware of the hazard of exposure to radioactivity.

To allow the appointment to be made when the department is quiet, thus ensuring waiting time is kept to a minimum and to minimize exposure to others (DH 1999: C).

(b) One porter and a nurse should accompany the patient in a wheelchair; two porters and a nurse should accompany the patient on a trolley. In the event of any delays, the nurse and porters should remain at the head and foot of the bed and at least 120 cm from the centre of the bed; if the source is intraoral, the nurse should stand at the foot of the bed.

To minimize the risk of exposure of staff to radiation (E).

(c) A radiation warning hazard sign should accompany the patient.

To warn all staff that the patient has a radioactive source in situ (DH 1999: C).

(d) Unless the patient is likely to be in the department for a long time the nurse and porter should stay with the patient.

To ensure time distance, shielding and segregation restrictions are maintained (E).

(e) If the source becomes dislodged during transfer, the porter must ring the switchboard who will send out an emergency call to the physics department. The nurse must ensure the area around the patient is kept clear of other patients, staff and visitors.

To minimize the risk of exposure to radiation (E).

(f) A member of staff from the ward should take a lead pot, forceps and a monitor to the nurse who will place the source in the lead pot and monitor the area to ensure it is free of radioactivity.

To contain the radioactive source and minimize the risk of exposure (Hart 2006: E).

(g) The Radiation Protection Adviser and supervisor should be informed of incident.

To evaluate the incident, and to prevent it recurring (DH 2000: C).

15 *In the event of a cardiac arrest*, an Ambu bag or similar device must be used, and the physics department must be informed immediately.

To minimize exposure (E).

16 *In the event of a fire*, the fire policy must be followed. Following evacuation, the appropriate distance between the radioactive patient and other staff should be maintained; help should be sought from the physics department.

To minimize exposure (E).

17 *In the event of a patient's death:*
Removable sources:
(a) The radiation sources should be removed by the radiotherapist. Inform the physics department.

Remove radioactivity to allow last offices to be undertaken as normal (E).

Non-removable sources:
(a) When a source cannot be removed, e.g. iodine-125 seeds, inform the physics department immediately.

In order for the physics department staff to begin making the necessary arrangements for removal of the body to the mortuary. Arrangements would include: segregated refrigerator, warning notices and use of body bag to contain seeds if they became dislodged (E).

703

Procedure guidelines *(cont.)*

(b) The body should be placed in a body bag.

To prevent loss of any sources that may become dislodged (E).

(c) Transfer of the body should be arranged by the physics department.

The physics staff will supervise the transfer of the body (E).

18 *In the event of bleeding*, in order to stem bleeding in the vicinity of the implant, apply pressure using at least four thick dressing pads. The padding should only be compressed for 15 minutes by any single person.

To minimize exposure (E).

19 In the event of a confused or agitated patient, premature removal of sources may be required.

To prevent overexposure to radiation of the nurses attending the patient, as well as to prevent the patient removing or dislodging sources (E).

20 Only staff who have received training and have been authorized may enter a controlled area. A list of suitably trained staff should be kept by the domestic and catering managers and by the ward's local Radiation Protection Supervisor. A domestic or catering supervisor should undertake tasks if the ward-based employee is not trained.

To keep all radiation exposure as low as can be reasonably achievable (DH 1999: C).

21 Domestic and catering staff should not remove items such as cleaning equipment and crockery until it has been monitored by a nurse and deemed safe.

To prevent sources being removed from the room before it is safe to do so (Hart 2006: E).

Procedure guidelines   Intraoral sealed radioactive sources: patient care

Preparation of patient

Dental assessment of the patient is usually carried out before oral brachytherapy so that caries, mouth infections and dental extractions may be dealt with in case of the oral blood supply being impaired by the treatment. The patient is usually admitted 24 hours before the implant, during which time the nature of the procedure and the implications of having a radioactive source should be explained to the patient. The patient will be nursed in a single controlled room away from other patients to reduce the amount of radiation exposure to other people. Only staff and visitors authorized to enter the controlled area should go into the room. Written arrangements for entering the room should be contained within the local rules and should be displayed at the door of the room.

Procedure

Action	Rationale
1 Encourage frequent mouth care. The patient should void the solution into a bowl and not into a handbasin.	To reduce the risk of infection. To prevent the loss of a dislodged source (DH Ionising Radiation Regulations 1999: C).
2 Provide a soft, puréed or liquid diet.	To reduce the risk of the patient biting into the source or tongue. Eating is often difficult when implants are present (E).
3 Avoid spicy and/or hot foods. Discourage the patient from smoking and/or drinking alcohol.	To prevent exacerbation of local reaction or soreness (E).
4 Encourage ingestion of carbonated drinks.	To alleviate dryness (E).

| 5 | Provide crushed ice for the patient to suck and/or soluble aspirin as a mouthwash. | To minimize oral pain and discomfort (E). |

| 6 | Give steroids as prescribed. | To prevent and/or minimize swelling (E). |

| 7 | Provide writing equipment for the patient. | To reduce the need for oral communication. This is liable to increase soreness and alter the distribution of the sources. The patient may have difficulty in swallowing due to soreness and oedema. |

| 8 | Provide paper tissues and a bowl for saliva. | The patient may have difficulty in swallowing due to soreness and oedema (E). |

| 9 | The sources should be checked at regular intervals, e.g. at the beginning of each shift. | To make sure that the sources have not become dislodged (E). |

| 10 | The patient should be confined to the room and only leave when necessary, e.g. to visit the X-ray department. | To minimize the risk of radiation exposure to other people on the ward (E). |

Discharge of the patient

The patient is usually discharged the day after the removal of the implant. The patient should be warned about the painful local reaction that may be experienced due to rapid cell breakdown induced by the radiation. In order to minimize the risk of infection or soreness, the patient should be taught how to care for the treated area (Hoskin & Coyle 2005).

Procedure guidelines **Iriduim and caesium gynaecological sources (manual and afterloaded): patient care**

Preparation of patient

The patient is usually admitted 12–48 hours before the procedure so that any preanaesthetic investigations may be performed. Full bowel preparation with a low-residue diet will reduce the chance of the patient having a bowel action while the sources are in place, which could dislodge the sources. Some patients, however, have diarrhoea on admission due to previous radiotherapy and will need regular medication, such as codeine phosphate, both before and during the application of the sources. A full explanation should be given to the patient along with information about the implications of having a radioactive source inside her and informed consent obtained. The patient should be bathed before any premedication is administered.

Procedure

Action | Rationale

| 1 | The patient must remain in bed in a recumbent or semi-recumbent position while the applicators or implants are in place. | To prevent the applicators becoming dislodged or changing their position in relation to the internal organs (E). |

| 2 | Log rolling from side to side is permitted and should be encouraged if the patient is at risk of developing a pressure sore. | To promote comfort and to relieve prolonged pressure on any one area (E). |

| 3 | On return from theatre, the following should be checked:
(a) The sanitary towel.
(b) Disposable pants in position.
(c) Urinary catheter in correct position and draining satisfactorily. | To contain any blood loss (E).
To secure the position of the sanitary towel (E).
To ensure that urine is draining freely (E). |

Procedure guidelines *(cont.)*

4 Observe for any blood or other discharge from the vagina. Ensure routine postoperative observations are performed until patient is stable. Continue to monitor temperature and pulse throughout treatment, at least 2 hourly.	To monitor haemorrhage, shock and other postoperative complications (E).
5 Administer prescribed analgesics, antiemetics and antidiarrhoeal agents.	For the patient's comfort (E).
6 Encourage fluid intake as soon as the patient is allowed to drink. (a) Encourage a fluid intake of 50–100% a day over and above the patient's normal intake. (b) A low-residue diet may be taken. Liaise with dietitian regarding suitable supplements.	To ensure adequate hydration. To reduce the risk of urinary tract infection (Beetz 2003: R 1a). To prevent the stimulation of a bowel action (E).

Procedure guidelines   Gynaecological caesium and iridium wires removal

The removal of applicators is usually performed by suitably qualified and competent nursing staff or a clinical oncologist.

Equipment

1 Sterile gynaecological pack containing large receiver, green towel, paper towel, long dissecting forceps, sanitary towel, cotton wool balls.
2 Equipment for the administration of Entonox.
3 Solutions of choice for swabbing, e.g. 0.9% sodium chloride.

4 Sterile gloves.
5 Sterile scissors or stitch cutter.
6 Contamination monitor.
7 Lead pot.
8 Alcoholic handrub.

Procedure

Action	Rationale
1 Explain and discuss the procedure with the patient.	To ensure that the patient understands the procedure and gives her valid consent (Faithfull & Wells 2003: E).
2 Check the date and time for removal on the form that was received from the physics department when sources were inserted.	The accurate timing of the removal is essential for the administration of the correct therapeutic dose of radiation (E).
3 Check that any pre-removal drugs (e.g. sedatives, analgesics) have been administered.	To reduce the risk of error (E).
4 Check, with another nurse, the exact time of removal and the number of applicators.	To reduce the risk of error (E).
5 Ensure that: (a) The lead shield is suitably positioned beside the patient. (b) The lead pot is also suitably positioned with the lid removed.	To shield the nurse from exposure to radiation (Hart 2006: E). So that sources can be placed in the pot immediately after removal (Hart 2006: E).

6 Begin the administration of Entonox at least 2 minutes before commencing the procedure.	To allow time for the effects of the gas to be felt. (For further information on Entonox administration, see Chapter 28.)
7 Prepare a trolley, clean hands, put on gloves and open the pack before going to the bedside.	Although this is a clinically clean, not an aseptic procedure, hands should still be cleaned before every patient contact. To reduce the time spent in close proximity to the source, all preparation of equipment should be undertaken away from the patient (DH 1999: C).
8 Working from behind the lead shield, assist the patient into the dorsal position with knees apart. Remove the sanitary towel.	To shield the nurse from exposure to radiation and to contain radioactivity (Hart 2006: E).
9 Remove any sutures, if present. Remove the vaginal packing.	To obtain access to the sources (E).
10 Remove the caesium sources in reverse order of insertion. Contact the clinical oncologist immediately if difficulty is encountered in removing a source. Place the removed sources in a lead pot immediately and cover with the lid.	To prevent damage to the vagina (E).
11 Remove the lead pot to a designated area, e.g. an isotope sluice or safe. Ensure that the lid of the pot or the sluice door is locked.	To remove the radioactive source from the ward area. To prevent unauthorized access to the source (DH 1999: C).
12 Monitor the patient's level of radioactivity.	To ensure that no sources remain inside the patient (E).
13 Remove gloves, clean hands then put on clean pair of gloves.	To reduce the risk of contamination from gloves that may have become contaminated whilst handling the lead pot (DH 2005: 1a).
14 Remove the urinary catheter.	The urinary catheter is no longer required (E).
15 Swab the vulva and perineal area with a solution such as 0.9% sodium chloride. Ensure that the patient has a clean sanitary towel in position and is made comfortable.	To promote patient hygiene and comfort (E).
16 Monitor the bed linen, paper bags, vaginal packing and other waste material. (Two nurses should monitor the patient independently.)	To ensure that no source has been lost or remains inside the patient (Hart 2006: E).
17 The patient should remain in bed until the physics department staff or other suitably trained staff member are satisfied that all sources are accounted for.	To ensure that all sources have been accounted for before the patient moves around (E).
18 Remove the radiation warning notice.	Radiation restrictions have ceased (E).

Problem solving: Gynaecological caesium and iridium wires

Problem	Cause	Suggested action
Patient has a bowel action.		Inform the radiotherapist (E).
Patient removes source herself.	Confusion, e.g. postanaesthetic	Using long-handled forceps place the source in the lead container or safe. Inform the radiotherapist and the physics department (Hart 2006: E).
Pyrexia.	Pelvic cellulitis or abscess. Reaction to the proflavine pack. Urinary infection. Physiological reaction to the breakdown of the tumour. Chest infection.	If the patient's temperature remains over 37.5°C for two consecutive readings, inform the radiotherapist. The source may have to be removed if the pyrexia persists (E).
	Peritonitis due to perforation of the uterus.	

Procedure guidelines Selectron treatment: patient care

Procedure

Action	Rationale
1 Ensure written consent has been obtained.	To ensure patient fully understands and agrees to the treatment planned (Faithfull & Wells 2003: E).
2 Ensure thorough nursing assessment of patient has been undertaken by nursing staff.	To ensure patient is suitable and will comply with treatment restrictions (Gosselin & Waring 2001: E).
3 Ensure full preoperative medical assessment has been undertaken, for example baseline blood tests, electrocardiogram (ECG) and X-ray.	To ensure patient is fit for treatment (E).
4 Administer antidiarrhoeal drugs the night before treatment. Patient to be monitored and if necessary treatment provided for radiation-induced enteritis.	To prevent bowel action dislodging applicators during treatment (E).
5 Nurse the patient on a pressure-relieving mattress or with a foam wedge under her buttocks or a pillow under knees to alter position.	To promote comfort and to relieve backache since rolling is not permitted (E).
6 Ensure the plastic transfer tubes are supported securely in the bed bracket, leaving slight slack.	To enable the patient to change position slightly without putting traction on the applicators (E).
7 Limit the frequency and duration of interruption to treatment. Visitors are discouraged unless the patient is markedly distressed.	To prevent unnecessary prolongation of treatment time (E).
8 Check patient's physical and psychological condition at least 2 hourly: (a) Temperature, pulse and vaginal loss. (b) Contents of catheter drainage bag. (c) Assist patient to adjust her position.	To monitor for haemorrhage, shock or other postoperative complications (E). To ensure urine is draining freely (E). To promote comfort and relieve prolonged pressure on any one area (E).

9 Check position of applicators. Marking the position of the applicators on the patient's legs can assist the checking of their position.	To ensure no movement of the applicators has occurred (E).
10 Administer prescribed analgesics, antiemetics, antidiarrhoeal and sedative agents as appropriate and evaluate effect.	To promote the patient's comfort and well-being (E).
11 Encourage fluid intake as soon as the patient is able to drink.	To ensure adequate hydration and reduce the risk of urinary tract infection (Beetz 2003: R 1a).
12 If the patient wishes to eat, a light, low-residue diet may be taken. Ideally food should be chosen which is easy to eat lying down.	To prevent stimulation of a bowel action (E).

Procedure guidelines   Selectron applicator removal

If two patients are being treated simultaneously, removal of the applicators may be delayed until both patients have finished treatment, depending on the individual treatment times. Monitor remaining treatment time of the second patient, to ensure that the applicators of both patients can be removed at the first possible opportunity.

Equipment

As for removal of other gynaecological applicators, see Procedure guidelines: Gynaecological caesium and iridium wires removal, above (items 1–7) plus:
  8 Rubber caps for the applicators.

Procedure

Action	Rationale
1 Check treatment has been terminated by: (a) Ensuring the appropriate channel lights are green. (b) Ensuring the time display on the Selectron unit reads zero for the appropriate channels. (c) Ensuring the print-out indicates treatment has stopped for those channels.	The applicators should be removed only on completion of treatment (E).
2 Check that the closed-circuit television camera is not focused on the patient.	To ensure privacy (E).
3 Explain and discuss the procedure with the patient.	To ensure that the patient understands the procedure and gives her valid consent (Faithfull & Wells 2003: E).
4 Ensure any pre-removal drugs have been administered.	To allow analgesic or sedative to be effective (E).
5 Assist the patient into a comfortable position with her knees apart.	To allow access to the applicators (E).
6 Uncouple the plastic transfer tubes by rotating the black coupling anticlockwise in the direction of the arrow and very carefully store the tubes on the plastic supporting mantle attached to the Selectron unit.	To prevent the plastic catheter becoming damaged or kinked (E).
7 Place rubber caps on the ends of the applicators.	To ensure no fluid or debris is allowed to enter the applicator tubes (E).

Procedure guidelines *(cont.)*

8	Commence administration of Entonox (see Chapter 28) at least 2 minutes before removal of the applicators.	To allow the effect of the gas to be felt (see Chapter 28).
9	Prepare the equipment and put on gloves.	The procedure is clinically clean and not aseptic (Rossoff *et al.* 1993: R1 b).
10	Remove the vulval dressing pads, any sutures and vaginal packing.	These must be removed before the applicators can be eased out (E).
11	Dismantle the applicators by loosening the screws holding them together.	To promote ease of removal. E
	Remove the uterine tube first, ensuring it is taken out complete with its small white flange, followed by the ovoids.	To prevent the flange being left in the patient's vagina (E).
12	Remove the catheter, swab the vulval area and ensure the patient has a clean sanitary pad and a fresh sheet.	To promote cleanliness and patient comfort (E).
13	The patient can then be assisted into a comfortable position and is permitted up to have a bath.	To reassure the patient that the procedure has been completed, that she is no longer radioactive and can resume normal activities (E).

Applicators are retained carefully for cleaning in accordance with local policies.

Problem solving: Selectron treatment

See also 'Problem solving' for conventional gynaecological sources, above.

Problem	Cause	Suggested action
Patient removes the applicators herself.	Confusion, e.g. postanaesthetic.	Check room for any sources that may have escaped, using contamination monitor. Sources that have escaped should be placed in lead pots using long-handled forceps. Remove applicators completely if partially removed.
Applicator is partially dislodged.	Patient may have moved too much or too vigorously.	Interrupt treatment. Inform physicist and radiotherapist. The applicator may have to be removed as above.
Alarm sounding at nurse station.	Treatment has been interrupted and inadvertently left off.	Check patient is unattended and recommence treatment.
Sources are not transferred to the applicators.	Incorrect coupling or loose connection.	Check print-out to identify which channel is at fault. Tighten appropriate coupling device.
Alarm activated at remote control unit.	Failure in the system.	Check the error code on the print-out with the Selectron user's manual. Rectify as indicated in the manual or seek technical assistance from the physics department.
Pellets stuck in the applicator or transfer tubing.	A damaged or kinked catheter.	A risk assessment to be completed regarding the likelihood of this occurrence (HSE 2003).

Procedure guidelines   Radioactive seeds (e.g. iodine-125): patient care

Preparation of the patient

The patient is usually admitted at least 1 day before treatment: patients do not necessarily need to be in a single room but, more importantly, in a bed, where observation of the patient's activity and in particular monitoring of urine can be achieved.

Seeds are implanted permanently into the tissue and therefore the patient must agree to stay in hospital until the physics staff state that the radioactivity is at a legally permissible level for discharge.

Breast and lymph node implantation
Procedure

Action	Rationale
1 Leave the dressing securely in position unless special instructions are given by the radiotherapist.	Sources may become detached, dressings will prevent them from becoming lost (E).
2 If dressing becomes dislodged, leave it at the bedside, preferably in a lead pot, and inform the physics staff.	If sources have become detached and are in the dressings physics staff will take the necessary action (Hart 2006: E).
3 If there is any possibility that the sources have become detached, inform physics department staff immediately and do not remove anything from the room.	It is important that the source is not lost as this could result in contamination of the environment. The patient's total dose will be altered and the medical staff will need to be informed (E).

Lung implantation
Procedure

Action	Rationale
1 Check all sputum and drainage from the chest with the contamination monitor. If no radioactivity is found the sputum and drainage may be disposed of in the usual way unless special instructions are given by the physics department or radiotherapy staff.	To check for radioactivity in case any sources are coughed up or expelled in the drainage (Hart 2006: E).
2 If radioactivity is detected, inform physics department staff immediately. Save the sputum or drainage for them to deal with.	To prevent contamination of the hospital environment (E).

Bladder and prostate implantation
Procedure

Action	Rationale
1 Check all urine with the contamination monitor. If no radioactivity is found the urine may be disposed of in the usual way.	To check for radioactivity in case any sources are expelled in the urine (E).
2 If radioactivity is detected, inform physics staff immediately and save urine for them to deal with.	To prevent contamination of the hospital environment (E).
3 Leave suspect urine in a safe place at the bedside, e.g. under the bed.	To prevent accidental disposal (E).

Procedure guidelines   Breast sealed radioactive sources: patient care

Preparation of the patient

The patient will usually be admitted for local excision of the breast tumour and an axillary clearance. Drains are inserted and these are usually removed before the iridium wire sources are loaded 24–48 hours after surgery. When the sources are loaded, the patient should be nursed in a single room.

Procedure

Action	Rationale
1 Leave any dressing undisturbed for the duration of treatment.	To minimize the time spent in proximity to the patient (E).
2 Confine the patient to the room.	To minimize the risk of radiation to other people on the ward (DH 1999: C).
3 Administer prescribed analgesia as required throughout the treatment period and before removal.	For the patient's comfort (see Chapter 29).

Discharge of the patient

The patient should normally be discharged the day after the removal of the implant. The patient should be warned about the painful local reaction which she may experience due to the rapid cell breakdown induced by the radiation. In order to minimize the risk of infection or soreness, the patient should be taught how to care for the treated area.

Procedure guidelines   Interstitial perineal template (Hammersmith hedgehog)

Care of patient with interstitial perineal template with insertion of radioactive sources (iridium-192). Please also refer to Procedure guidelines: Sealed radioactive sources insertion: patient care, above.

Procedure

Action	Rationale
1 Perform full preoperative nursing assessment (see Chapters 1 & 30).	To ensure patient is suitable for anaesthetic/spinal anaesthetic and suitable for treatment (E).
2 Assess for previous medical problems: (a) Deep vein thrombosis/pulmonary embolism. (b) Psychological problems. (c) Fear of isolation. (d) Pressure sores. (e) Back problems. (f) Any physical condition which may prevent patient from lying flat, e.g. chronic obstructive pulmonary disease, respiratory/cardiac problems.	To ensure patient can comply with approx. 5–7 days of complete bedrest in semi-recumbent position (see Action figure 2) (E).
3 Ensure informed consent has been obtained. Check patient's understanding of planned treatment.	To ensure that the patient understands the radiation protection restrictions associated with this treatment and the nature and outcome of surgery, to reduce anxiety and postoperative complications (Faithfull & Wells 2003: E).
4 Offer further explanation, verbal and written information.	It is important that patient fully understands the planned treatment to ensure compliance with treatment (Faithfull & Wells 2003: E).

5 Bowel preparation:
  (a) Ensure preoperative bowel preparation is carried out. *Note*: Consultant preference will dictate what bowel preparation is used. Generally this is either:
    ▪ Bowel preparation, e.g. Citramag given to ensure thorough bowel evacuation. Patient starts clear fluids while on bowel preparation or:
    ▪ A low-residue diet is commenced 2 days before treatment and phosphate enema is given the night before and on morning of surgery.

Treatment time is 5–7 days. Bowel action may dislodge applicator. Patient comfort is improved if bowel evacuation complete preoperatively (E).

Low-residue/light diet to prevent bowel stimulation and to prevent bloating and discomfort from constipation (E).

  (b) For duration of treatment, patient to receive codeine phosphate regularly to induce constipation. During treatment, patients to take a low-residue or light diet.

To reduce the likelihood of a bowel action which could cause the applicators to be moved (E).

  (c) Encourage good fluid intake, intravenous fluids if necessary.

To ensure adequate hydration (E).

  (d) Doctors and physics department to be contacted if patient has bowel action.

To assess whether applicators have been dislodged (E).

6 Observations:
  (a) Observations to be performed 2–4 hourly as patient's condition dictates during treatment.

To observe for bleeding/haemorrhage/infection/reaction to treatment (see Chapter 25).

  (b) Observe wires to check number and position.

To observe for accidental movement of wires, to prevent inappropriate treatment to surrounding tissues (DH 2000: C).

  (c) Ensure legs parted slightly using pillows to position.

Facilitates observation (E).

  (d) Monitor skin integrity around iridium wires.

Radiation skin reaction can occur and medical/nursing intervention may be required to relieve symptoms and promote comfort (E).

  (e) Monitor vaginal bleeding, changing pads as necessary.

Bleeding may occur which may require medical/nursing intervention to stop the bleeding (E).

  (f) Monitor pain and if necessary, provide prescribed analgesia and assess efficacy.

To minimize pain (see Chapter 27).

  (g) Monitor for nausea and vomiting and if necessary, provide prescribed antiemetics and assess efficacy.

To promote patient comfort, by reducing nausea (Windschall *et al.* 2005: R 1b).

  (h) Monitor for deep vein thrombosis. Ensure anti-thrombotic stockings are correctly fitted unless otherwise indicated. Deep vein thrombosis prophylaxis may be prescribed (e.g. Fragmin). Encourage gentle leg exercises, but avoid excessive movement.

To prevent deep vein thrombosis (Kehl-Pruett 2006: R 3a).

  (i) Monitor pressure areas.

To prevent development of pressure sores (Lyder 2006: E).

  (j) Patients can be log rolled onto side to allow assessment of pressure areas and hygiene needs and to relieve pressure areas.

To promote patient comfort (Lyder 2006: E).

7 Ensure access to radio, telephone, television with remote control, books, etc. as entry to radioactive patient's room is restricted.

To help patient deal with isolation by maintaining contact with outside world; prevent boredom (Stajduhar *et al.* 2000: R 1b).

8 Following removal of interstitial perineal template:
  (a) Encourage vulval douching/vaginal douching after removal of template. Use hairdryer to dry area.

To facilitate good hygiene and comfort and to prevent infection (So & Yuen 2006: R2 b). Hairdryer helps limit friction which can cause more discomfort (E).

  (b) Catheter to be removed after treatment.

Catheter no longer required (E).

  (c) Ensure normal urination recommences.

To ensure that retention of urine has not occurred following removal of catheter (see Chapter 18).

Procedure guidelines *(cont.)*

9 Encourage vaginal dilating 4–6 weeks post-procedure (length depending on postoperative recovery and other clinical and psychological factors) to be reassessed in the outpatient department.

To prevent vaginal stenosis, so facilitating patient comfort for future pelvic examinations and sexual intercourse (Ness *et al.* 2003: R 2b).

1 pillow approx. 45°

One pillow under head and a second under knees. Knees to be slightly apart

Action 2   Semi-recumbent position to be adopted during interstitial perineal template therapy.

Useful websites

www.doh.gov.uk/irmir.htm

www.legislation.hmso.gov.uk/si/si1999/19993232.htm

legislation.hso.gov.uk/si/si2000/20001059.htm

Training available on the web: www.iaea.or.at/ns/rasanet/training/index.htm

References and further reading

Advisory Group on Ionising Radiation (2003) Risk of leukaemia and related malignancies following radiation exposure: estimates for the UK population. National Radiation Protection Board **14**(1) www.nrpb.org. Accessed September 2007.

Agrawal, P.P. *et al.* (2005) The role of interstitial brachytherapy using template in locally advanced gynecological malignancies. *Gynecol Oncol*, **99**(1), 169–75.

Andreyev, H.J. *et al.* (2005) Gastrointestinal symptoms after pelvic radiotherapy: role for the gastroenterologist? *Int J Radiat Oncol Biol Phys*, **62**(5), 1464–71.

Anglesio, S. *et al.* (2005) Prostate brachytherapy with iodine-125 seeds: radiation protection issues. *Tumori*, **91**(4), 335–8.

Beetz, R. (2003) Mild dehydration: a risk factor for urinary tract infection? *Eur J Clin Nutr*, **57**(Suppl 2), S52–8.

Bergmark, K. *et al.* (1999) Vaginal changes and sexuality in women with a history of cervical cancer. *N Engl J Med*, **340**(18), 1383–9.

Blake, P.R. *et al.* (1998) *Gynaecological Oncology*. Oxford University Press, Oxford.

Blank, L.E. *et al.* (2000) Brachytherapy with transperineal [125]-iodine seeds for localized prostate cancer. *Radiother Oncol*, **57**(3), 307–13.

Bomford, K. (2002a) Radiation protection. In: *Walters & Miller Textbook of Radiotherapy* (eds C.K. Bomford & I.K. Kunkler), 6th edn. Churchill Livingstone, Edinburgh, **6**(1), pp. 69–88.

Bomford, K. (2002b) Brachytherapy. In: *Walters & Miller Textbook of Radiotherapy* (eds C.K. Bomford & I.K. Kunkler), 6th edn. Churchill Livingstone, Edinburgh, **14**(2), pp. 225–244.

Budrukkar, A.N. *et al.* (2001) Transperineal low-dose rate iridium-192 interstitial brachytherapy in cervical carcinoma state llB. *Strahlenther Onkol*, **177**(10), 517–24.

Chen, S.W. *et al.* (2004) Radiation injury to intestine following hysterectomy and adjuvant radiotherapy for cervical cancer. *Gynecol Oncol*, **95**(1), 208–14.

DH (1978) *The Medicine (Administration of Radioactive Substances) Regulations*. HMSO, London.

DH (1999) *The Ionising Regulations No. 3232*. HMSO, London.

DH (2000) *The Ionising Radiation (Medical Exposure) Regulations No. 1059*. HSMO, London.

DH (2005) *Saving Lives a Delivery Programme to Reduce Healthcare Acquired Infection Including MRSA*. Department of Health, London.

Faithfull, S. & Wells, M. (2003) *Supportive Care in Radiotherapy*. Churchill Livingstone, Edinburgh.

Farrell, E. (2002) Premature menopause. 'I feel like an alien'. *Aust Fam Physician*, **31**(5), 419–21.

Fung, A.Y. (2002) The syed temporary interstitial iridium gynaecological implant: an inverse planning system. *Phys Med Biol*, **47**(16), N203–8.

Gami, B. *et al.* (2003) How patients manage gastrointestinal symptoms after pelvic radiotherapy. *Aliment Pharmacol Ther*, **18**(10), 987–94.

Gosselin, T.K. & Waring, J.S. (2001) Nursing management of patients receiving brachytherapy for gynaecologic malignancies. *Clin J Oncol Nurs*, **5**(2), 59–63.

Grabenbauer, G.G. *et al.* (2001) Interstitial brachytherapy with Ir-192 low-dose-rate in the treatment of primary and recurrent cancer of the oral cavity and oropharynx. Review of 318 patients treated between 1985 and 1997. *Strahlenther Onkol*, **177**(7), 338–44.

Hart, S. (2006) Ionising radiation: promoting safety for patients, visitors and staff. *Nurs Stand*, **20**(47), 47–57.

Hoskin, P. & Coyle, C. (2005) *Radiotherapy in Practice: Brachytherapy*. Oxford University Press, Oxford.

HSE (2003) *Five Steps to Risk Assessment*. Health and Safety Executive Books, Norwich.

International Commission of Radiological Protection (2005) Radiation safety aspects of brachytherapy for prostate cancer using permanently implanted sources. A report of ICRP Publication 98. *Ann ICRP*, 35(3), iii–vi & 3–50.

IPEM/RCN (2002) Radiation. In: *Ionising Radiation Safety: A Handbook for Nurses*. York Publishing, York, pp. 1–7.

Jones, B. *et al.* (1999) High dose brachytherapy practice for the treatment of gynaecological cancers in the UK. *Br J Radiol*, 72(856), 371–7.

Karakoyun-Celik, O. *et al* (2005) Definitive radiotherapy with interstitial implant boost for squamous cell carcinoma of the tongue base. *Head Neck*, 27(5), 353–61.

Kehl-Pruett, W. (2006) Deep vein thrombosis in hospitalized patients: a review of evidence-based guidelines for prevention. *Dimens Crit Care Nurs*, 25(2), 53–9.

Kucera, H. *et al.* (2001) Radiotherapy alone for invasive vaginal cancer: outcome with intracavitary high dose rate brachytherapy versus conventional low dose rate brachytherapy. *Acta Obstet Gynecol Scand*, 80(4), 355–60.

Kuipers, T. *et al.* (2001) HDR brachytherapy applied to cervical carcinoma with moderate lateral expansion: modified principles of treatment. *Radiother Oncol*, 58(1), 25–30.

Lalos, A. (1997) The impact of diagnosis on cervical and endometrial cancer patients and their spouses. *Eur J Gynaecol Oncol*, 18(6), 513–19.

Lalos, A. *et al.* (1995) Experience of the male partner in cervical and endometrial cancer – a prospective interview study. *J Psychosom Obstet Gynaecol*, 16(3), 153–65.

Lapeyre, M. *et al.* (2004) Postoperative brachytherapy alone and combined postoperative radiotherapy and brachytherapy boost for squamous cell carcinoma of the oral cavity, with positive or close margins. *Head Neck*, 26(3), 216–23.

Leborgne, F. *et al.* (2002) Cesium-137 needle brachytherapy boosts after external beam irradiation for locally advanced carcinoma of the tongue and floor of the mouth. *Brachytherapy*, 1(3), 126–30.

Lyder, C.H. (2006) Assessing risk and preventing pressure ulcers in patients with cancer. *Semin Oncol Nurs*, 22(3), 178–84.

Montgomery, C., Lydon, A. & Lloyd, K. (1997) Psychological distress among cancer patients and informed consent. *J Psychosom Res*, 46(3), 241–5.

Muscari Lin, E., Aikin, J.L. & Good, B.C. (1999) Premature menopause after cancer treatment. *Cancer Pract*, 7(3), 114–21.

Nag, S. *et al.* (2002) Interstitial brachytherapy for salvage treatment of vaginal recurrences in previously unirradiated endometrial cancer patients. *Int J Radiat Oncol Biol Phys*, 54(4), 1153–9.

Nag, S. (2004) High dose rate brachytherapy: its clinical applications and treatment guidelines. *Technol Cancer Res Treat*, 3(3), 269–87.

Ness, R.B. *et al.* (2003) Why women douche and why they may or may not stop. *Sex Transm Dis*, 30(1), 71–4.

NICE (2005) Low dose rate brachytherapy for localised prostate cancer. National Institute for Health and Clinical Excellence, London. www.nice.org.uk/IPG132.

Nutting, C. *et al.* (2006) Manually after-loaded ^{192}Ir low-dose rate brachytherapy after subtotal excision and flap reconstruction of recurrent cervical lymphadenopathy from head and neck cancer. *Radiother Oncol*, 80(1), 39–42.

Petereit, D.G., Sarkaria, J.N. & Chappell, R.J. (1998) Perioperative morbidity and mortality of high dose rate gynecologic brachytherapy. *Int J Radiat Oncol Biol Phys*, 42(5), 1025–31.

RCN (2002) *Ionising Radiation Safety: A Handbook for Nurses*. Institute of Physics and Engineering in Medicine, York.

Robinson, J.W., Faris, P.D. & Scott, C.B. (1999) Psychoeducational groups increase vaginal dilation for younger women and reduce fears for women of all ages with gynecological carcinoma treated with radiotherapy. *Int J Radiat Oncol Biol Phys*, 44(3), 497–506.

Rossoff, L.J. *et al.* (1993) Is the use of boxed gloves in an intensive care unit safe? *Am J Med*, 94(6), 602–7.

Shang-Wen, C. *et al.* (2003) High dose-rate brachytherapy for elderly patients with uterine cervical cancer. *Jpn J Clin Oncol*, 33, 221–8.

So, W.K. & Yuen, J.K. (2006) Evaluation of an educational programme for Chinese women receiving internal radiation for uterine cervical cancer. *J Clin Nurs*. 15(3), 358–60.

Stajduhar, K.I. *et al.* (2000) Thyroid cancer patients experience of receiving iodine-131 therapy. *Oncol Nurs Forum*, 27(8), 1213–18.

Stock, R.G. *et al.* (2000) Postimplant dosimetry for ^{125}I prostate implants: definitions and factors affecting outcome. *Int J Radiat Oncol Biol Phys*, 48(3), 899–906.

Syed, A.M. *et al.* (2002) Long term results of low-dose-rate interstitial-intracavitary brachytherapy in treatment of carcinoma of the cervix. *Int J Radiat Oncol Biol Phys*, 54(1), 67–78.

Takacsi-Nagy, Z. *et al.* (2001) The importance of interstitial radiotherapy in the treatment of the base of tongue tumors : a retrospective analysis. *Neoplasma*, 48(1), 76–81.

Tan, L.T., Russell, S. & Burgess, L. (2004) Acute toxicity of chemo-radiotherapy for cervical cancer: the Addenbrooke's experience. *Clin Oncol (R Coll Radiol)*, 16(4), 255–60.

Teruya, Y. *et al.* (2002) High-dose intracavitary brachytherapy for carcinoma in situ of the vagina occurring after hysterectomy: a rational prescription of radiation dose. *Am J Obstet Gynecol*, 187(2), 360–4.

Tessa, M. *et al.* (2005) Concomitant chemotherapy and external radiotherapy plus brachytherapy for locally advanced esophageal cancer: results of a retrospective multicenter study. *Tumori*, 91(5), 406–14.

Ung, Y.C. *et al.* (2006) The role of high-dose-rate brachytherapy in the palliation of symptoms in patients with non-small-cell lung cancer: a systematic review. *Brachytherapy*, 5(3), 189–202.

Velji, K. & Fitch, M. (2001) The experience of women receiving brachytherapy for gynecologic cancer. *Oncol Nurse Forum*, 28(4), 743–51.

Wadsley, J.C. *et al.* (2003) Iridium-192 implantation for T1 and T2a carcinoma of the tongue and floor of mouth: retrospective study of the results of treatment at the Royal Berkshire Hospital. *Br J Radiol*, 76, 414–17.

Wallace, K. *et al.* (2006) Impact of a multi-disciplinary patient education session on accrual to a difficult clinical trial: the Toronto experience with the surgical prostatectomy versus interstitial radiation intervention trial. *J Clin Oncol*, 24(25), 4158–62.

Windschall, A. *et al.* (2005) Radiation therapy and simultaneous chemotherapy for recurrent cervical cancer. *Strhlenther Onkol*, 181(8), 545–50.

Wong, F.C. *et al.* (2003) Treatment results of high-dose-rate remote afterloading brachytherapy for cervical cancer and retrospective comparison of two regimens. *Int J Radiat Concol Biol Phys*, 55(5), 1254–64.

Wust, P. *et al.* (2004) Clinical and physical determinants for toxicity of 125-I seed brachytherapy. *Radiother Oncol*, 73(1), 39–48.

Zelefsky, M.J. (2006) Quality of life of patients after permanent prostate brachytherapy in relation to dosimetry. *Urol Oncol*, 24(4), 377–8.

715

Chapter 36

Radioactive source therapy and diagnostic procedures: unsealed sources

717 Reference material
726 *Procedure guidelines:* Iodine-131: pre-administration care
726 *Procedure guidelines:* Iodine-131 thyroid treatment: patient care
727 *Procedure guidelines:* Iodine-131 mIBG treatment: patient care
727 *Procedure guidelines:* Unsealed source therapy: patient care post-administration
730 *Procedure guidelines:* Unsealed radioactive sources for diagnostic investigations: patient care
731 *Procedure guidelines:* Unsealed radioactive sources: emergency procedures
733 Regulations
733 Web resources
733 References and further reading

Definition

Unsealed radioactive sources are radionuclides supplied in liquid or colloidal form, systemically administered orally or by injection. They are used in the diagnosis and treatment of disease (IPEM/RCN 2002).

Definition of terms

1   *Radiopharmaceutical*: this is a specially formulated sterile compound consisting of two main components: the pharmaceutical, which primarily determines the distribution profile of the compound around the body's organs, and a radionuclide, which enables the distribution of the radiopharmaceutical to be determined (Cherry *et al.* 2003).

2   *Radionuclide*: a nuclide of an element which possesses an unstable configuration of protons and neutrons within the nucleus, and which achieves stability by undergoing a radioactive decay process (Cherry *et al.* 2003).

3   *Imaging*: images that show the distribution of radiopharmaceutical within the patient and are obtained using a gamma camera (Ziessman *et al.* 2006).

4   *Scanning*: the measurement of the distribution of radioactivity over an area of the body by counting the rate at which the radiation is received (count rate) by a detector moved over the body surface (Cherry *et al.* 2003).

5   *Radiation protection adviser*: this is an individual who meets the Health and Safety Executive's (HSE's) criteria for competence (Ionising Radiations Regulations 1999 [IRR99] (regulation 2)). A radiation employer must appoint a radiation protection adviser in writing to advise him on the observance of the IRR99 (regulations 13(1), (2)) (DH 1999).

6   *Radiation protection supervisor*: this is a person appointed for the purpose of securing compliance with the IRR99 in respect of work carried out in any area subject to local rules (IRR99 regulation 17(4)).

7   *Controlled area*: this is any area where the effective dose to a person working in the area is likely to exceed 6 millisieverts (mSv) per year or an equivalent dose greater than three-tenths of any relevant dose limit (IRR99 regulation 16(1)). Entrance to controlled areas is restricted to classified workers and those entering under written arrangements (IRR99 regulation 18(2)).

8   *Supervised area*: this is any area not designated as a controlled area where any person is likely to receive an effective dose greater than 1 mSv per year or an equivalent dose greater than one-tenth of any relevant dose limit (IRR99 regulation 16(3)).

9   *Local rules*: these are documents that identify the key working instructions intended to restrict any exposure in controlled or supervised areas (IRR99 regulation 17(1), Approved Code of Practice (section 272)).

10   *Written arrangements*: these detail the conditions for access into controlled areas for non-classified employ-

ees to ensure adequate restriction of their exposure to ionizing radiation (IRR99 regulation 18(3), Guidance (section 314)).

11   *Classified persons*: these are employees who are likely to receive an effective dose in excess of 6 mSv per year or an equivalent dose which exceeds three-tenths of any relevant dose limit (IRR99 regulation 20).

12   *The Ionising Radiation (Medical Exposure) Regulations (IRMER) practitioner*: this is a registered medical practitioner, dental practitioner or other health professional who is entitled in accordance with the employer's procedures to take responsibility for an individual's medical exposure (IRMER regulation 2) (DH 2000).

13   *IRMER operator*: this is any person who is entitled, in accordance with the employer's procedure, to carry out practical aspects of medical exposures (IRMER regulations 2, 3).

14   *IRMER referrer*: this is a registered medical practitioner, dental practitioner or other health professional who is entitled, in accordance with the employer's procedures, to refer individuals for medical exposure to a practitioner (IRMER regulation 2).

15   *Radiation employer*: this is an employer who carries out work with ionizing radiation or who intends to carry out such work (IRR regulation 2) (DH 1999).

It is essential that nurses (Stajduhar *et al.* 2000) and doctors (Shiralkar *et al.* 2003) are provided with education, training and supervision so that they can provide comprehensive care to the patients, whilst ensuring that other patients, visitors, health care workers and the environment are not put at risk.

Reference material

Unsealed sources are used to concentrate a radioisotope in a particular part of the body. Unsealed sources carry an additional risk of environmental contamination and therefore protective measures are required to prevent contamination of staff, visitors, other patients and the environment (Sherry 2000). For example, unsealed sources may concentrate in body fluids, which will then contain radioactivity, and when eliminated reduce the amount of radioactivity in the patient (Henkin *et al.* 2006), but increase the risk of contamination to staff and the environment.

Radionuclides used for diagnosis of disease in the nuclear medicine department and four unsealed sources will be discussed here.

Radionuclides used in the nuclear medicine department

Unsealed radionuclides are used in nuclear medicine for the diagnosis and treatment of disease, during both imaging and non-imaging investigations. The important properties that make them useful for diagnostic purposes include:

- The physical half-life.
- Decay characteristics.
- Ease of incorporation into radiopharmaceuticals.
- Availability of radionuclide.

A desirable radionuclide should have a half-life just long enough to allow for the preparation, administration and concentration in the region of interest, but short enough for radiation to effectively disappear after the test (Cherry *et al.* 2003). Imaging studies commonly performed in a nuclear medicine department include:

- Assessment of structures and/or function of organs.
- Sites of infection.
- Presence of tumours.

Common non-imaging studies include investigations into red cell mass and plasma volume, gastrointestinal tract and renal function.

Radiopharmaceuticals are legally categorized as prescription only medicines (POMs), and, in addition to the standard legislation surrounding the administration of such drugs, are subject to regulations related to their radioactive content. In the UK, a statutory committee called the Administration of Radioactive Substances Advisory Committee (ARSAC) has been established to give ionizing radiation advice to health ministers and to manage the certification process for administration of radiopharmaceuticals. This committee issues certificates which authorize individuals to administer radiopharmaceuticals to patients. It also lists the maximum permissible doses of radioactivity that may be administered to adult patients, and appropriately reduced adult doses for children, according to a child's body weight or body surface area.

A radionuclide investigation involves administration of the appropriate radiopharmaceutical, and dynamic imaging or waiting a predetermined time to allow the dose to be taken up in the organ to be investigated. The patient is then positioned and is required to keep still during the scan, because movement causes artifacts which reduce diagnostic accuracy. The scan may last 15–60 minutes (Ziessman *et al.* 2006). Most procedures require little physical patient preparation (Table 36.1).

Four unsealed sources will be discussed:

- Rhenium-186 hydroxyethylidene diphosphonate (Re186 HEDP), used in the treatment of bone metastases.
- Iodine-131 (I-131), used in the treatment of thyroid disorders.
- Meta-iodobenzylguanidine (mIBG), used in the treatment and diagnosis of neuroblastoma and other neuroectodermal tumours.
- Sentinal node biopsy using technetium-99m colloid.

Rhenium-186 hydroxyethylidene diphosphonate (Re186 HEDP)

Definition

Rhenium-186 forms a stable diphosphonate chelate with hydroxyethylidene diphosphonate (HEDP) forming rhenium-186 hydroxyethylidene diphosphonate (Re186 HEDP). The linking of the radionuclide rhenium-186 to a suitable chemical compound produces a radiopharmaceutical which is localized in metastatic foci in bone (O'Sullivan *et al.* 2002). Re186 HEDP is a beta-gamma-emitting radionuclide with a maximum beta energy of 1.07 megaelectron volts (MeV), and has a gamma ray emission of 137 megakelvins volts (keV) (Maxon *et al.* 1992).

The beta particles travel only short distances and, therefore, their energy deposition is localized in metastatic foci in bone, delivering a therapeutic radiation dose directly to the metastases while delivering a much lower dose to normal bone marrow. Because Re186 HEDP also emits gamma rays, which can be located by diagnostic imaging techniques, it is possible to verify its location in areas of metastatic disease, and to measure the dose of radiation delivered to the tumour and bone marrow (McEwan 1998).

Use

Bone metastases are a common presentation of prostate, breast, lung and renal cancers, leading to various complications including pain, fractures and hypercalcaemia as well as reduced performance and quality of life, and are a significant cause of morbidity. A UK longitudinal study found that 18–29% of men with undiagnosed prostate cancer presented with metastatic disease by the time they attended a clinic appointment (Mokete *et al.* 2006). Eighty per cent of those patients with prostate cancer who develop clinical metastases will have bone metastases in spite of conventional therapy (Chung *et al.* 2005). Pain control is important; one study using Re186 HEDP to treat patients with bone metastases found a 67% improvement in pain (Liepe *et al.* 2005).

Studies using Re186 HEDP as targeted radiotherapy have shown that it can significantly reduce pain, improve quality of life, reduce management costs and may slow the progression of painful metastatic lesions (Liepe *et al.* 2005).

Re186 HEDP has advantages over conventional external beam radiotherapy because it is tumour specific with relative sparing of surrounding healthy tissue. While thrombocytopenia is a dose-limiting but short-lasting toxicity, leucopenia is less severe (Liepe *et al.* 2005). Re186 HEDP is administered by intravenous injection by an IRMER operator. Because Re186 HEDP is excreted in the urine, urinary catheterization is carried out prior to treatment to ensure that the bladder remains empty and the radiation dose to the bladder is minimized. Therefore caution must be exercised when emptying the catheter bag (see Preparation of therapy room section, below). Also as the half-life of Re186 HEDP is only 90 hours, patients only need to be segregated

Table 36.1 Radionuclide investigations. (Peter & Gambhir 2004; Henkin et al. 2006; Ziessman et al. 2006.)

Investigation/target organ	Radiopharmaceutical	Procedures and clinical interventions
Imaging studies		
Bone scan Used to assess bone function in which malignancy, fractures and diseases such as osteomalacia and Paget's disease can be diagnosed	Technetium (^{99m}Tc) phosphate and phosphonate compounds, including methylene diphosphonate (MDP) and hydroxymethylene diphosphonate (HDP)	Patient to drink 5–6 cups of fluid and to empty bladder regularly while waiting for scan. This is to enhance soft tissue clearance and minimize absorbed radiation dose to the bladder
Renogram (dynamic renal study) Used to assess renal function by monitoring clearance of radiopharmaceutical via kidneys	^{99m}Tc MAG$_3$ Benzoylmercaptoacetyltriglycine ^{99m}Tc DTPA Diethylenetriamine pentaacetic acid	Patients to drink approximately 600 ml of fluid and to empty bladder prior to scan, which takes approximately 1 hour Intravenous diuretic is to be administered to patient during the scan to diagnose obstructive uropathy (Russell 1998)
Static renal study Used to assess size, shape and position and function of kidneys. Used to diagnose renal scarring in children	^{99m}Tc DMSA Dimercaptosuccinic acid	No preparation
Perfusion lung scan Used to assess blood supply to alveolar tree. Provides complementary information to a ventilation lung scan. Used to diagnose pulmonary embolism	^{99m}Tc MAA Macroaggregated albumin	Radiopharmaceutical is administered as a slow bolus intravenous injection. Patient to lie supine and breathe deeply while injection is being given. This is to enhance even distribution of MAA through lung capillary bed. If patient is pregnant, administered activity needs to be reduced
Ventilation lung scan Provides complementary information to a perfusion lung scan in diagnosis of pulmonary embolism. Used to assess patency of airways	^{99m}Tc Technegas, ^{99m}Tc aerosol, ^{81m}Kr gas, ^{133}Xe gas	A chest X-ray performed within the preceding 24 hours is required prior to scan, to assist with interpretation of lung scan. Patient breathes the radiopharmaceutical through a special mouthpiece while scan is being performed
Cardiac studies: perfusion imaging Used to assess areas of viable perfused myocardium. This is a two-part test with myocardial perfusion monitored under stress and subsequently at rest. Stress may be exercise or pharmacologically induced. Often performed on patients with suspected coronary artery disease, recent myocardial infarction or those who have undergone coronary artery bypass surgery	^{99m}Tc MIBI, ^{99m}Tc tetrafosmin, ^{201}Tl thallous chloride	Patient needs to be closely monitored during post-exercise period because there is the potential risk of triggering a myocardial infarction after stress This test is usually performed within a cardiology unit with appropriately trained personnel and equipment. Patient is usually kept in the department until he/she has been assessed by a clinician
Cardiac – left ventricular ejection fraction/multiple gated acquisition scan Used to evaluate cardiac function in patients prior to and during courses of chemotherapy containing cardiotoxic agents	^{99m}Tc labelled red blood cells	Current weight of patient is required for calculation of dose of a red blood cell labelling agent, which ensures red blood cells are labelled with required radioactivity This volume calculated is then administered intravenously 20–30 minutes prior to scan. Patient lies supine for 30–40 minutes

(continued on p. 720)

Table 36.1   *(cont.)*

Investigation/target organ	Radiopharmaceutical	Procedures and clinical interventions
Thyroid scan May be used to confirm presence of one or more nodules within the thyroid, or to identify functional characteristics of nodule(s)	^{99m}Tc pertechnetate, ^{123}I/^{124}I/^{131}I sodium iodide	Patient to avoid foods containing iodine (including seasalt, seafood, cod liver oil, mineral tablets and kelp) for 3 days prior to test. These foods decrease uptake of radiopharmaceutical within thyroid bed. Patient to discontinue thyroid medication for between 3 days and 3 weeks prior to test, depending on specific instructions given by clinician
Parathyroid scan Used to diagnose parathyroid adenomas in patients with primary hyperparathyroidism	^{99m}Tc pertechnetate, ^{201}Tl thallous chloride	This is a two-part test, comprising a thyroid scan which is completed prior to the parathyroid scan. Patient should follow instructions for thyroid test
Tumour imaging Used to differentiate between metabolically active tumours and space-occupying lesions, or for the diagnosis of unknown primary tumours	^{18}F FDG 2-Fluorodeoxyglucose	Patient to fast for up to 6 hours prior to injection, with only water to be taken. Patients may experience a metallic taste in the mouth immediately after administration. Waiting interval between injection and scan is 30 minutes, scan being performed with a positron emission tomography (PET) camera
Used to diagnose infection and diagnose and stage cancers such as lung, Hodgkin's disease and lymphomas	^{67}Ga gallium citrate	Due to excretion of gallium citrate via the gastrointestinal tract, patients should be given laxatives or encouraged to increase fibre and fluid intake to avoid constipation. There are specific radiation protection precautions to be adhered to
Used to diagnose and assess patients with neuroectodermal tumours including phaeochromocytomas, neuroblastomas, carcinoid, medullary thyroid cancers and paragangliomas	^{123}I mIBG meta-iodobenzylguanidine	Patient must take Lugol's iodine or potassium iodide for 2 days prior to and for 3 days after day of administration. mIBG may cause hypertension and is administered slowly over a 10-minute period. On occasions, patients may experience some discomfort at the injection site. This may be relieved by applying heat to the area of discomfort and reducing rate of infusion. For paediatric patients, it is preferable to administer mIBG via a central venous catheter. Some drugs that act on the adrenergic system may interfere with uptake of mIBG
Often used in conjunction with mIBG scans to assist with localization of the primary tumour and sites of metastatic spread in the aforementioned diseases	^{111}In Octreotide DTPA-D-Phe-1-Octreotide	Patients with insulinoma should have their blood sugar levels monitored pre- and post-injection. An intravenous solution containing glucose should be available in case of hypoglycaemia. Patients should be encouraged to increase fluid and fibre intake to avoid constipation
Sites of infection To identify areas of lymphocyte localization in patients with either acute or chronic inflammatory infections	Labelled white blood cells	50 ml of blood is taken from patient using a 19 G needle. Labelled blood is reinjected after approximately 2 hours, following which patient is scanned later the same day and/or the following day

Table 36.2   *(cont.)*

Investigation/target organ	Radiopharmaceutical	Procedures and clinical interventions
Gastrointestinal tract To determine cause of gastrointestinal bleeding, including Meckel's diverticulum	^{99m}Tc pertechnetate	Patients (usually children) need to fast for 4–6 hours before scan; adults to fast from midnight
Non-imaging studies *Kidney function* Measurement of glomerular filtration rate (GFR) provides an assessment of renal function. Often used in renal transplant patients, in compromised renal function due to long-term use of certain drugs (e.g. cyclosporin) or in patients with systemic lupus erythematosus. Oncology patients often have renal function assessed prior to chemotherapy, particularly if regimen includes platinum-based cytotoxic agents	^{51}Cr EDTA Ethylenediaminetetra-acetic acid	Renal clearance of administered radiopharmaceutical is assessed from residual radioactivity in blood samples taken from patient at either 3 hours, or at 2, 3 and 4 hours post-injection. Patient's height and weight are required to enable GFR to be calculated accurately. It is important that no hydration or blood products are commenced during the test as this may alter results of test
Red cell mass/plasma volume Often used to diagnose polycythaemia vera in patients with cardiovascular disease	^{125}I human serum albumin, ^{51}Cr or ^{99m}Tc labelled red blood cells	10 ml of blood is taken from patient using a 19 G needle. Labelled blood is reinjected after approximately 1.5 hours, following which patient's blood is taken at 10-minute intervals for 40 minutes. Patient's height and weight are recorded

for a few days after it has been administered. In one study all patients were discharged within 4 days (O'Sullivan *et al.* 2002).

The Re186 HEDP treatment programme for carcinoma of prostate involves the following.

Preparation of patient prior to admission

- Complete assessment as an outpatient.
- At least 3 weeks before treatment: granulocyte-colony stimulating factor (G-CSF) growth factor (10 µg/kg) given over 4 days as an outpatient.
- At least 2 weeks before treatment: harvest of stem cells.

Admission and inpatient stay

- Admitted for up to 4 days into a controlled area.
- Re186 HEDP given intravenously on admission.
- Analgesics administered for initial increase in bone pain.

Following discharge of patient

- Fourteen days post-treatment: stem cells reinfused as a day patient.
- Analgesics administered as required for the expected initial increase in bone pain.

Iodine-131

Definition

Radioactive iodine-131 is a beta-gamma emitter with a half-life of 8 days, and is used mainly in the form of iodide solution. The beta radiation gives a high, local dose in iodine concentrating tissue. The gamma component is useful for external measurement and scanning (Bomford & Kunkler 2002).

Use

Thyroid cancer is one of the most common cancers in adolescents and young adults in the UK (BTA/RCP 2002; Pearce *et al.* 2005). Treatment with iodine-131 following surgery has been found to improve the patient's quality of life, with no further disease progression and a low mortality rate (Hod *et al.* 2005).

Thyroid tissue selectively concentrates iodide, which enables iodine-131 to be used in the diagnosis and treatment of thyroid disorders. These patients usually have a good prognosis (Harmer 1996):

- Thyrotoxicosis. Usually treatments of between 75 and 400 megabecquerels (MBq) activity of iodine-131 can be given, often on an outpatient basis.

- Well-differentiated thyroid cancers (papillary and follicular) and metastases that function similarly to the thyroid tissue. Treatment is usually on an inpatient basis because of the higher activities involved.

Iodine-131 is normally administered as a capsule taken orally by the patient, followed by a hot drink. It can also be administered in liquid form either intravenously or orally.

Treatment programme for carcinoma of the thyroid

Surgical removal of the thyroid

Normal thyroid tissue concentrates iodine more efficiently than malignant tissue, and some malignant tissues concentrate iodine-131 only after removal of normal tissue. It is recommended, therefore, that a surgical near-total thyroidectomy is performed before administration of iodine-131 (Beasley et al. 2002).

Iodine-131 treatment

This is one of the most specific therapies available that has few adverse effects. Following thyroidectomy an ablation dose of, typically, 3 gigabecquerel (GBq) of iodine-131 is administered to ablate the remnants of thyroid tissue. Further treatments of 5.5 GBq may be necessary to destroy deposits in local lymph nodes and distant metastases. Following treatment, patients will be followed up as outpatients (Pacini et al. 2002).

Preparation of patient before admission

- *Twenty-one days before admission*: patients taking tetraiodothyronine (T$_4$) (thyroxine) must stop taking this medication.
- *Ten days before admission*: patients taking triiodothyronine (T$_3$) must stop taking this medication.
- *Three days before admission*: occasionally, to enhance the uptake of iodine-131, three daily injections of thyroid-stimulating hormone (Thyrogen) are administered.

Principles of protection policies

Iodine-131 is excreted rapidly in patients who have had a thyroidectomy via all body fluids, especially the urine (Driver & Packer 2001). In those patients who have not undergone thyroidectomy, excretion is rapid initially, slowing as the iodine-131 is bound by the thyroid tissue. Consequently, great care must be taken with all body fluids, especially during the first few days.

Meta-iodobenzylguanidine (mIBG)

Definition

mIBG is a synthetic physiological guanethidine analogue which is structurally similar to both the neurotransmitter hormone nonadrenaline (norepinephrine) and the ganglionic blocking drug guanethidine. mIBG will localize in a wide variety of neuroendocrine tumours including neuroblastomas (Huang et al. 2006) and phaeochromocytomas (Manger 2006a) yet in relatively few normal cells (Brodeur et al. 2000).

mIBG can be linked to iodine-131 and iodine-123 (a radionuclide) to produce the radiopharmaceutical I-131 mIBG or I-123 mIBG. A radiopharmaceutical is a radionuclide linked to a suitable chemical compound whose biochemical properties allow the radionuclide to be localized in the desired tissue (Ziessman et al. 2006).

Use

Neuroblastoma is the most common extracranial solid tumour of childhood (Brodeur et al. 2000). Despite standard aggressive treatment including surgery, chemotherapy and radiotherapy the prognosis is poor (Brophy et al. 2004).

I-131 mIBG can be used as a safe, effective, non-invasive method of localizing both primary and metastatic neuroendocrine tumours (Okuyama et al. 2002). Therapeutic doses of I-131 mIBG can be given to patients in whom standard surgical and chemotherapeutic treatments have failed to control primary tumours, or can be used as an adjuvant to these treatments to prevent recurrence of the tumour (Brodeur et al. 2000). In the treatment of neuroblastoma, the combination of I-131 mIBG with chemotherapy has shown promising results (Matthay et al. 2006). Prior to therapy patients undergo scanning investigations using a tracer dose of I-123 or I-131 mIBG which allows calculation of the treatment dose. Therapeutic doses of I-131 mIBG are custom-synthesized for each patient and kept chilled or frozen from the time of synthesis until the dose is administered to reduce the risk of autoradiolysis. The solution is thawed and infused intravenously over 30–60 minutes using a shielded delivery system. During infusion patient monitoring is required (Brophy et al. 2004). This includes pulse and blood pressure monitoring due to the risk of rapid changes that may occur during and following treatment with I-131 mIBG (Manger 2006b). I-131 mIBG is a relatively non-toxic treatment (Brophy et al. 2004) but side-effects include anorexia and mild nausea and vomiting, which can be controlled with antiemetics and an adequate intake of fluids.

Preparation of patient

To prevent the uptake of any free iodine-131, the uptake of radioactive iodine by the thyroid gland is blocked by giving patients excess oral iodine (potassium iodate) prior to the infusion and up to 3 weeks after administration of mIBG for therapy doses, while for diagnostic investigations Lugol's iodine is taken before and after the injection of I-123 mIBG (Bomford & Kunkler 2002).

Parent and patient education on admission, during treatment and on discharge is important. To facilitate care, one centre in the USA has a multidisciplinary meeting 1 week before the patient's admission to discuss each child's specific needs so that a consistent plan can be agreed (Brophy *et al.* 2004).

Radioactive sentinel node biopsy using technetium-99m colloid

The pathological status of axillary lymph nodes is the most important prognostic indicator for patients with breast cancer (Luini *et al.* 2005). Intraoperative frozen section examination of sentinel nodes in breast cancer patients is associated with a high number of incorrect negative results, which can necessitate secondary axillary lymph node dissection (Schrenk *et al.* 2005). Sentinel node biopsy involves the use of technetium-99m colloid, a radiopharmaceutical, which is injected prior to the patient going to theatre. This nuclear medicine procedure assists the surgeon by identifying the nodes, thereby making removal of axillary sentinel lymph nodes easier and more accurate.

Sentinel lymph nodes receive drainage from the breasts (Luini *et al.* 2005). By undertaking biopsies of these nodes, the surgeon can predict the cancer status of all nodes in the axillary region. This procedure allows for accurate diagnosis of the patient's cancer status, as well as avoiding unnecessary axillary dissection (Schrenk *et al.* 2005), as axillary dissection can cause serious complications such as lymphoedema, scarring, numbness, pain and psychological distress (Mansel *et al.* 2006). Accurate diagnosis prevents understaging and inadequate treatment (Langer *et al.* 2004). During the procedure all staff must wear their film badges and those handling the specimen must wear finger dosimeters. The theatre door should be labelled with a warning controlled area sign and disposable drapes and gowns should be used. The specimen should be placed in a screw top container, which is labelled with the radioactive symbol and the details recorded in the log book. The specimen is then stored for 48 hours, after which time it is sent to histopathology in the normal way. The radioactive label is removed in histology after 1 week when the specimen is then considered non-radioactive.

On completion of the procedure, the used drapes, gown and gloves should be placed in a clinical waste bag and the environment and waste monitored to ensure no contamination is present. Any contaminated items should be marked radioactive and stored in a secure store, until sufficient radioactive decay has occurred. Only then should the warning symbols be removed by the physics department and the waste disposed of in the normal way.

On returning to the ward, the patient is cared for as described later.

Principles of radiation protection

Radiation is capable of being beneficial and harmful. It is essential that every effort is made to minimize the harmful effects of diagnostic and therapeutic radiation, whilst maximizing its benefits (Darby 1999). When setting standards for radiation protection, experience from atomic bomb survivors, accidents, and patients exposed to radiation therapeutically (Preston *et al.* 2003) as well as cohorts of workers in the nuclear industry are a consideration (Cardis *et al.* 2005).

The Health Protection Agency (HPA) has a statutory responsibility for advising UK government departments and those with responsibility for using ionizing radiation, on the risk to human beings caused by the use of radiation. This statutory responsibility applies to all medical, public health, occupational and environmental use of radiation. These responsibilities were passed to the HPA when the National Radiological Protection Board (NRPB) merged with the HPA on 1st April 2005 to form its Radiation Protection Division. Radiation protection is based on three principles:

- *Justification:* no practice should be adopted unless its introduction produces a net benefit.
- *Optimization:* all exposure shall be as low as reasonably practicable (ALARP).
- *Limitation:* the dose equivalent to staff and members of the public shall not exceed the dose limits.

The Ionising Radiation Regulations 1999, which came into force in 2000, set down requirements for the use of ionizing radiation and are enforced by the HSE. The regulations require that radiation safety standards be maintained. Requirements for procedures involving unsealed sources include:

- Those administering radioactive material must hold an approved Administration of Radioactive Substances Advisory Committee (ARSAC) certificate, for each radionuclide they intend to use.
- Administration of therapeutic and diagnostic radioactive substances can only be carried out in centres with appropriate facilities (Cormack *et al.* 1998).
- Risk assessments must be carried out prior to work with ionizing radiation, to ensure risks are properly controlled (Pearson *et al.* 2001).
- All controlled areas will have warning notices to restrict entry.
- All controlled and supervised areas have local rules and systems of work, summarizing the arrangements for controlling work with ionizing radiation. The radiation protection supervisor ensures the local rules are followed.
- Visitors are restricted. Doses received by relatives/friends of patients undergoing treatment or examination with ionizing radiation are restricted to the doses allowed to members of the public unless they are classified as comforters and carers when different rules and restrictions apply.
- Exposure is controlled by the use of time, distance and shielding.

723

- Personal protective clothing including gloves, aprons and overshoes used to limit the risk of contamination.
- Procedures are in place for reporting incidents (RIDDOR 1995).
- Adequate training is provided and only trained staff are allowed to work unsupervised.
- No pregnant or breastfeeding staff to enter the controlled area.
- Quality assurance initiatives have to be undertaken; these include clinical audit of procedures and standards.

Controlled area

The entrance to the controlled area must be marked with a warning sign. Information is displayed to indicate the following:

- The radioactive material and activity administered.
- That only essential nursing procedures should only be carried out and unnecessary time must not be spent in close proximity to the patient while the sign is displayed.

Appropriate barriers, i.e. lead shields, should be placed at the entrance to:

- Prevent inadvertent entry by unauthorized personnel.
- Reduce radiation exposure to visitors and staff.

Patients treated with unsealed radioactive sources should be confined to their rooms, except for special medical or nursing procedures, when they must be accompanied by suitably trained staff.

Therapeutic unsealed sources generate a significant amount of liquid radioactive waste. This can be from the patient's shower and toilet. However, the amount of radioactive waste that enters the sewage system is governed by local regulations. The impact on the river Thames, from radionuclide discharge from 86 authorized sites discharging liquid radioactive waste into the Thames, indicated that potential doses to the general public was significantly lower than the radiation dose limit of 1 mSv for a member of the public. Ingestion of fish and water from the river produced the highest dose to humans (Hilton *et al.* 2004). Multiple holding tank systems can be employed where waste can be held to allow decay to occur before being released into the main waste drainage system (Leung & Nikolic 1998).

Film badges

Film badges must be worn at all times when on duty (Figure 36.1). A digital dosimeter should be used when ongoing immediate dose records are required.

Contamination control

With unsealed sources, it is important to guard against contamination of both personnel and the hospital environment by the correct use of protective gloves, gowns and

Figure 36.1   Film badge.

overshoes. The patient's body fluids are highly radioactive, especially in the days immediately after iodine-131 has been administered. Any action that is likely to cause contamination of personnel, for example the application of cosmetics, eating, drinking or smoking when the health care worker's hands are contaminated with radioactivity, is prohibited.

In the event of any incident involving radioactive material, the physics department must be advised immediately, even if the incident occurs outside normal working hours.

Preparation of therapy room

Equipment

Equipment should be kept to a minimum. It must be checked to ensure that it is in working order, as maintenance staff will only be allowed into the room in exceptional circumstances.

Bed linen and disposable items (gloves, aprons, overshoes, cutlery and crockery) should be kept in a utility room or anteroom along with the patient's treatment chart and a radiation monitor.

Personal items

Nurses should be sensitive to the psychological implications for patients of being labelled 'radioactive' and confined in isolation. Although patients may want to bring some personal belongings with them, they should be advised to keep these to a minimum, as items may become contaminated and need to be stored until radioactivity has decayed. Generally patients will be supplied with disposable toothbrush and slippers and be asked to wear the hospital nightwear.

Protective floor covering

Plastic-backed absorbent paper, kept in place by adhesive tape, is used to retain accidental urine spills or splashes on the floor immediately surrounding the toilet. Each patient is assessed to decide whether further floor covering is necessary, e.g. catheterized patients will require floor covering below the catheter bag.

Cleaning the treatment room

During occupancy of the treatment room by the patient, cleaning of the room is kept to a minimum and should be supervised by the physics staff. After the patient is discharged, monitoring and any necessary decontamination of the room will be arranged by the physics department, which will inform the relevant personnel when this has been completed. Only then may the room be entered and thoroughly cleaned.

Preparation of patient

Consent

Every diagnostic or therapeutic use of radiation has an inherent risk. Awareness of the risk is essential for all staff who have to obtain informed consent from their patients (Picano 2004). A survey of patients and family members of patients receiving radioactive iodine found that many experienced psychological distress and few received adequate help (Fitch & McGrath 2003). Therefore careful preparation of the patient before the administration of unsealed source therapy is essential. Patients and relatives should be educated (Skalla et al. 2004) about the principles of radiation protection and the procedures with which the patient has to comply while in isolation. Psychosocial and physical needs must be addressed which require a collaborative approach between patients and nurses (Stajduhar et al. 2000). It is important to identify potential anxieties before administration while the nurse is able to reassure the patient and is unconstrained by time limits. Fully prepared, knowledgeable patients and visitors are the key to radiation safety and contamination control (Stajduhar et al. 2000; Thompson 2001). Incidents and accidents are less likely to occur if the patient fully understands the reasons for the restrictions being undertaken.

Patients are required to sign a consent form agreeing to treatment, following a full explanation from the treating clinician. This is to comply with medical, ethical and legal requirements and local hospital policy. Consent is usually obtained in the outpatient clinic before ordering the radioactive material. The patient must also agree to stay in hospital until the physics department advises that the level of radioactivity permits discharge (ICRP 2004).

On admission

Before the administration of unsealed sources, any symptoms of diarrhoea or constipation must be remedied. Diarrhoea could result in contamination of the treatment area. Constipation not only inhibits the elimination of radioactivity but also could obscure radiological investigations, e.g. scanning. All investigations including blood tests must be undertaken before administration of diagnostic and therapeutic unsealed sources. If essential specimens need to be processed after administration, the specimen and the request card must be labelled with a radiation warning sticker, and the laboratories must follow their standard operating procedures for processing and disposal of these specimens.

Although the patient will have been assessed in the outpatient department, it is important that the patient is reassessed on admission for their suitability for treatment, in case changes have occurred since their outpatient visit. In particular the needs of a debilitated patient must be assessed to ensure appropriate nusing care can be provided within the time constraints. A review of a patient who was quadriplegic, doubly incontinent and unable to swallow, found that nurses could provide appropriate care whilst following the recommended radiation protection restrictions (Williams & Woodward 2005). Multidisciplinary co-ordination of care is required in such cases.

Discharge of patient

A patient should not be discharged from hospital until the activity retained has fallen below recommended levels (ICRP 2004). This level will depend on several factors, including:

- Mode of transport on leaving hospital.
- Journey time involved.
- Personal circumstances, e.g. young children or pregnant women at home.

Patients will be assessed individually for radiation clearance by the physics department before discharge. The treating physician will then be advised of the results of the assessment. Advice will be given to patients on issues such as return to work and visits to public places. Patients who are discharged will be given appropriate information in the form of an instruction card carrying details of the precautions to be taken. This card must be signed by the treating clinician or the physics department staff.

It must be emphasized that this card must be carried and the instructions followed until the latest date shown so that, for instance, staff would be alerted should the patient be readmitted to hospital. Additional verbal instructions may be necessary.

725

Procedure guidelines   Iodine-131: pre-administration care

Procedure

Action	Rationale
1 Explain and discuss the procedure with the patient.	To ensure that the patient understands the procedure and gives his/her valid consent (O'Dwyer *et al.* 2003: R 1b).
2 The patient is to be fasted for 2 hours before and after administration of an iodine-131 dose. Offer a light diet for the remainder of the day.	To reduce the risk of nausea and/or vomiting (E).
3 Administer a prophylactic antiemetic 30 minutes before scheduled administration of the dose.	To prevent nausea and vomiting (E).
4 Check that the preparation of the room and the patient is complete. Ensure that any surplus items have been removed.	To prevent contamination of extraneous equipment (E).
5 Remove jewellery except wedding rings.	Jewellery may become contaminated (E).

Procedure guidelines   Iodine-131 thyroid treatment: patient care

Procedure

Action	Rationale
1 Explain and discuss the procedure with the patient.	To ensure that the patient understands the procedure and gives his/her valid consent (O'Dwyer *et al.* 2003: R 1b).
2 Assist the patient to remove dentures/bridges, if dose is administered in liquid form.	To prevent radioactive material being trapped behind dental plates (E).
3 The patient swallows the capsule or drinks the iodine-131 through a straw, physically directed by an authorized physicist in the presence of the clinician directing treatment.	Drinking through a straw reduces the amount of radioactive material left around the mouth. To meet current regulations (E).
4 Offer the patient a drink of water to rinse out the mouth. (This must be swallowed.) Assist the patient to replace dentures.	To remove any iodine-131 from inside the mouth (E).
5 Physics staff place the radiation warning sign at the entrance to the therapy room.	To identify the room as a controlled area (Ionising Radiation Regulations 1999: C).

Procedure guidelines   Iodine-131 mIBG treatment: patient care

Procedure

Action	Rationale
1 Explain and discuss the procedure with patient and/or parents if the patient is a child.	To ensure that the patient and/or parents understands the procedure and gives his/her consent (O'Dwyer *et al.* 2003: R 1b).
2 Apply a vital signs monitor with a variable time setting mode to the patient that will be visible to staff from outside the room.	Following the administration of mIBG, a transient rise in blood pressure and pulse may occur (Brophy *et al.* 2004: E).
3 Check that the patient has been cannulated or, for children, a central venous device is in place.	To ensure safe administration of mIBG (E).
4 The clinician will set up iodine-131 mIBG infusion and give it over 30–60 minutes.	To minimize transient rise in blood pressure and pulse (E).
5 Monitor blood pressure and pulse at least: (a) Every 5 minutes during infusion. (b) Monitor whole body retention measurements as directed by physics.	To detect and monitor any change (E).
6 Encourage the patient to take oral fluids.	To increase the urinary output and elimination of radioactivity from the bladder (E).
7 Avoid the patient becoming constipated.	To facilitate radioactivity being eliminated in faeces (E).

Procedure guidelines   Unsealed source therapy: patient care post-administration

Procedure

Entering the room of patient with unsealed radioactive soure

Action	Rationale
1 Collect digital dosimeter, record reading before entering and on leaving room.	Digital dosimeter provides ongoing and immediate indication of the amount of exposure received (Ionising Radiation Regulations 1999: C).
2 Put on disposable gloves.	To prevent contamination of the hands (HSE 2002: C).
3 Put on disposable overshoes.	To prevent spread of contamination outside the treatment area (HSE 2002: C).
4 Put on a suitable protective gown: (a) Long-sleeve cotton gown, e.g. for lifting patient. (b) Disposable plastic apron, e.g. for dealing with vomit or incontinence.	To protect against low levels of contamination, e.g. from the patient's skin (HSE 2002: C). To protect against high levels of contamination (HSE 2002: C).

Procedure guidelines *(cont.)*

5 Plan work before entering the controlled area and then work quickly and efficiently, keeping within the time allowance stated.	To minimize radiation exposure, as consistent with good nursing care (Ionising Radiation Regulations 1999: C).
6 Only use disposable crockery and cutlery to present meals to patients. Remove all fruit stones and fish and meat bones from diet.	China crockery and cutlery may become contaminated. Uneaten food and disposable cutlery and crockery are disposed of in a macerator. Fruit stones and bones will block the macerator (E).

Maintaining comfort and hygiene of patient with unsealed radioactive source

Action	Rationale
1 Encourage the patient to shower frequently, at least once a day.	To reduce any radioactive perspiration on the skin (E).
2 Encourage the patient to wash the hands thoroughly after each possible contact with bodily fluids, e.g. cleaning teeth, going to the toilet.	To remove radioactivity from the hands (E).
3 The patient should regularly remove any dentures and clean under running water.	To remove radioactive saliva from around dentures (E).
4 The patient should regularly remove any contact lenses and rinse in their usual cleaning fluid.	To remove any radioactive tears from lenses (E).
5 Encourage a good fluid intake of between 2 and 3 litres per day.	To increase the urinary output and elimination of radioactivity from the bladder (Thompson 2001: E).
6 Ensure that the patient has own personal toilet facilities and flushes the toilet twice after use.	To reduce contamination of others and of the environment. Urine of patients treated with iodine-131 is initially highly radioactive (Thompson 2001: E).
7 Bedbound patients should be catheterized before the dose is given. Empty the catheter bag every 4–6 hours, or more frequently if necessary.	Catheterization reduces the nursing time spent with the patient and the likelihood of contamination. Frequent emptying of the bag reduces the radiation level in the room (E).
8 If the patient requires a bedpan or urinal, this item must be kept solely for this patient's use. The bedpan or urinal must be handled carefully and the contents disposed of in the patient's toilet, which is flushed twice. The bedpan or urinal may be washed in the bedpan washer. It should be sealed in a plastic bag for the journey to and from the sluice.	To reduce contamination of the environment and of other patients and staff (E).
9 If leakage occurs from injection sites, wound sites, etc., the nurse should contact the medical staff and the physics department immediately. Any contact with the dressing should be done with long-handled forceps.	It must be remembered that all body fluids are potentially radioactive (E).
10 Gloves and a protective gown must be worn whenever handling soiled bed linen.	To prevent contamination (HSE 2002: C).

728

11 All used linen must be deposited in a special bag provided for this purpose.	Used linen must be monitored for contamination before going to the laundry (E).
12 Collection of laboratory specimens should, if possible, be deferred. If collections are unavoidable, a radiation warning sticker must be attached to the specimen and request card and the specimen delivered to the laboratory following consultations with the physics department.	To reduce the risk of contamination of the laboratory and its staff (Vialard-Miguel *et al.* 2005: E).

Visitors to patients with unsealed radioactive source

Action	Rationale
1 Visiting time is limited as advised by the physicist during the first day following administration of an unsealed source.	The patient is highly radioactive during this period (Ionising Radiation Regulations 1999: C).
2 On subsequent days, visiting is unlimited, providing visitors remain outside the room behind the lead screen, the exception being parents of young children who will need to be authorized by the physics department.	To minimize the exposure of visitors to radiation (Ionising Radiation (Medical Exposure) Regulations 2000: C).
3 Physical contact with the patient or bed linen is not allowed as protective clothing is not available to visitors.	To prevent contamination of visitors (E).
4 Children under 16 years of age and pregnant women will be discouraged from visiting.	Radiation exposure of children and the unborn must be kept as low as practicable (Ionising Radiation (Medical Exposure) Regulations 2000: C).

729

On leaving the room of patient with unsealed radioactive source

Action	Rationale
1 Remove overshoes, taking care not to touch the shoes worn underneath.	These are removed first while gloves are still being worn to prevent the spread of contamination to hands or the floor outside the room (E).
2 Remove the plastic apron, by holding the front of apron and breaking the neck and waist ties.	To prevent transfer of contamination from the gloves onto the uniform below (E).
3 Remove gloves by peeling them off the hands, taking care not to touch the outside surfaces with bare hands, and discard them in the clinical waste bag provided.	To prevent transfer of contamination from the gloves' outer surfaces to the hands (E).
4 Wash hands thoroughly using soap and water.	To remove any contamination (HSE 2003: C).
5 Use the radiation monitor each time when leaving the room and monitor for contamination of the hands, feet and clothing. If contamination has occurred, inform the physics department immediately and follow the decontamination procedure.	To ensure that the nurse is not contaminated (Ionising Radiation Regulations 1999: C).
6 The physics department will advise if further whole body monitoring is required.	To check for internal or external contamination (E).

Procedure guidelines   Unsealed radioactive sources for diagnostic investigations: patient care

Procedure

Action	Rationale
1 Explain and discuss the procedure with the patient, and, if relevant, with the relative accompanying the patient.	To ensure the patient is physically and psychologically prepared for the procedure and understands the procedure and gives his/her informed consent (O'Dwyer *et al.* 2003: E).

Action	Rationale
2 Preparation of patients (special considerations):	
(a) Provide effective pain control for those patients with pain.	Patients should be pain free so that immobility during scan time can be maintained (see Chapter 27) (E).
(b) Pregnant women will generally not be scanned. When essential tests must be undertaken, the patient must sign a consent form and receive a reduced dose of radionuclide.	To avoid unnecessary irradiation to the abdominal/pelvic region which will include the embryo or foetus (Ionising Radiation Regulations 1999: C).
(c) The person accompanying the patient should not be pregnant, or bring young children or babies with them.	To avoid unnecessary exposure in the time period immediately after the radionuclide administration (Ionising Radiation Regulations 1999: C).
(d) In women of reproductive age, the possibility of pregnancy must be excluded and the patient asked if her menstrual period is late. Patients receiving I-131 or other radioactive agent with a long half-life should not become pregnant for a minimum of 3 months (Sharp *et al.* 1998).	To avoid unnecessary irradiation to the abdomen of a woman who may be pregnant (Ionising Radiation Regulations 1999: C).
(e) With breastfeeding mothers, seek advice from the radiation protection adviser.	Radioactivity can be excreted in breast milk. Therefore breastfeeding may need to be suspended (Pomeroy *et al.* 2005: R 1b) and the mother encouraged to avoid unnecessary cuddling of the child during this time (E).
(f) If the patient is incontinent, incontinence pads should be worn and universal precautions are to be adopted.	To limit the spread of contamination. Disposable gloves and apron should be worn and handwashing performed following patient contact, as these will prevent contamination of staff in close contact with the patient (HSE 2002: C).
(g) Empty urine bags regularly.	To remove the radioactivity from the patient area (E).
(h) Debilitated patients may require prolonged close contact. Nursing staff should share the care of these patients, by regular rotation of staff.	To keep doses to staff as low as possible, by avoiding prolonged exposure to any one member of staff (E).

Action	Rationale
3 Administering radionuclides:	
(a) Follow guidelines for drug administration in Chapter 11.	To comply with national and professional guidelines for the administration of drugs (NMC 2008: C).
(b) Follow for guidelines aseptic technique in Chapter 5.	To reduce the risk of contamination (DH 2005: R 1a).
(c) Follow radiation protection precautions, which include:	To reduce the possible contamination of self and the environment (Ionising Radiation Regulations 1999: C).
▪ Wear thermoluminescent (TLD) finger-dose meter and film badge.	To measure radiation doses received by member of staff (Ionising Radiation Regulations 1999: C).
▪ Wear disposable gloves and plastic apron, which are discarded after use.	To reduce the risk of contamination (Ionising Radiation Regulations 1999: C).
▪ Draw up the dose behind a lead shield, and place the syringe in a lead syringe shield.	To reduce exposure to radiation (Ionising Radiation Regulations 1999: C).
▪ Dispose of all used syringes and needles in a designated radioactive sharps disposal bin which is stored within a lead shield.	To contain radioactivity and allow safe disposal (Ionising Radiation Regulations 1999: C).
▪ Wash hands at end of procedure.	To remove any possible radioactive contamination (Ionising Radiation Regulations 1999: C; DH 2005: R 1a).

■ Place yellow identity bracelet on the wrists of all inpatients, complete information card with the details of when precautions can be discontinued. Give the completed information card to the patient or the nurse accompanying the patient.

The yellow wrist band will provide visual warning to inform all health care workers of the patient's recent diagnostic investigation. The information card will inform ward staff of restrictions related to managing a patient, as well as when measures that have to be adopted in the event of the patient vomiting or being incontinent can be discontinued.

The card also states where to obtain help and advice related to the patient's diagnostic investigation (E).

■ Monitor hands at end of procedure and before leaving the room.

To check for possible radioactive contamination.

■ Monitor the room for radioactive contamination at the end of each day or if contamination may have occurred.

To establish whether contamination has occurred (Ionising Radiation Regulations 1999: C).

4 Avoid urine, faecal and blood sample collection for laboratories other than nuclear medicine for 24 hours. If collection is unavoidable, a radiation warning sticker must be attached to the specimen and request card, and the specimen taken to the laboratory under the supervision of the physics departmental staff (see Chapter 40).

To prevent contamination of the laboratory and its staff, as specimens taken within 24 hours of some scans may contain radioactivity (HSE 2003; Vialard-Miguel *et al.* 2005: C).

5 Avoid bone marrow and stem cell harvests for 24 hours. Seek advice from the physics department.

Cells may contain radioactivity (HSE 2003; Vialard-Miguel *et al.* 2005: C).

6 Seek advice from physics staff if the patient is to undergo a procedure in the operating theatre within 24 hours of a scan.

To prevent theatre equipment from becoming contaminated with radioactivity (E).

731

7 Place soiled bed linen used within the first 24 hours of certain scans, e.g. bone scan, within a purple plastic bag and inform the physics departmental staff.

To prevent contamination of the environment (E).

Procedure guidelines   Unsealed radioactive sources: emergency procedures

In an emergency, the safety and medical care of the patient must take precedence over any potential radiation hazards to staff. Written radiation safety instructions must be available in all radiation areas where an emergency may arise. These instructions must contain a detailed description of how to manage a patient in the event of a medical emergency and the action required in other emergency situations, such as fire. The course of action in an emergency procedure depends on local circumstances and the nature of the emergency.

An incident occurring within the first 24 hours of iodine-131 being administered is obviously a greater hazard than a similar incident on the day of discharge. Movement of the patient to other wards or areas, e.g. X-ray or coronary care unit (CCU), must only be undertaken following the physics department's advice.

Procedure

Major spillage of radioactive body fluids, i.e. incontinence and/or vomiting

Action
1 Inform the physics department immediately.

Rationale
So that the physics department can advise on radiation protection as soon as possible, to ensure local policy is adhered to (E).

2 If physics department staff are not immediately available, use a radiation monitor to assess the extent of the spillage.

To define extent of contamination and determine what further measures need to be taken (E).

3 Put some absorbent material on top of all the radioactive wet area.

To absorb contamination (E).

Procedure guidelines *(cont.)*

Action	Rationale
4 Any waste that cannot be flushed down the toilet or macerated must be placed in a purple polythene bag and the physics staff informed.	To prevent contamination of the environment (E).
5 Follow the advice of the physics department staff in clearing the spillage.	To prevent spread of contamination (E).

Contamination of bare hands by radioactive body fluids

Action	Rationale
1 Wash hands in warm soapy water, paying special attention to the areas around the fingernails, between the fingers and on the outer edges of the hands. Continue washing until contamination is below the permissible limits indicated by local monitoring protocols.	To remove radioactive material from any areas where it might be trapped (HSE 2002: C).
2 If the skin is broken in a contamination accident, wash thoroughly under running water, opening the edges of the cut. This should be continued until physics department staff can demonstrate that no residual radioactivity remains in the wound.	To stimulate bleeding and permit thorough flushing of the cut (E).

Death of patient who has received unsealed radioactive source therapy

Action	Rationale
1 Inform the physics department immediately.	So that the physics department staff can begin making the necessary arrangements for removal of the body to the mortuary (E).
2 Two nurses wearing gloves, plastic aprons, gowns and overshoes should perform last offices. All orifices must be packed carefully. Any vomit, blood, faeces or urine must be cleaned from the body.	To avoid contamination with body fluids. Minimal handling of the body reduces the risk of contamination (E).
3 The body should be totally enclosed in a plastic body bag.	To avoid contamination of the porters and the mortuary staff (Health Services Advisory Committee 1991: C).
4 Transfer of the body should be arranged with the physics department.	The physics department will supervise the transfer of the body (E).

Cardiac arrest of patient who has received unsealed radioactive source therapy

Action	Rationale
1 The switchboard must be told to inform the physics department as soon as possible after alerting the emergency resuscitation team.	So that the physics department can advise on radiation protection as soon as possible (E).
2 Do not use mouth-to-mouth resuscitation. All areas must be supplied with an Ambu bag for this purpose.	Mouth-to-mouth contact could result in contamination of the resuscitator (E).
3 Overshoes, gloves and gowns must be put on as soon as it is practicably possible.	To minimize personal contamination (HSE 2002: C).
4 All emergency equipment must be monitored and decontaminated as necessary before being returned to general use.	To prevent contaminated equipment leaving the controlled area (E).

Fire: evacuation of patients who have received unsealed radioactive source

Action	Rationale
1 Every effort should be made to contact the physics department without compromising the patient's safety.	To help in the evacuation of the patients treated with iodine-131 (E).
2 Following evacuation, patients treated with iodine-131 should be kept at a distance from other patients and staff.	To minimize exposure of others to radiation (E).

Regulations

Ionising Radiation Regulations (1999) HMSO, London.

Web resources

Ionising Radiation Regulations 1999 (SI 1999 No. 3232): www.legislation.hmso.gov.uk/si/si1999/19993232.htm.

Ionising Radiation (Medical Exposure) Regulations 2000 (SI 2000 No. 1059): www.legislation.hmso.gov.uk/si/si2000/20001059.htm.

References and further reading

Beasley, N.J. *et al.* (2002) Impact of nodal metastases on prognosis in patients with well-differentiated thyroid cancer. *Arch Otolaryngol Head Neck Surg*, **128**(7), 825–8.

Bomford, C.K. & Kunkler, I.H. (2002) *Walter & Miller's Textbook of Radiotherapy*, 6th edn. Churchill Livingstone, Edinburgh.

Brodeur, G.M. *et al.* (2000) *Neuroblastoma*. Elsevier, Edinburgh.

Brophy, P., Schmus, C. & Balistreri, L. (2004) Meeting the nursing challenge in treating children with 131 I-mIBG. *J Paed Oncol Nurs*, **21**(1), 9–15.

BTA/RCP (2002) *Guidelines for the Management of Thyroid Cancer in Adults*. Royal College of Physicians, London.

Cardis, E. *et al.* (2005) Risk of cancer after low doses of ionising radiation: retrospective cohort study in 15 countries. *BMJ*, **331**(7508), 77–82.

Cherry, S.R., Sorenson, J.A. & Phelps, M.E. (2003) *Physics in Nuclear Medicine*, 3rd edn. Saunders, Oxford.

Chung, L.W. *et al.* (2005) Molecular insights into prostate cancer progression: the missing link of tumor microenvironment. *J Urol*, **173**(1), 10–20.

Cormack, J., Towson, J.E.C. & Flower, M.A. (1998) Radiation protection and dosimetry in clinical practice. In: *Nuclear Medicine in Clinical Diagnosis and Treatment* (eds I.P.C. Murray & P.J. Ell), 2nd edn. Churchill Livingstone, Edinburgh, pp. 1651–77.

Darby, S. (1999) Radiation risks. *BMJ*, **319**(7216), 1019–20.

DH (1999) *The Ionising Regulations No. 3232*. HMSO, London.

DH (2000) *The Ionising Radiation (Medical Exposure) Regulations No. 1059*. HMSO, London.

DH (2005) *Saving Lives: a Delivery Programme to Reduce Healthcare Associated Infection Including MRSA*. Department of Health, London.

Driver, I. & Packer, S. (2001) Radioactive waste discharge quantities for patients undergoing radioactive iodine therapy for thyroid carcinoma. *Nucl Med Commun*, **22**(10), 1129–32.

Fitch, M.I. & McGrath, P.N. (2003) The needs of family members of patients receiving radioactive iodine. *Can Oncol Nurs*, **13**(4), 220–31.

Harmer, C.L. (1996) Radiotherapy in the management of thyroid cancer. *Ann Acad Med Singapore*, **25**(3), 413–19.

Health Services Advisory Committee (1991) *Safety in Health Service Laboratories. Safe Working and the Prevention of Infection in the Mortuary and Post Mortem Room*. HMSO, London.

Henkin, R.E. *et al.* (2006) *Nuclear Medicine*, 2nd edn., Mosby, St Louis.

Hilton, J., Harvey, M. & Simmonds, J. (2004) The combined impact on doses to man of multiple, authorized, radionuclide discharges for the year 1999 reaching the upper river Thames, UK. *Health Phys*, **87**(1), 33–45.

Hod, N., Hagag, P. & Baumer, M. (2005) Differentiated thyroid carcinoma in children and young adults: evaluation of response to treatment. *Clin Nucl Med*, **30**(6), 387–90.

HSE (2002) *Control of Substances Hazardous to Health Regulations (COSHH)*. Health and Safety Executive Books, Norwich.

HSE (2003) Safe working and the prevention of infection in clinical laboratories and similar facilities. Health and Safety Executive Books, Norwich.

Huang, S., Yang, H., Zhuang, H. (2006) Initial diagnosis and treatment follow up of neuroblastoma invasion of inferior vena cava with 1-131 mIBG. *Clin Nucl Med*, **31**(11), 718–20.

ICRP (2004) Release of patients after therapy with unsealed radionuclide. *Ann ICRP*, **34**(20), v–vi & 1–79.

IPEM/RCN (2002) Procedures involving radiation. In: *Ionising Radiation Safety. A Handbook for Nurses*. York Publishing, York, pp. 17–32.

Langer, S. *et al.* (2004) Lymphatic mapping improves staging and reduces morbidity in women undergoing total mastectomy for breast carcinoma. *Am Surg*, **70**(10), 881–5.

Leung, P.M. & Nikolic, M. (1998) Disposal of therapeutic 131-I waste using a multiple holding tank system. *Health Phys*, **75**(3), 315–21.

Liepe, K., Runge, R. & Kotzerke, J. (2005) Systematic radionuclide therapy in pain palliation. *Am J Hosp Palliat Care*, **22**(6), 457–64.

Luini, A. *et al.* (2005) The sentinel node biopsy after previous breast surgery: preliminary results on 543 patients treated at the European Institute of Oncology. *Breast Cancer Res Treat*, **89**(2), 159–63.

Manger, W.M. (2006a) Diagnosis and management of pheochromocytoma – recent advances and current concepts. *Kidney Int Suppl*, **12**(104), S30–5.

Manger, W.M. (2006b) An overview of pheochromocytoma: history, current concepts, vagaries, and diagnostic challenges. *Ann N Y Acad Sci*, **1073**, 1–20.

Mansel, R.E. *et al.* (2006) Randomized multicenter trial of sentinel node biopsy versus standard axillary treatment in operable breast cancer: the ALMANAC Trial. *J Natl Cancer Inst*, **98**(9), 599–609.

Matthay, K.K. *et al.* (2006) Phase 1 dose escalation of iodine 131. *J Clin Oncol*, **24**(3), 500–6.

733

Maxon, H.R. *et al.* (1992) Rhenium-186 hydroxyethylidene diphosphonate for the treatment of painful osseous metastases. *Semin Nucl Med*, **22**(1), 33–40.

McEwan, A.J. (1998) Palliation of bone pain. In: *Nuclear Medicine in Clinical Diagnosis and Treatment* (eds I.P.C. Murray & P.J. Ell), 2nd edn. Churchill Livingstone, Edinburgh, pp. 1083–1100.

Mokete, M. *et al.* (2006) The increased rate of prostate specific antigen testing has not affected prostate cancer presentation in an inner city population in the UK. *BJU Int*, **97**(2), 266–72.

NMC (2008) *Standards for Medicines Management*. Nursing and Midwifery Council, London.

O'Dwyer, H.M. *et al.* (2003) Informed consent for interventional radiology procedures: a survey detailing current European practice. *Cardiovas Intervent Radiol*, **26**(5), 428–33.

Okuyama, C. *et al.* (2002) Utility of follow up studies using meta-[123-I]iodobenzylguanidine scintigraphy for detecting recurrent neuroblastoma. *Nucl Med Commun*, **23**(7), 663–72.

O'Sullivan, J.M. *et al.* (2002) High activity rhenium-HEDP with autologous peripheral blood stem rescue: a phase I study in progressive hormone refractory prostate cancer metastatic to bone. *Br J Cancer*, **86**(11), 1715–20.

Pacini, F. *et al.* (2002) Diagnostic 131-iodine whole body scan may be avoided in thyroid cancer patients who have undetectable stimulated serum Tg levels after initial treatment. *J Clin Endocrinol Metabol*, **87**(4), 1499–501.

Pearce, M.S. *et al.* (2005) Cancer in adolescents and young adults aged 15–24 years: a report from the north of England young malignant disease registry, UK. *Pediatr Blood Cancer*, **45**(5), 687–93.

Pearson, D., Rogers, A.T. & Moss, E. (2001) A generic approach to risk assessment for the Ionising Radiation Regulations 1999. *Br J Radiol*, **74**(877), 62–8.

Peter, J.E. & Gambhir, S. (2004) *Nuclear Medicine in Clinical Diagnosis and Treatment*, 3rd edn. Churchill Livingstone, Edinburgh.

Picano, E. (2004) Informed consent and communication of risk from radiological and nuclear medicine examination: how to escape from a communication inferno. *BMJ*, **329**(7470), 849–51.

Pomeroy, K.M., Sawyerm, L.J. & Evans, M.J. (2005) Estimated radiation dose to breast feeding infants following maternal administration of 57Co labelled to vitamin B12. *Nucl Med Commun*, **26**(9), 839–41.

Preston, D.L. *et al.* (2003) Studies of mortality of atomic bomb survivors. Report 13: Solid cancer and noncancer disease mortality: 1950–1997. *Radiat Res*, **160**(4), 381–407.

RIDDOR (1995) *The Reporting of Injuries, Diseases and Dangerous Occurrences Regulations*. HMSO, London.

Russell, C. (1998) Measurement and interpretation of renal transit times. In: *Nuclear Medicine in Clinical Diagnosis and Treatment* (eds I.P.C. Murray & P.J. Ell), 2nd edn. Churchill Livingstone, Edinburgh, pp. 257–62.

Schrenk, P. *et al.* (2005) The use of sentinel node biopsy in breast cancer patients undergoing skin sparing mastectomy and immediate autologous reconstruction. *Plas Reconstr Surg*, **116**(5), 1278–86.

Sharp, C., Shrimpton, J.A. & Bury, R.F. (1998) *Diagnostic Medical Exposures: Advice on Exposure to Ionising Radiation during Pregnancy*. National Radiological Protection Board, Didcot.

Sherry, I. (2000) Nuclear medicine: will I glow in the dark, Nurse? *Nurs Stand*, **14**(19), 48–53.

Shiralkar, S. *et al.* (2003) Doctors' knowledge of radiation exposure: questionnaire study. *BMJ*, **327**(7411), 371–2.

Skalla, K.A. *et al.* (2004) Patients' need for information about cancer therapy. *Oncol Nurs Forum*, **31**(2), 313–19.

Stajduhar, K.I. *et al.* (2000) Thyroid cancer: patients' experience of receiving iodine-131 therapy. *Oncol Nurs Forum*, **27**(8), 1213–18.

Thompson, M.A. (2001) Radiation safety precautions in the management of the hospitalized 131-I therapy patient. *Nucl Med Technol*, **29**(2), 61–6.

Vialard-Miguel, J. *et al.* (2005) I131 in blood samples: management in the laboratory. *Ann Biol Clin (Paris)*, **63**(5), 561–5.

Williams, C.E. & Woodward, A.F. (2005) Management of the hapless patent after radioiodine ablation therapy. Are we being too strict? *Nucl Med Commun*, **26**(10), 925–8.

Ziessman, H.A., O'Malley, J.P. & Thrall, J.H. (2006) *Nuclear Medicine*, 3rd edn. Mosby, St Louis.

Chapter 37

Renal replacement therapy: peritoneal dialysis and continuous venovenous haemodiafiltration

Reference material **736**
Peritoneal dialysis **736**
Reference material **736**
Continuous renal replacement therapy **739**
Reference material **739**
Procedure guidelines: Peritoneal dialysis **740**
Problem solving: Peritoneal dialysis **742**
Procedure guidelines: CVVHDF: utilizing a CVVHDF device **744**
References and further reading **747**

Definition

Renal replacement therapies such as peritoneal dialysis, haemodialysis and continuous filtration methods are interventions used when patients have inadequate renal function and can no longer filter the blood and excrete waste products. This malfunction may be temporary, as in acute renal failure, or permanent when patients are in end-stage renal disease (ESRD) (Levy *et al.* 2005).

Reference material

In health the kidneys are the main excretory organ of the body. Every day they filter approximately 180 litres of fluid from the blood. Less than 1%, i.e. 1.0–1.5 litres, is excreted as urine while the remainder is reabsorbed. This fluid contains toxins, metabolic waste and excess ions and leaves the body as urine. As the kidneys excrete this fluid they are maintaining the volume and electrolyte balance of the blood by balancing water and salts, and the pH of the blood by balancing acids and bases (Marieb 2004; Waugh & Grant 2006).

When renal replacement therapy is required the kidneys are temporarily replaced by using an alternative membrane or filter. In peritoneal dialysis (PD) the membrane used is the peritoneum itself; in all other forms of renal replacement therapy an artificial membrane or filter is used. Therefore renal replacement therapies may be instituted when the patient is in end-stage renal failure (ESRF), the main causes of which are diabetes, uncontrolled hypertension, glomerulonephritis, polycystic kidney disease and trauma (Marieb 2004). For ESRF the therapies of choice will be transplant where possible, haemodialysis or PD. In 2001, the median age of those receiving renal replacement therapy in the UK was 64 years, and 21% were over 75 years (Levy *et al.* 2005).

In the setting of a critical illness, acute renal failure (ARF) can be caused by a number of insults to the body, including sepsis, nephrotoxic drugs or other compounds, severe burns, hypovolaemic shock, tumour lysis syndrome, rhabdomyolysis and multiorgan failure (Block & Manning 2002). An elevated blood urea nitrogen (BUN) and serum creatinine (Cr) are evident during ARF (Quan & Quigley 2005). When the patient is critically ill and in acute renal failure, haemodynamic instability is common and life threatening so the treatment of choice in this setting is continuous venovenous haemodiafiltration (CVVHDF) (Toft *et al.* 1999).

Types of renal replacement therapy

There are three main types of therapy available:

- Peritoneal dialysis (PD).
- Haemodialysis.
- Continuous filtration and diafiltration methods.

The choice of therapy will depend first on whether the patient's kidneys are likely to recover and second on their current condition. If the patient is in ESRF then the optimum therapy is a renal transplant; however, the need for organs constantly outpaces the supply and many patients require

haemodialysis while they are awaiting a transplant (Briggs *et al.* 1997). Haemodialysis is usually performed 2–3 times a week either in a regional renal centre or in the patient's home. The patient is connected up to a renal dialysis machine via an arteriovenous shunt which is formed usually between the artery and vein at their wrist (Marieb 2004). For these patients each day's treatment takes about 4–8 hours and patients have to adhere to a special diet and a restricted fluid intake (Oreopoulos 1998).

Many patients elect to utilize PD as opposed to haemodialysis in the chronic setting as, when it is working effectively, it has less impact on their quality of life than haemodialysis (Cameron *et al.* 2000; Shu-Fen & Chuan Li 2004). As PD and the slow continuous filtration methods of renal replacement therapy are used outside specialist centres, they will be described in greater detail.

Peritoneal dialysis

Indications

Patients and their clinicians may select peritoneal dialysis (PD) for the following reasons:

- Widespread availability.
- Technical simplicity.
- The greater stability of biochemical parameters.

The use of continuous ambulatory peritoneal dialysis (CAPD) devices means that the patient can remain ambulant, at home and achieve greater independence (Oreopoulos 1998).

Because the patient can use PD every day or every night, they have greater freedom with diet and fluid intake and often feel better (CANUSA 1996).

However a meta-analysis conducted by Selgas *et al.* (2001) on survival, morbidity, hospitalization and quality of life between patients receiving haemodialysis and CAPD was not able to demonstrate significant differences. Local circumstances and the patient's individual clinical needs should therefore be addressed in deciding which therapy to choose.

Reference material

In 1926 Rosenak, basing his work on that of Ganter, saw the possibility of using the peritoneum of humans as a dialysing membrane (Blumenkrantz & Roberts 1979). Gunther is described as the first to introduce 2 litres of fluid into the peritoneal cavity of a patient with acute renal failure (Oreopoulos 1998). The use of PD steadily increased and in 1959 came the introduction of commercial dialysis solutions and tubing. The 1960s saw advances made in the catheters designed by Tenckhoff, thus ensuring the long-term access needs of patients on PD. The technique of CAPD is attributed to Popovich *et al.* (1978). In the middle to late 1980s the Italian group described the use of the Y set for PD, a technique that, whilst modified, is still widely used today (Buoncristiani 1989; Daly *et al.* 2001). In the 1990s the first papers

736

were published highlighting that malnutrition was a significant problem for over 40% of patients on CAPD (Jones 1994; CANUSA 1996). This has since improved with multi-disciplinary input and nutrition guidelines (Thomas 2006).

In the late 1980s the technique of haemodialysis had been introduced and towards the late 1990s the first papers comparing outcomes from the two techniques were published (Bloembergen *et al.* 1995; Fenton *et al.* 1997; Selgas *et al.* 2001). Clinical practice guidelines under the auspices of the National Kidney Foundation of the United States were then introduced which covered areas such as haemodialysis, PD, vascular access, anaemia and nutrition (KDOQI 2000). In the UK, guidelines for the identification, management and referral of chronic kidney disease in adults has also been developed by the Royal College of Physicians of London and the Renal Association Joint Speciality Committee (2006).

Anatomy and physiology

The peritoneum in the abdominopelvic cavity is the most extensive of the body's serous membranes. In adults it has a surface area of approximately 2.2 m^2 (Marieb 2004). The peritoneum consists of two layers:

- The visceral peritoneum that covers the surface of most of the organs within the abdominal and pelvic cavities.
- The parietal peritoneum that lines the abdominal wall.

Although the peritoneum has these two layers, they are continuous with each other and surround the peritoneal cavity. The peritoneal cavity is a narrow potential space containing fluid secreted by the serous membranes. This serous fluid is used to lubricate the mobile digestive organs, allowing them to glide easily across one another and along the body wall as they perform their digestive functions. The visceral peritoneum is formed of areolar connective tissue covered with

mesothelium, which is a single layer of squamous epithelial cells (Marieb 2004; Waugh & Grant 2006).

The process of osmosis and diffusion and solution concentrations

Osmosis is the process by which a solvent such as water diffuses through a selectively permeable membrane. Osmosis will occur whenever the water concentration is different on either side of the membrane. When the concentration on either side of the membrane is equal, osmosis will cease (Marieb 2004).

Diffusion refers to the tendency of molecules or solutes to scatter evenly throughout their environment. All molecules possess kinetic energy and are in constant motion. Molecules generally move away from areas where they are in higher concentrations to areas where their concentration is lower. Therefore molecules diffuse along their concentration gradient (Marieb 2004).

Finally filtration is the process by which water and solutes are forced through a membrane by fluid or hydrostatic pressure (Marieb 2004) (Figure 37.1).

All types of renal replacement therapy rely on osmosis, diffusion and to some degree filtration.

The osmotic pressure of dextrose is utilized in PD to remove water and solutes from the patient. The composition of most commonly available and prescribed PD solutions are three strengths of glucose (Thomas 2006):

a. 1.36%;
b. 2.27%;
c. 3.86%.

However, the long-term disadvantages of utilizing glucose based fluids, such as hyperglycaemia, are now becoming more evident (Thomas 2004). The ideal PD solution is one that does not affect the structure and function of the

737

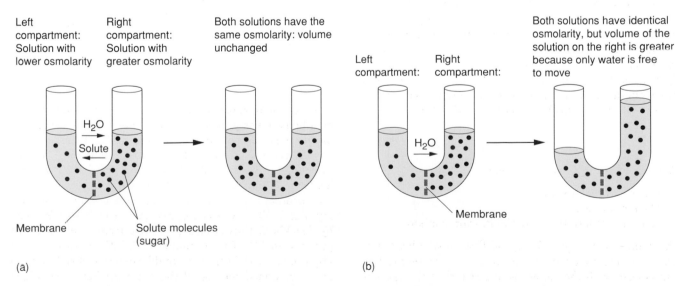

| Left compartment: Solution with lower osmolarity | Right compartment: Solution with greater osmolarity | Both solutions have the same osmolarity: volume unchanged |

H$_2$O
Solute

Membrane

Solute molecules (sugar)

(a)

| Left compartment: | Right compartment: | Both solutions have identical osmolarity, but volume of the solution on the right is greater because only water is free to move |

H$_2$O

Membrane

(b)

Figure 37.1 Influence of membrane permeability on diffusion and osmosis. (a) Membrane permeable to both solute molecules and water. (b) Membrane impermeable to solute molecules, permeable to water. (Redrawn from Marieb 2004, with permission.)

peritoneum. Research into new solutions has focused on two areas: an improved more biocompatible osmotic agent, and a better pH and buffer (Mahon 2002). Other solutions available include bicarbonate/lactate-based solutions, glucose-polymer-based solutions and amino-acid-based solutions. It is thought that a combination of all available solutions is of benefit to patients (Thomas 2006). Double and triple chamber solution bags have been developed with the top chamber containing a solution of dextrose, calcium chloride and magnesium chloride. The bottom chamber contains a solution of sodium bicarbonate, sodium lactate and sodium chloride (Levy *et al.* 2005). When the seal between the two chambers is broken the contents are mixed together and can be infused into the patient. Decisions concerning which solutions to use will depend on the clinical needs of the patient and whether they are sensitive to lactate-buffered solutions (Carrasco *et al.* 2001; Mahon 2002).

Dialysis cycle

Normally, a cycle consists of three steps (Levy *et al.* 2005; Saunorus Baird *et al.* 2005; Thomas 2006) (Figure 37.2) as follows.

Step 1 (inflow)

The dialysis solution at body temperature is infused into the peritoneal cavity to initiate the dialysis. The fluid infuses by gravity and its rate can be controlled by raising or lowering the container in relation to the patient's abdomen or by releasing or compressing the occluding clamp on the tubing.

Step 2 (dwell time)

The dwell time is the time that the fluid remains in the peritoneal cavity to allow for equilibration. Different dwell times may be established to remove substances of differing molecular weights. The dwell time is relevant to the molecular weight of the solute and how much needs to be removed.

Step 3 (drainage)

The drainage stage is that of emptying the equilibrated solution from the peritoneal cavity to complete dialysis or to prepare for the infusion of fresh solution. Drainage is also dependent on gravity.

Procedure

Step 1 Open clamp A and B to commence infusion of dialysate. Close clamps when required volume through

Step 2 Open clamp C when dialysate is infusing– or when draining– and it will remain closed during the 'dwell' period

Step 3 Clamp D is only opened during the drainage period

Figure 37.2   Using the Y-type administration set for peritoneal dialysis.

Technique

In PD the patient's own peritoneum is used as the dialysing membrane. A cuffed long-dwelling dialysis catheter is introduced into the lower abdomen through the rectus muscle and is secured with three purse-string sutures (Stegmayr 2002). It is important that the catheter produces balance among deep pelvic position, has an exit site that is manageable for the patient and causes the least amount of tubing stress through the abdominal wall (Crabtree *et al.* 2005). A Y set is then connected to the dialysis catheter and iso-osmotic fluid is introduced into the peritoneal cavity. The fluid is left to equilibrate for 15–60 minutes in acute therapy and several hours in chronic treatments; this is known as the 'dwell time' (Saunorus Baird *et al.* 2005). The fluid is then allowed to drain out through the same dialysis catheter and the procedure is repeated. The cycles then may be repeated until the patient's blood biochemistry has returned to agreed parameters (Levy *et al.* 2005). For PD to achieve maximum efficacy, fresh solutions must be instilled at equilibration to prevent reabsorption of water and uraemic toxins (Marieb 2004).

Continuous renal replacement therapy

Reference material

The use of continuous renal replacement therapy (CRRT) was first reported by Kramer *et al.* (1977). The use of CRRT has increased markedly since the late 1980s with advances in technology that have ensured safe user-friendly devices. In many critical care units CRRT can now be provided by critical care or appropriately trained nurses. The main advantage of CRRT for the acutely ill patient is its ability to provide excellent clearance of solutes and water whilst avoiding the haemodynamic instability that can result from haemodialysis, although more research is needed in this area (Kellum *et al.* 2002). CRRT provides a more precise control over fluid and metabolic abnormalities compared to intermittent haemodialysis (IHD) in the critically ill (Sasaki *et al.* 2001). CRRT can also be instituted in a patient who has a lowered mean arterial pressure, a condition which is common in critical care.

Continuous arteriovenous haemofiltration (CAVH) and continuous venovenous haemodiafiltration (CVVHDF) are used more than the filtration methods, with CVVHDF being the most common as it has the advantage that only one vessel needs to be cannulated (Thomas 2006). As CVVHDF is the therapy with the widest application to a variety of clinical situations, it is examined in greater detail here.

Vascular access

Temporary vascular access should be utilized if the period of CRRT is less than 3 weeks. The device may be tunneled or non-tunneled. The preferred access site is the right internal jugular vein, as it has been shown to have low rate of complications, and longer patency (Iovino *et al.* 2001; Maya & Allon 2005). If this is not possible the subclavian or femoral veins may be used. Femoral access should only be used when the patient is immobile as movement will occlude the vascular access device. This route is also utilized if lying the patient flat is contraindicated during internal jugular catheter placement (Levy *et al.* 2005). Ultrasound guidance (two dimensional) is recommended as the preferred method for the elective insertion of all central venous catheters (NICE 2002).

Continuous venovenous haemodiafiltration (CVVHDF)

CVVHDF is beneficial for critically ill patients with ARF (Sasaki *et al.* 2001). CVVHDF combines convection and diffusion. The convection of ultrafiltration utilizes a large hydrostatic pressure gradient which means that 1–2 litres of fluid an hour can be removed from the patient via the filter. Removal of the solutes (i.e. urea, creatinine and potassium) is achieved by blood flow through the filter, while dialysate is administered in a countercurrent flow (Murray & Hall 2000) (Figure 37.3).

Figure 37.3 Fluid pathway for continuous venovenous haemodiafiltration (CVVHDF). Redrawn with permission from HOSPAL (2000).

Manufacturers of CRRT devices supply biocompatible filters with different clearance specificities. Generally the filters clear molecules with small and medium size molecular weights but there are high-flux filters being tested which may be useful in the treatment of severe sepsis (Cole *et al.* 2001).

Because the patient's blood flows through an extracorporeal circuit and over a filter, there is a danger of blood clotting in the circuit. Unless the patient is auto-anticoagulated,

an anticoagulant should be administered continuously (Levy *et al.* 2005).

Note: because the filters used in CVVHDF filter out some drugs it is essential to calculate concomitant drug therapy utilizing the literature available (Tsubo *et al.* 2001). Some drugs are effectively cleared by the filter while others are only partially cleared (Pittrow & Penk 1998; Bunn & Ashley 1999).

Procedure guidelines   Peritoneal dialysis

Equipment

1 Dialysis Y-type administration set and drainage bag.
2 Sterile paracentesis abdominus set containing forceps, scalpel, topical swabs, towels, suturing equipment.
3 Sterile gown, gloves.
4 Peritoneal catheter stylet or trocar and drainage bag.
5 Local anaesthetic (1–2% lidocaine).
6 Syringe, needle.
7 Chlorhexidine in 70% alcohol.
8 Supplementary drugs as prescribed.
9 Peritoneal dialysis fluid, as prescribed, warmed to 36°C.

Procedure

Action	Rationale
1 Wash hands with antibacterial detergent and running hand hot water. Ensure hands are dried with disposable paper hand towels.	To reduce the risk of contamination and cross infection (DH 2005: C; RCN 2005: C).
2 Explain and discuss the procedure with the patient. An acutely ill patient may be confused and restless, but every effort should be made to ensure the patient is informed.	To ensure that the patient understands the procedure and gives his/her valid consent. Some hospitals require a patient to sign a consent form before the procedure can be carried out (NMC 2006: C; NMC 2008: C).
3 Ask the patient to micturate and defecate before the procedure begins.	To avoid perforation of the bladder and/or rectum when the trocar is introduced into the peritoneum (Levy *et al.* 2005: E).
4 Record the patient's vital signs before the procedure begins.	To assess physical/psychological state and to monitor changes (Zabat 2003: E).
5 Weigh the patient before the procedure begins and then daily.	To assess hydration and to monitor any fluid losses (Zabat 2003: E).
6 Assist the patient to lie flat with one pillow.	To ensure that the patient is in the safest position for the insertion of the trocar (Levy *et al.* 2005: E).
7 Continue to observe and reassure the patient throughout the procedure.	To assess and monitor any physical/psychological changes (Zabat 2003: E).
8 Assist the doctor as required.	To facilitate a smooth and effective procedure for the patient (E).

Insertion of peritoneal dialysis catheter

Action	Rationale
1 Using aseptic technique, the abdomen is prepared and local anaesthetic injected subcutaneously.	To reduce the risk of contamination and infection (DH 2005: C; RCN 2005: C). To minimize the pain of the incision (Levy *et al.* 2005: E).

2 A small incision is made in the abdominal wall 2–3 cm below the umbilicus. A 16–18-gauge trocar is inserted through the incision. The patient is asked to raise their head from the pillow after the trocar is introduced.

This tightens the abdominal muscles and permits easier penetration of the trocar without danger of injury to the internal organs (Levy *et al*. 2005: E).

3 When the peritoneum is punctured, the trocar is directed to the left side of the pelvis. The stylet is removed and the catheter is inserted through the trocar and gently manoeuvred into position.

To prevent the omentum from adhering to the catheter or occluding its opening (Levy *et al*. 2005: E).

4 The exit site is normally 3 cm from where the distal cuff will be in the subcutaneous tunnel.

To prevent the loss of the catheter in the abdomen (Levy *et al*. 2005: E).

5 A small incision is made for the exit site. A tunneling device is attached to the catheter to create a tunnel and expose the catheter.

To prevent fluid leakage and the need for sutures (Levy *et al*. 2005: E).

6 The original incision site will be sutured, but other sutures are not required.

To prevent early exit site infection (Levy *et al*. 2005: E).

7 The tubing is flushed with the dialysis fluid.

To prevent air from entering the peritoneal cavity (Zabat 2003: E).

Preparation of peritoneal dialysis fluid

Action

1 Wash hands with antiseptic detergent and running hand hot water. Ensure hands are dried with disposable paper.

Rationale

To reduce the risk of infection (DH 2005: C; RCN 2005: C).

2 Apply gloves, apron and eye shield. Proceed using aseptic technique.

To reduce the risk of infection (DH 2005: C; RCN 2005: C).

3 The dialysis fluid should have been warmed to body temperature (36°C).

For the patient's comfort. To prevent abdominal pain. Heating causes dilatation of the peritoneal vessels and increases clearance of urea. Cold fluid would decrease rate of removal of large molecular solutes and can cause abdominal cramp pain (Adam & Osborne 2005: E).

4 Add any drugs, e.g. heparin or potassium, to the dialysis fluid if prescribed.

Heparin prevents fibrin clots from occluding the catheter, potassium to regulate body potassium (Adam & Osborne 2005: E).

5 Attach the dialysis fluid to the administration set via Luer–Lok connections.

To prevent disconnection (E).

6 Attach the administration set to the catheter connection.

To prevent disconnection.

7 Allow the dialysis fluid to flow freely into the peritoneal cavity. (This normally takes from 5 to 10 minutes.)

To ascertain whether the catheter is in the required position. The flow should be steady and brisk. If not, the tip of the catheter may be buried in the omentum or it may have been occluded by a blood clot (Hudak *et al*. 1998: E).

8 Allow fluid to remain in the peritoneal cavity for the prescribed time. Prepare the next exchange while the first container of fluid is in the peritoneal cavity.

The fluid must remain in the peritoneal cavity for the prescribed dwell time so that potassium, urea and other waste products may be removed. The solution is most effective over the first 5–10 minutes when the concentration gradient is at its greatest (De Fijter *et al*. 1994: E).

741

Procedure guidelines (*cont.*)

9	Unclamp the peritoneal drainage tube. Drainage time will vary with each patient but, on average, should be completed in 10 minutes.	To rid the body of the required products. The abdomen is drained by a siphon effect through the closed system (Hudak *et al.* 1998: E).
10	Clamp off the drainage tube when outflow ceases and begin infusing the next exchange, again using aseptic technique.	To enable the next cycle to begin. To reduce the risk of local and/or systemic infection (DH 2005: C; RCN 2005: C).
11	Record the following: (a) Time of commencement and completion of each exchange and the start and finish of the drainage stage. (b) Amount of fluid infused and recovered. (c) Fluid balance after each complete exchange. (d) Any medication added to the dialysis fluid.	To detect and monitor trends and fluctuations and to identify any outflow obstruction (Zabat 2003: E).
12	Take and record the vital signs: (a) Blood pressure and pulse every 15 minutes during the first exchange and hourly thereafter, depending on the patient's condition. (b) Temperature every 4 hours, or more frequently if condition demands.	Hypotension may be indicative of excessive fluid loss due to the glucose concentration of the dialysis fluid. Changes in pulse may indicate impending shock or overhydration (Swearingen & Hicks Keen 2001: E). To monitor for any signs of infection. Infection is more likely to become evident after dialysis has been discontinued (Hudak *et al.* 1998: E).
13	Record fluid balance accurately.	To prevent complications such as circulatory overload and hypertension that may occur if most of the fluid is not recovered during the drainage stage. The fluid balance should be even or slightly negative unless the reason for treatment was to remove excess fluid (Hudak *et al.* 1998: E).
14	Dialysis is usually continued until blood chemistry levels are satisfactory.	The duration of dialysis is related to the severity of the condition and the size and weight of the patient. The usual time is about 12–36 hours, giving between 24 and 28 exchanges (Hudak *et al.* 1998: E).
15	Ensure that the patient is comfortable during dialysis by attending to pressure area care and altering the patient's position as required. Assist the patient to sit in a chair for short periods as their condition allows.	The period of dialysis is lengthy and often exhausts the patient (Hudak *et al.* 1998: E).
16	Send a specimen of drained peritoneal fluid for microscopy and culture if peritonitis is suspected.	To monitor for any infections (Levy *et al.* 2005: E).

Problem solving: Peritoneal dialysis

Problem	Cause	Suggested action
Peritonitis, indicated by fever, persistent abdominal pain and cramping, abdominal fullness, abdominal rigidity, slow dialysis drainage, cloudy and offensive-smelling drainage, swelling and tenderness around the catheter and increased white blood cell count.	Poor aseptic technique during catheter insertion or dialysis, or poor nutritional/immune state.	If peritonitis is suspected, notify the doctor immediately. Send a peritoneal fluid sample to the laboratory for fluid analysis, culture and sensitivity testing, Gram staining and cell count. Antibiotics may be prescribed by the doctor either locally or systemically in severe cases. Monitor vital signs; optimal pain control is required.

Problem	Cause	Suggested action
Infection at the site of entry, indicated by redness, swelling, rigidity, tenderness and purulent drainage around the catheter.	Poor aseptic technique during catheter insertion or dialysis, or incomplete healing around the site of entry.	Discuss with medical team. Obtain a specimen of the drainage fluid and send it to the laboratory. Antibiotics and pain control may be prescribed as above. Monitor vital signs.
Subcutaneous tunnel infection with cuffed catheter indicated by redness, rigidity and tenderness over subcutaneous tunnel.	Poor aseptic technique during catheter insertion or dialysis, or incomplete healing in subcutaneous tunnel.	Notify a doctor. Antibiotics may be prescribed as above. Monitor vital signs.
Perforation of the bladder or the bowel, indicated by signs and symptoms of peritonitis, bright yellow dialysis fluid drainage (if bladder is perforated) or faeces in drainage (if bowel is perforated).	Catheter inserted when the patient had a full bladder or bowel.	If perforation is suspected, stop dialysis and notify a doctor immediately. Monitor vital signs. Only minimal oral fluids should be given in case surgery is required.
Bleeding through the catheter.	Minor trauma to the abdomen or minor trauma to the subcutaneous tunnel (with a cuffed catheter) or perforation of a major abdominal blood vessel during surgery.	Bleeding usually stops spontaneously. If it does not, notify the doctor, who may order a full blood count and/or blood transfusion. One-litre hourly dialysis exchanges may be ordered until the drainage fluid is clear.
Dialysis fluid leaking around the catheter.	Excessive instillation of dialysis fluid. Incomplete healing around the cuff of the catheter. Catheter obstruction. Catheter dislodged or positioned improperly.	Instil less dialysis fluid at exchanges. Drain the patient's abdomen completely during outflow. Use small volumes of dialysis fluid in exchanges through a new catheter. Irrigate the catheter with sterile 0.9% sodium chloride solution. Inform a doctor, who will replace the catheter or revise its position surgically.
Kinking of the cuffed catheter.	Subcutaneous tunnel too short or scarring in the subcutaneous tunnel.	Discuss with medical team, who will remove the catheter and implant a new one.
Lower back pain.	Pressure and weight of dialysis fluid in the abdomen (particularly so in CAPD patients).	Doctor may order analgesics. Exercises to strengthen the patient's muscles and improve posture may also be ordered.
Abdominal or rectal pain (with possible referred pain in shoulder).	Improperly positioned catheter tip causing irritation.	Catheter position to be revised surgically.
	Dialysis fluid accumulating under the diaphragm.	Drain the abdomen completely during outflow.
	Dialysis fluid not at 36°C. With 2 litres of 6.36% solution, severe shoulder pain can occur.	Ensure that the fluid is infused at the correct temperature. If hypertonic dialysis fluid is used, only one container should be used per cycle.
	If air enters the peritoneal cavity, pain may occur.	Maintain a closed system.
Paralytic ileus indicated by sharp pain in abdomen, constipation, abdominal distension, nausea and vomiting, and diarrhoea.	Catheter manipulated excessively during insertion.	Notify the doctor immediately as signs and symptoms may indicate peritonitis. Administer fluids, electrolytes and pain management as prescribed. If general condition allows, encourage patient to walk, unless advised otherwise by the doctor. Prepare the patient for surgery, as advised by the doctor. The condition may disappear spontaneously after 12 hours.

743

Problem solving (cont.)

Problem	Cause	Suggested action
Cramping.	Dialysis fluid warmer or cooler than 36°C.	Adjust the temperature of the dialysis fluid to 36°C before infusion.
	Too rapid infusion or drainage.	Decrease the infusion or drainage rate to a speed the patient can tolerate.
	Pressure from excess dialysis fluid in the abdomen.	Infuse less dialysis fluid at exchanges to a total volume that the patient can tolerate.
	Chemical irritation.	Use a dialysis fluid with a dextrose concentration lower than 7%.
	Air in the abdomen.	Clamp off the dialysis tubing before the dialysis fluid empties completely into the abdomen.
Excessive fluid loss.	Use of dialysis fluid with too great a dextrose concentration for the patient or inadequate sodium intake or inadequate fluid intake.	Monitor the patient's weight and blood pressure. Ensure that the patient is receiving dialysis fluid with the correct dextrose concentration. The doctor may prescribe a reduced dextrose concentration.
Fluid overload.	Use of dialysis fluid with an osmotic pressure that is too low for the patient or excessive sodium intake or excessive fluid intake.	Monitor the patient's weight and blood pressure. The doctor will order a reduced fluid and sodium intake. The doctor may also order increased use of dialysis fluid with a 4.25% dextrose concentration.
Metabolic disturbance usually affects plasma levels of glucose, potassium or sodium.	Continued use of inappropriate dialysate fluid.	Monitor relevant plasma levels pre- and post-dialysis. If patient has pre-existing diabetes mellitus or insulin deficiency, insulin dosage should be titrated carefully.
Respiratory difficulties.	Pressure from the fluid in the peritoneal cavity and upward displacement of the diaphragm or 'splinting' of the diaphragm, resulting in shallow breathing.	Elevate the head of the bed. Encourage breathing exercises and coughing, in discussion with medical and multidisciplinary teams.

744

Procedure guidelines CVVHDF: utilizing a CVVHDF device

Note: when using the CVVHDF method of filtration, venous access is obtained by the insertion of a double- or preferably a triple-lumen catheter. This will be inserted into a central vein, usually the internal jugular, subclavian or femoral vein. The catheter will then be flushed with a heparinized solution and capped off ready to commence CVVHDF.

Preparation of equipment for CVVHDF

Equipment

1 Volumetric infusion pump × 1.
2 CVVHDF machine.
3 Set of dialysate tubing and filter.
4 10 ml Luer–Lok syringe × 2.
5 Plastic clamps × 3.
6 Non-sterile gloves.
7 Chlorhexidine 0.5% in 70% alcohol.
8 Low-linting gauze swabs.
9 Disposable apron.
10 Eye protective shield.

Procedure

Action	Rationale
1 Discuss patient's condition with the multidisciplinary team and establish treatment plan.	To ensure all medical and nursing teams are aware of patient's biochemistry and haematological profiles and the plan for treatment (Levy *et al.* 2005: E).

2 Collect all equipment together as above.

To ensure that all the equipment is available before commencing the procedure (Levy *et al*. 2005: E).

3 Instill 5000 units heparin (or as per manufacturer's instructions) into 1 litre of 0.9% sodium chloride.

To anticoagulate the tubing and the filter to provide prophylaxis against clotting in the extracorporeal circuit (HOSPAL 2000: C).

4 Load the CVVHDF device following the automated instructions on the electronic screen of the device.

To form the CVVHDF circuit (HOSPAL 2000: C).

5 When the circuit has been primed, ensure that the patient is ready for connection to the CVVHDF device.

The first 15–30 minutes can cause a period of haemodynamic instability and it is therefore important to ensure that the patient is comfortable (i.e. does not want to use the commode) and ready to commence therapy (Palevsky *et al*. 2005: R 5).

6 If the patient is not connected to the set shortly after priming, flush the set with at least 500 ml priming solution (step 3) before connecting to the patient. A new priming solution and empty collection bag will be required.

To ensure anticoagulation of the tubing and the filter to provide prophylaxis against clotting in the extracorporeal circuit (HOSPAL 2000: C).

Commencement of CVVHDF

Procedure

Action	Rationale
1 Explain and discuss the procedure with the patient and his/her family.	To ensure that the patient understands the procedure and gives his/her valid consent (NMC 2006: C; NMC 2008: C & P).
2 Ensure that all information concerning the patient's blood biochemistry, full blood count and clotting profile is available.	To have a baseline from which to work and to monitor any change in the patient (Levy *et al*. 2005: E).
3 Ensure that the patient's mean arterial pressure is above 60 mmHg or that the physician's guidelines have been agreed.	Upon commencement of CVVHDF there is usually a large fluid drainage, which can result in a sudden drop in blood pressure especially in the critically ill (Palevsky *et al*. 2005: R 5).
4 Ensure that baseline recordings of weight, temperature, heart rate, blood pressure, respiratory rate, tissue oxygen saturation (SaO_2) and central venous pressure (CVP) have been recorded.	To have a baseline from which to work and to monitor any change in the patient (Levy *et al*. 2005: E).
5 Ensure that the patient is attached to a haemodynamic monitor.	CVVHDF can cause cardiac instability, although this is rare (Toft *et al*. 2000: R 5).
6 Ensure that a treatment programme has been agreed with the multidisciplinary team and review regularly.	To ensure that the plan for cycling and the total fluid removal has been discussed and that it is altered according to patient status (Levy *et al*. 2005 : E).
7 Prepare the appropriate fluid replacement.	There is a rapid fluid loss with CVVHDF and patients often require replacement of this loss (Levy *et al*. 2005: E).
8 Wash hands with antiseptic detergent and running hand-hot water. Ensure hands are dried with disposable paper.	To reduce the risk of infection and provide universal protection for the nurse (RCN 2005: C).

Procedure guidelines (*cont.*)

9 Prepare a sterile field and apply gloves, apron and eye shield.	To reduce the risk of infection and provide universal protection for the nurse (RCN 2005: C).
10 While keeping the patient's catheter clamped, remove the injection caps from both lumens and clean the lumens with chlorhexidine 0.5% in 70% alcohol.	To prevent haemorrhage and to reduce the risk of infection (DH 2005: C).
11 Flush each lumen with heparinized saline.	To ensure that the patient's catheter is patent.
12 Apply plastic clamps to the patient ends of the red and blue tubing and separate from each other. Clean the ends of the tubing with chlorhexidine 0.5% in 70% alcohol.	To prevent air entering the tubing (HOSPAL 2000: C) and to reduce the risk of infection (DH 2005: C).
13 Connect red tubing to the red lumen and blue tubing to the blue lumen of the catheter.	To complete patient circuit (HOSPAL 2000: C).
14 Undo catheter clamps and plastic clamp on tubing.	To ensure free flow (HOSPAL 2000: C).
15 Ensure that there are no clamps left closed and that all connections are secure.	To ensure that there is no obstruction to flow and no risk of fluid leakage (HOSPAL 2000: C).
16 Turn on machine and start blood pump at 75–100 ml/hour.	To commence CVVHDF at a gentle speed.
17 Observe the patient and monitor the dialysis circuit carefully.	To ensure that any alteration in patient condition is noted immediately (HOSPAL 2000: C).
18 If the vital signs are stable, increase speed to appropriate level, between 100 and 150 ml/hour.	To ensure good filtration (Levy *et al.* 2005: E).
19 Commence dialysate fluid infusion at appropriate rate, usually between 1 and 2 litres/hour.	To provide the counter-current and achieve movement of solutes (HOSPAL 2000: C).
20 Continue monitoring patient with continuous electrocardiogram (ECG), heart rate, rhythm, blood pressure, CVP, SaO_2 and respiratory rate hourly or more frequently if required.	To ensure any change in patient condition is noted immediately and dealt with as appropriate (Levy *et al.* 2005: E).
21 Maintain accurate fluid balance.	To ensure patient is protected from large positive or negative fluid shifts (Levy *et al.* 2005: E).
22 Send regular blood samples for biochemical analysis.	To adjust dialysate fluid and electrolyte replacement therapy as appropriate (Levy *et al.* 2005: E).
23 Send regular blood samples for clotting profile.	To provide appropriate anticoagulant therapy (Levy *et al.* 2005: E).
24 Ensure patient tubing and circuit are easily visible and free from obstruction.	To protect patient from sudden disconnection or obstruction to tubing (HOSPAL 2000: C).
25 Review patient's condition regularly with multidisciplinary team.	To ensure optimum patient monitoring and evaluation of care to enable appropriate treatment (Levy *et al.* 2005: E).
26 Ensure optimum recording in documentation of venous pressure, pump speeds and drainage.	To ensure information exchange between members of the nursing team (Levy *et al.* 2005: E; NMC 2008: C).

References and further reading

Adam, S.K. & Osborne, S. (2005) *Critical Care Nursing: Science and Practice*, 2nd edn. Oxford University Press, Oxford.

Block, C.A. & Manning, H.L. (2002) Prevention of acute renal failure in the critically ill. *Am J Respir Crit Care Med*, 165(3), 320–4.

Bloembergen, W.E. *et al.* (1995) A comparison of mortality between patients treated with hemodialysis and peritoneal dialysis. *J Am Soc Nephrol*, 6(2), 177–83.

Blumenkrantz, M.J. & Roberts, M. (1979) Progress in peritoneal dialysis: an historical prospective. *Contrib Nephrol*, 17, 101–10.

Briggs, J.D. *et al.* (1997) Organ donation in the UK: a survey by a British Transplantation Society working party. *Nephrol Dial Transplant*, 12(11), 2251–7.

Bunn, R. & Ashley, C. (1999) *The Renal Drug Handbook*. Radcliffe Medical Press, Oxford.

Buoncristiani, U. (1989) The Y set with disinfectant is here to stay. *Peritoneal Dialysis Int*, 9(3), 149–50.

Cameron, J.I. *et al.* (2000) Differences in quality of life across renal replacement therapies: a meta-analytic comparison. *Am J Kidney Dis*, 35, 629–37.

CANUSA (1996) Adequacy of dialysis and nutrition in continuous peritoneal dialysis: association with clinical outcomes. *J Am Soc Nephrol*, 7(2), 198–207.

Carrasco, A.M. *et al.* (2001) Acidosis correction with a new 25 mmol/l bicarbonate/15 mmol/l lactate peritoneal dialysis solution. *Peritoneal Dialysis Int*, 21, 546–53.

Chitalia, V.C. *et al.* (2002) Is peritoneal dialysis adequate for hypercatabolic acute renal failure in developing countries? *Kidney Int*, 61(2), 747–57.

Cole, L. *et al.* (2001) High volume haemofiltration in human septic shock. *Intens Care Med*, 27, 978–86.

Crabtree, J.H., Burchette, R.J. & Siddiqi, N.A. (2005) Optimal peritoneal dialysis catheter type and exit site location: an anthropometric analysis. *ASAIO J*, 51, 743–7.

Daly, C. *et al.* (2001) Double bag or Y-set versus standard transfer system for continuous ambulatory peritoneal dialysis in end-stage renal disease: review. *Cochrane Database Systematic Review (2): CD003078*.

De Fijter, C.W. *et al.* (1994) Morbidity associated with continuous cyclic compared with continuous ambulatory peritoneal dialysis. *Ann Intern Med*, 120(4), 264–71.

DH (2005) *Saving Lives: a Delivery Programme to Reduce Healthcare Associated Infection Including MRSA: Skills for Implementation*. Department of Health, London.

Fenton, S.S. *et al.* (1997) Hemodialysis versus peritoneal dialysis: a comparison of adjusted mortality rates. *Am J Kidney Dis*, 30(3), 334–42.

HOSPAL (2000) *PRISMA System: an Integrated System for Continuous Fluid Management and Renal Replacement Therapies*. HOSPAL Renal Intensive Care, Switzerland.

Hudak, C.M., Gallo, B.M. & Gonce Morton, P. (1998) *Critical Care Nursing: a Holistic Approach*, 7th edn. Lippincott, New York.

Hyman, A. & Mendelssohn D.C. (2002) Current Canadian approaches to dialysis for acute renal failure in the ICU. *Am J Nephrol*, 22(1), 29–34.

Iovino, F. *et al.* (2001) Central venous catheterisation: complications of different placements. *Ann Chir*, 126(10), 1001–6.

Jones, M.R. (1994) Etiology of severe malnutrition: results of an international cross-sectional study in continuous ambulatory peritoneal dialysis. *Am J Kidney Dis*, 23(3), 412–20.

KDOQI (2000) The National Kidney Foundation – DOQI – clinical practice guidelines. www.kidney.org. Accessed 14/8/2006.

Kellum, J.A. *et al.* (2002) Continuous versus intermittent renal replacement therapy: meta-analysis. *Intens Care Med*, 28(1), 29–37.

Kramer, P. *et al.* (1977) Arteriovenous haemofiltration: a new and simple method for treatment of over-hydrated patients resistant to diuretics. *Klin Wochenschr*, 55(22), 1121–2.

Levy, J., Morgan, J. & Brown, E. (2005) *Oxford Handbook of Dialysis*, 2nd edn. Oxford University Press, Oxford, pp. 3–5.

Mahon, A. (2002) Advances in bicarbonate peritoneal dialysis solutions. www.nephronline.org/management/advances. Accessed 08/5/2002.

Marieb, E.N. (2004) The urinary system. In: *Human Anatomy and Physiology*, 6th edn. Benjamin Cummings, New York, pp. 996–1032.

Maya, I.D. & Allon, M. (2005) Outcomes of tunneled femoral hemodialysis catheters: comparison with internal jugular vein catheters. *Kidney Int*, 68(6), 2886–9.

Murray, P. & Hall, J. (2000) Renal replacement therapy for acute renal failure. *Am J Respir Crit Care Med*, 162, 777–81.

NICE (2002) Final appraisal determination: ultrasound locating devices for placing central catheters. www.nice.org.uk. Accessed 14/8/2006.

NMC (2006) *A–Z Advice Sheet Consent*. www.nmc.org.

NMC (2008) *The Code: Standards of Conduct, Performance and Ethics for Nurses and Midwives*. Nursing and Midwifery Council, London.

Oreopoulos, D.G. (1998) Shaping the future of peritoneal dialysis. Satellite Symposium, 18th International CAPD Meeting, Nashville, pp. 1–10.

Palevsky, P.M. *et al.* (2005) Renal replacement therapy and the kidney: minimizing the impact of renal replacement therapy on recovery of acute renal failure. *Curr Opin Crit Care*, 11, 548–54.

Pittrow, L. & Penk, A. (1998) Pharmacokinetics and dosage of fluconazole in continuous haemofiltration and haemodialysis. *Mycoses*, 41(Suppl 2), 86–8.

Popovich, R.P. *et al.* (1978) Continuous ambulatory peritoneal dialysis. *Ann Intern Med*, 88(4), 449–56.

Quan, A. & Quigley, R. (2005) Renal replacement therapy and acute renal failure. *Curr Opin Pediatr*, 17, 205–9.

RCN (2005) *Good Practice in Infection Control: Guidance for Nursing Staff*. Royal College of Nursing, London.

Royal College of Physicians of London and the Renal Association Joint Speciality Committee (2006) *Chronic Kidney Disease in Adults: UK Guidelines for Identification, Management and Referral*. Royal College of Physicians of London, London.

Sasaki, S. *et al.* (2001) Predictors of mortality in patients treated with continuous hemodiafiltration for acute renal failure in an intensive care setting. *American Society of Artificial Internal Organs*, 47(1), 86–91.

Saunorus Baird, M., Hicks Keen, J. & Swearingen, P.L. (2005) *Manual of Critical Care Nursing: Nursing Interactions and Collaborative Management*, 5th edn. Elsevier Mosby, St Louis, MI.

Selgas, R. *et al.* (2001) Comparisons of hemodialysis and CAPD in patients over 65 years of age: a meta-analysis. *Int Urol Nephrol*, 33(2), 259–64.

Shu-Fen, N. & Chuan Li, I. (2004) Quality of life of patients having renal replacement therapy. *J Adv Nurs*, 51(1), 15–21.

Stegmayr, B. (2002) Various clinical approaches to minimise complications in peritoneal dialysis. *Int J Artif Organs*, 25(5), 365–72.

Swearingen, P.L. & Hicks Keen, J. (2001) *Manual of Critical Care Nursing: Nursing Interventions and Collaborative Management*, 4th edn. Mosby, London.

747

Thomas, N. (ed.) (2004) *Advanced Renal Care*. Blackwell Publishing, Oxford.

Thomas, N. (ed.) (2006) Renal nutrition. In: *Renal Nursing*, 2nd edn. Bailliere Tindall, London, pp. 267–310.

Toft, P. *et al.* (1999) The immunological effects of continuous venovenous haemodiafiltration in critically ill patients. *Crit Care*, 3, 159–65.

Toft, P., Felding, M. & Tonnesen, E.K. (2000) Continuous venovenous hemodiafiltration in critically ill patients with acute renal failure. *Ugeskr Laeger*, **162**(20), 2868–71.

Tsubo, T. *et al.* (2001) Ketamine and midazolam kinetics during continuous hemodiafiltration in patients with multiple organ dysfunction syndrome. *Intensive Care Med*, **27**(6), 1087–90.

Waugh, A. & Grant, A. (2006) The urinary system. In: *Ross and Wilson Anatomy and Physiology in Health and Illness*, 10th edn. Churchill Livingstone Elsevier, Edinburgh, pp. 335–54.

Zabat, E. (2003) When your patient needs peritoneal dialysis. *Nursing*, **33**(8), 52–4.

Chapter 38

Respiratory therapy

Reference material **750**
Continuous positive airway pressure **756**
Reference material **756**
Hazards of oxygen therapy **758**
Procedure guidelines: Pre-continuous positive airway pressure (pre-CPAP) **760**
Procedure guidelines: Continuous positive airway pressure (CPAP): setting up **761**
Procedure guidelines: Humidification for respiratory therapy **761**
Problem solving: Oxygen therapy by nasal cannulae or oxygen mask **762**
Problem solving: Continuous positive airway pressure (CPAP) **763**
References and further reading **765**

Definition

The principle of respiratory therapy is the application of pharmacological and non-pharmacological means to improve breathing and therefore improve gaseous exchange. This will include an assessment of the cause of the impaired breathing, reversal of causes where possible, and therapies to optimize respiratory function.

Indications

- Respiratory failure, of which there are two types, is characterized by problems with some or all of the four functions listed below:
  - *Type 1*, referred to as hypoxaemic respiratory failure (failure to oxygenate the tissues). The PaO_2 is <8 kPa (60 mmHg) while the carbon dioxide (PCO_2) is normal or low. Common causes include infectious conditions, pneumonia, pulmonary oedema and adult respiratory distress syndrome.
  - *Type 2*, referred to as hypercapnic (raised carbon dioxide) or respiratory pump failure. Alveolar ventilation is insufficient to excrete carbon dioxide accompanied by hypoxaemia (deficiency of oxygen in the arterial blood). The PCO_2 is >6 kPa (45 mmHg). Common causes include chronic obstructive pulmonary disease (COPD), chest wall deformities, drug overdose and chest injury.
- Acute myocardial infarction.
- Cardiac failure.
- Shock–haemorrhagic, bacteraemic and cardiogenic.
- Conditions in which there is a reduced ability to transport oxygen, e.g. anaemia.
- During anaesthesia.
- Postoperatively.
- Sleep apnoea.
- Severe pain.
- Asthma.
- Pulmonary embolus.
- Conditions that affect the neuromuscular control of breathing such as muscular dystrophy, Guillain Barré.
- Severe trauma affecting the diaphragm, ribs, lungs, or trachea.
- Tension pneumothorax.
- Pleural effusion.

Reference material

Physiology (see also Chapter 25)

The respiratory system is a complex system that is responsible for the efficient exchange of the respiratory gases primarily oxygen and carbon dioxide. The respiratory system is responsible for ensuring a continuous optimum supply of oxygen to the tissues and the elimination of carbon dioxide during expiration. Four separate functions are necessary to achieve optimal respiration (Marieb 2006):

1 Pulmonary ventilation: adequate breathing ensuring movement of air in and out of the lungs ensuring a fresh supply of oxygen to the alveoli;
2 External respiration: ensuring adequate gas exchange oxygen uptake and carbon dioxide unloading between the blood and the alveoli of the lungs.
3 Transport of respiratory gases: oxygen and carbon dioxide between the lungs and the body tissues. Transport is affected by the cardiovascular system and uses the blood as a carrying mechanism.
4 Cellular respiration: oxygen delivery and carbon dioxide uptake between the systemic blood and tissue cells.

The respiratory system is composed of the following structures:

- The two respiratory centres in the medulla oblongata and pons of the brain.
- The nose, mouth and connecting airways.
- The trachea, main bronchus, bronchioles and alveoli.
- The respiratory muscles: the diaphragm and the intercostal muscles.
- The respiratory nerves: the subphrenic nerve and the intercostal nerves.
- The bone structure of the thorax: the ribs, vertebrae and sternum.
- The lung parenchyma.
- The pleura.

Alteration, damage or blockage to any of the structures listed above may result in either respiratory impairment or respiratory failure. It is essential when considering respiratory function to remember the close association and dependence between the cardiovascular, neurological, musculoskeletal and respiratory system.

Tissue oxygenation

All the cells of the body require a continuous supply of oxygen to ensure growth and repair of tissues and optimum metabolism. Oxygen is drawn into the body through the nose and mouth; it then travels down the trachea and into the smaller airways and alveoli of the lungs. Once it has reached the alveoli oxygen in solution is able to transfer into the network of capillaries and from there travels via the venous network to all cells of the body. This tissue oxygenation is known as cellular oxygenation. Low oxygen levels are called hypoxia. In low oxygen conditions anaerobic cellular oxygenation will occur generating the waste product lactic acid. If the low oxygen state is allowed to continue lactic acid will accumulate leading to a metabolic acidosis and cell death (West 1995; Oh 1997; Berne & Levy 1998; Guyton 2000; Hess 2000; Pierson 2000; Kumar & Clark 2005; Marieb 2006; Tortora & Derrickson 2008).

There are three components to oxygenation: oxygen uptake, oxygen transportation and oxygen utilization. *Oxygen uptake* is the process of extracting oxygen from the environment. *Oxygen transportation* is the mechanism by which the uptake of oxygen results in the delivery of oxygen to the cells. *Oxygen utilization* is the metabolic need for molecular oxygen by the cells of the body.

In order for oxygenation to take place there needs to be an adequate cardiac output.

Oxygen uptake

The air that we breathe in during normal conditions from the atmosphere is composed of the following gases:

- oxygen 21%;
- carbon dioxide 0.03%;
- nitrogen 79%;
- rare gases 0.003%.

Inspired air at sea level has a total atmospheric pressure of 760 mmHg. According to Dalton's law, where there is a mixture of gases each gas exerts its own pressure as if there were no other gases present. The pressure of an individual gas in a mixture is called the partial pressure and is denoted as P, which is then followed by the type of gas so that the partial pressure of oxygen is written PO_2 (Tortora & Derrickson 2008):

- Oxygen $0.21 \times 760 = 159$ mmHg (21 kPa).
- Carbon dioxide $0.03 \times 760 = 22.8$ mmHg (3.0 kPa).
- Nitrogen $0.79 \times 760 = 600$ mmHg (80 kPa).

The partial pressure of gases controls the movement of oxygen and carbon dioxide through the body between the atmosphere and the lungs, the lungs and the blood and finally the blood and the cells. Movement of gases is by diffusion. Diffusion is the movement of gas molecules from an area of relatively high partial pressure to one of lower partial pressure.

Diffusion of oxygen takes place from the alveolus into the pulmonary capillaries and movement of carbon dioxide from the capillary into the alveolus. From the alveolus the oxygen diffuses from the capillaries into the tissues and mitochondria of the cells (Figure 38.1).

The alveolar oxygen partial pressure is higher than the arterial oxygen partial pressure in order to push the oxygen through the alveolar membrane into the interstitial spaces and from there into the pulmonary capillaries. Oxygen continues to diffuse from the capillaries into the tissues then to the mitochondria of the cells for metabolism (Carpenter

Table 38.1 Oxygen cascade. Pressure gradients for oxygen transfer from inspired gas to tissue cells.

	mmHg	kPa
Inspired air	150	20.0
Alveolar	103	13.7
Arterial	100	13.3
Capillary	51	6.8
Tissue	20	2.7
Mitochondrial	1–20	0.13–1.30

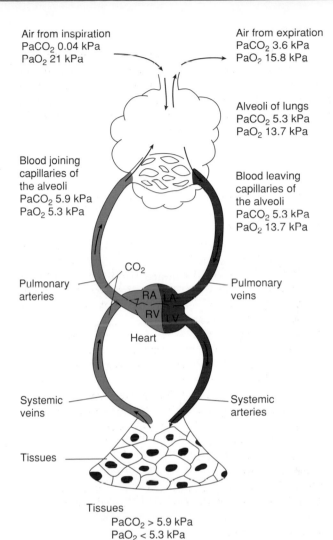

Figure 38.1 Gas movement in the body is facilitated by partial pressure differences. Top of figure illustrates pressure gradients that facilitate oxygen and carbon dioxide exchange in the lungs. Bottom of figure shows pressure gradients that facilitate gas movements from systemic capillaries to tissues.

1991; Pierce 1995; Oh 1997; Berne & Levy 1998; Esmond 2000; Guyton 2000; Marieb 2006; Tortora & Derrickson 2008).

As inspired air enters the respiratory tract it encounters water vapour present in the upper airways which warms and humidifies it. Water vapour exerts its own partial pressure of 47 mmHg. The partial pressure of the water vapour must be subtracted from the total atmospheric pressure to give a corrected atmospheric pressure and partial pressure of each gas:

- Corrected total atmospheric $760 - 47 = 713$ mmHg.
- Oxygen $0.21 \times 713 = 150$ mmHg (20 kPa).
- Carbon dioxide $0.03 \times 713 = 21$ mmHg (2.8 kPa).

As oxygen continues to pass down the respiratory tract to the alveolus it encounters carbon dioxide leaving the respiratory tract which also exerts a partial pressure, equal to 40 mmHg. This in turn must be subtracted to determine the correct values. Oxygen has a corrected value of 150 − 40 = 110 − 100 mmHg (14.6 − 13.3 kPa).

Oxygen transportation

Oxygen is carried in the blood in two ways:

- *Dissolved in the plasma (serum)*: only 2–3% is carried in this way as oxygen is not very soluble (Aherns & Tucker 1999; Marieb 2006). This is measured as the PaO_2. There is 0.003 ml of blood for each 1 mmHg partial pressure oxygen. At 100 mmHg partial pressure, only 0.3 ml of oxygen would be carried per 100 ml of plasma.
- *Bound to haemoglobin in the red blood cells*: 95–98% of oxygen is carried in this way and is measured as the percentage of oxygen saturated (SaO_2). Each gram of haemoglobin can carry 1.34 ml of oxygen per 100 ml blood.

Haemoglobin is composed of haem (iron) and globulin (protein). Each haemoglobin molecule has four binding sites each able to carry one molecule of oxygen. A haemoglobin molecule is said to be fully saturated with oxygen when all four haem sites are attached to oxygen. When fewer than four are attached the haemoglobin is said to be partially saturated.

The bond between haemoglobin and oxygen is affected by various physiological factors that shift the oxygen dissociation curve to the right or left (Figure 38.2).

Oxyhaemoglobin curve shift to the right

When a shift occurs to the right there is reduced binding of oxygen to haemoglobin and oxygen is given up more easily to the tissues. The saturation will be lower.

Figure 38.2 Oxyhaemoglobin dissociation curve. With a PaO_2 of 8 kPa and more, saturations will remain high (flat portion of curve). NB. The middle red line is the normal position of the curve.

Factors that cause the curve to shift to the right are:

- Increase in body temperature due to infection, sepsis.
- Increase in hydrogen ion content (acidaemia), known as the Bohr effect due to infection, sepsis or other shock conditions.
- Increase in carbon dioxide due to sepsis, pulonary disease, postoperatively.
- Increase in 2-3-DPG (2-3-DPG is an enzyme found in the red blood cells that affects haemoglobin and oxygen binding).

Oxyhaemoglobin curve shift to the left

When a shift occurs to the left there is an increase in the binding of oxygen to the haemoglobin, oxygen is given less easily to the tissues and cellular hypoxia can occur.

Factors that cause the curve to shift to the left are:

- Decrease in body temperature due to exposure, near drowning, trauma.
- Decrease in hydrogen ion content (alkalaemia).
- Decrease in carbon dioxide.
- Decrease in 2-3-DPG.

Oxygen utilization

The relationship between the PaO_2 and the SaO_2 is represented as the oxygen dissociation curve. Oxygen uptake in the lungs is shown by the upper flat part of the curve. When the PaO_2 is between 8.0 and 13.3 kPa (60–100 mmHg) the haemoglobin is 90% or more saturated with oxygen. At this point of the curve, large changes in the PaO_2 lead to small changes in the SaO_2 of haemoglobin, because the haemoglobin is almost completely saturated. Release of oxygen to the tissues is shown by the lower part of the curve. There is easy removal of oxygen from the haemoglobin for use by the cells. It is at this part of the curve that small changes in the PaO_2 cause major changes in the SaO_2. This is important clinically.

A patient's oxygen level must be kept at 8.5 kPa or above (60 mmHg). Below this level desaturation can occur at a rapid rate, resulting in tissue hypoxia and cell death.

Oxygen consumption

At rest the normal oxygen consumption is approximately 200–250 ml/minute. As the available oxygen per minute in a normal man is about 700 ml, this means there is an oxygen reserve of 450–500 ml/minute. Factors that increase the above consumption of oxygen include fever, sepsis, shivering, restlessness and increased metabolism (Oh 1997). It is difficult to say at which absolute level oxygen therapy is necessary as each situation should be judged by the requirements for oxygen and the availability of oxygen. Therefore, all of the above information needs to be taken into account together with the measurement of the arterial blood gases.

Generally, additional oxygen will be required when the PaO_2 has fallen to 8.5 kPa (60 mmHg) or less (Oh 1997). Oxygen saturation level in the tissues can be measured using a pulse oximeter, which works by emitting narrow shafts of red and infrared light through the tissue of a finger, toe or earlobe. Different amounts of light rays are absorbed by the arterial blood depending on its saturation with oxygen. The final oxygen saturation (SaO_2) is then calculated by computer (Ehrhardt & Graham 1990).

Carbon dioxide excretion

The second function of the respiratory system is to excrete carbonic acid from the lungs during expiration. The normal level of carbon dioxide in the blood is 3.5–5.3 kPa. Carbon dioxide has a direct effect on the respiratory centres in the brain. As the carbon dioxide level rises and diffuses from the blood into the cerebrospinal fluid (CSF) it is hydrated and carbonic acid is formed. The acid then dissociates and hydrogen ions are liberated as there are no proteins in the CSF to buffer the hydrogen ions, the pH of the CSF falls which excites the central chemoreceptors, and the respiratory rate is increased (Marieb 2006).

Respiratory assessment

When assessing respiratory function it is essential to include all of the respiratory tree cited above in the evaluation. Having received information about the person's past medical history one of the most reliable and important assessments is to closely observe and talk to the patient. Normal respiration is effortless and almost unconscious, and the person can eat, drink and speak in full sentences without appearing breathless. Essential first steps in respiratory assessment are therefore to observe the person's breathing for the following:

- Ease and comfort.
- Rate.
- Pattern.
- Position the patient has adopted: for example does the patient need to sit at 90° upright to breathe effectively?
- Rate and ease of breathing during speaking or movement.
- General colour and appearance: is there any evidence of greyness, cyanosis, pallor, sweating?
- Additional audible breath sounds: wheezing or stridor?

Having rapidly made this assessment other essential assessments are a chest X-ray and arterial blood gas, and a computed tomography (CT) scan or ventilation/perfusion (V/Q) scan may also be necessary.

Having made a comprehensive assessment the immediate cause should be corrected where possible. It is important to recognize that this may result from interruption to any part of respiration; for example, the patient may be in severe pain and appropriate pain management may improve their respiratory function, or conversely an opioid overdose may result in decreased or absent respiration and the antidote to an opioid will then need to be given. There may be a mechanical obstruction to respiration such as an infective obstruction like epiglottitis and the treatment is therefore

directed at treating the infection whilst also oxygenating the patient.

Respiratory therapy therefore covers a wide area and will include any manipulation or management of alteration to any part of the respiratory tree. It may include: pharmacological management including pain management, antidotes to drug toxicity, antimicrobials for infections of the respiratory tract, or respiratory stimulants; surgery to repair a ruptured diaphragm, to manage trauma, the insertion of a tracheostomy, the insertion of chest drains, or a thoracoabdominal shunt for superior vena cava obstruction. Finally positioning and physiotherapy play a major role in improving respiratory function.

Any person who is unable to maintain tissue oxygenation will need to receive supplemental oxygen until they are able to manage again on room air. This oxygen may be delivered in different ways depending on the severity of the condition and the level of hypoxia.

General considerations

- Oxygen is an odourless, tasteless, colourless, transparent gas that is slightly heavier than air.
- Oxygen supports combustion; therefore, there is always a danger of fire when oxygen is being used. The following safety measures should be remembered:

  (a) Oil or grease around oxygen connections should be avoided.
  (b) Alcohol, ether and other inflammatory liquids should be used with caution in the vicinity of oxygen.
  (c) No electrical device must be used in or near an oxygen tent.
  (d) Oxygen cylinders should be kept secure in an upright position and away from heat.
  (e) There must be no smoking in the vicinity of oxygen.
  (f) A fire extinguisher should be readily available.
  (g) Care should be taken with high concentrations of oxygen when using the defibrillator in a cardiorespiratory arrest, or during elective cardioversion.

Equipment necessary to administer respiratory therapy

Any oxygen delivery system will include these basic components:

- Oxygen supply, from either a piped supply or a portable cylinder. All medical gas cylinders have to conform to a standardized colour coding: oxygen cylinders are black with a white shoulder and are labelled 'Oxygen' or 'O_2'. Since 2004, small portable oxygen cylinders have been in use: these are totally white and are a C-size cylinder.
- A reduction gauge: to reduce the pressure to that of atmospheric pressure.
- Flowmeter: a device that controls the flow of oxygen in litres per minute.

Figure 38.3 Nasal cannula.

- Tubing: disposable tubing of varying diameter and length.
- Mechanism for delivery: a mask or nasal cannulae.
- Humidifier: to warm and moisten the oxygen before administration.
- Water trap if humidifier in use.

Oxygen delivery systems

Nasal cannulae catheter (Figure 38.3)

Nasal cannulae consist of two prongs that are inserted inside the anterior nares and supported on a light frame. Advantages to the patient are that they may seem less claustrophobic and do not interfere with eating, drinking and communication. Nasal cannulae catheters provide an alternative to a mask, but can only be used where the patient only requires a low percentage of added oxygen. Nasal cannulae are usually used with flow rates of 1–4 litres of oxygen per minute and probably provide approximately 28–35% oxygen. Nasal cannulae cannot be attached satisfactorily to an external humidification device but in many cases the oxygen will be humidified as it passes through the nasal passages into the trachea (Table 38.2). Nasal cannulae are generally well tolerated and are useful postoperatively or where the patient requires minimal support. They are also used in the

Table 38.2 Oxygen flow rates for nasal cannulae.

Oxygen flow rate (l/min)	% Oxygen delivered
1	24
2	28
3	32
4	36
5	40
6	44

Figure 38.4 Semi-rigid plastic mask.

chronic setting where a patient at home requires long-term oxygen therapy.

Simple semi-rigid plastic masks (Figure 38.4)

Simple semi-rigid plastic masks are low-flow masks which entrain the air from the atmosphere and therefore are able to deliver a variable oxygen percentage (anything from 21 to 60%) (Table 38.3). Large discrepancies between the delivered fractional inspired oxygen (FiO_2) and the actual amount received by the patient will occur, dependent on the patient's rate and depth of breathing. These masks are useful for patients who need a higher percentage of oxygen temporarily whilst the cause for their hypoxia is treated. This type of mask may be worn for hours or several days, but they should be used in conjunction with a humidifier if used for more than 12 hours. If the patient requires 60% added oxygen or more this is the threshold for requiring more invasive respiratory support and expert help should be sought.

Partial rebreathing masks

These are similar to the simple semi-rigid plastic masks with the addition of a reservoir bag. The reservoir bag allows the oxygen delivered to increase beyond 60%. During

Table 38.3 Approximate oxygen concentration related to flow rates of semi-rigid masks.

Oxygen flow rate (l/min)	% Oxygen delivered
2	24
4	35
6	50
8	55
10	60
12	65
15	70

inspiration the patient draws air and oxygen from the mask, bag and through the holes in the side of the mask. When the patient expires the initial one-third of the expired gases will flow back into the reservoir bag. The expired gas is rich in oxygen and contains very little carbon dioxide. The patient is able to breathe the previously expired gas along with the oxygen from the source.

Note: if the oxygen flow is too low the carbon dioxide can accumulate in the reservoir bag and fail to meet the patient's requirement, resulting in an increase in carbon dioxide (Pierce 1995). This device should only be used in the presence of expert nursing and medical support and usually during emergency intervention or before more invasive ventilatory therapy is instituted.

Non-rebreathing mask

Oxygen delivery of greater than 80% can be achieved. The semi-rigid mask has the addition of a reservoir bag with a one-way valve between the reservoir bag and mask, preventing accumulation of expired gases in the reservoir bag and retention of carbon dioxide (Pierce 1995).

Fixed performance masks or high-flow masks (*Venturi-type masks*) (Figure 38.5)

With fixed performance masks it is possible to achieve an unvarying mixture of gases and a known concentration of oxygen using the high air flow oxygen enrichment principle (Table 38.4). These masks derive their name from the Venturi barrel in which a relatively low-flow rate of oxygen is forced through a narrow jet. There are side holes in the barrel and this jet causes the air to be drawn in at a high rate. As the mixture of gas created is at a flow rate above that of inspiration, the mixture will be constant (Foss 1990). There are many Venturi-type masks available, but the larger-capacity masks are the most accurate and therefore the safest when a known concentration of oxygen is required or when

Figure 38.5 High-flow mask with venturi barrel.

Table 38.4 Fixed performance mask oxygen flow rates.

Oxygen flow rate (l/min)	% Oxygen delivered
2	24
6	31
8	35
10	40
15	60

efficient elimination of carbon dioxide is essential, for example, to provide respiratory therapy for the patient with chronic respiratory disease (Fell & Boehm 1998).

Tracheostomy mask

Tracheostomy masks perform in a similar way to the simple semi-rigid plastic face mask, outlined above. The mask is placed over the tracheostomy tube or stoma (see also Chapter 42).

T-piece circuit

The T-piece circuit is a simple, large-bore, non-rebreathing circuit which is attached directly to an endotracheal or tracheostomy tube. Humidified oxygen is delivered through one part of the T, and expired gases leave through the other part. This device may be used as part of the weaning process when a patient has been ventilated previously by a mechanical ventilator (Oh 1997).

Domiciliary oxygen and portable oxygen

Some patients are so disabled by chronic respiratory disease that they require continual supplementary oxygen at home. Low-flow oxygen given over a period of time improves the prognosis of some patients (Benditt 2000).

Long-term oxygen may be prescribed for treatment of COPD, cystic fibrosis, interstitial lung disease, neuromuscular and skeletal disorders, pulmonary hypertension and palliation in lung cancer. Long-term oxygen may be provided in the form of cylinders. The problem with this supply is that the cylinders need changing frequently. Oxygen condensers (concentrators) are far more economical than cylinders. A condenser consists of a compressor powered by electricity. The condenser works by drawing in room air that is passed through a bacterial filter and a sieve bed. The sieve bed contains zeolite which has an affinity with nitrogen and when under pressure works by removing nitrogen and other gases, concentrating oxygen and delivering it through a meter at the front of the compressor.

The oxygen can be delivered to the patient by nasal cannulae or mask (Esmond 2000).

Liquid oxygen

The use of liquid oxygen in a portable cylinder has been developed for portable oxygen delivery. The patient is provided with a large tank in their own home from which smaller cylinders can be filled.

Continuous positive airway pressure

Definition

Continuous positive airway pressure (CPAP) therapy is the maintenance of a positive airway pressure greater than ambient pressure throughout inspiration and expiration. It can be delivered through a face mask, nasal mask or mouthpiece, or through an endotracheal or tracheostomy tube (Oh 1997).

Indications

- In acute respiratory failure in a spontaneously breathing patient who is able to maintain his or her own airway.
- As a method of weaning a patient from mechanical ventilation.
- After major surgery as a means of improving gaseous exchange.
- As a supportive measure in patients where intubation and mechanical ventilation are not considered appropriate (Greenbaum et al. 1976).
- Acute hypoxia with a normal $PaCO_2$.
- Acute respiratory distress syndrome (ARDS)
- Postoperatively (following major abdominal or thoracic surgery) prophylactically to prevent atelectasis.
- Pulmonary oedema.
- In patients with sleep apnoea.
- In neonates with respiratory distress syndrome/hyaline membrane disease.

Reference material

Use of the CPAP circuit dates back at least to 1912, when Bunnell used a primitive circuit during thoracic surgery. The first recorded use in intensive care was by Poulton and Oxon in 1936. In the 1940s increased interest in CPAP was prompted by research into respiratory support in high altitude flying. Further developments occurred in the 1950s and 1960s, and in 1976 Greenbaum et al. reported the use of CPAP with a face mask in ARDS. In 1972 Williamson & Modell successfully used CPAP for selected spontaneously breathing patients with acute respiratory failure.

The aim of CPAP therapy is to improve gas exchange (oxygen and carbon dioxide) within the lungs and improve the work of breathing. CPAP is able to do this by:

- Increasing the functional residual capacity (FRC), which is the amount of gas left in the lungs at the end of normal expiration available for pulmonary gas exchange. In acute lung injury where gaseous exchange is severely inhibited CPAP increases the FRC by improving ventilation in poorly or non-ventilated alveoli (Miller & Semple 1991).
- Improving the ventilation/perfusion ratio. Decreased intrapulmonary shunting with hypoxia could cause ventilation to the lungs to be reduced or blood flow to them impaired. Intrapulmonary shunting can then occur with under ventilation of the lungs. CPAP helps to decrease the intrapulmonary shunting by improving the ventilation to perfusion mismatch (Lenique et al. 1997).
- Improved lung compliance (elasticity) of the lungs. In respiratory failure the lungs become much stiffer and less compliant and breathing can become more difficult. Reduction in lung volume below a certain level results in airway collapse and under ventilation. The pressure required to overcome this can be achieved by CPAP.
- Increasing lung volume (alveolar volume) for gaseous exchange to take place. The factors above enable the work of breathing to be reduced plus a decrease in the percentage of oxygen that might be required.

Disadvantages of CPAP therapy

- With any circuit that includes the use of positive end expiratory pressure (PEEP) there is the possibility of reduction in cardiac output; however, spontaneous ventilation decreases both the incidence and severity of this complication (Oh 1997).
- There is a danger of vomiting and aspiration of gastric contents due to gastric insufflation, although this is minimized when used in awake patients, or by the insertion of an oro/nasogastric tube (Schumaker et al. 1996).
- Damage to skin integrity due to pressure from the tightly fitting face mask; the sites particularly vulnerable are the bridge of the nose and over the ears.

Non-invasive ventilation

Non-invasive ventilation refers to mechanical ventilatory support applied without an artificial airway (endotracheal tube or tracheostomy). It can be delivered to the patient via a nasal or face mask. The patient must be conscious and co-operative for this type of ventilation to be effective. It is particularly useful in patients with chronic respiratory disease:

- In restrictive pulmonary disease, e.g. muscular dystrophy.
- In progressive neuromuscular disease, e.g. motor neurone disease.
- In obstructive pulmonary disease, e.g. COPD, bronchiectasis, cystic fibrosis.
- In nocturnal hypoventilation.
- In patients with acute exacerbation of chronic respiratory disease.
- In patients where endotracheal intubation and ventilation may not be considered appropriate or where difficulties may be anticipated in weaning a patient from a ventilator.

Non-invasive ventilators generally fall into two categories (Esmond 2000):

- Pressure preset machines.
- Volume preset machines.

Mechanical ventilation

A mechanical ventilator is a device used to replace or assist breathing in order for satisfactory gas exchange to take place. The decision to ventilate a patient will be made after careful clinical examination including assessment of respiratory mechanics, oxygenation and ventilation.

Ventilators are able to control tidal volume, respiratory rate, time of inspiration against time of expiration, inspired flow rate and inspired oxygen concentration (Pierce 1995; West 1995; Hinds 1997; Bersten & Soni 2003).

Ventilators are divided into two main categories: negative pressure ventilators and positive pressure ventilators.

Negative pressure ventilators

These devices are now rarely used. They mimic normal breathing (negative pressure) and are known as iron lungs. The patient is enclosed in an airtight tank and a negative pressure is created by a separate pump which causes the alveolar pressure to fall within the lungs so a pressure gradient results, with air flowing into the lungs along the pressure gradient in order for ventilation to take place. An adaptation from the tank ventilator is the cuirass shell, which surrounds the thorax and abdomen, which works on the same principle. The rare use of these devices would be in patients with chronic respiratory failure (neuromuscular disease, skeletal deformity or sleep-related respiratory problems).

Positive pressure ventilators

These devices provide a satisfactory gas exchange when inflating the lungs with a positive pressure via an endotracheal tube or tracheostomy.

Positive pressure ventilators have four main functions to perform during each respiratory cycle:

- Inflate the lungs.
- Cycle from inspiration to expiration.
- Allow expiration to take place.
- Cycle from expiration to inspiration.

They have a driving mechanism and can cycle from one phase of the respiratory cycle to another by a preset pressure, preset time or preset volume.

Varying modes of ventilation can be used:

- Intermittent mandatory ventilation (IMV).
- Pressure support.
- Pressure control.
- Simulated intermittent mandatory ventilation (SIMV).
- Continuous positive airway pressure (CPAP).

Hyperbaric respiratory therapy

Hyperbaric respiratory therapy is used mainly in the treatment of carbon monoxide poisoning, burns, gas gangrene, skin lesions, soft tissue injury, decompression sickness (the bends) and in multiple sclerosis. The therapy is designed to give 100% oxygen at a range of pressures greater than atmospheric pressure. Oxygen is dissolved in the plasma, increasing the oxygen tension in the tissues (Bersten & Soni 2003).

Humidification

Humidity is the amount of water vapour present in a gas. The terms used to define humidity are absolute humidity, maximum capacity and relative humidity. Absolute humidity is the mass of water vapour that a given volume of gas can carry at a set temperature. When a gas is at its maximum capacity it is said to be fully saturated. Relative humidity is the ratio of the absolute humidity to the maximum capacity.

The warmer the gas, the more vapour it can hold but if the temperature of the gas falls, water held as vapour will condense out of the gas into the surrounding atmosphere.

In normal health the nasal passages and upper airways are able to warm, moisten and filter the inspired gases very effectively. The process of humidification is necessary to compensate for the normal loss of water from the respiratory tract which, under resting conditions, is about 250 ml per day. This can increase in patients who are unwell.

Normal room air has an approximate temperature of 22°C with a relative humidity of 50% and a water content of 10 mg H_2O. For effective gas exchange to occur in the lungs, the air would need to be at a temperature of 37°C with 100% humidity and a water content of 44 mg H_2O per litre by the time it reaches the bifurcation in the trachea, which is referred to as the isothermic point.

When the temperature falls below 37°C and humidity falls below 100% several changes take place in the airways. The respiratory tract is lined with ciliated epithelial cells that secrete mucus. Each cell has about 200 hair-like structures known as cilia, whose role is to remove unwanted mucus and secretions. With a drop in temperature and humidity, the mucus that collects in the airways thickens and movement of the cilia is reduced. If there is no improvement the mucus will become thicker and immobile; the cilia will also lose their mobility so clearance of all secretions will stop and infection can set in.

If there is a continuing lack of humidity further damage occurs. The cilia can break off, causing damage to the mucosal lining of the respiratory tract. The isothermic point of saturation moves from the bifurcation of the trachea to a lower point in the lungs, resulting in further damage which can lead to collapse of the alveoli, decrease in lung function and hypoxaemia (Carroll 1997b; Fell & Boehm 1998; Ward & Park 2000).

Inhalation of oxygen used during respiratory therapy, which is a dry gas, can cause evaporation of water from the respiratory tract and lead to the consequences above if humidification is not provided.

In patients who are intubated or have a tracheostomy the natural pathway of humidification is bypassed.

Methods of humidification

Many devices can be used to supply humidification; the best of these will fulfil the following requirements:

- The inspired gas must be delivered to the trachea at a room temperature of 32–36°C with 100% humidity and should have a water content of 33–43 g/m^3 (Oh 1997).
- The set temperature should remain constant; humidification and temperature should not be affected by large ranges of flow.
- The device should have a safety and alarm system to guard against overheating, overhydration and electric shocks.
- It is important that the appliance should not increase resistance or affect the compliance of respiration.
- It is essential that whichever device is selected, wide-bore tubing (elephant tubing) is used to allow efficient formation of water vapour.

Devices for humidification (see Table 38.5)

- *Heat and moisture exchanger (HME).* In this situation an HME performs the function of the nose and pharynx in conditioning the inspired air. It retains heat and moisture in the expired air and returns them to the patient in the next inspired breath. Many HMEs contain a bacterial filter.

The HME consists of spun, pleated, highly thermal conductive material. It can be used in a self-ventilating patient with a tracheostomy who is being weaned from oxygen (Fig. 38.6a). It is also known as an artificial or 'Swedish' nose. It

Table 38.5 A comparison of devices for humidification.

Device	Advantages	Disadvantages
HME	Simple Cheap Short term	Inadequate humidity Risk of airway obstruction Can become waterlogged Infection risk
Cold water humidifier	Simple Cheap	Inadequate humidity Infection risk
Hot water humidifier	Delivers maximal humidification	Infection risk Overhumidification Risk of aspiration water/drowning Excessive condensation in circuit Overheating causing damage to trachea Resistance in circuit Restriction of gas flow

HME, heat and moisture exchanger.

can also be used in ventilated patients, inserted between the patient's airway and the ventilator circuit (Figure 38.6b).

- *Cold water bubble humidifier.* This device delivers partially humidified oxygen at about 50% relative humidity. Gas is either forced across or bubbled through water at room temperature (Figure 38.6c). This method is not advised as it is so inefficient (Oh 1997).
- *Water bath humidifiers.* With these devices, inspired gas is forced over or through a heated reservoir of water (Figure 38.6d). To achieve an adequate humidity for the patient, the water bath must reach a set temperature. The gas will then cool as it moves down the breathing circuit to the patient, and a relative humidity of 100% will be reached. Hot water bath humidifiers are therefore very efficient and useful for humidification for the immobile patients particularly if they are receiving mechanical ventilatory support. However, they have four main disadvantages:

(a) Danger of overheating and causing damage to the trachea.
(b) Their efficiency can alter with changes in gas flow rate, surface area and the water temperature.
(c) Condensation and collection of water in the oxygen delivery tubes.
(d) The possibility of microcontamination of stagnant water (Tinker & Zapol 1992).

- *Aerosol generators.* These devices are not governed by temperature, but provide microdroplets of water suspended in the gas (Bersten & Soni 2003). The gas provided through aerosol devices can be very highly saturated with water. There are three main types of aerosol humidifier:

(a) Gas-drive nebulizer.
(b) Mechanical (spinning disc) nebulizer.
(c) Ultrasonic nebulizer.

These devices are useful for the spontaneously breathing patient with chronic chest disease.

Hazards of oxygen therapy

Carbon dioxide narcosis

Carbon dioxide is the chemical that most directly influences respiration by its direct effect on the efficiency of alveolar ventilation. The normal partial pressure of carbon dioxide in the blood is 4.0–6.0 kPa (30–45 mmHg). When this level rises, the pH of the CSF drops which in turn causes excitation of the central chemoreceptors, and hyperventilation occurs (Marieb 2006).

In people who always retain carbon dioxide, and are therefore usually hypercapnic because of chronic pulmonary disease such as chronic bronchitis, the chemoreceptors are no longer sensitive to a raised level of carbon dioxide. In these

Figure 38.6 (a) Heat and moisture exchanger. (b) Cross-section of a heat and moisture exchanger (HME) used with a ventilator circuit. (c) Cold water bubble humidifier. (d) Hot water bath humidifier.

cases the falling PaO_2 becomes the principal respiratory stimulus (the hypoxic drive) (Marieb 2006). Therefore, if a high level of supplementary oxygen was delivered to such patients, severe respiratory depression would ensue and ultimately unconsciousness and death.

Oxygen toxicity

Pulmonary toxicity following prolonged higher percentages of oxygen therapy is recognized clinically, but there is still much to be learnt about the condition. The degree of injury is related to the length of time of exposure and percentage of oxygen to which the individual is exposed. The pattern is one of decreasing lung compliance as a result of a sequence of events, tracheal bronchial inflammation, haemorrhagic

interstitial and intra-alveolar oedema, leading ultimately to fibrosis (Pierce 1995; Oh 1997; Pierson 2000).

Where possible, long periods (i.e. 24 hours or more) of oxygen therapy above 50% should be avoided.

Retrolental fibroplasia

Retrolental fibroplasia is a disease affecting premature babies that weigh under 1200 g (about 28 weeks' gestation) if they are exposed to high concentrations of oxygen within the first 3–4 weeks of life. It appears that the oxygen stimulates immature blood vessels in the eye to vasoconstrict and obliterate, which results in neovascularization, accompanied by haemorrhage, fibrosis and then retinal detachment and blindness (Pierce 1995; Bersten & Soni 2003).

Procedure guidelines   Pre-continuous positive airway pressure (pre-CPAP)

Procedure

Action	Rationale
1 Assess patient's conscious level.	To obtain a baseline and to be able to assess for change in condition (see Chapter 26) (E).
2 Explain the principles of CPAP to the patient and family and demonstrate the system to them. Observe and record the following:	To gain consent, minimize anxiety, increase knowledge and aid in patient compliance (E).
(a) Patient's respiratory function.	To obtain a baseline of respiratory function (E).
(b) Respiratory rate.	To observe for any change in respiratory function (E).
(c) Work of breathing.	
(d) Colour, skin, etc.	
(e) Tissue oxygen saturation (SaO_2).	
3 Decide whether it is appropriate to insert an arterial cannula.	In order to monitor the acid base balance (E).
4 Observe and record the patient's cardiovascular function, including:	To obtain a baseline in order to assess any change in conditions (see Chapter 25) (E).
(a) Heart rate.	
(b) Blood pressure.	
(c) Temperature.	
(d) Central venous pressure (if patient has a central line).	
5 Accurate assessment of fluid balance including:	To obtain a baseline of fluid balance.
(a) Input.	To enable assessment of dehydration or fluid overload.
(b) Output.	
(c) Accumulative balance.	
(d) Overall fluid balance.	
(e) Daily weight.	
6 Assess patient's level of anxiety and compliance with treatment (the patient's ability to cope with the treatment).	To enable an assessment to be made and an evaluation of the suitability of CPAP therapy (E).

760

Procedure guidelines   Continuous positive airway pressure (CPAP): setting up

Equipment

1 Oxygen supply.
2 Compressed air supply.
3 Flow generator.
4 Oxycheck.
5 Prepared CPAP circuit.
6 Humidifier.
7 Temperature probe.
8 Water trap.
9 CPAP helmet/mask/nasal mask.
10 Headstrap.
11 PEEP valves (2.5/5.0/7.5/10.0 cm).

Procedure

Action	Rationale
1 Set up CPAP circuit.	
2 Ensure patient is in a comfortable position, sitting up in bed at a 45° angle or more or chair well supported by a pillow.	To promote comfort and aid lung expansion and breathing (E).
3 Ensure patient is comfortable in surrounding environment.	To promote comfort and aid in compliance with using CPAP (E).
4 Explain to patient how the helmet or mask is to be applied. Apply helmet/mask gently, applying pressure as the patient adapts to the tight-fitting mask. Hold mask until patient is comfortable and settled.	To relieve anxiety and to reassure patient (E). To aid patient's compliance with CPAP (E).
5 Once the patient is settled with mask/helmet, apply the headstrap or shoulder straps. Ensure mask/helmet and headstrap are comfortable for the patient; alter position as required.	To retain mask in place and aid patient comfort (E).
6 Ensure a good seal and that no leaks are present.	To ensure a tight seal in order that the system functions optimally (E).
7 Apply tissue protective dressing around vulnerable pressure points: nose, ear, back of head and neck.	To alleviate pressure and prevent tissue breakdown (E).
8 Give further explanation to family/next of kin of how CPAP works and the importance of their presence and participation in communication.	To relieve anxiety and support and reassure family and patient (E).
9 Reassure the patient constantly.	To relieve patient anxiety and promote co-operation (E).
10 Discuss with doctor use of medication that might aid the patient in compliance with CPAP therapy.	

Procedure guidelines   Humidification for respiratory therapy

Various humidifiers exist. Select the system most appropriate for the patient.

Procedure

Action	Rationale
1 Discuss with the team the choice of system to be used.	The most appropriate device is selected to meet the patient's needs (E).

Procedure guidelines (*cont.*)

2 Explain to patient the reason for use of the humidifier and how it works.

So patient understands what is happening and thus to help the patient tolerate the humidification (E).

3 Prepare the device to be used.
  (a) Some circuits are ready prepared with humidifier.
  (b) Prepare humidifier and circuit.
  (c) Humidifier/wide-bore oxygen tubing: ensure minimal length of tubing, water trap and mask.

4 Once circuit is set up, run system to check it is functioning correctly and the circuit is intact.

To ensure that oxygen is being delivered through the circuit as set (E).
To ensure the system is humidifying the oxygen and that no leaks exist (E).

5 If hot water system is in use check it is running within recommended temperature range.

To ensure no damage to the patient's lungs if temperature above range (E).

6 Ensure water is present in water source of system; do not allow to run dry.

Aid adequate delivery of humidity to the patient. Prevent damage to the humidifier (E).

7 Ensure circuit tubing is positioned below patient.

To ensure collection of humidity in the circuit is able to drain into the water trap or circuit rather than into the patient (E).

8 Ensure the patient finds the humidification comfortable.

9 Continually check running of system.

To ensure the system is functioning adequately and delivering humidity (E).

10 Ensure the patient is well informed and continuously reassured. The patient may find the system noisy and may be distressed by excessive moisture in the circuit.

11 Change the humidification and circuit on a weekly basis.

Problem solving: Oxygen therapy by nasal cannulae or oxygen mask

Problem	Cause	Suggested action
Maintenance of airway.	Position of patient. Airway secretions.	Position patient preferably sitting up at an angle of greater than 45°. Encourage patient to cough and expectorate if able or remove secretions by suction if patient unable to do so (E).
Maintenance of adequate oxygenation.	Inadequate oxygen delivery, patient's condition deteriorating. More breathless. Oxygen saturation decreased. Deteriorating blood gases.	Assess level of oxygen support required by assessing previous medical history and current respiratory assessment. Increase oxygen delivery using the lowest percentage of oxygen to achieve the individual goal for the patient (E).
Dry mouth.	Oxygen therapy drying mouth.	Add humidification to the circuit (see Procedure guidelines: Humidification, above). Give regular mouth care (E).

Problem	Cause	Suggested action
Nasal cannulae or mask discomfort.	Position or use of cannulae and oxygen mask.	Ensure correct placement and that the patient is comfortable (E).
Development of pressure points on nose/ears.	Incorrect placement of cannulae support or mask headstrap.	Change position of cannulae or mask (E). Apply padding around headstrap or to bridge of nose to relieve pressure (F).
Intolerance of oxygen therapy.	Fear and anxiety. Confusion. Hypoxia.	Assess patient for change. Ensure continual reassurance given to patient. Ensure patient remains orientated to the environment and oxygen device. If intolerant of mask, nasal cannulae may be tolerated. If hypoxic, oxygen may need to be increased (E).
Communication.	Mask makes communication difficult; patient may not hear carer and nurse may not hear patient.	Assist patient to move around bed area if not able to go far. Mobilize patient with portable oxygen cylinder if appropriate (E).
Inability to maintain personal hygiene.	Immobility. On bedrest. Mask restricting independence.	Provide reassurance for patient to remain independent where able. Allow them to carry out their own hygiene if able or to help patient with hygiene if not (E).
Maintenance of safety.	Detachment of oxygen from flow meter. Kinked or looped oxygen tubing. Mask removed by patient.	Ensure oxygen attached to flow meter. Check patient regularly. Ensure no kinks or loops arise. Ensure patient is attached to oxygen.
Documentation.	Rapidly changing situation.	Ensure all changes to oxygen therapy or patient are documented in nursing care plan (E).

763

Problem solving: Continuous positive airway pressure (CPAP)

Problem	Cause	Suggested action
Maintenance of airway.	Deteriorating respiratory function. Physical tiring.	Regular monitoring of respiratory function including skin colour; breathing pattern; respiratory rate; oxygen saturation; blood gases. Discuss changes with medical or anaesthetic staff (E).
Cardiovascular instability.	Hypotension. Arrhythmias. Decreasing central venous pressure. Decreasing cardiac output due to CPAP.	Continuously monitor cardiovascular function: heart rate; blood pressure. Continuously monitor central venous pressure (E). Report changes to medical staff (E).
Dehydration.	Decreased oral intake. Decreased circulating volume. Nausea and vomiting.	Maintain an accurate fluid balance chart measuring input and output of both enteral and intravenous fluids and urinary and other fluid output (E). Take into account fluid loss from vomit/diarrhoea or wound drainage. Check overall balance on an hourly basis. Administer prescribed antiemetic if patient feels nauseated.

Problem solving (*cont.*)

Problem	Cause	Suggested action
Fluid overload: May present with pulmonary oedema. Retention of urine.	Sepsis. Cardiac failure.	Observe and assess patient. Maintain accurate fluid balance chart. Discuss any changes with medical staff, who may prescribe a diuretic (E). Undertake further assessment of fluid balance (E). Catheterize patient if unable to pass urine (E). Carry out accurate assessment of output (E).
Inadequate dietary intake.	Gastric distension due to CPAP. Loss of appetite. Difficulty in eating; distress caused by respiratory status and CPAP. Nausea and vomiting.	Encourage diet and oral supplementary fluids. If unable to take orally, refer to dietitian an alternative method of feeding may be considered, e.g. enteral feeding via nasogastric or jejunal tube, or intravenous feeding (TPN). Administer antiemetic. Encourage and reassure patient (E).
Aspiration, if unable to maintain own airway.	Inability to maintain own airway. Continuous pressure from CPAP system. Insufflation of air.	Observe and assess patient closely. After discussion with medical staff a nasogastric tube may be inserted (E).
Gastric distension and discomfort may cause nausea and vomiting.	Continuous pressure from CPAP system. Insufflation of air.	Encourage patient to belch to relieve air if it aids comfort. Insert nasogastric tube and leave on free drainage (E).
Dry mouth.	CPAP system utilizes a very high oxygen flow which has a drying effect.	Carry out regular mouth care (see Chapter 32). Give patient regular sips of water, ice to suck or drinks as patient is able to take. Humidify, as in CPAP circuit (E).
Eyes (only applies to face mask CPAP): Dry. Sore. Conjunctival oedema.	Mask: air leak. High-flow oxygen. Facial pressure from mask: causing oedema.	Ensure mask/helmet is well sealed with no leaks. Apply pressure-relieving padding around mask. Apply regular eye care (see Chapter 31) (E). Adjust mask to facial contour. Alter and position mask as comfortable. Position padding around the headstrap to relieve pressure (E).
Tissue integrity problems with sacrum, elbows, heels.	Continued bedrest. Difficulty in moving. Fear of moving.	Change patient's position in bed regularly (E). Nurse patient on alternate sides (E). Patient may sit out of bed if able (E). Consider alternative pressure-relieving mattress (E). if patient immobile or has high Waterlow score (see Chapter 48).
Mask/helmet incorrectly sealed.		Alter mask/helmet position to correct and ensure comfort (E). Ensure mask/helmet is correct size. Alter position to ensure correct seal (E).
Anxiety.	Tight-fitting mask/ helmet. Feeling of claustrophobia and isolation. Fear of dying.	Reassure patient (E). Inform patient that nurse is present at all times and able to see patient (E). Inform patient of any changes taking place. Communicate with the patient's family, keep them informed and involve them in care and communication with patient (E). Inform doctor of patient's anxiety level. Administer prescribed anxiolytic agent if required (E).

Problem	Cause	Suggested action
Maintenance of safety of patient and environment.		Ensure nurse present with patient at all times. Observe patient and CPAP system closely to ensure equipment is working optimally and there is no failure of the system (E).
Communication: Inability to communicate effectively. Feelings of isolation.	Mask/helmet restriction.	Reassure patient and ensure he or she is comfortable (E). Encourage patient to communicate and explain how he or she can use letterboard to do so. Reassure patient (E).

References and further reading

Aherns, T. & Tucker, K. (1999) Pulse oximetry. *Crit Care Clin North Am*, **11**(1), 87–97.

Allan, D. (1988) Making sense of oxygen delivery. *Nurs Times*, **83**(18), 40–2.

Allison, R.C. (1991) Initial treatment of pulmonary oedema: a physiological approach. *Am J Med Sci*, **302**(6), 385–91.

Ball, C. (1999) Optimising oxygen delivery: haemodynamic workshop, part 1. *Intensive Crit Care Nurs*, **15**, 371–3.

Ball, C. (2000a) Optimising oxygen delivery: haemodynamic workshop, part 2. *Intensive Crit Care Nurs*, **16**, 33–44.

Ball, C. (2000b) Optimising oxygen delivery: haemodynamic workshop, part 3. *Intensive Crit Care Nurs*, **16**, 84–7.

Beaumont, M. *et al.* (1997) Effects of chest wall counter pressure on lung mechanics under high level CPAP in humans. *J Physiol*, **83**(2), 591–8.

Benditt, J.W. (2000) Adverse effects of low flow oxygen therapy. *Respir Care*, **45**(1), 54–80.

Berne, R.M. & Levy, M.N. (1998) *Physiology*, 4th edn. Mosby, St. Louis, MO.

Bersten, A & Soni, N. (2003) *Oh's Intensive Care Manual*, 5th edn. Butterworth Heinemann, Sydney.

Byron Brow, C.W. & Dracup, K. (2000) Too much of a good thing. *Am J Crit Care*, **9**(5), 300–2.

Carpenter, D. (1991) Oxygen transport in the blood. *Crit Care Nurse*, **11**(9), 20–31.

Carroll, P. (1997a) Pulse oximetry at your fingertips. *RN Magazine*, **60**(2), 22–7.

Carroll, P. (1997b) When you want humidity. *RN Magazine*, **60**(5), 30–4.

Cooper, N. (2002) Oxygen therapy: myths and misconceptions. *Care Crit Ill*, **18**(3), 74–7.

Coull, A. (1992) Making sense of pulse oximetry. *Nurs Times*, **88**(32), 42–3.

Dunn, L. & Chrisholm, H. (1998) Oxygen therapy. *Nurs Stand*, **13**(7), 57–64.

Ehrhardt, B.S. & Graham, M. (1990) Pulse oximetry. An easy way to check oxygen saturation. *Nursing*, **20**(3), 50–4.

Esmond, G. (2000) *Respiratory Nursing*. Bailliere Tindall, London.

Fell, H. & Boehm, M. (1998) Easing the discomfort of oxygen therapy. *Nurs Times*, **94**(38), 56–8.

Foss, M.A. (1990) Oxygen therapy. *Prof Nurse*, January, **5**(4), 180–90.

Goldhill, D. (2001) Postoperative oxygen. *Care Crit Ill*, **17**(5), 154–5.

Greeg, R.W. *et al.* (1990) Continuous positive airway pressure by face mask in *Pneumocystis carinii* pneumonia. *Crit Care Med*, **18**(1), 21–4.

Greenbaum, D.M. *et al.* (1976) Continuous positive airways pressure without tracheal intubation in spontaneously breathing patients. *Chest*, **69**, 615–20.

Guyton, A. (2000) *A Textbook of Medical Physiology*, 10th edn. W.B. Saunders, Philadelphia.

Hess, D. (2000) Detection and monitoring of hypoxaemia and oxygen therapy. *Respir Care*, **45**(1), 65–80.

Hinds, C.J. (1997) *Intensive Care. A Concise Textbook*, 2nd edn. Bailliere Tindall, London.

Keen, A. (2000) Continuous positive airway pressure in the intensive care unit: uses and implications for nursing management. *Nurs Crit Care*, **5**(3), 137–41.

Keilty, S.E. & Bott, J. (1992) Continuously positive airway pressure. *Physiotherapy*, **78**(2), 90–2.

Kumar, P. & Clark, C. (2005) *Clinical Medicine*, 5th edn. W.B. Saunders, London.

Lenique, F. *et al.* (1997) Ventilatory and haemodynamic effects of continuous positive airway pressure in heart failure. *Am J Respir Crit Care Med*, **155**, 500–5.

Marieb, E.N. (2006) *Human Anatomy and Physiology and Brief Atlas of the Human Body*, 7th edn. Benjamin Cummings, New York.

Miller, R. & Semple, S. (1991) Continous positive airway pressure ventilation for respiratory failure associated with *Pneumocystis carinii* pneumonia. *Respir Med*, **85**, 133–8.

Oh, T.E. (1997) *Intensive Care Manual*. Butterworth-Heinemann, Sydney.

Petty, T.L. (2000) Historical highlights of long-term oxygen therapy. *Respir Care*, **45**(1), 29–38.

Pierce, L.N.B. (1995) *Guide to Mechanical Ventilation and Intensive Respiratory Care*. W.B. Saunders, London.

Pierson, D.J. (2000) Pathophysiology and clinical effects of chronic hypoxia. *Respir Care*, **45**(1), 39–51.

Place, B. (1998) Pulse oximetry in adults. *Nurs Times*, **94**(50), 48–9.

Romand, J.A. & Donald, E. (1995) Physiological effects of continuous positive airway pressure ventilation in the critically ill. *Care Crit Ill*, **11**(6), 239–42.

Schumaker, W.C. *et al.* (1996) *Textbook of Critical Care*. W.B. Saunders, Philadelphia, pp. 628–952.

Tinker, J. & Zapol, W. (1992) *Care of the Critically Ill Patient*. Springer, New York.

Tortora, G.J. & Derrickson, B.H. (2008) *Principles of Anatomy and Physiology*, 12th edn. John Wiley & Sons, Inc., New York.

Ward, B. & Park, G.R. (2000) Humidification of inspired gases in the critically ill. *Clin Intensive Care*, **11**(4), 169–76.

West, J.B. (1995) *Pulmonary Pathophysiology: The Essentials*. Williams and Wilkins, Baltimore.

Williamson, D.C. & Modell, J.H. (1972) Intermittent continuous airways pressure by mask – its use in the treatment of atelectasis. *Arch Surg*, **177**, 970–2.

765

Chapter 39

Scalp cooling

767   Reference material
770   *Procedure guidelines:* Scalp cooling
772   *Problem solving*: Scalp cooling
772   References and further reading

Definition

Scalp cooling is a method of preventing chemotherapy-induced alopecia. It works in three ways (Bulow *et al.* 1985; Batchelor 2001):

1 Reducing perfusion of scalp of hair follicles by vasoconstriction thus limiting the amount of exposure of chemotherapy (an intradermal scalp temperature of 30°C decreases scalp blood flow by 25%).
2 Reduced temperature dependent cellular uptake of chemotherapy.
3 Reduced intrafollicular metabolic rate.

Indications

The effectiveness of scalp cooling has been demonstrated satisfactorily with doxorubicin, epirubicin, docetaxel and paclitaxel (Dean *et al.*1979; Robinson 1987; Lemanager *et al.* 1995; Katsimbri 2000). Patients receiving other cytotoxic drugs which may cause alopecia, such as vindesine and vincristine, have undergone the procedure, although there is insufficient data to evaluate its effectiveness with these drugs. However, scalp cooling requires the consultant's permission as the procedure may protect micrometastases in the scalp from chemotherapy, especially where there is the possibility of circulating cancer cells, e.g. in cases of leukaemia and lymphoma (Witman *et al.* 1981). In spite of this, scalp cooling has been used successfully in patients with relapsed lymphoma (Purohit *et al.* 1992). Dean *et al.* (1983), drawing on evidence from 7800 women with breast cancer, found that only two experienced recurrence of disease on the scalp, suggesting that the risk of scalp metastases was minimal. They concluded that scalp cooling should not be contraindicated and could be used routinely with a wide variety of solid tumours. Nevertheless, patients with advanced metastatic disease have been found to develop scalp metastases during scalp cooling and Middleton *et al.* (1985) argued strongly against the use of scalp cooling in this group. Other studies have found no scalp metastases at follow-up (Ron *et al.* 1997). The potential risk of scalp metastases, albeit remote, should be addressed and demands discussion by health care professionals and patients (Peck 2000; Batchelor 2001).

The issues relating to scalp metastases are controversial. This dilemma, along with the media coverage regarding preventive measures for chemotherapy-induced alopecia (Carr 1998; Kendell 2001), have led some practitioners to question whether scalp cooling should be offered. Patients have highlighted how they feel about hair loss (Carr 1998) and also the need to provide more comfortable and effective scalp cooling in all cancer units and centres (Wilson 1994). In addition, an extensive review of the literature concluded that scalp cooling was effective and should be offered to all patients for whom it was appropriate (Crowe *et al.* 1998; Batchelor 2001). This was supported by the views of many nurses who felt that the use of scalp cooling with chemotherapy protocols which are associated with hair loss can effectively prevent alopecia and result in improved quality of life for patients (Lemanager *et al.* 1998). Patients also feel it is worthwhile to undergo scalp cooling regardless of how successful it is (Dougherty 2006).

Reference material

Alopecia is a common consequence of many chemotherapeutic regimens and is one of the most devastating effects of cancer chemotherapy (Pickard-Holley 1995; Williams *et al.* 1999). Chemotherapy-induced alopecia is the temporary loss of all body hair (Dougherty 2005) and it has been identified as such a devastating prospect that some patients may refuse to accept treatment (Williams *et al.* 1999). Hair loss can also result in changes to the patient's body image (Freedman 1994; Gallagher 1996; Williams *et al.* 1999) which may not be reversed by the regrowth of hair (Munstedt *et al.* 1997).

Prevention of chemotherapy-induced alopecia

Several techniques have been tested to prevent chemotherapy-induced hair loss, the first being scalp tourniquets. These were used to minimize the contact the drug had with the hair follicles by occluding, using pressure, the superficial blood vessels supplying the scalp (Maxwell 1980). However, while some investigators found scalp tourniquets effective, others reported this method to be time-consuming, uncomfortable or ineffective (Parker 1987). Research findings indicate that scalp hypothermia may be simpler, less traumatic and more effective as a means of preventing alopecia when compared with the scalp tourniquet (David & Speechley 1987). Scalp cooling has an advantage over the scalp tourniquet in that it inhibits the cellular uptake of a drug that is temperature dependent (Dean *et al.* 1979).

More recently, biological methods of preventing hair loss have focused on promoting hair growth or protecting the hair follicles (Batchelor 2001). For example:

- Minoxidil 2% topical solution applied twice a day (Shapiro & Price 1998).
- Topical topitriol (Hidalgo *et al.* 1999).
- Application of a steroid 5-α reductase inhibitor (Uno & Kurata 1993).
- Immunosuppressive immunophilin ligands such as cyclosporin (Maurer *et al.* 1997), immunomodulators, AS101 (Sredni *et al.* 1996), CDK2 inhibitors (Davis *et al.* 2001) and P53 (a mediator of cellular response which is essential for chemotherapy-induced hair loss) (Vladimir *et al.* 2000).

The scientific rationale for scalp cooling

The rationale is based on characteristics of hair growth, the effect of cytotoxic drugs on hair follicles, physiological changes in scalp circulation and pharmacokinetics (Keller & Blausey 1988). Ninety per cent of all scalp hair is in an active phase of growth. The growth phase is characterized by significant mitotic activity; this means the hair bulb is especially sensitive to chemotherapeutic agents (Parker 1987). Scalp hypothermia produces changes in the scalp circulation by causing vasoconstriction of superficial vessels. Decreased blood flow to the scalp reduces the amount of the drug reaching the hair follicles and thus minimizes damage to the scalp hair (Kennedy *et al.* 1983; Parker 1987). Its success is also related to the metabolic effects of cooling, i.e. slowing the metabolic rate (Bulow *et al.* 1985), and it also appears that the degree of hair loss is temperature dependent. In order to prevent alopecia the temperature of the scalp must be reduced to at least 24°C but preferably 22°C (Gregory *et al.* 1982). Caps have to be kept in a freezer in order to reach temperatures of −18 to −20°C (Anderson *et al.* 1981; Kennedy *et al.* 1983; Giacone *et al.* 1988). Then when the cap is placed on the head the scalp temperature will drop from 37°C to 23–24°C within the first 15 minutes (Guy *et al.* 1982; Tollenaar *et al.* 1994). This is why a preinjection scalp cooling time of 20–30 minutes is said to be required (Anderson *et al.* 1981; Kennedy *et al.* 1983; Satterwhite & Zimm 1984; Middleton *et al.* 1985; Robinson 1987; Giacone *et al.* 1988).

Scalp cooling has been used in an attempt to reduce hair loss with palliative whole-brain radiotherapy. However, a pilot study (Shah *et al.* 2000) found that all patients still lost their hair and there was evidence that the cold cap application increased the dose of radiotherapy to the scalp.

Types of drugs

Doxorubin is commonly used in cancer chemotherapy and has a uniquely short half-life of approximately 30 minutes (compared to other drugs, such as cyclophosphamide which has a plasma half-life of over 6 hours) (Priestman 1989). This factor makes prophylactic scalp cooling feasible because it need only be utilized during peak plasma levels (Cline 1984). This is particularly important since doxorubicin results in a consistently high incidence of alopecia (80–90% of all patients), often leading to total hair loss (Dean *et al.* 1983). The involvement of doxorubicin, whether used alone or in combination, is a feature of most of the reported scalp cooling studies. In some studies, there was less success in maintaining hair with increasing doses of doxorubicin and/or liver metastases (Dean *et al.* 1983; David & Speechley 1987), but this may be resolved by extending the time the cap remains in place following chemotherapy administration.

Scalp cooling has also been used during the administration of epirubicin, as a single agent, with good results (Robinson 1987), although doses may influence outcomes (Adams *et al.* 1992). Subsequent studies have investigated combination regimens containing epirubicin and other drugs such as cyclophosphamide and 5-fluorouracil, with results of mild to moderate hair loss. However, when intravenous cyclophosphamide is added to any single agent anthracycline, the success rate is reduced from 80% of patients keeping most of their hair to about 50–60% of patients (Middleton

et al. 1985; David & Speechley 1987). Some authors have therefore concluded that when combinations of cyclophosphamide and anthracyclines are given, scalp cooling has no place at all (Tollenaar *et al.* 1994). The group of drugs known as the taxanes also have the unfortunate side-effect of total alopecia; however, there is now evidence that using scalp cooling in patients receiving docetaxel and paclitaxel can prevent complete hair loss (Lemanager *et al.* 1995, 1997; Katsimbri 2000; MacDuff *et al.* 2003).

Techniques

Most of the studies that used an ice cap method of scalp cooling used a 'homemade' or commercial cap (Anderson *et al.* 1981; Dean *et al.* 1983; David & Speechley 1987; Lemanager *et al.* 1997).

Homemade caps

Initially scalp cooling was achieved using crushed ice in plastic bags (Dean *et al.* 1979). A study of the efficacy of using a moulded prefrozen ice cap handmade from cryogel bags was conducted at The Royal Marsden Hospital (Anderson *et al.* 1981; David & Speechley 1987).

Cryogel caps

The first commercial cap (Kold Kap) was successful in reducing hair loss, particularly with higher doses of doxorubicin (Dean *et al.* 1983). A three-layer cap (inner cotton, middle cryogel, outer lamb's wool) was also reported to prevent total hair loss (Howard & Stenner 1983). However, Wheelock *et al.* (1984) found that most patients suffered from severe hair loss even with the use of the Kold Kap. The most recent work has involved the use of cryogel caps such as the Chemocap and Penguin caps, which have been used for patients receiving single agents and combinations of anthracyclines (Peck 2000; Katsimbri 2000; Christodoulou *et al.* 2002) as well as in the use of docetaxel (Lemanager *et al.* 1995, 1997).

A large (170 patients) randomized study comparing Chemocap with the gelpack method found no statistical difference in efficacy between the two caps but Chemocap was shown to be more comfortable and offered a better fit, as well as being easier to use (Dougherty 2006).

Scalp cooling machines

Attempts have been made to produce an alternative type of cap that would improve effectiveness of scalp cooling, in particular to achieve a temperature that ensures a sufficiently low and constant reduction in scalp temperature that would endure during the entire procedure. Two types of scalp cooling machine have been designed:

1 Refrigerated cooling systems where liquid coolant is pumped via a cap and maintains a more reliable temperature. Guy *et al.* (1982) reported encouraging results when the thermocirculator was first introduced, although

Tollenaar *et al.* (1994) found that when used with patients receiving fluorouracil, epirubicin and cyclophosphamide (FEC), there was still a 50% chance of total alopecia occurring.

2 The other scalp cooling machines appear to provide a more comfortable and effective system, e.g. Paxman (Massey 2004) and digitized systems (Ridderheim *et al.* 2003). The use of refrigerated air passed over the patient's scalp via a hair-drying helmet was reported to be beneficial in over 50% of patients, with most experiencing no hair loss or slight hair loss and six requiring a wig (Symonds & McCormick 1986). However, other authors found that the system was only successful at lower doses of epirubicin (Adams *et al.* 1992).

There have also been good results using an electrically cooled cap in patients receiving cyclophosphamide, methotrexate and fluorouracil (CMF) chemotherapy (Ron *et al.* 1997).

Limitations of scalp cooling studies

Despite the large number of studies on scalp cooling they are difficult to compare with one another, owing to the multiple variables: different types of scalp cooling caps, varying methods of applying the caps, different chemotherapy regimens, tools for assessment of hair loss and who performs the assessment. Also sample numbers are often small and few studies are randomized or have a control group (Grevelman & Breed 2005; Dougherty 2006). This results in difficulties when making decisions related to selection of scalp cooling systems, discussing the risk of scalp metastases, or even whether to offer scalp cooling at all (Breed 2004; Christodoulou *et al.* 2005; Grevelman & Breed 2005; Randall & Ream 2005).

Factors which influence success

The success of all these methods in preventing hair loss varies and the amount of hair loss experienced by the patient is dependent on a number of factors:

■ Involvement of the liver with metastatic disease leads to elevated plasma levels of doxorubicin for a longer period. Early studies seemed to indicate that extension of the cooling period did not seem to improve the results (Satterwhite & Zimm 1984) but more recent studies are finding longer cooling times in general improve success rates (Massey 2004).
■ Inadequate cooling because of exceptionally thick hair may lead to partial loss. It has been demonstrated that maximum cooling occurs 20 minutes after the cap has been placed in position.
■ The weight of the cap (as well as the temperature) may be a factor, as this ensures that the contact is maintained over the complete scalp (Hunt *et al.* 1982).
■ Success does not appear to be dose dependent, as was first thought (David & Speechley 1987; Dougherty 2006).

■ It seems likely that when anthracyclines are used in combination with other drugs that cause alopecia (e.g. etoposide and cyclophosphamide) the success rate is not as high as with anthracyclines alone (Middleton *et al.* 1985). It has also been found that the type of anthracycline used will affect success rates as hair loss is greater in doxorubicin and cyclophosphamide than when using epirubicin and cyclophosphamide (Dougherty 2006).

Patient selection

All patients with solid tumours receiving doxorubicin, epirubicin or docetaxel as a single agent or in combination should be offered scalp cooling. However, scalp cooling should not be offered to (Dougherty 2005):

■ Patients with haematological disease unless the consultant feels it is appropriate to offer scalp cooling on the basis of quality of life.
■ Patients receiving drugs that cause hair loss, e.g. vincristine, where there is no research or evidence of the effectiveness of scalp cooling.
■ Patients who have already received a first course of chemotherapy which may induce hair loss but who were not offered or declined scalp cooling.

Patients must give consent for the procedure but must first be fully informed about the nature and length of the procedure, the chances of success and, where appropriate, the risk of scalp metastases (Peck 2000). Scalp cooling can be a long and uncomfortable procedure and should not be offered unless it is beneficial or the patient insists on undergoing the procedure. Patients must also be informed that they may discontinue the procedure at any time if they find it too physically or psychologically traumatic (Tierney 1987) or if they fail to retain hair.

Research shows that scalp cooling can be very distressing (Tierney *et al.* 1989), although patients still find it a worthwhile procedure to undergo regardless of whether or not it is successful and would have it again if necessary (Dougherty 1996, 2006). It has also been shown that the severity and distress associated with hair loss may be less for those who use scalp cooling (Protiere *et al.* 2002). Patients have reported adverse effects during and following treatment such as headaches, claustrophobia and ice phobias (Tierney *et al.* 1989; Dougherty 2006). Nurses need to understand the meaning that hair loss has for the patient. Alopecia can cause depression, loss of self-confidence and humiliation: it is a very visible sign of cancer. Patients who have relapsed and are undergoing further chemotherapy which causes alopecia may find the loss of hair a second time to be more devastating (Gallagher 1996).

Supporting the patient

It is important to ensure that if a patient fails to retain hair or decides not to undergo scalp cooling, adequate time is spent helping the patient to adapt to the hair loss physically, psychologically and socially. It is recommended that nursing interventions be directed towards helping the patient and family to adapt to alopecia by using patient education, available resources and supportive listening (Pickard-Holley 1995). This can be partly achieved by ensuring that the patient sees the surgical appliance officer as soon as possible, in order to obtain a wig that can be matched to the patient's desired hair style and colour. Advice can be given on hair care such as the type of shampoo. There is a misconception that a mild shampoo such as baby shampoo is best, but this kind of shampoo is alkaline and it is recommended that a neutral pH shampoo be used (Dougherty 2005, 2006). Using a wide-toothed comb can prevent pulling on hair but the patient should not be afraid to comb hair daily (Dougherty 2006). Patients should be advised to avoid anything that can dry out their hair such as using hair dryers, curlers, etc., or using chemicals such as perming lotions or hair dyes, and should seek advice from a hairdresser. Finally the patient should be given advice about the use of head covering such as hats, turbans and scarves. All verbal information should be reinforced with a hair care information booklet (Pickard-Holley 1995; Batchelor 2001).

Procedure guidelines   Scalp cooling

Equipment

1 A scalp cooling cap, e.g. Chemocap.
2 Overcap.
3 Skin protection, e.g. gauze, cotton wool pads.

4 Comfortable chair (recliner) or bed.
5 Extra pillows and blankets as required.

Procedure

Action	Rationale
1 Before beginning, it is important to explain and discuss the procedure fully with the patient. Explain that the coldest and most uncomfortable time is the first 15 minutes after the cap has been applied. The patient should understand that the scalp cooling can be discontinued at any time and that it will not jeopardize the chemotherapy.	To ensure that the patient understands the procedure and what the success rate is likely to be depending on the type of chemotherapy regimen he/she is receiving (Dougherty 2006: R 2b). Patients who have undergone scalp cooling highlighted this as important knowledge to share when first undergoing scalp cooling (Dougherty 2006: P). To ensure that the patient gives his/her valid consent and knows that if the scalp cooling does not work, he/she can obtain a wig (E; NMC 2006: C).
2 Check the cap has been in the freezer for a minimum of 12 hours (temperature −25 to −32°E).	To ensure the cap is cold enough to be effective (C).
3 Place the cap on the patient's head, making sure it fits closely and covers the whole hairline (see Action figure 3).	To ensure cooling over the head, including all the hair roots (E).
4 Apply the overcap to the patient's head (see Action figure 4).	To ensure even and close contact of the cap to the scalp (C; Dougherty 2006, R 2b).
5 Place protection in any areas where the cap touches the skin.	To prevent cold injury and improve the patient's comfort (E; P) .
6 Place a pillow behind the patient's head if required.	To provide support for the patient's head and neck and to reduce the effect of the heaviness of the cap (P; Dougherty 1996: R 2b).
7 Offer the patient the use of a blanket.	To provide the patient with some protection against the feeling of cold (P; Dougherty 1996 R2b).
8 Leave the patient for at least 15 minutes before injection of the drug.	To obtain initial cooling of the scalp (Hunt *et al.* 1982: R 4; Lemanager *et al.* 1997: R 2b; Dougherty 2006: R 2b).

9 Administer the drug by intravenous injection as per prescription.	To administer treatment as appropriate (E).
10 The cap must be changed after 30 minutes regardless of the stage of administration.	To maintain adequate cooling (C; Hunt *et al.* 1982 R 4; Lemanager *et al.* 1997: R 2b; Dougherty 2006: R 2b).
11 If a drug takes longer than 30 minutes to administer the cap will need to be changed after 45–60 minutes and then every hour thereafter depending on the type of drug and the temperature of the freezer.	To maintain adequate cooling (C; Dougherty 2006: R 2b).
12 On completion of the drug (i.e. the one likely to cause alopecia, e.g. doxorubicin), leave the patient for a further 45 minutes.	To maintain cooling until the plasma levels of drug have fallen (Hunt *et al.* 1982: R 4; Lemanager *et al.* 1997: R 2b; Dougherty 2006 R 2b).
13 When sufficient time has elapsed, remove the cap.	To prevent damage to the scalp and hair (E, P).
14 Encourage the patient to rest, if desired.	To prevent the patient feeling faint when the cap is lifted off the head (P, E).
15 Wash the cap, dry and store on cardboard insert.	To minimize cross-infection and to maintain shape (E).
16 Ensure the patient is given the booklet 'Hair care and hair loss' (Patient information series).	To reinforce verbal information given during procedure (E, P, E).

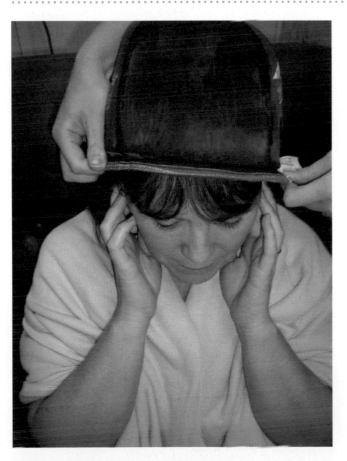

Action 3 Placing cap on the patient's head.

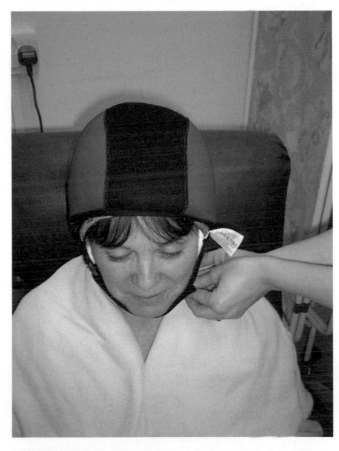

Action 4 Applying the over cap.

Problem solving: Scalp cooling

Problem	Cause	Suggested action
Inadequate cooling.	Poorly fitting cap. Cap not sufficiently cooled.	Follow the procedure carefully. Ensure the cap size is correct and that the hair roots are covered. Ensure the cap is changed at correct times. Check the cap has been cooled to the correct temperature.
Excess cooling.	Thin hair.	Use plenty of gauze between the cap and scalp. If it is still painful then discontinue the procedure.
Complaints of headache.	Weight and coldness of cap.	Provide physical support to the neck and shoulders and blankets as required.
Distressed patient.	Claustrophobia.	Support and reassure the patient. If necessary, remove the cap.
	Ice phobia.	Be aware of this possible problem; encourage the patient to discuss their feelings.
Hair loss.	Scalp cooling was not successful.	Offer the patient the opportunity to discontinue the scalp cooling. Make arrangements for the patient to see the appliance officer and obtain a wig. Discuss care of hair and scalp and give patient information booklet.

References and further reading

Adams, L. *et al.* (1992) The prevention of hair loss from chemotherapy by the use of cold air scalp cooling. *Eur J Cancer Care*, **15**, 16–18.

Anderson, J. *et al.* (1981) Prevention of doxorubicin-induced alopecia by scalp cooling in patients with advanced breast cancer. *Br Med J*, **282**, 423–4.

Batchelor, D. (2001) Hair and cancer chemotherapy. *Eur J Cancer Care*, **10**, 147–63.

Breed, W.P. (2004) What is wrong with the 30 year old practice of scalp cooling for prevention of chemotherapy induced alopecia. *Support Care Cancer*, **12**(1), 3–5.

Bulow, J. *et al.* (1985) Frontal subcutaneous blood flow and epiand subcutaneous temperatures during scalp cooling in normal man. *Scand J Clin Lab Invest*, **45**, 505–8.

Burdine, S.A. (2001) *Who Needs Hair–The Flipside of Chemotherapy*. Saba Books, Florida.

Carr, K. (1998) How I survived the fall out. *You Magazine, Mail on Sunday*, 10 May, pp. 61–7.

Christodoulou, C. *et al.* (2002) Effectiveness of the MSC cold cap system in the prevention of chemotherapy induced alopecia. *Oncology*, **62**(2), 97–102.

Christodoulou, C. *et al.* (2005) Scalp metastases and scalp cooling for chemotherapy induced alopecia prevention. *Ann Oncol*, **17**(2), 350.

Cline, B.W. (1984) Prevention of chemotherapy-induced alopecia; a review of the literature. *Cancer Nurs*, **7**(3), 221–8.

Crowe, M., Kendrick, M. & Woods, S. (1998) Is scalp cooling a procedure that should be offered to patients receiving alopecia induced chemotherapy for solid tumours? Proceedings of 10th International Conference on Cancer Nursing, Jerusalem, Abstract, p. 64.

David, J.A. & Speechley, V. (1987) Scalp cooling to prevent alopecia. *Nurs Times*, **83**(32), 36–7.

Davis, S.T. *et al.* (2001) Prevention of chemotherapy induced alopecia in rats by CDC inhibitors. *Science*, **5**(291), 25–6.

Dean, J.C. *et al.* (1979) Prevention of doxorubicin-induced hair loss with scalp hypothermia. *N Engl J Med*, **301**, 1427–9.

Dean, J.C. *et al.* (1983) Scalp hypothermia: a comparison of ice packs and the Kold Kap in the prevention of doxorubicin-induced alopecia. *J Clin Oncol*, **1**(1), 33–7.

Dougherty, L. (1996) Scalp cooling to prevent hair loss in chemotherapy. *Prof Nurse*, **11**(8), 1–3.

Dougherty, L (2005) Alopecia. In: *The Royal Marsden Hospital Handbook of Cancer Chemotherapy* (eds D. Brighton & M. Wood). Elsevier Churchill Livingstone, Edinburgh, pp. 197–200.

Dougherty, L. (2006) A study to compare two methods of scalp cooling to prevent chemotherapy induced alopecia. *Cancer Nurs Pract*, **6**, 25–31.

Freedman, T.G. (1994) Social and cultural dimensions of hair loss in women treated with breast cancer. *Cancer Nurs*, **174**, 334.

Gallagher, J. (1996) Women's experiences of hair loss associated with chemotherapy – longitudinal perspective. Proceedings of 9th International Conference on Cancer Nursing, Brighton, Abstract, p. 52.

Gallagher, J. (1997) Chemotherapy induced hair loss – impact on a woman's quality of life. *Qual Life*, **5**(4), 75–8.

Giacone, G. *et al.* (1988) Scalp hypothermia in the prevention of doxorubicin induced hair loss. *Cancer Nurs*, **11**(3), 170–3.

Gregory, R.P. *et al.* (1982) Prevention of doxorubicin induced alopecia by scalp hypothermia: relation to degree of cooling. *Br Med J*, **284**, 1674.

Grevelman E.G. & Breed W.P. (2005) Prevention of chemotherapy induced hair loss by scalp cooling. *Ann Oncol*, **16**, 352–8.

Guy, R. *et al.* (1982) Scalp cooling by thermocirculator. *Lancet*, **1**(8278), 937–8.

Hidalgo, G.M. *et al.* (1999) A phase I trial of topical topitriol. *Anticancer Drugs*, **10**(4), 393–5.

Howard, N. & Stenner, R.W. (1983) Technical notes – an improved 'ice cap' to prevent alopecia caused by adriamycin (doxorubicin). *Br J Radiol*, **56**, 963–4.

Hunt, J. *et al.* (1982) Scalp hypothermia to prevent adriamycin-induced hair loss. *Cancer Nurs*, **5**(1), 25–31.

Katsimbri, P. (2000) Prevention of chemotherapy induced alopecia using an effective scalp cooling system. *Eur J Cancer Care*, **36**, 766–71.

Keller, J.F. & Blausey, L.A. (1988) Nursing issues and management in chemotherapy-induced alopecia. *Oncol Nurs Forum*, **15**(5), 603–7.

Kendell, P. (2001) Magic gel that helps cancer patients hold onto their hair. *Daily Mail*, 6 January, p.19.

Kennedy, M. *et al.* (1983) The effects of using Chemocap on occurrence of chemotherapy induced alopecia. *Oncol Nurs Forum*, **10**(1), 19–24.

Lemanager, M. *et al.* (1995) Docetaxel induced alopecia can be prevented. *Lancet*, **346**, 371–2.

Lemanager, M. *et al.* (1997) Effectiveness of cold cap in the prevention of docetaxel induced alopecia. *Eur J Cancer*, **33**(2), 297–300.

Lemanager, M. *et al.* (1998) Alopecia induced by chemotherapy – a controllable side effect. *Oncol Nurs Today*, **3**(2), 18–20.

MacDuff, C. *et al.* (2003) The effectiveness of scalp cooling in preventing alopecia for patients receiving epirubicin and docetaxel. *Eur J Cancer Care*, **12**, 154–61.

Massey, A. (2004) A multicentre study to determine the efficacy and patient acceptability of the Paxman scalp cooler to prevent hair loss in patients receiving chemotherapy. *Eur J Oncol Nurs*, **8**(2), 121–30.

Maurer, M. *et al.* (1997) Hair growth modulation by topical immunophilin ligands. *Am J Pathol*, **150**(4), 1433–41.

Maxwell, M.B. (1980) Scalp tourniquets for chemotherapy-induced alopecia. *Am J Nurs*, **5**, 900–2.

Middleton, J. *et al.* (1985) Failure of scalp hypothermia to prevent hair loss when cyclophosphamide is added to doxorubicin and vincristine. *Cancer Treat Rep*, **69**(4), 373–5.

Munstedt, K. *et al.* (1997) Changes in self concept and body image during alopecia induced cancer chemotherapy. *Support Care Cancer*, **5**, 139–43.

NMC (2006) *A–Z Advice Sheet Consent.* www.nmc.org.

Parker, R. (1987) The effectiveness of scalp hypothermia in preventing cyclophosphamide induced alopecia. *Oncol Nurs Forum*, **14**(6), 49–53.

Peck, H.J. (2000) Evaluating the efficacy of scalp cooling using Penguin cold caps. *Eur J Cancer Care*, **4**(4), 246–8.

Pickard-Holley, S. (1995) The symptom experience of alopecia. *Semin Oncol Nurs*, **11**(4), 235–8.

Priestman, T.J. (1989) *Cancer Chemotherapy: an Introduction*, 3rd edn. Springer, Berlin.

Protiere, C. *et al.* (2002) Efficacy and tolerance of a scalp cooling system for prevention of hair loss and the experience of breast cancer patients treated by adjuvant chemotherapy. *Support Care Cancer*, **10**, 529–37.

Purohit, O.P. *et al.* (1992) A 6 week chemotherapy regimen for relapsed lymphoma efficacy results and the influence of scalp cooling. *Ann Oncol*, **3**(Suppl 5), 126.

Randall, J. & Ream, E. (2005) Hair loss with chemotherapy: at a loss over its management. *Eur J Cancer Care*, **14**, 223–31.

Ridderheim, M., Bjurburg, M. & Gustavsson, A. (2003) Scalp hypothermia to prevent chemotherapy-induced alopecia is effective and safe: a pilot study of a new digitized scalp-cooling system used in 74 patients. *Support Care Cancer*, **11**, 371–7.

Robinson, M.H. (1987) Effectiveness of scalp cooling in reducing alopecia caused by epirubicin treatment of advanced breast cancer. *Cancer Treat Rep*, **71**, 913–14.

Ron, I.G. *et al.* (1997) Scalp cooling in the prevention of alopecia in patients receiving depilating chemotherapy. *Support Care Cancer*, **5**, 136–8.

Satterwhite, B. & Zimm, S. (1984) The use of scalp hypothermia in the prevention of doxorubicin-induced hair loss. *Cancer*, **54**, 34–7.

Shah, N. *et al.* (2000) A pilot study to assess the feasibility of prior scalp cooling of palliative whole brain radiotherapy. *Br J Radiol*, **73**, 514–16.

Shapiro, J. & Price, V.H. (1998) Hair regrowth: therapeutic agents. *Dermatol Clin*, **16**(2), 341–56.

Sredni, B. *et al.* (1996) The protective role of the immunomodulator AS101 against chemotherapy induced alopecia: studies on humans and animals. *Cancer Res*, **65**, 97–103.

Symonds, R.P. & McCormick, C.V. (1986) Adriamycin alopecia prevented by cold air scalp cooling. *Am J Clin Oncol*, **9**(5), 454–7.

Tierney, A.J. (1987) Preventing chemotherapy-induced alopecia in cancer patients: is scalp cooling worthwhile? *J Adv Nurs*, **12**, 303–10.

Tierney, A.J. *et al.* (1989) *A Study to Inform Nursing Support of Patients Coping with Chemotherapy for Breast Cancer.* Report prepared for the Scottish Home and Health Department. Nursing Research Unit, Department of Nursing Studies, University of Edinburgh.

Tollenaar, R.A.E.M. *et al.* (1994) Scalp cooling has no place in the prevention of alopecia in adjuvant chemotherapy in breast cancer. *Eur J Cancer*, **30A**(10), 1448–53.

Uno, H. & Kurata, S. (1993) Chemical agents and peptide affect hair growth. *J Invest Dermatol*, **101**(1), S143–8.

Vladimir, A.B. *et al.* (2000) P53 is essential for chemotherapy induced hair loss. *Cancer Res*, **60**, 5002–6.

Wheelock, J.B. *et al.* (1984) Ineffectiveness of scalp hypothermia in the prevention of alopecia in patients treated with doxorubicin and cisplatin combinations. *Cancer Treat Rep*, **68**, 1387–8.

Williams, J. *et al.* (1999) A narrative study of chemotherapy induced alopecia. *Oncol Nurs Forum*, **26**(9), 1463–8.

Wilson, C. (1994) The ice cap that could help save your hair. *Daily Mail*, 20 September, pp. 36–7.

Witman, G. *et al.* (1981) Misuse of scalp hypothermia. *Cancer Treat Rep*, **65**(5–6), 507–8.

Chapter 40

Specimen collection for microbiological analysis

775 Reference material
781 *Procedure guidelines:* Specimen collection: section swabs
784 *Procedure guidelines:* Specimen collection: body fluid
789 *Procedure guidelines:* Cervical uterine smear or Pap smear
793 References and further reading

Definition

Specimen collection is the collection of a required amount of tissue or fluid for laboratory examination, to allow for the isolation and identification of micro-organisms that cause disease, and to determine their antimicrobial sensitivity to guide the doctor with the selection of appropriate antimicrobial therapy (Mims *et al*. 2004).

Indications

Specimen collection is required when microbiological, biochemical or other laboratory investigations are indicated. Nursing staff should be able to identify the need for microbiological investigations and, if appropriate, initiate the taking of specimens (Papasian & Kragel 1997; Higgins 2007). Specimen collection is often a first crucial step in investigations that define the nature of the disease and determine diagnosis and the mode of treatment.

The clinical microbiology laboratory plays a fundamental role in the diagnosis of infection and an increasingly important role in reducing new antibiotic resistance (Peterson *et al*. 2001). Its importance increases in immunosuppressed and myelosuppressed cancer patients because the usual signs and symptoms of infection may be absent (Shelton 1999) and due to the significant associated morbidity and mortality (Sandin & Rinaldi 1996).

Reference material

General principles

Successful laboratory diagnosis depends on the collection of specimens at the appropriate time, using the correct technique and equipment and transporting them to the designated laboratory safely without delay. For this to be achieved, good liaison is essential between medical, nursing, portering and laboratory staff (Higgins 2007).

The first step in the accurate diagnosis of infectious disease is to recognize the need to obtain adequate specimens for microbiological examination. Signs of infection such as fever should trigger a careful clinical assessment to ensure unnecessary tests are avoided and the most useful laboratory samples are obtained to identify therapeutic options (O'Grady *et al*. 1998).

The nurse's role is:

- To identify the need for and importance of microbiological investigation.
- To initiate, if appropriate, the taking of a swab or specimen, e.g. during wound dressing it is usually the nurse who identifies signs of infection (Gilchrist 2000).
- To know the appropriate investigation to be undertaken so as to avoid indiscriminate specimen collection which wastes time and money.
- To collect the desired material in the correct container.
- To arrange prompt delivery to the laboratory.

Close communication between the doctor and the laboratory is important, especially when unusual infections are suspected or the patient is immunosuppressed, as the infection may be caused by unusual organisms whose identification requires special techniques (Thomson 2002).

Collection of specimens

If specimens of poor quality are sent to the microbiology department, then the results may be of little or no clinical utility (Wilson 1996; Higgins 2007). The greater the quantity of material sent for laboratory examination, the greater the chance of isolating a causative organism. Other considerations include the type of organisms and their growth requirements. Aerobic bacteria will grow in the presence of air (Gold & Eisenstein 2000). Anaerobic bacteria fail to grow in air, preferring an atmosphere reduced of oxygen. Facultative bacteria can grow in either the presence or absence of air. Fastidious bacteria require selective plating media to encourage growth (Finegold 2000), and may not survive prolonged storage or may be overgrown with less fastidious organisms, before cultures can be made (Gill *et al*. 2004). A delay in transporting a specimen to the laboratory can compromise the specimen integrity and cause a false negative or positive result (Peterson *et al*. 2001).

There are many types of specimen collection tools, for example, swabs and pots. Advice should be sought from the microbiology department with regard to the best type of container required for unusual specimens. It is essential that the specimen and its transport container are appropriate for the infection being investigated, to ensure that adequate quantity of material is obtained to allow complete microbiological examination. Material from skin and mucous membranes can be collected by a swab, which generally contains a transport medium. This is designed to preserve micro-organisms, while preventing the multiplication of rapidly growing organisms, which makes identification easier. Unfortunately only a limited amount of material can be collected by this means; therefore pus should be collected in a syringe which can be transferred to a sterile container (Wilson & Jenner 2006). Biopsy material, pus, fluid or tissue removed surgically provide ideal material in adequate quantities for appropriate microbiological smears and cultures (Gill *et al*. 2004).

Specimens are readily contaminated by poor technique. Cultures taken from such specimens often result in confusing or misleading results. Aseptic technique must be used when collecting specimens to avoid inadvertent contamination of the site of sample or the specimen (Macleod 1992). Specimens must be collected in sterile containers with close-fitting lids and swabs must never be removed from their sterile containers until everything is ready for taking the sample.

Ideally, samples should be collected before beginning any treatment, e.g. antibiotics or antiseptics. If the patient is receiving such treatment at the same time the specimen is collected, the laboratory staff must be informed. Both antibiotics and antiseptics may destroy organisms that are, in fact, active in the patient and will affect the outcome of the laboratory test. Specimens should also be obtained using safe technique and practices (Higgins 2007). For example, gloves should always be worn when handling all body fluids. Cross-infection precautionary measures should always be undertaken if an infection is suspected until a full microbiology report has been given and the causative agent confirmed (Wilson & Jenner 2001).

Documentation

Requests for microbiological investigations must include the following information:

- Patient's name, ward and/or department.
- Hospital number.
- Date specimen collected.
- Time specimen collected.
- Diagnosis.
- Relevant signs and symptoms.
- Relevant history, e.g. recent foreign travel.
- Any antimicrobial drug being taken by the patient.
- Type of specimen.
- Consultant's name.
- Name of the doctor who ordered the investigation, as it may be necessary to telephone the result before the typed report is dispatched.
- If the specimen is high risk, it should be labelled with a 'danger of infection' label (Health Services Advisory Committee 2003).

Without full information, it is impossible to examine a specimen adequately or to report it accurately. The most common reason for specimens to be rejected by the laboratory is improper labelling of the specimen (Malarkey & McMorrow 2005). Incorrectly or unlabelled specimens will normally be discarded (Health Services Advisory Committee 2003).

Transportation of specimens

Guidelines are now available on the labelling, transport and reception of specimens (Health Services Advisory Committee 2003). Specimens that need to be transported outside the hospital, e.g. by van, car, taxi or by post, must be transported in an adequate leak-proof primary container, a leak-proof secondary container and an outer box to comply with British Standards ISO 6710 (British Standards Institute 1995). Laboratory technicians will undertake this task, following local written instructions relating to containment, labelling and transport boxes (Health Services Advisory Committee 2003).

The sooner a specimen arrives in the laboratory, the greater is the chance of organisms present surviving and being identified. Delays will cause changes that may radically alter the result. The laboratory count of bacteria in a de-

layed specimen could be significantly different from that of the specimen when it was collected (Shanson 1999; Higgins 2007).

If specimens cannot be sent to a laboratory immediately, they should be stored as follows:

- Blood culture samples in a 37°C incubator (Higgins 2007).
- All other specimens in a specimen refrigerator at a temperature of 4°C, where the low temperature will slow the bacterial growth (Higgins 2007).

In diagnostic pathology it is likely that at any given time there will be a number of specimens that present a risk of infection. Every health authority, therefore, must ensure that medical, nursing, phlebotomy, laboratory, portering and any other staff involved in handling specimens are trained to do so (RCN 2005). The person collecting the specimen must ensure that the specimen container used is an appropriate one for the purpose, is properly closed and has not been externally contaminated by the contents (Health Services Advisory Committee 2003). Any accidental spillage must be cleaned up immediately by staff, who should wear gloves and other appropriate protective clothing to prevent contamination. Ideally, all specimens should be placed in a double self-sealing bag with one compartment containing the request form and the other the specimen. Specimens should be transported to the laboratory in boxes or deep-sided trays which are not used for any other purpose, are disinfected weekly and whenever contaminated (Health Services Advisory Committee 2003).

It is essential to remember that there will always be patients or specimens that have not been identified as presenting a particular risk of infection. If a specimen is suspected or known to present an infectious hazard, the person taking the specimen has the responsibility to ensure that the form and containers are correctly labelled with a biohazard label, to enable those handling the specimen to take appropriate precautions (Health Services Advisory Committee 2003).

Specimens from patients who have recently been treated with toxic therapy, i.e. gene therapy, drugs, radioactivity or active metabolites, need to be handled with caution. (See Chapter 19 for further information related to gene therapy specimen collection). Local rules must be compiled, which will outline how such specimens should be labelled, bagged and transported to the laboratory. For example, in the case of gene therapy the specimen must be labelled with a biohazard label, double bagged and transported to the laboratory in a secure transport box with a fastenable lid. Each box must carry a warning label, and be made of smooth impervious material such as plastic or metal which will retain liquid and can be easily disinfected and cleaned in the event of leakage of the specimen (Health Services Advisory Committee 2003). (See Chapter 36 for further information related to unsealed sources and specimen collection.)

Types of investigation

Bacterial

A wide range of methods are available for obtaining cultures and identifying organisms from a specimen or swab. To employ all these tests would be time consuming and costly. Testing, therefore, tends to be selective. It is at this stage that the laboratory request form plays a particularly important part. A faecal specimen, for example, from a patient with diarrhoea who also has a recent history of foreign travel, would be investigated for organisms not normally looked for in faecal specimens from patients without such a history.

The majority of specimens undergo microscopic investigation. This is valuable as an early indication of the causative organisms in an infection. The specimen is often cultured for 24–48 hours longer in the case of blood cultures. Prolonged incubation (up to 21 days) may be required for growth of some organisms, e.g. *Brucella* species (Mims *et al.* 2004). This is followed by antibiotic sensitivity testing on any pathogenic organisms that are isolated. This involves the application of paper discs impregnated with antibiotics onto the agar plates. After overnight incubation during which time the growth of bacteria may be inhibited by the antibiotic disc, the zones of inhibition can be observed for the degree of sensitivity of the organism (Mims *et al.* 2004).

Viral

In order to interpret positive viral specimens, the choice of specimen and time of collection in relation to the onset of the patient's illness and transportation to the laboratory are all of prime importance (Baker *et al.* 1998). The collection of specimens for virology investigations should ideally be discussed with the microbiology laboratory beforehand (Shanson 1999). There are three main laboratory techniques available for the diagnosis of viral infections (Baker *et al.* 1998):

- Direct microscopy.
- Culture (isolation of growth in living cell systems).
- Serology.

For culture specimens the use of viral transport media and speed of delivery to the laboratory are important as viruses do not survive well outside the body. With good liaison, the nurses should obtain the specimen when the laboratory staff have the transport ready to take it to the virus laboratories. If delays occur, the specimen should be refrigerated at a temperature of 4°C, but never frozen in normal refrigerator freezers, where the temperature is around −20°C, as viruses may die rapidly at this temperature (Shanson 1999).

The time at which specimens are collected for viral investigations is important. Many viral illnesses have a prodromal phase during which the multiplication and shedding of the virus are at a peak and the patient is most infectious (Mims *et al.* 2004). Immunocompromised patients are particularly susceptible to viral respiratory tract infections. When an upper respiratory specimen is collected it is important to ensure the recovery of respiratory epithelial cells from the lining of the upper part of the nasal passage. To obtain an adequate number of cells nasopharyngeal swabs, aspirates and washes need to be undertaken correctly (Buller 2000). See procedure guidelines for nasopharyngeal specimen collection, below.

Serological

Serological testing for the presence of antigens and antibodies is used when it is not possible to isolate the organism easily from the patient's tissue. By demonstrating serum antibodies to suspected organisms it is inferred that the patient is, or has been, infected with the organism. Despite the disadvantage of the test being performed retrospectively, antibody testing is the main method of diagnosing viral infections (Mims *et al.* 2004). A single test is inadequate as if the titres (the concentration of the substance being measured) are raised it is impossible to determine whether this is due to past or present infection. Two tests need to be carried out, both of which involve the collection of 10 ml of blood once at the beginning of the illness and again 10–14 days later. If a rising titre level is demonstrated it suggests the patient's infection is current (Mims *et al.* 2004).

Mycosis

Although many pathogenic fungi will grow on ordinary bacteriological culture media, they grow better and with less risk of bacterial overgrowth on special mycological media. The presence of fungi in clinical specimens is difficult to interpret, as *Candida albicans*, for example, is commonly present in the upper respiratory, alimentary and female genital tract and on the skin of healthy people. However in people where immune function has been affected by disease or treatment, such as cancer, this fungi can lead to systemic disease (Baker *et al.* 1998).

Mycobacteriological

For further information, please refer to the procedure on tuberculosis (see Chapter 6).

Protozoa

Most protozoa do not cause disease, but those that do, e.g. malaria, make a formidable contribution to human illness (Armitage & King 2000). Laboratory investigations depend on direct microscopy which necessitates specimens being delivered to the laboratory as quickly as possible, while the protozoa are mobile and therefore visible.

Blood

Blood specimens are obtained for several reasons (Weinstein 2007):

- To indicate relatively common disorders.
- To make a diagnosis.

- To follow the course of a disease.
- To regulate therapy and drug dosage.

Wherever possible, blood should be obtained peripherally (see Chapter 46). Blood samples can be obtained from central venous access devices (CVADs); however, the first sample must be discarded to ensure accurate results and the device must then be flushed directly after obtaining the blood sample to avoid an occlusion (Gabriel 2008) (see Chapter 45).

Blood cultures

Bacteraemia and fungaemia are frequent complications in immunocompromised and critically ill patients; the accurate and timely detection of these remains one on the most important functions of clinical microbiology (Wilson 1996). Intravenous antibiotic therapy needs to be started within the first hour of recognition of severe sepsis after cultures have been obtained (Dellinger *et al.* 2004). Accurate and speedy microbiological detection of infection using blood cultures is of paramount importance to determine the cause and guide the treatment (see Chapter 6). Success in gaining information from blood cultures relies on the accurate timing of the specimen and obtaining the correct volume of blood. The volume is critial to ensure the optimum blood to broth ratio, so the manufacturer's instructions should be followed as to the total volume required for each bottle. However the potential to cause anemia also needs to be considered, so a smaller volume (1–5 ml) for infants and small children should be obtained from each venepuncture site (Wilson 1996; Gill *et al.* 2004). As there are a number of systems in use it is essential that maufacturers' guidelines are followed. Most bacteraemias are intermittent, so blood cultures should be taken when the signs of infection are present (Gill *et al.* 2004). These may include fever, chills, rigors, changes in mental status and lethargy (Shelton 1999).

Blood for culture should be sampled before administration or modification of antibiotic therapy, as antibiotics may delay or prevent bacterial growth, causing false negative results (Engervall & Bjorkholm 1996; Higgins 2007).

One of the most important aspects of identifying a causative agent using blood cultures is the level of contamination of the blood samples which remains a common problem with rates varying from 2 to 10% (Madeo *et al.* 2003; DH 2007). Failure to use aseptic technique when obtaining blood cultures can result in diagnosis of a pseudobacteraemia, due to contamination of the culture by bacteria originating outside the patient's bloodstream. As the majority of this contamination comes from endogenous microbial flora on the skin, preparation is very important in reducing the number of false positive blood cultures (Traunter *et al.* 2002; DH 2007). This could result in inappropriate antibiotic therapy being administered and a significant waste of health care resources (Jumaa & Chattopadhyay 1994).

The use of needles to decant into the bottles is now largely redundant due to the common use of vacuumed blood collection systems to acquire blood samples (Rushing 2004). However, if a needle is used then it must be changed prior to decanting the blood into the blood culture bottle, as studies have indicated an increase in contamination rates when the needle is not changed (Spitalnic *et al.* 1995).

Catheter-related sepsis is the main risk factor when using central venous catheters and has an incidence of between 4 and 14% (Theaker 2005). CVAD-related infection and its morbidity and mortality associated with sepsis are often underestimated in clinical practice (Moller *et al.* 2005). Studies have found that between 16 and 44% of bone marrow transplant patients with CVAD experience catheter-related infections (Zitella 2003). When it is suspected that the CVAD is the source of infection, a blood culture sample must be obtained from all lumens of the device and a peripheral vein (Gabriel 2008; Dellinger *et al.* 2004; DH 2007). If there are signs of infection, e.g. redness and/or discharge around the site of insertion, a swab should also be taken for microbiological culture but at the same time the patient should be assessed for any other source of infection. Controversy continues about the sensitivity and specificity between catheter-drawn and peripheral blood cultures; some studies suggest that peripheral cultures are more reliable when the results of paired cultures are different (McBryde *et al.* 2005; Safdar *et al.* 2005), whereas others conclude the sensitivity from either route is not adequate to eliminate the need to take samples from the other site (Beutz *et al.* 2003).

Quantitative analysis of drugs in blood

Therapeutic drug monitoring by blood analysis is important to determine the correct optimal dosage, while avoiding dangerous side-effects. For most drugs used in clinical practice this type of monitoring is unnecessary. However, there are a limited number of drugs that must be frequently monitored in clinical practice. These include: lithium, digoxin, theophylline, phenytoin, cyclosporin and a number of antibiotics, for example the aminoglycoside antibiotics and vancomycin (Higgins 2007). The use and monitoring of vancomycin has increased due to the emergence of methicillin-resistant *Staphylococcus aureus* (MRSA); however, there remains little concensus in the UK about postdose sampling times, target ranges and what constitutes a toxic level (Tobin 2002), and the emergence of vancomycin-resistant MRSA further complicates this clinical issue. The advances in rapid polymerase chain reaction (PCR) testing for MRSA may also affect how monitoring of vancomycin is used in the future (Cunningham *et al.* 2007; Thomas *et al.* 2007).

The aminoglycoside antibiotics and vancomycin possess a narrow therapeutic range, so if the serum levels are too low the efficacy of the drug is decreased (Tam *et al.* 1999). These antibiotics are potentially nephrotoxic and ototoxic, but with the more pure drug formulation of vancomycin used today its toxicity is not as common or severe as originally reported. In spite of this it has been suggested that all patients receiving these drugs should have serum sent regularly for antimicrobial assay (Downie *et al.* 2000). The primary purpose is to avoid toxic accumulation, but it is also important to obtain good therapeutic levels, particularly in patients with a Gram-negative sepsis (Shirrel *et al.* 1999).

Analysis involves laboratory testing of blood serum. Although this knowledge can be gained from random sampling, most benefit will be obtained by the correct timing of sample collection. This will provide a direct relationship to drug administration, and therefore give the correct interpretation of the serum concentration results.

Ideally, a trough sample just before the next scheduled dose, plus a peak level at a set time following the administration of the drug, will provide the most useful information (Mims *et al.* 2004). The post-dose peak level timing will vary depending on the drug; in the case of vancomycin which has a slow distribution phase it is recommended the sample is taken at least 1–2 hours after the infusion ends (Tobin 2002). Abnormally elevated drug levels may be obtained if the blood samples are taken from a CVAD through which the drug has been administered. This is more likely when residual drug remains in the catheter if it has not been flushed correctly following administration of the drug or the first 5–10 ml of blood has not been discarded (Himberger & Himberger 2001). Occasionally the CVAD may have to be used, for example, for paediatric patients or when only poor or limited venous access is available. If a multilumen CVAD is in place, a different lumen from the one used to administer the drug must be used to obtain the blood specimen. If scrupulous attention to policy is adhered to, blood levels obtained from CVAD can compare favourably with specimens taken from peripheral veins (Shulman *et al.* 1998).

If blood samples have to be taken from a CVAD because peripheral vein access is not available, this information must be written onto the microbiology request card (Shulman *et al.* 1998).

Gentamicin is commonly prescribed to treat Gram negative infections but requires careful attention to patient specific dosing and monitoring although this is not always achieved (Leong *et al.* 2006). A 6-year audit of gentamicin drug monitoring to establish optimal regimens found that in those patients who achieved therapeutic drug levels, the average duration of antibiotic therapy was statistically shorter than in those patients who failed to achieve therapeutic peak concentrations, thereby preventing toxicity and improving outcome (Ismail *et al.* 1997).

In the procedure guidelines below two examples of drug analysis are discussed; the laboratory will supply specific times for blood sampling for other drugs.

For further information on the collection of blood see the procedure for venepuncture (see Chapter 46).

Urine

The correct collection of urine specimens is very important as urinary tract infections are considered to be the most common bacterial infection (Foxman 2002). Urinary catheter associated infections are the most common type of noscomial infection (Godfrey & Evans 2000), and have been associated with both morbidity and mortality (Wazait *et al.* 2003). Urine is normally sterile, while the distal urethra of both men and women is normally colonized with a large number of bacteria (Gill *et al.* 2004; Higgins 2007) and even a carefully taken urine specimen may contain a number of bacteria. As urine is such a good culture medium, any bacteria present at the time of collection will continue to multiply in the specimen container, resulting in a falsely raised bacteriuria (Higgins 2007), which will then result in misleading information (Gill *et al.* 2004).

It was thought that cleaning of the area around the urinary meatus prior to the collection of a midstream specimen of urine makes no difference to contamination rates (Holliday *et al.* 1991), although perineal and penile cleaning was potentially beneficial to those patients whose personal hygiene was poor (Holliday *et al.* 1991). Higgins (2007) now suggests that to collect a specimen uncontaminated by bacteria, which may be present on the skin, peri-anal region, external genital tract or distal third of the urethra, patients should be encouraged to wash their hands prior to collecting a 'clean catch' midstream urine specimen and to clean around the urinary meatus prior to sample collection. Female patients should also be instructed to part the labia while passing urine to avoid possible contamination (Graham & Galloway 2001; Higgins 2007).

The principle for obtaining midstream collection of urine is that any bacteria present in the urethra are washed away in the first portion of urine voided (Higgins 2007).

Cytology

Cervical smear or 'pap' smear

In the UK 80% of cervical smears are taken in the primary care setting and most are taken by practice nurses. Screening is recommended in the UK for all women between the ages of 25 and 65 years and is an investigation to confirm the cervix is healthy; it is not a test for diagnosing cervical cancer (NHS Cancer Screening Programmes 2006; Higgins 2007).

The intention of a smear test is to collect squamous epithelial cells and some endocervical cells from the transformation zone and squamo-columnar junction of the cervix (Figure 40.1) The sampling technique must take into consideration that the position of the squamo-columnar junction changes with age, contraception and parity (WHO 2006; Higgins 2007) (Box 40.1).

779

Figure 40.1 The cervix.

Figure 40.2 The different types of sampling devices.

Box 40.1 Common reasons why cervical smears require repeating when using the conventional method of smear sampling

(a) The cervix has not been scraped firmly enough to obtain adequate epithelial cells (WHO 2006).
(b) The sample on the spatula was not completely transferred to the slide or applied too thinly or too thickly (Higgins 2007).
(c) Fixative not applied immediately allowing the sample to dry and causing the cells to become misshapen (WHO 2006).
(d) Sample contaminated with lubricants, spermicide or blood (Higgins 2007).

There are several devices which are used in sampling the uterine cervix (Figure 40.2). These are:

- Wooden spatula (Aylesbury spatula).
- Plastic spatula/brush/broom.
- Endocervical brush.

Cotton-tipped swabs are no longer recommended (NHS Cancer Screening Programmes 2006). Whichever device is used, once the sample is taken it is vital that the cells collected are transferred onto a glass slide and preserved immediately or placed into the correct vial containing liquid preservative and fixative. Slides must not be placed in a refrigerator (NHS Cancer Screening Programmes 2006; Higgins 2007).

The ideal time for obtaining a cervical smear is mid-cycle if the woman is premenopausal; this prevents contamination from menstrual flow and allows for accuracy of results (WHO 2006; Higgins 2007). It is not ideal to take a cervical smear if a woman is pregnant or immediately postpartum as results obtained can be misleading. Higgins (2007) suggests delaying the procedure for a few months following childbirth; however, the World Health Organization (WHO) suggest that if a woman is in the target age group and there are concerns about access to screening postpartum, then a cervical smear should be taken after consent is obtained (WHO 2006).

In order to obtain an adequate cervical smear the following procedure will guide the practitioner through the practical detail and technique recommended to gain an adequate sample for analysis.

Web resources

www.cancerscreening.nhs.uk/cervical (a full list of NHS Cancer Screening Programmes publications related to cervical screening)
www.ic.nhs.uk

Liquid-based cytology

Liquid-based cytology (LBC) technology has been used in Europe and the USA since 1996. After extensive clinical trials in 2003 using LBC for cervical smears, the National Institute for Health and Clinical Excellence (NICE) recommended that LBC should replace the conventional cervical smear test by 2008 as part of the National Health Service (NHS) Cervical Screening Programmes. The change to LBC for smear taking has resulted in the reduction of reported 'inadequate smears', women's anxieties, and in the workload for primary care and laboratory personnel (Karnon *et al.* 2004; NHS Cancer Screening Programmes 2004).

Procedure guidelines   Specimen collection: section swabs

Procedure

Action	Rationale
1 Explain and discuss the procedure with the patient and ensure privacy while the procedure is being carried out.	To ensure that the patient understands the procedure and gives his/her valid consent (NMC 2006: C; NMC 2008: C).
2 Wash hands using bactericidal soap and water or bactericidal alcoholic handrub before and after obtaining specimen.	Hand washing greatly reduces the risk of infection transfer (DH 2005: C).
3 On completion of procedure, place specimens and swabs in the appropriate, correctly labelled containers.	To ensure that only organisms for investigation are preserved (Health Services Advisory Committee 2003: C).
4 Dispatch specimens promptly to the laboratory with the completed request form.	To ensure the best possible conditions for any laboratory examinations (Baker *et al.* 1998: R 5; Higgins 2007: E).

Ear swab

Action	Rationale
1 No antibiotics or other chemotherapeutic agents should have been used in the aural region 3 hours before taking the swab.	To prevent collection of traces of such therapeutic agents (Mims *et al.* 2004: E).
2 Place the swab into the outer ear as shown in Action figure 2. Rotate the swab gently.	To avoid trauma to the ear. To collect any secretions (Mims *et al.* 2004: E).

Pinna
Inner ear
Outer ear
Ear canal
Ear swab
Ear drum
Middle ear
Eustachian tube

Action 2   Area to be swabbed when sampling the outer ear.

Eye swab

Action	Rationale
1 Seek advice from microbiology about what type of culture medium and swab is required.	Different culture media and swabs are required for bacteria, viruses and chlamydia (Stollery *et al.* 2005: E).
2 Using a cotton wool swab, hold the swab parallel to the cornea and gently rub the conjunctiva in the lower eyelid from the nasal side outwards.	To ensure that a swab of the correct site is taken. To avoid contamination by touching the eyelid (Buller 2000: E; Marsden & Shaw 2003: E; Stollery *et al.* 2005: E).
3 If both eyes are to be swabbed, ensure the specimens are labelled 'right' and 'left'.	To prevent cross-infection (Stollery *et al.* 2005: C).

Procedure guidelines (*cont.*)

Nose swab

Action	Rationale
1 Moisten the swab beforehand with sterile water.	To prevent discomfort to the patient. The healthy nose is virtually dry and a dry swab may cause discomfort (Tortora & Derrickson 2006: C).
2 Move the swab from the anterior nares and direct it upwards into the tip of the nose (see Action figure 2).	To swab the correct site and to obtain the required sample (E).
3 Gently rotate the swab.	

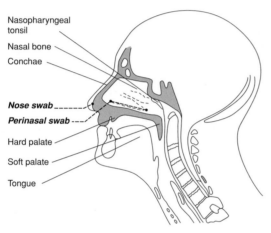

Action 2   Area to be swabbed when sampling the nose.

Penile swab

Action	Rationale
1 Retract prepuce.	To obtain maximum visibility of area to be swabbed (E).
2 Rotate swab gently in the urethral meatus.	To collect any secretions (Malarkey & McMorrow 2005: E).

Rectal swab

Action	Rationale
1 Pass the swab, with care, through the anus into the rectum.	To avoid trauma. To ensure that a rectal and not an anal sample is obtained (E).
2 Rotate gently.	To avoid trauma (E).
3 In patients suspected of suffering from threadworms, take the swab from the perianal region.	Threadworms lay their ova on the perianal skin (Mims *et al*. 2004: E).

Throat swab

Action	Rationale
1 Ask the patient to sit in such a position that he/she is facing a strong light source. Depress the patient's tongue with a spatula.	To ensure maximum visibility of the area to be swabbed. The procedure is one that is likely to cause the patient to gag and the tongue will move to the roof of the mouth, contaminating the specimen (Parini 2000: E).

2 Quickly, but gently, rub the swab over the prescribed area, usually the tonsillar fossa or any area with a lesion or visible exudate (see Action figure 2).

To obtain the required sample (Parini 2000: E).

3 Avoid touching any other area of the mouth or tongue with the swab.

To prevent contamination by other organisms (Mims *et al.* 2004: E).

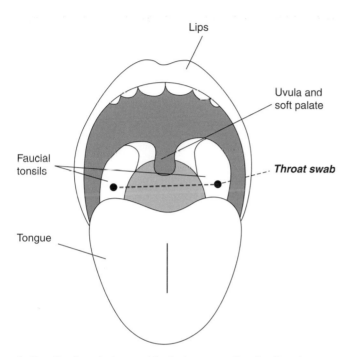

Action 2   Area to be swabbed when sampling the throat.

Labels in figure: Lips; Uvula and soft palate; Faucial tonsils; *Throat swab*; Tongue

Vaginal swab
Action
1 Introduce a speculum into the vagina to separate the vaginal walls. Take the swab as high as possible in the vaginal vault.

Rationale
To ensure maximum visibility of the area to be swabbed. To ensure that the swab is taken from the best site (Malarkey & McMorrow 2005: E). If infection by *Trichomonas* species is suspected, a charcoal-impregnated swab is recommended as this organism survives longer in this medium (Mims *et al.* 2004: E).

Wound swab
Action
1 Take any swabs required before cleaning procedure begins.

Rationale
To collect the maximum number of micro-organisms and to prevent collection of any therapeutic agents that may be employed in the dressing procedure (Gilchrist 2000: E).

2 Rotate the swab gently.

To collect samples. It is preferable to send samples of purulent discharge instead of swabs (Parini 2000: E).

Note: the use of disposable gloves is recommended in the following procedures in order to prevent cross-infection.

Procedure guidelines   Specimen collection: body fluid

Blood cultures

Blood cultures should always be collected by members of staff who have been trained in the collection procedure and whose competence in blood culture collection has been assessed (DH 2007). The femoral vein should also be avoided as the skin is difficult to clean adequately and disinfect (DH 2007).

Procedure

Action	Rationale
1 Explain and discuss the procedure with the patient and ensure privacy while the procedure is being carried out.	To ensure that the patient understands the procedure and gives his/her valid consent (NMC 2006: C; NMC 2008: C).
2 Wash hands using bactericidal soap and water or bactericidal alcoholic handrub before and after obtaining specimen. Apply non-sterile gloves.	Hand washing greatly reduces the risk of infection transfer (DH 2005a: C).
3 Clean both bottle tops with 2% chlorhexidine in alcohol swabs and allow to dry.	To reduce the risk of false positive results (DH 2007: C).
4 If taking blood from a peripheral vein, clean the skin area with a 2% chlorhexidine in alcohol solution and leave to dry. Do not repalpate the area.	To reduce risk of contamination of the site and to prevent cross-contamination from practitioner's fingers (DH 2007: C).
5 If taking blood from a central venous access device (CVAD), clean the lumen ends with a 2% chlorhexidine in alcohol solution and then take a vacuum bottle of blood and dispose of it prior to attaching blood culture bottles. Take sample from each lumen.	To reduce risk of contamination (DH 2007: C). To remove saline and heparin that may be present in catheter (E).
6 Take blood sample following manufacturer's guidelines.	To ensure blood sample is collected using correct method and in correct volume (Manufacturer's guidelines: C).
7 If vacuum system is not used then change needle to decant blood into bottles.	To prevent cross-contamination (Rushing 2004: E).
8 Record the procedure with indication for culture, time, site of venepuncture and any complications in patient's record.	To ensure continuity of care and accurate record keeping (NMC 2008: C; DH 2007: C).

Drug levels in blood

Procedure

Action	Rationale
1 Following venepuncture guidelines (see Chapter 46), withdraw 10 ml of blood and place in appropriate blood specimen container.	To ensure blood is obtained correctly and safely (Himberger & Himberger 2001: R 3).
2 Clearly label blood specimen container 'pre-drug administration blood'.	To ensure that there is no confusion between the pre-drug and post-drug serum level specimens (E).
3 Administer intravenous antibiotic as patient's prescription states (following procedure for administration of drugs; see Chapter 11) via the patient's established vascular access device.	To continue with patient's prescribed drug regimen (E).

4 Within an allotted time after administration of drug withdraw 10 ml of blood to obtain specimen to provide peak-level serum following venepuncture guidelines (see Chapter 46). Clearly label blood specimen container 'post-drug administration blood'.	Time gap allows for even distribution of the drug through the blood and for peak blood levels to be achieved (Tobin 2002: R 2).
5 Rarely, but occasionally, when only poor and limited venous access is available, the blood specimens may have to be obtained from the patient's existing device. The device must be flushed thoroughly before taking the blood sample (see Chapter 45). The blood specimen container and request form must be labelled to indicate this deviation from the usual procedure.	The possibility of these specimens being contaminated with residue drug is high (Shulman *et al.* 1998: R 2b). Contamination can be reduced by thorough flushing of the device (E). The clinician interpreting the result will then be aware of the method of obtaining the blood specimen (E).

Faecal collection

Action	Rationale
1 Ask the patient to defecate into a clinically clean bedpan.	To avoid unnecessary contamination from other organisms (Parini 2000: E).
2 Scoop enough material to fill a third of the specimen container using a spatula or a spoon, often incorporated in the specimen container.	To obtain a usable amount of specimen. To prevent contamination (Malarkey & McMorrow 2005: E).
3 Examine the specimen for such features as colour, consistency and odour, and record your observations.	To monitor any fluctuations and trends (Gill 1999: E).
4 Segments of tapeworm are seen easily in faeces and any such segments should be sent to the laboratory for identification.	Unless the head is dislodged, the tapeworm will continue to grow. Laboratory confirmation of the presence of the head is essential (Gill 1999: E).
5 Patients suspected of suffering from amoebic dysentery should have any stool specimens dispatched to the laboratory immediately.	The parasite causing amoebic dysentery exists in a free-living non-motile cyst. Both are characteristic in their fresh state but are difficult to identify when dead (Baker *et al.* 1998: E).
6 Patients with diarrhoea and especially in the presence of a fever should have samples taken to the laboratory immediately.	Due to the risk of *Clostridium difficile* (Poutanen & Simor 2004: R 2a).

Nasopharyngeal specimen collection: nasal wash: syringe method

Equipment

1 5 ml 0.9% sodium chloride.
2 5 ml syringe or wide-bore bladder syringe.
3 Filling tube (or cut-off tip from a suction catheter if using 5 ml syringe).

4 Viral transport medium (VTM) (if required by laboratory).
5 Specimen container.

Procedure

Action	Rationale
1 Fill a syringe with 0.9% sodium chloride and attach a filing tube to the syringe tip.	To facilitate instillation of 0.9% sodium chloride high into the patient's nostril (E).

Procedure guidelines (*cont.*)

2 (a) Ask the patient to tilt their head slightly back whilst sitting upright.	To promote the flow of 0.9% sodium chloride into the nostril (E).
(b) Quickly instil 0.9% sodium chloride into one nostril.	To facilitate maximum recovery of epithelial cells (E).
3 (a) Aspirate the recoverable nasal specimen.	Recovery must occur immediately as the instilled saline will rapidly drain (E).
(b) Alternatively, where appropriate, patients may tilt head forward and gently push the fluid out of the nostril into the specimen container.	To allow specimen to drain into suitable sterile container. Patient may feel more comfortable (E).
4 If aspirated: inject aspirated specimen from syringe into suitable dry, sterile container or one containing viral transport medium, according to virology laboratory requirements.	To ensure a good-quality specimen is transported safely to the laboratory (E).
5 Repeat procedure on other nostril (see Action figure 5).	To promote optimal combined specimen (E).

Action 5   Nasopharyngeal specimen collection. Nasal wash: syringe method.

Nasopharyngeal specimen collection: vacuum-assisted nasal aspirate method

Equipment

1 Suction pump.
2 Sterile suction catheter.

3 Mucus trap (i.e. Lukens tube).
4 Viral transport medium (VTM) (if required by laboratory).

Procedure

Action	**Rationale**
1 Attach mucus trap to suction pump and appropriate sized catheter (Table 40.1), leaving wrapper on suction catheter.	To ensure catheter stays clean while getting equipment ready (E).
2 Turn on suction and adjust to suggested pressure (Table 40.1).	To ensure suction machine is working correctly and pressure is set at the appropriate level (E).

3 Without applying suction, insert catheter into the nose, directed posteriorly and towards the opening of the external ear (see Action figure 3). *Note*: depth of insertion necessary to reach posterior pharynx is equivalent to distance between anterior naris and external opening of ear.	To prevent damaging the nasopharynx (E). To minimize patient discomfort (E).
4 Apply suction. Using a rotating movement, slowly withdraw catheter. *Note*: catheter should remain in nasopharynx no longer than 10 seconds.	To prevent damaging nasopharynx (E).
5 Hold trap upright to prevent secretions from going into pump.	To prevent loss of specimen (E).
6 Rinse catheter (if necessary) with approximately 20 ml viral transport medium.	To ensure maximum recovery of epithelial cells (E).
7 Disconnect suction; connect tubing to arm of mucus trap to seal.	To prevent contamination and/or loss of specimen (E).

Action 3   Nasopharyngeal specimen collection. Vacuum-assisted nasal aspirate method.

Table 40.1   Catheter sizes and suction pressures.

Patient age	Catheter size (French)	Suction pressure (mmHg)
Premature infant	6	80–100
Infant	8	80–100
Toddler/preschooler	10	100–120
School age	12	100–120
Adolescent/adult	14	120–150

Semen

Action

Rationale

1 Sexual intercourse should not have taken place for 3–4 days before the specimen is collected.	To ensure the sperm count will be at maximum levels. It takes between 3 and 4 days for the sperm count to return to normal after ejaculation (National Collaborating Centre for Women's and Children's Health 2004: C).
2 A fresh masturbated specimen must be collected in a sterile container and delivered to the laboratory within 2 hours of the collection of the specimen.	Sperm will die if there is a delay in testing. Specimens must not be collected in a condom as sperm die when in contact with materials such as rubber (E).
3 The specimen must be kept warm.	To ensure viability of the sperm (E).

Procedure guidelines (*cont.*)

Sputum collection

Action	Rationale
1 Use a sterile specimen container with a leakproof top.	Sputum is never free from organisms since material originating in the bronchi and alveoli has to pass through the pharynx and mouth, areas that have a normal commensal population of bacteria (Thomson 2002: E).
2 Care should be taken to ensure that the material sent for investigations is sputum, not saliva.	To obtain the required sample (Health Services Advisory Committee 2003: C).
3 Encourage patients who have difficulty producing sputum to cough deeply first thing in the morning. Alternatively, a physiotherapist should be called to assist.	To facilitate expectoration (E).
4 Send any sputum specimen to the laboratory within 1 hour.	The bacterial population alters rapidly and rapid dispatch should ensure accurate results (Thomson 2002: R 5).

Urine specimen

Action	Rationale
1 Specimens of urine should be collected as soon as possible after the patient wakes in the morning and at the same time each morning if more than one specimen is required.	The bladder will be full of concentrated urine which has accumulated overnight (Malarkey & McMorrow 2005: E). If specimens are taken at other times, the urine may be diluted (E).
2 Dispatch all specimens to the laboratory as soon after collection as possible.	Urine specimens should be examined within 2 hours of collection or 24 hours if kept refrigerated at a temperature of 4°C. At room temperature overgrowth will occur and lead to misinterpretation (Buller 2000: E).

Midstream specimen of urine (MSU): male

Action	Rationale
1 Retract the prepuce and clean the skin surrounding the urethral meatus with soap and water, 0.9% sodium chloride solution or a solution that does not contain a disinfectant.	To prevent other organisms contaminating the specimen. Disinfectants may irritate or be painful to the urethral mucous membrane (Malarkey & McMorrow 2005: E; Higgins 2007: E).
2 Ask the patient to direct the first and last part of his stream into a urinal or toilet but to collect the middle part of his stream into a sterile container.	To avoid contamination of the specimen with organisms normally present on the skin (Parini 2000: E; Higgins 2007: E).

Midstream specimen of urine (MSU): female

Action	Rationale
1 Part the labia, clean the urethral meatus with soap and water, 0.9% sodium chloride solution or a solution that does not contain a disinfectant.	To prevent other organisms contaminating the specimen (Parini 2000: E). Disinfectants may irritate or be painful to the urethral mucous membrane (Malarkey & McMorrow 2005: E).
2 (a) If using a cotton swab, use a separate cotton-wool swab for each wipe.	To prevent cross-infection (Parini 2000: E).
(b) Wipe in a downwards motion from the front to the back encourage the patient to still separate the labia with one hand while micturating.	To prevent perianal contamination (Parini 2000: E). To avoid contamination of the specimen with organisms normally present on the skin (Higgins 2007: E; Graham & Galloway 2001: E).

3   Place sterile receiver or a wide-mouthed sterile container under the stream of urine and remove before micturation finishes.

To prevent contamination of specimen (Parini 2000: E).

4   Transfer the specimen into a sterile universal container and screw the cap on immediately. Care should be taken not to touch inside of cap or rim of the universal container.

To prevent contamination with bacteria in the environment (Higgins 2007: E).

Specimen of urine from an ileal conduit

For further information see the relevant section in the procedure on stoma care (see Chapter 17).

Catheter specimen of urine

For further information see the relevant section in the procedure on urinary catheterization (see Chapter 18).

Twenty-four-hour urine collection

Action

1   Request the patient to void the bladder at the time appointed to begin this procedure. Discard this specimen.

Rationale

To ensure the urine collected is that produced in the 24 hours stated (Malarkey & McMorrow 2005: E).

2   All urine passed in the next 24 hours is collected in a large specimen bottle. The final specimen is collected at exactly the same time the bladder was voided 24 hours earlier.

Body chemistry alters constantly. A 24-hour collection will accommodate all the variables within a representative period (Thomson 2002: E).

3   Care must be taken to ensure the patient understands the procedure in order to eliminate the risk of an incomplete collection.

A 24-hour collection will not be obtained if one sample is lost, and the results will be invalid (Malarkey & McMorrow 2005: E).

Procedure guidelines   Cervical uterine smear or Pap smear

Equipment

1   Alcoholic handrub.
2   Light source.
3   An examination couch.
4   Disposable clean paper couch covers.
5   Various sized speculum (disposable or reusable).
6   Disposable clean gloves.
7   Wooden spatula or sampling device.
8   A glass slide with frosted edge.
9   A pencil for labelling slide.
10 Fixative solution.
11 Plastic slide container.
12 Specimen form and plastic specimen bag.
13 A container of warm water.
14 Box of tissue paper.
15 A collecting container for Central Sterile Services (CSS).
16 Clinical waste container.
17 Trolley.

Procedure

Action

1   Discuss benefits and limitations of screening and significance of smear results. Explain the purpose of procedure and explain what will occur at each step of the procedure. Document the woman's clinical and screening history, specifically:
  (a) Date of last menstruation.
  (b) Any abnormal bleeding.
  (c) Any unusual vaginal discharge.
  (d) Contraception.
  (e) Date of last cervical smear.
  (f) Any abnormal smear results.
  (g) Any treatment to the cervix.

Rationale

To ensure that the woman understands the procedure involves removing underwear and that the speculum will be inserted into her vagina, and consents to the procedure (NMC 2006: C; NMC 2008: C).
Allows the woman time to ask any questions (E).

Procedure guidelines (cont.)

2 Wash hands before and after the procedure. Place all the equipment you require for the procedure on the trolley.

To minimize the risk of infection (DH 2005a: C).
To facilitate the efficient taking of the smear (E).

3 Close room door or curtains and ask the woman to remove her underwear.

To provide privacy and comfort for the woman (E).

4 Turn the light source on and position at end of examination table.

To provide illumination of the cervix and increase the accuracy of the smear taking (NHS Cancer Screening Programmes 2004, 2006: C).

5 Assist the woman into the appropriate position on the examination couch in a supine position with knees drawn up and legs parted. Keep the women as covered as possible.

To facilitate easy access of the vaginal speculum and the taking of the cervical smear (NHS Cancer Screening Programmes 2004, 2006: C; WHO 2006: C, E).

6 Wash hands thoroughly or use an alcohol-based handrub.

To reduce the risk of contamination (DH 2005a: C).

7 Select the appropriate size speculum, from very small, small, medium, large including a long bladed narrow speculum if the vagina is long or the cervix is lying posterior. The sterilized speculum can be warmed or cooled using clean tap water.

To promote patient comfort and reduce anxiety (NHS Cancer Screening Programmes 2006: C). If removed from a sterilizer may need to be cooled down, if cold then warmed up to reduce patient discomfort. It must be explained to patient that the speculum has been sterilized but the water will not contaminate it (E).

8 Apply gloves. Part the labia and holding the speculum blades together sideways, slip the speculum into the vagina.

To insert the speculum reducing patient discomfort (DH 2005a: C, E; WHO 2006: C).

9 When the speculum is halfway into the vagina turn the speculum so that the handle is facing down. If insertion is difficult apply a small amount of water based lubricant to the sides of the speculum avoiding the tip of the speculum.

To promote patient comfort and reduce contamination of the cervix with lubricants (NHS Cancer Screening Programmes 2006: C, E).

10 Gently open the blades of the speculum and look for the cervix. It may be necessary to move the speculum up or down until the entire cervix is visible.

To reduce patient discomfort and visualize the cervix (WHO 2006: C, E).

11 Once the cervix is visible tighten the screw or lock the speculum in the open position so it remains in place. Adjustment of the light source may be required. Reassure the woman and allow time for her to relax.

To keep the speculum in the correct position and visualize the cervix (WHO 2006: C, E).
To reduce patient discomfort and anxiety (E).

12 Take the spatula and insert the long tip into the cervical os; rotate it through 360°.

To ensure an adequate cell sampling is obtained from the transformation zone (WHO 2006: C, E; Higgins 2007: C).

13 Remove the spatula from the vaginal cavity then smear both sides of the wooden spatula onto the glass slide using straight sweeps.

To ensure maximum collection of cells (WHO 2006: C, E).

14 Apply fixative immediately.
   (a) Spray fixative is used at right angles to the slide and at a distance of 15–20 cms.
   (b) If immersing the slide in 95% ethanol, then leave for 5 minutes, remove from solution and allow to air dry.

To preserve the specimen and ensure accurate results (NHS Cancer Screening Programmes 2006: C; WHO 2006: C; Higgins 2007: C).

(c) If using 90% ethanol, then leave for 10–15 minutes, remove from solution and allow to air dry.

(d) If using 'Cytofixx' (95% industrial methylated spirit), apply a few drops to the slide and allow to dry for 5 minutes.

15 If using an endocervical brush in conjunction with a spatula, insert into the cervical os and rotate it through 360° in a clockwise direction. *(Laboratories may prefer both spatula and brush samples on the same slide, check with laboratory services).*	To ensure an adequate cell sample is obtained from the endocervical canal (NHS Cancer Screening Programmes 2006: C; WHO 2006: C, E; Higgins 2007: C).
16 Remove the brush from the vaginal cavity then gently roll the brush along the glass slide.	To ensure maximum collection of cells (NHS Cancer Screening Programmes 2006: C, E; WHO 2006: C; Higgins 2007: C).
17 Apply fixative immediately. **(a)** Spray fixative is used at right angles to the slide and at a distance of 15–20 cm. **(b)** If immersing the slide in 95% ethanol, then leave for 5 minutes, remove from solution and allow to air dry. **(c)** If using 90% ethanol, then leave for 10–15 minutes, remove from solution and allow to air dry. **(d)** If using 'Cytofixx', apply a few drops to the slide and allow to dry for 5 minutes.	To ensure correct preservation of the specimen and ensure accurate results (NHS Cancer Screening Programmes 2004, 2006: C; WHO 2006: C, E; Higgins 2007: C).
18 If there are clinical signs of possible infection then a high vaginal swab is recommended prior to removal of speculum. *(If active infection is present, the cervical smear should be delayed until infection has been treated and resolved).*	To ensure the swab is taken from the best site (Higgins 2007: C). A charcoal-impregnated swab is recommended if *Trichomonas* species is suspected as these organisms survive longer in this medium (Mims *et al.* 2004: R 5; Higgins 2007: C).
19 Place the swab into the medium.	To ensure specimen is correctly placed in the culture medium to ensure accuracy of results (E).
20 Gently pull the speculum out until the blades are clear of the cervix, then close blades and remove speculum, placing in clinical waste bin if disposable or into CSS container if a reusable speculum.	Prevent pinching the cervix or vaginal walls and to ensure safe disposal of contaminated equipment (DH 2005b: C; NHS Cancer Screening Programmes 2006: C; WHO 2006: C).
21 Cover the woman and offer tissue paper to wipe away any excess vaginal discharge.	To ensure dignity and privacy while promoting hygiene and comfort (E).
22 Dispose of the waste into clinical waste receiver.	Safe disposal of clinical waste (DH 2005b: C).
23 Assist the woman off the examination table and allow her to redress.	To ensure safety and promote dignity and privacy (E).
24 Using a pencil label the frosted end of the slide with woman's name, clinic number, date of birth and date sample taken. Using a black ball point pen label the vaginal swab.	To ensure patient details are documented correctly on specimen. *Note that ballpoint pens do not work on glass slides* (E).
25 Place the slide into transport container.	To prevent the slide from being damaged and safe transportation of specimen to the laboratory for analysis (E).

791

Procedure guidelines (*cont.*)

Action	Rationale
26 Remove gloves and dispose in clinical waste container.	Safe disposal of clinical waste (DH 2005: C).
27 Place the container and any swabs into plastic specimen bag with the correctly labelled specimen form/s and send to laboratory.	To ensure safe handling and transportation of a biohazard (DH 2005b: C).

Cervical uterine smear using liquid-based cytology

Procedure

Action

Following steps 1–11 as for conventional smear sampling.

Rationale

Action	Rationale
12 Using the Cervex-Brush®, insert the central bristles of the brush into the endocervical canal so that the shorter, outer bristles fully contact the ectocervix.	To ensure accuracy of site sampled (NHS Cancer Screening Programmes 2004, 2006: C).
13 Using pencil pressure, rotate the brush in a clockwise direction five times. *Note*: the plastic fronds of the brush are bevelled for rotation in a clockwise direction only.	To ensure good contact with the ectocervix and gather a high cellular yield (NHS Cancer Screening Programmes 2004, 2006: C).
(a) *Using Thinprep®*. Using a swirling motion rinse the brush into the fixative vial; then push the brush into the base of the vial at least 10 times forcing the bristles apart.	Firm pressure is required to ensure the cells do not cling to the brush (NHS Cancer Screening Programmes 2004, 2006: C).
Inspect the brush for any residual material and remove any remaining material by passing the brush over the edge of the fixative vial.	To ensure a usable amount of cellular material is collected (NHS Cancer Screening Programmes 2004, 2006: C).
Ensure that the material reaches the liquid. Then tighten the cap so that the torque line passes the torque line on the vial and give the vial a shake.	To ensure the cellular material reaches the preservative solution (NHS Cancer Screening Programmes 2004, 2006: C, E).
(b) *Using SurePath™*. Remove head of the brush from the stem and place into the vial of fixative. Then screw lid on tightly and shake the vial.	To ensure that the cells do not cling to the device (NHS Cancer Screening Programmes 2004, 2006: C).
Note: it is essential that the sample is placed into the vial in order to achieve immediate fixation.	To ensure accurate preservation of cervical material (NHS Cancer Screening Programmes 2004, 2006: C).
14 Gently pull the speculum out until the blades are clear of the cervix, then close blades and remove speculum, placing in clinical waste bin if disposable or into Central Sterile Services (CSS) container if reusable.	Prevent pinching cervix or vaginal walls and safe disposal of contaminated equipment (NHS Cancer Screening Programmes 2006: E; WHO 2006: C).
15 Cover the woman and offer tissue paper to wipe away any excess vaginal discharge.	To ensure dignity and privacy while promoting hygiene and comfort (E).
16 Remove gloves and dispose of waste in clinical waste receiver.	Safe disposal of clinical waste (DH 2005b: C).
17 Assist the woman off the examination table and allow her to redress.	To ensure safety and promote dignity and privacy (E).
18 Using a black ballpoint pen label the vial with woman's name, clinic number or date of birth.	To ensure patient details are documented correctly (E).
19 Place the vial into plastic specimen bag with the correctly labelled specimen form and send to laboratory.	To ensure safe handling and transportation of a biohazard (DH 2005b: C).

References and further reading

Armitage, K.B. & King, C.H. (2000) Malaria. In: *Principles and Practice of Infectious Diseases* (eds G. Mandell, J. Bennett & R. Dolin). Churchill Livingstone, Philadelphia, pp. 2817–31.

Baker, F.J., Silverton, R.E. & Pallister, C.J. (1998) Microbiology. In: *Introduction to Medical Laboratory Technology*. Butterworth Heinemann, Oxford, pp. 251–325.

Beutz, M. *et al.* (2003) Clinical utility of blood cultures drawn from central vein catheters and peripheral venipuncture in critically ill medical patients. *Chest*, **123**, 854–61.

Bille, J. (2000) Microbiologic diagnostic procedures. In: *Management of Infection in Immunocompromised Patients* (eds M. Glauser & P. Pizzo). W.B. Saunders, London, pp. 230–65.

British Standards Institute (1995) *BS ISO 6710. Single-use Containers for Venous Blood Specimen Collection*. British Standards Institute, London.

Buller, R. (2000) Specimen collection and transport. In: *Diagnostic Virology* (ed. G.A. Storch). Churchill Livingstone, New York, pp. 25–36.

Cunningham, R. *et al.* (2007) Effect on MRSA transmission of rapid PCR testing of patients admitted to critical care. *J Hosp Infect*, **65** (1), 24–8.

Dellinger, R.P. *et al.* (2004) Surviving sepsis campaign guidelines for management of severe sepsis and septic shock. *Intens Care Med*, **30**, 536–55.

DH (2005a) *Saving Lives: A Delivery Programme to Reduce Healthcare Associated Infection including MRSA: Skills for Implentation*. Department of Health, London.

DH (2005b) *Hazardous Waste (England) Regulations*. Department of Health, London.

DH (2007) *Saving Lives: a Delivery Programme to Reduce Healthcare Associated Infection Including MRSA: Taking Blood Cultures – a Strategy for NHS Trusts, a Summary of Best Practice*. Department of Health, London.

Downie, G., Mackenzie, J. & Williams, A. (2000) Drug treatment of infections. In: *Pharmacology and Drug Management for Nurses*. Churchill Livingstone, Edinburgh, pp. 189–206.

Durnell Schuiling, K. & Likis, F.E. (2006) *Women's Gynecologic Health*. Jones and Bartlett Publishers, Sudbury, MA.

Engervall, P. & Bjorkholm, M. (1996) Infections in neutropenic patients II: management. *Med Oncol*, **13**(1), 63–9.

Finegold, S.M. (2000) Anaerobic bacteria: general concepts. In: *Principles and Practice of Infectious Diseases* (eds G. Mandell, J. Bennett & R. Dolin). Churchill Livingstone, Philadelphia, pp. 1805–62.

Foxman, B. (2002) Epidemiology of urinary tract infections: incidence, morbidity, and economic costs. *Am J Med*, **113**(1, Suppl 1), 5–13.

Gabriel, J. (2008) Long-term central venous access. In: *Intravenous Therapy in Nursing Practice* (eds L. Dougherty & J. Lamb), 2nd edn, Blackwell Publishing, Oxford.

Gilchrist, B. (2000) Taking a wound swab. *Nurs Times*, **96**(4), 2.

Gill, D. (1999) Stool specimen part 1. *Nurs Times*, **95**(25), 1–2.

Gill, V.J., Fedorko, D.P. & Witebsky, F.G. (2004) The clinician and the microbiology laboratory. In: *Principles and Practice of Infectious Diseases* (eds G. Mandell, J. Bennett & R. Dolin). Churchill Livingstone, Philadelphia, pp. 203–41.

Godfrey, H. & Evans, A. (2000) Catherization and urinary tract infections: microbiology. *Br J Nurs*, **9**(11), 682–4.

Gold, H.S. & Eisenstein, B.I. (2000) Introduction to bacterial diseases. In: *Principles and Practice of Infectious Diseases* (eds G. Mandell, J. Bennett & R. Dolin). Churchill Livingstone, Philadelphia, pp. 2065–9.

Graham, J.C. & Galloway, A. (2001) The laboratory diagnosis of urinary tract infections. *J Clin Pathol*, **54**, 911–19.

Hazardous Waste (England and Wales) Regulations (2005) HMSO, London.

Health Services Advisory Committee (2003) *Safe Working and the Prevention of Infection in Clinical Laboratories and Similar Facilities*. HMSO, London.

Henderson, D.K. (2000) Bacteraemia due to percutaneous intravenous devices. In: *Principles and Practice of Infectious Diseases* (eds G. Mandell, J. Bennett & R. Dolin). Churchill Livingstone, Philadelphia, pp. 3005–3020.

Henker, R. (2000) Infection control. Use of blood cultures in critically ill patients. *Crit Care Nurs*, **20**(1), 45–9.

Higgins, C. (2007) *Understanding Laboratory Investigations for Nurses and Health Professionals*, 2nd edn. Blackwell Publishing, Oxford.

Himberger, J.R. & Himberger, L.C. (2001) Acuracy of drawing blood through infusing intravenous lines. *Heart Lung*, **30**(1), 66–73.

Holliday, G., Strike, P.N. & Masterton, R.G. (1991) Perineal cleansing and midstream urine specimen in ambulatory women. *J Hosp Infect*, **18**(1), 71–5.

Ismail, R. *et al.* (1997) Therapeutic drug monitoring of gentamicin: a 6-year follow-up audit. *J Clin Pharm Ther*, **22**(1), 21–5.

Jumaa, P.A. & Chattopadhyay, B. (1994) Pseudobacteraemia. *J Hosp Infect*, **27**(3), 167–77.

Karnon, J. *et al.* (2004) Liquid-based cytology in cervical screening: an updated rapid and systematic review and economic analysis. Executive summary. *Health Technol Assess*, **8**(20).

Leong, C.L. *et al.* (2006) Providing guidelines and education is not enough: an audit of gentamicin use at The Royal Melbourne Hospital. *Intern Med J*, **36**(1), 37–42.

Macleod, J.A. (1992) Collecting specimens for the laboratory tests. *Nurs Stand*, **6**(20), 36–7.

Madeo, M. *et al.* (2003) Reduction in the contamination rate of blood cultures collected by medical staff in the accident and emergency department. *Clinical Effectiveness in Nursing*, **7**, 30–2.

Magadia, R.R. & Weinstein, M.P. (2001) Laboratory diagnosis of bacteremia and fungemia. *Infect Dis Clin North Am*, **15**(4), 1009–24.

Malarkey, L.M. & McMorrow, M.E. (2005) *Saunders Nursing Guide to Laboratory and Diagnostic Tests*. Elsevier Saunders, St Louis, MO.

Marsden, J. & Shaw, M. (2003) Correct administration of topical eye treatment. *Nurs Stand*, **17**(30), 42–4.

McBryde, E.S. *et al.* (2005) Comparison of contamination rates of catheter-drawn and peripheral blood cultures. *J Hosp Infect*, **60**, 118–21.

Mead, M. (1999) High vaginal swab. *Practice Nurse*, **17**(9), 642.

Mims, C. *et al.* (2004) *Medical Microbiology*, 3rd edn. Elsevier Mosby, Edinburgh.

Moller, T. *et al.* (2005) Patient education – a strategy for prevention of infections caused by permanent central venous cathethers in patients with haematological malignancies: a randomized clinical trial. *J Hosp Infect*, **61**, 330–41.

National Collaborating Centre for Women's and Children's Health (2004) *Fertility: Assessment and Treatment for People with Fertility Problems. Clinical Guidelines*. Royal College of Obstetricians and Gynaecologists (RCOG) Press, London.

NHS Cancer Screening Programmes (2003) *Inequalities of Access to Cancer Screening: a Literature Review*. Series No 1. NHS Cancer Screening Programmes Publication, Sheffield.

NHS Cancer Screening Programmes (2004) *Colposcopy and Programme Management Guidelines for the NHS Cervical Screening*

793

Programmes. No. 20. NHS Cancer Screening Programmes Publication, Sheffield.

NHS Cancer Screening Programmes (2006) *An Easy Guide to Cervical Screening*. NHS Cancer Screening Programmes Publication, Sheffield.

NHS Screening Programmes (2004) *Training in Taking Samples for Liquid Based Cytology*. Implementation Guide No 4, Version 1. National Health Service Screening Programmes Publication, Sheffield.

NHS Screening Programmes (2006) *Taking Samples for Cervical Screening: a Resource Pack for Trainers*. No 23 April. National Health Service Screening Programmes Publication, Sheffield.

NICE (2004) *Referral for Suspected Cancer: NICE Guideline*. National Institute for Health and Clinical Excellence, London.

NMC (2006) *A–Z Advice Sheet Consent*. www.nmc.org.

NMC (2008) *The Code: Standards of Conduct, Performance and Ethics for Nurses and Midwives*. Nursing and Midwifery Council, London.

O'Grady, N.P. *et al.* (1998) Practice guidelines for evaluating new fever in critically ill adult patients. *Clin Infect Dis*, **26**(5), 1042–59.

Papasian, C.J. & Kragel, P.J. (1997) The microbiology laboratory's role in life-threatening infections. *Crit Care Nurse*, **20**(3), 44–59.

Parini, S. (2000) How to collect specimens. *Nursing*, **30**(5), 66–7.

Peterson, L.R. *et al.* (2001) Role of clinical microbiology laboratories in the management and control of infectious diseases and the delivery of health care. *Clin Infect Dis*, **32**, 605–11.

Poutanen, S.M. & Simor, A.E. (2004) *Clostridium difficile*-associated diarrhoea in adults. *Can Med Assoc J*, **171**(1), 51–68.

RCN (2005) *Good Practice in Infection Prevention and Control – Guidance for Nursing Staff*. Royal College of Nursing, London.

Rushing, J. (2004) Drawing blood with vacuum tubes. *Nursing*, **34**(1), 26.

Safdar, N. *et al.* (2005) Meta-analysis: methods for diagnosing intravascular devise-related bloodstream infection. *Ann Intern Med*, **142**(6), 451–66.

Sandin, R.L. & Rinaldi, M. (1996) Special consideration for the clinical microbiology laboratory in the diagnosis of infections in the cancer patient. *Infect Dis Clin North Am*, **10**(2), 413–30.

Shanson, D.C. (1999) Use of the microbiology laboratory – general principles. In: *Microbiology in Clinical Practice*. Butterworth-Heinemann, Oxford, pp. 24–36.

Shelton, B.K. (1999) Sepsis. *Semin Oncol Nurs*, **15**(3), 209–21.

Shirrel, D.J. *et al.* (1999) Understanding therapeutic drug monitoring. *Am J Nurs*, **99**(1), 42–4.

Shulman, R.J. *et al.* (1998) Central venous catheter versus peripheral veins for sampling blood levels of commonly used drugs. *J Parenteral Enteral Nutr*, **22**(4), 234–7.

Spitalnic, S.J., Woolard, R.H. & Mermel, L.A. (1995) The significance of changing needles when inoculating blood cultures: a meta-analysis. *Clin Infect Dis*, **21**(5), 1103–6.

Stollery, R., Shaw, M. & Lee, A. (2005) *Ophthalmic Nursing*. Blackwell Publishing, Oxford, p. 27.

Tam, V.H. *et al.* (1999) Vancomycin peak serum concentration monitoring. *J Intraven Nurs*, **22**(6), 336–42.

Theaker, C. (2005) Infection control issues in central venous catheter care. *Intensive Crit Care Nurs*, **21**, 99–109.

Thomas, L.C. *et al.* (2007) Development of a real-time *Staphylococcus aureus* and MRSA (SAM) PCR for routine blood culture. *J Microbiol Methods*, **68**(2), 296–302.

Thomson, R.B. (2002) Use of microbiology laboratory tests in the diagnosis of infectious diseases. In: *Expert Guide to Infectious Diseases* (ed. J. Tan). American College of Physicians, Philadelphia, pp. 1–41.

Tobin, C.M. (2002) Vancomycin therapeutic drug monitoring: is there a consensus view? The results of a UK National External Quality Assessment Scheme (UK NEQAS) for antibiotic assays questionnaire. *J Antimicrob Chemother*, **50**(5), 713–18.

Tortora, G.J. & Derrickson, B.H. (2006) *Introduction to the Human Body: the Essentials of Anatomy and Physiology*, 7th edn. John Wiley & Sons, New Jersey, pp. 900–52.

Traunter, W.B. *et al.* (2002) Skin antisepsis kits containing alcohol and chlorhexidinegluconate or tincture of iodine are associated with low rates of blood culture contamination. *Infect Control Hosp Epidemiol*, **23**, 397–401.

Wazait, H.D. *et al.* (2003) Catheter-associated urinary tract infections: prevalence of uropathogens and pattern of antimicrobial resistance in a UK hospital (1996–2001). *Br J Urol*, **91**(9), 806–9.

Weinstein, S.M. (2007) Laboratory tests. In: *Plumer's Principles and Practice of Intravenous Therapy*. J.B. Lippincott, Philadelphia, pp. 63–93.

Wilson, J. & Jenner, E.A. (2006) Understanding the microbiology laboratory. In: *Infection Control in Clinical Practice*. Bailliere Tindall, Edinburgh, pp. 19–33.

Wilson, M.L. (1996) General principles of specimen collection. *Clin Infect Dis*, **22**(5), 766–77.

WHO (2006) *Comprehensive Cervical Cancer Control: a Guide to Essential Practice*. World Health Organization Press, Switzerland.

Zitella, L. (2003) Central venous catheter care for blood and marrow transplant recipients. *Clin J Oncol Nurs*, **7**(3), 289–97.

Chapter 41

Spinal cord compression management

Reference material **796**
Procedure guidelines: Moving and handling a person with suspected **800**
spinal cord compression
Procedure guidelines: Spinal cord compression (suspected): assessment **801**
Procedure guidelines: Spinal cord compression (suspected): treatment **803**
Procedure guidelines: Spinal cord compression (suspected): rehabilitation **804**
Problem solving: Spinal cord compression (suspected) **806**
References **807**

Definition

Spinal cord compression is compression of the spinal cord and nerve roots.

Reference material

Spinal cord compression (SCC) is an oncological emergency that requires prompt assessment and treatment in order to minimize neurological deterioration and consequently optimize functional mobility and quality of life. It is therefore imperative that professionals dealing with such patients are knowledgeable of the condition (British Association of Surgical Oncology 1999) and ensure that they educate those at risk of SCC about the signs and symptoms and the action to take if any are noted.

SCC may be attributable to a number of causes including disease processes, intradural or extradural tumours. Involvement of specific spinal tracts will determine presentation of symptoms, with nerve root involvement resulting in symptoms which are motor, sensory or a combination of both in origin. Myelopathy refers to presenting symptoms as a consequence of compression of the spinal cord, whereas radiculopathy relates to compression of the nerve roots.

Despite the similarities of SCC and spinal trauma, for the purpose of this chapter the former will be dealt within the context of cancer therapy and rehabilitation.

Incidence and aetiology

The spine is one of the most common sites for bone metastases and it is estimated that SCC develops in 3–5% of patients with cancer (Quinn & DeAngelis 2000), with postmortem revealing a further 5% of undiagnosed cases (Posner 1995). In the adult population, approximately 60% of all cases of SCC occur as a result of carcinoma of the breast, lung or prostate (Loblaw & Laperriere 1998), with primary malignancies in the spinal cord being extremely rare (Solberg & Bremnes 1999). In children, pathologies such as Ewing's sarcoma and neuroblastoma may predispose to the condition (Britton & Ng 1998).

Classification

SCC may occur as a result of the following:

Tumours (Figure 41.1)

The position of the spinal cord tumour to the spinal cord and dura determines its classification, and the three main types are:

1 Extradural tumours: occurring outside of the dura, this is the most common position for tumours (Flounders & Ott 2003). An example of this type of tumour is bone metastases within the vertebrae.

Figure 41.1 Spinal cord compression.

2 Intradural extramedullary tumours: inside the dura but outside of the spinal cord, for example neurofibromas and meningiomas (Lohani & Sharma 2004).
3 Intramedullary tumours: situated within the spinal cord, such as in the case of ependymomas and low-grade astrocytomas (Britton & Ng 1998).

Degeneration

Conditions such as osteoporosis and spondylosis may result in vertebral fractures potentially leading to SCC (Mann *et al.* 2000).

Haematoma

Traumatic, spontaneous or congenital, may be of epidural or subdural haematoma origin (Kalina *et al.* 1995).

796

Trauma

For example, vertebral fractures, which may result in compression or severing of the spinal cord (Schafer 1997).

Clinical presentation

Clinical presentation of SCC is dependent on the location of the compression, the duration of its presence and consequently the level of neural function that is spared. Although treatment is generally palliative, early diagnosis is crucial in order to at best prevent and otherwise minimize irreversible neurological damage. Participation in activities of daily living and functional mobility will be indicated by the neurological symptoms and corresponding mobility level, and these symptoms are described further in Table 41.1.

Pain

Radiating back pain is the most common symptom, often beginning mildly and worsening with time (DeMichele & Glick 2001). Although pain is cited as the first presenting symptom in 96% of this patient group (Quinn & DeAngelis 2000), it is important to consider that an absence of pain does not automatically eliminate SCC diagnosis (Posner 1995).

Motor deficits

Presenting features of motor deficiency may encompass muscle weakness initially presenting distally, ataxia, impaired co-ordination and paralysis (Hillier & Wee 1997), dependent on the location of the compression, the duration of its

presence and consequently the level of neural function that is spared (Keller & Benton 2001). Hemiparesis or hemiplegia may result from oedema and decreased blood supply to the spinal cord and mechanical damage to the neural tissue (Dyck 1991).

Altered sensation

Presenting distally and progressing proximally, altered sensation manifests as numbness, paraesthesia and insensitivity to temperature and pain (DeMichele & Glick 2001).

Disturbances to the autonomic nervous system

Bowel and bladder symptoms such as incontinence, urinary retention or constipation may occur as a result of disturbances to the autonomic nervous system, and indicate advanced SCC (DeMichele & Glick 2001). Opiates may aggravate constipation (Posner 1995).

Investigations

There are a variety of diagnostic tools that can be used to identify or eliminate a diagnosis of SCC, and the literature recommends that patients are managed in accordance with local spinal cord policy until the condition is confirmed (Bucholtz 1999).

Figure 41.2 shows the The Royal Marsden Protocol (Royal Marsden NHS Foundation Trust 2006) for managing patients with suspected SCC.

Magnetic resonance imaging (MRI) is cited as the investigation of choice (Husband *et al.* 2001), and is a non-invasive investigation that provides a detailed picture of

Table 41.1 Grading of neurological symptoms to indicate level of functional mobility and independence with activities of daily living (ADLs) (Royal Marsden NHS Foundation Trust 2006).

Neurological symptoms	Mobility level	ADLs & functional mobility
Mild symptoms Pain Mobile No focal neurological deficits Bladder and/or bowel symptoms	1	■ Continue to mobilize ■ Self caring for ADLs, i.e. eating and drinking, washing/bathing, dressing, toileting, transfers, walking, walking up/down stairs
Moderate symptoms Pain Weakness of trunk or limbs Decreased sensation ±Pins and needles Bladder and/or bowel symptoms	2	■ Position according to symptoms, i.e. pain, motor or sensory loss ■ Patient to mobilize for practical care, e.g. toileting if tolerated and has no deterioration in neurological symptoms ■ Assist with ADLs as necessary, e.g. sitting and moving in bed, transfers
Severe symptoms ± unstable spine Severe pain Numbness Pins & needles ±Paraplegia/quadriplegia Bladder and/or bowel symptoms	3	■ Lie flat (one pillow only) ■ Log roll: supporting the neck, keep the spine in alignment and the legs straight when rolling ■ Assist with ADLs, e.g. feeding, personal care ■ Assist with toileting using slipper bed pan ■ Pressure area care

Figure 41.2 Management of spinal cord compression (Royal Marsden NHS Foundation Trust 2006).

spinal stability and tumour presence in order to guide treatment rationale (Levack *et al*. 2001). Indications for its use include (Royal Marsden NHS Foundation Trust 2006):

- Back pain with progressive power loss in the lower limbs or all limbs.

- Back pain associated with power loss and spasticity in all limbs.
- Back pain associated with lower motor neurone signs including flaccid paraparesis.
- Severe back pain associated with radicular pain.
- Sphincter disturbance of recent onset.
- Sensory level.

However, in some cases the patient may be unable to tolerate an MRI scan, so a computed tomography (CT) scan or plain X-ray is indicated (Bucholtz 1999). Once these investigations have diagnosed the level and extent of SCC, further treatment and rehabilitation plans can be established.

Treatment

In order to maximize recovery and minimize functional deficits, treatment should be commenced as soon as possible once a diagnosis has been established (Janjan 1996). Bucholtz (1999) suggests that the main aims of treatment are pain management, maintenance or improvement in neurological status, and spinal stabilization. Treatments may include the following and are indicated by the type and location of the tumour, its rapidity of onset and the overall prognosis:

Steroid therapy

The aim of steroids is to reduce oedema within the brain and spinal cord (Quinn & DeAngelis 2000; Keller & Benton 2001). Due to the glucocorticoid (anti-inflammatory) and mineralcorticoid (water and mineral) components of steroids there are side-effects which must be considered both prior and during their administration (Bucholtz 1999). Glucocorticoid side-effects may include diabetes, osteoporosis and Cushing's syndrome, and the mineralcorticoid side-effects can include hypertension, decrease in potassium and sodium and water retention (BNF 2002).

Analgesia

An accurate assessment should be carried out to determine the type and severity of pain and its effects on the patient (Scottish Intercollegiate Guidelines Network 2000). Assessment should include the quality, intensity, duration and location of back pain and any radicular or referred pain, as well as noting the type and dose of any analgesics used, their effectiveness and any related side-effects (see Chapter 27).

Radiotherapy

In patients who have been paraplegic at presentation for greater than 24-hours duration, radiotherapy is unlikely to reverse neurological deficit to regain ambulation, with a success rate of 11% (Maranzano & Latini 1995).

Keller & Benton (2001) suggest radiotherapy is used for patients with:

- Radiosensitive cancer.
- Lesions below the conus medullaris.
- Slow onset of compression.
- Medical contraindications to surgery.
- Surgically unapproachable tumours.

Surgical resection/decompression

Surgery is usually indicated for:

- Epidural SCC where there is no history of cancer or a remote history of cancer.
- The level of SCC is in an area previously irradiated.
- There is neurological deterioration during radiotherapy.
- Where patients have spinal instability or bony compression of their spinal cord (Quinn & DeAngelis 2000).

Adjuvant chemotherapy or hormonal therapy

Due to the chemoresponsiveness of the primary lung cancer or lymphoma diagnosis, treatment with tumour specific cytotoxic drugs is indicated (Guerrero 1998) in these cases.

Prognosis and predictors

There are a number of prognostic indicators identified within the literature that can assist in determining outcome both in terms of life span and function:

- Stage of primary tumour.
- Neurological status of the patient at the time of diagnosis (Maranzano & Latini 1995).
- Speed of onset of symptoms, with patients of gradual onset of symptoms (more than 14 days) maintaining or regaining more function than those patients with acute neurological onset (less than 14 days) (Rades *et al*. 2002).
- Functional mobility was maintained or improved post-treatment from 80% if ambulatory to less than 10% if paraplegic prior to treatment (Pigott *et al*. 1994).
- One-year survival post-spinal cord diagnosis was 73% for ambulant patients as opposed to only 9% for non-ambulant patients (Ruff & Lanska 1989).

799

Rehabilitation programme

Rehabilitation of the individual with SCC necessitates a multiprofessional approach co-ordinated by the nurse to optimize effectiveness through peer support and advice (Robinson 1998), and each profession's role is broadly described in Box 41.1. However, the approach that the team should take is very much dependent on whether the patient is to receive palliative care or active treatment, particularly as those patients within the former category generally have a poor prognosis. In these situations, the goal is to optimize the quality of life for both patient and carer. This may include specialist equipment and liaison with community palliative care teams and should be commenced as early as possible. Additionally, appropriate support should be provided to address psychosocial and sexual needs, which may take the form of counselling. Following consent from the patient, carers should be encouraged to actively participate in care including, where appropriate, catheter and bowel care and administering medication in an attempt to increase familiarity and prevent crisis upon discharge home.

Box 41.1   Referral criteria to the multiprofessional team

Occupational therapist (OT)

If patient:

- Has difficulties with activities of daily living (i.e. washing, dressing, cooking, etc.).
- Requires rehabilitation regarding personal care, leisure or work issues.
- Has difficulties with transfers.
- Has difficulties with access into and around home.
- Requires a wheelchair and pressure-relieving cushion.
- Is anxious and has problems relaxing.

Physiotherapist

If patient:

- Has altered neurological symptoms.
- Has difficulties with transfers.
- Has difficulties with mobilizing safely and independently.
- Requires rehabilitation and ongoing therapeutic input in the community.

Complex discharge coordinator/specialist sister palliative care (discharge planning)

- Patient who has had a significant change in functional ability and who will need a comprehensive care package.
- If patient requires continuing care level 1, i.e. prognosis < 3 months (different criteria apply for each Primary Care Trust (PCT), but normally < 3 months).
- Advice and guidance on discharge planning.

Social services

- If patient/carer is considered to have social care needs (irrespective of section 2 notification).
- If patient has functional problems, e.g. personal care.
- Community social service referrals and/or section 2 notification, i.e. patient is at risk on discharge if services are not arranged.

Welfare benefits

- If the patient requires benefits advice/financial or housing advice.

Other referrals as appropriate

- Hospital services, e.g. palliative care regarding symptom management; therapeutic massage; psychological support (psychological medicine, chaplain; art therapy).
- Community services, e.g. district nurses, community OT, community social services regarding provision of bed, pressure-relieving cushions, hoist and commode at home.

Adapted from Royal Marsden NHS Foundation Trust (2006).

Procedure guidelines   Moving and handling a person with suspected spinal cord compression

Procedure

Action	Rationale
1 Ensure that an assessment for manual handling is completed and documented (Griffiths & Gallimore 2005).	To maintain staff and patient safety. To prevent further complications resulting from injury (C).

2 A thorough assessment of the patient's condition and ability to mobilize should be made by the multidisciplinary team, involving the physiotherapist, medical team, nurse and, most importantly, the patient.

A multiprofessional perspective of the patient's ability to mobilize is needed to agree on safe practice which should include patient transfer and positioning. This will aid patient comfort (E).

3 A risk of falls care plan should be instigated as necessary.

To alert all staff and promote patient safety (E).

4 Mobilize if neurological symptoms allow (see Table 41.1). If neurological symptoms deteriorate at any time reassess patient and establish level of functional mobility. **If there is any doubt be cautious and seek medical advice**.

To monitor and recognize the neurological symptoms that may determine the functional mobility of a patient (E).

5 Antiembolic socks should be worn by all patients with spinal cord compression requiring admission to the hospital. Additional factors such as the patient's past medical history and recent drug history must also be considered (Falanga & Rickles 1999).

To reduce the risk of deep vein thrombosis (E).

6 The use of subcutaneous low molecular weight or unfractionated heparin may be required. If a patient receives heparin their platelet count should be carefully monitored (Royal Marsden NHS Foundation Trust 2006).

To reduce the risk of deep vein thrombosis (E).

Procedure guidelines   **Spinal cord compression (suspected): assessment**

Procedure

Action

1 Complete a comprehensive nursing assessment. (See Chapter 2.) Respiratory function and vital signs require monitoring to enable complications such as spinal shock and respiratory failure to be identified. (See Chapters 25 & 38.) All abnormal findings need to be reported to the appropriate members of the multidisciplinary team.

Rationale

To provide information on the current condition of the patient allowing treatment and care to be planned and implemented. Spinal shock requires immediate review by the medical team. These complications are more commonly associated with spinal injury patients, but may also exist with patients with spinal cord compression (C).

2 Refer to the neurological assessment and risk assessment for activities of daily living and functional mobility (see Table 41.1). By careful observation, monitor the patient and report any changes to the medical staff immediately.

To establish a baseline which will enable early detection of any deterioration at the earliest opportunity (E).

3 After careful assessment, urinary catheterization may be indicated if urinary retention is present. If required, a urinary catheter should be inserted using strict aseptic technique. Catheter care must be provided. (See Chapter 14.)

To allow voiding of urine. To reduce the risk of infection (E).

4 Monitor blood chemistry and the patient for signs of hypercalcaemia such as confusion, drowsiness and lethargy. If patient has hypercalcaemia refer to care plan (Royal Marsden NHS Foundation Trust 2006).

Hypercalcaemia may be associated with bone metastases causing the spinal cord compression (Falk & Fallon 1997: R 4).

Procedure guidelines *(cont.)*

5 Assess patient's pain. (See Chapter 27.) The type, duration, location and intensity of pain should be clearly documented.

To assist in identifying the possible level of spinal cord involvement and helping to prescribe the most appropriate analgesia and interventions to minimize pain. An accurate pain assessment may provide an indication of underlying pathology. For example, local pain occurs over the area of the tumour and may be constant. Radicular pain (pain caused by nerve root compression) may travel down the extremity associated with the area of compression. This may be worsened by sneezing, coughing and straining. Thoracic pain is often described as a tight band around the chest or upper abdomen. Medullary pain is referred pain which can be described as 'burning' or 'shooting' in nature and may be difficult to locate. An accurate assessment of a patient's pain will greatly assist in its management (Bostrom *et al.* 2004: R 4).

6 Use of a pain assessment chart.

Comprehensive documentation will provide for continuity of care and review. This will allow accurate assessment and evaluation of all pharmacological and non-pharmacological interventions (C).

7 Administer analgesia as required noting effects and side-effects. Report to medical team as necessary. Consider use of non-pharmacological therapy such as relaxation, therapeutic massage and simple repositioning when in bed.

Adequate pain relief is important for mobilization (E).

8 Refer all patients who do not have adequate pain relief to the palliative care team.

To utilize the knowledge and expertise of appropriate members of the multidisciplinary team (E).

9 Assess and document the understanding of the patient and their family.

This is significant as spinal cord compression may be identified at diagnosis or it may indicate the progression of their disease. Both will come as a great shock to the patient and the family (P).

10 Assess the need to facilitate discussions between medical staff, patient and family.

To promote honesty and openness, to aid understanding. Good communication is essential (E).

11 Assess and discuss care needs of patient at the weekly multidisciplinary team meetings.

To ensure all the support needs of the patient are met and appropriate referrals are made to members of the multidisciplinary team (see Box 41.1) (Purdue 2004; Royal Marsden NHS Foundation Trust 2006: C).

12 Assess social support at home and document needs.

To enable discharge planning to commence as early as possible, the needs of family members must not be forgotten and they must be involved in all aspects of the discharge planning process (E).

13 Assess the patient's expectation of recovery.

Patients should not be left without all hope but equally they should not be given false hope, or be encouraged to have unrealistic expectations of recovery (Twycross 2003: R 4; E, P).

14 Assess the patient's psychological well-being making appropriate referrals as needed. Many patients will benefit from a referral to the hospital's pastoral care team, the psychological care department, therapeutic massage and the occupational therapist for relaxation techniques.

Spinal cord compression can have a sudden and sometimes permanent effect on a patient's mobility and therefore independence. This, as well as the knowledge that spinal cord compression can indicate progressive disease raising the issue of mortality, can cause considerable psychological distress to the patient and their family (Purdue 2004: R 4; E).

Procedure guidelines   Spinal cord compression (suspected): treatment

Procedure

Preparation for neurosurgery

Action

1 Pre- and postoperative care is required. (See Chapter 30.)

Rationale

Surgical intervention with a decompression and or/stabilization of the spine or spinal cord. Combining surgery + radiotherapy has been shown to be of significant benefit versus radiotherapy alone (Regine *et al.* 2003: R 4). Also see Figure 41.2 noting indications for referral to a neurosurgical unit (Royal Marsden NHS Foundation Trust 2006: C).

Preparation for radiotherapy

Action

1 Prepare the patient for radiotherapy by providing written and verbal information.

Rationale

The basis for treatment of cancer-related spinal cord compression is radiotherapy and this may be commenced as an emergency treatment to conserve as much neurological function as possible (Neal & Hoskin 2003: R 4).

2 Prepare patient for daily treatments, considering the need for analgesia before therapy.

The Royal Marsden Hospital's policy is to offer 20 Gy in 5# over an average over 1 week (Royal Marsden NHS Foundation Trust 2006: C).

3 Monitor and manage side-effects depending on area affected as follows (Summers 2005):
   (a) Skin: erythema at treatment area (see Chapter 48).
   (b) Oesophagitis: administer analgesia and antacids as prescribed. Patient may require a soft diet and/or referral to a dietician.
   (c) Nausea and vomiting: administer antiemetics as prescribed.
   (d) Diarrhoea: administer antidiarrhoeal agents.
   (e) Dysuria: exclude the possibility of urinary tract infection. Encourage oral fluids and set an acceptable intake daily.
   (f) Fatigue: provide and encourage rest periods.

A number of side-effects may occur due to the radiotherapy treatment and will vary depending on the area treated, i.e. cervical/thoracic/lumbar area of spine (E).

4 Radiotherapy is used in conjunction with steroids.

Steroids are usually beneficial and should be commenced as soon as spinal cord compression is suspected and before a confirmed diagnosis is obtained. Steroids should be weaned as appropriate (Pease *et al.* 2004: R 4).

Preparation for chemotherapy

Action

1 Prepare the patient for chemotherapy by providing written and verbal information. (See Chapter 12.)

Rationale

Chemotherapy can be given as a primary treatment for chemosensitive tumours such as small cell lung cancer (Siegal *et al.* 2002: R 4).
Chemotherapy may cause side-effects which could impact on the rehabilitation process (E).

Procedure guidelines   Spinal cord compression (suspected): rehabilitation

Procedure

Action

Rationale

1 Refer the patient to the appropriate multiprofessional teams. This should include:
  - Physiotherapy.
  - Occupational therapy.
  - Social worker.
  - Community liaison nurse specialist.
  - Specialist palliative care physicians and nurse.

Nurses play a key role in facilitating effective teamwork (Webster 2002: E).

2 Await written confirmation from medical/surgical team regarding stability of spine before commencing rehabilitation programme and mobilization.

If the spine is unstable and medical stabilization procedures are inappropriate the patient may need to have completed radiotherapy (to reduce tumour mass and improve pain) before mobilization. Close liaison with medical, physiotherapy and occupational therapy team is necessary to plan rehabilitation programme and avoid further damage to spine (Hillier & Wee 1997: E).

3 Ensure goal setting is carried out in collaboration with the patient and carers.

Goal setting should be patient-centred, flexible, realistic and achievable, taking into account what is meaningful and pertinent to the individual patient (Law *et al.* 1995: E). This allows the patient to express his/her own wishes and choices (Lindsell 2006: E).

4 Ensure all team members and patients are aware of goals. In particular, if mobilization is not realistic, the team must ensure that everyone works towards same goals.

Communication amongst team and patients must be honest and false hope should not be given. However, the approach needs to allow patient and carers time to fully comprehend the magnitude of the disability at their own pace (E, P).

5 Goal setting needs to be flexible.

The flexible nature of rehabilitation allows for alteration in approach dependent on patient's response to treatment and primary disease. For example, patient and therapists may be aiming for improved mobility and transfers. However, in the case of treatment being ineffective, rehabilitation may require a compensatory approach if there is no return of function (Cooper 2006: E).
The patient's choices and autonomy may need to be balanced with resources available regarding rehabilitation staff, equipment and options available in the community (Eva 2006: E).

6 Ensure that regular multiprofessional team meetings are held to assess the patient's progress.

Team meetings aid good communication (Opie 1997: E).

7 The rehabilitation programme requires regular assessment and review.

The patient's response to treatment is never predictable or textbook case, and adjustments to aims and goals of rehabilitation need to be made in line with patient's capabilities (Cooper 2006: E).

8 Assess and monitor patients' and carers' psychological status and coping mechanisms relating to diagnosis of spinal cord compressions and its implications. Encourage patient to express feelings, communicate with them with empathy and promote the use of a variety of coping techniques.

Rehabilitation encompasses helping the patient acknowledge the disability and address the range of feelings including the grief process. Patients may or may not lack motivation and the rehabilitation programme will be influenced by this (E, P).

9 Optimize potential for independence both in mobility and function. Work as an integral part of the rehabilitation team to ensure rehabilitation is continuous.

The aim is to:
- Maintain and increase patient's independence in activities requiring motor performance.
- Help adjust and adapt to altered functional performance.
- Facilitate participation in social and occupational activities (E).

10 Assist the patient to perform an active or passive range of movement exercises, based on physiotherapy assessment and treatment plan.

Active and passive range of movement exercises help to prevent complications relating to decreased movement and may increase muscle strength (E).

11 Reinforce transfer techniques advised following physiotherapy and occupational therapy assessment.

To ensure safety of patient and health care team and to ensure consistency of approach across the multiprofessional team (Freeman et al. 2000: E).

12 Encourage optimum independence in self-care and other activities following occupational therapy assessment.

To restore confidence and self-esteem, to give structure and routine to patient's day and to increase the understanding of realistic aims of rehabilitation (Law et al. 1995: E).

13 The occupational therapist may assess the need for a home assessment prior to discharge from hospital to ensure correct equipment is in place.

For safety and independence (Bray & Cooper 2004: E).

14 Begin discharge planning as soon as level of functioning is established. Work closely with rehabilitation team, patient and carers, community support team, health care professionals and social services.

To offer thorough package of care to enable patient and carers to return home (if they wish) safely, with adequate care to support them and rehabilitation follow up to optimize independence (Bray & Cooper 2004: E).

15 Assess the patient's long-term care needs, making appropriate referrals to community services for ongoing rehabilitation and adaptations to housing.

Long-term needs and potential rehabilitation will be dependent on:
- The level of malignant spinal cord compression.
- The response to treatment.
- Function outcome in terms of return to mobility and managing activities of daily living.
- The services available in the individual patient's demographic area (E).

16 Monitor pressure areas regularly; provide pressure-relieving mattress and cushion as required following thorough ongoing assessment.

It is essential to be aware that this group of patients differ from spinal injury patients, due to immunosuppressive treatments and overall physical condition. The predisposition towards shearing forces and pressure sores may be greater (Cooper 2006: E).

Problem solving: Spinal cord compression (suspected)

Problem	Cause	Preventive action	Suggested action
Altered respiratory status.	Diaphragmatic paralysis can be associated with cervical and/or thoracic spine involvement. (NB. breathing pattern may be altered due to pain.)	On admission record vital signs documenting rate and pattern of respirations. Assess patient and establish baseline measurement for comparison with future measurements. Encourage patient to report any altered sensation or difficulty with breathing immediately.	Respiratory function monitoring should be recorded and documented as often as clinical assessment demands. The recording of a respiratory rate is one of the most important observations (Goldhill *et al.* 1999: R 4). Reduced respiratory function is often linked with adverse events (Considine 2004: R 4). It is therefore important that a patient is given the opportunity to make a decision about any future management, should respiratory failure result. If the patient is for full resuscitation it is important that there is good communication between ward staff and the critical care outreach teams (DH 2000: C). If the emphasis of treatment is palliative then good communication with the patient and family is vital (Crossno, 2004: R 4).
Neurogenic or 'spinal' shock, characterized by hypotension and bradycardia (Hughes 2003). This is rare in patients with spinal cord compression and more common in patients with spinal injury associated with cord transection.	Spinal shock is caused by a disruption of sympathetic outflow and manifests as low vascular resistance with increased intravascular capacity. The patient is functionally hypovolaemic even if no blood has been lost (Barker 1995).	Care with manual handling to prevent spinal injury as outlined previously.	Assess vital signs and ensure the medical team and the critical care outreach team is contacted urgently. The patient may require transfer to a critical care unit. Intravenous fluid resuscitation is required to correct hypovolaemia. Careful monitoring is needed as fluid overload may precipitate pulmonary oedema, particularly as fluid volume has not been lost. Central venous access for drug administration and fluid balance monitoring is indicated. Urinary catheterization may be necessary to record output accurately (E).
'Autonomic dysreflexia' is a medical emergency and is indicated by an acute rise in blood pressure. The systolic pressure can exceed 200 mmHg. Other symptoms are bradycardia, severe headache, visual blurring and flushing above injury level and pallor below. Seizures are also possible (Hughes 2003).	Complications associated with compression of spinal cord at T6–8 or higher, caused by an imbalance between sympathetic and parasympathetic response and usually triggered by an internal stimulus, such as a distended bladder or bowel and or pressure sores.	If left untreated this condition can be fatal due to the risk of a cerebral haemorrhage. The first line of treatment is prevention or removal of the stimulus. The medical team and outreach team should be contacted immediately.	Ensure a vasodilator is used and the patient should be kept as calm as possible. If a blocked urinary catheter is suspected this must be changed. A bladder washout should not be attempted as there may be a risk of fluid retention. Refer to the local spinal injury unit for advice (E).

References

Barker, S.J. (1995) Anaesthesia in the high risk patient. In: *Textbook of Critical Care*, 3rd edn (eds W.C. Shoemaker, M.A. Ayres, A. Grenvik & P.R. Holbrook). W.B. Saunders, Philadelphia.

BNF (British National Formulary) (2002) British Medical Association and Royal Pharmaceutical Society of Great Britain, London.

Bostrom, B. *et al.* (2004) Cancer-related pain in palliative care: patients' perceptions of pain management. *J Adv Nurs*, 45(4), 410–19.

Bray, J. & Cooper, J. (2004) The contribution of occupational therapy to palliative medicine. In: *The Oxford Textbook of Palliative Medicine* (eds D. Doyle *et al.*), 3rd edn. Oxford University Press, Oxford, pp. 1035–41.

British Association of Surgical Oncology (1999) The management of metastatic bone disease in the United Kingdom. The Breast Speciality Group of the BASO. *Eur J Surg Oncol*, 25(1), 3–23.

Britton, J. & Ng, V. (1998) Clinical neuro-imaging. In: *Neuro-Oncology for Nurses* (ed. D. Guerrero). Whurr, London, pp. 81–123.

Bucholtz, J. (1999) Metastatic epidural spinal cord compression. *Semin Oncol Nurs*, 15, 150–9.

Considine, J. (2004) Who, when and where? Identification of patients at risk of an in-hospital adverse event: implications for nursing practice. *Int J Nurs Pract*, 10(1), 21–31.

Cooper, J. (2006) *Occupational Therapy in Oncology and Palliative Care*. John Wiley & Sons, Ltd, Chichester.

Crossno, R. (2004) Dying in the emergency department: what emergency physicians should know about palliative medicine. *Top Emerg Med*, 26(1), 19–28.

DeMichele, A. & Glick, J. (2001) Oncologic emergencies. In: *Clinical Oncology* (eds R. Lenhard, R. Osteen & T. Gansler). American Cancer Society, Atlanta, pp. 733–64.

DH (2000) *Comprehensive Critical Care: A Review of Adult Critical Care Services*. Department of Health, London.

Dyck, S. (1991) Surgical instrumentation as a palliative treatment for spinal cord compression. *Oncol Nurs Forum*, 18(3), 515–21.

Eva, G. (2006) *Spinal Cord Compression Secondary to Cancer: Disability and Rehabilitation*. Sir Michael Sobell House, Churchill Hospital, Oxford.

Falanga, A. & Rickles, F.R. (1999) Pathophysiology of the thrombophilic state in the cancer patient. *Semin Thromb Hemos*, 25, 173–82.

Falk, S. & Fallon, M. (1997) ABC of palliative care: emergencies. *BMJ*, 315, 1526–1528.

Flounders, J. & Ott, B. (2003) Oncology emergency modules: spinal cord compression [online exclusive]. *Oncol Nurs Forum*, 30, E17–23. www.ons.org/publications/journals/ONF/Volume30/Issue1/pdf/34.pdf. Accessed 7/7/06.

Freeman, M., Miller, C. & Ross, N. (2000) The impact of individual philosophies of teamwork on multiprofessional practice and the implications for education. *J Interprof Care*, 14(3), 237–48.

Goldhill, D., White, S. & Sumner, A. (1999) Physiological values and procedures in the 24 hours before ICU admission from the ward. *Anaesthesia*, 54(6), 529–34.

Griffiths, H. & Gallimore, D. (2005) Positioning critically ill patients in hospital. *Nurs Stand*, 19(42), 56–64.

Guerrero, D. (1998) *Neuro-Oncology for Nurses*. Whurr, London.

Hillier, R. & Wee, B. (1997) Palliative management of spinal cord compression. *Eur J Palliat Care*, 4(6), 189–92.

Hughes, R. (2003) The management of patients with spinal cord injury. *Nurs Times*, 99(50), 38–41.

Husband, D.J., Grant, K.A. & Romaniuk, C.S. (2001) MRI in the diagnosis and treatment of suspected malignant spinal cord compression. *Br J Radiol*, 74, 15–23.

Janjan, N.A. (1996) Radiotherapeutic management of spinal metastases. *J Pain Symptom Manage*, 8(1), 1–7.

Kalina, P. *et al.* (1995) Spinal cord compression by spontaneous spinal subdural haematoma in polycythemia vera. *Postgrad Med J*, 71(836), 378–9.

Keller, J.W. & Benton, J.B. (2001) Oncologic emergencies. In: *Clinical Oncology: a Multidisciplinary Approach for Physicians and Students* (ed. P. Rubin). W.B. Saunders, London, pp. 208–19.

Law, M., Baptiste, S. & Mills, J. (1995) Client-centred practice: what does it mean and does it make a difference. *Can J Occup Ther*, 62(5), 250–6.

Levack, P. *et al.* (2001) A prospective audit of the diagnosis, management and outcome of malignant cord compression (CRAG 97/08). www.show.scot.nhs.uk/crag/committees/CEPS/reports/F%20Report%20copy%206-2-02.PDF. Accessed 7/7/06.

Lindsell, G. (2006) Client-centred approach of occupational therapy programme: case study. In: *Occupational Therapy in Oncology and Palliative Care* (ed. J. Cooper), 2nd edn. John Wiley & Sons, Ltd, Chichester, pp. 83–105.

Loblaw, D. & Laperriere, N. (1998) Emergency treatment of malignant extradural spinal cord compression: an evidence-based guideline. *J Clin Oncol*, 16, 1613–24.

Lohani, B. & Sharma M.R. (2004) Patterns of spinal tumors in Nepal: a clinico-radiological study. *Nepal Journal of Neurosciences*, 1, 113–19.

Mann, F.A., Kubal, W.S. & Blackmore, C. (2000) Improving the diagnosis of cervical spine injury in the very elderly: implications of epidemiology of injury. *Emerg Radiol*, 7(1), 35–41.

Maranzano, E. & Latini, P. (1995) Effectiveness of radiation therapy without surgery in metastatic spinal cord compression: final results from a prospective trial. *Int J Radiat Oncol Biol Phys*, 32(4), 959–67.

Neal, A.J. & Hoskin, P.J. (2003) *Clinical Oncology: Basic Principles and Practice*. Edward Arnold, London.

Opie, A. (1997) Effective teamwork in healthcare: a review of issues discussed in recent research literature. *Health Care Annal*, 5(1), 62–73.

Pease, N., Harris, R. & Finlay, I. (2004) Development and audit of a care pathway for the management of patients with suspected malignant spinal cord compression. *Physiotherapy*, 90, 27–34.

Pigott, K.H., Baddeley, H. & Maher, E.J. (1994) Patterns of disease in spinal cord compression on MRI scan and implications for treatment. *Clin Oncol*, 6(1), 7–10.

Posner, J. (1995) *Neurologic Complications of Cancer*. F.A. Davis, Philadelphia.

Purdue, C. (2004) Diagnosis and treatment of malignant spinal cord compression. *Nurs Times*, 100(38), 38–41.

Quinn, J.A. & DeAngelis, L.M. (2000) Neurologic emergencies in the cancer patient. *Semin Oncol*, 27(3), 311–21.

Rades, D., Heidenreich, F. & Karstens, J.H. (2002) Final results of a prospective study of the prognostic value of the time to develop motor deficits before irradiation in metastatic spinal cord compression. *Int J Radiat Oncol Biol Phys*, 53(4), 975–9.

Regine, W.F., Tibbs, P.A. & Young, A. (2003) Metastatic spinal cord compression: a randomized trial of direct decompressive surgical resection plus radiotherapy vs radiotherapy alone. *Int J Radiat Oncol Biol Phys*, 57(suppl 2), S125.

Robinson, S. (1998) Multidisciplinary teamwork. In: *Neuro-Oncology for Nurses* (ed. D. Guerrero). Whurr, London, pp. 221–52.

Royal Marsden NHS Foundation Trust (2006) *Spinal cord compression guidelines*. Royal Marsden NHS Foundation Trust, London. [unpublished.]

Ruff, R.L. & Lanska, D.J. (1989) Epidural metastases in prospectively evaluated veterans with cancer and back pain. *Cancer*, **11**, 2234–41.

Schafer, S. (1997) Oncologic complications. In: *Oncology Nursing* (ed. S. Otto), 3rd edn. Mosby, St. Louis, MO, pp. 406–74.

Scottish Intercollegiate Guidelines Network (2000) *Control of Pain of Patients with Cancer: a National Clinical Guideline*. Scottish Executive Health Department, Edinburgh.

Siegal, T., Siegal, T. & Brada, M. (2002) Spinal metastatic disease. In: *Oxford Textbook of Oncology*, Vol. I (eds R.L. Souhami *et al.*), 2nd edn. Oxford University Press, Oxford, pp. 977–93.

Solberg, A. & Bremnes, R.M. (1999) Metastatic spinal cord compression: diagnostic delay, treatment, and outcome. *Anticancer Res*, **19**, 677–84.

Summers, E. (2005) Understanding the nature of cancer-related fatigue. *Nurs Times*, **101**(40), 30–2.

Twycross, R. (2003) *Introducing Palliative Care*. Radcliffe Medical Press, Oxford.

Webster, J. (2002) Teamwork: understanding multiprofessional working. *Nurs Older People*, **14**(3), 14–19.

Chapter 42

Tracheostomy care and laryngectomy care (including voice rehabilitation)

Tracheostomy and laryngectomy care **810**
Reference material **810**
Laryngectomy voice rehabilitation **819**
Reference material **820**
Procedure guidelines: Tracheostomy dressing change **822**
Procedure guidelines: Tracheostomy suction **823**
Humidification **824**
Procedure guidelines: Humidification of patient with tracheostomy **825**
Procedure guidelines: Tracheostomy tube change **825**
Problem solving: Tracheostomy **827**
Procedure guidelines: Changing a Blom–Singer type non-indwelling **828**
voice prosthesis
References and further reading **829**

(a)   (b)   (c)   (d)

Figure 42.3   Shiley's tracheostomy tubes. **(a)** Shiley plain tube. **(b)** Shiley cuffed tube (courtesy of Tyco Healthcare). **(c)** Shiley plain fenestrated tube. **(d)** Shiley cuffed fenestrated tube (courtesy of Tyco Healthcare).

tracheostomy tube for lengthy periods, a cuff manometer should be used to check cuff pressure. In order to prevent tracheal tissue necrosis, stenosis and/or fistula formation (Mol *et al*. 2004; Russell 2004a) cuff pressure should not exceed 18 mmHg (Russell 2004b; Edgtton-Winn & Wright 2005; Clotworthy *et al*. 2006b).

Cuff pressure should be checked every shift (Clotworthy *et al*. 2006b) and each time the cuff is re-inflated (Woodrow 2002).

Shiley fenestrated tube (Figure 42.3c)

This is a plastic tube with an introducer and three inner tubes. One inner tube has no hub jutting out, is less obtrusive and is suitable for those patients not requiring attachment to other equipment (Russell 2004a). The other two inner tubes have the universal 15 mm extension at the upper aspect to facilitate connection to other apparatus, and one of these (with a green coloured hub) also has a fenestration midway down the tube. This is to encourage the passage of air and secretions into the oral and nasal passages. It is useful when attempting to encourage a return to normal function follow-

ing long-term use of a temporary tracheostomy, e.g. enabling the patient to communicate verbally.

The fenestrations enable this type of tube to be most suitable for the weaning method. A cap is inserted onto the tube, occluding the artificial airway. This enables the patient to become used to breathing via the oral and nasal passages again. The cap can be left in situ for certain periods of time until the patient can tolerate the tube occluded for a full uninterrupted 24 hours. Only then can removal of the entire tube, known as decannulation, be considered (Serra 2000; Harkin 2004). The decannulation procedure should take place in the morning, during the week to ensure that a specialist assessment can be sought in the unlikely event that the patient requires tracheostomy tube reinsertion (Harkin 2004).

Shiley cuffed fenestrated tube (Figure 42.3d)

This is a plastic tube with an introducer and two inner tubes. Both inner tubes have the universal 15 mm extension at the upper aspect to facilitate connection to other apparatus, and one of these (with a green coloured hub) also has a fenestration midway down the tube. The fenestrated tube can also be occluded with a cap, to assess the patient's oral and nasal

(a)   (b)

Figure 42.4 (a) Jackson's silver tube. (b) Negus's silver tube.

airway, first ensuring that the cuff has been completely de-flated and that the fenestrated inner tube is in situ. The outer tube has a fenestration in the middle of the cannula, again to encourage a return to normal function. The outer tube also has an inflatable cuff to give an airtight seal. The cuff prevents secretions from reaching the lungs. This tube is particularly useful for patients who require both periods of cuff inflation (to protect the airway) and cuff deflation (to enable a speaking valve to be used) (Russell 2004a).

Jackson's silver tracheostomy tube

This is a silver tube with an introducer and inner tube (Figure 42.4a). The inner tube is locked in position by a small catch on the outer tube and may be removed and cleaned as necessary without disturbing the outer tube.

Negus's silver tracheostomy tube

This is a silver tracheostomy tube with an introducer and a choice of inner tubes, with and without speaking valves (Figure 42.4b). The outer tube does not have a safety catch; consequently the inner tube may be coughed out inadvertently.

Speaking valve

This is a plastic device with a two-way valve which fits onto the 15 mm hub of the fenestrated inner tube (Figure 42.5). Distinction should be made between open and closed position valves:

The open position speaking valve (e.g. *Rusch* valve) is open by default and closes with positive pressure (expiration)

Figure 42.5 Rusch speaking valve.

813

which diverts air through the upper airways past the vocal cords, therefore allowing production of a voice. The closed position speaking valve (e.g. *Passy Muir* valve) is closed by default and requires negative pressure (patient's inspiratory effort) to open; as soon as expiration starts it closes which causes air to be diverted as described above. This type of valve can be used in ventilator circuits for patients who are mechanically ventilated.

If a non-fenestrated cuffed tube is in situ, the cuff should always be deflated before a speaking valve is fitted as the patient will not be able to exhale (Clotworthy *et al.* 2006b). Ordinarily, practitioners will also consider changing a non-fenestrated tube for a fenestrated tube (double lumen, with fenestrated inner tube). This will allow air to be diverted through the fenestrations of the tube in addition to air already diverted past the cuff to the upper airways. If a non-fenestrated tube is in situ, depending on the size of the tracheostomy tube and the diameter of the patient's trachea, sufficient air may not be diverted past the cuff. This will result in pressure building up because the patient will not be able to breathe out and the valve will not be tolerated. In this case it will be necessary for a complete outer tube change to a fenestrated tube.

However, anecdotal evidence from practice would suggest that in some instances cuff deflation alone (without changing a non-fenestrated tube for a fenestrated tube) may be sufficient to allow air diversion past the cuff through the upper airways as described above. It is important that each individual case is considered carefully and that practitioners weigh up the potential discomfort and distress a complete tracheostomy tube change may cause against the potential risks of fitting a speaking valve on a non-fenestrated tube. It is therefore imperative that when a speaking valve is used for the first time, the patient is carefully monitored for any signs of respiratory distress.

Kapitex Tracoetwist fenestrated tube

This is a plastic tube with an introducer and two inner tubes (Figure 42.6a). One of these inner tubes has an extension at its upper end to facilitate connection to other apparatus. The other inner tube has a fenestration midway down the tube. The outer tube also has a fenestration consisting of a series of small holes. This helps to reduce the risk of granulation tissue growing through the fenestration. The neck plate or flange moves in a vertical and horizontal direction enabling the plate to move as the patient moves. An inner tube with integrated speaking valve can be ordered separately.

A variety of other tubes are available in this series, including both cuffed and plain tracheostomy tubes.

Decannulation plug

This is a small plastic plug which fits into the outer fenestrated tube (Figure 42.6b). It is used to encourage patients to breathe via the oral and nasal air passages before removal of the tracheostomy tube. Alternatively, a small plastic plug (Kapitex) or a blind hub (Shiley) can be fitted into or over the inner fenestrated tube. This is particularly useful for patients who are still producing tenacious secretions as the plug or hub can be removed to enable the inner tube to be cleaned (Harkin 2004).

Colledge silver laryngectomy tube

This is a silver laryngectomy tube with an introducer (Figure 42.7a). It is often used to dilate a laryngectomy stoma which has stenosed. These tubes can be cleaned, autoclaved and reused.

Shiley laryngectomy tube

This is a plastic tube with an introducer and inner tube (Figure 42.7b). The inner tube has the universal 15 mm hub enabling the attachment to other equipment. It is shorter in length than a tracheostomy tube, thereby conforming to the slightly shorter trachea in the patient who has undergone a total laryngectomy. The inner tube may be removed and cleaned frequently without disturbing the outer tube. It is sometimes worn postoperatively while the stoma is healing to help facilitate a good shaped stoma.

(a)

(b)

Figure 42.6   (a) Kapitex Tracoetwist cuffed fenestrated tube. (b) Decannulation plug.

Figure 42.7 Tubes for permanent tracheostomies. **(a)** Colledge silver tube. **(b)** Shiley laryngectomy tube. **(c)** Shaw's laryngectomy tube. **(d)** Stoma button. **(e)** Laryngectomy tube.

Shaw's silver laryngectomy tube

This is a silver laryngectomy tube with an introducer and an inner tube beyond both lower and upper aspects of the outer tube (Figure 42.7c). Thus pressure dressings may be secured without occluding the stoma. The silver catch on the outer tube keeps the inner tube in position.

Stoma button

This is a soft Silastic 'button' (Figure 42.7d). It may be used in place of a laryngectomy tube. It is very light and comfortable to wear and can be used in conjunction with a Blom–Singer speaking valve. In order to facilitate the use of the Blom–Singer speaking valve a diamond-shape is cut out of the Silastic (see Laryngectomy voice rehabilitation section, below, for specific information on surgical voice restoration).

Laryngectomy tube

This is a slightly opaque Silastic tube which is longer in length in comparison to the stoma button. These tubes are 36 and 55 mm in length and are available in a variety of different sizes (Figure 42.7e). This tube is most suitable for patients who experience a degree of stenosis further down the trachea

(see Stoma buttons and vents, in Laryngectomy voice rehabilitation section, below, for further information).

Heat and moisture exchange filters

Following a tracheostomy or a laryngectomy, patients lose normal nasal airway functions. The air they breathe is no longer warmed, humidified and filtered by the nasal passages as they now breathe directly in and out of the tracheostomy. Drying of the airway impairs mucous and cilia function resulting in thickened airway secretions (Woodrow 2002). The amount of secretions produced will vary from patient to patient but is greater in the immediate and early postoperative period and gradually improves over the ensuing months. Patients find that any sharp change in temperature stimulates excessive mucus production (Mathieson 2001).

Prior to the development of heat and moisture exchange (HME) filters, patients coped with this by spraying the tracheostomal area with water, using a Roger's spray or equivalent and wearing either a small foam pad, a 'bib' or specially designed cravat or scarf over the stoma. HME filters are now widely available on prescription in many different styles enabling the patient and/or the nurse to decide on the appropriate method of humidification, depending on

Figure 42.8   A trachphone.

the individual patient's circumstances (Billau 2004). The importance of systemic hydration of the patient via a feeding tube, intravenous fluids or oral fluids must not be overlooked (Clotworthy *et al.* 2006c) as this can impact on the tenacity of secretions.

HME filters for laryngectomy use consist of a self-adhesive baseplate, which is placed around the stoma and a specially treated foam filter which is clipped into the centre. This enables the patient to breathe more easily while the air is warmed, humidified and filtered by the foam. For a minority of patients who cannot tolerate the baseplate on the skin or maintain a good seal, the filter section can also be clipped into a flexible Silastic laryngectomy tube, vent or stoma button. It is the role of the speech and language therapist and/or clinical nurse specialist and/or physiotherapist to assess and fit the HME filter in the initial stages of care (Pathways in Cancer Care 2001).

HME filters for tracheostomy use follow the same rationale as those for laryngectomy use. The filter is attached directly onto the tracheostomy tube and some have an integral speaking valve and enable suctioning to be performed and/or oxygen to be administered whilst still in situ, e.g. trachphone (Figure 42.8).

Communication for the patient with a tracheostomy

The presence of a cuffed tracheostomy tube can impair verbal communication as air can no longer flow over the vocal cords. Loss of speech can be both frustrating and frightening (Serra 2000) and it is essential for the nurse to encourage both the patient and family to use other forms of communication during this time. The ultimate goal is to restore the

patient's ability to communicate verbally, consistently and effectively (Hales 2004a). The call bell must be within reach at all times and pen and paper or a magic slate should be provided. The latter enables the patient to erase previous conversations enabling some confidentiality to be maintained. For those patients unable to read or write and/or understand written English a picture board or alphabet board combined with phrases can be useful. This is where laminate A4 sheets displaying the alphabet in large letters, or simple pictures depicting basic activities (e.g. drink, toilet) supplemented with useful phrases are used (Clotworthy *et al.* 2006d). Those proficient at using a keyboard can communicate using a laptop or an electronic communication aid. The latter enables the individual to type in a phrase to obtain an automated voice repeating the phrase. The importance of a thorough nursing assessment on admission to hospital and the provision of patient information cannot be overestimated as this will help to identify communication issues early as well as patient and family concerns regarding the tracheostomy (Serra 2000).

Extra attention should be given to non-verbal communication, such as facial expression, hand and body positions and movement (Serra 2000). Lip reading may be appropriate for some patients. The patient is encouraged to exaggerate lip movements and use short but complete sentences in order to make the message clearer (Clotworthy *et al.* 2006d). Whichever communication method is utilized by the patient it is essential that all recipients (hospital staff, friends or relatives) allow the patient time to express him or herself.

Communication for the patient with a laryngectomy

The same strategies for effective communication can also be used for the patient who has undergone a total laryngectomy. This is particularly important in the early postoperative days and for those patients who have not undergone surgical voice restoration (see Laryngectomy voice rehabilitation section, below, for specific information on surgical voice restoration). An electro-larynx can be used in the short- and long-term period. This device vibrates the air in the airway (in place of the vocal cords) creating a sound which can be shaped into speech sounds by the palate, tongue, cheeks, teeth and lips (Hales 2004a). Some patients prefer to use oesophageal speech. This is produced by inhaling or injecting air into the pharynx and upper oesophagus and then releasing it in a controlled fashion through the pharynx into the mouth (Rhys Evans & Blom 2003). All patients who have undergone total laryngectomy require immense support and encouragement to persevere with communication whichever method is chosen to enable them to achieve intelligible speech (Hahn & Jones 2000).

Swallowing for the patient with a tracheostomy

The presence of a tracheostomy tube can impair swallowing and consequently compromise the patient's nutritional status

(Bond *et al.* 2003). The presence of a tracheostomy tube can cause tethering of the larynx, hindering the normal swallowing mechanism, particularly movement of the epiglottis over the airway to prevent aspiration (Hales 2004b). Assessment by a speech and language therapist is an essential part of these patients' care (Serra 2000). It is now recommended that patients should be nil by mouth when the cuff is inflated on the tracheostomy tube (Hales 2004b). There are two reasons for this: firstly, the inflated cuff does not offer complete protection from aspiration and can potentially disguise obvious signs of aspiration; and secondly, the cuff puts additional pressure on the larynx reducing laryngeal elevation needed for the normal swallowing mechanism (Hales 2004b).

Swallowing for the patient with a laryngectomy

Following the total laryngectomy procedure the patient is usually nil by mouth for 7 days if no previous radiotherapy has been given (Rhys Evans & Blom 2003) to enable healing in the pharynx. Once oral diet and fluids commences, the patient's stoma site should be observed closely for any evidence of leaking which might indicate a pharyngocutaneous fistula. Patients who have undergone previous radiotherapy are nil by mouth for 10 days and commence oral diet following a satisfactory barium swallow (Rhys Evans & Blom 2003). Patients who have a tracheo-oesophageal puncture as a primary procedure for the fitting of a voice valve may be fed immediately postoperatively via a catheter inserted through the puncture site (Shaw 2003) (see Laryngectomy voice rehabilitation section, below, for specific information on surgical voice restoration). A nasogastric, gastrostomy or jejenostomy tube will be used to provide nutrition to those without a tracheo-oesophageal puncture (see Chapter 24 for specific information).

At times a speaking valve may leak or fall out (see Laryngectomy voice rehabilitation section, below, for specific information on surgical voice restoration). A leaking valve can usually be replaced fairly quickly by a speech and language therapist or surgical doctor or a nurse who has undergone training. It may be necessary to insert a cuffed tracheostomy tube to prevent the patient aspirating diet/fluids and/or saliva until the valve is replaced. If a valve has fallen out, it is essential to check clinically and if necessary with a chest X ray that this has not fallen into the trachea or bronchus, and a temporary catheter should be inserted into the tracheo-oesophageal puncture promptly to ensure that the tract remains patent and to ensure that food and fluids do not leak into the stoma causing aspiration. Some patients are capable of effectively coughing the prosthesis out, while others require endoscopic retrieval (Singer & Deschler 1998).

General care of tracheostomy patients

- When caring for a tracheostomy patient the following should always be at the bedside or accessible if the patient is self-caring or ambulant:

(a) Humidified oxygen with tracheostomy mask.
(b) Suction machine with a selection of suction catheters.
(c) Sterile water (Serra 2000) can be used to help clear suction tubing of secretions after suctioning has been performed.
(d) Clean disposable gloves and individually packaged, sterile, disposable gloves (Edgtton-Winn & Wright 2005).
(e) Disposable plastic apron and goggles (Day *et al.* 2002).
(f) Two cuffed tracheostomy tubes, one the same size as the patient is wearing, the other a size smaller, in the event of an emergency tracheostomy tube change (Serra 2000; Tamburri 2000).
(g) One 10 ml syringe to inflate cuff on tracheostomy tube.
(h) Tracheal dilators, in the event of tracheostomy tube falling out or being removed and inability to insert another tube. Tracheal dilators can be used to keep stomal opening patent until medical assistance arrives.
(i) Cuff pressure manometer (Serra 2000).

- Outer tube changes are mostly dependent on the type of secretions the patient has, for example, a patient with copious, tenacious secretions will need a daily tube change, sometimes twice a day, as this will be the only way of ensuring that the stoma and tube are free from any accumulation of secretions. If the patient has minimal secretions then the necessity to change the tube decreases until some patients need to have their tube changed only weekly. Sometimes if the patient has a wound area up to the stoma edge, the entire tracheostomy tube has to be removed to gain access for cleaning the wound and observing its general status.
- The frequency of inner tube changes depends on the volume, tenacity and viscosity of secretions and the comfort of the patient. In the immediate postoperative phase it may be necessary to change the inner tube half hourly. Any nurse starting a span of duty should perform a baseline assessment of the airway and tube to check on the type and amount of secretions and the need for humidification (Rhys Evans 2003).

The tracheostomy dressing can be renewed without removing the tube which should be done twice a day or more frequently if necessary (Serra 2000). Changing the dressing will ensure that the surrounding skin remains clean, dry and free from irritation and infection (Edgtton-Winn & Wright 2005).

General care of patients with a total laryngectomy

- When caring for the patient who has undergone a total laryngectomy, the following should always be at the bedside or accessible if the patient is self-caring or ambulant:

817

(a) Humidified oxygen with tracheostomy mask.

(b) Suction machine with a selection of suction catheters.

(c) Sterile water (Serra 2000) can be used to help clear suction tubing of secretions after suctioning has been performed.

(d) Clean disposable gloves and individually packaged, sterile, disposable gloves (Edgtton-Winn & Wright 2005).

(e) Disposable plastic apron and goggles (Day *et al.* 2002).

(f) Two cuffed tracheostomy tubes, one the same size as the patient is wearing, the other a size smaller, in the event of an emergency tube change (Serra 2000; Tamburri 2000).

(g) One 10 ml syringe to inflate cuff on tracheostomy tube.

(h) Tilley's forceps: these are angled forceps that can be used to remove crusts or plugs of mucous from in and around the stoma.

(i) Pen torch (or access to a light source).

(j) Micropore or Elastoplast tape for those with a tracheo-oesophageal puncture, to ensure that the catheter keeping the puncture patent is secured firmly with tape or a suture (see Laryngectomy voice rehabilitation section, below, for specific information on surgical voice restoration).

■ Patients who have undergone a total laryngectomy may require a cuffed tracheostomy tube for the first 24–48 hours. The tube stents the often oedematous stoma and the inflated cuff prevents blood-stained secretions from entering the lungs. The frequency of inner tube changes depends on the volume, tenacity and viscosity of secretions and the comfort of the patient. In the immediate postoperative phase it may be necessary to change the inner tube half hourly. Any nurse starting a span of duty should perform a baseline assessment of the airway and tube to check on the type and amount of secretions and the need for humidification (Rhys Evans 2003).

■ The dressing around the tracheostomy tube can be renewed without removing the tube which should be done twice a day or more frequently if necessary (Serra 2000). Changing the dressing will ensure that the surrounding skin remains clean, dry and free from irritation and infection (Edgtton-Winn & Wright 2005).

■ During the immediate postoperative phase the decision on whether a tube is required and which type is required is made by the surgeon (Clotworthy *et al.* 2006a). For those patients with no tube in situ, the nurse must be extremely vigilant, assessing the bare stoma frequently to ensure that the stoma is not at risk of stenosis. A stenosed stoma will restrict the patient's breathing, hinder the removal of secretions and prevent the insertion of a cuffed tube in an emergency situation. Stoma size should be sufficiently large, ideally 20–25 mm in diameter (Rhys Evans & Blom 2003) in order to insert a size 6

or above Shiley tracheostomy tube or equivalent. In the longer term, many patients no longer require a tube of any type in situ.

■ Stoma sutures are removed on day 7. If the patient has previously received external beam radiotherapy to the neck, stoma sutures are removed on day 10.

■ A moisturizing cream, such as E45, can be applied twice daily to the stoma once the tracheostomy tube and associated dressing is removed. For those patients with secretions that tend to accumulate around the stoma, a Cavilon wand can be used to prevent the skin becoming red and excoriated (Hampton 1998).

Suctioning via a tracheostomy or a laryngectomy

Patients with a tracheostomy or a laryngectomy will often require suctioning due to their impaired ability to clear tracheo-bronchial secretions. The function of the upper airways is to filter, warm and humidify inspired air. When a patient breathes through a tracheostome the upper airways are bypassed and cold, unfiltered and unhumidified air reaches the tracheo-bronchial tree. This is thought to impair the normal beating action of the cilia on the mucosal lining of the trachea which under normal circumstances causes an upward stream of mucous and foreign bodies (Pilbeam 1998). Furthermore, patients with a tracheostomy may have a reduced ability to generate a forceful cough and, in addition may experience an increased production of bronchial secretions due to irritation of the trachea caused by the tracheostomy tube (Hooper 1996). These factors all contribute to the potential for the patient with a tracheostomy to develop sputum retention which could be detrimental and result in an increased risk of infection and impaired gas exchange, due to the plugging of airways and airflow limitation.

Indications for suctioning

The use of routine suctioning should be avoided and careful assessment of the patient's respiratory function should be carried out instead. Inspection, auscultation, percussion and palpation will help to determine the following (Pryor & Prasad 2001; Hough 2001):

■ Patient's ability to clear his or her own secretions.
■ Location of any secretions.
■ Whether these secretions could be reached by the catheter.
■ How detrimental these secretions might be for the patient.

Despite the benefits of suctioning, this action can also be hazardous for the patient:

■ *Hypoxia*: the act of suctioning reduces vital lung volume from the lungs and upper airways. Each suctioning procedure should last no longer than 10–15 seconds to decrease the risk of trauma, hypoxia and other side-effects

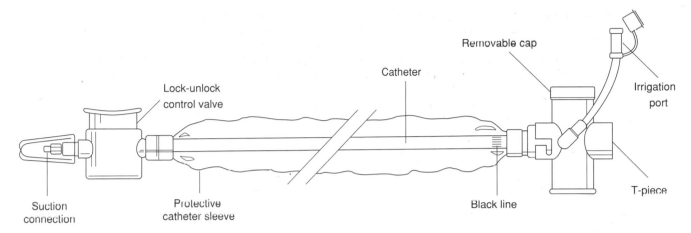

Figure 42.9 Components of a closed-circuit catheter. The control valve locks the vacuum on or off. The catheter is protected inside an airtight sleeve. A T-piece connects the device to the tracheal tube. The irrigation port allows saline instillation for irrigating the patient's airway or for cleaning the catheter (Hough 2001).

(The Joanna Briggs Institute 2000; Day 2000). Ventilator disconnection or the removal of the oxygen supply will also add to the risk of hypoxia prior to suctioning. Within a critical care setting this risk can be avoided by hyperoxygenating the lungs with 100% oxygen, either manually or via a ventilator (Glass & Grap 1995; Hough 2001).

- *Mucosal trauma*: an incorrect choice of catheter, poor technique and the use of an excessively high suction pressure may all lead to mucosal trauma. The recommended suction pressure is 80–150 mmHg or 11–20 kPa for adults (Day 2000; Day *et al.* 2002).
- *Cardiac arrhythmias*: arrhythmias may be brought about by the onset of hypoxaemia or a vagal reflex instigated by tracheal stimulation by the catheter (MacIntyre & Branson 2001).
- *Raised intracranial pressure*: this may occur if the suction catheter causes excessive tracheal stimulation and result in coughing and an increase in the patient's intrathoracic pressure, both of which compromise cerebral venous drainage (Pryor & Prasad 2001).
- *Infection risk*: both care giver and patient are at risk of infection when suctioning is performed. In order to minimize this, examination gloves should be worn and an aseptic technique should be used, decontaminating hands with an alcoholic handrub before and after the suction procedure (DH 2005).

Suction catheters

Choosing the correct suction catheter size depends on the size of the tracheostomy tube. As a guide, the diameter of the suction catheter should not exceed one-half of the internal diameter of the tracheostomy tube (Griggs 1998; Hough 2001). The following formula can be used to determine the correct size catheter: divide the internal diameter of the tracheostomy tube by two and multiply this by three to obtain the French gauge of the suction catheter (Billau 2004).

Within a critical care setting, a closed-circuit suction system is an alternative method to the open suction system for patients being mechanically ventilated. This closed system has the catheter sealed in a protective plastic sleeve, which is connected permanently into a standard ventilator circuit thus preventing the catheter becoming contaminated (Figure 42.9). This also reduces the number of times the patient is disconnected from the ventilator, avoiding further hypoxia and cross-infection. Other patient groups who may benefit from its use include those who are immunosuppressed, actively infectious patients or those who require high levels of positive end expiratory pressure (PEEP) (Billau 2004).

Resuscitation

In the event of a patient with a tracheostomy needing resuscitation, the nurse should ensure that the tracheostomy is clear then connect an artificial ventilation device (for example, an Ambu bag with a connector or catheter mount attached) to the tracheostomy tube in order to perform manual ventilation. The cuff of the tracheostomy tube must be inflated to prevent air leakage, thus ensuring adequate oxygenation and ventilation.

Laryngectomy voice rehabilitation

Definition

A voice prosthesis is a one-way silicone valve that slots into a surgically created fistula reconnecting the trachea to the pharynx following surgical removal of the larynx (Delassus Gress & Singer 2005). The valve, once fitted, allows air to be directed from the lungs and trachea into the pharynx when the patient wishes to speak. This airflow causes the pharyngeal muscles to vibrate, producing the sound or voice for speech. Since the valve is one-way it also prevents food and drink passing from the pharynx forward into the trachea

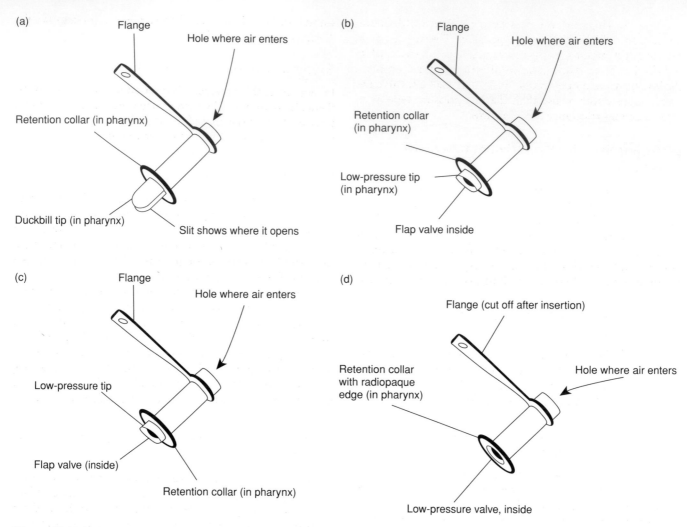

(a)
Flange
Hole where air enters
Retention collar (in pharynx)
Duckbill tip (in pharynx)
Slit shows where it opens

(b)
Flange
Hole where air enters
Retention collar (in pharynx)
Low-pressure tip (in pharynx)
Flap valve inside

(c)
Flange
Hole where air enters
Low-pressure tip
Flap valve (inside)
Retention collar (in pharynx)

(d)
Flange (cut off after insertion)
Hole where air enters
Retention collar with radiopaque edge (in pharynx)
Low-pressure valve, inside

Figure 42.10   Laryngectomy voice rehabilitation. **(a)** Duckbill valve. **(b)** Low-pressure valve, 16 Fr gauge. **(c)** Low-pressure valve, 20 Fr gauge. **(d)** Indwelling valve, 20 Fr gauge.

820

and down the airway. A valve which begins to leak food and/or drink may be defective, worn-out or ill-fitting.

The fistula, also known as a tracheo-oesophageal puncture for the voice valve may be created at the time of the total laryngectomy operation. This is a surgically created puncture, which means that this will close in the absence of a catheter or voice prosthesis. Hence the terms primary surgical voice restoration (at the time of laryngectomy) and secondary surgical voice restoration (procedure carried out later) are used.

Reference material

Voice prostheses for patients undergoing laryngectomy have been available in Britain since the early 1980s (Blom 1998). There are a number of different types of prosthesis on the market, including Blom–Singer, Provox and Gröningen. All work according to the same principle. The Blom–Singer prosthesis, developed in the USA by Eric Blom, a speech pathologist, and Mark Singer, an otolaryngologist, will be described in detail here.

Types of valve (Figure 42.10)

There are different makes of voice valve. The Blom–Singer range usually have a diameter of either 16 or 20 Fr. Other diameters are found in other makes. All makes of valve are available in a series of different lengths (Blom–Singer prostheses range from 4–22 mm) to fit the depth of the tracheopharyngeal wall, which varies from patient to patient. Initially, the patient should be measured and fitted with a prosthesis by an experienced and specialized practitioner who will select the most suitable type of valve, taking into account the patient's fitness and individual needs (Leder & Blom 1998).

Duckbill valve Blom–Singer type voice prosthesis

This prosthesis is named after its design: the valved end of the prosthesis opens like a duck's bill to allow air to pass into the pharynx. Talking with the prosthesis requires a little more effort than talking prior to laryngectomy. The device has a rounded end, making it easy to insert, and is less susceptible to infection by *Candida albicans* affecting its function than the low-pressure model (Blom 1998). The duckbill valve requires more effort to use than the low-pressure type as it creates greater resistance to the airflow.

Low-pressure valve Blom–Singer type voice prosthesis

The Blom–Singer low-pressure device has a flatter posterior aspect than the duckbill with a small hinged flap acting as the one-way valve. The gel cap insertion technique is standard practise for inserting these valves (Leder & Blom 1998). Its design makes it more susceptible to infection with *Candida albicans*. Talking with the prosthesis requires approximately the same amount of effort as talking prior to laryngectomy.

Low-pressure valve Blom–Singer type voice prosthesis (20 Fr gauge)

This is a special wide-diameter prosthesis recommended for patients with specialized needs. The decision to fit this lies with the specialist ears, nose and throat (ENT) doctor and/or specialist speech and language therapist.

Indwelling valve Blom–Singer advantage prosthesis (16 Fr gauge)

This has been developed in recent years in response to specific needs of stable patients who find that they have very resistant *Candida albicans*. The silicone flap valve and internal barrel incorporate silver oxide, known to counteract *Candida albicans* (Blom 1998). It has to be inserted and removed by a specialist speech and language therapist, an ENT doctor experienced in fitting and managing voice prostheses or a nurse trained in the procedure.

Indwelling valve Blom–Singer type voice prosthesis (20 Fr gauge)

The main advantage of this valve is that it can last for about 6 months, providing the patient uses prophylactic antifungal treatment to counteract fungal infection of the valve. It has to be inserted and removed by a specialist speech and language therapist, ENT doctor experienced in fitting and managing voice prostheses or a nurse trained in the procedure.

Provox type indwelling voice prosthesis

This device is more difficult to insert as it has to be passed through the mouth and pharynx. This can be done under local anaesthetic, although for some patients a general anaesthetic is preferable. Once inserted it remains in place for an average of 4–6 months. This device is susceptible to infection by *Candida albicans*. The Provox 2 voice prosthesis has more recently become available and can be inserted and removed

via the tracheostoma. It can have a wider diameter than the Blom–Singer type prosthesis.

Gröningen type voice prosthesis

In most cases this prosthesis is inserted under general anaesthetic. It continues to be used at one centre in the UK. Once inserted it remains in place for approximately 6 months. This device is susceptible to infection by *Candida albicans*.

Stoma buttons and vents

If they experience stenosis of the stoma created for the voice prosthesis, patients may need to wear a stoma button, especially in the first few weeks after surgery. Although the stoma would not close completely, it may become so narrow that breathing is restricted and care of the voice prosthesis difficult (Singer & Deschler 1998).

Stoma buttons, made of soft Silastic, are available in a range of diameters: 10, 12 and 14 mm. For patients with voice prostheses, 12 or 14 mm is most suitable, so that the stoma is wide enough for the patient to clean the prosthesis. If a voice prosthesis is used with a stoma button, a hole is cut in the button to allow air to pass through the valve during speech. If the button is adapted in this way it should only be done by an experienced, specialized practitioner.

Silastic laryngectomy tube for use with a voice prosthesis

These devices are made of a softer plastic than the traditional Shiley type laryngectomy tube, making them more comfortable and more appropriate for long-term use (beyond the postoperative period and on a continuing basis providing they are kept clean). Some patients find the stoma consistent enough in diameter to dispense completely with a vent or button during the first year after the laryngectomy. Other patients need to continue wearing either a vent or a button all the time. They are available in a range of three diameters, and two different lengths: 36 or 55 mm. If a voice prosthesis is used at the same time as either of these two devices, an aperture is made in the upper side to allow air to pass through the valve. The tube is made with an indentation to mark the site of the aperture. If the tube is adapted in this way it should only be done by an experienced, specialized practitioner. (For further information see Stoma buttons and vents section, above.)

Indications for replacing a voice prosthesis

- *Voice prosthesis showing signs of wear and tear*. In most cases, experience indicates that a voice prosthesis can last anything from 6 to 12 weeks. After that time patients may find it harder to use it to make voice, when previously they had no difficulty. This deterioration is gradual.
- *Voice prosthesis is leaking*. Valves are made of silicone and are therefore susceptible to fungal infection by

Candida albicans. Micro-organisms burrow into the silicone and interfere with the functioning of the posterior (internal) end of the prosthesis. The effect of this is to cause saliva and drinks to leak in small drops through it, causing the patient to cough (Leder & Blom 1998). Leakage such as this is a very common problem and can shorten the life of the prosthesis considerably.

- *Drink and/or food are leaking around the valve.* This problem is less common (Lewin 1998). It indicates that the diameter of the fistula or tracheo-oesophageal puncture has become greater than the diameter of the valve, probably as a result of infection. A specialist speech and language therapist or a nurse or doctor with the ENT training required to fit and manage voice prostheses should be contacted for advice.
- *Patient cannot make any sound with the voice prosthesis.* It is possible that patients may suddenly find that they can no longer make any sound with the prosthesis, or sound may be intermittent. The prosthesis must be removed and inspected, and will almost certainly need to be changed. A specialist speech and language therapist, or a nurse or

doctor with the ENT training required to fit and manage voice prostheses should be contacted for advice.

Indications for replacing a 'lost' or dislodged voice prosthesis

The voice prosthesis is held in position by a silicone retention collar which is an integral part of the whole device. It is therefore possible for it to become accidentally dislodged. Patients are told that this might happen, and shown how to insert their dilator, a Jacques 14 Fr red rubber catheter, through the fistula to keep it open. The patients need to understand the importance of being able to do this. If patients are able to perform this procedure when a voice prosthesis is accidentally dislodged, the fistula remains open and a new prosthesis is inserted after removal of the dilator or catheter. If the voice prosthesis is ejected and the patient is unable to insert a catheter satisfactorily a speech and language therapist or doctor with experience in fitting and managing voice prostheses should be contacted for advice (Leder & Blom 1998).

Procedure guidelines   Tracheostomy dressing change

Equipment

1 Sterile dressing pack.
2 Tracheostomy dressing or a keyhole dressing.
3 Cleaning solution, such as 0.9% sodium chloride.

4 Tracheostomy tape.
5 Bactericidal alcohol handrub.

Procedure

Action	Rationale
1 Explain and discuss the procedure with the patient.	To ensure that the patient understands the procedure and gives his/her valid consent (DH 2001: C).
2 Screen the bed or cubicle.	To ensure the patient's privacy (E).
3 Wash hands using bactericidal soap and water or bactericidal alcohol handrub, and prepare the dressing tray or trolley.	To minimize the risk of infection (DH 2005: C).
4 Perform the procedure using aseptic technique.	To minimize the risk of infection (E).
5 Remove the soiled dressing from around the tube, clean around the stoma with 0.9% sodium chloride using low-linting gauze.	To reduce the risk of dressing fragments entering the altered airway (Russell 2005: E) and to remove secretions and any crusts.
6 Replace with a tracheostomy dressing or a comfortable keyhole dressing.	To ensure the patient's comfort (E). To avoid pressure from the tube (Scase 2004: E).
7 Renew tracheostomy tapes, checking that 1–2 fingers can be placed between the tapes and neck.	To secure the tube (E). To ensure that the tapes are not too tight (Woodrow 2002: E; Scase 2004: E) or too loose, thus decreasing the chance of necrosis caused by excessive pressure from the tapes (Serra 2000: E).

Procedure guidelines   Tracheostomy suction

Equipment

1 Suction source (wall or portable), collection container and tubing, changed every 24 hours to prevent growth of bacteria (Billau 2004).
2 Sterile suction catheters (assorted sizes; see Action 7).
3 A selection of non-sterile, clean boxed gloves.
4 Sterile bottled water (labelled 'suction' with opening date), changed every 24 hours to prevent the growth of bacteria (Billau 2004).

5 Disposable plastic apron.
6 Eye protection, e.g. goggles.
7 Bactericidal alcohol handrub.

Procedure

Action	Rationale
1 If secretions are tenacious, consider using, as prescribed, 2 hourly or more frequently 0.9% sterile sodium chloride nebulizers or other mucolytic agents such as acetylcisteine.	Suctioning may not be as effective if the secretions become too tenacious or dry. Anecdotal evidence through practice suggests that frequent 0.9% sterile sodium chloride or acetylcisteine nebulizers may assist in loosening dry and thick secretions (E).
2 Explain procedure to patient and ensure upright position if possible. If the patient is able to perform his/her own suction, self-suction should be taught.	To obtain the patient's co-operation and to help him or her relax (E). The procedure is unpleasant and can be frightening for the patient (Billau 2004: E). Reassurance is vital (E). Selfcontrol of the patient's suction is preferable if the patient is able to manage it (E).
3 If a patient has a fenestrated outer tube, ensure that a plain inner tube is in situ, rather than a fenestrated inner tube (Russell 2005).	Suction via a fenestrated inner tube allows a catheter to pass through the fenestration and cause trauma to the tracheal wall (Billau 2004: E).
4 Wash hands with bactericidal soap and water or bactericidal alcohol handrub, and put on a disposable plastic apron, disposable gloves and eye protection.	To minimize the risk of cross-infection (E). Some patients may accidently cough directly ahead at the nurse; standing to one side with tissues at the patient's tracheostomy minimizes this risk (E).
5 If patient is oxygen dependent, hyperoxygenate for a period of 3 minutes.	To minimize the risk of acute hypoxia (Billau 2004: E).
6 Check that the suction pressure is set to the appropriate level.	Recommended suction pressure is 80–150 mmHg or 11–20 kPa for adults (Day 2000: E; Day et al. 2002: C).
7 Select the correct size catheter. As a guide, the diameter of the suction catheter should not exceed one-half of the internal diameter of the tracheostomy tube (Griggs 1998; Hough 2001). To ensure the correct catheter size use the formula: divide the internal diameter of the tracheostomy tube by two and multiply by three (Billau 2004).	This ensures that hypoxia does not occur while suctioning: the larger the volume, the greater the bore of the tube (E).
8 Open the end of the suction catheter pack and use the pack to attach the catheter to the suction tubing. Keep the rest of the catheter in the sterile packet.	To reduce the risk of transferring infection from hands to the catheter and to keep the catheter as clean as possible (E).

823

Procedure guidelines (*cont.*)

9 For new surgically formed tracheostomy and laryngectomy stomas, use an individually packaged, sterile disposable glove on the hand manipulating the catheter (Ward *et al.* 1997). For subsequent admissions use clean, disposable gloves on both hands. To facilitate easy disposal of the suction catheter after suction, an additional clean, disposable glove can be used on the dominant hand.

Gloves minimize the risk of infection transfer to the catheter or from the sputum to the nurse's hands (DH 2005: C).

10 Remove the catheter from the sleeve and introduce the catheter to about one-third of its length, until the resistance of the carina is felt or until the patient coughs. If resistance is felt, withdraw catheter approximately 1 cm before applying suction by placing the thumb over the suction port control and withdraw the remainder of the catheter gently (Dean 1997; Wood 1998).

Gentleness is essential; damage to the tracheal mucosa can lead to trauma and respiratory infection (E). The catheter should go no further than the carina to prevent trauma (E). The catheter is inserted with the suction off to reduce the risk of trauma (Clotworthy *et al.* 2006e: C).

11 Do not suction the patient for more than one breath cycle, 10–15 seconds (MacIntyre & Branson 2001).

Prolonged suctioning may result in acute hypoxia, cardiac arrhythmias (Day *et al.* 2002: C), mucosal trauma, infection and the patient experiencing a feeling of choking.

12 Wrap catheter around dominant hand, then pull back glove over soiled catheter, thus containing catheter glove, then discard.

Catheters are used only once to reduce the risk of introducing infection (E).

13 If the patient is oxygen dependent, reapply oxygen immediately.

To prevent hypoxia (E).

14 Rinse the suction tubing by dipping its end into the sterile water bottle and applying suction until the solution has rinsed the tubing through.

To loosen secretions that have adhered to the inside of the tube (E).

15 If the patient requires further suction, repeat the above actions using new gloves and a new catheter. Allow the patient sufficient time to recover between each suction (Billau 2004), particularly if oxygen saturation is low or if patient coughs several times during the procedure. The patient should be observed throughout the procedure.

To ensure general condition is stable.

16 Repeat the suction until the airway is clear. No more than three suction passes should be made during any one suction episode (Glass & Grap 1995; Day 2000) unless an emergency such as tube occlusion (Nelson 1999).

To minimize the risk of hypoxaemia (Day 2000: E).

17 Where appropriate, reconnect the patient to oxygen.

To minimize the risk of hypoxaemia within 10 seconds post-suctioning (Day 2000: E).

Humidification

Definition

Humidification can be defined as increasing water content, the moisture or dampness in the atmosphere or a gas (Hough 2001; Pryor & Prasad 2001). In health, inspired air is filtered, warmed and moistened by the ciliated lining, and mucus is produced in the upper respiratory pathways. Because the upper respiratory pathways are bypassed in patients with a tracheostomy, they need artificial humidification to ensure that these pathways remain moist (Pryor & Prasad 2001).

Procedure guidelines   Humidification of patient with tracheostomy

Procedure

Action	Rationale
1 **For patients requiring oxygen therapy** fill a suitable nebulizer with sterile water and attach it to the oxygen supply, then set the gas rate for the liquid to form into humidification droplets.	Constant humidification is required while the new stoma adapts to the outside environment. Humidification also prevents the formation of crusts which are liable to obstruct the airway. The use of sterile water reduces the risk of infection (Hough 2001: E). Any liquid remaining after 24 hours should be replaced.

Subsequent care

Action	Rationale
1 **For patients no longer requiring oxygen therapy** give humidification as required. Usually, patients need about 10–15 minutes of humidification every 4 hours. This may be adapted according to the patient's needs, e.g. throughout the night, according to time.	Patients begin to adapt to breathing through their tracheostomy after the first 24–48 hours. Some humidification is required according to individual needs and to prevent crust formation in the airway (E).
2 Provide laryngeal stoma protectors, e.g. Laryngofoam, Buchanan bib, Romet or heat and moisture exchangers.	To protect and humidify the airway (E).

Procedure guidelines   Tracheostomy tube change

With a newly formed tracheostomy, tube changing should be avoided where possible for the first 5 days to enable the tract to become well established (Seay *et al.* 2002).

Equipment

1 Sterile dressing pack.
2 Tracheostomy dressing or a keyhole dressing.
3 Tracheostomy tape.
4 Cleaning solution, such as 0.9% sodium chloride.
5 Barrier cream.
6 Lubricating jelly.
7 Disposable plastic apron.
8 Bactericidal alcohol handrub.
9 Eye protection.

Procedure

Action	Rationale
1 Explain and discuss the procedure with the patient.	To ensure that the patient understands the procedure and gives his/her valid consent (DH 2001: C).
2 Wash hands using bactericidal soap and water or bactericidal alcohol handrub, and prepare a dressing trolley.	To minimize the risk of infection (DH 2005: C).
3 Screen the patient's bed.	To ensure the patient's privacy (E).
4 Perform the procedure using clean technique.	To minimize the risk of contamination (E).
5 Assist the patient to sit in a semi-recumbent position (Clotworthy *et al.* 2006f) with the neck extended.	To ensure the patient's comfort and to maintain a patent airway. Extending the neck will make removal and insertion of the tube easier (Clotworthy *et al.* 2006f: C).
6 Remove the dressing pack from its outer wrappings and open the tracheostomy dressing.	To reduce the risk of cross-infection (DH 2005: C).

825

Procedure guidelines (*cont.*)

7	Put on a disposable plastic apron and eye protection, e.g. goggles.	Some patients may accidently cough directly ahead at the nurse; standing to one side and wearing a disposable apron and eye protection will minimize transfer of secretions on to the nurse (E).
8	Clean hands with bactericidal alcohol handrub.	To minimize the risk of infection (DH 2005: C).
9	Put on clean disposable plastic gloves.	Gloves minimize the risk of infection from the sputum to the nurse's hands (DH 2005: C).
10	Prepare the tracheostomy tube as outlined in steps 11–14.	So that the tube is ready for immediate insertion when required (E).
11	Thread on piece of tape through the slits in the flanges so that the tape passes behind the flange next to the stoma. Alternatively, secure tracheostomy ties to both flanges.	The tape is kept behind the flange to prevent it occluding the passage of air into the tracheostomy tube (E). These are made of Velcro and are more comfortable to wear and easy to adjust (E).
12	Put the tracheostomy dressing around the tube.	To prevent abrasion of the patient's skin by the tube (E).
13	If the new tracheostomy is cuffed, check the cuff by inflating it with air (according to manufacturer's instructions) then fully deflate the cuff.	To check for air leaks and spontaneous deflation (Clotworthy *et al.* 2006f: C).
14	Insert the introducer or obturator, checking that it can be easily removed.	To become familiar with removing the introducer or obturator prior to insertion (Clotworthy *et al.* 2006f: C).
15	Lubricate the tube sparingly with a lubricating jelly and place on the sterile dressing surface.	To facilitate insertion and maintain sterility (E).
16	If the old tube is cuffed slowly deflate the cuff, suctioning patient if required.	Pooled secretions above the cuff may enter the lungs when the cuff is deflated (Clotworthy *et al.* 2006f: C).
17	Remove the soiled tube from the patient's neck while asking the patient to breathe out.	Conscious expiration relaxes the patient and reduces the risk of coughing (E). Coughing can result in unwanted closure of the tracheostomy (E).
18	Clean around the stoma with 0.9% sodium chloride and dry gently. Apply barrier cream with topical swabs. (An aqueous cream may be used if the patient is having the site irradiated.)	To remove superficial organisms and crusts. Skin around the stoma is at risk of breakdown due to the constant presence of moisture in this area (Serra 2000: C). Meticulous skin care is therefore essential in order to prevent infection. Creams containing metallic compounds must not be used on irradiated skin as metal will worsen any skin reaction (Holmes 1996: C).
19	Insert a clean tube with introducer in place, using an 'up and over' action.	Introduction of the tube is less traumatic if directed along the contour of the trachea (E).
20	Remove the introducer immediately.	The patient cannot breathe while the introducer is in place (E).
21	Place the inner tube in position.	The inner tube can be changed as necessary when the outer tube is in position, thus minimizing the risk of trauma to trachea and stoma (E). The quantity of secretions present will determine the frequency with which the inner tube is changed (E).

22 Tie the tape securely at the side of the neck.

To secure the tube (E). Place the tie in an accessible place, at the same time ensuring that it will not cause discomfort to the patient (E).

23 Remove gloves and ask the patient to breathe out onto the palm of your hand.

Flow of air will be felt if the tube is in the correct position (E).

24 Ensure that the patient is comfortable.

The procedure can be traumatic for some patients resulting in coughing and even discomfort. It is important for the nurse to stay with the patient until coughing has resolved, provide reassurance and administer analgesia where appropriate (E).

25 Clear away the trolley and equipment.

26 Clean the soiled tube under running water, in line with the manufacturer's recommendations. If the tube is very soiled then use sodium bicarbonate to remove debris. The tube must be rinsed thoroughly and stored dry at the patient's bedside.
Note: plastic tubes should not be soaked in solutions as there is a danger that the material may absorb the solution which could then cause irritation of the trachea.

To remove debris that may occlude the tube and/or become a source of infection (E).

Problem solving: Tracheostomy

Problem	Cause	Suggested action
Profuse tracheal secretions.	Local reaction to tracheostomy tube.	Suction frequently, e.g. every 1–2 hours.
Lumen of tracheostomy tube occluded.	Tenacious mucus in tube.	Change the inner tube. Use 0.9% sodium chloride nebulizers, heat and moisture exchangers and suction.Continue to change the inner tube regularly, e.g. 1–3-hourly.
	Dried blood and mucus in the tube, especially in the postoperative period.	Provide humidified air. (For further information, see Procedure guidelines: Humidification, administering air if there is no need for oxygen.)
Tracheostomy tube dislodged accidentally.	Tapes not secured adequately.	Put in spare tube. This should be clean and ready at the bedside (Serra 2000). *Note*: tracheal dilators must be kept at the bedside of patients with tracheostomies (Serra 2000).
Unable to insert clean tracheostomy tube.	Unpredicted shape or angle of stoma.	Remain calm since an outward appearance of distress may cause the patient to panic and lose confidence. Lubricate the tube well and attempt to reinsert at various angles. If unsuccessful, attempt to insert a smaller-size tracheostomy tube. If this is impossible, keep the tracheostomy tract open using tracheal dilators and inform the doctor.
	Tracheal stenosis due to patient coughing, patient being very anxious or because the tube has been left out too long.	Insert a smaller-size tracheostomy tube. If insertion still proves difficult, do not leave the patient but ask for a tube to be brought to the bed. Keep the tracheostomy patent with tracheal dilators if stenosis is pronounced until the tube is reinserted.

Problem solving (cont.)

Problem	Cause	Suggested action
Tracheal bleeding following or during change of the tube.	Trauma due to suction or to the tube being changed. Presence of tumour. Granulation tissue forming in fenestration of tube.	Change the tube as planned if bleeding is minimal. For profuse bleeding, insert a cuffed tube and inflate the cuff (Clotworthy *et al.* 2006f). Inform the doctor. Perform tracheal suction to remove the blood from the trachea.
Infected sputum.	Nature of surgery and condition of patient often predispose to infection.	Encourage the patient to cough up secretions and/or suction regularly. Change the tube and clean the stoma area frequently, e.g. 4-hourly. Protect permanent stomas with a bib or gauze. Following result of sputum specimen, commence appropriate antibiotics as needed.

Procedure guidelines   Changing a Blom–Singer type non-indwelling voice prosthesis

Nurses must wear gloves and eye protection (to prevent phlegm/blood entering the eyes) when carrying out this procedure. The area must be well lit to illuminate the stoma.

Equipment

1 Clinically clean tray or receiver.
2 Correct replacement voice prosthesis and introducer.
3 Red rubber Foley catheter (14 Fr gauge).
4 White plastic dilator with correct diameter.
5 Lubricant jelly, e.g. KY jelly or similar.
6 Tissues.
7 Blenderm transparent hypoallergenic tape or Micropore tape.

Procedure

Action	Rationale
1 Explain and discuss the procedure with the patient.	To ensure that the patient understands the procedure and gives his/her valid consent (DH 2001: C).
2 Settle the patient in a chair and arrange lighting to illuminate stoma.	To ensure the patient is comfortable and well supported (E).
3 Place a little lubricating jelly on the tip of the red rubber catheter and/or dilator, and on the voice valve and introducer.	To ease insertion (E).
4 Ask the patient to swallow then keep his/her lips apart as the old valve is removed; hold flange where it joins the body of the valve.	To minimize amount of saliva entering fistula and reduce the risk of coughing (E).
5 Swiftly insert red rubber catheter (or dilator) 20 cm into the fistula.	To keep fistula open (E). To ascertain the shape and direction of the fistula (E).
6 Place valve on introducer, securing with flange.	To prevent valve dislodging from introducer during insertion (E).
7 Remove catheter or dilator and replace with valve. A slight click will be felt as the retention collar on the valve passes into the pharynx.	To insert valve (E).

8 Check valve is correctly inserted by pulling it gently: it will move slightly, then resist. The valve should rotate freely within the puncture.	To ensure valve is correctly positioned (E).
9 Place 5 cm length of Blenderm tape over flange to secure it to the patient's neck.	To keep flange neatly out of way (E).

References and further reading

Billau, C. (2004) Suctioning. In: *Tracheostomy. A Multiprofessional Handbook* (eds C. Russell & B. Matta). Greenwich Medical, London, pp. 157–71.

Blom, E.D. (1998) Evolution of tracheo-oesophageal voice prosthesis. In: *Tracheoesophageal Voice Restoration Following Total Laryngectomy* (eds E.D. Blom, M.I. Singer & R.C. Hamaker). Singular Publishing Group, San Diego, pp. 1–8.

Bond, P. *et al.* (2003) Best practice in the care of patients with a tracheostomy. *Nurs Times*, 90(30), 24–5.

Brown, I. (1982) Trach care? Take care – infection on the prowl. *Nursing*, 6, 70–1.

Clotworthy, N. *et al.* (2006a) Post-operative care of the patient following a laryngectomy. In: *Guidelines for the Care of Patients with Tracheostomy Tubes*. St George's Healthcare NHS Trust. Smiths Medical International Limited, Watford, pp. 15–16.

Clotworthy, N. *et al.* (2006b) Tracheostomy tubes. In: *Guidelines for the Care of Patients with Tracheostomy Tubes*. St George's Healthcare NHS Trust. Smiths Medical International Limited, Watford, pp. 9–14.

Clotworthy, N. *et al.* (2006c) Humidification. In: *Guidelines for the Care of Patients with Tracheostomy Tubes*. St George's Healthcare NHS Trust. Smiths Medical International Limited, Watford, pp. 17–18.

Clotworthy, N. *et al.* (2006d) Communication. In: *Guidelines for the Care of Patients with Tracheostomy Tubes*. St George's Healthcare NHS Trust. Smiths Medical International Limited, Watford, pp. 27–32.

Clotworthy, N. *et al.* (2006e) Suctioning. In: *Guidelines for the Care of Patients with Tracheostomy Tubes*. St George's Healthcare NHS Trust. Smiths Medical International Limited, Watford, pp. 23–6.

Clotworthy, N. *et al.* (2006f) Tube changes. In: *Guidelines for the Care of Patients with Tracheostomy Tubes*. St George's Healthcare NHS Trust. Smiths Medical International Limited, Watford, pp. 39–42.

Day, T. (2000) Tracheal suctioning: when, why and how. *Nurs Times*, 96(20), 13–15.

Day, T., Farnell, S. & Wilson-Barnett, J. (2002) Suctioning: a review of current research recommendations. *Intens Crit Care Nurs*, 18, 79–89.

Dean, B. (1997) Evidence based suction management in accident and emergency: a vital component of airway care. *Accid Emerg Nurs*, 5(2), 92–8.

Delassus Gress, C. & Singer, M.I. (2005) Tracheoesophageal voice restoration. In: *Contemporary Considerations in the Treatment and Rehabilitation of Head and Neck Cancer. Voice, Speech and Swallowing* (eds P.C. Doyle & R.L. Keith) PRO-ED Incorporated, Austin, Texas, pp. 431–52.

DH (2001) *Good Practice in Consent Implementation Guide: Consent to Examination or Treatment.* www.dh.gov.uk. Accessed 24/9/07.

DH (2005) *Saving Lives: A Delivery Programme to Reduce Healthcare Associated Infection including MRSA.* Department of Health, London.

Dropkin M. (1996) Nursing Research. SOHN's 20 year experience. *ORL Head and Neck Nursing,* 14(3), 14–16.

Edgtton-Winn, M. & Wright, K. (2005) Tracheostomy: a guide to nursing care. *Aust Nurs J*,13(5), 17–20.

Gibson, I.M. (1983) Tracheostomy management. *Nursing*, 2(18), 538.

Glass, C. & Grap, M. (1995) Ten tips for safe suctioning. *Am J Nurs*, 5(5), 51–3.

Griggs, A. (1998) Tracheostomy: suctioning and humidification. *Nurs Stand*, 13(2), 49–56.

Hahn, M.J. & Jones A. (2000) Psychosocial problems. In: *Head and Neck Nursing* (eds M.J. Hahn & A. Jones). Churchill Livingstone, London, pp. 137–42.

Hales, P. (2004a) Communication. In: *Tracheostomy. A Multiprofessional Handbook* (eds C. Russell & B. Matta). Greenwich Medical, London, pp. 211–34.

Hales, P. (2004b) Swallowing. In: *Tracheostomy. A Multiprofessional Handbook* (eds C. Russell & B. Matta). Greenwich Medical, London, pp. 187–208.

Hampton, S. (1998) Film subjects win the day. *Nurs Times*, 94(24), 80–2.

Harkin, H. (2004) Decannulation. In: *Tracheostomy. A Multiprofessional Handbook* (eds C. Russell & B. Matta). Greenwich Medical, London, pp. 255–69.

Hess, D.R. (2005) Tracheostomy tubes and related appliances. *Respir Care*, 50(4), 497–510.

Holmes, S. (1996) *Radiotherapy. Radiation Induced Side Effects.* Austin Cornish, London, pp. 67–78.

Hooper, M. (1996) Nursing care of the patient with a tracheostomy. *Nurs Stand*, 10(340), 40–3.

Hough, A. (2001) *Physiotherapy in Respiratory Care. An Evidence-Based Approach to Respiratory and Cardiac Management*, 3rd edn. Nelson Thornes, Cheltenham.

Leder, S.B. & Blom, E.D. (1998) Tracheoesophageal voice prosthesis fitting and training. In: *Tracheoesophageal Voice Restoration Following Total Laryngectomy* (eds E.D. Blom, M.I. Singer & R.C. Hamaker). Singular Publishing Group, San Diego, pp. 57–65.

Lewarski, J.S. (2005) Long-term care of the patient with a tracheostomy. *Respir Care*, 50(4), 535–7.

Lewin, J.S. (1998) Maximising tracheo-oesophageal voice and speech. In: *Tracheoesophageal Voice Restoration Following Total Laryngectomy* (eds E.D. Blom, M.I. Singer & R.C. Hamaker). Singular Publishing Group, San Diego, pp. 67–72.

MacIntyre, N.R. & Branson, R.D. (2001) *Mechanical Ventilation.* W.B. Saunders, Philadelphia.

Mathieson, L. (2001) Physiological effects of laryngectomy. In: *The Voice and its Disorders* (ed. L. Mathieson). Whurr, London, pp. 597–600.

Mol, D.A. *et al.* (2004) Use and care of an endotracheal/tracheostomy tube cuff – are intensive care unit staff adequately informed? *SAJS*, 42(1), 14–16.

Nelson, L. (1999) Points of friction. *Nurs Times*, **95**(34), 72–5.

Patel, J. & Matta, B. (2004) Percutaneous dilatational tracheo-stomy. In: *Tracheostomy. A Multiprofessional Handbook* (eds C. Russell & B. Matta). Greenwich Medical, London, pp. 59–68.

Pathways in Cancer Care (2001) *Head and Neck Cancer Care Pathway*. NHS Executive Northwest. SC Research, London.

Pilbeam, S.B. (1998) Physiological effects and complications of positive pressure ventilation. In: *Mechanical Ventilation: Physiological and Clinical Applications*, 3rd edn (ed. S.B. Pilbeam). Mosby, St Louis, pp. 161–2.

Price, P. (2004a) Surgical tracheostomy. In: *Tracheostomy. A Multiprofessional Handbook* (eds C. Russell & B. Matta). Greenwich Medical, London, pp. 35–58.

Price, P. (2004b) What is a tracheostomy? In: *Tracheostomy. A Multiprofessional Handbook* (eds C. Russell & B. Matta). Greenwich Medical, London, pp. 29–34.

Prior, T. & Russell, S. (2004) Tracheostomy and head and neck cancer. In: *Tracheostomy. A Multiprofessional Handbook* (eds C. Russell & B. Matta). Greenwich Medical, London, pp. 269–83.

Pryor, J.A. & Prasad, S.A. (2001) *Physiotherapy for Respiratory and Cardiac Problems: Adult and Paediatric*, 3rd edn. Churchill Livingstone, Edinburgh.

Rhys Evans, F. (2003) Nursing care of head and neck cancer patients. In: *Principles and Practice of Head and Neck Oncology* (eds P.H. Rhys Evans, P.Q. Montgomery & P.J. Gullane). Taylor & Francis, London, pp. 115–26.

Rhys Evans, P.H. & Blom, E.D. (2003) Functional restoration of speech. In: *Principles and Practice of Head and Neck Oncology* (eds P.H. Rhys Evans, P.Q. Montgomery & P.J. Gullane) Taylor & Francis, London, pp. 571–602.

Rossoff, L.J. *et al.* (1993) Is the use of boxed gloves in an intensive care unit safe? *Am J Med*, **94**(6), 602–7.

Russell, C. (2004a) Tracheostomy tubes. In: *Tracheostomy. A Multiprofessional Handbook* (eds C. Russell & B. Matta). Greenwich Medical, London, pp. 85–114.

Russell, C. (2004b) Tracheostomy tube changes. In: *Tracheostomy. A Multiprofessional Handbook* (eds C. Russell & B. Matta). Greenwich Medical, London, pp. 235–54.

Russell, C. (2005) Providing the nurse with a guide to tracheostomy care and management. *Br J Nurs*, **14**(8), 428–33.

Scanlan, C.L., Wilkins, R.L. & Stoller, J.K. (1999) *Fundamentals of Respiratory Care*, 7th edn. Mosby, St. Louis, MO.

Scase, C. (2004) Wound care. In: *Tracheostomy. A Multiprofessional Handbook* (eds C. Russell & B. Matta). Greenwich Medical, London, pp. 173–87.

Seay, S.J., Gay, S.L. & Strauss, M. (2002) Tracheostomy emergencies correcting accidental decannulation or displaced tracheostomy tube. *Am J Nurs*, **102**(3), 59–63.

Serra, A. (2000) Tracheostomy care. *Nurs Stand*, **14**(42), 45–52.

Shaw, C. (2003) Nutritional support of head and neck cancer patients. In: *Principles and Practice of Head and Neck Oncology* (eds P.H. Rhys Evans, P.Q. Montgomery & P.J. Gullane). Taylor & Francis, London, pp. 127–35.

Singer, M.I. & Deschler, D.G. (1998) Complications of primary and secondary tracheo-oesophageal voice restoration. In: *Tracheo-esophageal Voice Restoration Following Total Laryngectomy* (eds E.D. Blom, M.I. Singer & R.C. Hamaker). Singular Publishing Group, San Diego, pp. 51–5.

Tamburri, L.M. (2000) Care of the patient with a tracheostomy. *Orthop Nurs*, **19**(2), 49–60.

The Joanna Briggs Institute (2000) Tracheal suctioning of adults with an artificial airway. *Best Practice*, **4**(4), 1–6.

Ward, V. *et al.* (1997) *Supplement to Hospital Acquired Infection: Surveillance, Policies and Practice. Preventing Hospital-Acquired Infection. Clinical Guidelines*. Public Health Laboratory Service, London.

Wood, C.J. (1998) Endotracheal suctioning: a literature review. *Intens Crit Care Nurs*, **14**, 124–36.

Woodrow, P. (2002) Managing patients with a tracheostomy in acute care. *Nurs Stand*, **16**(44), 39–48.

Chapter 43

Transfusion of blood and blood products

Reference material **832**
Procedure guidelines: Blood product request **843**
Problem solving: Requesting a blood product **843**
Procedure guidelines: Blood sampling: pre-transfusion **844**
Problem solving: Blood sampling: pre-transfusion **844**
Procedure guidelines: Transfusion of blood components **845**
Problem solving: Transfusion of blood components **847**
References and further reading **847**

Definition

The administration of whole blood or any of its components into the bloodstream to correct or treat a clinical abnormality (Anderson *et al*. 1994).

Reference material

Blood safety and quality in the UK

Approximately 3.4 million blood products are administered in the UK every year (Gray & Illingworth 2006). The transfusion of blood and its components is usually safe and uneventful; however, there are associated risks and there have been significant developments over recent years to improve the quality and safety of transfusion practice in the UK. The Blood Safety and Quality Regulations came into effect in February 2005 and were fully implemented on 8 November 2005. These regulations cover the collecting, testing, processing, storing and distributing of blood and blood components (Crown 2005). The official government agency with jurisdiction for these regulations is the Medicines and Healthcare Products Regulatory Agency (MHRA) who are the competent authority.

The principal requirements of these regulations in relation to transfusion practice are:

(a) *Traceability* whereby hospitals must have a system to record and retain information on the fate of each unit of blood/blood component for a period of 30 years.

(b) *Haemovigilance*, an organized surveillance procedure relating to serious adverse or unexpected events or reactions. The reporting of such events can be done via the on-line Serious Adverse Blood Reactions and Events (SABRE) reporting system which is maintained by the medical device adverse incident reporting centre. This will usually be done by a designated member of laboratory staff and therefore clinical staff must ensure all incident reporting is conducted in line with hospital policy.

The MHRA define such events as follows:

A **serious adverse event** is defined as an unintended occurrence associated with the collection, testing, processing, storage and distribution of blood or blood components that might lead to death or life threatening, disabling or incapacitating conditions for patients or which results in, or prolongs, hospitalisation or morbidity.

A **serious adverse reaction** is defined as an unintended response in a donor or in a patient associated with the collection or transfusion of blood components that is fatal, life-threatening, disabling or incapacitating, or which results in or prolongs hospitalisation or morbidity.

(MHRA 2006)

Prior to these regulations, Better Blood Transfusion initiatives aimed to ensure that such guidance became an integral part of National Health Service (NHS) care making blood transfusion safer, ensuring that all blood used in clinical practice is necessary and improve the information both patients and the public receive about blood transfusion (DH 2002). Therefore it is a key requirement that all staff involved in the process of transfusion maintain their awareness of all appropriate guidance.

Blood donation and testing

All blood donated in the UK is given voluntarily. The successful selection of a donor must protect them from any harm that may be caused by the donation process and also protect the possible recipient of products derived from the donor's blood. Donors of blood for therapeutic use should be in good health; if there is any doubt about their suitability the donation should be deferred and they should be fully assessed by a designated medical officer. All donors of blood or its components (via apherisis) should be assessed in accordance with the Joint UKBTS/NIBSC Professional Advisory Committee (JPAC) donor selection guidelines (JPAC 2005). The assessment of fitness to donate includes a questionnaire relating to general health, lifestyle, past medical history and medication. Donation may be temporarily or permanently deferred for a variety of reasons including cardiovascular disease, central nervous system diseases, malignancy and some infectious diseases, all of which are detailed in the JPAC (2005) guidelines. Donors are also screened for risk of exposure to transmissible infectious diseases, and specific guidance is provided for donors receiving therapeutic drugs. Prevention of transmission of infection is determined by donor selection criteria and laboratory testing. In the UK, all blood donations are tested for infections which could be passed on to the recipient. However, concern about transfusion-related variant Creutzfeldt–Jakob disease (vCJD) transmission is now supported by clinical evidence (Ludlam & Turner 2006) and, despite continuing research, a screening test for preclinical human infection has yet to be developed (Brown 2005). Therefore, donor exclusion criteria remain an ever important precautionary measure (Cervenakova & Brown 2004; Brown & Cervenakova 2004). When a donor has been successfully screened, they must validate the information they have provided and record that they have given consent to proceed.

Autologous donation

Since the 1980s there has been interest in autologous donation. This has largely been attributed to high profile infection risks; human immunodeficiency virus (HIV), hepatitis C and more recently vCJD (James & Harrison 2002). However, autologous donation is not risk free and is contraindicated in certain circumstances. Furthermore, there has been significant concern about the efficacy of some methods (Henry *et al*. 2001; Carless *et al*. 2004). Three principal methods of autologous donation exist:

Preoperative autologous donation (PAD)

This requires the patients to donate up to 4 units of blood whilst simultaneously taking iron supplements in the month preceding surgery. However, the efficacy of this method has been questioned by systematic review (Henry *et al.* 2001) and is only indicated in very specific circumstances such as patients with very rare blood types, patients donating bone marrow, and fit patients who have a significant fear of receiving allogeneic blood products such that it is preventing them from seeking necessary surgery (James 2004).

Acute normovolaemic haemodilution (ANH)

This involves the donation of up to 3 units of blood immediately prior to surgery. The patient is then given crystalloids to dilute the circulating volume. This method is only indicated for surgery where considerable blood loss is expected on the principle that the number of red cells lost will be reduced and the patient's autologous whole blood can be returned after surgery; however, little evidence exists to support the efficacy of ANH (Harrison 2004).

Intra-operative cell salvage (ICS)

Blood loss during surgery is collected, anticoagulated, filtered and held in a sterile reservoir. The collected blood is then processed, washed and suspended in saline for return. Although ICS is not without risks such as embolism, bacterial contamination and enhanced inflammatory responses through reinfusion of inflammatory mediators (Harrison 2004), it has been recommended as the most effective form of autologous transfusion to assist in the conservation of blood supplies (James 2004). However, it is not currently recommended in surgery for malignant disease, gastrointestinal surgery or postpartum haemorrhage (Harrison 2004).

Blood component donation

Donors of blood components by automated apherisis are subject to the same selection criteria used for donating whole blood and any exception to this must be decided by a designated medical officer. Apherisis can be used to collect plasma, red cells and platelets. Leukapheresis procedures are used for the collection of granulocytes, lymphocytes and peripheral blood progenerator cells (James 2005).

ABO blood groups and rhesus types

In 1901, Landsteiner discovered that human blood groups existed and developed the ABO system which marked the start of safe blood transfusion (Bishop 2008). There are four principal blood groups: A, B, AB and O. Each group relates to the presence or absence of surface antigens on the red blood cells and antibodies in the serum which dictate blood compatibility (Table 43.1).

People with the blood group **AB** have red cells with A and B surface antigens, but they do not have any anti-A or

Table 43.1 Blood group compatability.

Group	Antigens	IgM antibodies	Compatible donor for	Compatible recipient of
A	A	Anti B	A AB	A O
B	B	Anti A	B AB	B O
AB	A & B	None	AB	A B AB O
O	None	Anti A Anti B	A B AB O	O

anti-B immunoglobulin M (IgM) antibodies in their serum. Therefore they are able to receive blood from any group, but can only donate to other people from group AB.

People with group **O** red cells do not have either A or B surface antigens, however they do have anti-A and anti-B IgM antibodies in their serum. They are only able to receive blood from group **O**, but can donate to A, B, O and AB groups.

People with group **A** red cells have type A surface antigens, and they have anti-B IgM antibodies in their serum. They are only able to receive blood from groups **A** or **O** and can only donate blood to people from A and AB groups.

People with group **B** red cells have type B surface antigens and they have anti-A IgM antibodies in their serum. They are therefore only able to receive blood from groups **B** or **O** and can only donate blood to people from B and AB groups.

In addition to the ABO system described above the rhesus (Rh) system was discovered in 1940; again these are surface antigens and they are another essential system used in transfusion therapy (Mollison *et al.* 1997). The Rh D antigen is the most immunogenic of the Rh antigens (Porth 2005). However, many other red cell antigens exist and exposure to them may stimulate the development of corresponding antibodies (McClelland 2007).

Blood group incompatibility

The transfusion of ABO incompatible red cells can lead to intravascular haemolysis where the recipient's IgM antibodies bind to the corresponding surface antigens of the transfused cells (McClelland 2007). Complement activation results in lysis of the transfused cells and the haemoglobin that is released precipitates renal failure with the fragments of the lysed cells activating the clotting pathways, which in turn leads to the development of disseminated intravascular coagulation (DIC) (Mollison *et al.* 1997). Transfusion of rhesus positive cells to a rhesus negative individual will result in immunization and the appearance of anti-D antibodies

(Hoffbrand *et al.* 2001). However, on any subsequent exposure extravascular haemolysis occurs when rhesus antibody coated red cells are destroyed by macrophages in the liver and spleen (McClelland 2007). A patient's rhesus status is of particular note in pregnancy as haemolytic disease of the newborn (HDN) can occur when the mother is rhesus negative and the developing foetus is rhesus positive as exposure to foetal blood can stimulate anti-D activation in the mother which in turn can cross the placenta causing haemolysis (McClelland 2007).

Blood groups in haemopoietic stem cell transplantation

The human leucocyte antigen (HLA) is used to determine compatibility for organ transplantation including bone marrow and peripheral blood stem cells. However, because ABO blood groups and HLA tissue types are determined genetically, it is not uncommon to find a suitable HLA donor who is ABO and/or rhesus incompatible with the recipient. In such circumstances, major transfusion reactions can be avoided by red cell and/or plasma depletion of the donor cells in the laboratory before reinfusion (Mollison *et al.* 1997). Occasionally, if the recipient has a very high titre of anti-A or anti-B lytic antibody and the donor marrow or peripheral blood stem cells are blood group A, B or AB, then plasmapheresis of the recipient may be performed to lower the titre of this antibody to safe limits. This is necessary because it is not possible to remove all the red cells from the donor product and those remaining may cause a major transfusion reaction in this situation (Mollison *et al.* 1997).

Appropriate use of blood and blood products

The impetus from recent publications and legislation has created greater awareness of the need to continue to improve transfusion practice in many ways. Blood and blood products are no longer regarded as safe unlimited resources. There are risks that are inherent to transfusion practice and therefore unnecessary exposure to blood products should be avoided. This is of particular importance for patients who may only have one transfusion in their lifetime, such as surgical patients. Therefore, these patients should only receive a transfusion when it is absolutely necessary. Furthermore the appropriate use of products is essential for the conservation of blood supplies. Regularly updated guidance on the safe appropriate use of blood and blood products is now available online at www.transfusionguidelines.org.uk and these should be consulted in collaboration with local hospital and blood transfusion service guidelines.

Infusion of cryopreserved bone marrow and peripheral blood stem cells

Stem cells from either the bone marrow or peripheral blood are cryopreserved between collection (harvesting) and rein-

fusion. Stem cells can be either administered/used as an autologous or an allogeneic transfusion. Thawing of the cells is carried out using a large-volume water bath. Care should be taken as heating may cause cellular damage. As there is an increased risk of bacterial contamination, aseptic techniques should be adopted during administration to reduce any possibility of contamination (McClelland 2007) in a recipient group that is already immunocompromised.

Indications

Blood and blood products have varying shelf lives and storage requirements. The range of products currently available, indications for use and recommendations for administration are listed in Table 43.2.

The process of transfusion

Errors made in the process of transfusion present a significant risk to patients. Although there is little evidence to support the efficacy for set procedures to manage this risk, current professional opinion has been provided by the British Committee for Standards in Haematology (BCSH) in collaboration with The Royal College of Nursing (RCN) and the Royal College of Surgeons for England (RCS) (BCSH 1999; Gray & Illingworth 2006). As a result of this guidance every hospital should have a policy in place for the administration of blood and blood components including identification of the patient, blood sampling, special blood requirement requests, processing of blood samples, the storage, collection and transportation of blood products, administration of blood products and the care and monitoring of the transfused patient. Furthermore, hospitals are also required to manage and report any adverse event or near misses with a statutory requirement to hold a record of every step of the transfusion process including the final fate of each blood product for 30 years (James 2005). Only staff authorized to do so should be involved at any stage in the transfusion process.

Caring for the patient receiving a blood transfusion

Patients who are to receive a transfusion of blood products must always wear an identity wristband with their full name, date of birth and unique hospital number clearly written or printed. The nurse caring for the patient should clearly explain the procedure ensuring that the patient fully understands the information they have been given. The patient should be asked to inform a member of staff if they complain of any symptoms which may indicate a transfusion-related adverse event such as complaining of feeling anxious, rigors (shivering), flushing, pain or shortness of breath. The patient should be cared for where they can be visually observed and the patient should be shown how to use the nurse call system. The patient should have vital signs monitored as indicated in the procedure guidelines below; however, it may be necessary

Table 43.2   Blood and blood products used for transfusion.

Type	Description	Indications	Cross-matching	Shelf life	Average infusion time	Technique	Special considerations
Red cells in optimal additive solutions (SAGM)*	Red cells with plasma removed: 100 ml additive fluid used as replacement to give optimal red cell preservation; haematocrit 60–65% Leucodepleted	Correction of anaemia	ABO and Rh compatible (not necessarily identical)	35 days at 2–6°C	1–2 hours/unit	Give via a blood administration set	If more than half blood volume is replaced with red cells in SAGM, use of FFP should be considered to replace clotting factors
Washed red blood cells	Red cells centrifuged and resuspended twice in 0.9% sodium chloride Leucodepleted	Correction of anaemia where patient may react to plasma components. For example in IgA deficiency	As above	Prepared by non-sterile process, therefore to be used within 24 hours	1–2 hours/unit	As above	–
Frozen red blood cells	Red cells of very rare phenotype Leucodepleted	To treat patients with very rare antibody	As above	Stored frozen cells: 3 years. Use within 12 hours of thawing	2–3 hours/unit	As above	–
White blood cells (buffy coat or apheresed granulocytes)[†]	Mainly granulocytes obtained by leucophoresis or by 'creaming off' the white blood cell layer from fresh blood	To treat patients with life-threatening granulocytopenia	As above	24 hours after preparation. Stored at room temperature	60–90 minutes/unit	Administer via a blood administration set	White blood cell infusion induces fever, may cause hypotension, rigors and confusion. Treat symptoms and reassure patient Preparation is always irradiated to prevent initiation of transfusion-associated graft-versus-host disease (TA-GVHD). *Do not* give to patients receiving amphotericin B. Indications for granulocyte transfusions should be when possible benefits are thought to outweigh considerable hazards of the treatment option (Brozovis *et al.* 1998)
Platelets*	Platelets in 200–300 ml plasma. May be pooled from 5 donors or apheresed from a single donor Leucodepleted	To treat thrombocytopenia	No crossmatching necessary	Up to 7 days after collection. Storage is at 22 °C, with continuous gentle agitation	20–30 minutes/unit	Administration using a platelet administration set. Use a new set for each transfusion. Do not use micro-aggregate filters	General guide to use: 1 Count less than $10 \times 10^9/l$ 2 Count $10–20 \times 10^9/l$ with haemorrhage and/or persistent pyrexia 3 Count $20–50 \times 10^9/l$ in special cases or pre-invasive procedure

835

(continued on p. 836)

Table 43.2   (continued)

Type	Description	Indications	Cross-matching	Shelf life	Average infusion time	Technique	Special considerations
Fresh frozen plasma (FFP)	Citrated plasma separated from whole blood	To treat a deficiency in clotting factors due to dilution effects, consumption (in disseminated intravascular coagulation [DIC]), liver failure or overdose of coumarin anticoagulant	No crossmatching necessary	2 years at −30°C. Once thawed, kept at 4°C, to be used as soon as possible but within 24 hours	15–45 minutes/unit (approx. 250 ml)	Administer rapidly via a blood administration set	FFP should be considered if patient has received more than half their blood volume in red cells, to prevent dilutional hypocoagulability
Albumin 4.5% (HAS)	Solution of albumin from pooled plasma in a buffered, stabilized 0.9% sodium chloride diluent. Supplied in 250 ml or 500 ml bottle	To treat hypovolaemic shock or hypoproteinaemia due to burns, trauma, surgery or infection Sourced outside UK to reduce risk of transmission of variant Creutzfeldt–Jakob disease (vCJD)	Unnecessary. Not blood group specific	5 years at room temperature Kept in dark	30–60 minutes/unit	Administer via a standard solution administration set	The solution should be crystal clear with no deposits
Albumin 20% (HAS)	Heat-treated, aqueous, chemically processed fraction of pooled plasma	To treat hypovolaemic shock or hypoproteinaemia due to burns, trauma, surgery or infection. To maintain appropriate electrolyte balance	Unnecessary	5 years at room temperature Kept in dark	30–60 minutes/unit	Administer via a blood administration set undiluted or diluted with 0.9% sodium chloride or 5% glucose solution. Slower administration is advised if a cardiac disorder is present to avoid gross fluid shift	The solution should be crystal clear with no deposits
Cryoprecipitate	Cold-insoluble portion of plasma recovered from FFP: rich in factor VIII, von Willebrand's disease and fibrinogen. Available as single packs (20–40 ml) or 5 units pooled (120–140 ml)	To control bleeding disorders due to lack of factor VIII or fibrinogen, e.g. haemophilia, von Willebrand's disease, DIC	No crossmatchng necessary	2 years at −30°C. Use immediately after thawing.	15–30 minutes via infusion, 10–15 minutes via intravenous push	Administer rapidly via syringe or blood administration set	
Cryo-depleted plasma	FFP with cryoprecipitate removed	Useful in treating thrombotic thrombocytopenic purpura: patients are plasma-exchanged daily to reduce circulating von Willebrand's disease	No crossmatching necessary	2 years at −30°C. Once thawed, kept at 4°C, to be used as soon as possible but within 24 hours	Time varies on machine average ±2.5 hours	Via apheresis machine	

*Most commonly used blood products.
†See leucocyte depletion.

to take additional observations if clinically indicated, such as if the patient complains of feeling unwell or they develop signs of a transfusion reaction (Gray & Illingworth 2006). As many drugs may cause a pyretic hypersensitivity reaction (Mehta 2006), nurses caring for patients receiving the transfusion of blood and blood products should ensure that they do not simultaneously administer drugs such as antifungals or first- or second-course antibiotics.

Jehovah's Witnesses and blood transfusion

The role of blood in Jehovah's Witnesses' spiritual belief is based on scripture and followers are usually well informed both of their beliefs and their rights. Many Jehovah's Witnesses carry information with them regarding any objection and therefore the need to ensure informed consent is very important. Staff caring for patients must ensure that decisions to consent to or refuse treatment are respected and recorded appropriately (McClelland 2007). Furthermore, in individual circumstances, practitioners should endeavour to consider non-blood or autologous methods described above where appropriate (McClelland 2007).

Transfusion reactions and complications

In November 1996 the Serious Hazards of Transfusion (SHOT) scheme was launched. This voluntary and anonymized reporting scheme collected data from participating hospitals across the UK and Ireland. The purpose of SHOT is to collect data on the serious morbidity related to the transfusion of blood and blood products. These data have since been utilized to inform education programmes, policy development, guideline development, ultimately improving hospital transfusion practice (SNBTS 2004). Although the Blood Safety and Quality Regulations have now made the reporting of such events via SABRE mandatory (see above), the SHOT scheme remains active and important and has presented yearly retrospective reports of data collected since its inception. These data demonstrate improved performance in recognizing reporting of transfusion-related incidents and continue to generate key recommendations to improve all transfusion practice (SNBTS 2004). Despite significant improvement in the reduction of risk from transfusion transmitted infection, human error which results in the Incorrect Blood Component Transfused (IBCT) remains the greatest risk to patients (SNBTS 2004). An IBCT is the transfusion of a blood product that is not suitable for or not intended for the recipient. Most IBCT incidents are the result of one or more errors in the transfusion pathway (SHOT 2005).

Managing adverse transfusion events

The prompt management of any adverse transfusion reaction can reduce associated morbidity and can be life saving. Therefore staff caring for patients receiving transfused products must be fully familiar with the immediate management of any suspected reaction. However, specialist advice should always be sought for the diagnosis and ongoing management of transfusion reactions, such as haemolytic, anaphylactic and septic reactions (SNBTS 2004; McClelland 2007).

Minor transfusion reactions

It should always be remembered that the symptoms of a 'minor' transfusion reaction may be the prelude to a major, life-threatening reaction. It is essential that staff take any transfusion reaction seriously. Symptomatic patients should have their vital signs monitored closely and they should be clearly observable. Patients with persistent or deteriorating symptoms should always be managed as a major reaction and urgent medical and specialist support should be sought (SNBTS 2004; McClelland 2007).

Symptoms of minor reactions include: a temperature rise of up to $1.5°C$, rash without systemic disturbance and moderate tachycardia without hypotension (SNBTS 2004). Such reactions may be caused by an immunological reaction to components of the blood product. Whilst it may be possible to manage such symptoms and continue with the transfusion the following action should always be taken (Contreras & Mollison 1998):

- Stop the transfusion and inform the responsible medical team.
- Confirm the patient's identity and re-check their details against the product compatibility label.
- Antihistamines should be considered for skin rashes or urticarial itch.
- Antipyretic agents can be considered for mild fever.

It may be possible to continue with the transfusion at a reduced rate once the patient's symptoms are controlled; however, it may be necessary to increase the frequency of observations until the transfusion is completed. Some patients who have regular transfusions may experience recurrent febrile reactions and may benefit from an antipyretic pre-medication. *Note*: aspirin and other non-steroidal anti-inflammatory drugs (NSAIDs) are contraindicated in patients with a thrombocytopenia or coagulopathy (Mehta 2006).

Major transfusion reactions

Major transfusion reactions include anaphylaxis, haemolysis and sepsis and may present as a fever of $>38.5°C$, tachycardia $\pm$ hypotension. In such circumstances a severe reaction should always be considered and the transfusion should be stopped until a specialist assessment has been conducted (Box 43.1).

Box 43.1   Initial management of a suspected transfusion reaction

- Stop the transfusion and seek urgent medical help.
- Initiate appropriate emergency procedures, e.g. call resuscitation team.
- Depending on venous access withdraw the contents of the lumen being used and disconnect the blood product.
- Keep venous access patent.
- Confirm the patient's identity and re-check their details against the product compatibility label.
- Keep the patient and relative informed of all progress and reassure as indicated.
- Initiate close and frequent observations of temperature, pulse, blood pressure, fluid balance.
- Inform the transfusion laboratory and seek the urgent advice of the haematologist for further management.
- Return the transfused product to the laboratory with new blood samples (10 ml clotted and 5 ml ethylenediamine tetraacetic acid (EDTA)) from the patient's opposite arm (SNBTS 2004) with a completed transfusion reaction notification form (if available) or note the patient's details, the nature and timing of the reaction and details of the component transfused.

Care should be taken when returning the blood product to the laboratory, to ensuring that the product does not leak and that no needles remain attached. Any further products being held locally for the patient should also be returned to the hospital transfusion laboratory for assessment. The events surrounding the reaction should be clearly documented and reported in the following ways:

- Record the adverse event in the patient's clinical record.
- Complete a detailed incident form as per local policy.

- Follow local, regional and national criteria for reporting via SABRE and SHOT.

Reactions and complications

Acute haemolytic reactions

These are usually directly related to ABO incompatibilities due to an IBCT where antigen/antibody reactions occur when the recipient's antibodies react with surface antigens on the donor red cells. This reaction causes a cascade of events within the recipient as described above. Such reaction can present with chills/rigor, facial flushing, pain/oozing at cannula site, burning along the vein, chest pain, lumbar or flank pain, or shock (Gillespie & Hillyer 2001; McClelland 2007). Patients may express a feeling of anxiety or doom, which may be associated with cytokine activity. Haemolytic shock can occur after only a few millilitres of blood has been infused. Treatment is often vigorous to reverse hypotension, aid adequate renal perfusion and renal flow to reduce potential damage to renal tubules, and appropriate therapy for DIC reactions (Provan *et al.* 1998). It is important to remember that most acute haemolytic reactions are preventable as they are usually caused by clerical or checking errors at the bedside, and as this is the final check before administration it presents the last opportunity to identify and avert an error, thus emphasizing the importance of the final check before transfusion (McClelland 2007) (Figure 43.1).

Acute anaphylactic reactions

These are rare and usually occur after only a few millilitres of blood or plasma has been infused (Weinstein 2007) and present with bronchial spasm, respiratory distress, abdominal cramps, shock and potential loss of consciousness.

BLOOD PACK   **PATIENT'S WRISTBAND**

SURNAME

FORENAME

DATE OF BIRTH

HOSPITAL NUMBER

Always involve the patient by asking them to state their name and date of birth, where possible.

Figure 43.1   Check the compatability label or tie-on-tag against the patient's wristband.

Air embolism

Air embolism is a risk with any intravenous therapy (Shamash 2002) and care should be taken throughout the transfusion process.

Circulatory overload (transfusion-associated circulatory overload [TACO])

Circulatory overload can occur when blood or any of its components are infused rapidly or administered to a patient with an increased plasma volume, causing hypervolaemia. Patients at risk are those with renal or cardiac deficiencies, the young and elderly (Weinstein 2007). Patients with signs of cardiac failure should receive their transfusion slowly with diuretic support (McClelland 2007). The need for concomitant drugs such as diuretics should always be assessed before commencing treatment (SNBTS 2004).

Febrile non-haemolytic reactions

These reactions are due to an immunological response to the transfusion of cellular components such as donor leucocytes. Specific patient groups are at risk of greater sensitization to leucocytes, for example, critically ill patients, those receiving anticancer therapies or patients requiring multiple transfusion therapy (Williamson *et al.* 1998). Such reactions present with a mild fever (up to 1.5°C), rash without systemic disturbance and moderate tachycardia without hypotension (SNBTS 2004).

Hypothermia

Infusing large quantities of cold blood rapidly can cause hypothermia. Patients likely to suffer from this reaction are those who have suffered massive blood loss due to trauma, haemorrhage, clotting disorders or thrombocytopenia (McClelland 2007). Such reactions present with alteration in vital signs, and development of pallor and chills.

Blood warming devices

The warming of blood and blood products is generally not recommended as it is of limited benefit and can be dangerous. Blood warmers are only indicated when:

- Massive, rapid transfusion could result in cooling of cardiac tissue, causing potentially fatal dysrythmia (McClelland 2007). If the rate of transfusion is greater than 100 ml per minute blood warming devices should be used (McClelland 2007).
- Transfusion is required by patients with cold agglutination disease (Gray & Illingworth 2006).
- Exchange transfusion is indicated in the newborn (Weinstein 2007).
- Thawing of cryopreserved stem cells prior to transfusion (blood or marrow).

Both water baths and dry heat blood warmers are available. However, whichever device is chosen the temperature should be maintained below 38°C. Warming in excess of this can cause haemolysis of red cells and can denature proteins and increase the risk of bacterial infection. Blood warmers must always be used and maintained according to the manufacturer's guidelines. Blood products must **never** be warmed by improvisation, such as putting the pack into hot water, in a microwave or on a radiator, as uncontrolled heating can damage the contents of the pack (Gray & Illingworth 2006; McClelland 2007). The use of water baths also increases the risk of bacterial contamination. Therefore certain safety measures must be adhered to:

- Water baths must be drained after each use and must be stored dry and empty.
- The blood warmer should be drained after each use and must be stored dry and empty.
- When needed, they should be refilled with sterile water.
- A protective sterile over-bag to thaw blood and blood products reduces the entry of contaminants through microscopic punctures or breaks in the seal.
- The product should be used immediately after it has been thawed.

All devices should be serviced as per hospital health and safety policies, Medicines and Healthcare Products Regulatory Agency (MHRA) and manufacturers' guidelines.

Sepsis

Sepsis occurs when bacteria enter the blood or blood product that is to be infused. Bacteria can enter at any point from the time of collection, during storage through to administration to the patient. Organisms implicated in transfusion-related sepsis include Gram-negative *Pseudomonas*, *Yersinia* and *Flavobacterium* (Provan *et al.* 1998). Septic reactions usually present with a fever, tachycardia and/or hypotension, and can lead rapidly to systemic inflammatory response syndrome (SIRS) (Porth 2005). This is a serious life-threatening condition, sometimes referred to as septic shock, and requires urgent medical attention.

Transfusion-related acute lung injury (TRALI)

TRALI is usually caused by anti-leucocyte antibodies reacting against donor leucocytes. This reaction can result in 'leucoagglutination'. Leucoagglutinins can in turn become trapped in the pulmonary microvasculature, causing severe respiratory distress without evidence of circulatory overload or cardiac failure (Contreras & Mollison 1998). TRALI presents with a rapid onset of breathlessness, a nonproductive cough, distress, chills or fever, cyanosis, hypotension and coma. A chest X-ray will show bilateral nodular infiltrates in a characteristic 'bat wing' presentation (McClelland 2007). TRALI is usually treated as any adult respiratory distress syndrome (ARDS) and therefore patients that develop TRALI may require ventilatory support (SNBTS 2004) and should be treated as an emergency. As TRALI is donor related it is essential that cases are reported to the blood transfusion services so that donors can be contacted and removed from the donor panel (McClelland 2007).

Urticaria

This uncommon reaction is caused by the recipient reacting to protein in the donor plasma (Davies & Williamson 1998). Urticaria is characterized by localized oedematous plaques, hives and itching and is usually mediated by histamines (Porth 2005). Therefore urticarial reactions usually respond well to antihistamines and they should be administered once the patient has been assessed and antihistamine therapy has been prescribed (SNBTS 2004). The infusion can then be recommenced; however, if symptoms return, the infusion should be discontinued.

Delayed effects

These reactions may occur days, months or even years after transfusion.

Delayed haemolytic reactions

These reactions are caused when immune antibodies react to a foreign antigen. Reactions are classified as primary or secondary. A *primary* reaction is often mild, occurring days or weeks after initial transfusion, and may be indicated by no clinical alteration in haemoglobin following transfusion therapy (Cook 1997a). *Secondary* reactions occur with re-exposure to the same antigen, and on rare occasions may be associated with ABO incompatibilities (Cook 1997a). The patient may present with a fever, mild jaundice and unexplained decrease in haemoglobin value and may require antiglobulin testing (McClelland 2007).

Hyperkalaemia

Hyperkalaemia is a rare complication associated with trauma and the subsequent infusion of large quantities of blood. Potassium is known to leak out of red cells during storage, thereby increasing circulatory levels in recipients receiving blood products (Cook 1997b). The process is exacerbated if products are kept too long at room temperature or gamma irradiated (Davies & Williamson 1998). From starting the infusion to completion, the infusion should take a maximum of 4 hours (McClelland 2007). The patient may present with irritability, anxiety, abdominal cramps, diarrhoea and weakness in the extremities (Cook 1997b). The patient's medical team should be contacted to assess the patient.

Iron overload

Patients who are dependent on frequent transfusion, such as those with thalasemic, sickle cell and other transfusion-dependent disorders can become overloaded with iron (McClelland 2007). A unit of red blood cells contains 250 mg iron, which the body is unable to excrete, and as a result

patients receiving large volumes of blood are at risk of iron overload (Davies & Williamson 1998). This can result in poor growth, pigment changes, hepatic cirrhosis, hypoparathyroidism, diabetes, arrhythmia, cardiac failure and death. Chelation therapy through the use of desferrioxamine, which induces iron excretion, is used to minimize the accumulation of iron (Mehta 2006).

Transfusion-associated graft-versus-host disease (TA-GVHD)

Although rare, TA-GVHD is a serious complication for recipients and is often fatal. TA-GVHD is usually caused by an IBCT incident where non-irritated blood components containing immunocompetent T lymphocytes are given to severely immunocompromised recipients. The donor T lymphocytes engraft and multiply, reacting against the recipient's 'foreign' tissue causing a graft-versus-host reaction (Davies & Williamson 1998). It is not commonly associated with fresh frozen plasma (FFP) or cryoprecipitate. Onset occurs 1–2 weeks after transfusion and the condition is predominantly fatal (McClelland 2007). Irradiation (25 gray) of blood and blood products, to inactivate T lymphocytes (McClelland 2007) is essential in the prevention of TA-GVHD and is especially important in the following recipients:

- Foetuses receiving intrauterine transfusions.
- Patients undergoing or who have undergone blood or bone marrow progenitor cell transplantation.
- Immunocompromised recipients.

Infectious complications of blood products
Bacterial infections

Contamination of blood and blood products can occur during donation, collection, processing, storage and administration. Despite strict guidelines and procedures, the risk of contamination remains. Most common contaminating organisms are skin contaminants such as staphylococci, diphtheroids and micrococci, which enter the blood at the time of venesection (Barbara & Contreras 1998; Provan *et al.* 1998). Bacterial contamination can lead to severe septic reaction as discussed above.

Viral infections

Viruses transmissible via blood transfusions can be either plasma borne or cell associated (Barbara & Contreras 1998; Williamson *et al.* 1998). Plasma-borne viruses include hepatitis B, hepatitis C, hepatitis A (rarely), serum parvovirus B19, and human immunodeficiency viruses (HIV-1 and HIV-2). Cell-associated viruses include cytomegalovirus (CMV), Epstein–Barr virus, human T-cell leukaemia/lymphoma viruses (HTLV-1/HTLV-2) and HIV-1/HIV-2.

Human T-leukaemia/lymphoma virus type 1 (HTLV-1)

HTLV-1 is an oncogenic retrovirus, associated with the white cells that cause adult T-cell leukaemia, and is connected with several degenerative neuromuscular syndromes. The enzyme-linked immunosorbent assay (ELISA) has been recommended because of concerns relating to the transmission of the virus via blood transfusion, and the associated long incubation period of adult T-cell leukaemia. In the UK all blood is tested for HTLV (JPAC 2005).

Cytomegalovirus (CMV)

CMV is classified as part of the herpes family and hence has the ability to establish latent infection with reactivation during periods of immunosuppression (Barnes 1992; Barbara & Contreras 1998). Approximately 50% of the population in the UK has antibodies to CMV. Therefore it is recognized that the virus may be transmitted by transfusion. Although it poses little threat to immunologically competent recipients, CMV infection in vulnerable patient groups can cause significant morbidity and mortality. For example, CMV pneumonitis carries an 85% mortality rate in blood and bone marrow transplant recipients (Mollison et al. 1997). Screening of donors and the use of CMV-seronegative or leucocyte-depleted blood and blood products are seen as essential for neonates and immunocompromised recipients who have tested negative to CMV (Prentice et al. 1998).

Hepatitis B virus (HBV)

Screening for hepatitis B surface antigen (HBsAg) in donor blood is mandatory as it is estimated that approximately 180 000 people in the UK currently suffer from chronic hepatitis B (Foundation for Liver Research 2004).

Hepatitis C virus (HCV)

Screening for hepatitis C using the ELISA is mandatory in the UK. Hepatitis C is transmitted primarily via contact with blood or blood products (Friedman 2001).

Human immunodeficiency virus (HIV-1 and HIV-2)

HIV is a retrovirus that infects and kills helper T cells, also known as CD4-positive lymphocytes. Transmission of the virus can be via most blood products including red cells, platelets, FFP, and factor VIII and IX concentrates. These viruses are not known to be transmitted in albumin, immunoglobulins or antithrombin III products (Barbara & Contreras 1998). The retrovirus invades cells and slowly destroys the immune system, rendering the individual susceptible to opportunistic infections. Since 1983, when it was recognized that the virus could be transmitted via transfusion, actions were developed to safeguard blood supplies from transmitting the virus that caused acquired immune deficiency syndrome (AIDS). These include the careful screening of donors and the testing of donated blood.

Other infective agents

Parasites

Plasmodium falciparum is the most dangerous of the human malarial parasites (Barbara & Contreras 1998). Prevention is maintained by questioning donors about foreign travel, in particular those who have visited areas where the disease is prevalent (Bishop 2008).

Prion diseases

Known as transmissible spongiform encephalopathies (TSEs), these are a rare group of conditions which cause progressive neurodegeneration in humans and some animal species. Prion diseases are believed to be caused by the presence of an abnormal form of a cellular protein (Aguzzi & Collinge 1997; Barbara & Contreras 1998; Vamvakas 1999). These abnormal proteins have an altered cellular shape, and become infectious and multiply by converting normal cellular protein to the irregular form. This irregular form is resistant to digestion and breakdown, and, once accumulation occurs, can result in the formation of plaque in brain tissue. Transmission is thought to be by direct contact with infected brain or lymphoreticular tissue (Aguzzi & Collinge 1997; Barbara & Contreras 1998; Vamvakas 1999).

1 Prion diseases in animal species:
   (a) Scrapie, a disease of sheep.
   (b) Bovine spongiform encephalopathy (BSE).
   (c) Feline spongiform encephalopathy (FSE).
   (d) Chronic wasting disease of deer, mule and elk.
2 Prion diseases in humans:
   (a) Sporadic: classic Creutzfeldt–Jakob disease (CJD).
   (b) Inherited: CJD, Gerstmann–Sträussler–Scheinker disease, fatal familial insomnia (FFI).
   (c) Acquired: kuru, variant Creutzfeldt–Jakob disease (vCJD).

There is evidence to suggest that in TSEs, of which vCJD is one, leucocytes, particularly lymphocytes, are the key cells in the transportation of the putative infectious agent to the brain (Aguzzi & Collinge 1997; Bradley 1999). Leucodepletion of all blood and blood components is viewed as a sensible yet precautionary action to reduce any risk of blood-borne infection. All products in the UK are now leucodepleted at source. Currently, all plasma products are brought in from the USA, except FFP and cryoprecipitate which are leucodepleted at source in the UK.

Procedure

The transfusion of any blood product carries with it the potential of reaction and risk (SHOT 2005). All staff involved in the process of the transfusion of blood and/or blood products must have the knowledge and skills to ensure the process is completed safely. Therefore the nurse caring for those receiving transfusion therapy must do so within his or her sphere of competence, always acting to minimize risk to the patient (NMC 2008). A guide to the necessary elements of blood pack labelling is shown in Figure 43.2.

STOP, SEE BACK OF THIS TAG BEFORE TRANSFUSION

NHS
SCOTLAND
©Scottish National Blood Transfusion Service 2005 V9

Donation No: G101 606 597 229 N	
Component: Red Cells	
Signature 1:	Date Given:
Signature 2:	Time Given:

Peel off label above and place in patient's Medical Records

Surname: MACDONALD	Forename: MORAG
DOB: 11/07/1956	Gender: FEMALE

**25 HILL STREET
TOWN CENTRE**

Patient Identity No: 100198E	Date/Time Required: 20/12/2006
Patient Blood Group: O Rh POS	Component: Red Cells

Donation Number: **G101 606 597 229 N**

Special Requirements:

Once transfusion has been started, you must send the completed section below to the Hospital Transfusion Laboratory. This is a legal requirement

Surname: MACDONALD	Forename: MORAG
Patient Identity No: 100198E	Lab Sample No: 1803905

Donation Number: **G101 606 597 229 N**

Component: **Red Cells**

Date Given:	Time Given:

I confirm that the above patient received this blood component
Sign and Print Name

Compatibility label or tie-on tag

The compatibility label is generated in the hospital transfusion laboratory. It is attached to the blood bag and contains the following patient information; *Surname, First Name(s), Date of Birth, Gender, Hospital Number/Patient Identification Number, Hospital* and *Ward*.
The *blood group*, *component type* and *date requested* are also included on the label. The *unique donation number* is printed on the compatibility label; this number must match exactly with the number on the blood bag label.

Unique donation number

This is the unique number assigned to each blood donation by the transfusion service and allows follow-up from donor to patient. From April 2001 all donations bear the new 14 digit (ISBT 128) donation number.
The unique donation number on the blood bag must match exactly the number on the compatibility label.

Blood group

Shows the blood group of the component.

This does not have to be identical with the patient's blood group but must be compatible.

Group O patients must receive group O red cells.

Expiry date

The expiry date must be checked – do not use any component that is beyond the expiry date.

Cautionary notes

This section of the label gives instructions on storage conditions and the checking procedures you are required to undertake when administering a blood component. It also includes information on the component type and volume.

Special requirements

This shows the special features of the donation, e.g. CMV negative.

G101 606 597 229   N

DCYTE DEPLETED

RED CELLS IN ADDITIVE SOLUTION
STORE AT 4°C±2°C (SAGM)

Volume 275ml

INSTRUCTION
Always check patient/component compatibility/identity
Inspect pack for signs of deterioration or damage
Risk of adverse reaction/infection

O
Rh O POSITIVE
Do Not Use After
31 Dec 2006 22:59

CMV Negative

SHOTS
Date 29 Oct 2005

LOT B1080210629+68

REF C0010510Z8   REF

Figure 43.2   Blood pack labelling.

842

Procedure guidelines   Blood product request

Equipment

1 Blood request form.

Procedure

Action	Rationale
1 Complete the following patient information: 　(a) First name. 　(b) Surname. 　(c) Date of birth. 　(d) Gender. 　(e) Hospital identification number. 　(f) Ward or department.	Full demographics are required to minimize the risk of patients with the same or similar names being given the incorrect blood component (SNBTS 2004: C; McClelland 2007: C). Details on the request form must match the enclosed blood sample. Discrepant samples should not be processed (James 2005: C).
2 Complete the following clinical information: 　(a) Diagnosis. 　(b) Reason for request; this should include details of any surgical procedure. 　(c) Number and type of components requested. 　(d) Any special requirements such as irradiated, CMV negative. 　(e) If group and screen only. 　(f) Date and time required.	Enables laboratory staff to assess need against the surgical blood ordering schedule (E). Some vulnerable patient groups may have a fatal reaction to wrongly transfused non-irradiated or CMV-positive products (McClelland 2007: C). Negative and positive status should always be written in full and not as + or − as they may get defaced and be incorrectly processed (SNBTS 2004: C). This allows laboratory staff to plan ahead for complex cross-matches to ensure the required products are available at the correct time (SNBTS 2004: C).
3 Each request should also include: 　(a) The name of the doctor/nurse requesting the products. 　(b) The name and signature of the person who has taken the blood sample.	Every step of the transfusion must be fully traceable and the record held for 30 years (James 2005: C).
4 The following information can also be included if it is available in the patient's clinical record: 　(a) Patient's blood group. 　(b) Presence of known antibodies. 　(c) Date of last transfusion.	This information is useful to laboratory staff (E). Negative and positive should always be written in full and not as + or − as they may get defaced and be incorrectly processed (SNBTS 2004: C).

Problem solving: Requesting a blood product

Problem	Cause	Suggested action
Unable to collect patient information.	Unknown unconscious patient.	Assign unique hospital identification number to all requests and sample (E).
	Major incident.	Use unique major incident identification number to all requests and sample (E).

Procedure guidelines   Blood sampling: pre-transfusion

Equipment

1 For a full equipment list refer to Chapter 46.

Procedure

Action	Rationale
1 Take pre-transfusion blood from one patient at a time.	It is possible to get samples for different patients confused which can have fatal consequences (P). Therefore, it is vital to sample one patient at a time to minimize this risk (E).
2 Before taking the sample ask the patient to state their first name, surname and date of birth. Cross-check these details against the blood request form.	Ensure that the sample obtained corresponds with the request (P, E).
3 Check these details against the patient's identity wristband.	Ensure that the sample obtained corresponds with the request and the patient's stated identity (P, E).
4 Check the patient's hospital number on the wristband with the blood request form.	Ensure that the sample obtained corresponds with the request (P, E).
5 Follow the procedure for venepucture in Chapter 46 obtaining 5 ml of blood in the appropriate tube.	To ensure the correct procedure is followed and adequate sample is obtained (P, E).
6 Handwrite the sample tube clearly and accurately ensuring all names are spelt correctly. This should only be done once the sample has been successfully obtained and should be done at patient's bedside or before the patient leaves the department: (a) First name. (b) Surname. (c) Date of birth. (d) Gender. (e) Hospital identification number. (f) Ward or department. (g) Date.	BCSH guidelines do not recommend the use of addressograph (BCSH 1999: C). Blood tubes should never be completed in advance as this has been identified as a major cause of patient identification errors (SNBTS 2004: C).

Problem solving; Blood sampling: pre-transfusion

Problem	Cause	Suggested action
Unable to obtain verbal confirmation.	Patient unconscious.	Confirm identity with a relative or use unique patient identifier as above.
	Patient unable to verbally communicate.	Confirm identity with a relative or second member of staff (SNBTS 2004: C). **Always** follow local policy and **never** use secondary identifiers such as bed numbers, notes or request forms that the patient may be carrying (BCSH 1999: C).
Patient does not have a name band.	Name band has been removed or is no longer legible.	All inpatients are required to wear a name band; therefore, replace name band and reconfirm identity as above.
	Patient is in an outpatient setting.	Follow local hospital policy (E).

Procedure guidelines   Transfusion of blood components

Blood administration sets should be changed at least every 12 hours or after every second unit for a continuing transfusion (Gray & Illingworth 2006). Platelet transfusions may be administered using a standard blood administration set or a dedicated platelet administration set (McClelland 2007). Platelets should not be administered through an administration set that has been used for red cells or other blood components as this may cause aggregation and retention of platelets in the set/device (McClelland 2007).

Equipment

1 Blood administration giving set with 170–200 μm macroaggregate filter.
2 Equipment for patient's intravenous access requirements (if necessary).

3 Blood product to be transfused.
Note: all blood products that require leucocyte depletion are leucodepleted at source by the blood transfusion service (SNBTS 2004).

Procedure

Action	Rationale
Pre-administration check:	
1 Ensure that the component has been correctly prescribed, including any special requirements such as irradiated or CMV-negative blood and if the patient requires any other medications, e.g. diuretic, pre-medication.	Prevention of Incorrect Blood Component Transfused (IBCT) error: ABO incompatibility or non-irradiated CMV-positive products may cause a fatal reaction if transfused (McClelland 2007: C). Negative and positive status should always be written in full and not as + or − as they may get defaced and be incorrectly processed (E).
2 Record the patient's baseline vital signs, temperature, pulse, blood pressure and respirations.	To ensure that any transfusion reaction can be immediately identified and managed appropriately (SNBTS 2004: C) due to changes in baseline (E).
3 Check the expiry date of the component to be used.	To prevent the administration of expired blood products (E).
4 Conduct a visual inspection of the component to be used for signs of clumping, discoloration damage or leaks. *Note*: **if there are any discrepancies at this point do not proceed until they have been resolved.**	Expired or damaged products must not be used (E). To ensure an Incorrect Blood Component Transfused (IBCT) event does not occur (E).
5 Positively identify the patient by asking him/her to state the following information: (a) First name. (b) Surname. (c) Date of birth.	This is the final check of identity prior to transfusion and is absolutely vital in minimizing the risk of Incorrect Blood Component Transfused (IBCT) errors (SNBTS 2004: C).
6 Check the details given against the patient's name band and the patient details on the blood product.	To minimize the risk of error (SNBTS 2004: C).
7 Check that the information on the compatibility label matches the details on the blood component. *Note*: **if there are any discrepancies at this point do not proceed until they have been resolved.**	To minimize the risk of error (SNBTS 2004: C).
8 Where necessary obtain venous access (see Chapter 46).	To enable transfusion to be administered (E).
9 No agent other than 0.9% saline should be administered through the same lumen as a blood product.	Other agents may damage the product components and precipitate transfusion complications (SNBTS 2004: C).
10 Prime the blood administration set with the required product.	It is not necesarry to prime the device with saline unless there is a concern about device patency. Dextrose should never be used to prime a set or flush the blood administration set following a transfusion as this can cause haemolysis (SNBTS 2004: C).

11 Set up infusion via a volumetric infusion pump if appropriate.

Some older infusion pumps can damage the red cells. Blood administration sets for specific infusion pumps must always be used. If none are available the standard blood administration set should be used via gravity and the rate monitored as necessary (E).

12 Set the desired infusion rate as indicated by the blood product being used and the patient's condition:
    (a) Red-cell administration can range from 5–10 minutes in acute blood loss to the maximum time of 4 hours in elderly patients (SNBTS 2004).
    (b) Platelets, fresh frozen plasma and cryoprecipitate should be transfused over 30–60 minutes and must be completed within 4 hours of puncturing the blood component.

The rate of administration is indicated by the patient's clinical condition (SNBTS 2004: C; Weinstein 2007: E). Dictated by current guidelines (SNBTS 2004: C).

13 Take and record the patient's temperature and pulse 15 minutes after commencing each unit.

Adverse reactions will often occur during the first 15 minutes of transfusion (Gray & Illingworth 2006 : C). Complaints of serious anxiety, transfusion site pain, loin pain, backache, fever, skin flushing or urticaria could be indicative of a serious transfusion reaction (McClelland 2007: C). In such cases the transfusion should be stopped immediately and urgent medical advice sought (SNBTS 2004: C).

14 Record the start and finish times of each unit. All units must be completed within 4 hours of commencing.

Continuation of a transfusion beyond 4 hours increases the risk of transfusion reaction and complications (E).

15 Take and record the patient's vital signs on completion of each unit.

This forms a record of the patient's progress and acts as a baseline for subsequent units (E).

16 Record the volume of the product transfused on the patient's fluid balance chart.

Monitoring of fluid balance can demonstrate fluid overload in at-risk patients (Weinstein 2007: E).

17 Carefully file all transfusion documentation in the patient's clinical record. In line with local policy return information on the final fate of each blood product to the hospital laboratory manager.

To maintain the clinical record for patient safety. To comply with *Statutory Instrument 2005 No. 50. The Blood Safety and Quality Regulations 2005* where the final fate of all blood products must be held for a duration of 30 years (Crown 2005: C).

18 Return any unused blood products to the laboratory promptly.

Unused products may be re-allocated if returned in time. Refer to local guidelines (E).

19 Keep all empty blood component bags in the clinical area until the transfusion is completed. Once the transfusion is completed, dispose of in clinical waste.

Access to transfused bags is generally only useful for acute reactions (SNBTS 2004: C).

20 For patients receiving ongoing transfusion support the blood administration set should be changed every 12 hours.

Minimize risk from macroaggregates and bacterial contamination (SNBTS 2004:C).

Problem solving: Transfusion of blood components

Problem	Cause	Suggested action
Unable to obtain verbal confirmation.	Patient unconscious.	Confirm identity with a relative or use unique patient identifier as above.
	Patient unable to verbally communicate.	Confirm identity with a relative or second member of staff (SNBTS 2004). Always follow local policy and never use secondary identifiers such as bed numbers, notes or request forms that the patient may be carrying (BCSH 1999).
Patient does not have a name band.	Name band has been removed or is no longer legible.	All inpatients are required to wear a name band. Therefore replace name band and reconfirm identity as above.
	Patient is in an outpatient setting.	Follow local hospital policy.
Infusion slows or stops.	Venous spasm due to cold infusion. Occlusion.	Apply warm compress to dilate the vein and increase the blood flow. Flush gently with 0.9% sodium chloride and resume infusion. If occlusion persists consider resiting canula.
Elevation in temperature after commencing a unit of blood with no other symptoms. Temperature falls if the blood is slowed/stopped.	Pyrogenic reaction.	Observe the patient's temperature, pulse and blood pressure during the transfusion as indicated. If the patient has received multiple transfusions or previous history ensure that appropriate medication is prescribed before commencing transfusions.
Complaints of serious anxiety, transfusion site pain, loin pain, backache, fever, skin flushing or urticaria.	Adverse reaction to transfusion/transfusion error.	Stop infusion immediately and seek urgent medical advice.

References and further reading

Aguzzi, A. & Collinge, J. (1997) Post exposure prophylaxis after accidental prion inoculation. *Lancet*, 350, 1519–20.

Anderson, K.N., Anderson, L.E. & Glanze, W.D. (eds) (1994) *Mosby's Medical, Nursing, and Allied Health Dictionary*, 4th edn. Mosby, St. Louis, MO.

Barbara, J.A.J. & Contreras, M. (1998) Infectious complications of blood transfusion: bacteria and parasites. In: *ABC of Transfusion* (ed. M. Contreras), 3rd edn. British Medical Journal Publishing, London, pp. 58–61.

Barnes, R. (1992) Infections following bone marrow transplantation. In: *Bone Marrow Transplantation in Practice* (eds J. Treleavan & J. Barrett). Churchill Livingstone, Edinburgh, pp. 281–8.

BCSH (1999) Guidelines on the administration of blood components and the management of transfused patients. Blood Transfusion Task Force. *Transfus Med*, 9, 227–38.

Bishop, E. (2008) Blood transfusion therapy. In: *Intravenous Therapy in Nursing Practice* (eds L. Dougherty & J. Lamb), 2nd edn. Blackwell Publishing, Oxford.

Bradley, R. (1999) BSE transmission studies with particular reference to blood. *Dev Biol Stand*, 99, 35–40.

Brown, P. (2005) Blood infectivity, processing and screening tests in transmissible spongiform encephalopathy. *Vox Sanguinous*, 89(2), 63–70.

Brown, P. & Cervenakova, L. (2004) The modern landscape of transfusion-related iatrogenic Creutzfeldt–Jakob disease and blood screening tests. *Curr Opin Hematol*, 11(5), 351–6.

Brozovic, B., Hows, J. & Contreras, M. (1998) Platelet and granulocyte transfusion. In: *ABC of Transfusion* (ed. M. Contreras), 3rd edn. British Medical Journal Publishing, London, pp. 17–23.

Carless, P. *et al.* (2004) Autologous transfusion techniques: a systematic review of their efficacy. *Transfus Med*, 14(2), 123–44.

Cervenakova, L. & Brown, P. (2004) Advances in screening test development for transmissible spongiform encephalopathies. *Expert Review in Anti-infective Therapy*, 2(6), 873–80.

Contreras, M. & Mollison, P.L. (1998) Immunological complications of transfusion. In: *ABC of Transfusion* (ed. M. Contreras), 3rd edn. British Medical Journal Publishing, London, pp. 53–7.

Cook, L.S. (1997a) Blood transfusion reactions involving an immune response. *J Intraven Nurs*, 20(1), 5–14.

Cook, L.S. (1997b) Non-immune transfusion reactions: when type and crossmatch aren't enough. *J Intraven Nurs*, 20(1), 15–22.

Crown (2005) *The Blood Safety and Quality Regulations 2005.* HMSO, London. Available at www. opsi.gov.uk.

Davies, S.C. & Williamson, L.M. (1998) Transfusion of red cells. In: *ABC of Transfusion* (ed. M. Contreras), 3rd edn. British Medical Journal Publishing, London, pp. 10–17.

DH (2002) *Better Blood Transfusion: Appropriate Use of Blood, HSC 2002/009.* Department of Health, London. Available at www.transfusionguidelines.org.uk.

Friedman, D. (2001) Hepatitis. In: *Handbook of Transfusion Medicine.* Academic Press, New York, pp. 275–84.

Foundation for Liver Research (2004) *Hepatitis B: Out of the Shadows, a Report into the Impact of Hepatitis B on the Nation's Health.* Foundation for Liver Research, London.

Gillespie, T. W. & Hillyer, D. (2001) Granulocytes. In: *Handbook of Transfusion Medicine.* Academic Press, New York, pp. 63–8.

Gray, A. & Illingworth, J. (2006) *Right blood, Right Patient, Right Time.RCN Guidance for Improving Transfusion Practice.* Royal College of Nursing, London.

Harrison, J. (2004) Getting your own back – an update on autologous transfusion. *Blood Matters*, 16, 7–9.

Henry, D.A. *et al.* (2001) Pre-operative autologous donation for minimising perioperative allogeneic blood transfusion. *Cochrane Database Syst Rev*, 4, CD003602. DOI: 10.1002/14651858.CD003602.

Hewitt, P.E. & Wagstaff, W. (1998) The blood donor and tests on donor blood. In: *ABC of Transfusion* (ed. M. Contreras), 3rd edn. British Medical Journal Publishing, London, pp. 1–5.

Hoffbrand, A.V., Pettit, J.E. & Moss, P.A.H. (2001) *Essential Haematology.* Blackwell Science, Oxford.

James, V. (2004) *A National Blood Conservation Strategy for NBTC and NBS: Report from the Working Party on Alternatives to Transfusion.* National Blood Service, London.

James, V. (ed.) (2005) *Guidelines for the Blood Transfusion Services in the United Kingdom*, 7th edn. HMSO, London.

James, V. & Harrison, J. (2002) The pros and cons of predeposit autologous donation & transfusion (PAD). *Blood Matters*, 11, 4–5.

JPAC (Joint UKBTS/NIBSC Professional Advisory Committee) (2005) JPAC Donor Selection Guidelines, available at www. transfusionguidelines.org.uk.

Ludlam, C.A. & Turner, M. (2006) Managing the risk of transmission of variant Creutzfeldt Jakob disease by blood products. *Br J Haematol*, 132(1), 13–24.

MacLennan, S. (2003) Transfusion related acute lung injury (TRALI). NBS Transfusion Medicine Clinical Policies Group. www.blood.co.uk/hospitals/library/pdf/TRALI.pdf. Accessed 06/08/06.

McClelland, D.B.L. (ed) (2007) *Handbook of Transfusion Medicine.* HMSO, London.

Mehta, D. (2006) *British National Formulary*, V.51. BMJ Publishing, London.

MHRA (2006) Haemovigilance – how we monitor the safety of blood and blood components. www.mhra.gov.uk/home/idcplg? IdcService=SS_GET_PAGE&nodeId=282. Accessed 30/7/06.

Mollison, P.L., Engelfriet, C.P. & Contreras, M. (1997) *Blood Transfusion in Clinical Medicine.* Blackwell Science, London.

NMC (2008) *The Code: Standards of Conduct, Performance and Ethics for Nurses and Midwives.* Nursing and Midwifery Council, London.

Porth, C.M. (2005) *Pathophysiology: Concepts of Altered Health States*, 7th edn. Lippincott, Williams & Wilkins, Philadelphia.

Prentice, G., Grundy, J.E. & Kho, P. (1998) Cytomegalovirus. In: *The Clinical Practice of Stem Cell Transplantation* (eds J. Barrett & J. Treleaven). Isis Medical Media, Oxford, pp. 697–708.

Provan, D. *et al.* (1998) *Oxford Handbook of Clinical Haematology.* Oxford University Press, Oxford.

Shamash, J. (2002) Blood counts. *Nurs Times*, 98(45), 23–6.

SHOT (2005) *Annual Report 2004.* Serious Hazards of Transfusion, London.

SNBTS (2004) Better blood transfusion level 1 safe transfusion practice. self-directed learning pack. Effective Use of Blood Group, Scottish National Blood Transfusion Service. www.learnbloodtransfusion.org.uk/Level_1_SDL.pdf. Accessed 06/08/06.

Vamvakas, E.C. (1999) Risk of transmission of Creutzfeldt–Jakob disease by transfusion of blood, plasma, and plasma derivatives. *J Clin Apher*, 14(3), 135–43.

Weinstein, S. (2007) *Plumer's Principles and Practices of Intravenous Therapy*, 8th edn. Lippincott, Philadelphia.

Williamson, L.M. *et al.* (1998) *Serious Hazards of Transfusion (SHOT). Summary of Annual Report 1996–97.* Serious Hazards of Transfusion Office, Manchester.

Chapter 44

The unconscious patient

Reference material 850
Procedure guidelines: Unconscious patient care 852
References and further reading 853

Definition

Consciousness is a state of awareness of self, environment and one's response to that environment. To be fully conscious means that the individual appropriately responds to the external stimuli. An altered level of consciousness represents a decrease in this full state of awareness and response to environmental stimuli (Boss 1998).

Unconsciousness is a physiological state in which the patient is unresponsive to sensory stimuli and lacks awareness of self and the environment (Hickey 2003a). There are many central nervous system conditions that can result in the patient being in an unconscious state. The depth and duration of unconsciousness span a broad spectrum of presentations from fainting, with a momentary loss of consciousness, to prolonged coma lasting several weeks, months or even years. If a patient is unconscious and in the terminal phase of an illness, the focus will be on the general care of any person who is dying. Care of the dying encompasses an integrated model of care between health care professionals, the patient and family (Seymour & Ingleton 2004).

In the critically ill patient sedation is an essential part of the management. Sedation helps to minimize anxiety, promote sleep and keep the patient comfortable. It facilitates mechanical ventilation, helps to control physiological reactions to stress such as hypertension, tachycardia and raised intracranial pressure (Adam & Osborne 2005). A sedation scoring system such as the Riker scale should be used to achieve a therapeutic sedation level. This scale is a numerical scale from one to seven with one equivalent to unrousable and seven equivalent to dangerously agitated (Janz *et al.* 2005).

The nurse often cares for those who are unconscious for prolonged periods of time. In addition to managing the primary neurological problem, the nurse must also incorporate a rehabilitation framework to maintain intact function, prevent complications and disabilities, and restore lost function to the maximum that is possible. Total care of the patient involves communicating with families and friends on a regular basis to ensure they are supported and are able to participate in patient care if they wish to, and if this is appropriate (Geraghty 2005). There is evidence that unconscious patients are aware of what is happening to them and can hear conversations around them (Lawrence 1995; Jacobson 2000). Being aware of what the unconscious patient may be experiencing will add to the ongoing holistic approach to the needs of the patient physically, psychologically and spiritually.

Reference material

Assessment of level of consciousness

There are many methods available to measure a patient's level of consciousness. The most commonly used and universally accepted tool is the Glasgow Coma Scale (GCS) (Hickey 2003a; Geraghty 2005). A detailed explanation of examination techniques and correct evaluation of this tool is vital to ensure accuracy of rating of the GCS by nurses (Heron

et al., 2001; Geraghty 2005). However, the use of the GCS to assess the sedated and intubated patient is thought to be inappropriate. Sedation influences the patient's level of consciousness and is likely to impede the patient's eye opening and motor responses whereas the presence of an endotracheal tube will hinder assessment of the patient's verbal response (Price *et al.* 2000) (see Chapter 26). The unconscious patient is a medical emergency. Assessment of the patient's airway, breathing and circulation is vital (Geraghty 2005) (see Chapter 8).

Physiological changes in the unconscious patient

The physiological changes that occur in unconscious patients will depend on the cause of unconsciousness, on the length of immobility while unconscious, outcome and quality of care. It is not only being unconscious that will have a deleterious effect on the body but also drugs, e.g. some muscle relaxants such as those used in intensive care, can contribute to muscle weakness, raised intraocular and intracranial pressure, electrolyte imbalances and airway tone (Booij 1996). Unconsciousness can lead to changes and problems for the patient which have implications for nursing interventions. The discussion below is not exhaustive but offers an insight into the effects of unconsciousness on the main systems of the body.

Immobility

The human body is designed for physical activity and movement. Therefore any lack of exercise, regardless of reason, can result in multisystem deconditioning, anatomical and physiological changes. Involvement of a physiotherapist for passive exercises early in the period of unconsciousness may help in the prevention of further complications.

- *Decreased muscle strength*: the degree of loss varies with the particular muscle groups and the degree of immobility. The antigravitational muscles of the legs lose strength twice as quickly as the arm muscles and recovery takes longer.
- *Muscle atrophy*: this alludes to loss of muscle mass. When the muscle is relaxed, it atrophies about twice as rapidly as in a stretched position. As increased muscle tone prevents complete atrophy, patients with upper motor neurone disease lose less muscle mass than those with lower motor neurone disease (Hickey 2003b).

Gastrointestinal function

Bowel action is likely to become irregular in the unconscious patient, thus monitoring and observation are a priority (Geraghty 2005). Gastric complications can develop in the unconscious patient for a variety of reasons. Gastric ulcers, bleeding, constipation and faecal impaction can be identified as causing symptomatic problems. Nutrition is commonly provided by enteral tube feeding (see Chapter 24) which does not generally stimulate peristalsis. Loose stool can be a result of poorly tolerated enteral feeding or antibiotics. In contrast to this, some pharmacological interventions can lead to constipation. It is imperative that a diagnosis is made to differentiate between true diarrhoea and faecal impaction as they can occasionally be misinterpreted as being one and the same thing (see Chapter 15).

Genitourinary function

An unconscious state can induce urinary incontinence or retention of urine. The unconscious patient is at risk of two problems: urinary tract infections and kidney or bladder stones. On admission an unconscious patient will usually have an indwelling catheter (see Chapter 18). This is necessary for accurate fluid monitoring and to prevent skin breakdown.

Respiratory function

Due to the immobile nature of the unconscious patient, there is an increased threat of developing respiratory complications such as, atelectasis, pneumonia, aspiration and airway obstruction. If the patient is intubated with an endotracheal tube they are at increased risk of developing nosocomial infections (Hickey 2003b).

Respiratory assessment should include checking patency of the airway, monitoring the rate, pattern and work of breathing, pulse oximetry to check oxygen saturations and blood gases to assess adequacy of gaseous exchange. If the patient is intubated and ventilated then lung volumes and respiratory mechanics should be continuously monitored (Hickey 2003b).

Cardiovascular function

Immobility can cause changes in cardiovascular function, for example increased cardiac workload, decreased cardiac output and decreased blood pressure. In addition, the positioning of the unconscious patient causes central fluid shift, from the legs to the thorax and head, so the head of the unconscious patient with raised intracranial pressure may need to be elevated to 30° (Hickey 2003b).

Changes in cardiovascular function may be secondary to neurological changes; therefore the patient's neurological function should be monitored. Hypovolaemia, sepsis or cardiogenic shock are other factors that should be considered as they will cause cardiovascular instability and should be treated accordingly (Geraghty 2005).

The risk of deep vein thrombosis and pulmonary embolism is increased in the unconscious patient. This is due to several factors: blood pooling in the legs, hypercoagulability and prolonged pressure from immobility in bed (Hickey 2003b).

Impaired tissue integrity

Skin

Direct pressure to the skin and friction during movement of patients are two of the most common causes of injury to the skin that can result in pressure ulcers. Correct moving and handling of the patient will minimize the risk of pressure ulcer formation (see Chapter 48). Other contributing factors include incontinence, profuse perspiration, poor nutrition and obesity (Hickey 2003b). Use of special beds may be required depending on individual assessment. Skin integrity should be assessed using the Waterlow Scale (see Chapter 48).

Eyes

The blink reflex is absent in the unconscious patient and tear production may be reduced (Carpenito 2002). Assessment of the eyes for signs of oedema, irritation, corneal drying or abrasions is essential. Application of an eye patch may protect the eye from injury (Hickey 2003b) (see Chapter 31).

Mouth

The lips, oral mucosa and tongue must be assessed for signs of dryness, irritation and infection (see Chapter 32).

Self-care

The fluid unconscious patient will require nursing care for all self-care needs. The nurse's role is to ensure that the patient's hygiene needs are met and that the patient is clean and comfortable (see Chapter 33)

Fluid/electrolyte imbalance

The fluid volume and electrolyte composition within the extracellular and intracellular compartments in the healthy patient are generally static. Different states may bring about changes in fluid volume or electrolye composition within the compartments (Kumar & Clark 2001). Therefore, serum electrolytes will require regular monitoring in the acute period of unconsciousness. Monitoring of fluid balance is important and correct fluid balance will assist in the prevention of deep vein thrombosis, pulmonary embolism, pressure ulcers and constipation.

Ethical considerations

There are many ethical considerations when nursing the unconscious patient, e.g. consent, organ donation, advance directives and termination of life support. It is not within the scope of this manual to discuss these in detail. However, consenting adults who lack capacity, e.g. unconscious patients, can be given treatment under the doctrine of necessity under common law (Leung 2002).

Advance directives enable people to document their wishes regarding refusal of medical treatment in the event of their being unable to make decisions about their medical and nursing care (UK Clinical Ethics Network 2003). These are legally binding documents; nevertheless, in practice these may be difficult to interpret and of little value in the acute setting (Travis et al. 2001; Leung 2002).

851

Procedure guidelines   Unconscious patient care

Equipment

1 Airway of correct size.
2 Suction.
3 Oxygen mask.
4 Intravenous infusion equipment.
5 Personal hygiene equipment (measures for eye, oral and catheter care).

6 Cotsides (to be assessed on an individual basis, according to hospital policy).
7 Observation charts (neurological, fluid balance).
8 Feeding equipment.
9 Pen torch.

Procedure

Action	Rationale
1 Introduce yourself. Call the patient by their preferred name, as discussed with family/carer. Explain each procedure before starting.	Hearing often remains intact and recognition of a familiar word may assist in orientation of the unconscious patient (Elliott & Wright 1999: R 4; Leigh 2001: R 5).
2 Orientate the patient to day, date, time and place.	To promote orientation (Elliott & Wright 1999: R 4; Leigh 2001: R 5).
3 Remove dentures, note any loose teeth caps or crowns. Insert oropharyngeal or nasopharyngeal airway if appropriate. Monitor rate, rhythm and pattern of breathing.	To obtain and maintain a patent airway. To assess condition of the mouth and teeth. To assess breathing pattern and note changes (Geraghty 2005: E).
4 Monitor and document the patient's vital signs. Monitor electrolytes and full blood count as appropriate. Administer intravenous fluids as required. Monitor fluid balance.	To detect any changes in the patient's condition and manage as required. To detect potential fluid or electrolyte imbalances (Geraghty 2005: E).
5 Positioning of the unconscious patient: (a) Head: maintain proper alignment of head and neck; support with pillow, towel roll or soft collar.	Helps to maintain a patent airway (P).
(b) Elevate the head of the bed by 30°.	Helps reduce the risk of nosocomial pneumonia (Drakulovic *et al*. 1999: R 1b). It facilitates the drainage of secretions from the oropharynx, minimizes the risk of aspiration, assists the maintenance of adequate cerebral perfusion pressure and promotes an effective breathing pattern (Hickey 2003b: E).
(c) Body: position in alignment with spine (utilize towels and pillows).	This helps to maintain proper alignment of the body and helps minimize complications such as contractures and helps maintain musculoskeletal function (Geraghty 2005: E).
(d) Limbs: *Upper*. Support arms and wrists on pillows and flex the arms at the elbow. *Lower*. Place a pillow between the knees, use pillows or splints to flex the ankles parallel to the feet, align the hips with the head.	To prevent shoulder drag and wrist drop (Geraghty 2005: E). To prevent skin breakdown and footdrop (Geraghty 2005: E). To prevent internal rotation of the upper leg (Hickey 2003b: E).
(e) Fit antiembolic stockings on the patient if appropriate.	Helps reduce the risk of venous thromboembolism (Geraghty 2005:E).
(f) Liaise with the physiotherapist about positioning/exercises for the patient. Monitor colour, temperature and pulses of the limbs.	To enhance pulmonary function, prevent atelectasis and hypostatic pneumonia (Geraghty 2005: E) and to help preserve musculoskeletal function and prevent deep vein thrombosis (Hickey 2003b: E).

6 Perform neurological assessment as frequently as patient condition dictates using Glasgow Coma Scale or appropriate tool (see Chapter 26).

To note changes in patient's condition and respond appropriately (NICE 2003: R 1a).

7 Assess skin integrity using Waterlow Scale or appropriate tool. Change position every 2 hours or sooner if condition indicates (see Chapter 48)

To prevent and monitor for signs of pressure ulcers (Waterlow 1998: C).

8 Carry out oral care as frequently as patient's condition indicates (see Chapter 32).

To maintain a clean and healthy mouth and to promote comfort.

9 Carry out eye care as frequently as patient's condition indicates. Place eye patch if appropriate (see Chapter 31).

To prevent corneal scratches, dryness or ulceration, which can lead to blindness.

10 Assess bowel pattern as per hospital policy (colour, frequency, consistency and size).

To prevent diarrhoea, constipation, abdominal discomfort, bloating and to promote comfort (Klaschik *et al.* 2003: R 5).

11 Catheterize as per hospital policy (see Chapter 18).

To promote comfort and prevent stasis of urine, infection and renal calculi (Geraghty 2005: R 5).

12 Move patient as indicated by their condition. Choose type of pressure relieving mattress according to the patient needs.
Passive exercises as discussed with physiotherapist.

To prevent complications associated with bedrest, e.g. pressure sores, deep vein thrombosis. To prevent muscle wasting and contractures (Cullum *et al.* 2004: R 1a).

Conclusion

For the nurse there are physical, psychological and ethical considerations when caring for the unconscious patient. The preservation of life and avoidance of further disabilities are priorities of care, but the psychological effects on the patient's family and carers also require sensitivity and open communication. Patients' psychological needs should be addressed and Leigh (2001) suggests that these can be met through communication about their environment and through touch. Nursing this group of patients can be complex and challenging; however, being proactive to the needs of the unconscious patient can result in positive outcomes for the patient, family and health care professional.

References and further reading

Adam, S.K. & Osborne, S. (2005) *Critical Care Nursing: Science and Practice*, 2nd edn. Oxford University Press, Oxford.

Booij, L. (1996) Muscle relaxants and concurrent diseases. In: *Neuromuscular Transmission* (eds L. Booij *et al.*). BMJ Books, London, pp. 124–59.

Boss, B.J. (1998) Nursing management of adults with common neurologic problems. In: *Adult Health Nursing*, 3rd edn (eds P. Gauntlett Beare & J.L. Myers). Mosby, St. Louis, MO, pp. 904–47.

Carpenito, L.J. (2002) *Nursing Diagnosis: Application to Clinical Practice*, 9th edn. Lippincott, Philadelphia.

Cullum, N. *et al.* (2004) Support surfaces for pressure ulcer prevention. *Cochrane Database Syst Rev*, **3**, CD001735. DOI: 10.1002/14651858.CD001735.pub2.

Drakulovic, M.B. *et al.* (1999) Supine body positions as a risk factor for nosocomial pneumonia in mechanically ventilated patients: a randomised trial. *Lancet*, **354**, 1851–8.

Elliott, R. & Wright, L. (1999) Verbal communication: what do critical care nurses say to their unconscious or sedated patients? *J Adv Nurs*, **29**(6), 1412–20.

Geraghty, M. (2005) Nursing the unconscious patient. *Nurs Stand*, **20**(1), 54–66.

Heron, R. *et al.* (2001) Interrater reliability of the Glasgow Coma Scale scoring among nurses in subspecialities of critical care. *Aust J Crit Care*, **14**(3), 100–5.

Hickey, J.V. (2003a) Neurological assessment. In: *The Clinical Practice of Neurological and Neurosurgical Nursing*, 5th edn. Lippincott, Williams & Wilkins, Philadelphia, pp. 159–84.

Hickey, J.V. (2003b) Management of the unconscious neurological patient. In: *The Clinical Practice of Neurological and Neurosurgical Nursing*, 5th edn. Lippincott, Williams and Wilkins, Philadelphia, pp. 345–57.

Jacobson, A.F. (2000) Caring for unconscious patients. *Am J Nurs*, **100**(1), 69.

Janz B.A. *et al.* (2005) *A Multivariable Analysis of Sedation, Activity and Agitation in Critically Ill Patients Using the Riker Scale, ECG, Blood Pressure, and Respiratory Rate.* Harvard–MIT Division of Health Sciences and Technology, Cambridge MA.

Klaschik, E., Nauck, F. & Ostgathe, C. (2003) Constipation – modern laxative therapy. *Support Care Cancer*, **11**, 679–85.

Kumar, P. & Clark, M. (2001) *Clinical Medicine*, 4th edn. W.B. Saunders, Edinburgh.

Lawrence, M. (1995) The unconscious experience. *Am J Crit Care*, 4(3), 227–32.

Leigh, K. (2001) Communicating with unconscious patients. *Nurs Times*, 97(48), 35–6.

Leung, W.C. (2002) Consent to treatment in the A&E department. *Accident Emerg Nurs*, 10, 17–25.

NICE (2003) *Head Injury, Triage, Assessment, Investigation and Early Management of Head Injury in Infants, Children and Adults*. National Institute for Health and Clinical Excellence, London.

Price, T., Miller, L. & Descissa, M. (2000) The Glasgow Coma Scale in intensive care: a study. *Crit Care Nurs*, 5(4), 170–3.

Seymour, J. & Ingleton, C. (2004) Transitions into the terminal phase: overview. In: *Palliative Care Nursing: Principles and Evidence for Practice* (eds S. Payne, J. Seymour & C. Ingleton). Open University Press, Milton Keynes, Berks, pp. 187–9.

Travis, S. *et al.* (2001) Guidelines in respect of advance directives. *Int J Palliat Nurs*, 7(10), 493–500.

UK Clinical Ethics Network (2003) Advance directives (online version). www.ethics-network.org.uk/Ethics/eendlife.htm#advance. Accessed 29/6/06.

Waterlow, J. (1998) The treatment and use of the Waterlow Card. *Nurs Times*, 94(7), 63–7.

Chapter 45

Vascular access devices: insertion and management

Reference material	856
Peripheral cannulae	**860**
Reference material	860
Midline catheters	**865**
Reference material	865
Central venous access devices	**866**
Peripherally inserted central catheters	**866**
Reference material	866
Short-term percutaneous central venous catheters (non-tunnelled)	**869**
Reference material	869
Skin-tunnelled catheters	**872**
Reference material	872
Implantable ports	**874**
Reference material	874
Discharging patients home with a VAD in situ	**876**
Quality-of-life issues: living with a VAD	**877**
Procedure guidelines: Peripheral cannula insertion	878
Procedure guidelines: Midline catheter insertion	882
Procedure guidelines: Peripherally inserted central catheter (PICC) insertion and removal	884
Procedure guidelines: Central venous catheter insertion site dressing change	887
Procedure guidelines: Central venous access device: maintaining patency	888
Procedure guidelines: Central venous access device: taking blood samples	889
Procedure guidelines: Central venous access device: unblocking an occlusion	891
Procedure guidelines: Implanted ports: insertion and removal of non-coring needles	894
Procedure guidelines: Central venous catheter (non-cuffed/tunnelled): removal	896
Procedure guidelines: Central venous catheter (skin-tunnelled): surgical removal	897
Problem solving: Central venous access devices	899
Arterial cannulae	**902**
Reference material	902
Procedure guidelines: Arterial puncture: radial artery	904
Procedure guidelines: Arterial cannula insertion: preparation and setting up of monitoring set	907
Procedure guidelines: Arterial cannula: taking a blood sample	909
Procedure guidelines: Arterial cannula: removal	911
Problem solving: Arterial cannulation	912
References and further reading	913

Definition

A vascular access device (VAD) is a device that is inserted into either a vein or an artery, via the peripheral or central vessels, to provide for either diagnostic (blood sampling, central venous pressure [CVP] reading) or therapeutic (administration of medications, fluids and/or blood products) purposes. There is now a comprehensive range of VADs available which allow for patient device, therapy and quality-of-life needs. Table 45.1 lists the main types of VADs.

Reference material

Principles of care

Regardless of the type of VAD used, the principles of care for the device remain the same:

- To prevent infection.
- To maintain a 'closed' intravenous system with few connections to reduce risk of contamination.
- To maintain a patent device.
- To prevent damage to the device and associated intravenous equipment.

Each of these principles will be discussed generally and then in more detail under each type of access device.

Prevention of infection

Aseptic technique and compliance with recommendations for equipment and dressing changes are essential if microbial contamination is to be prevented (RCN 2005; INS 2006; Pratt *et al.* 2007) (see Chapter 5). Whenever the insertion site is exposed or the intravenous system is broken, aseptic technique should be practised. Where blood or body fluids may be present, gloves should be worn to comply with safe practice (Rowley 2001).

Cleaning solutions

Most transient flora can be removed from the skin with soap and water using mechanical friction (Carlson *et al.* 2001). Chlorhexidine 2% in 70% alcohol has been shown to be the most effective agent for skin cleaning around the VAD insertion site prior to insertion and between dressing changes (Maki *et al.* 1991; Ryder 2001; DH 2007; RCN 2005; Pratt *et al.* 2007). Seventy per cent alcohol acts by denaturing protein and so has excellent properties for destruction of Gram-positive and -negative bacteria, as well as being active

Table 45.1   Vascular access devices.

Type of device	Material	Features	Common insertion site (veins)	Recommended indwelling life and common uses
Peripheral cannulae	Teflon Vialon	Winged Non-winged Ported	Cephalic Basilic Dorsal venous network	48–96 hours for short-term access
Midline catheters	Silicone Polyurethane	Single lumen Dual lumen	Basilic Median cubital Cephalic	Used for 1–6 weeks or longer for short to intermediate-term access
Peripherally inserted central catheters	Polyurethane Silicone	Dual lumen Single lumen Valved	Antecubital fossa Basilic Cephalic	Used primarily for patients requiring several weeks or months of intravenous access
Short-term percutaneous central venous catheters (non-tunnelled)	Polyurethane Silicone	Heparin, antibiotic and antiseptic coatings, multiple lumen	Jugular Subclavian Femoral	Intended for days to weeks of intravenous access
Skin-tunnelled catheters	Polyurethane Silicone	Valved Antimicrobial/silver cuff Multiple lumen	Jugular Axillary Subclavian Femoral	Indefinite. Used for long-term intermittent, continuous or daily intravenous access. May be appropriate for short-term use if reliable access needed
Implanted ports	*Catheter* Silicone *Port* Titanium Stainless steel Plastic	Dual ports Peripheral ports Valved	Antecubital fossa Subclavian Femoral	Indefinite. Used for long-term intermittent, continuous or daily intravenous access

against fungi and viral organisms. Alcohol concentration between 70 and 92% provides the most rapid and greatest reduction in microbial counts on skin but does not have any residual activity (Larson 1988). This is where chlorhexidine has an advantage over alcohol used alone, as it has excellent residual activity for 4–6 hours after application (Carlson *et al.* 2001; Pratt *et al.* 2007). Solutions should be applied with friction for up to 1 minute and allowed to air dry for 30–60 seconds (Springhouse 2002; INS 2006). It has been found that 1 minute of application with alcohol is as effective as 12 minutes of scrubbing and reduces bacterial counts by 75%. A quick wipe fails to reduce bacterial counts prior to peripheral cannulation (INS 2006; Weinstein 2007). Allowing any cleaning solution to dry is vital in order for disinfection to be completed, and in the case of alcohol, which is a plasticizer, it ensures that plastic equipment will not 'glue together' (Dougherty 2006).

Inspection of insertion site and cleaning of equipment

Cleaning solutions should be used not only on insertion sites, but also to clean junctions and connections, etc. It is recommended that injection caps should be cleaned vigorously with appropriate cleaning agents such as chlorhexidine 0.5% in alcohol (Brown *et al.* 1997; Pratt *et al.* 2007). The frequency of cleaning the insertion site is debatable; peripheral sites are rarely cleaned once the device is sited because the device is in situ for such a short period of time. However, central venous access sites, e.g. peripherally inserted central catheters (PICCs), may be cleaned weekly (at dressing change) and short-term central venous catheters (CVCs) may be cleaned daily or more frequently (being associated with the highest infection risk). The insertion site should be checked regularly for signs of phlebitis (erythema, pain and/or swelling) or for signs of infection (for further actions see Chapter 12) (DH 2003). Complaints of soreness, unexpected pyrexia and damaged, wet or soiled dressing are reasons for immediate inspection and renewal of the dressing.

Securement of device and dressings

Devices are secured to prevent movement, which reduces the risk of phlebitis, infiltration, infection and migration (Yamamoto *et al.* 2002; Moureau & Iannucci 2003; Schears 2005; INS 2006). This can be achieved by suturing, taping or use of securing devices. These all require a dressing over them. The choice of dressing is usually based upon which is most suitable for a particular VAD site or type of skin. An intravenous dressing is applied to minimize the contamination of the insertion site and provide stability of the device (Dougherty 2006). Therefore the ideal intravenous dressing should provide an effective barrier to bacteria; allow the catheter to be securely fixed; be sterile and easy to apply and remove; be waterproof and adhere well; and finally be comfortable for the patient (Finlay 2004). There are two main

types of dressing: dry, sterile low-linting gauze and transparent dressings. A dry, sterile, low-linting dressing secured with the minimum of hypoallergenic tape is most suitable for patients with skin that is prone to allergy or is thin and tears easily, as transparent dressings can damage the skin if not removed correctly.

The benefits of transparent dressings (Springhouse 2002) are that they allow inspection of the insertion site while the dressing is in situ and therefore do not require removal; they are waterproof and many are also moisture permeable. This means that the dressing allows moisture vapour transmission, an important factor related to infection as collection of moisture enhances the proliferation of micro-organisms.

When transparent dressings have been compared with sterile gauze it has been shown that there is no significant difference and that infection rates may have been reduced (Maki & Ringer 1987; DH 2007; RCN 2005). All CVC dressings must be removed and replaced within 24 hours following insertion of the catheter (Ryder 2001; RCN 2005; Dougherty 2006). This is due to the bacterial colonization, 'biofilm', which occurs 6–18 hours following insertion (Ryder 2002). If gauze is used it must be replaced when the dressing becomes damp, loosened, soiled or when inspection of the site is necessary (RCN 2005; Pratt *et al.* 2007). Transparent dressings should be changed every 7 days unless manufacturers recommend otherwise or the integrity is compromised, i.e. when damp, loose or soiled (RCN 2005; INS 2006; Pratt *et al.* 2007). When the dressing is changed the insertion site should be inspected for inflammation and/or discharge and the condition of the skin noted (DH 2007).

Maintaining a closed intravenous system

If equipment becomes accidentally disconnected, air embolism or profuse blood loss may occur, depending on the condition and position of the patient (Perucca 2001). Accidental disconnection poses a greater risk in patients with central venous access devices (CVADs) than in those with peripheral devices. This is because of the amount of air that could be introduced via a CVAD and the speed with which it could enter the pulmonary vessels. Luer-Lok provide a more secure connection and all equipment should have these fittings, i.e. administration sets, extension sets, injection caps (Dougherty 2006). Needle-free systems provide a closed environment, which further reduces the risk of air entry (Perucca 2001). Care should be taken to clamp the catheter firmly when changing equipment. Connections must be double checked and precautions taken to prevent the introduction of air into the system when making additions to, or taking blood from, a CVC (Dougherty 2006).

Maintaining patency

Patency is defined as the ability to infuse through and aspirate blood from a VAD (Dougherty 2006). It is important at all times for the patency of the device to be maintained. Blockage predisposes to device damage, infection, inconvenience to patients and disruption to drug delivery. Occlusion of the device is usually the result of:

- Clot formation due to: (a) an administration set or electronic infusion device being turned off accidentally and left for a prolonged period; or (b) insufficient or incorrect flushing of the device when not in use.
- Precipitate formation due to inadequate flushing between incompatible medications (Dougherty 2006).

Kinking or pinch-off syndrome may also impair patency of the device. Meticulous intravenous technique will prevent the majority of these problems.

Two main types of solutions are used to maintain patency in VADs; heparin inhibits the conversion of prothrombin to thrombin and fibrinogen to fibrin thus inhibiting coagulation and is therefore used to prevent the build-up of fibrin, and sodium chloride is used to clean the internal diameter of the device of blood and drugs (Camp Sorrell 2005). All devices should be flushed with 10–20 ml 0.9% sodium chloride after blood withdrawal (RCN 2005; Dougherty 2006; INS 2006; Dougherty 2008).

Maintaining patency can be achieved by: (a) a continuous infusion to keep the vein open (KVO), either by the patient being attached to an infusion of 0.9% sodium chloride via a volumetric pump, which reduces comfort and mobility, or by use of an elastomeric device, which is less restrictive and has been able to reduce loss of patency by 50% (Heath & Jones 2001); or (b) intermittent flushing (previously known as a 'heparin lock'). The advantages of intermittent flushing compared with a continuous infusion are:

- It reduces the risk of circulatory overload.
- It reduces the risk of vascular irritation.
- It decreases the risk of bacterial contamination as it eliminates a continuous intravenous pathway.
- It increases patient comfort and mobility.
- It may reduce the cost of intravenous equipment (Phillips 2005).

One of the disadvantages is the necessity for constant vigilance and regular flushing (Weinstein 2007).

When used for intermittent therapy, the device should be flushed after each use with the appropriate flushing solution. (Guidelines for volumes, concentrations and frequency of flushing are commonly established within individual institutions.) It is now well-established that flushing with 0.9% sodium chloride can also adequately maintain the patency of the cannula (Goode *et al.* 1991). This avoids side-effects such as local tissue damage, drug incompatibilities and iatrogenic haemorrhage, which can occur with heparin (Goode *et al.* 1991). As well as being cost effective, it appears that daily or twice daily flushing with a volume of 2–5 ml 0.9% sodium chloride is acceptable (Goode *et al.* 1991).

Solutions and frequency of flushing may depend on whether the catheter is either open ended or valved. Heparinized saline is still the accepted solution for maintaining the patency of CVCs for intermittent use or infrequent use (RCN 2005; Pratt *et al.* 2007). Use of 0.9% sodium chloride alone is not yet widespread (except with certain types of catheters such as the Groshong valve [INS 2006]). Flushing regimens ranging from once daily to once weekly have been found to be effective. Implanted drug delivery systems such as implanted ports are flushed using a stronger solution of heparin, usually 500 IU heparin in 5 ml 0.9% sodium chloride (Perucca 2001). Recommendations range from monthly (RCN 2005) to every 3–4 months when not in use (Hayden & Goodman 2005).

Using the correct techniques to flush the VAD has been highlighted as one of the key issues in maintaining patency (Baranowski 1993; Goodwin & Carlson 1993). There are two stages in flushing:

1 Using a pulsated (push pause) flush to create turbulent flow when administering the solution, regardless of type and volume. This removes debris from the internal catheter wall (Goodwin & Carlson 1993; Macklin & Chernecky 2004; Phillips 2005).
2 The procedure is completed using the positive pressure technique. This is accomplished by maintaining pressure on the plunger of the syringe while disconnecting the syringe from the injection cap, which prevents reflux of blood into the tip, reducing the risk of occlusion (Moureau 1999; Phillips 2005; INS 2006).

Manufacturers have now produced needleless injection caps which enable a positive 'displacement' flush and achieve positive pressure without practitioners being required to actively achieve the positive pressure (Weinstein 2007). They have been shown to significantly reduce the incidence of catheter occlusions (Berger 2000; Lenhart 2000; Mayo 2001a; Rummel *et al.* 2001).

Excessive force should never be used when flushing devices. However, when the catheter lumen is totally patent, internal pressure will not increase during flushing (Hadaway 1998a). If resistance is felt (due to partial occlusion), and a force is applied to the plunger, this could result in a high pressure within the catheter, which may then rupture (Conn 1993; Hadaway 1998a; Macklin 1999). It is, therefore, recommended that the device is checked first with a 10 ml or larger syringe containing 0.9% sodium chloride (Hadaway 1998a; Macklin 1999; RCN 2005). However, smaller syringes should only be used to administer drugs where there is no pressure or occlusion and where it is not possible to further dilute drugs and administer in a large syringe (Hadaway 1998a; Macklin 1999). The composition of the individual device determines the maximum pressure that can be exerted. If a catheter becomes occluded the nurse should establish the cause of the clot: occlusion or precipitation (INS 2006). If precipitation occurs, then instillation of hydrochloric acid or ethyl chloride may be required (Holcombe *et al.* 1992; LSC 2002). There are two types of thrombotic occlusion:

- *Partial withdrawal occlusion (PWO)* (Figure 45.1): this is usually caused by fibrin sheath formation and identified by the absent or sluggish blood return whilst fluids can be

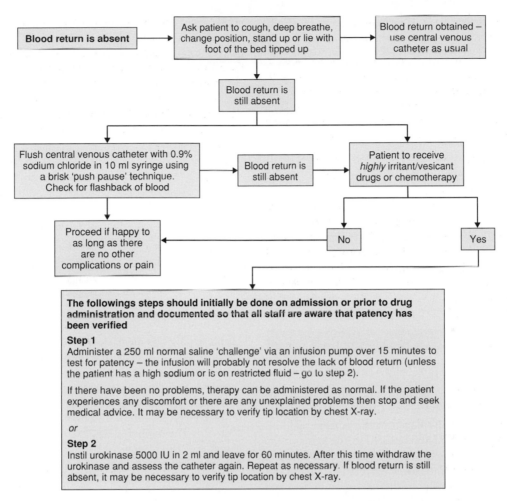

Figure 45.1 Algorithm for persistent withdrawal occlusion, i.e. fluids can be infused freely by gravity but blood cannot be withdrawn from the catheter. (Adapted from UCL Hospital Central Venous Catheter Policy.)

infused. Fibrin sheaths can result in seeding of bacteria and drug extravasation (Mayo 2000, 2001a) and can be resolved by the instillation of a thrombolytic agent such as urokinase or alteplase (Haire & Herbst 2000; Rinn 2001; Dougherty 2006; Weinstein 2007).

■ *Total occlusion*: when there is an inability to withdraw blood or infuse fluids or medications. This can be resolved by instillation of a thrombolytic agent (Ponec *et al.* 2001; Dietcher *et al.* 2002; Timoney *et al.* 2002) or by use of an endoluminal brush (Archis *et al.* 2000; Weinstein 2007).

If the occlusion is caused by a clot, gentle pressure and aspiration may be sufficient to dislodge the clot. Silicone catheters expand on pressure and allow fluid to flow around the clot, facilitating its dislodgement. This should only be attempted using a 10 ml or larger syringe. Smaller syringes should never be used as they create a greater pressure (Perdue 2001; Springhouse 2002; Camp Sorrell 2005) of mmHg or pounds per square inch (psi). This can result in rupture of the catheter, resulting in loss of catheter integrity, or dislodge the clot (Perucca 2001). Instillation of thrombolytic agents

should be performed using a three-way tap and negative pressure (Simcock 2001a; Dougherty 2006; Gabriel 2008).

Preventing damage of the VAD and performing a repair

If damage occurs to peripheral devices, they are usually removed and replaced. Most CVCs are made of silicone which is prone to cracking or splitting if handled incorrectly (Tingey 2000), but both temporary and permanent repairs can be performed depending on where the catheter is damaged and the type of catheter (Dougherty 2006). However, prevention of this occurrence is preferred.

Clamping

Artery forceps or sharp-edged clamps should not be used to clamp the catheter. A smooth clamp should be placed on the reinforced section of the catheter provided for clamping (Dougherty 2006). If a reinforced section is not present, placing a tape tab over part of the catheter can create one. A second alternative is to move the clamp up or down the catheter at regular intervals to reduce the risk of wear and tear at one point.

Use of the correct syringe size in accordance with manufacturer's guidelines will reduce the risk of catheter rupture (INS 2006). However, syringe size alone will not be sufficient to prevent catheter rupture. If resistance is felt and more pressure is applied to overcome it, catheter fracture could result regardless of syringe size (Hadaway 1998a; Macklin 1999). The nurse must be familiar with the action to be taken to minimize any risk to patient safety in this event. Immediate clamping of the catheter proximal to the fracture or split is essential to prevent blood loss or air embolism. The split area should be covered with an alcohol swab and emergency repair equipment collected, together with sterile gloves to ensure that all manipulations are aseptic. A permanent repair should be performed as soon as possible using the specific equipment provided by the manufacturer. A member of the medical staff or other designated personnel should do this (Dougherty 2006).

Peripheral cannulae

Definition

A cannula is a flexible tube containing a needle (stylet) which may be inserted into a blood vessel (Phillips 2005; Weller 2005). Cannulae are usually placed in the peripheral veins in the lower arm but may also be placed in the veins of the foot (an area used particularly in paediatric care) (Weinstein 2007). However, veins of the lower extremities should not be routinely used in adults due to the risk of embolism and thrombophlebitis (RCN 2005; INS 2006).

Indications

- Short-term therapy of 3–5 days.
- Bolus injections or short infusions in the outpatient/day unit setting (Perucca 2001; RCN 2005).

Reference material

The advantages of using a peripheral cannula are that they are usually easy to insert and have few associated complications; however, they are associated with phlebitis (either mechanical or chemical) and require constant resiting (RCN 2005; INS 2006; Dougherty 2008).

Device information

A number of different types of peripheral cannula are available. It has been shown that the incidence of vascular complications increases as the ratio of cannula external diameter to vessel lumen increases. Therefore most of the literature recommends the smallest, shortest gauge cannula in any given situation (Macklin & Chernecky 2004; RCN 2005)

Table 45.2 Gauge sizes and average flow rates (using water).

Gauge (G)	Flow rate (ml/min)	General uses
14	350	Used in theatres or emergency for rapid transfusion of blood or viscous fluids
16	215	As 14 G
18	104	Blood transfusions, parenteral nutrition, stem cell harvesting and cell separation, large volumes of fluids
20	62	Blood transfusions, large volumes of fluids
22	35	Blood transfusions, most medications and fluids
24	24	Medications, short-term infusions, fragile veins, children

(Table 45.2). The measurement used for needle and cannulae is standard wire gauge (swg), which measures the internal diameter; the smaller the gauge size, the larger the diameter. Standard wire gauge measurement is determined by how many cannulae fit into a tube with an inner diameter of 1 inch (25.4 mm) and uses consecutive numbers from 13 to 24. The diameter, e.g. 1.2 mm, may be expressed as a gauge, e.g. 18 G (Nauth Misir 1998). Needles are odd numbers, e.g. 19 G, 21 G, while cannulae are even numbers, e.g. 18 G, 20 G (Weinstein 2007).

The walls of the device should, therefore, be thin to provide the largest internal diameter without increasing the external diameter. This is to ensure that maximum flow rates may be achieved while reducing complications such as mechanical irritation. Flow rates vary with equipment from different manufacturers. Flow rate through a cannula is related to its internal diameter and is inversely proportional to its length. However, as the length of the cannula increases, so does the likelihood of vascular complications, for example a large-gauge device of longer length (1.6–2.0 cm) will fill the vessel, preventing blood flow around it, which could result in mechanical trauma to the vessel and encourage the development of phlebitis (Tagalakis et al. 2002; Dougherty 2008).

The most suitable material is one that is non-irritant and does not predispose to thrombus formation (Dougherty 2008). The material should also be radiopaque or contain a stripe of radiopaque material for radiographic visualization in the event of catheter embolus (Perucca 2001; Dougherty 2008). Types of material include polyvinylchloride, Teflon, Vialon, and various polyurethane and elastomeric hydrogel materials. Studies have compared the different types of material available such as Teflon and Vialon, to ascertain which is most likely to be associated with the lowest potential risk of phlebitis (Karadag & Gorgulu 2000). When considering the results of these studies, however, it must be noted that investigators often use different phlebitis scales and calculations for creating a total score for each device. Other inconsistencies relate to the differences in catheter size, skin preparation, the use of dressings and the type of solution being infused. This makes comparison between catheter materials difficult.

The 'over the needle' type of cannula is the most commonly used device for peripheral venous access and is available in various gauge sizes, lengths, composition and design features (Dougherty 2008). The cannula is mounted on the needle (known as the stylet) and once the device is pushed off the needle into the vein, the stylet is removed. A sharp-tipped stylet facilitates penetration into the vein and the type of graduation from the cannula to the needle can affect the degree of trauma to the vessel and the cannula tip (Perucca 2001). A thin smooth-walled cannula tapering to a scalloped end causes less damage than one that is abruptly cut off (Macklin & Chernecky 2004; Dougherty 2008).

Some peripheral cannulae have wings which help with the securing of the device to the skin in order to prevent a piston-like movement within the vein and accidental removal (Dougherty 2008). Some devices may have small ports on the top (these are favoured more in Europe than in the USA) (Figure 45.2). The advantage of a ported device is the ability to administer drugs without interfering with continuous infusion. However, the caps are often not replaced correctly, which leaves the system exposed to contamination and the possible risk of air entering. It has also been found that the ports cannot be adequately sterilized with a swab, as there is no flat surface. The use of ports may encourage the practitioner not to remove the dressing and inspect the site but merely to administer the drug via the port (Dougherty 2008). Safety cannulae are now available and have either active or passive mechanisms. The active devices are where the practitioner has to push a button in order to activate the safety feature whilst the passive devices are where the stylet has a blunting or shielding facility which is automatically

Figure 45.3   Example of a safety non-ported cannula.

activated on removal from the cannula (RCN 2005; Dougherty 2008) (Figure 45.3).

Choice of vein

The main factors to consider prior to inserting a peripheral cannula are the location for siting, condition of the vein, purpose of the infusion (that is the rate of flow required and the solution to be infused) and the duration of therapy (Phillips 2005; Dougherty 2008).

The suitable vein should always be selected prior to selection of the device. The veins should feel bouncy, refill when depressed, should be straight and free of valves to ensure easy advancement of the cannula. Valves can be felt as small lumps in the vein, some may be visualized at bifurcations, some may be visible to the naked eye in certain vessels (see below). It is best to avoid siting a cannula over a joint as this will lead to an increased risk of mechanical phlebitis and an infusion that will infuse intermittently due to the patient's movement (RCN 2005; INS 2006; Dougherty 2008; Weinstein 2007). It can also be very awkward for the patient and may restrict his or her ability to carry out activities (Marsigliese 2001; Macklin & Chernecky 2004).

The veins of choice are either the cephalic or basilic veins, followed by the dorsal venous network (see Figure 46.1 in Chapter 46). The practitioner should start distally and cannulate at proximal points (Perucca 2001; INS 2006). The best vein should always be used (Weinstein 2007).

The cephalic vein

The size and position of the cephalic vein make it an excellent vessel for administration of transfusions. It readily accommodates a large-gauge cannula and, by virtue of its position on the forearm, provides a natural splint (Weinstein 2007). However, its position at a joint may increase complications such as mechanical phlebitis and even general discomfort.

Figure 45.2   Example of a ported cannula.

The tendons controlling the thumb obscure the vein during insertion (Hadaway 2001), and care must be taken not to touch the radial nerve (Dougherty 2008).

The basilic vein

The basilic vein is a large vessel, which is often overlooked due to its inconspicuous position on the ulnar border of the hand and forearm. It is found on palpation when the patient's arm is placed across the chest, with the practitioner opposite the patient (Hadaway 2001). Cannulation can be awkward because of its position, mobility and tendency to have many valves (Hadaway 2001; Springhouse 2002; Dougherty 2008).

The dorsal venous network

Using the veins of the dorsal venous network of the hand will allow for cannulation proximally along the veins when resiting the device (Weinstein 2007). They can usually be visualized and palpated easily:

- The digital veins are small and may be prominent enough to accommodate a small-gauge needle as a last resort for fluid administration. With adequate taping the fingers can be immobilized, making it more comfortable as well as also preventing the cannula from piercing the posterior wall of the vein (leading to bruising or infiltration) (Springhouse 2002).
- The metacarpal veins are accessible, and easily visualized and palpated. They are well-suited for cannulation as the cannula lies flat and the metacarpal veins provide a natural splint (Weinstein 2007). The veins tend to be smaller than the forearm and therefore may prove difficult to access in infants because they have higher amounts of subcutaneous fat than older children and adults. The use of these veins is contraindicated in the elderly as there is diminished skin turgor and loss of subcutaneous tissue, making the vein difficult to stabilize. They are also more fragile and venous distension is slower (Powers 1999; Hadaway 2001; Walther 2001; Springhouse 2002). Metacarpal veins are a better option for short-term or outpatient intravenous therapy.

Improving venous access (see Chapter 46 for methods to improve venous access)

Insertion

As the most common cause of VAD infection is the patient's own skin flora, it is important to adequately clean the skin prior to cannulation. The patient's skin should be washed with soap and water if visibly dirty which will remove most transient flora (Carlson *et al.* 2001; Perucca 2001). Then an antiseptic solution such as chlorhexidine solution or 70% alcohol should be applied in an area of 4–5 cm in diameter with friction for 30–60 seconds. A quick wipe fails to reduce bacterial count (Weinstein 2007). It should be allowed to air dry for up to 1 minute to ensure coagulation of the organism and to prevent stinging as the needle pierces the skin (RCN 2005; INS 2006; Weinstein 2007). Once the skin has been cleaned it must not be touched or repalpated (Dougherty 2008). If it is necessary to repalpate, then the cleaning regimen should be repeated.

Shaving the skin prior to cannulation is not recommended (RCN 2005; INS 2006; Weinstein 2007) as the need to remove hair has not been substantiated by scientific evidence (Weinstein 2007). Shaving with a razor should not be performed because of the potential for causing micro-abrasions, which increase the risk of infection (Carlson *et al.* 2001; RCN 2005; INS 2006). Depilatories should not be used because of the potential for allergic reaction or irritation (Perucca 2001; RCN 2005). If hair removal is necessary then this can be accomplished by clipping with scissors or clippers (Carlson *et al.* 2001; RCN 2005). These should be cleaned between patients or only used once to prevent cross-infection (RCN 2005).

Skin stabilization is one of the most important elements for successful venepuncture or cannulation (Perucca 2001; Springhouse 2002). Superficial veins tend to roll; to prevent this the vein must be stabilized by applying traction to the side of the insertion site or below it, using the practitioner's non-dominant hand. This also facilitates a smoother needle entry. Various methods are used (Springhouse 2002; Dougherty 2008):

- The thumb can be used to stretch the skin downwards.
- The hand of the practitioner can be placed under the patient's arm and traction applied with the thumb and forefinger on either side, creating an even traction.
- The vein can be stretched between forefinger and thumb.

Stabilization of the vein must be maintained throughout the procedure until the needle or cannula is successfully sited. If the tension is released half way through the procedure, it can result in the needle penetrating the opposite wall of the vein, resulting in a haematoma formation (Dougherty 2008).

It is important that the needle enters the skin with the bevel up, as this results in a smooth venepuncture as the sharpest part of the needle will penetrate the skin first, and this also reduces the risk of piercing the posterior wall of the vein (Weinstein 2007). The angle the needle enters the skin varies, with the type of device used and the depth of the vein in the subcutaneous tissue, from 10 to 45° (Perucca 2001; Springhouse 2002; Dougherty 2008; Weinstein 2007). Once the device is in the vein, the angle should always be reduced in order to prevent puncturing the posterior wall of the vein (Perucca 2001).

There are two main methods for approaching the vein:

- The direct method is when the device enters through the skin and immediately enters the vein. However, with smaller veins this method may result in puncture of the posterior wall (Dougherty 2008).

- The indirect method is when the device is inserted through the skin and then the vein is relocated and the device advanced into the vessel. This method enables a more gentle entry and may be useful in veins which are palpable and visible for only a short section (Hadaway 2000; Perucca 2001; Dougherty 2008; Weinstein 2007).

When blood appears in the chamber of a cannula, known as 'flashback', this indicates that the initial entry into the vein has been successful. This may be accompanied by a 'giving way' sensation felt by the practitioner, which occurs due to resistance from the vein wall as the device enters the lumen of the vein. This usually occurs with thicker walled cannulae (Springhouse 2002; Weinstein 2007). If the device punctures the posterior wall, the flashback will stop. However, the flashback may be slow with small-gauge cannulae or hypotensive patients.

The cannula should be advanced gently and smoothly into the vein and a number of techniques are used by practitioners. One method which provides the least risk of through puncture but which is more difficult to learn initially is the one-handed technique (Hadaway 2000; Perucca 2001). If one hand is not used to apply traction then on cannula advancement there may be unnecessary damage to the endothelium, resulting in phlebitis (Hadaway 2001). The same hand that performs cannulation also withdraws the stylet and advances the cannula into the vein. This allows skin traction to be maintained while the device is advanced and if the patient is unable to co-operate allows the practitioner to hold onto the patient's arm (Hadaway 2000; Dougherty 2008).

The one-step technique is when the cannula has entered the vein and the practitioner can slide the cannula off the stylet in one movement. The disadvantage with this method is that the stylet must remain completely still in order to prevent damage to the vein. It is best accomplished on a straight vein and when the cannula has a small fingerguard which can be used to 'push' the cannula off (Dougherty 2008). The two-handed technique is where the practitioner performs the cannulation with one hand but releases the skin traction in order to advance the cannula off the stylet. This method prevents blood spill, but as it necessitates the release of skin traction, it can often lead to the puncturing of the vein wall (Millam 1992).

If the cannulation is unsuccessful the stylet should not be reintroduced as this could result in catheter fragmentation and embolism (Perucca 2001). A practitioner should not have more than two attempts before passing the patient onto a more experienced colleague (Perucca 2001; INS 2006; Dougherty 2008).

Pain relief

There are a number of methods for releiving pain both pharmacological and non-pharmacological (which includes distraction such as cough trick (Usichenko et al. 2004); massage (Wendler 2003) and transcutaneous electrical nerve stimu-

lation (TENS) (Coyne et al. 1995). The use of local anaesthetic prior to insertion of peripheral cannulae has been advocated to reduce pain and anxiety in children and selected adults (Scales 2005); it is recommended if the cannula is larger than 18 G, dependent on site and also at the patient's request (Moureau & Zonderman 2000; Dougherty 2008). When required the agent that is the least invasive and/or carries the least risk for allergic reaction should be considered first (RCN 2005).

Local anaesthetic may be applied in a cream/gel, given as an intradermal injection or administered by iontophoresis: a painless dry electrode pushing the local anaesthetic into the skin within 7–10 minutes to a depth of 10 mm (Moureau & Zonderman 2000; Macklin & Chernecky 2004; Dougherty 2008).

The most commonly used local anaesthetic creams are EMLA (eutectic mixture of local anaesthetics: lidocaine and prilocaine) and Ametop (topical amethocaine). These are applied to the skin 30–60 minutes prior to cannulation and covered with an occlusive dressing. A recent meta-analysis showed that EMLA cream significantly decreased the pain of intravenous cannulation in 85% of adults and children (Fetzer 2002). However, it causes vasoconstriction, making cannulation more difficult. Ametop has been shown to be more effective than EMLA and to cause significantly less vasoconstriction (Browne et al. 1999). However, it can result in an erythematous rash if left in situ longer than the recommended time (BMA & RPS 2008).

Intradermal lidocaine 1% can be slowly injected around the vein to be cannulated after skin sterilization to minimize the discomfort of the procedure. Intradermal injection of lidocaine has been shown to reduce the pain of intravenous cannulation and be less painful than placement of the cannula itself (Brown & Larson 1999). However, it should be used with caution because of the potential to cause an allergic reaction, tissue damage and inadvertent injection of the drug into the vascular system, and it can even obliterate the vein (Perucca 2001; INS 2006). It is not recommended for routine use (Perucca 2001; RCN 2005; INS 2006).

Iontophoresis uses a painless electrical current to facilitate the movement of solute ions across the skin. It has been used to administer lidocaine prior to intravenous cannulation without the need for intradermal injection and has been shown to be as effective as EMLA (Galinkin et al. 2002; Dougherty 2008).

Although local anaesthetic reduces the pain of intravenous cannulation, it is not without complications. Irrespective of the method of anaesthesia there is a risk that the symptoms of extravasation may be obscured or may even influence the risk of injury occurring (Stanley 2002).

Care and management in situ

Once sited the peripheral cannula should be flushed using a pulsatile flush, ending with positive pressure (RCN 2005; Weinstein 2007; Dougherty 2008). The cannula should be

863

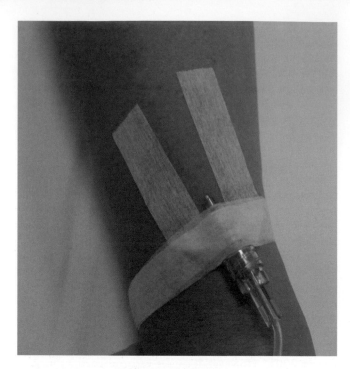

Figure 45.4   Example of a cannula in situ.

secured using clean tape. Non-sterile tape should not cover the insertion site and taping should enable the site to remain visible and the cannula stable (Figure 45.4). The procedure shown in Figure 45.5 is recommended (Hadaway 2000; Perucca 2001; Springhouse 2002; Dougherty 2008).

Other securement devices are now available and reduce the risk of dislodgement and other complications (Moureau & Iannucci 2003). A dressing should be applied: this can be either a transparent dressing or low-linting gauze (Madeo *et al*. 1997). Once the gauze is in place a bandage may be applied. However, transparent dressings, particularly moisture-permeable dressings, should not be bandaged as the visibility and moisture permeability are obscured.

Removal

It has been recommended that peripheral devices should be resited every 48–72 hours (Barker *et al*. 2004; DH 2003; RCN 2005) but some literature supports dwell times of up to 96 hours with no significant complications providing that non-irritants are administered (Homer & Holmes 1998). Other studies have found that drug irritation is the most significant predictor of phlebitis and infiltration, rather than dwell time, and that extending the dwell time up to 144 hours could be considered under certain circumstances (Bregenzer 1998; Catney *et al*. 2001). Removal of the intravenous device or cannula should be an aseptic procedure. The device should be removed carefully using a slow, steady movement and pressure should be applied until haemostasis is achieved. This pressure should be firm and not involve any rubbing movement. A haematoma will occur if the device is carelessly removed, causing discomfort and a focus for infection (Perdue 2001). The site should be inspected to ensure bleeding has stopped and the site should then be covered with a sterile dressing (INS 2006). The cannula integrity should be checked to ensure the complete device has been

Figure 45.5   Method of taping a peripheral cannula.

removed (RCN 2005; INS 2006; Dougherty 2008). The date, time and reason for removal of the cannula must then be documented in the patient's notes (DH 2003; RCN 2005; Dougherty 2008).

Midline catheters

Definition

A midline catheter can be defined as one that is between 7.5 and 20 cm in length (Perucca 2001; RCN 2005; Dougherty 2008). It provides vascular access in a larger peripheral vein without entering the central venous circulation. It is inserted into an antecubital vein and the tip is extended into the vein of the upper arm for about 20 cm, but it is not extended past the axilla (Perucca 2001; RCN 2005).

Indications

Midline catheters are indicated in the following circumstances:

- When patients do not have accessible peripheral veins in the lower arm.
- When patients will be undergoing therapy for 1–4 weeks (Carlson 1999), in order to preserve the integrity of the veins and increase patient comfort by removing the need for resites, e.g. antibiotics.
- Patient preference (Dougherty 2008).

Reference material

The midline catheter offers an alternative to peripheral and central venous access. Where patients present with poor peripheral venous access and when the use of a CVC is contraindicated, the midline catheter provides venous accessibility along with easy, less hazardous insertion at the antecubital fossa (Goetz *et al.* 1998; Weinstein 2007). Because the tip of the catheter does not extend beyond the extremities in which it is placed, radiographic confirmation of tip placement is optional and recommended only when there is difficulty in insertion or flushing (Carlson 1999; Weinstein 2007). The insertion is performed using either an over-the-needle or Seldinger technique: venous access is established with a needle, a guidewire is threaded though the needle, the needle is removed and the catheter is threaded over the guidewire (Weinstein 2007). Benefits to the patient include less frequent resiting of the catheter and a subsequent reduction in associated venous trauma (Weinstein 2007). However, mechanical phlebitis is a common side-effect and close observation and appropriate management are indicated. Once in situ, the catheter should be managed exactly as a CVC. The following therapies are not appropriate for administration via a midline catheter: vesicant medications, especially by continuous infusion; parenteral nutrition, solutions and/or medications with pH less than 5 or greater than 9 and those with osmolarity greater than 500 mOsm/l (Banton & Leahy 1998; Hadaway 2000; Frey 2001; INS 2006).

Device information

Silicone and polyurethane are the most frequently used materials in the manufacture of midline catheters (Kupensky 1998; Hadaway 2000) and they are available as single and double lumen catheters in lengths of up to 20 cm, which can be cut to the desired length following measurement of the arm from the selected vein towards the axilla. They are available in various gauges (16–24) (Perucca 2001; Dougherty 2008).

Choice of vein

The basilic vein is the vein of choice due to its larger size, straighter course for catheter advancement and improved haemodilution capability (Perucca 2001; Weinstein 2007). The cephalic and median cubital veins would be the second and third choices (INS 2006).

Insertion

The procedure should only be performed by competent nurses with excellent insertion skills (Weinstein 2007). Adequate assessment of the patient's veins is vital and given the choice the non-dominant arm should be used. The procedure requires a sterile approach and it is recommended that sterile gloves are worn. These should be powder-free, as powder on the catheter can result in mechanical phlebitis (Hayden & Goodman 2005).

Care and management in situ

It is not usually appropriate to suture these devices in situ, as they can be adequately secured with Steristrips or catheter securement devices such as a Statlock (Perucca 2001). The insertion site can then be covered with a moisture-permeable transparent dressing and changed according to the manufacturer's recommendations, e.g. once a week. The device should be flushed with 0.9% sodium chloride after each use and then with a heparinized solution according to the manufacturer's recommendations, e.g. weekly. Midline catheters can be left in situ for extended periods of time; the optimal time interval for removal of a midline catheter is unknown. Therefore it is recommended that maximum dwell times should be limited to 2–4 weeks (INS 2006). Longer dwell times should be decided on site assessment, length of maintaining therapy and patient condition (Kupensky 1998; INS 2006).

Removal

Removal requires gentle firm traction and the catheter will slide out from the insertion site. Pressure should be applied for at least 3–4 minutes and the site inspected prior to applying a dressing to ensure bleeding has stopped. The catheter integrity should be checked and its length measured to ensure that a complete device has been removed (RCN 2005).

Central venous access devices

Definition

A central venous access device (CVAD) is one where the catheter is threaded into the central vasculature. If inserted by direct skin puncture into a vein it is percutaneous, e.g. non-tunnelled or PICC; it can also be tunnelled under the skin (INS 2006). A CVC tip will always be in the superior vena cava (SVC) or right atrium (Galloway & Bodenham 2004; Dougherty 2006).

Indications

- To monitor CVP in seriously ill patients.
- For the administration of large amounts of intravenous fluid or blood, e.g. in cases of shock or major surgery.
- To provide long-term access for (Springhouse 2002; Dougherty 2006; Weinstein 2007):

  (a) Hydration or electrolyte maintenance.
  (b) Repeated administration of drugs, such as cytotoxic and antibiotic therapy.
  (c) Repeated transfusion of blood or blood products.
  (d) Repeated specimen collection.
  (e) Parenteral nutrition.

Hazards of insertion

See Box 45.1.

Box 45.1   Hazards of central venous catheter insertion

- Sepsis
- Hydrothorax
- Brachial plexus injury
- Catheter embolism
- Arterial puncture and malposition
- Air embolism
- Haemorrhage
- Thoracic duct trauma
- Thrombosis
- Pneumothorax
- Haemothorax
- Misdirection or kinking
- Cardiac tamponade
- Cardiac arrhythmias

Dougherty 2006; INS 2006; Weinstein 2007.

Complications associated with indwelling CVCs

The complications associated with indwelling CVCs are: dislodgement or twiddler's syndrome; catheter migration or occlusion; pinch-off syndrome; catheter-related thrombosis; SVC syndrome; damaged catheter; site infection or erosion (Dougherty 2006; INS 2006).

Peripherally inserted central catheters

Definition

A peripherally inserted central catheter (PICC) is a catheter that is inserted via the antecubital veins in the arm and is advanced into the central veins, with the tip located in the SVC (usually the lower third) (NAVAN 1998; RCN 2005; INS 2006). It is not to be confused with a midclavicular catheter (often referred to as a 'long line') where the tip is located in a central vein leading to the SVC such as the subclavian or proximal axillary vein (Carlson 1999; Dougherty 2006). Because of the increasing evidence that midclavicular catheters are associated with a high incidence of thrombotic complications (up to 60%), mid-clavicular placement should only be considered if there are anatomical or pathophysiological reasons, e.g. SVC syndrome (Carlson 1999; Dougherty 2006).

Indications

- Lack of peripheral access.
- Infusions of vesicant, irritant, parenteral nutrition or hyperosmolar solutions.
- Intermediate to long-term venous access.
- Patient preference.
- Patients with needle phobia, to prevent repeated cannulation.
- Clinician preference if patients are at risk of complications associated with CVAD insertion, e.g. haemorrhage or pneumothorax or if other types of devices are contraindicated (Philpott & Griffiths 2003; Dougherty 2006).

PICCs should not be considered as a last resort, but introduced early in treatment (Springhouse 2002).

Reference material

The PICC has many advantages over the other central venous access devices: firstly, it eliminates the risks associated with CVC placement, particularly pneumothorax (Perucca 2001; Dougherty 2006). Secondly, PICCs have been shown to be associated with a reduction in catheter sepsis when using these devices. This may be related to the temperature of the skin and it has been reported that peripheral sites rarely have more than 50–100 colony-forming units (cfu) of bacteria per 10 cm² of skin compared with 1000–10 000 cfu/cm² on the neck and chest (Carlson 1999; Carlson *et al.* 2001; Philpott & Griffiths 2003). Thirdly, it is easy to use for both staff and patients (Dougherty 2006) as well as helping to preserve peripheral veins (Gabriel 2000; Oakley *et al.* 2000; Philpott & Griffiths 2003). It has been shown to reduce patient discomfort and provide a reliable form of access (Oakley *et al.* 2000; Costa & Ferguson 2002). It has also been shown to be cost effective when compared with other long-term and short-term catheters and can be inserted at the bedside (Snelling *et al.* 2001; Springhouse 2002; Hayden & Goodman 2005). Disadvantages include an increase in self-care; blood withdrawal is not always easy with the smaller gauges and they may occlude (Dougherty 2006). Over time multiple insertions can cause venous scarring and decrease the ability to reuse the site (Hayden & Goodman 2005). It has also been found that compared with skin-tunnelled catheters in patients with gastrointestinal cancers, the advantages of a PICC decrease significantly if treatment lasts more than 120 days (Snelling *et al.* 2001).

Contraindications for using a PICC include the inability to locate suitable antecubital veins; anatomical distortions from surgery, injury or trauma, e.g. scarring from mastectomy, lymphoedema or burns, which may prevent advancement of the catheter to the desired tip location; if a patient is unable to carry out catheter care or is confused; if the patient is unable to lie supine for the insertion period (Philpott & Griffiths 2003; Dougherty 2006).

Device information

PICCs are available as single- and double-lumen catheters, open-ended or valved, and may be made of silicone or polyurethane (Springhouse 2002; Dougherty 2006). Catheters measure 50–65 cm long, with a diameter of 2–7 Fr. PICCs can be cut to the required length, except for valved catheters (Dougherty 2006). The catheter may be inserted through a breakaway needle or peel-away introducer with or without a guidewire (Perucca 2001). With the breakaway needle design the catheter is passed through a splittable needle (Weinstein 2007) and the peel-away introducer is plastic, peeling away once the catheter is inserted. A guidewire within the catheter adds firmness to a silicone catheter, enhancing its advancement. Guidewires are not usually required with a polyurethane catheter (Perucca 2001).

A microintroducer technique can be used to facilitate placement in a smaller difficult vein (Perucca 2001) and improves success (Sansivero 2000). A cannula is inserted and once the needle has been removed, a guidewire is advanced, the cannula is removed, an introducer is passed over the wire. Once the wire has been removed, the catheter can be advanced via the introducer into the vein (Sansivero 2000; Dougherty 2006; Gabriel 2008).

Choice of vein

Careful evaluation and adequate assessment of the patient prior to attempting catheter placement go a long way to ensuring success. Examine both arms with a tourniquet in place, palpate for the healthiest, largest vein, and preferably use the non-dominant arm. Problems associated with vein location have been overcome with the use of a hand-held Doppler, which can identify forearm veins larger than 2 mm in diameter (Whitely *et al.* 1995). In patients with limited venous access, PICCs may be introduced using ultrasound technology. It has been shown that ultrasonography can increase the chance of successful cannulation of the vein on the first attempt (La Rue 2000) compared with using the traditional landmark method. This method is described as using surface anatomical landmarks and knowing the expected anatomical relationship of the vein to its palpable companion artery (NICE 2002; Dougherty 2006). However, by using ultrasound, the nurse may identify arterial vessels and ultrasound can facilitate visualization of solid material, such as a thrombus, in the lumen of the vessel (Weinstein 2007).

The basilic vein

The median basilic vein is the vein of choice for PICC insertions owing to its larger size, straighter course for catheter advancement and improved haemodilution capability (NAVAN 1998; Perucca 2001; Springhouse 2002; RCN 2005) (see Figure 45.6).

The basilic vein begins in the ulnar (inner aspect) part of the forearm, runs along the posterior, medial surface (back of the arm) and then curves towards the antecubital region, where it is joined by the median cubital vein. It then progresses straight up the upper arm for approximately 5–8 cm and enters the deep tissues. It ascends medially to form the axillary vein (Hadaway 2001; Dougherty 2006).

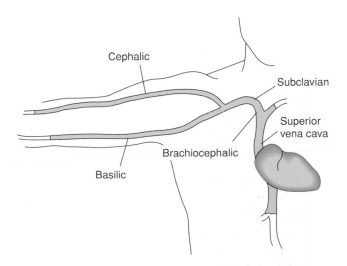

Figure 45.6   Veins of the thorax. (Redrawn from BD First PICC Clinical Education Class Manual D11 952B 5/98.)

The median cubital vein

The median cubital vein ascends from just below the middle of the antecubital region and commonly divides into two vessels, one of which joins the basilic and the other the cephalic vein. The median cubital vein is commonly used for blood sampling owing to its size and ease of needle entry. If a practitioner is having difficulty locating and/or cannulating the basilic vein, then the median cubital vein may be used as an alternative insertion route (Egan Sansivero 1998). The catheter will then advance into the basilic (or cephalic) vein.

The cephalic vein

The cephalic vein begins in the radial side (thumb side) of the hand and ascends laterally (along the outer region of the forearm) into the antecubital region, where it forms a junction with the axillary vein. This vein is usually more accessible than the basilic but its size and the sharp angle where it anastomoses with the subclavian make it more difficult to advance the catheter (Perucca 2001; Springhouse 2002; Dougherty 2006) and therefore presents a greater potential for catheter tip malposition (Dougherty 2006; Weinstein 2007).

Insertion

Venous assessment and selection play key roles in the successful insertion of a PICC, along with the correct positioning of the patient and careful measurement of the patient and the device. To obtain the correct measurement of the length of catheter to be inserted, using a tape measure, measure diagonally from the selected point for venepuncture with the arm at 45°, to the middle of the clavicle, and then add the length of the clavicle: this gives the measurement for right-sided placement. For left-sided placement add the width of the manubrium (about 2–4 cm) (Lum 1999) (see Action figure 6 in the Procedure guidelines: Peripherally inserted central catheter (PICC) insertion and removal, below). Lum (2004) has since developed a formula-based measurement guide based on a patient's height which provides a more accurate assessment to achieve optimal tip placement (Dougherty 2006) (see Box 45.2).

The use of local anaesthetic either topically or by injection should be considered to reduce the pain associated with the initial venepuncture with the introducer. It has been found that lidocaine intradermally is superior to EMLA prior to insertion of PICCs (Fry & Aholt 2001). The position of the tip of the PICC should be verified immediately after insertion before any infusion. This is done by a chest X-ray. Ascertaining correct placement is the major reason for ordering a chest X-ray, but a chest X-ray also rules out malposition and pneumothorax and confirms acceptable tip location for the type of medication being administered (Royer 2001; Wise *et al.* 2001; RCN 2005; Dougherty 2006; INS 2006).

Care and management in situ

Most PICCs are designed with suture wings, so the PICC can be sutured to the patient's skin. However, patients have reported long-term suturing to be uncomfortable; scarring when the device is removed (Gabriel 2000; Gabriel 2001); and inflammation and bacterial colonization of the exit site (Schears 2005). So suturing is no longer recommended (Maki 2002). PICCs can be adequately secured using Steristrips or securement devices (self-adhesive anchoring devices applied to the skin such as Statlocks (Figure 45.7). These have been shown to result in significantly longer catheter dwell times and fewer total complications (Gabriel 2001; Maki 2002; Yamamoto *et al.* 2002; Schears 2005). Bleeding occurs in the first 24 hours so a fold of sterile gauze should be placed over the site under the dressing (Philpott & Griffiths 2003). The insertion site is then covered with a moisture-permeable transparent dressing and the initial dressing changed at 24 hours and then changed according to manufacturer's recommendations, e.g. once a week, to minimize the potential for infection and catheter migration (NICE 2003; RCN 2005; Pratt *et al.* 2007).

Flushing solution and frequency are usually dependent on the type of catheter and so manufacturer's recommendations should be followed, e.g. valved catheters are usually flushed once a week with 0.9% sodium chloride, while open-ended catheters are flushed with a heparinized solution (Dougherty 2006; Pratt *et al.* 2007). Care should be taken when using devices such as power injectors for administering intravenous contrast agents via a PICC as the pressure created may lead to catheter rupture. This will depend on the gauge and manufacturer of the catheter (Williamson & McKinney 2001); however, the Medicines and Healthcare Products Regulatory Agency (MHRA 2004) recommendations are that computed tomography (CT) contrast using a pressure injector should not be performed via any CVAD.

Removal

Removal requires gentle firm traction and the catheter will slide out from the insertion site. A PICC may resist removal because of venous spasm, vasoconstriction, phlebitis, valve inflammation, thrombophlebitis or when a fibrin sheath is

---

Box 45.2   Formula to calculate measurement for length of peripherally inserted central catheter (PICC) (with PICC located 2.5 cm below the antecubital fossa)

Right PICC

   Height in cm $\times$ 3 $\div$ 10

Left PICC

   Height in cm $\times$ 3 $\div$ 10 + 4 cm

Adapted from Lum 2004.

Figure 45.7   PICC in situ with securing device.

present (Perucca 2001). Difficulty may occur in 1% of removals (Drewett 2000). Gentle traction and a warm moist compress can be applied to alleviate venous spasm, resulting in easier removal of the catheter (Marx 1995; Perucca 2001). If there is difficulty with removal then wait 20–30 minutes and try again or leave for 12–24 hours (Dougherty 2006). Other interventions to aid removal include smooth muscle relaxants or relaxation techniques (Marx 1995).

Following removal of the PICC, pressure should be applied for at least 3–4 minutes and the site inspected prior to applying a sterile transparent dressing to ensure bleeding has stopped. The catheter integrity should be checked and its length measured to ensure an intact device has been removed (Springhouse 2002; Dougherty 2006).

Short-term percutaneous central venous catheters (non-tunnelled)

Definition

A short-term non-tunnelled percutaneous central venous catheter (CVC) is a device that enters through the skin directly into a central vein (Dougherty 2006).

Indications

- Short-term therapy of a few days up to several weeks.
- CVP readings.
- Emergency use, e.g. fluid replacement.
- Absence of peripheral veins (Simcock 2001b; Dougherty 2006).

Reference material

Percutaneous non-tunnelled CVCs are commonly used for patients in acute settings and insertion may be in response to an emergency or planned event (Simcock 2001b; Springhouse 2002). This catheter is made of polyurethane which is stiff, and aids in CVP monitoring. In addition, its configuration as a multilumen catheter allows administration of several solutions at once and it is easy to remove (Dougherty 2006). However, these catheters are associated with an increased risk of complications such as pneumothorax and infection (Perucca 2001) and the catheter material results in irritation of the inner lumen of the vessel and is more thrombogenic (Springhouse 2002; Dougherty 2006).

Device information

Most catheters are made of polyurethane and range from single- to multi- (up to five) lumen devices (Figure 45.8). There are a variety of lumen gauges and the catheters vary in length. The catheters are usually open ended, but lumens can exit at staggered points along the catheter (Figure 45.9a, b) (Dougherty 2006). Multilumen catheters

869

Figure 45.8   Non-tunnelled multilumen central venous catheter.

carry a high risk of infection, which has resulted in the manufacture of coated and impregnated catheters. These can have antimicrobial agents such as chlorhexidine or silver sulphadiazine bonded onto the surface. It has been shown that this can reduce the incidence of catheter-related bloodstream infections and their use is strongly recommended by the Department of Health (DH) (Pratt *et al.* 2007) (Bassetti *et al.* 2001; Sampath *et al.* 2001; RCN 2005).

(a)

(b)

Figure 45.9   Types of catheter tips. (a) Open-ended catheter (single and double lumen). (b) Staggered exit open-ended catheter.

Choice of vein

These catheters are usually placed in the jugular, subclavian or femoral veins. The preferred vein for most CVCs is the subclavian (Perucca 2001; Springhouse 2002; Weinstein 2007). The shortest catheters and the most direct route are required to create a rapid blood flow around the catheter, which reduces irritation and obstructions, the risk of complications and increases the dwell time of the catheter (Springhouse 2002; Weinstein 2007). This route also has the lowest risk of infection (Mermel *et al.* 2000) and allows greatest patient mobility after insertion (Springhouse 2002). Disadvantages are an increased risk of pneumothorax and a difficulty controlling bleeding (Springhouse 2002). Its use is contraindicated in patients with radiation burns to the insertion site, fractured clavicle, malignant lesion at base of neck or apex of lungs (Dougherty 2006; Scales 2008), SVC syndrome or a history of central placement problems. The jugular vein approach can be via the internal or external jugular vein. The anatomical location of the internal jugular vein makes it easier to catheterize than the subclavian vein and there is less risk of pneumothorax (Springhouse 2002). The external jugular vein is observable and easily entered and insertion complications are rare (Springhouse 2002; Weinstein 2007). Disadvantages include catheter occlusion and venous irritation as a result of head movement, difficulty in maintaining an intact dressing, and the position of the catheters being disturbing for patient and family (Perucca 2001; Springhouse 2002; Dougherty 2006; Weinstein 2007). The femoral veins are primarily used for short-term access when other sites are not suitable (Springhouse 2002). This route is associated with an increased risk of infection difficulty in maintaining an intact dressing and inhibiting the patient's mobility (Perucca 2001; Springhouse 2002; Dougherty 2006).

Insertion

CVC insertion is a sterile procedure and the insertion requires use of a mask, sterile gloves, a gown and sterile drapes (RCN 2005; INS 2006; Pratt *et al.* 2007). These catheters may be inserted at the patient's bedside, but it is recommended that the procedure is performed in a controlled environment to reduce the risk of contamination (Perucca 2001). This procedure is usually performed by doctors although more nurses are expanding their roles to include this procedure. In general the nurse's responsibilities include the following:

- To ensure, where possible, that the patient understands and has been given a full explanation of the procedure and had the opportunity to discuss any aspects.
- To explain any specific pre- and post-procedure instructions and the appearance and function of the catheter or device.
- To teach the patient techniques that may be required during insertion, the Valsalva manoeuvre and being placed in the Trendelenburg position (where the patient lies flat with their head lowered; knees may be bent) (Perucca 2001; Springhouse 2002; Dougherty 2006; Weinstein 2007) (Figure 45.10).
- To assemble the equipment requested.
- To prepare local anaesthesia and dressing materials.
- To ensure the correct positioning of the patient during insertion, that is, in the supine or Trendelenburg position.

Figure 45.10 Ways of achieving the Trendelenburg position.

- To attend to the physical and psychological comfort of the patient during and immediately following the procedure.
- To ensure that no fluid or medication is infused before the correct position of the catheter is confirmed on X-ray by medical staff and documented.

The Valsalva manoeuvre and Trendelenburg position

Placing the patient in the Trendelenburg position facilitates entry to the vein by distending the vein, increasing CVP and venous blood supply, making veins more usable and accessible. It also reduces the chance of air embolism because the venous pressure is higher than atmospheric pressure. This is especially important when the catheter is placed using the subclavian approach (Dougherty 2006). A rolled towel may be placed under the back along the spinal cord and between the shoulders to hyperextend the neck and clavicle (Weinstein 2007). The Valsalva manoeuvre can be performed by conscious patients to aid insertion of the catheter and also to prevent air embolism (Verghese *et al.* 2002; Dougherty 2006; Weinstein 2007). The patient is asked to breathe in and then try to force the air out with the mouth and nose closed (i.e. against a closed glottis). This increases the intrathoracic pressure so that the return of blood to the heart is reduced momentarily and the veins in the neck region become engorged (Dougherty 2006).

Insertion can be aided by the use of two-dimensional imagery. Ultrasound guidance should be used routinely when a CVC is being inserted whether in an elective or emergency situation (NICE 2002). Ultrasound has been shown to increase success, decreasing failure by 83% and reducing complications by 57% (NICE 2002).

It is recommended that these types of catheter remain in for 10–14 days. They can then be removed or the site rotated (Timsit 2000) or they can be replaced over a guidewire (Cook *et al.* 1997). The catheter is easily removed by either nursing or medical staff, using aseptic technique. The site should be cleaned prior to catheter removal to prevent a false-positive result if the catheter tip needs to be sent for microbiological examination (Perucca 2001). CVC removal is associated with air embolism (Scales 2008). Precautions are required to prevent this: position the patient in the Trendelenburg position and ask the patient to perform the Valsalva manoeuvre while the catheter is being withdrawn (Perucca 2001; Springhouse 2002). Patients should remain flat for a short time after catheter removal to maintain positive intrathoracic pressure and allow the tissue tract time to seal (Perucca 2001).

Care and management in situ

The catheter may be sutured in place but this is no longer recommended due to the risk of infection (Crnich & Maki 2002; Maki 2005). The use of other securement devices is

871

recommended. Flushing is recommended after each use of the catheter. Since these devices are usually in constant use, 0.9% sodium chloride is the flushing solution of choice to reduce the risk of occlusion (Pratt *et al.* 2007). It may be appropriate to use continuous infusions to keep the vein open. The types of dressings used at the insertion site may vary according to the type of patient and unit. Staff in some critical care units do not dress the site but clean the insertion site every 4 hours whilst other units may use a moisture-permeable dressing which is changed as necessary (Scales 2008). This enables the staff to observe the site regularly for any signs of infection.

Removal

Major vessels usually heal quickly, but direct pressure must be applied to the site until cessation of bleeding confirms this (Dougherty 2006; INS 2006). A sterile transparent occlusive dressing should be applied (RCN 2005; Scales 2008), and the site assessed daily until the site has epithelialized (INS 2006), usually within 72 hours (Springhouse 2002). The integrity of the catheter should be ascertained and documented (RCN 2005).

Skin-tunnelled catheters

Definition

A skin-tunnelled catheter is a long-term catheter that lies in a subcutaneous tunnel before entering a central vein (usually subclavian). The tunnel commonly exits between the sternum and the nipple. The tip lies at the junction of the SVC and right atrium or within the lower portion of the SVC or the upper right atrium (Galloway & Bodenham 2004; Dougherty 2006) (see Figure 45.11).

Indications

A skin-tunnelled catheter is used when long-term venous access is required or if peripheral vascular access is problematic (Dougherty 2006).

Reference material

Tunnelled silicone catheters were first described by Broviac in Seattle in 1973 and were modified by Hickman and his colleagues, creating a larger lumen of 1.6 mm internal diameter (Bjeletich & Hickman 1980). Their special features included an inert anti-thrombogenic flexible material and a subcutaneous Dacron cuff attached to the catheter. The cuff has two functions. First, the cuff is used to secure the catheter as fibrous tissue grows around it and obliterates part of the subcutaneous tunnel within 1–2 weeks of insertion. Second, the cuff impedes the migration of micro-organisms, creat-

(a)

(b)

Figure 45.11   (a) Anatomical positioning of tunnelled catheter. (b) Patient with tunnelled catheter in situ.

ing a 'barrier' along the subcutaneous tract and therefore reducing the incidence of catheter-related infection (Perucca 2001; Wilson 2001; Springhouse 2002; Dougherty 2006; Weinstein 2007). The cuff is about 1 cm wide (Perucca 2001) and is usually located about 3–5 cm from the exit site (Stacey *et al.* 1991; Weinstein 2007).

The catheter currently used at The Royal Marsden Hospital has a cuff that is situated 20–22 cm from the top of the bifurcation (Figure 45.12). This measurement may assist

22 cm

Figure 45.12   Distance from cuff to bifurcation of skin-tunnelled catheter.

the practitioner in locating the cuff during removal of the catheter. However, the distance of the cuff from the bifurcation may vary according to the type of catheter.

Device information

Polyurethane or silicone skin-tunnelled catheters present as single-, double- or triple-lumen catheters and the tip may be open ended or closed with a slit valve (Dougherty 2006). The disadvantage of an open-ended catheter is the problem of blood reflux, resulting in occlusion. Catheters such as the Groshong catheter have a round closed tip which incorporates a two-way valve that remains closed at normal vena caval pressure. Application of a vacuum in order to withdraw blood enables the valve to open inwards; positive pressure into the catheter forces the valve to open outwards (Figure 45.13) (Dougherty 2006). The advantages of valved catheters are the reduced risk of bleeding or air emboli on insertion and during subsequent care; the elimination of catheter clamping; and the elimination of the need for heparin along with a reduction in the frequency of flushing (Hoffer *et al.* 1999; Inwood 1999; Weinstein 2007). However, if a thrombus forms around the tip it can result in malfunction and loss of valve competence (Dougherty 2006).

Another type of catheter is the pressure-activated safety valve (PASV). The valve opens with minimal positive pressure for infusion but requires four times as much negative pressure for aspiration (Weinstein 2007). This feature reduces the risk of air embolism or bleeding resulting from accidental disconnection. The valve is incorporated within the hub and not the tip and reduces the risk of reflux even during periods of raised CVP (Weinstein 2007).

Choice of vein

The aim of the insertion is to place the catheter tip in the right atrium via the subclavian vein and SVC (Galloway & Bodenham 2004). When there is an SVC obstruction from thrombosis or compression, the femoral vein can be used to access the inferior vena cava. Selection of vessels is as for non-tunnelled CVC.

Insertion

The insertion of a skin-tunnelled catheter is a surgical procedure usually carried out in an operating theatre or designated area, under aseptic conditions, using fluoroscopy and monitoring of the patient by pulse oximetry and electrocardiogram (ECG) to detect arrhythmias (Benton & Marsden 2002; Galloway & Bodenham 2004; Dougherty 2006; Weinstein 2007). The procedure is now also performed by nurse specialists at the bedside and within radiology departments (Hamilton *et al.* 1995; Fitzsimmons *et al.* 1997; Benton & Marsden 2002; Boland *et al.* 2003). The procedure is usually performed under sedation along with the use of local anaesthesia (Dougherty 2006). In some patients, e.g. children, this procedure would be carried out under general anaesthesia.

Access may be gained percutaneously using a needle and a guidewire or via an open surgical cutdown procedure. The percutaneous insertion involves the subclavian vein being accessed using a guidewire and Seldinger technique. After the catheter has been tunnelled subcutaneously, a vein dilator is passed over the guidewire and the catheter is cut to length and introduced using a 'peel-away' sheath (Davidson & Al Mufti 1997; Galloway & Bodenham 2004). Position is confirmed by the easy aspiration of blood from each lumen and these are then flushed with heparin or a slow infusion of 0.9% sodium chloride (10–20 ml/hour) until correct tip placement has been confirmed. A chest X-ray should be performed 2 hours after insertion to check for correct placement and pneumothorax (Stacey *et al.* 1991; Davidson & Al Mufti 1997).

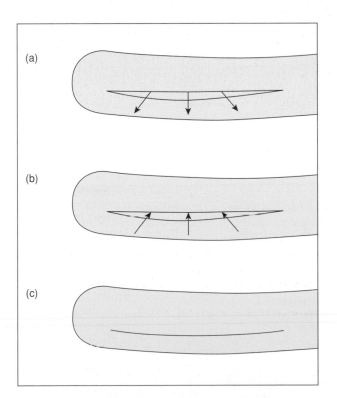

Figure 45.13   The Groshong two-way valve catheter. **(a)** Infusion (positive pressure). **(b)** Aspiration (negative pressure). **(c)** Closed (neutral pressure). (Groshong is a registered trademark of C.R. Bard, Inc. or an affiliate.)

Care and management in situ

Following healing of the skin tunnel, which takes approximately 7 days, sutures at the entry site may be removed (Dougherty 2006). The exit sutures should be retained until the fibroblastic response to the Dacron cuff is adequate to secure the catheter, usually in 2–3 weeks (Stacey *et al.* 1991; Perucca 2001; Weinstein 2007). A transparent dressing should cover the site and be changed weekly until removal of sutures. Thereafter a dressing is not usually required unless the patient requests one (Dougherty 2006).

Removal

Removal techniques for skin-tunnelled catheters vary. Removal should only be performed by specially trained nurses or doctors. It is recommended that the patient is placed supine and that aseptic technique is used throughout. There are two methods for removal:

Surgical excision

This method involves locating the cuff and performing a minor surgical excision under local anaesthetic. A small incision is made over the site of the cuff and blunt dissection, i.e. using forceps, is carried out to prise apart tissues (Galloway & Bodenham 2004); this causes less damage to the tissues than using a scalpel. The cuff and the catheter are freed from the surrounding fibrous tissue (Dougherty 2006). The catheter is then cut in order to remove the distal end via the exit site and the proximal end through the incision. Once the catheter has been removed, the wound is sutured using interrupted sutures, which can be removed after 7 days (Galloway & Bodenham 2004).

Traction method

With the traction method there is a greater risk of the catheter breaking, which could result in a catheter embolism. The catheter is gripped firmly and constant traction applied until the cuff is loosened in the tunnel (Hayden & Goodman 2005). It may take a few minutes for the catheter and cuff to become loose before sliding free. Constant steady pressure will remove the complete catheter; however, the catheter should be checked on removal to ensure it is complete as breakage and splitting can occur (Hayden & Goodman 2005; INS 2006). The catheter and cuff may be pulled through, but the cuff may remain attached to tissue. This is thought to be of no significance and may be left in place, although some suggest that if the cuff is not removed it could become infected later (Drewett 2000; Galloway & Bodenham 2004). Difficulty with removal or a break in the catheter will require surgical intervention.

Since the vein closes following removal of the catheter there is usually no bleeding. However, there may be slight bleeding at the exit site immediately after removal because of the passage of the cuff.

Following either removal method, pressure should be applied to the site until the bleeding stops, and a dressing may be required for up to 24 hours. The patient should be encouraged to rest flat for 30–60 minutes to allow the tissue tract time to seal (Galloway & Bodenham 2004).

If the tip is required for microbiological examination, care should be taken to clean the exit site with chlorhexidine in 70% alcohol, prior to removal, to prevent a false positive tip culture. The tip should be placed into a sterile container im-

mediately upon removal and sent to the laboratory (Perucca 2001).

Implantable ports

Definition

An implanted port is a totally implanted VAD made of two components: a reservoir with a self-sealing septum which is attached to a silicone catheter (Figure 45.14). The port is inserted on either the chest or the arm and is accessed using a special non-coring needle (Hayden & Goodman 2005; Dougherty 2006; Weinstein 2007).

Indications

An implanted port can be used for long-term venous access for all types of therapies, both continuous and intermittent, and if patients have problematic venous access (Springhouse 2002; Dougherty 2006).

Reference material

Ports are implanted subcutaneously to provide repeated long-term access (Weinstein 2007) to the vascular system (other ports include arterial, epidural and peritoneal ports).

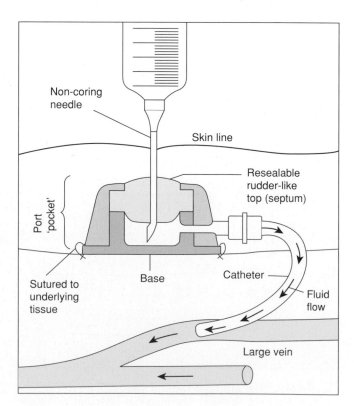

Figure 45.14   Cross-section of an implantable port, accessed with non-coring needle.

Implanted ports require little care of the site because of the intact skin layer over the accessible port, except when accessed. When not in use, the only care required is a monthly flush (Weinstein 2007). Other benefits include a reduced risk of infection (Mirro *et al.* 1989; Bow *et al.* 1999; Moureau 1999) and less interference with daily activities such as bathing or swimming (Hayden & Goodman 2005), and body image is less threatened than by the presence of an external catheter (Mirro *et al.* 1989; Bow *et al.* 1999). Patients with ports are often very satisfied with their access devices (Chernecky 2001).

Disadvantages of the port include discomfort when accessing is performed (particularly if placed deeply or in a difficult area to access). This can be overcome with the use of topical local anaesthetic. However, the tissue over the septum becomes calloused or scarred and over time there is loss of sensitivity (Moureau 1999; Perucca 2001). Needle dislodgement with resulting extravasation or needlestick injury are well-documented problems associated with ports (Nesti & Kovac 2000; Schulmeister & Camp Sorrell 2000; Hallquist Viale 2003). There are also issues related to occlusion and 'sludge' build-up and newer designs are attempting to reduce this (Stevenis *et al.* 2000). Finally there are often problems with obtaining blood return (Moureau 1999).

Device information

A variety of ports are available and the one chosen is dependent on a number of factors; for example, whether the patient is a child or an adult, the amount of access required and where it is located (Perucca 2001). Ports are usually single lumen, although double-lumen ports are available (Dougherty 2006). However, double-lumen ports have two septums and therefore require needle access into each septum (Hayden & Goodman 2005). Port reservoirs (Figure 45.15) are about 2.5 cm in height and 0.625 cm in diameter and can weigh from 21 to 28 g; low-profile ports are smaller and often placed in the arm (Perucca 2001). Entry can be gained via the side or top but most are accessed by top entry (Hayden & Goodman 2005; Weinstein 2007). Catheters are made of silicone and may be open ended or have a Groshong valve (Biffi *et al.* 2001; Perucca 2001). The portal body may be made of stainless steel, plastic or titanium, although steel is not often used any more as it interferes with electromagnetic imaging procedures and is quite heavy in comparison with other materials (Perucca 2001; Dougherty 2006). The self-sealing silicone septum can be accessed 1000–3600 times, often dependent upon the size of the needle used (Hayden & Goodman 2005). Non-coring needles have the penetration of a knife so when the needle is removed the septum closes behind it. The bevel opens on the side of the needle instead of the end (Perucca 2001; Weinstein 2007; Gabriel 2008). They are available in straight or 90° angle configuration with or without extension sets. The needle is available with a metal or plastic hub in gauges 19–24 and lengths from 0.65 to 2.5 cm. Needle gauge is selected dependent on type and rate of infusate as well as the location of the port (Dougherty 2006; Weinstein 2007).

Figure 45.15   Examples of implanted ports.

Choice of vein

The most common veins used are subclavian, internal or external jugular veins, cephalic or femoral vein. Ports can also be inserted in the antecubital area of the arm (Perucca 2001; Hayden & Goodman 2005; Weinstein 2007).

Insertion

Implantation is a surgical procedure usually carried out under general anaesthetic. Some catheters are preattached to the reservoir whilst others require attachment on insertion (Hayden & Goodman 2005; Dougherty 2006). The catheter is introduced into the SVC via the subclavian, jugular or cephalic vein and fluoroscopy verifies the placement of the tip and the catheter is tunnelled to the pocket (Perucca 2001; Springhouse 2002; Dougherty 2006). The pocket is made just under the skin, usually on a bony area prominence for stabilization (Springhouse 2002). The port is then sutured into place to the underlying fascia. The suture line should be lateral, medial, superior or inferior to the port septum because repeated access could cause stress to the suture line (Dougherty 2006; Weinstein 2007). The area is tender and oedematous for up to a week following implantation and any manipulation/accessing may be painful. When immediate use is indicated the port should be accessed and dressed in theatre (Hayden & Goodman 2005).

Care and management in situ

When the port is accessed the needle can remain in situ for 7 days (Springhouse 2002; Dougherty 2006). Accessing should always be performed by specifically trained nurses owing to the risk of extravasation if the needle is incorrectly placed (Hayden & Goodman 2005). Patients can also be taught to access their own ports. The needle should be supported with gauze and covered with a transparent dressing to minimize the risk of needle dislodgement. Regular assessment of the port when accessed is essential to check for signs of erthyema, swelling or discomfort, which could indicate infection, infiltration or extravasation (Springhouse 2002; INS 2006). Most manufacturers recommend that only syringes 10 ml or larger should be used for drug administration or when flushing to prevent excessive pressure which could result in separation of the catheter from the reservoir or rupture if the catheter is occluded (Conn 1993). When not in use the port only requires flushing once a month with a concentrated solution of heparin (100 IU in 1 ml); usually a total of 5–6 ml (Perucca 2001; Springhouse 2002; Weinstein 2007).

Removal

Implanted ports may be surgically removed and after removal the site must be assessed for any signs of inflammation (Galloway & Bodenham 2004).

Discharging patients home with a VAD in situ

Patients may be discharged home with a VAD in situ which will allow them to receive treatment at home (e.g. continuous chemotherapy or intermittent antibiotics) or allow for easier access on each admission (e.g. via implantable ports). An early referral to the district nurse is crucial to ensure adequate support for the patient once at home (Dougherty 2006).

Patients may now receive daily treatment over a 3–5 day period with an indwelling peripheral cannula (Shotkin & Lombardo 1996). The degree of care is minimal compared with a CVC, but patients should receive adequate information about the early signs of phlebitis, i.e. pain, redness and swelling, and what to do in the case of accidental dislodgement or removal of the cannula.

Patients with long-term CVADs in situ such as PICCs or skin-tunnelled catheters will require instruction and supervision to ensure adequate understanding of the care and maintenance of their devices (Dougherty 2006). This must start early within the discharge planning process along with an assessment of the home environment, the patient's manual dexterity, physical and medical condition (Weinstein 2007; Kayley 2008). Patient education is one of the most important aspects of care, but to make teaching effective it is essential to recognize each patient's needs and limitations. It is also vital to acknowledge each patient's past experiences and readiness to learn (Cole 1999; Lonsway 2001). Education of the patient should encompass care and maintenance of the device as well as signs and symptoms of complications (RCN 2005; Kayley 2008). Educational packages should be prepared in the form of practical demonstrations and clear, succinct handouts (NICE 2003; INS 2006; Kayley 2008) (Figure 45.16). It is also important to recognize the need to prepare patients carefully to participate in their own self-care and therapy treatment. The patient, relative and/or friends should understand the following:

- The frequency of changing the dressing and how to care for the site.
- How to maintain patency.
- How to inspect for signs of infection or other complications.
- How to problem solve and where to seek help (RCN 2005).

Care of the site/dressing changes

The dressing of choice for PICC and skin-tunnelled insertion sites is one that is moisture permeable and transparent (NICE 2003; Pratt et al. 2007), which usually requires changing, following the initial change within first 24 hours, once a week (Ryder 2001; RCN 2005). This type of dressing may make it difficult for the patient to change the dressing themselves and so a carer or district nurse will need to be involved.

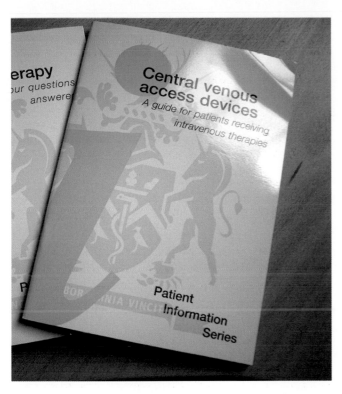

Figure 45.16 Patient information booklet on central venous access devices.

At the dressing change the site should be inspected and any signs of erythema or inflammation should be reported to the hospital at once in order for appropriate treatment to be prescribed (DH 2007). The area should be cleaned using an aseptic technique with a 2% chlorhexidine-based solution (NICE 2003; DH 2007; Pratt *et al.* 2007).

Maintaining patency and handling of equipment

If a patient wishes to be self-caring, the nurse should observe them carrying out the flushing procedure, either in hospital or in the home setting, until competent to do so without supervision of a nurse (Dougherty 2006; INS 2006). However, some patients prefer the district nurse to take responsibility for maintaining patency. Sufficient equipment must be supplied to enable the patient or nurse to care for the CVAD from the time of discharge until the patient's next admission. A kit should be assembled containing the following when a patient has a skin-tunnelled catheter or PICC in situ:

- Needleless injection caps.
- Ampoules of heparinized saline (50 IU heparin in 5 ml 0.9% sodium chloride).
- Chlorhexidine 0.5% in 70% alcohol or 70% isopropyl alcohol swabs.
- Sterile 10 ml syringes.
- 21 and 23 G needles.

- Instruction leaflet to provide both the community nurse and patient with a point of reference, e.g. your hospital patient information leaflet on central venous access devices.
- Sharps container.

Early recognition of complications

Patients should be taught what early signs and symptoms to look out for and who and when to contact. The most common complications associated with CVADs are infection and thrombosis (RCN 2005; Dougherty 2006; Kayley 2008). The patients should be told to report signs of redness and tracking at the exit site, along the skin tunnel or up the arm, any oozing at the exit site and fevers or rigors. Patients are no longer routinely prescribed prophylactic warfarin as this has been shown to have no apparent benefit in the prevention of thrombosis (Couban *et al.* 2005; Young *et al.* 2005). Therefore it should be stressed to the patient that any of the following signs or symptoms should be reported immediately: pain and/or swelling over the shoulder, across the chest and into the neck and arm. Early reporting may enable effective treatment and avoid removal of the device.

Problem solving and who and when to ask for help

Patients must be informed what to do if the catheter becomes occluded or damaged and given a contact name and number in order to be able to seek professional advice. This will help to alleviate any anxiety (Dougherty *et al.* 1998). Most problems can be managed at home with the involvement of the community nurses and general practitioner.

Quality-of-life issues: living with a VAD

Body image and a patient's lifestyle can be issues when living with a CVAD (Dougherty 2006). This is particularly true with an external catheter, which can be distressing and embarrassing for some patients (Hayden & Goodman 2005). It can result in restrictions to normal daily activities, e.g. bathing or involvement in sporting activities such as swimming (Gabriel 2000; Robbins *et al.* 2000); some of these can be resolved by the use of an implantable device (Chernecky 2001).

The following have been listed as ways in which a CVAD can affect body image:

- Physical presence and alteration of body appearance and invasion of body integrity.
- It influences the type of clothes that can be worn.
- It may interfere with bodily expressions of closeness and sexuality (Daniels 1995).

The presence of a CVAD could also have implications on how others view the role function of the individual, particularly if the patient is attached to an infusion pump (Thompson *et al.* 1989). The psychological impact of an indwelling catheter on body image should not be overlooked, especially when patients are sexually active (Gabriel 2000; Oakley *et al.* 2000).

Patients may be well-informed about access devices from the media or via the Internet. They may also have gained knowledge from friends or family experiences. Therefore, involving the patient in the decision-making process is vital (Dougherty 2006). Patient choice about the device or even the site of insertion, e.g. use of the non-dominant arm, results in better compliance with care of the device and monitoring of problems (Gabriel 2008). It also enables patients to cope better with the changes to their normal activities (Daniels 1995) and the impact on body image can be reduced by involving the individual in the choice and management of the device (Daniels 1995; Dougherty 2006).

Procedure guidelines Peripheral cannula insertion

Equipment

1 Sterile dressing pack.
2 Various gauge sizes of cannula.
3 Alcohol-based hand scrub.
4 Alcohol-based skin cleaning preparation, e.g. 2% chlorhexidine in 70% alcohol.
5 Extension set.
6 Needleless injection cap.
7 Non-sterile well-fitting gloves.
8 Hypoallergenic tape.
9 Bandage.
10 5 ml syringe.
11 21 G needle.
12 0.9% sodium chloride 5 ml.

Procedure

Action	Rationale
1 Explain and discuss the procedure with the patient.	To ensure that the patient understands the procedure and gives his/her valid consent (DH 2001: C).
2 If he/she requires topical local anaesthetic, then apply it to chosen venepuncture sites for 30–60 minutes prior to cannulation.	In order to give adequate time for local anaesthetic to be effective (BMA & RPS 2008: C).
3 Assemble all the equipment necessary for cannulation.	To ensure that time is not wasted and that the procedure goes smoothly without unnecessary interruptions (E).
4 Check all packaging before opening and preparing the equipment to be used.	To maintain asepsis throughout and check that no equipment is damaged or out of date (E).
5 Carefully wash hands using bactericidal soap and water or bactericidal alcohol handrub before commencement, and dry.	To minimize the risk of infection (DH 2007: C).
6 Check hands for any visibly broken skin, and cover with a waterproof dressing.	To minimize the risk of contamination of the nurse by the patient's blood (Pratt *et al.* 2007: C).
7 In both an inpatient and outpatient situation, the correct lighting, ventilation, privacy and position of the patient must be ascertained.	To ensure that the operator and patient are comfortable and that adequate light is available to illuminate the procedure (E).
8 Support the chosen limb on a pillow.	To ensure the patient's comfort and ease of access (P; E).
9 Apply the tourniquet to the chosen limb.	To dilate the veins by obstructing the venous return. If necessary, use other methods to encourage venous access (Dougherty 2008: E).
10 Assess and select the vein (see Action figure 10).	

11 Release the tourniquet.	To ensure that the patient does not feel discomfort while the device is selected and equipment prepared (Dougherty 2008: E).
12 Select the device based on the vein size.	To reduce damage or trauma to the vein. To reduce the risk of phlebitis (RCN 2005: C; Dougherty 2008: E).
13 Wash hands using bactericidal soap and water or bactericidal alcohol handrub.	To minimize risk of infection (DH 2007: C).
14 Open a pack, empty all equipment onto the pack and place a sterile dressing towel under the patient's arm (see Action figure 14).	To create a clean working area. (E)
15 Reapply the tourniquet.	To promote venous filling (Dougherty 2008: E).
16 Clean the patient's skin and the selected vein for at least 30 seconds using an appropriate preparation and allow to dry. Do not repalpate the vein or touch the skin (see Action figure 16).	To maintain asepsis and remove skin flora (RCN 2005; DH 2007: C; Dougherty 2008: E).
17 Put on gloves.	To prevent contamination of the nurse from any blood spill (DH 2007: C).
18 Remove needle guard and inspect the device for any faults (see Action figure 18).	To detect faulty equipment, e.g. bent or barbed needles. If these are present, do not use and report to company as faulty equipment (MHRA 2005; RCN 2005: C).
19 Anchor the vein by applying manual traction on the skin a few centimetres below the proposed site of insertion.	To immobilize the vein. To provide countertension, which will facilitate a smooth needle entry (Dougherty 2008: E).
20 Ensure the cannula is in the bevel-up position and place the device directly over the vein; insert the cannula through the skin at the selected angle according to the depth of the vein (see Action figure 20).	To ensure a successful, pain-free cannulation (Dougherty 2008: E).
21 Wait for the first flashback of blood in the flashback chamber of the stylet (see Action figure 21).	To indicate that the needle has entered the vein (Dougherty 2008: E).
22 Level the device by decreasing the angle between the cannula and the skin and advance the cannula slightly to ensure entry into the lumen of the vein.	To avoid advancing too far through the vein wall and causing damage to the vein wall. To stabilize the device (Dougherty 2008: E).
23 Withdraw the stylet slightly and a second flashback of blood will be seen along the shaft of the cannula (see Action figure 23).	To ensure that the cannula is still in a patent vein. This is called the hooded technique (Dougherty 2008: E).
24 Maintaining skin traction with the non-dominant hand, and using the dominant hand, slowly advance the cannula off the stylet and into the vein.	To ensure the vein remains immobilized and thus reducing the risk of a 'through puncture' (Dougherty 2008: E).
25 Release the tourniquet.	To decrease the pressure within the vein (E).
26 Apply digital pressure to the vein above the cannula tip and remove the stylet (see Action figure 26).	To prevent blood spillage (E).
27 Immediately dispose of the stylet into an appropriate sharps container (see Action figure 27).	To reduce the risk of accidental needlestick injury (NHS Employers 2007: C).

Procedure guidelines *(cont.)*

28 Attach an extension set, needleless injection cap or an administration set and flush the cannula with 0.9% sodium chloride (see Action figure 28).

To ascertain and maintain patency (Goode *et al*. 1991: R 1b).

29 Observe the site for signs of swelling or leakage and ask the patient if any discomfort or pain is felt.

To check that the device is positioned correctly (RCN 2005: C).

30 Tape the cannula using the method illustrated in Figure 45.5.

To ensure the device will remain stable and secure (Dougherty 2008: E).

31 Cover with low-linting swabs and bandage firmly.

To ensure patient comfort and security of device (P; E; Dougherty 1994 R 5).

32 Discard waste, making sure it is placed in appropriate containers.

To ensure safe disposal in the correct containers and avoid laceration or injury of other staff. To prevent reuse of equipment (NHS Employers 2007: C).

33 Document date and time of insertion; site and size of cannula in patient's notes or care plan.

To ensure adequate records and to enable continued care of device and patient (DH 2003: C; NMC 2005: C).

Action 10   Palpating a vein.

Action 14   Opening equipment.

Action 16   Cleaning the skin.

Action 18   Checking needle tip.

Action 20 and 21   Inserting the cannula. Wait for first flashback.

Action 23   Second flashback.

Action 26   Applying digital pressure and removing stylet.

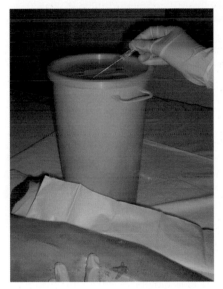

Action 27   Disposing of stylet into sharps bin.

Action 28   Flushing the cannula.

Procedure guidelines Midline catheter insertion

Equipment

1 Sterile minor operation pack.
2 Sterile powder-free gloves.
3 Alcohol-based hand scrub.
4 Alcohol-based skin cleaning preparation, e.g. 2% chlorhexidine in 70% alcohol.
5 Extension set and needleless injection cap.
6 Midline catheter.

7 Introducer.
8 Transparent dressing, securing device and sterile tapes.
9 10 ml syringes.
10 0.9% sodium chloride.
11 21 G needle.
12 Tape measure.

Procedure

Action	Rationale
1 Explain and discuss the procedure with the patient.	To ensure that the patient understands the procedure and gives his/her valid consent (DH 2001: C).
2 Apply tourniquet to the arm. Assess venous access in both arms and locate veins by sight and palpation.	To ensure the patient has adequate venous access and to select the vein for catheterization (RCN 2005:C).
3 Apply local anaesthetic cream/gel to chosen venepuncture site and leave for allotted time.	To minimize the pain of insertion (BMA & RPS 2008: C).
4 Draw screens and position patient in a comfortable position.	To ensure privacy. To aid insertion and correct placement (E).
5 Measure using the tape measure from the selected venepuncture site up the arm, to just below the axilla.	To enable selection of the most suitable catheter length and to know how far to advance the catheter in order for its tip to be located in the correct position (E).
6 Take equipment required to patient's bedside. Open outer pack.	
7 Wash hands using a bactericidal handrub.	To minimize the risk of infection (Pratt *et al.* 2007: C).
8 Put on powder-free sterile gloves; open sterile pack, arranging the contents as required. Prefill the syringe with 0.9% sodium chloride.	To prevent contamination. Powder on gloves can increase the risk of mechanical phlebitis (E).
9 Remove the cap from the extension set and attach 0.9% sodium chloride; gently flush with 2 ml and leave syringe attached.	To check that the catheter is patent and to enable easy removal of guidewire (E).
10 If the catheter tip can be trimmed, using the graduated markings along the catheter, select the marking required and pull back guidewire 1 cm from desired new tip, and using sterile scissors trim the catheter. *Never trim the guidewire!*	To ensure the catheter will be the correct length for placement and to prevent damage to the vein if the guidewire is damaged (E).
11 Place sterile towel under patient's arm.	To provide a sterile field to work on (E).
12 Clean the skin at the selected site with an appropriate disinfectant, e.g. chlorhexidine in 70% alcohol, using concentric circles with friction and prepare an area of 15–25 cm.	To ensure skin flora is destroyed and to minimize the risk of infection (RCN 2005: C).

882

13 Allow the solution to dry thoroughly.	To ensure coagulation of bacteria and completion of disinfection process (Pratt *et al.* 2007: C).
14 Drape the patient with a fenestrated towel.	To provide a sterile field (Pratt *et al.* 2007: C).
15 Inject local anaesthetic if required using a 25 G needle to area intradermally and wait for a few minutes for it to take effect.	To enable adequate anaesthesia (BMA & RPS 2008: C).
16 Reapply tourniquet.	To aid venous distension (Dougherty 2008: E).
17 Perform venepuncture with introducer by entering the skin, 1 cm from desired point of entry, at a 15–30° angle. Advance 0.5–1.0 cm once flashback is seen.	To gain venous access (Dougherty 2008: E).
18 Release tourniquet.	To prevent blood loss and 'through puncture' and enable advancement of catheter (Dougherty 2008: E).
19 Position fingers in a V, with index finger on wings and middle finger above sheath tip, and gently remove stylet. Apply pressure.	To contain flashback, prevent contamination of the area with blood and minimize the amount of blood loss from patient (Dougherty 2008: E).
20 Grip catheter 1 cm from the tip and thread through the introducer sheath.	To ensure tip is not contaminated (Dougherty 2008: E).
21 Continue slow advancement of the catheter to the desired length.	To minimize damage to intima of vein (Dougherty 2008: E).
22 Apply pressure above introducer and carefully withdraw the introducer and peel apart.	To ensure there is no movement of the catheter. To remove peel-away introducer (Dougherty 2008: E).
23 Aspirate for blood return and flush catheter with 0.9% sodium chloride.	To check patency of device and ensure continued patency (Dougherty 2008: E).
24 Apply gentle pressure on catheter and slowly withdraw the guidewire.	To ensure there is no withdrawal of catheter (Dougherty 2008: E).
25 Attach needleless injection cap and flush as per midline guidelines.	To ensure patency of the device (Dougherty 2008: E).
26 Secure the catheter with sterile tape or other securing device. Apply a transparent dressing. Apply gauze and a bandage.	To ensure stability of device and protection of the site (Dougherty 2008: E).
27 Dispose of equipment appropriately. Dispose of sharps and clinical waste.	To prevent risk of sharps injurys (NHS Employers 2007: C).
28 Document the procedure in the patient's notes: type, length and gauge of catheter, where it was inserted, any problem, how it was secured.	To ensure adequate records and enable continued care of device and patient (NMC 2005: C).

Procedure guidelines   Peripherally inserted central catheter (PICC) insertion and removal

Equipment

1 Sterile minor operations pack.
2 Two pairs of sterile powder-free gloves.
3 Alcohol-based hand scrub.
4 Alcohol-based skin cleaning preparation, e.g. 2% chlorhexidine in 70% alcohol.
5 Extension set and needleless injection cap.
6 Sterile low-linting gauze.
7 Peripherally inserted central catheter.
8 Introducer.
9 Transparent dressing, securing device and sterile tapes.
10 21 G needle.
11 10 ml syringes.
12 0.9% sodium chloride.
13 Tape measure.

Procedure

Action	Rationale
1 Gain consent from doctor and assess patient's medical and intravenous device history.	To ensure the patient has no underlying medical problems and is suitable to undergo the procedure (E).
2 Explain and discuss the procedure with the patient.	To ensure that the patient understands the procedure and gives his/her valid written consent (DH 2001: C).
3 Apply tourniquet and assess venous access, assessing both extremities, and locate veins by sight and palpation.	To ensure the patient has adequate venous access and to select the vein for catheterization (Gabriel 2008: E).
4 Apply local anaesthetic cream/gel to chosen venepuncture site and leave for allotted time.	To minimize the pain of insertion (BMA & RPS 2008: C).
5 Draw screens and position patient in a supine position, with patient's arm at a 45° angle, with ability to move arm to a 90° angle.	To ensure privacy. To aid insertion of introducer and then advancement of catheter (Gabriel 2008: E).
6 Measure using the tape measure from the selected venepuncture site diagonally across to the middle of the clavicle, then measure total distance of clavicle. Added together, these will give catheter measurement (see Action figure 6) or use the formula (see Box 45.2).	To enable selection of the most suitable catheter length and to establish how far to advance the catheter in order for its tip to be located in the correct position, i.e. the SVC (Lum 1999: E; Lum 2004: R 5).
7 Take equipment required to patient's bedside. Open outer pack.	To ensure appropriate equipment is available for procedure (E).
8 Wash hands using a bactericidal handrub.	To minimize the risk of infection (Pratt *et al.* 2007: C).
9 Put on sterile gown and powder-free sterile gloves; open sterile tray, arranging the contents as required. Prefill the syringe with 0.9% sodium chloride.	To prevent contamination. Powder on gloves can increase the risk of mechanical phlebitis (Elliott 1993; Pratt *et al.* 2007: C).
10 Remove the cap from the extension set and attach 0.9% sodium chloride; gently flush with 2 ml and leave syringe attached.	To check that the catheter is patent and to enable easy removal of guidewire (Manufacturer's guidelines: C).
11 If the catheter tip can be trimmed, using the graduated markings along the catheter, select the marking required and pull back guidewire 1 cm from desired new tip, and using sterile scissors trim the catheter. *Never trim the guidewire!*	To ensure the catheter will be the correct length for SVC tip placement and to prevent damage to the vein if the guidewire is damaged (Manufacturer's guidelines: C).
12 Place sterile towel under patient's arm.	To provide a sterile field to work on (E).

13 Clean the skin at the selected site with an appropriate disinfectant, e.g. 2% chlorhexidine in 70% alcohol, with friction and prepare an area of 15–25 cm.

To ensure the removal of skin flora and to minimize the risk of infection (Pratt *et al.* 2007: C).

14 Allow the solution to dry thoroughly.

To ensure coagulation of bacteria and disinfection (Pratt *et al.* 2007: C).

15 Drape the patient with a fenestrated towel.

To provide a sterile field (Pratt *et al.* 2007: C).

16 Inject local anaesthetic if required using a 25 G needle to area intradermally and wait a few minutes for it to take effect.

To enable adequate anaesthesia (BMA & RPS 2008: C).

17 Reapply tourniquet.

To aid venous distension (Dougherty 2008: E).

18 Remove gloves and discard. Put on a new pair of sterile gloves.

To minimize risk of contamination of venepuncture site or catheter (Pratt *et al.* 2007: C).

19 Perform venepuncture with introducer by entering the skin, 1 cm from desired point of entry, at a 15–30° angle. Advance 0.5–1.0 cm once flashback is seen.

To gain venous access (Gabriel 2008: E).

20 Release tourniquet.

To prevent blood loss and 'through puncture' and enable advancement of catheter (Gabriel 2008: E).

21 Position fingers in a V, with index finger on wings and middle finger above sheath tip, and gently remove stylet. Apply pressure.

To contain flashback, prevent contamination of the area with blood and minimize the amount of blood loss from the patient (Gabriel 2008: E).

22 Grip catheter 1 cm from the tip and thread through introducer sheath.

23 Advance the catheter 10–15 cm.

To ensure the catheter is securely within the vein before moving the patient's arm (Gabriel 2008: E).

24 Ask the patient (assisted) to move the arm to a 90° angle if necessary.

To enable further advancement of catheter (Gabriel 2008: E).

25 Turn patient's head towards the arm of insertion and place the chin on the clavicle if possible.

To prevent the catheter entering the jugular vein and to ensure correct advancement of catheter downwards to the SVC (Gabriel 2008: E).

26 Continue slow advancement of the catheter to the desired length.

To minimize damage to intima of vein (Gabriel 2008: E).

27 Apply pressure above introducer and carefully withdraw the introducer and peel apart.

To ensure there is no movement of the catheter. To remove peel-away introducer (Gabriel 2008: E).

28 Aspirate for blood return and flush catheter with 0.9% sodium chloride.

To check patency of device and ensure continued patency (Pratt *et al.* 2007: C; Gabriel 2008: E).

29 Apply gentle pressure on catheter and slowly withdraw the guidewire.

To ensure there is no withdrawal of catheter (Gabriel 2008: E).

30 Attach a needleless injection cap and flush as per local policy.

To ensure patency of the device (Pratt *et al.* 2007: C; Gabriel 2008: E).

31 Secure the catheter with a securing device such as Statlock. Apply a small pad of low-linting gauze directly over the insertion site and secure with sterile tape.

To ensure stability of device and to minimize blood leakage at the site which occurs following insertion (Moureau & Lannucci 2003; RCN 2005: C; Gabriel 2008: E).

Procedure guidelines *(cont.)*

32 Apply a transparent dressing. Apply low-linting gauze under the extension set and cap, then bandage.	To ensure protection of the site. To prevent the tubing pressing into the patient's skin (RCN 2005: C; Gabriel 2008: E).
33 Dispose of equipment appropriately. Dispose of sharps and clinical waste.	To prevent sharps injury (NHS Employers 2007: C).
34 Send patient for chest X-ray. Position of catheter to be assessed and documented by the doctor.	To allow position of tip to be assessed. To ensure correct tip location (Wise *et al.* 2001: E).
35 Document the procedure in the patient's notes: type, length and gauge of cannula, where it was inserted, tip confirmation, any problem, how it was secured and patient education.	To ensure adequate records and enable continued care of device and patient (NMC 2005: C).

Removal of PICC

Action	Rationale
1 Wash hands using a bactericidal handrub and gather equipment required (dressing pack, dressing, tape).	To minimize the risk of infection (DH 2007: C).
2 Remove transparent dressing and gently remove securing devices and/or sterile tapes.	To prepare for catheter removal (E).
3 Apply a pair of gloves and, using a steady and constant motion, gently pull catheter until completely removed from exit site.	To remove the catheter and prevent vein damage (E).
4 Apply digital pressure over exit site for about 2–3 minutes or until bleeding stops, and apply dressing.	To minimize blood loss and bruising. To provide protection of the entry site (E).
5 Check marking of length removed and check it is same as the length inserted. Document in care plan.	To ensure that complete catheter has been removed (RCN 2005: C).
6 If the catheter is removed because of infection, carefully cut off the tip (approximately 5 cm) of the catheter using sterile scissors and place it in a sterile container for microbiological investigation.	To detect any infection related to the catheter and thus provide necessary treatment (DH 2007: C).

Right-sided placement

Measure total distance to end of clavicle and add measurement from intended entry site of PICC to midclavicle

Left-sided placement

Measure total distance of clavicle and manubrium and add to measurement from intended entry site of PICC to midclavicle

Action 6 Preinsertion measurement of a peripherally inserted central catheter (PICC).

Procedure guidelines   Central venous catheter insertion site dressing change

Equipment

1 Sterile dressing pack (contains gloves).
2 Alcohol-based handrub.
3 Alcohol-based skin cleaning preparation, e.g. 2% chlorhexidine in 70% alcohol.
4 Semi-permeable transparent dressing or other appropriate dressing.

5 Hypoallergenic tape.
6 Bacteriological swab.
7 Pair of non-sterile gloves.

Procedure

Action	Rationale
1 Explain and discuss the procedure with the patient.	To ensure that the patient understands the procedure and gives his/her valid consent (DH 2001: C).
2 Perform the dressing using an aseptic technique.	To prevent infection (DH 2007: C). (For further information on asepsis, see Chapter 5.)
3 Screen the bed. Assist the patient into a supine position, if possible.	To allow dust and airborne organisms to settle before the insertion site and the sterile field are exposed (E).
4 Wash hands with bactericidal soap and water or bactericidal alcohol handrub. Place all equipment required for the dressing on the bottom shelf of a clean dressing trolley.	To reduce the risk of cross-infection (DH 2007: C).
5 Take the trolley to the patient's bedside, disturbing the screens as little as possible.	To minimize airborne contamination (DH 2007: C).
6 Open the sterile dressing pack.	
7 Attach a yellow clinical waste bag to the side of the trolley below the level of the top shelf.	So that contaminated material is below the level of the sterile field (DH 2007: C).
8 Open the other sterile packs, tipping their contents gently onto the centre of the sterile field. Pour lotions into gallipots or an indented plastic tray.	To reduce risk of contamination of contents (E).
9 Wash hands with bactericidal alcohol handrub.	Hands may have become contaminated by handling the outer packs, etc. (DH 2007: C).
10 Loosen the old dressing gently.	So that the dressing can be lifted off easily (E).
11 Put on clean gloves.	To protect the nurse from any contact with the patient's blood (E).
12 Using gloved hands, remove the old dressing and discard it.	To remove old dressing without contaminating hands (DH 2007: C).
13 If the site is red or discharging, take a swab for bacteriological investigation.	For identification of pathogens. To select appropriate treatment (DH 2007: C).
14 Remove gloves and put on sterile gloves from pack.	To minimize the risk of introducing infection (DH 2007: C).

887

Procedure guidelines *(cont.)*

15 Clean the wound with 2% chlorhexidine in 70% alcohol, with friction. Allow area to dry prior to applying the dressing.	To minimize the risk of infection spread from a 'dirty' to a 'clean' area. To enable disinfection process to be completed. To prevent skin reaction in response to the application of a transparent dressing to moist skin (Pratt *et al.* 2007: C).
16 Apply appropriate dressing, moulding it into place so that there are no folds or creases.	To minimize skin irritation and reduce risk of dressing peeling or becoming damaged (E).
17 Remove gloves.	
18 Fold up the sterile field, place it in the yellow clinical waste bag and seal it before moving the trolley. Draw back the curtains. Dispose of waste in appropriate containers.	To prevent environmental contamination (DH 2007: C).
19 Document date and time of dressing and any relevant changes.	To ensure adequate records and to enable continued care of device and patient (NMC 2005: C).

Procedure guidelines   Central venous access device: maintaining patency

This is a simple procedure which may be performed after each use or once weekly when no therapy is necessary. For implanted ports the procedure requires the port to be accessed and flushed once a month (see Procedure guidelines: Implantable ports: insertion and removal of non-coring needles, below).

Equipment

1 Flushing solution ready prepared in a 10 ml syringe in a clinically clean container.

2 Chlorhexidine in 70% alcohol/swab saturated with 70% isopropyl alcohol.

Procedure

Action	Rationale
1 Explain and discuss the procedure with the patient.	To ensure that the patient understands the procedure and gives his/her valid consent (DH 2001: C).
2 Wash hands thoroughly or use an alcohol-based handrub.	To reduce the risk of contamination (DH 2007: C).
3 Clean the needleless injection cap using chlorhexidine in 70% alcohol/swab saturated with 70% isopropyl alcohol and apply with friction, rubbing the cap in a clockwise and anticlockwise manner at least five times.	To minimize the risk of contamination at the connections (Pratt *et al.* 2007: C).
4 Attach the syringe to the needleless injection cap.	To establish connection between cap and syringe (E).
5 Using a push–pause method, inject the contents of the syringe (inject 1 ml at a time).	To create turbulence in order to flush the catheter thoroughly (Goodwin & Carlson 1993: E).
6 Maintain pressure on the plunger as the syringe is disconnected from the cap then clamp catheter if necessary.	To maintain positive pressure and prevent back-flow of blood into the catheter, and possible clot formation (Dougherty 2006: E).
7 Dispose of equipment safely.	To prevent contamination of others (DH 2007: C).
8 Demonstrate the procedure clearly and methodically. If the patient is to undertake the procedure, ensure patient receives written instructions.	To ensure the patient is aware of each step, and the need for good hand washing/drying techniques, etc., if he/she may be performing this procedure on discharge (P; E).

Procedure guidelines   Central venous access device: taking blood samples

Obtaining blood samples from a central venous access device can lead to inaccurate results, especially coagulation values, if the correct method is not followed to ensure removal of any drug/solution prior to sampling (Frey 2002).
A number of methods may be used to withdraw samples:

1 The discard method: this is the standard accepted method (recommended by The Royal Marsden Hospital) where the first 6–10 ml of blood is withdrawn and discarded (Cosca *et al.* 1998; Holmes 1998). This ensures removal of any heparin or saline solution but may result in excessive blood removal in small children or those requiring multiple samples, e.g. for pharmacokinetic tests (Cosca *et al.* 1998).

2 Push–pull/mixing method: a syringe is attached to the catheter, the catheter is flushed with 0.9% sodium chloride, then 6 ml is withdrawn and pushed back without removing the syringe; this is repeated three times. This removes any residual solution and reduces exposure to blood and there is no blood wastage (Holmes 1998).

This method supposes that mixing of blood eliminates intravenous fluids and heparin from the catheter lumen (Cosca *et al.* 1998). However, it may be difficult to obtain enough blood for 3–4 times push/pull and there is a chance for haemolysis with agitation of blood (Frey 2002).

3 Reinfusion method: this method is performed by taking the first 6 ml of blood, capping off the syringe, taking the samples and then reinfusing the blood first taken (Keller 1994). It does not result in depleted blood volume but there is a risk of blood exposure, the discard syringe could be confused with the specimen sample and there could be contamination or clots in the sample for reinfusion (Frey 2002).

Whichever method is used, once the samples have been taken it is vital that the catheter is adequately flushed with sodium chloride to reduce the risk of clot formation and subsequent infection and/or occlusion (Dougherty 2006).

It is preferable to use the proximal lumen of a multilumen catheter when obtaining a sample and where these catheters have different-sized lumens, the largest should be reserved for blood sampling (Dougherty 2006).

Equipment

1 Sterile dressing pack.
2 Alcohol-based hand wash solution.
3 Extra 10 ml blood bottle without heparin or sterile 10 ml syringe.
4 Vacuum system container holder (shell).
5 Vacuum system adaptor.
6 Appropriate vacuumed blood bottles (*or*)
7 Sterile syringe of appropriate size for sample required.
8 Needleless injection cap (as necessary).
9 10 ml syringe of 0.9% sodium chloride.
10 Flushing solution, as per policy.

Procedure

Action	Rationale
1 Explain and discuss the procedure with the patient. Check forms to ascertain sample bottles required and bottles are check patient's identity.	To ensure that the patient understands the procedure and gives his/her valid consent (DH 2001: C). To ensure correct used and blood is taken from correct patient.
2 Perform procedure using an aseptic technique.	To reduce the risk of infection (DH 2007: C). (For further information on asepsis see Chapter 5.)
3 Wash hands with bactericidal soap and water or bactericidal alcohol handrub.	To reduce the risk of cross-infection (DH 2007: C).
4 Prepare a tray or trolley and take it to the bedside. Clean hands as above. Open sterile pack and prepare equipment.	To reduce the risk of contamination of contents (DH 2007: C).
5 If intravenous fluid infusion is in progress, switch it off.	To prevent spillage of fluid following disconnection (E).
6 Where required, disconnect the administration set from the catheter and cover the end of the set with sterile cap.	To reduce the risk of contaminating the end of the administration set (E).

Procedure guidelines *(cont.)*

7 Clean hands with a bactericidal alcohol handrub. Put on non-sterile gloves. Clean hub thoroughly with chlorhexidine. Allow to dry.	To minimize the risk of introducing infection into the catheter, and prevent contamination of practitioner's hands with blood. To enable disinfection process to be completed (DH 2007: C).
8 For vacuum sampling (method of choice):	
(a) Attach vacuum container holder and adaptor via the needleless injection cap and release clamp.	To maintain a closed system and prevent contamination of practitioner or air entry (E).
(b) Attach extra sample bottle: fill and discard.	To remove blood, heparin and intravenous fluids from the 'dead space' of the catheter. Samples from this 'dead space' are likely to cause inaccuracies in blood tests, because of the risk of contamination of the sample with heparin, sodium or dextrose, etc. (Cosca *et al.* 1998: R 5; Holmes 1998: R 4).
(c) Attach required sample bottles for requested specimens.	To obtain sample. It is not necessary to clamp the catheter when changing collection bottles, as the system is not open (C; E).
(d) Re-clamp catheter and detach vacuum container holder.	To prevent blood loss or air embolism (E).
9 For syringe sampling:	
(a) Attach a 10 ml syringe to the needleless injection cap. Release the clamp and withdraw 5–10 ml of blood.	To remove blood, heparin and intravenous fluids from the 'dead space' of the catheter. Samples from this 'dead space' are likely to cause inaccuracies in blood tests (Holmes 1998: R 4; Cosca *et al.* 1998: R 5).
(b) Clamp and remove syringe and discard.	To discard contaminated sample and prevent mixing (Cosca *et al.* 1998: R 5; Holmes 1998: R 4).
(c) Attach a new syringe of appropriate size. Unclamp and withdraw the required amount of blood.	To obtain the sample (E).
(d) Clamp and detach the syringe.	
(e) Decant blood into sample bottles.	
10 Flush with 10 ml 0.9% sodium chloride, using the push–pause method (i.e. 1 ml at a time).	To create turbulence, ensure removal of all blood in the catheter and prevent occlusion (INS 2006: C).
11 Reconnect the administration set, unclamp the catheter and recommence infusion or attach new needleless injection cap. Release clamp and flush catheter through injection cap using the push–pause method and finishing with the positive pressure technique.	To prevent the catheter clotting between use (Moureau 1999: E; Dougherty 2006: E).
12 Ensure that blood samples have been placed in the correct containers and agitated as necessary to prevent clotting. Label them with patient's name, number, date of birth, etc., and send them to the laboratory with the appropriate forms.	To make certain that the specimens, correctly presented and identified, are delivered to the laboratory, enabling the requested tests to be performed and the results returned to the correct patient's records (RCN 2005: C).

Difficulty may be encountered when taking blood samples. This is more common when the central venous catheter is made of silicone and has been in place for a long period of time. One of the causes is that the tip of the soft catheter lies against the wall of the vessel and the suction required to draw blood brings this into close contact, leading to temporary occlusion. There could also be a collapse of the catheter walls when using the vacuum system which may necessitate the use of syringes to obtain the blood.

Measures to try to dislodge the tip include asking the patient to:

1 Cough and breathe deeply.
2 Roll from side to side.
3 Raise his/her arms.
4 Perform the Valsalva manoeuvre, if possible.
5 Increase general activity, e.g. walk up and down stairs.

Pinch-off syndrome occurs when a central venous catheter inserted via the percutaneous subclavian site is compressed by the clavicle and first rib and aspirating blood becomes difficult (Andris & Krzywda 1997; Verhage & van Bommel 1999). The tip of the catheter may be covered in a fibrin sheath. This may be resolved with rapid flushing of the catheter with 0.9% sodium chloride or a dilute solution of heparin. Occasionally this results in persistent withdrawal occlusion (PWO) and may require a fibrinolytic agent (Ponec *et al.* 2001; Dietcher *et al.* 2002) to remove the fibrin (Mayo 1998). However, it may be necessary to take blood from a peripheral vein (see Chapter 46).

Procedure guidelines Central venous access device: unblocking an occlusion

Catheters may become occluded for a number of reasons, e.g. not being flushed adequately or using the incorrect flushing technique, infusion being switched off or running too slowly or precipitation formation due to inadequate flushing between solutions/drugs. Clearance of a catheter occlusion is best performed using a negative pressure approach. The establishment of negative pressure within a catheter means creating a vacuum by aspiration of the air or dead space within a catheter (Moureau *et al.* 1999; Dougherty 2006; Gabriel 2008). Unblocking a catheter is not a quick procedure and can take up to 30 minutes to achieve success.

Equipment

1 Sterile dressing pack.
2 Bactericidal handrub.
3 Alcohol-based skin cleaning preparation, e.g. chlorhexidine in 70% alcohol.
4 Extension set or needleless injection cap.
5 10 ml syringes.
6 0.9% sodium chloride.
7 Three-way tap.
8 Heparin 50 IU in a saline solution.

Procedure

Action	Rationale
1 Explain and discuss the procedure with the patient.	To ensure that the patient understands the procedure and gives his/her valid consent (DH 2001: C).
2 Perform the procedure using an aseptic technique.	To minimize the risk of infection (DH 2007: C). (For further information on asepsis see Chapter 5.)
3 Wash hands with bactericidal soap and water or bactericidal alcohol handrub. Place all equipment required on bottom shelf.	To minimize the risk of cross-infection (DH 2007: C).
4 Open a sterile pack and empty other equipment onto it.	To create a clean working area (DH 2007: C).
5 Wash hands with bactericidal alcohol handrub.	Hands may have become contaminated by handling the outer packs, etc. (DH 2007: C).
6 Clean connections thoroughly with chlorhexidine in 70% alcohol before disconnection.	To minimize infection risk at connection site (DH 2007: C).

891

Procedure guidelines *(cont.)*

7 Remove any extension sets or injection caps.	Occlusion may be in extension set/cap and not in catheter (E).
8 Attempt to flush with 0.9% sodium chloride using a 10 ml syringe.	Smaller syringes create excessive pressure which could result in catheter rupture (Conn 1993: E).
9 If there is pressure within the catheter lumen, attempt to gently instil the 0.9% sodium chloride using a 'to and fro' motion (push–pull) over a few minutes.	To attempt to clear the catheter (Gabriel 2008: E).
10 If nothing can be aspirated, attach a three-way tap and to this add an empty 10 ml syringe and a 10 ml syringe containing heparin 50 IU in 5 ml saline.	To commence the negative pressure technique (see Action figure 10) (Gabriel 2008: E).
11 Attempt to unblock catheter using the negative pressure technique (see Action figure 11a, b).	This enables the solution to be drawn into catheter without creating any pressure which could result in catheter rupture (Gabriel 2008: E).
12 If still unable to aspirate, then determine the cause of the occlusion: (a) Blood: discuss with doctors who may prescribe a fibrinolytic agent, e.g. urokinase (5000 IU/ml), alteplase. (b) Precipitation: discuss with pharmacy for best antidote, e.g. ethyl alcohol or hydrochloric acid.	To break down fibrin (RCN 2005: C; BMA & RPS 2008). To break down drug precipitate or fat emulsion (BMA & RPS 2008: C).
13 Draw up prescribed solution in a 10 ml syringe.	To prepare appropriate treatment (E).
14 Put on clean gloves.	To minimize the risk of introducing infection (DH 2007: C).
15 Instil via a three-way tap using negative pressure technique (see above).	To prevent catheter rupture (Conn 1993: E).
16 Cap off catheter and leave for allotted time, e.g. 2–4 hours or overnight.	To allow the drug to destroy fibrin (Gabriel 2008: E; BMA & RPS 2008: C).
17 Attach an empty syringe to catheter and attempt to aspirate any clots and solution.	To unblock catheter and ensure no clots are administered into the patient (Gabriel 2008: E).
18 If blood returns, withdraw at least 10 ml and discard.	To ensure no fibrinolytic agent or clots are flushed into the patient (Gabriel 2008: E).
19 Flush catheter with 10 ml 0.9% sodium chloride using a pulsatile flush and then flush with heparinized saline.	To ensure the catheter is flushed and patent (RCN 2005: C).
20 Dispose of waste.	To prevent contamination of others (DH 2007: C).

21 If still unable to aspirate, discuss the use of a second instillation of fibrinolytic agent. It may be necessary to remove the catheter if a single lumen or if multilumen, to refrain from using the occluded lumen.

To maintain some venous access for the patient. If occlusion cannot be removed the catheter is no longer patent. In multilumen catheters there may be another patent lumen for use (Gabriel 2008: E).

Action 10   Turn tap to close off prefilled syringe and open it to empty syringe.

(a)

(b)

Action 11   Unblocking an occluded catheter. (a) Aspirate on empty syringe, which creates a negative pressure. (b) Turn tap to close off empty syringe and open to prefilled syringe. The medication will automatically be aspirated into the catheter. Repeat as necessary. (Modified from BD First PICC Clinical Education Class Manual D11952B 5/98.)

Procedure guidelines   Implanted ports: insertion and removal of non-coring needles

Placement of a non-coring 'Huber' point needle into the implanted port should be performed by a nurse who has been specifically assessed as being competent to access ports. The needle may be connected to an extension set and a needle-free injection cap placed at the end of this. The needle and extension set can remain in position for 7 days but will then need to be changed.

Equipment

1 Plastic apron.
2 Sterile gloves.
3 Dressing pack.
4 10 ml syringes containing 0.9% sodium chloride ×2.
5 Non-coring (Huber point) needle with extension set.
6 2% Chlorhexidine in 70% alcohol.
7 Heparinized saline in 10 ml syringe.
8 Plaster.

Procedure

Action	Rationale
1 Explain and discuss the procedure with the patient.	To ensure the patient understands the procedure and gives his/her valid consent (DH 2001: C).
2 If required, apply topical local anaesthetic cream for 30–60 minutes.	To reduce the feeling of pain on insertion of the needle (E).
3 Place the patient in a comfortable position.	
4 Locate the port and identify the septum; assess the depth of the port and thickness of the skin.	In order to select correct length of needle (Dougherty 2006: E).
5 Check length and type of therapy.	In order to select correct gauge and configuration of needle (Camp Sorrell 2005: C; Dougherty 2006: E).
6 Wash hands using a bactericidal hand soap or rub.	To minimize the risk of contamination (DH 2007: C).
7 Put on sterile gloves.	To minimize the risk of contamination (DH 2007: C).
8 Flush port needle and extension set with 0.9% sodium chloride.	To check patency of needle and set (Dougherty 2006: E).
9 Clean the skin over the port with 2% chlorhexidine in 70% alcohol with friction. Allow to dry.	To minimize the risk of contamination and destroy skin flora (DH 2007: C). To ensure disinfection (DH 2007: C).
10 Holding the needle in the dominant hand, stabilize the port between the forefinger and index finger of the non-dominant hand (see Action figure 10).	To ensure the port is stabilized and will not move on insertion of the needle (Dougherty 2006: E).
11 Inform the patient you are about to insert the needle.	To prepare the patient for a pushing sensation (P; E).
12 Using a perpendicular angle, push the needle through the skin until the needle hits the back plate.	To ensure the needle is well inserted into the portal septum (E).
13 Draw back on the syringe and check for blood return.	To check the needle is correctly placed and the port is patent (Camp Sorrell 2005: C; Dougherty 2006: E).
14 Flush with 0.9% sodium chloride and observe the site for any swelling or pain.	To check for patency and correct positioning (Camp Sorrell 2005: C; Dougherty 2006: E).

15 Administer the drug as required.	To carry out instructions as per prescription (E).
16 Flush with 10 ml 0.9% sodium chloride.	To ensure all of the drug is administered (RCN 2005: C).
17 If the needle is to remain in situ, attach an injection cap and flush with heparinized saline using a pulsatile flush and ending with positive pressure.	To maintain patency (Camp Sorrell 2005: C; Dougherty 2006: E).
18 Secure the needle by placing gauze under the needle if necessary and cover with transparent dressing.	To ensure the needle is well supported and will not become dislodged (Camp Sorrell 2005: C; Dougherty 2006: E).
19 If needle is to be removed, then heparinize using 500 IU heparin in 5 ml 0.9% sodium chloride.	To maintain patency over a longer period of time, e.g. 1 month (Camp Sorrell 2005: C; Dougherty 2006: E).
20 Maintain pressure on the plunger as syringe is disconnected from injection cap.	To prevent back-flow of blood and possible clot formation (Camp Sorrell 2005: C; Dougherty 2006: E).
21 Press down on either side of the portal of the implanted port with two fingers.	To support the port while removing the needle (P; Camp Sorrell 2005: C; Dougherty 2006: E).
22 Withdraw the needle using steady traction Discard needle in appropriate sharps container.	To prevent trauma to the skin and the risk of needlestick injury (NHS Employers 2007: C).
23 No dressing is usually required, but a small plaster may be applied.	To prevent oozing at the site (E).
24 Document date of access, size and length of needle and number of attempts in patient's notes or care plan.	To ensure adequate records and to enable continued care of device and patient (NMC 2005: C).

(a)

(b)

Action 10   Flushing a port.

Procedure guidelines Central venous catheter (non-cuffed/tunnelled): removal

Equipment

As for Procedure guidelines: Central venous catheter insertion site dressing change (above) items 1–6, plus:

7 Sterile scissors.
8 Small sterile specimen container.
9 Stitch cutter.

10 Additional sterile low-linting gauze swab and sterile transparent dressing.

Procedure

Place patient flat in the Trendelenburg position, i.e. head slightly lower than feet (to prevent air entering vein on catheter removal) and then proceed as for Procedure guidelines: Central venous catheter insertion site dressing change (above), steps 1–13, then continue as follows:

Action	Rationale
14 Clean the insertion site.	To prevent contamination of the catheter on removal, and a false-positive culture result (DH 2007: C).
15 Discontinue the infusion, if in progress, and disconnect the infusion system from the catheter. Clamp the catheter.	To prevent entry of air or leakage of blood when the catheter is disconnected (E).
16 Put on clean gloves.	To minimize the risk of infection after handling unsterile parts of the system (DH 2007: C).
17 Cut and remove any skin suture securing the catheter.	To facilitate removal (E).
18 Ask the patient to perform the Valsalva manoeuvre.	To reduce the risk of air embolus (Drewett 2000: E).
19 Cover the insertion site with low-linting gauze.	Swabs are used to discourage the entry of organisms into the insertion site and to absorb any leakage of blood (E).
20 Hold the catheter with one hand near the point of insertion and pull firmly and gently. As the catheter begins to move, press firmly down on the site with the swabs. Maintain pressure on the swabs for about 5 minutes after the catheter has been removed.	Pressure is applied to prevent haemorrhage and to encourage resealing of the vein wall. It also prevents the entry of air into the vein (E). Continued pressure is necessary to allow time for the puncture in the vein to close (E).
21 If the catheter is removed because of infection, carefully cut off the tip (approximately 5 cm) of the catheter using sterile scissors and place it in a sterile container for microbiological investigation.	To detect any infection related to the catheter, and thus provide necessary treatment (DH 2007: C).
22 When bleeding has stopped (approximately 5 minutes), cover site with transparent dressing.	To detect any infection at exit site. To prevent air entering the vein via the site (Scales 2008: E).
23 Fold up the sterile field, place it in the yellow clinical waste bag and seal it before moving the trolley. Dispose of the equipment in the appropriate containers.	To reduce the risk of environmental contamination (DH 2007: C).
24 Make the patient comfortable.	To ensure patient comfort (E).
25 Document date and time of removal in patient's notes or care plan.	To ensure adequate records and to enable continued care of device and patient (NMC 2005: C).

896

Procedure guidelines   Central venous catheter (skin-tunnelled): surgical removal

Equipment

1 Plastic apron.
2 Sterile gloves.
3 Minor operations set.
4 10 ml Luer–Lok syringe.
5 25 G needle.
6 21 G needle.
7 10 ml plain lidocaine 1%.
8 10 × 10 cm low-linting gauze swabs × 5.
9 3/0 Mersilk suture on a curved needle.
10 2 cm hypoallergenic tape.
11 Chlorhexidine in 70% alcohol.
12 Steristrips (to be used if necessary).

Procedure

Action	Rationale
1 Check the patient's full blood count and clotting profile for that day.	To ensure that the patient is not at risk of bleeding or infection from this invasive procedure. The platelets should be above 100×10^9/litre, the white blood count >2 and the international normalized ratio (INR) <1.3 (Dougherty 2006: E).
2 Explain and discuss the procedure with the patient.	To ensure that the patient understands the procedure and gives his/her valid consent (DH 2001: C).
3 Screen the bed and ask patient to remove clothing down to the waist.	To ensure ease of access to the patient's chest (E).
4 Ask patient to lie as flat as possible with his/her arms by his/her sides.	To minimize the risk of bleeding from gravitational pressure and to dissuade the patient from touching the sterile field (Dougherty 2006: E).
5 Palpate and identify the position of the cuff in the patient. This can be done by gently pulling on the catheter and observing for skin pucker.	To locate the area for the incision (Galloway & Bodenham 2004: E).
6 If the cuff cannot easily be felt, measure 22 cm up from the bifurcation at the end of the catheter distal to the patient dependent on the type of catheter in situ (see Figure 45.12), then palpate again. If it still cannot be felt ask for assistance from a more experienced colleague.	To locate the probable site of the cuff. To guard against malplaced incisions (Dougherty 2006: E).
7 Open the outer bag of the minor operation pack. Put on plastic apron and wash hands, then dry hands on sterile towel provided in the pack.	To reduce risk of infection (DH 2007: C).
8 Accept and put on sterile gloves from assistant and assemble all necessary equipment on the sterile pack.	To maintain asepsis and to prepare for the procedure and maximize efficiency (DH 2007: C).
9 Advise the patient that you will explain each step of the procedure as you go along if the patient wishes.	This should take into account the patient's individual wish for information (E).
10 Clean the area directly over the cuff with swabs soaked in chlorhexidine in 70% alcohol. Use a circular motion working out from the centre directly over the cuff. Allow the area to dry.	To reduce the risk of infection. To enable disinfection process to be completed. To prevent stinging on insertion of the needle (Dougherty 2006: E).

Procedure guidelines *(cont.)*

11 Position the two sterile towels: one horizontally across the waist and the other longitudinally down the side of the patient between you and the patient.	To create a sterile field to operate within and therefore reduce the risk of infection (Dougherty 2006: E).
12 Inform the patient that you are about to administer the local anaesthetic and that this will cause a stinging sensation.	To prepare the patient. The first injection can be painful and causes a stinging sensation (BMA & RPS 2008: C; P).
13 With a 25 G needle, administer the first millilitre of local anaesthetic intradermally directly over the cuff site causing a raised bleb.	To commence the numbing of the area to be incised. To provide a raised area for the next injection and identification of the site (Macklin & Chernecky 2004: E).
14 Give a further 1–2 ml of local anaesthetic subcutaneously using the bleb as the area for the insertion of the needle, but directing the needle out and around the area of the cuff site area.	To reduce pain for the patient with repeated injections. To ensure all the incision area is numb (Macklin & Chernecky 2004: E).
15 Attach the 21 G needle and with the last remaining 4 ml of local anaesthetic give two deeper injections to either side of the cuff area.	To ensure anaesthesia at a deeper level during the blunt dissection around the cuff (Macklin & Chernecky 2004: E).
16 Test the area above the cuff for numbness and then make the incision over the cuff site. The incision should be longitudinal and about 2 cm in length. Ensure that the incision is through the epidermis and dermis.	To ensure that the patient will not experience any pain. To facilitate identification and removal of the cuff. To allow access to the cuff which is situated below the dermis. To reduce the risk of cutting through the cuff before the cuff has been identified (Dougherty 2006: E).
17 With one pair of the small artery forceps, commence blunt dissection of tissue from around the cuff. At intervals place your finger into the site and feel the cuff.	To free the cuff from the surrounding fibrous tissue. To assess the mobility of the cuff (Dougherty 2006: E).
18 Continue with blunt dissection around and under the cuff until it feels mobile.	To facilitate the loosening of the cuff (Dougherty 2006: E).
19 With one pair of artery forceps, clamp onto the cuff and lift it up out of the incision while looking down the incision to identify the catheter distal to the cuff.	To identify the catheter to allow the distal portion to be severed (Dougherty 2006: E).
20 Once the catheter is clearly visible, maintaining your grip on the cuff with the forceps, cut through the full thickness with the blade. Then pull the portion of the catheter distal to the cuff out through the exit site.	To remove the distal half of the catheter below the cuff (Dougherty 2006: E).
21 Still maintaining your grip on the cuff, gently dissect away the fibrous tissue from around the cuff and the first 5 mm of the catheter immediately above the catheter.	To free the cuff in readiness for removal of the proximal portion of the catheter (Dougherty 2006: E).
22 Once the cuff is free, still maintaining your grip on the cuff, gently and carefully peel away the thin straw-coloured tissue from the catheter with the blade, ensuring the blade is pulled away from the catheter.	To free the catheter from the anchoring fibrous bands to enable removal. To reduce the risk of accidental incision of the catheter (Dougherty 2006: E).
23 As the last strands of fibre are separated you should feel the catheter becoming free and you should be able to see the white material of the catheter.	To ensure that you have completely freed the catheter for removal (Dougherty 2006: E).

24 While holding a low-linting swab to the incision site, gently pull out the catheter and apply pressure.	To remove the catheter and be prepared to stop any bleeding (Dougherty 2006: E).
25 If the catheter is removed because of infection, carefully cut off the tip (approximately 5 cm) of the catheter using sterile scissors and place it in a sterile container for microbiological investigation.	To detect any infection related to the catheter and thus provide necessary treatment (DH 2007: C).
26 Close the incision with three sutures. Commence the first suture in the middle of the incision, the remaining sutures evenly on either side.	To close the incision efficiently. To ensure that the skin edges and insert are brought together in alignment (Dougherty 2006: E).
27 If there continues to be any bleeding, Steristrips can be applied across the incision over the sutures.	To minimize blood loss (Dougherty 2006: E).
28 Apply a small pressure dressing and cover with a transparent dressing.	To absorb any slight bleed and to maintain a clean site (Scales 2008: E).
29 Advise patient that there might be some oozing and to reapply a dry dressing after 24 hours and thereafter once a day until the sutures are removed. Advise the patient that the sutures should be removed in 7 days.	To ensure that the incision has fully closed and healed (Dougherty 2006: E).
30 Ask the patient to rest on the bed for the next 30–60 minutes, or longer if required; especially patients who are prone to bleeding.	To reduce the risk of bleeding as the patient sits or gets up (Dougherty 2006: E).
31 Liaise with the nursing team and document the removal and findings in the nursing and medical notes.	To ensure there is good communication between all teams and a written record of the procedure (NMC 2005: C).

Problem solving: Central venous access devices

Problem	Cause	Suggested action
Venous obstruction during advancement of midline or peripherally inserted central catheter (PICC).	Valves. Bifurcations. Scarring. Sclerosed veins. Venospasm. Patient position. Muscle spasm in neck.	Midline or PICC can be flushed as it is advanced. Rotate patient's arm and move further round to a right angle. Check patient has not had any surgery/fractures, etc., which could cause scarring. Ask patient to relax neck and wait for spasm to resolve. Open and close fist to change pressure within vein and open valves.
Malposition of PICC tip.	Incorrect measurement of patient. Abnormal anatomy. Incorrect positioning of patient.	With the patient sitting upright, inject 20–50 ml 0.9% sodium chloride rapidly. If advanced too far, the catheter may need to be retracted several centimetres. If curled in a knot, the radiologist should attempt to straighten or remove it. Insert guidewire and attempt to realign or remove and replace catheter. If jugular placement with consent of medical team, leave overnight and re-X-ray to see if tip has repositioned.

Problem solving (cont.)

Problem	Cause	Suggested action

Mast cell activation syndrome:
Major:
  Generalized urticaria.
  Angioedema.
  Bronchospasm.
  Hypotension.
  Syncope.
  Upper airway obstruction.
Minor:
  Abdominal pain.
  Nausea and vomiting.
  Diarrhoea.
  Flushing.
  Conjunctivitis.
  Rhinitis.
	Basophil mast cell system is activated by a non-antigen-dependent mechanism, 'trauma' of touch, vibrations, pressure, heat and cold.	Maintain airway, breathing and circulation; call for medical assistance.

Mechanical phlebitis (redness, warmth, inflammation, pain).	Traumatic insertion of catheter. Rapid advancement of catheter.	Apply heat to affected area as soon as phlebitis is observed. Rest and elevate the arm. Catheter may be used during this time, but the patient should be observed for improvement in symptoms. Continue heat until complete resolution (should be resolved within approximately 72 hours). If it does not resolve then catheter should be removed.
Dyspnoea, chest pain or cyanosis (may be slow in onset).	Hydrothorax, pneumothorax or haemothorax due to insertion technique.	Inform a doctor. Arrange for a chest X-ray. Assist with any immediate treatment and with chest drainage if necessary.
Change in pulse rate and rhythm after insertion of catheter.	Cardiac irritability.	Inform a doctor. May require withdrawal of catheter by a few centimetres.
Dyspnoea, chest pain, tachypnoea, disorientation, cyanosis, raised central venous pressure (CVP), coma, cardiac arrest.	Air embolism due to air entering circulation during the insertion procedure or via the catheter.	Monitor the patient. If signs or symptoms develop, clamp the catheter to prevent further air entry. Lay the patient on the left side in Trendelenburg position. Inform a doctor. Give oxygen or external cardiac compression in the event of cardiac arrest.
Change in pulse rate, rhythm, dyspnoea, cyanosis, cardiac arrest.	Ventricular rupture due to insertion.	Observe patient closely. Inform doctor immediately. Prepare to commence cardiac massage.
Tingling in fingers, shooting pain down arm, paralysis.	Injury to brachial plexus during insertion.	Inform a doctor. Treatment is based on symptoms experienced by patient. Physiotherapy may be necessary.
Oedema of the arm on the side of the catheter insertion, may be associated with pain or limb discoloration.	Thoracic duct injury at insertion, resulting in alterations in lymph flow.	Inform a doctor. Removal of the catheter is usually necessary.

Problem	Cause	Suggested action
Oedema/pain and tenderness of arm, neck and/or chest. Engorged peripheral veins or feelings of tightness.	Thrombosis in major vessel due to irritation/damage by foreign body (catheter).	Report to doctor. Ultrasound and/or venogram may be performed and anticoagulant therapy. May necessitate removal of catheter.
Pyrexia, tachycardia, rigors indicating systemic infection.	Infection.	Culture of the blood is required from the catheter and patient's peripheral blood. Take a swab of the insertion site, employing strict asepsis. Administer antimicrobials as prescribed. Observe the patient closely. Removal of the catheter is sometimes indicated.
Leakage of fluid onto the dressing.	Loose connection in the system. Cracking of catheter or hub.	Check and tighten connections. Report to the relevant nursing staff and/or doctors. Repair may be possible.
Catheter required for many functions, e.g. blood sampling and extra drug administration.	Limited routes of access available to satisfy the patient's requirements.	Consider multilumen catheter before insertion. Use simple regimens and methods of administration. Use extension sets and administration sets available for this purpose. May require additional peripheral access.
Fluid overload resulting in dyspnoea, oedema, raised pulse rate and blood pressure.	Infusion is too fast. Inaccurate fluid monitoring.	Revise the patient's fluid intake regimen. Use flow control devices. Keep accurate records of the patient's fluid balance and weight. Inform a doctor. Patient may require diuretics.
Potential pulmonary embolus due to catheter tip embolus. Symptoms include chest pain, cool clammy skin, haemoptysis, tachycardia, hypotension.	Occasionally occurs after the removal of the catheter especially when using traction method for removal of skin-tunnelled catheter.	Check catheter length where possible and check integrity of catheter on removal. Avoid using the traction method. Notify a doctor immediately if the patient develops any of the related symptoms.
Bleeding at the insertion site following removal of the catheter.	Opening in the vein wall. Low platelets, anticoagulant therapy.	Apply pressure over the site with sterile low-linting swabs, until bleeding has stopped. Patients prescribed warfarin or heparin will require a longer period of pressure to compensate for the prolonged clotting time. Apply sterile transparent dressing. If bleeding persists, the doctor must be informed.
Pyrexia of unknown origin.	Could be related to central venous access device (CVAD).	Do not remove catheter until site of infection confirmed (unless clinical condition dictates otherwise). Inform doctors. Carry out investigations such as 'blood cultures' (from catheter and peripheral vein), swab of entry site, full blood count, midstream urine, chest X-ray, swabs of areas that could be the source of infection, e.g. throat or wound swabs. If catheter removed, tip should be sent for bacteriological examination.

In addition, the problem solving list associated with intravenous management (see Chapter 11) may contain useful and relevant information.

Arterial cannulae

Definition

An arterial cannula is a cannula inserted and secured in a peripheral or central artery. When the cannula is electronically transduced arterial waveforms can be observed in conjunction with continuous blood pressure readings.

An arterial cannula is generally inserted into a peripheral artery, most commonly the radial or dorsalis pedis. It provides an invaluable tool in providing continuous monitoring of systemic blood pressure and facilitates frequent arterial blood gas (ABG) and laboratory sampling. Arterial cannulation is most commonly achieved and maintained in the critical care and theatre setting (Mignini *et al.* 2006).

Indications for arterial cannulation

- During and following major anaesthesia.
- Monitoring of acid base balance and respiratory status in (Adam & Osborne 2005):
  (a) Acute respiratory failure.
  (b) Mechanical ventilation, especially in response to alteration of support and oxygenation.
  (c) The period during and after cardio-respiratory arrest.
  (d) Severe sepsis.
  (e) Shock conditions.
  (f) Major trauma.
  (g) Acute poisoning.
  (h) Acute renal failure.
  (i) Severe diabetic ketoacidosis.
  (j) Critically ill patients.

In critical care, continuous arterial monitoring is invaluable in optimizing and evaluating treatments, particularly in patients receiving intravenous nitrates and inotropes where their effects on mean blood pressure (MBP) can be instantaneous, necessitating appropriate titration (Mignini *et al.* 2006). Arterial devices must be cared for, managed and interpreted by skilled personnel who are able to regularly assess areas distal to the cannula, identify accurate waveforms, distinguish artefact, troubleshoot complications and maintain safe practice. The hazard of disconnection, the necessary monitoring systems, the potential consequence of severe haemorrhage and risks associated with accidental intra-arterial drug administration limit its use out of specialized areas.

Reference material

Radial arterial cannulation

Cannulation of the radial artery is the most common placement of arterial cannulae (Mignini *et al.* 2006) and is performed in most acute care settings (Box 45.3). The hand

has a good collateral blood supply, as the radial artery is near the skin surface, it is readily accessible, easily secured, and the patient is disturbed less (Wallach 2004; Adam & Osborne 2005). However, radial cannulation is not without risk (Wallach 2004); there is an estimated 0.2% risk of serious complications associated with the procedure. In response to these risks, cannulation of the non-dominant hand should be attempted whenever possible (Wallach 2004). Ideally the cannula should not be positioned close to any intravenous cannula as this may compromise blood flow around the adjoining structures.

Box 45.1   Contraindications of radial arterial cannulation

- Previous upper extremity surgery (harvested for pedicled/free flaps)
- Previous axillary clearance
- Peripheral vascular disease
- Raynaud's disease
- Diabetes
- Collagen vascular disease
- Active upper extremity infection

The radial artery arises at the bifurcation of the brachial artery, most commonly distal to the antecubital fossa, and then transverses distally along the radial side of the forearm under the brachioradial muscle and the radial flexor muscle of the wrist (Wallach 2004). The radial artery gives off multiple fasciocutaneous perforators until it reaches the wrist where it forms the deep palmar arch. The radial artery contributes to the main artery of the thumb and index finger (Wallach 2004). The radial pulse can be easily palpated at the wrist where the radial artery contacts the distal end of the radius, and is covered by fascia and skin.

It is important prior to any cannulation that the circulation of the hand is assessed: temperature, capillary refill and the colour of the hand (RCN 2005). More than 97% of patients have adequate flow through collateral supply, which prevents ischaemia, should either the radial or ulner artery be interrupted (Durbin 2001). Although not fully reliable, the Allen test should be completed prior to radial arterial cannulation in order to establish whether there is adequate blood supply to the hand (Figure 45.17). This test consists of simultaneously compressing both the radial and ulner arteries for approximately 1 minute (Tegtmeyer *et al.* 2006). During this time the conscious patient rapidly opens and closes the hand to promote local exsanguination. Approximately 5 seconds after release of one of the arteries (usually the ulner), the extended hand should blush owing to capillary refilling. If blanching occurs, palmar arch circulation is inadequate and a radial cannula could lead to ischaemia of the hand (Pierce 1998). Evaluation by a Doppler probe may be carried out as a more reliable alternative (Adam & Osborne 2005).

(a)

(b)

Figure 45.1   The Allen test.

Dorsalis pedis cannulation

The dorsalis pedis route for arterial cannulation is, according to Martin *et al*. (1995), equally as risky as radial cannulation, more technically difficult but provides a safe and easy available alternative when radial arteries are not appropriate.

Blood pressure measured from the dorsalis pedis and radial artery typically have a higher systolic and lower diastolic than centrally measured blood pressure, although the mean blood pressure is identical and clinically interchangeable (Mignini *et al*. 2006); this is described as distal pulse amplification (Dorman *et al*. 1998).

Femoral artery cannulation

The femoral artery may be cannulated if it is not possible to cannulate a peripheral artery, particularly if the patient is haemodynamically compromised. The femoral artery is accessible and there is relative ease in palpating even a weak pulse (Adam & Osborne 2005). If a patient has a femoral catheter in place and is required to be positioned at a 45° angle there is an increased risk of catheter fracture (Ho *et al*. 2003). This is particularly serious as there is no collateral blood supply to the leg and lower limb, and as such may have long-term consequences for the patient (Box 45.4).

Box 45.2   Contraindications of femoral arterial cannulation

- Diabetes
- Peripheral vascular disease
- Collegan vascular disease
- Active lower limb infection

Complications

There are a number of complications that can occur as a result of arterial cannulation: see Box 45.5.

Box 45.3   Complications of arterial cannulation

- Vascular thrombosis
- Distal embolization (see Box 45.6 for treatment of distal embolization)
- Proximal embolization: digital ischaemia
- Local/systemic infection
- Vascular spasm
- Skin necrosis of catheter site due to accidental intra-arterial injection
- Hypovolaemia secondary to accidental disconnection
- Cannula fracture/breakage
- Pseudo-aneurysm formation
- Median nerve palsy (Ho *et al*. 2003)
- Damage to nearby structures

Hypovolaemia

Accidental disconnection of tubing from the cannula or from one of the connections within the system can result in severe haemorrhage and hypovolaemia. The flow from an 18 gauge cannula can result in blood loss of 250 ml per minute (Oh 2003). Unconscious or delirious patients and children are at particular risk. The risk can be minimized by clear labelling of the arterial cannula (Zideman & Morgan 1981), and arterial tubing and sets should be predominantly red in colour, and alarm settings on the monitor must be turned on and audible (Adam & Osborne 2005). The use of Luer–Lok connections, ensuring visibility of the cannula, appropriate nurse/patient ratios and adequate training and competency of nurses caring for patients with arterial cannulae, will also help reduce this complication.

Accidental intra-arterial injection of drugs

Accidental intra-arterial injection of drugs intended for administration through a central or peripheral venous device may cause distal ischaemia and necrosis, sometimes resulting in permanent damage (Teplitz 1990; Tinker & Zapol 1991; Marieb 2001). Careful labelling and appropriate training can minimize this risk.

Local damage to the artery

Local damage to the artery is the most common complication of arterial cannulation (Marieb 2001). Regular close inspection and assessment of the limb and areas distal to the cannula must be carried out as there is a risk of thrombosis and embolism. Signs and symptoms include pain, a change in temperature in the distal limb, mottling and blanching of the limb when the cannula is flushed. The medical team should be informed if any of the above are discovered (Adam & Osborne 2005). If a distal embolism is suspected, the

903

cannula may have to be removed and limb warming attempted in order to avoid permanent damage (Box 45.6). The risk of ischaemia distal to the cannula is increased when associated with low cardiac output, shock, sepsis and prolonged cannulation (Gamby & Bennett 1995; Oh 2003).

Box 45.4 Treatment of distal embolism

- Remove the cannula
- Arrange for Doppler imaging
- After consultation with consultant, heparinize (if no contraindications)
- Consider a peripheral vasodilator

Nursing considerations

The arterial device is attached to a transducer that enables the mechanical energy of the arterial pressure to be transformed into an electrical signal. This is displayed as a waveform by a haemodynamic monitoring system. An amplifier enhances the signal, which is converted into a digital display and oscilloscope trace (Hazinski 1992). Arterial device tubing should be stiff with low compliance as this prevents the loss of pressure signals through tube expansion, and it must not exceed 120 cm in length because this may alter pressure readings (Daily & Schroeder 1995).

The arterial waveform has three separate components that reflect the cardiac cycle (Ciano 2001):

1 The upstroke: the positive deflection occurs at the peak of systole.
2 The dicrotic notch occurs with aortic valve closure and reflects the beginning of diastole.
3 The lowest point of the waveform is end-diastole.

Pulsus paradoxus is a term used when the difference in peak systolic pressure is greater than 10 mmHg between inspiration and expiration. This accentuates the normal pattern and an exaggerated *swing in systolic pressure* is seen on the monitor. This is caused by:

- Pericardial disease, e.g. cardiac tamponade causing impeded ventricular filling.
- Exaggerated inspiration by the patient.

- Changes in intrathoracic pressure, caused by lung pathology, i.e. asthma.
- Hypovolaemia can also produce this respiratory *swing*, particularly when the patient has concurrent high airway pressures.

If the arterial device is inserted under emergency conditions and asepsis has been compromised the Communicable Diseases Centre (2002) recommends the cannula should be replaced within 24 hours. Colonization and infection of arterial devices are rare (Minnaganti 2000) and is usually related to duration of cannulation. Data suggests arterial cannulae may be associated with a substantially lower risk of local cannula-related infection when compared to short-term peripheral venous cannulae which have been left in situ for the equivalent length of time (RCN 2005). This reduced risk of colonization may be related to exposure to high vascular pressures and subsequent local turbulence experienced in arterial cannulae (Communicable Diseases Centre 2002). There is also no evidence suggesting any difference in infection rates between femoral or peripheral arterial cannulation (Communicable Diseases Centre 2002). However, regular observation of the arterial cannula insertion site is imperative: signs of inflammation may predispose patients to cannula-related infection. Cannulation for more than 4 days also increases this risk (Communicable Diseases Centre 2002).

Arterial punctures

It is worth noting that morbidity associated with arterial cannulation is less than that associated with five or more arterial punctures (Oh 2003). However, arterial punctures are important and useful in the initial and short-term assessment of acid base balance. Multiple puncture attempts will increase the risk of injury, not only due to the direct trauma but also associated with vasospasm (Lipsitz 2004). If the patient requires repetitive blood sampling it may be more appropriate to admit the patient into a more clinically suitable area where arterial cannulation is possible. This not only minimizes both the distress to the patient and time taken by skilled personnel in obtaining each sample, but reduces the risks associated with multiple punctures.

Ideally prior to obtaining any arterial blood gas sample the patient should be in a respiratory steady state for 15–20 minutes. The oxygen should not be titrated, and if ventilated, suction should not be attempted and ventilation parameters not adjusted (Weinstein 2007).

Procedure guidelines   Arterial puncture: radial artery

Equipment

1 Intravenous sterile dressing pack.
2 Gloves.
3 Hypoallergenic tape.

4 Chlorhexidine in 70% alcohol.
5 Arterial blood gas syringe.
6 18 G needle.

Procedure

Action	Rationale
1 Explain and discuss the procedure with the patient.	To ensure the patient understands the procedure and gives his/her valid consent (DH 2001: C). To minimize anxiety which may distort analysis or exacerbate symptoms (E).
2 Check the concentration of oxygen the patient is breathing and body temperature at time of sampling.	Inspired oxygen concentration and temperature parameters are required to interpret arterial blood gases accurately (Weinstein 2007: E).
3 Check the patient's current coagulation screen, platelet count, medical history and prescription chart for anti-coagulation therapy.	To identify possible risk of bleeding and haematoma formation post-procedure, and, where appropriate, to prevent puncture until coagulation is corrected (E).
4 Prepare trolley as described in Procedure guidelines: Aseptic technique in Chapter 5.	To reduce the risk of cross-infection (DH 2007: C).
5 Wash hands with bactericidal soap and water or bactericidal alcohol handrub.	To reduce the risk of cross-infection (DH 2007: C).
6 Perform the Allen test.	To confirm patency of ulnar artery circulation and assess collateral circulation to the hand in the event of radial artery damage, e.g. thrombosis (White 2003: E)
7 Locate and palpate the radial artery with the middle and index fingers of the non-dominant hand.	To assess maximum pulsation to ensure radial artery is optimum site for successful puncture. The dominant hand will be used to perform puncture (Weinstein 2007: E).
8 Inspect and assess the surrounding tissues and anatomical structures.	Check and assess surrounding tissues for excoriation/infection, poor perfusion or other puncture sites. If any of these are present the site should not be used (Weinstein 2007: E).
9 Prepare the patient position: gently extend the wrist over a rolled towel (ask for assistance if required).	To reduce the risk of the patient moving unexpectedly which could result in through puncture (Lipsitz 2004: R 5; Hudson 2006; E). To flex the hand/foot slightly to facilitate insertion (E).
10 Open the pack and equipment onto it. Withdraw the plunger of the syringe 1–2 ml before the puncture.	To reduce blood haemolysis. Arterial pressure causes a brisk pulsatile reflux of blood into the syringe (unless the patient is severely hypotensive) (Weinstein 2007: R 5).
11 Place a sterile field under the patient's wrist and maintain aseptic technique throughout the procedure.	To minimize the risk of infection (DH 2007: C).
12 Clean site with chlorhexidine in 70% alcohol.	To minimize the risk of infection (DH 2007: C).

Procedure guidelines (cont.)

13 Administer subcutaneous local anaesthetic.	To minimize pain during the procedure. Local vasodilation effects of the local anaesthetic may reduce vasospasm, making for a successful puncture (Lipsitz 2004: R 5).
14 Clean hands with bactericidal skin cleaning solution.	To minimize the risk of infection (DH 2007: C).
15 Apply sterile gloves.	To minimize the risk of infection and prevent contamination of hands with blood (Pratt *et al.* 2007: C).
16 Re-identify the point of maximum pulsation, hold position with index/middle finger.	To guide position of radial artery and aid successful puncture (E).
17 Angle the needle 30–45° angle, with the bevel of the needle up just distal to the finger position. Advance needle slowly into the artery until a flashing pulsation is seen in the hub of the needle.	To minimize trauma to the artery (E). Rapid insertion may result in a through puncture (White 2003: E). Pulsatile flow indicates access to radial artery (E). Arterial pressure causes blood to pulsate spontaneously back into the syringe (Weinstein 2007: E).
18 Slowly aspirate by gently pulling the plunger of the arterial gas syringe to a minimum of 0.6 ml of blood for the sample (check recommended amount of blood as directed by manufacturer's guidelines).	To minimize vasospasm (E). To ensure optimal volume is obtained in order to ensure an appropriate mix of blood with heparin (see manufacturer's guidelines: C).
19 Withdraw the needle, immediately followed by application of pressure using a low linting dressing. Promptly return the wrist to the neutral position following sampling.	To prevent haematoma formation and excessive bleeding (E). Prolonged hyperextension may be associated with changes in median nerve conduction (Chowet *et al.* 2004: R 4).
20 Apply pressure for a minimum of 5 minutes or until no signs of bleeding are observed. Ask for assistance from another nurse if necessary.	To minimize blood loss (Ciano 2001: R 5) and to ensure pressure exerted to prevent haematoma and blood loss (RCN 2005: C). Assistance with pressure application enables the sample to be analysed swiftly (Bucher 2001: E).
21 Dispose of equipment safely.	To prevent contamination of others (DH 2007: C).
22 Expel any air bubbles from the syringe, and cap the arterial syringe and label according to hospital policy.	To keep sample airtight and avoid inaccuracies (White 2003: E).
23 Check puncture site and apply a clean, sterile, low linting gauze dressing using a non-touch technique. Secure with tape.	To maintain pressure and prevent haematoma formation (E).
24 Clearly document rationale for procedure in patient's notes and verbally communicate arterial analysis findings to relevant medical and nursing teams.	To acknowledge accountability for actions and ensure effective comunication. To ensure prompt and appropriate treatment (NMC 2005: C; NMC 2008: C).

Procedure guidelines   Arterial cannula insertion: preparation and setting up of monitoring set

Equipment

1 500 ml pressure infuser cuff.
2 500 ml bag of 0.9% sodium chloride.
3 Designated arterial cannula.
4 Sterile intravenous pack.
5 Non sterile gloves.
6 Chlorhexidine in 70% alcohol.

7 Transparent dressing.
8 Syringes: various sizes.
9 A label to identify arterial device.
10 1% lidocaine injection.
11 Pressure monitoring system equipment.

Procedure

Action	Rationale
1 Explain the procedure with the patient.	To ensure the patient understands the procedure and gives valid consent wherever appropriate (DH 2001: C; NMC 2008: C). *Note*: many patients are anaesthetized when arterial devices are inserted.
2 Prepare infusion and transducer sets using aseptic technique.	Minimize risk of infection (DH 2007: C).
3 Check that all Luer–Lok connections are secure.	To prevent disconnection, as equipment is often loose when taken straight from package (E).
4 Connect transducer to bag of 500 ml 0.9% NaCl.	To prepare infusion, saline is more effective than heparinized flush (Kulkarni *et al*. 1994: R 3; Gamby & Bennett 1995: R 3; Communicable Diseases Centre 2002: C). To prime the administration set and three-way tap ports (E).
5 Open roller clamp fully, squeeze the flush device-actuator (see instructions with set).	To reduce the risk of air embolus, although retrograde air embolus is a rare event after routine radial artery cannula flushing (E).
6 Check thoroughly for air bubbles in the circuit.	To reduce the risk of inaccurate pressure readings caused by bubbles in the set (Daily & Schroeder 1995: R 4).
7 Insert bag into pressure infuser, inflate the pressure bag to 300 mmHg.	To prevent back pressure of blood into the transducer set by ensuring pressure is higher than arterial blood pressure (Hudak*et al*. 1998: R 5). An automatic flush mode is activated within the system which delivers 3 ml per hour, which maintains patency of cannula (Morven 1995: R 4).
8 Wash hands with bactericidal soap and water or bactericidal handrub.	To reduce the risk of cross-infection (DH 2007: C).
9 Prepare trolley near the patient as described in Chapter 4 Aseptic technique.	To reduce the risk of cross-infection (DH 2007: C).
10 Complete the Allen test if radial artery is used.	To assess whether palmar arch circulation is adequate, although not completely reliable (Wallach 2004: R 4).
11 Prepare the insertion site with chlorhexidine in 70% alcohol and place a sterile towel under the appropriate area.	To maintain asepsis. To provide a clean working area (DH 2007: C).

Procedure guidelines *(cont.)*

12 Administer adequate local anaesthetic.	To minimize pain during the procedure, this may reduce the sudden movement which could result in through puncture (Lipsitz, 2004: R). Local vasodilation effects of the local anaesthetic may reduce vasospasm, making a successful cannulation more likely (Lipsitz 2004: R 5).
13 The practitioner applies gloves (see Chapter 5).	To prevent contamination of hands if blood spillage occurs (Pratt *et al.* 2007: C).
14 The nurse may act as an assistant and holds the patient's foot or arm. If the radial artery is cannulated the wrist must be hyperextended.	To prevent movement and to flex the hand/foot slightly to facilitate insertion (E). Prolonged hyperextension may be associated with changes in median nerve conduction, promptly return the wrist to the neutral position following cannulation (Chowet *et al.* 2004: R 4).
15 The cannula is inserted by the practitioner, blood flash back is observed.	To ascertain the cannula is in the artery (E).
16 Attach transducer set and fully open roller clamp.	To commence flush infusion system, and prevent backflow of blood (E).
17 Apply transparent dressing over the cannula and tape tubing securely.	To leave the site visible and secure and to allow the observer to recognize immediately any dislodgement, inflammation or disconnection (E).
18 Clearly label the device as arterial.	To ensure the device is not mistaken for a venous cannula, preventing accidental intra-arterial injection of drugs (E).
19 Loop the tubing around the thumb, ensuring this is not too tight (see Action figure 19).	To minimize movement of cannula and damage to the vessel, to prevent ulcer formation (E).
20 Connect transducer to monitoring equipment.	Allows to check arterial waveform and obtain continuous blood pressure measurements (E).
21 Calibrate the arterial device.	The transducer will read an arterial pressure calibrated to atmospheric air which offsets the extraneous atmospheric and hydrostatic pressures (E).

Cannula in position
with criss-cross strapping

Arterial
label

Loop tube loosely
around thumb

Transparent dressing

Action 19   Positioning, securing and labelling of cannula.

Procedure guidelines   Arterial cannula: taking a blood sample

The following volumes of blood should be withdrawn and discarded in order to clear saline, old blood and small emboli from the dead space, the cannula and the three-way tap.

  Discarded volumes vary according to arterial cannula placement:

- Peripheral artery cannula: take 3 ml and discard.
- Femoral artery cannula: take 5 ml and discard.

When using a vacuum system, take one bottle and discard prior to obtaining formal samples.

Equipment

1 Intravenous sterile pack.
2 Gloves.
3 Appropriate syringes and blood sampling bottles.
4 Chlorhexidine in 70% alcohol.
5 Bactericidal alcohol handrub.

Procedure

Action	Rationale
1 Explain and discuss the procedure with the patient.	To ensure the patient understands the procedure and gives their valid consent (DH 2001: C).
2 Prepare the trolley.	To ensure all the equipment is ready (E).
3 Wash hands with bactericidal soap and water or bactericidal alcohol handrub.	To minimize the risk of cross-infection (DH 2007: C).
4 Check the three-way tap is closed to port (see Action figure 4).	To prevent back-flow of blood and blood spillage (E).
5 Clean hands with bactericidal alcohol handrub.	To prevent cross-infection (DH 2007: C).
6 Prepare trolley as in Procedure guidelines: Aseptic technique in Chapter 5.	Minimize the risk of cross-infection (DH 2007: C).
7 Press silence button on arterial monitor for duration of sampling.	The continual alarm disturbs both the patient and others in the unit. Alarms of no clinical significance should be minimized (Chambrin 2001: R 5).
8 Apply gloves (see Safe technique section and Procedure guidelines: Aseptic technique in Chapter 5).	To prevent contamination of hands with blood (DH 2007: C).
9 Remove cap from three-way tap and clean port with a swab soaked in chlorhexidine in 70% and allow to dry.	To minimize the risk of infection (DH 2007: C).
10 Turn three-way tap to artery and port (see Action figure 10).	To prevent contamination of blood with flush solution (E).
11 Slowly withdraw appropriate volume of blood.	To prevent the artery going into spasm (Lipsitz 2004: R 5).
12 Turn three-way tap diagonally to close off both the artery and flush (see Action figure 12).	To enable the syringe to be removed without blood loss, to prevent back flow from artery (E).
13 Remove syringe and discard.	To discard the contaminated sample (E).

909

Procedure guidelines *(cont.)*

14	Connect the blood gas syringe.	The gas syringe is open to the artery in order to withdraw the sample (E).
15	Turn three-way tap on to artery and port (see Action figure 10).	To open the syringe directly onto the artery (E).
16	Slowly remove the recommended amount of blood (as specified on manufacturer's instructions).	To prevent the artery going into spasm ensuring the correct volume of blood mixes with the recommended heparin in the gas syringe (Lipsitz 2004: R 5).
17	Turn three-way tap diagonally to close off both the artery and flush (see Action figure 17).	To prevent haemorrhage or blood spillage (E).
18	Remove the gas syringe, gently rotate syringe.	Send for analysis, and ensure the blood and heparin contained within the syringe are mixed (E).
19	Turn three-way tap onto flush and port, apply a sterile swab to the port flush squeezing the actuator (see manufacturer's instructions) (see Action figure 19).	The swab will absorb the blood, preventing contamination (E). Blood is cleared from the port, reducing risk of thrombosis and micro-emboli (Hazinski 1992: R 5).
20	Turn three-way tap onto flush and artery, flush cannula by gently squeezing actuator. As cannula is flushed observe digits for signs of blanching, discoloration, or complaints of pain from the patient.	Blood is cleared from the cannula and arterial tubing (E). To ensure early recognition of proximal or distal embolism (E).
21	Clean port with chlorhexidine in 70% alcohol swab.	To minimize the risk of infection (DH 2007: C).
22	Apply sterile Luer–Lok cap and check it is secure.	To minimize infection and prevent exsanguination (Hart 2008: E).
23	Check pressure infuser cuff is inflated to 300 mmHg.	To prevent back flow of blood into circuit (E).
24	Analyse or send to nearest blood gas analyser and document result.	To obtain result (E).

Action 4   Three-way tap: closed to port.

Action 10   Three-way tap: turned to artery and port.

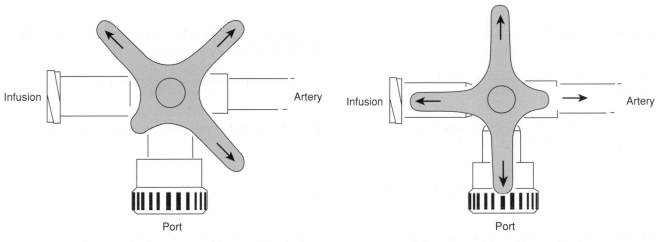

Action 17   Three-way tap: turned diagonally to close off infusion, artery and port.

Action 19   Three-way tap: turned to infusion and port.

Procedure guidelines   Arterial cannula: removal

Equipment

1 Sterile dressing pack.
2 Non sterile gloves.

3 Hypoallergenic tape.
4 Chlorhexidine in 70% alcohol.

Procedure

Action	Rationale
1 Explain and discuss the procedure with the patient.	To ensure the patient understands the procedure and gives his/her valid consent (DH 2001: C).
2 Check platelet and coagulation screen.	To prevent delay in removal whilst coagulation is corrected (E).
3 Prepare trolley as described in Procedure guidelines: Aseptic technique in Chapter 5.	To reduce the risk of cross-infection (DH 2007: C).
4 Wash hands with bactericidal soap and water or bactericidal alcohol handrub before leaving the clinical room.	To reduce the risk of cross-infection (DH 2007: C).
5 Prepare the trolley as described in Procedure guidelines: Aseptic technique in Chapter 5.	To reduce the risk of cross-infection (DH 2007: C).
6 Turn three-way tap diagonally.	To prevent back-flow of blood into cannula (E).
7 Turn off flush set.	To prevent spillage when removing cannula (E).
8 Deflate pressure cuff.	Pressure is no longer required (E).
9 Loosen transparent dressing and tape from the cannula site.	To facilitate removal of cannula (E).

Procedure guidelines *cont.*

10	Clean hands with bactericidal skin cleaning solution.	To minimize the risk of infection (DH 2007: C).
11	Apply gloves.	To prevent contamination of hands with blood (Pratt *et al.* 2007: C).
12	Remove dressing and tape. Clean cannula site area with chlorhexidine in 70% alcohol.	To reduce the risk of infection (DH 2007: C).
13	Place sterile piece of gauze over area and gently remove cannula.	To minimize bleeding and blood spillage (Pratt *et al.* 2007: C).
14	Apply pressure for a minimum of 5 minutes.	To prevent haematoma and blood loss (RCN 2005: C).
15	Apply a clean, sterile, low linting gauze dressing.	To maintain asepsis and minimize blood loss (Ciano 2001: R 5).
16	Secure with tape.	To ensure pressure and prevent haematoma or blood loss (E).

Following the procedure, check the patient's hand, assessing and documenting the temperature, colour, swelling and any signs of bleeding (Ciano 2001). Ask the patient to inform staff if there is any oozing from the dressing. Avoid blood pressure measurement being taken manually on the arm where the arterial cannula was removed for 12–24 hours to minimize bleeding or haematoma formation. Medical staff must be informed immediately if the hand or forearm becomes discoloured or swollen, or if the patient complains of pain in the limb. In the event of any complication careful documentation is essential; consider a request for medical photography to photograph area.

Problem solving: Arterial cannulation

Problem	Cause	Suggested preventive care
Haemorrhage. Severe haemorrhage (hypovolaemia).	Luer–Lok connections are loose or cracked. Blood will be lost from open connection. Blood may ooze around the cannula site.	Check that Luer–Loks are fitted securely. Do not force because the connections may crack.
	Accidental disconnection.	Use Luer–Lok devices, expose the site, educate staff.
	Cannula may have become dislodged.	Inform the patient about the danger of dislodging the cannula and amount of movement that is preferred. Take care when moving the patient. Avoid putting stress on the arm and connections. Secure the cannula (see Action figure 19 in Procedure guidelines: Arterial cannula insertion: preparation and setting up of monitoring set, above).
Back-flow of blood into the cannula.	The pressure infusor cuff may not be inflated to the optimal pressure.	Ensure that the pressure infusor cuff is inflated to 300 mmHg. This pressure is higher than arterial blood pressure and an automatic flush mode is activated in the system which delivers 3 ml per hour. This maintains patency of circuit, cannula and artery (Allan 1984).

Problem	Cause	Suggested preventive care
Ischaemia.	A thrombosis may have formed in the circuit cannula or artery.	Ensure that heparin is added to the saline infusion (Clifton *et al.* 1991). Assess limb pulse, colour and temperature hourly, or more frequently as required. Absent pulses, pallor, cyanosis and coldness denote occlusion. If this occurs, medical advice must be sought and the cannula removed promptly (Hinds 1987).
Erythema or inflammation around the insertion site.	Phlebitis due to sepsis, chemical irritation or mechanical irritation.	Refer to the Problem-solving list in Chapter 11.
Hypotension, tachycardia, cyanosis, unconsciousness.	Embolism: Air. Particle.	Refer to the Procedure guidelines in Chapter 11.
Arterial spasm.	Forceful flushing or forceful aspiration when withdrawing blood.	Avoid forceful flushing or aspiration and maintain a slow even pressure when withdrawing blood.
Necrosis.	Accidental injection of a drug into the artery, causing local necrosis to vessel wall.	Label the arterial cannula and circuit clearly (see Action figure 19 in Procedure guidelines: Arterial cannula insertion: preparation and setting up of monitoring set, above). In the event of accidental injection of any drug, report the error immediately to medical staff and the senior nurse and perform the following: (a) Gently withdraw blood from the three-way tap to try to withdraw the drug. (b) Stop administering the drug. (c) Assess limb pulse, colour and temperature hourly, or more frequently if required. (d) Complete an accident form and/or other relevant documentation.

References and further reading

Adam, S. & Osborne, S. (2005) *Critical Care Nursing: Science & Practice.* Oxford University Press, Oxford.

Allan, D. (1984) Care of the patient with an arterial catheter. *Nurs Times,* 80(46), 40–1.

Andris, D.A. & Krzywda, E.A. (1997) Catheter pinch off syndrome: recognition and management. *J Intraven Nurse,* 20(5), 233–7.

Archis, C.A., Black, J. & Brown, M.A. (2000) Does an endoluminal catheter brush improve flows or unblock haemodialysis catheters? *Nephrology,* 5, 55–8.

Bagnell Reeb, H. (1998) Diagnosis of central venous access device occlusions: implications for nursing practice. *J Intraven Nurse,* 21(Suppl 5), S115–21.

Bahruth, A.J. (1996) PICC insertion problems associated with topical anesthesia. *J Intraven Nurse,* 19(1), 32–4.

Banton, J. & Leahy Cross, K. (1998) Assessing catheter performance – 4 years of tracking patient outcomes of midline, midclavicular and PICC line program. *J Vasc Access Device,* 3(3), 19–25.

Baranowski, L. (1993) Central venous access devices – current technologies, uses and management strategies. *J Intraven Nurse,* 16(3), 167–94.

Barker, P., Anderson, A.D.G. & MacFie, J. (2004) Randomised clinical trial of elective re-siting intravenous cannulae. *Ann R Coll Surg Engl,* 86, 281–93.

Bassetti, S. *et al.* (2001) Prolonged antimicrobial activity of a catheter containing chlorhexidine silver sulfadiazine extends protection against catheter infection in vivo. *Antimicrob Agents Chemother,* 45, 1535–8.

Benton, S. & Marsden, C. (2002) Training nurses to place tunnelled central venous catheters. *Prof Nurse,* 17(9), 531–5.

Berger, L. (2000) The effects of positive pressure devices on catheter occlusions. *J Vasc Access Devices,* 5(4), 31–3.

Biffi, R. *et al.* (2001) A randomised prospective trial of central venous ports connected to standard open ended or groshong catheters in adult oncology patients. *Cancer,* 92(5), 1204–12.

Bjeletich, J. & Hickman, R.O. (1980) The Hickman indwelling catheter. *Am J Nurs,* 80(1), 62–5.

BMA & RPS (2008) *British National Formulary.* British Medical Association & Royal Pharmaceutical Society, London.

Boland, A. *et al.* (2003) A randomised controlled trial to evaluate the clinical and cost effectiveness of Hickman line insertion in adult cancer patients by nurses. *Health Technology Assessment,* 7, 36.

Bow, E.J., Kirkpatrick, M.G. & Clinch, J.J. (1999) Totally implantable venous access ports systems for patients receiving chemotherapy for solid tissue malignancies. *J Clin Oncol,* 17(4), 1267.

Bregenzer, T. (1998) Is routine replacement necessary? *Arch Intern Med,* 158, 151–6.

Brown, J. & Larson, M. (1999) Pain during insertion of peripheral intravenous catheters with or without intradermal lidocaine. *Clin Nurse Specialist*, 13, 283–5.

Brown, J.D. *et al.* (1997) The potential for catheter microbial contamination from a needleless connector. *J Hosp Infect*, 36, 181–9.

Browne, J. *et al.* (1999) Topical ametocaine (Ametop) is superior to EMLA for intravenous cannulation. *Can J Anesth*, 46, 1014–18.

Bucher, L. (2001) Arterial puncture. In: *AACN Procedure Manual for Critical Care* (eds L. McHale & K.K. Carlson), 4th edn. W.B. Saunders, London, pp. 496–503.

Camp Sorrell, D. (2005) *Oncology Nursing Society Access Device Guidelines: Recommendations for Nursing Practice and Education*. Oncology Nursing Society, Pittsburgh.

Carlson, K., Perdue, M.B. & Hankins, J. (2001) Infection control. In: *Infusion Therapy in Clinical Practice* (eds J. Hankin *et al.*), 2nd edn. W.B. Saunders, Philadelphia, pp. 126–40.

Carlson, K.R. (1999) Correct utilisation and management of PICCs and midline catheters in the alternate care setting. *J Intraven Nurse*, 22(Suppl 6), S46–50.

Catney, M.R. *et al.* (2001) Relationship between peripheral IV catheter dwell time and the development of phlebitis and infiltration. *J Intraven Nurse*, 24(5), 332–41.

Chambrin, M.C. (2001) Alarms in the intensive care unit, how can the number of false alarms be reduced. *Crit Care*, 5(4), 184–8.

Chernecky, C. (2001) Satisfaction versus dissatisfaction with venous access devices in outpatient oncology: a pilot study. *Oncol Nurs Forum*, 28(10), 1613–16.

Chernecky, C. *et al.* (2002) The need for shared decision making in the selection of VADs: an assessment of patient and clinicians. *JVAD*, 7(3), 34–9.

Chowet, A.L. *et al.* (2004) Wrist hyperextension leads to median nerve conduction block: implications for intra-arterial catheter placement. *Anaesthesiology*, 100(2), 287–91.

Ciano, B.A. (2001) Hemodynamic monitoring. In: *Infusion Therapy in Clinical Practice* (eds J. Hankin *et al.*), 2nd edn. W.B. Saunders, Philadelphia, pp. 404–17.

Clifton, G.D. *et al.* (1991) Comparison of 0.9% sodium chloride and heparin solutions for maintenance of arterial catheter patency. *Heart Lung*, 20(2), 115–18.

Cole, D. (1999) Selection and management of central venous access devices in the home setting. *J Intraven Nurse*, 22(6), 315–19.

Collin, G.R. (1999) Decreasing catheter colonisation through the use of an antiseptic impregnated catheter: a continuous quality improvement project. *Chest*, 115, 1632–40.

Communicable Diseases Centre (2002) Guidelines for the prevention of intravascular catheter-related infections. *MMWR Morb Mortal Wkly Rep*, 51(RR10), 1–29.

Conn, C. (1993) The importance of syringe size when using an implanted vascular access device. *J Vasc Access Networks*, 3(1), 11–18.

Cook, D. *et al.* (1997) Central venous catheter replacement strategies: a systemic review of the literature. *Crit Care Med*, 25(8), 1417–24.

Cosca, P.A. *et al.* (1998) Reinfusion of discard blood from venous access devices. *Oncol Nurs Forum*, 25(6), 73–6.

Costa, N. & Ferguson, E. (2002) Placement of triple lumen – peripherally inserted central catheters in critical patients. *J Vasc Access Devices*, 7(4), 27–32.

Couban, S. *et al.* (2005) Randomised placebo controlled study of low dose warfarin for the prevention of CVC associated thrombosis in patients with cancer. *J Clin Oncol*, 23(18), 4063–9.

Coyne, P.J. *et al.* (1995) Transcutaneous electrical nerve stimulator for procedural pain associated with intravenous needlesticks. *J Intraven Nurs*, 18(5), 263–7.

Crawford, M. *et al.* (2000) Peripherally inserted central catheter program. *Nurs Clin North Am*, 35(2), 349–59.

Crnich, C.J. & Maki, D.G. (2002) The promise of novel technology for the prevention of intravascular device-related blood stream infections. II. Long term devices. *Healthcare Epidemiology, Clinical Infectious Diseases*, 34(10), 1362–8.

Daily, E. & Schroeder, J. (1995) *Techniques in Bedside Haemodynamic Monitoring*, 5th edn. Mosby, St. Louis, MO.

Daniels, L.E. (1995) The physical and psychosocial implications of central venous access devices in cancer patients: a review of the literature. *J Cancer Care*, 4, 141–5.

Darouiche, R.O. (1999) A comparison of two antimicrobial impregnated central venous catheters. *N Engl J Med*, 340, 1–8.

Davidson, T. & Al Mufti, R. (1997) Hickman central venous catheters in cancer patients. *Cancer Topics*, 10(8), 10–14.

Dennis, A.R. *et al.* (1995) Local anaesthesia for cannulation – has practice changed? *Anaesthesia*, 50, 400–2.

DH (2001) *Good Practice in Consent Implementation Guide: Consent to Examination and Treatment*. www.dh.gov.uk. Accessed 24/9/07.

DH (2003) *Winning Ways Working Together to Reduce Healthcare Associated Infection in England*. Department of Health, London.

DH (2007) *Saving Lives: reducing infection, delivering clean and safe care. High impact intervention No. 1 (central venous care bundle) and No. 2 (peripheral IV cannula care bundle)*. Department of Health, London.

Dietcher, S.R. *et al.* (2002) Safety and efficacy of alteplase for restoring function in occluded central venous catheters: results of the Cardiovascular Thrombolytic to Open Occluded Lines Trial. *J Clin Oncol*, 20(1), 317–24.

Dorman, T., Breslow, M.J. & Lipsett, P. (1998) Radial artery pressure monitoring underestimates central arterial pressure during vasopressor therapy in critically ill surgical patients. *Crit Care Med*, 26(10), 1623–4.

Dougherty, L. (1994) A study to discover how cancer patients perceive the intravenous cannulation experience. Unpublished MSc thesis, University of Surrey, Guildford.

Dougherty, L. (2006) *Central Venous Access Devices*. Blackwell Publishing, Oxford.

Dougherty, L. (2008) Obtaining peripheral vascular access. In: *Intravenous Therapy in Nursing Practice* (eds L. Dougherty & J. Lamb), 2nd edn. Blackwell Publishing, Oxford.

Dougherty, L., Viner, C. & Young, J. (1998) Establishing ambulatory chemotherapy at home. *Prof Nurse*, 13(6), 356–60.

Drewett, S. (2000) Central venous catheter removal: procedures and rationale. *Br J Nurs*, 9(22), 2304–15.

Durbin, C.G. (2001) Radial arterial lines and sticks: what are the risks? *Repair Care*, 46(3), 229–31.

Egan Sansivero, G. (1998) Venous anatomy and physiology. Considerations for vascular access device placement and function. *J Intraven Nurs*, 21(Suppl 5), S107–14.

Elliott, T.S. (1993) Line associated bacteraemias. *Public Health Laboroatory Services Communicable Disease Report*, 3(7), R91–R96.

Fetzer, S.J. (2002) Reducing venipuncture and intravenous insertion pain with eutectic mixture of local anesthetic: a meta analysis. *Nurs Res*, 51, 119–24.

Finlay, T. (2004) *Intravenous Therapy*. Blackwell Publishing, Oxford.

Fitzsimmons, C.L. *et al.* (1997) Central venous catheter placement: extending the role of the nurse. *J R Coll Phys London*, 31(5), 533–5.

Fletcher, S.J. & Bodenham, A.R. (1999) Catheter related sepsis: an overview – part 1. *Br J Intensive Care*, 9(2), 46–53.

Frey, A.M. (2001) IV therapy in children. In: *Infusion Therapy in Clinical Practice* (eds J. Hankin *et al.*), 2nd edn. W.B. Saunders, Philadelphia, pp. 561–91.

Frey, A.M. (2002) Drawing labs from venous access devices. Presentation at NAVAN 15th Annual Conference, Virginia, January.

Fry, C. & Aholt, D. (2001) Local anaesthetic prior to insertion of a PICC. *J Intraven Nurse*, 24(6), 404–8.

Fuller, A. & Winn, C. (1999) Selecting equipment for peripheral intravenous cannulation. *Prof Nurs*, 14(4), 233–6.

Gabriel, J. (2000) What patients think of a PICC. *J Vasc Access Devices*, 5(4), 26–9.

Gabriel, J. (2001) PICC securement: minimising potential complications. *Nurs Stand*, 15(43), 42–4.

Gabriel, J. (2008) Long term central venous access. In: *Intravenous Therapy in Nursing Practice* (eds L. Dougherty & J. Lamb), 2nd edn. Blackwell Publishing, Oxford.

Galinkin, J.L. *et al.* (2002) Lidocaine iontophoresis versus eutectic mixture of local anaesthetics (EMLA) for IV placement in children. *Anesth Analg*, 94(6), 1484–8.

Galloway, S. & Bodenham, A. (2004) Long term central venous access. *Br J Anaesth*, 92, 722–34.

Gamby, A. & Bennett, J. (1995) A feasibility study of the use of non-heparinised 0.9% sodium chloride for transduced arterial and venous lines. *Intensive Crit Care Nurs*, 11(3), 148–50.

Goetz, A.M., *et al.* (1998) Complications related to intravenous midline catheter usage. *J Intraven Nurs*, 21(2), 76–80.

Goode, C.J. *et al.* (1991) A meta analysis of effects of heparin flush and saline flush – quality and cost implications. *Nurs Res*, 40(6), 324–30.

Goodwin, M. & Carlson, I. (1993) The peripherally inserted catheter: a retrospective look at 3 years of insertions. *J Intraven Nurs*, 16(2), 92–103.

Hadaway, L. (1998a) Catheter connection. *J Vasc Access Devices*, 3(3), 40.

Hadaway, L. (1998b) Major thrombotic and non thrombotic complications: loss of patency. *J Intraven Nurs*, 21(Suppl 5), S143–60.

Hadaway, L. (2000) Peripheral IV therapy in adults. In: *Self Study Workbook*. Hadaway Associates, Georgia.

Hadaway, L. (2001) Anatomy and physiology related to intravenous therapy. In: *Infusion Therapy in Clinical Practice* (eds J. Hankin *et al.*), 2nd edn. W.B. Saunders, Philadelphia, pp. 65–97.

Haire, W.D. & Herbst, S.F. (2000) Use of alteplase. *J Vasc Access Devices*, 5(2), 28–36.

Hallquist Viale, P. (2003) Complications associated with implantable vascular access devices in the patient with cancer. *J Intraven Nurs*, 26(2), 97–102.

Hamilton, H., O'Byrne, M. & Nicholai, L. (1995) Central lines inserted by clinical nurse specialists. *Nurs Times*, 91(17), 38–9.

Hanchett, M. (1999) Science of IV securement. *J Vasc Access Devices*, 4(3), 9–15.

Hart, S. (2008) Infection control. In: *Intravenous Therapy in Nursing Practice* (eds L. Dougherty & J. Lamb), 2nd edn. Blackwell Publishing, Oxford.

Hayden, M.K. & Goodman, M. (2005) Chemotherapy: principles of administration. In: *Cancer Nursing* (eds C. Henke Yarbro *et al.*). Jones & Bartlett, Boston, pp. 351–411.

Hazinski, M.F. (1992) *Nursing Care of the Critically Ill Child*, 2nd edn. Mosby, St. Louis, MO.

Heath, J. & Jones, S. (2001) Utilisation of an elastomeric continuous infusion device to maintain catheter patency. *J Intraven Nurs*, 24(2), 102–6.

Hinds, C.J. (1987) *Intensive Care*. Balliere Tindall, London.

Ho, K.S., Chia, K.H. & Teb, L.Y. (2003) An unusual complication of radial artery cannulation and its management; a case report. *J Oral Maxillofac Surg*, 61, 955–7.

Hoffer, E.K. *et al.* (1999) Prospective randomised comparison of valved vs non-valved peripherally inserted central venous catheters. *Am J Radiol*, 173, 1393–8.

Holcombe, B.J. *et al.* (1992) Restoring patency of long term central venous access devices. *J Intraven Nurs*, 15, 36–41.

Holmes, K. (1998) Comparison of push–pull versus discard method from central venous catheters for blood testing. *J Intraven Nurs*, 21(5), 282–5.

Homer, L.D. & Holmes, K.R. (1998) Risks associated with 72 and 96 hour peripheral IV catheter dwell times. *J Intraven Nurs*, 21(5), 301–5.

Hudak, C.M., Gallo, B.M. & Morton, P.G. (1998) *Critical Care Nursing; A Holistic Approach*, 7th edn. Lippincott, New York.

Hudson, T.L. (2006) Use of local anaesthesia for arterial puncture. *Am J Crit Care*, 15(6), 595–9.

ICNA (2003) Reducing Sharps Injury – Prevention and Risk Management. Infection Control Nurses Association, London.

INS (2006) Standards for Infusion Therapy. *Journal of Infusion Nurses Society*, 29(1) supplement.

Inwood, S. (1999) A preliminary assessment of an innovative valved catheter. *J Vasc Access Devices*, 4(2), 30–2.

Jackson, D. (2001) Infection control principles and practices in the care and management of VADs: alternate care settings. *J Intraven Nurse*, 24(Suppl 3), S28–34.

Kamimoto, V. & Olson, K. (1996) Using normal saline to lock peripheral intravenous catheters in ambulatory cancer patients. *J Intraven Nurse*, 19(2), 75–8.

Karadag, A. & Gorgulu, S. (2000) Vialon better than Teflon? *J Intraven Nurse*, 23(3), 158–66.

Kayley, J. (2008) IV therapy in the community. In: *IV Therapy in Nursing Practice* (eds L. Dougherty & J. Lamb), 2nd edn. Blackwell Publishing, Oxford.

Keenleyside, D. (1993) Avoiding an unnecessary outcome. A comparative trial between IV 3000 and a conventional film dressing to assess rates of catheter related sepsis. *Prof Nurse*, 8, 288–91.

Keller, C.A. (1994) Method of drawing blood samples through central venous catheters in paediatric patients undergoing bone marrow transplants – results of a national survey. *Oncol Nurs Forum*, 21(5), 879–84.

Kerrison, T. & Woodhull, J. (1994) Reducing the risk of thrombophlebitis – comparison of Teflon and Vialon cannulae. *Prof Nurse*, 9(10), 662–6.

Kulkarni, M., *et al.* (1994) Heparinised saline vs normal saline in maintaining patency of the radial artery catheter. *Can J Surg*, 37(1), 37–42.

Kupensky, D.T. (1998) Applying current research to influence clinical practice – utilization of midline catheters. *J Intraven Nurse*, 21(5), 271–4.

Larson, E. (1988) Guidelines for use of topical antimicrobial agents (review). *Am J Infec Control*, 16(6), 253–66.

La Rue, G.D. (2000) Efficacy of ultrasonography in peripheral venous cannulation. *J Intraven Nurse*, 23(1), 29–34.

Lenhart, C. (2000) Prevention vs treatment of vascular access devices occlusions. *J Vasc Access Devices*, 5(4), 34–5.

Lipsitz, E.C. (2004) Cannulation injuries of the radial artery. *Am J Crit Care*, 13(4), 314–19.

Lonsway, R.A. (2001) IV therapy in the home. In: *Infusion Therapy in Clinical Practice* (eds J. Hankin *et al.*), 2nd edn. W.B. Saunders, Philadelphia.

LSC (2002) *Standards of Care of External Central Venous Catheters in Adult Cancer Patients*. London Standing Committee, London.

Lum, P. (1999) Techniques for optimising catheter tip position. Presentation at NAVAN 13th Annual Conference, Orlando, September.

Lum, P. (2004) A new formula based measurement guide for optimal positioning of central venous catheter. *JAVA*, **9**(2), 80–6.

Macklin, D. (1999) A review of the physical principles of fluid administration. *J Vasc Access Devices*, **4**(2), 7–11.

Macklin, D. & Chernecky, C. (2004) *IV Therapy*. W.B. Saunders, St. Louis, MO.

Macrae, K. (1998) Hand held Dopplers in central catheter insertion. *Prof Nurse*, **14**(2), 99–102.

Madeo, M. *et al.* (1997) A randomised study comparing IV 3000 (transparent polyurethane dressing) to a dry gauze dressing for peripheral intravenous catheter sites. *J Intraven Nurse*, **20**(5), 253–6.

Maki, D.G. (2002) The promise of novel technology for prevention of intravascular device related blood stream infections, NAVAN conference, San Diego.

Maki, D.G. (2005) Reknowned expert Dennis Maki addresses catheter related infections. *Infection Control Today*, **9**(1): www.infectioncontroltoday.com. Accessed 20/9/07

Maki, D.G. & Ringer, M. (1987) Evaluation of dressing regimes for prevention of infection with peripheral IV catheters. *JAMA*, **258**(17), 2396–403.

Maki, D.G. *et al.* (1991) Prospective randomized trial of povidone iodine, alcohol and chlorhexidine for prevention of infection associated with CVC and arterial catheters. *Lancet*, **338**, 339–43.

Maki, D.G. *et al.* (1997) Prevention of central venous catheter related bloodstream infection by the use of an antiseptic impregnated catheter. *Ann Intern Med*, **127**(4), 257–66.

Marieb, E. (2001) *Human Anatomy and Physiology*, 5th edn. Benjamin Cummings, San Francisco, CA.

Marsigliese, A.M. (2001) Evaluation of comfort level and complication rates as determined by peripheral intravenous catheter sites. *CINA*, 26–39.

Martin, S.D. *et al.* (1995) Do arterial lines equal unnecessary testing. *Chest*, **108**(1), 7–8.

Marx, M. (1995) The management of the difficult peripherally inserted central venous catheter line removal. *J Intraven Nurse*, **18**(5), 246–9.

Mayo, D.J. (1996) The effects of heparin flush on patency of Groshong catheter: a pilot study. *Oncol Nurs Forum*, **23**(9), 1401–5.

Mayo, D.J. (1998) Fibrin sheath formation and chemotherapy extravasation: a case report. *Support Care Cancer*, **6**, 51–6.

Mayo, D.J. (2000) Catheter-related thrombosis. *J Vasc Access Devices*, **5**(2), 10–20.

Mayo, D.J. (2001a) Catheter related thrombosis. *J Intraven Nurse*, **24**(Suppl 3), S13–22.

Mayo, D.J. (2001b) Reflux in vascular access devices – a manageable problem. *J Vasc Access Devices*, **6**(4), 39–40.

McDermott, M.K. (1995) Patient education and compliance issues associated with access devices. *Semin Oncol Nurs*, **11**(3), 221–6.

MHRA (2004) *Medical Device Alert MDA/2004/010 Central venous catheters (all manufacturers (25/2/04), 1–3*. Medcines and Healthcare Products Agency, London.

MHRA (2005) *Alert MDA 2005/01 and Device Bulletin DB 2005 (01), Reporting Adverse Incidents and Disseminating Medical Device Alerts*. Medicines and Healthcare Products Agency, London.

Mermel, L.A. *et al.* (2000) Guidelines for management of intravascular catheter related infections. *J Intraven Nurse*, **24**(3), 180–205.

Mignini, M.A., Piacentini, E. & Dubin, A. (2006) A peripheral arterial blood pressure monitoring adequately tracks central arterial blood pressure in critically ill patients: an observational study. *Crit Care*, **10**(2) R43.

Millam, D. (1992) Starting IVs – how to develop your venepuncture skills. *Nursing*, **92**, 33–46.

Minnaganti, V.R. (2000) Acintobacter baumanii-associated arterial line infection. *Am J Infect Control*, **28**, 376–7.

Mirro, J. *et al.* (1989) A prospective study of Hickman/Broviac catheters and implanted ports in paediatric oncology patients. *J Clin Oncol*, **7**, 214–22.

Morven, H. (1995) The first years of continuing arterial pressure measurement. *Br J Anaesth*, **67**, 353–9.

Moureau, N. (1999) Practicing prevention with implanted ports. *J Vasc Access Devices*, **4**(3), 30–5.

Moureau, N. & Iannucci, A.L. (2003) Catheter securement: trends in performance and complications associated with the use of either traditional methods or adhesive anchor device. *J Vasc Access Devices*, **8**(3), 29–33.

Moureau, N. & Zonderman, A. (2000) Does it always have to hurt? *J Intraven Nurse*, **23**(4), 213–19.

Moureau, N. *et al.* (1999) Multidisciplinary management of thrombotic catheter occlusions in VADs. *J Vasc Access Devices*, **4**(2), 22–9.

Murphy, G.S. *et al.* (2006) Retrograde blood flow in the brachial and axillary arteries during routine radial arterial catheter flushing. *Anesthesiology*, **105**(3), 492–7.

Nauth Misir, N. (1998) Intravascular catheters. *Prof Nurse*, **13**(7), 463–71.

NAVAN (1998) Tip location of peripherally inserted central catheters. *J Vasc Access Devices*, **3**(2) 8.

Nesti, S.P. & Kovac, R. (2000) 5-FU extravasation following port failure. *J Intraven Nurse*, **23**(3), 176–80.

NHS Employers (2007) Needlestick injury. In: *The Healthy Workplace Handbook*. National Health Service Employers, London.

NICE (2002) *Ultrasound Imaging for Central Venous Catheter Placement*. National Institute for Health and Clinical Excellence, London.

NICE (2003) *Infection Control – Prevention of Healthcare Associated Infection in Primary and Community Care. Clinical Guideline 2*. National Institute for Health and Clinical Excellence, London.

NMC (2008) *The Code: Standards of Conduct, Performance and Ethics for Nurses and Midwives*. Nursing and Midwifery Council, London.

NMC (2005) *Records and Record Keeping*. Nursing and Midwifery Council, London.

Oakley, C., Wright, E. & Ream, E. (2000) The experiences of patients and nurses with a nurse led peripherally inserted central venous catheter line service. *Eur J Oncol Nurs*, **4**(4), 207–18.

Oh, T.E. (2003) *Intensive Care Manual*, 5th edn. Butterworth Heinemann, Oxford.

Parker, L. (2002) Management of IV devices to prevent infection. *Br J Nurs*, **11**(4), 240–5.

Payne-James, J.J. *et al.* (1991) Development of thrombophlebitis in peripheral veins with Vialon and PTFE–Teflon cannulas: a double blind randomised controlled trial. *Ann R Coll Surg Engl*, **73**, 322–5.

Pearson, M.L. (1996) Guideline for prevention of intravascular device-related infections: part one an overview. *Am J Infect Control*, **24**, 262–93.

Perdue, M.B. (2001) Intravenous complications. In: *Infusion Therapy in Clinical Practice* (eds J. Hankin *et al.*), 2nd edn. W.B. Saunders, Philadelphia, pp. 418–45.

Perucca, R. (2001) Obtaining vascular access. In: *Infusion Therapy in Clinical Practice* (eds J. Hankin *et al.*), 2nd edn. W.B. Saunders, Philadelphia, pp. 375–88.

916

Phillips, L. (2005) *Manual of IV Therapeutics*, 4th edn. F.A. Davis, Philadelphia.

Philpott, P. & Griffiths, V.R. (2003) The peripherally inserted central catheter. *Nurs Stand*, 17(44), 39–46.

Pierce, L.R. (ed.) (1998) Non invasive respiratory monitoring and invasive monitoring of direct and derived tissue oxygenation variables. In: *Guide to Mechanical Ventilation and Intensive Respiratory Care*. W.B. Saunders, Philadelphia, p. 259.

Ponec, D. *et al.* (2001) Recombinant tissue plasminogen activator (Alteplase) for restoration of flow in occluded central venous access devices: a double blind placebo controlled trial – the Cardiovascular Thrombolytic to Open Occluded Lines (COOL) efficacy trial. *J Vasc Interv Radiol*, 12, 951–5.

Powers, F.A. (1999) Can you keep her safe? *Nursing*, 99, 54–5.

Pratt, R.J. *et al.* (2007) Epic 2: national evidence-based guidelines for preventing healthcare-associated infections in NHS hospitals in England. *J Hosp Infect*, 655(suppl), S1–64.

Randolph, A.G. *et al.* (1998) Benefit of heparin use in central venous catheters and pulmonary artery catheters – a meta analysis of randomised controlled trials. *Chest*, 113, 165–71.

RCN (2005) *Standards for Infusion Therapy*. Royal College of Nursing, London.

RCN & Infection Control Nurses' Association (1992) *Intravenous Line Dressings – Principles of Infection Control*. Smith & Nephew Medical, Hull. Rickard, N.A.S. (2001) Central venous catheter – infection and patient susceptibility. *Br J Nurs*, 10(16), 1044–53.

Rinn, T.L. (2001) Fibrinolytic therapy in CVC occlusion. *J Intraven Nurse*, 24(Suppl 3), S9–12.

Robbins, J., Cromwell, P. & Korones, D.N. (2000) Swimming and central venous catheter related infections in children with cancer. In: *Measuring Patient Outcomes* (eds M. Nolan & V. Mock). Sage Publications, Thousand Oaks, CA, pp. 169–84.

Rowley, S. (2001) Theory to practice: aseptic non touch technique. *Nurs Times*, 97(7), 6–8.

Royal College of Anaesthetists (1990) *The Working Party of the Commission on the Provision of Surgical Services*. Royal College of Surgeons and College of Anaesthetists, London.

Royer, T. (2001) A case for post, anterior and lateral CXR being performed following each PICC placement. *J Vasc Access Devices*, 6(4), 9–11.

Rummel, M.A., Donnelly, P.J. & Fortenbaugh, C.C. (2001) Clinical evaluation of a positive pressure device to prevent central venous catheter occlusion: results of a pilot study. *Clin J Oncol Nurs*, 5(6), 261–5.

Ryder, M. (2001) The role of biofilm in vascular catheter related infections. *New Dev Vasc Dis*, 2(2), 15–25.

Ryder, M. (2002) Biofilm – unlocking the mystery of catheter-related infections. Presentation at NAVAN 15th Annual Conference, Virginia, January.

Sampath, L.A. *et al.* (2001) Safety and efficacy of an improved antiseptic catheter impregnated intraluminally with chlorhexidine. *J Intraven Nurse*, 24(6), 395–403.

Sansivero, G.E. (1998) Venous anatomy and physiology. *J Intraven Nurse*, 21(Suppl 5), S107–14.

Sansivero, G.E. (2000) Microintroducer techniques for PICC placement. *J Intraven Nurse*, 23(6), 345–51.

Santolla, A. & Weckel, C. (1983) A new closed system for arterial lines. *Reg Nurse*, 46(6), 49–52.

Scales, K. (2005) Vascular access: a guide to peripheral venous cannulation. *Nurs Stand*, 19(49), 48–52.

Scales, K. (2008) Anatomy and physiology. In: *IV Therapy in Nursing Practice* (eds L. Dougherty & J. Lamb), 2nd edn. Blackwell Publishing, Oxford.

Schears, G.J. (2005) The benefits of a catheter securement device on reducing patient complications. *Manag Hosp Infect*, 5(2), 14–20.

Schulmeister, L. & Camp Sorrell, D. (2000) Chemotherapy extravasation from implanted ports. *Oncol Nurs Forum*, 27(3), 531–60.

Sheppard, K. *et al.* (1999) A prospective study of two intravenous catheter securement techniques in a skilled nursing facility. *J Intraven Nurse*, 22(3), 151–6.

Shotkin, J.D. & Lombardo, F. (1996) Use of an indwelling peripheral catheter for 3–5 day chemotherapy administration in the outpatient setting. *J Intraven Nurse*, 19(6), 315–20.

Simcock, L. (2001a) Managing occlusion in central venous catheters. *Nurs Times*, 97(21), 36–8.

Simcock, L. (2001b) The use of central venous catheters for IV therapy. *Nurs Times*, 97(18), 34–5.

Snelling, R. *et al.* (2001) CVC for infusion therapy in GI cancer. *J Intraven Nurse*, 24(1), 38–47.

Springhouse Corporation (2002) *Intravenous Therapy Made Incredibly Easy*. Springhouse, Lippincott, Williams & Wilkins, Philadelphia.

Stacey, R.G.W. *et al.* (1991) Percutaneous insertion of Hickman type catheters. *Br J Hosp Med*, 46, 396–8.

Stanley, A. (2002) Managing complications of chemotherapy administration. In: *The Cytotoxic Handbook* (eds M. Allwood *et al.*). Radcliffe Medical Press, Oxford, pp. 119–93.

Stevenis, B. *et al.* (2000) A randomised prospective trial of conventional vascular ports vs the vortex 'clear-flow' reservoir ports in adult oncology patients. *J Vasc Access Devices*, 5(2), 37–40.

Tagalakis, V. *et al.* (2002) The epidemiology of peripheral vein infusion thrombophlebitis: a critical review. *Am J Med*, 113, 146–51.

Taylor, M.J. (2000) A fascination with phlebitis. *J Vasc Access Devices*, 5(3), 24–8.

Tegtmeyer, K. *et al.* (2006) Placement of an arterial line; videos in clinical medicine. *N Engl J Med*, 354(15), e13. www.NEJM.org. Accessed 24/09/07.

Teplitz, L. (1990) Arterial line disconnection: first aid procedure. *Nursing*, 20(5), 33.

Thompson, A. *et al.* (1989) Long-term central venous access: the patient's view. *Intensive Ther Clin Monit*, 10(5), 142–5.

Timoney, J.P. *et al.* (2002) Safe and effective use of Alteplase for the clearance of occluded central venous access devices. *J Clin Oncol*, 20(7), 1918–22.

Timsit, J.F. (2000) Rotation of central venous catheter sites. *Infect Control Hosp Epidemiol*, 21(6), 371–4.

Tingey, K.G. (2000) Desirable properties for vascular catheter materials. *J Vasc Access Devices*, 5(3), 14–16.

Tinker, J. & Zapol, W. (1991) *Care of the Critically Ill Patient*. Springer, London.

Tortora, G. & Grabowski, S.R. (2003) The cardiovascular system, blood vessels and haemodynamics. In: *The Principles of Anatomy and Physiology*, 10th edn. John Wiley & Sons, Inc., New York, pp. 696–756.

Usichenko, T. I. *et al.* (2004) Reducing venipuncture pain by a cough trick: a randomized crossover volunteer study. *Anesth Analg*, 98, 343–5.

Veenstra, D.L. *et al.* (1999) Efficacy of antiseptic impregnated central venous catheters in preventing catheter related blood stream infection: a meta analysis. *JAMA*, 281(3), 261–7.

Verghese, S.T. *et al.* (2002) The effects of the simulated Valsalva maneuver liver compression and/or Trendelenburg position on the cross sectional area of the internal jugular vein in infants and young children. *Anesthes Analg*, 94(2), 250–4.

Verhage, A.H. & van Bommel, E.P.H. (1999) Catheter fracture: an under recognised and serious condition. *JVAD*, 4(2), 33–4.

Wallach, S.G. (2004) Cannulation injury of the radial artery: diagnosis and treatment algorithm. *Am J Crit Care*, 13(4), 315–19.

917

Walther, K. (2001) Intravenous therapy in the older adult. In: *Infusion Therapy in Clinical Practice* (eds J. Hankin *et al.*), 2nd edn. W.B. Saunders, Philadelphia, pp. 592–603.

Weinstein, S. (2007) *Plumer's Principles and Practices of Intravenous Therapy*, 8th edn. Lippincott, Philadelphia.

Weller, B.F. (2005) *Bailliere's Nurses Dictionary*, 24th edn. Elsevier, Edinburgh.

Wendler, M.C. (2003) Effects of Tellington touch in healthy adults awaiting venipuncture. *Res Nurs Health*, **26**, 40–52.

White, G.C. (2003) *Basic Clinical Lab Competencies for Respiratory Care: an Integrated Approach*, 4th edn. Delmar Publishing, London.

Whitely, M.S., Change, B.Y.P. & Marsh, H.P. (1995) Use of hand held Doppler to identify 'difficult' forearm veins for cannulation. *Ann R Coll Surg Engl*, **77**, 224–6.

Whitson, M. (1996) Intravenous therapy in the older adult: special needs and considerations. *J Intraven Nurse*, **19**(5), 251–5.

Williamson, E.E. & McKinney, J.M. (2001) Assessing the adequacy of PICCs for power injection of intravenous contrast agents for CT. *J Comput Assist Tomogr*, **25**(6), 932–7.

Wilson, J. (2001) Preventing infection associated with intravenous therapy. In: *Infection Control in Clinical Practice*, 2nd edn. Bailliere Tindall, London.

Wilson, K.J. & Waugh, A. (1996) *Ross and Wilson's Anatomy and Physiology and Illness*, 8th edn. Churchill Livingstone, Edinburgh.

Wise, M. *et al.* (2001) Catheter tip position. *J Vasc Access Devices*, **6**(2), 18–27.

Xu, Q.A. *et al.* (2000) Adequacy of a new chlorhexidine bearing polyurethane central venous catheter for administration of 82 selected parenteral drugs. *Ann Pharmacother*, **34**, 1109–16.

Yamamoto, A.J. (2002) Sutureless securement devices reduces the complications of peripherally inserted central venous catheters. *J Vasc Interv Radiol*, **13**(1), 77–81.

Young, A.M. *et al.* (2005) WARP: a multi centre prospective randomized controlled trial of thrombosis prophylaxis with warfarin in cancer patients with central venous catheters, ASCO meeting abstracts.

Zideman, D.A. & Morgan, M. (1981) Inadvertent intra-arterial injection of flucloxacillin. *Anaesthesia*, **36**(6), 296–8.

Chapter 46

Venepuncture

Reference material 920
Procedure guidelines: Venepuncture 924
Problem solving: Venepuncture 928
References and further reading 931

Definition

Venepuncture is the procedure of entering a vein with a needle.

Indications

Venepuncture is carried out for two reasons:

- To obtain a blood sample for diagnostic purposes.
- To monitor levels of blood components.

Reference material

Venepuncture is one of the most commonly performed invasive procedures (Castledine 1996) and is now routinely being undertaken by nurses (Ernst 2005). In order to perform venepuncture safely the nurse must have basic knowledge of the following:

- The relevant anatomy and physiology.
- The criteria for choosing both the vein and device to use.
- The potential problems which may be encountered, how to prevent them and necessary interventions.
- The health and safety/risk management of the procedure, as well as the correct disposal of equipment (RCN 2005).

Certain principles, such as adherence to an aseptic technique, must be applied throughout (see Chapter 5). The circulation is a closed sterile system and a venepuncture, however quickly completed, is a breach of this system providing a means of entry for bacteria.

The nurse must be aware of the physical and psychological comfort of the patient (Hoeltke 2006). He or she must appreciate the value of adequate explanation and simple measures to prevent the complications of venepuncture, such as haematoma formation, when it is neither a natural nor acceptable consequence of the procedure (Hoeltke 2006).

Anatomy and physiology

The superficial veins of the upper limb are most commonly chosen for venepuncture. These veins are numerous and accessible, ensuring that the procedure can be performed safely and with minimum discomfort (Ernst 2005). In adults veins located on the dorsal portion of the foot may be selected but there is an increased risk of deep vein thrombosis (Garza & Becan McBride 2005) or tissue necrosis in diabetics (Ernst 2005). Therefore, veins in the lower limbs should be avoided where possible.

The veins commonly used for venepuncture are those found in the antecubital fossa because they are sizeable veins capable of providing copious and repeated blood specimens (Weinstein 2007). However, the venous anatomy of each individual may differ. The main veins of choice are (Figure 46.1a):

- The median cubital veins.
- The cephalic vein.

(a)

(b)

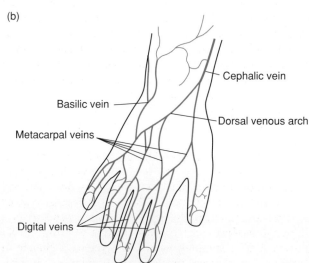

Figure 46.1   (a) Superficial veins of the forearm. (b) Superficial veins of dorsal aspect of the hand. (Reproduced with permission from Becton Dickinson and Company.)

- The basilic vein.
- The metacarpal veins (used only when the others are not accessible) (Figure 46.1b).

The median cubital vein may not always be visible, but its size and location make it easy to palpate. It is also well supported by subcutaneous tissue, which prevents it from rolling under the needle.

On the lateral aspect of the wrist, the cephalic vein rises from the dorsal veins and flows upwards along the radial border of the forearm as the median cephalic, crossing the antecubital fossa as the median cubital vein. Care must be taken to avoid accidental arterial puncture, as this vein crosses the brachial artery. It is also in close proximity to the radial nerve (Masoorli 2002; Dougherty 2008).

The basilic vein is often overlooked as a site for venepuncture and has its origins in the ulnar border of the hand and forearm (Waugh & Grant 2006). It may well be prominent but is not well supported by subcutaneous tissue, making it roll easily, which can result in difficult venepuncture. Owing to its position, a haematoma may occur if the patient flexes the arm on removal of the needle, as this squeezes blood from the vein into the surrounding tissues (McCall & Tankersley 2003; Weinstein 2007). Care must also be taken to avoid accidental puncture of the median nerve and brachial artery (Garza & Becan McBride 2005).

The metacarpal veins are easily visualized and palpated. However, the use of these veins is contraindicated in the elderly where skin turgor and subcutaneous tissue are diminished (Weinstein 2007).

Veins consist of three layers: the tunica intima is a smooth endothelial lining, which allows the passage of blood cells. If it becomes damaged, the lining may become roughened and there is an increased risk of thrombus formation (Weinstein 2007). Within this layer are folds of endothelium called valves, which keep blood moving towards the heart by preventing back flow of blood. Valves are present in larger vessels and at points of branching and are present as noticeable bulges in the veins (Weinstein 2007). However, when suction is applied during venepuncture, the valve can compress and close the lumen of the vein, thus preventing the withdrawal of blood (Weinstein 2007). Therefore, if detected, venepuncture should be performed above the valve in order to facilitate collection of the sample (Weinstein 2007).

The tunica media, the middle layer of the vein wall, is composed of muscular tissue and nerve fibres, both vasoconstrictors and vasodilators, which can stimulate the vein to contract or relax. This layer is not as strong or stiff as an artery and therefore veins can distend or collapse as the pressure rises or falls (Waugh & Grant 2006; Weinstein 2007). Stimulation of this layer by a change in temperature, mechanical or chemical stimulation can produce venous spasm, which can make a venepuncture more difficult.

The tunica adventitia is the outer layer and consists of connective tissue, which surrounds and supports the vessel.

Arteries tend to be placed more deeply than veins and can be distinguished by the thicker walls, which do not collapse, the presence of a pulse and the blood is bright red. It should be noted that aberrant arteries may be present. These are arteries that are located superficially in an unusual place (Weinstein 2007).

Choosing a vein

The choice of vein must be that which is best for the individual patient. The most prominent vein is not necessarily the most suitable vein for venepuncture (Weinstein 2007). There are two stages to locating a vein:

1 Visual inspection.
2 Palpation.

Visual inspection is the scrutiny of the veins in both arms and is essential prior to choosing a vein. Veins adjacent to foci of infection, bruising and phlebitis should not be considered, owing to the risk of causing more local tissue damage or systemic infection (Dougherty 2008). An oedematous limb should be avoided as there is danger of stasis of lymph, predisposing to such complications as phlebitis and cellulitis (Smith 1998; Hoeltke 2006). Areas of previous venepuncture should be avoided as a build-up of scar tissue can cause difficulty in accessing the vein and can result in pain due to repeated trauma (Hoeltke 2006).

Palpation is an important assessment technique, as it determines the location and condition of the vein, distinguishes veins from arteries and tendons, identifies the presence of valves and detects deeper veins (Dougherty 2008). The nurse should use the same fingers for palpation as this will increase the sensitivity and ability of the nurse to know what she or he is feeling. The less dominant hand should be used for palpation so that in the event of a missed vein the nurse can repalpate and realign the needle (Hoeltke 2006). The thumb should not be used as it is not as sensitive and has a pulse, which may lead to confusion in distinguishing veins from arteries in the patient (Weinstein 2007).

Thrombosed veins feel hard and cord-like, and should be avoided along with tortuous, sclerosed, fibrosed, inflamed or fragile veins, which may be unable to accommodate the device to be used and will result in pain and repeated venepunctures (Dougherty 2008). Use of veins which cross over joints or bony prominences and those with little skin or subcutaneous cover, e.g. the inner aspect of the wrist, will also subject the patient to more discomfort (Dougherty 2008). Therefore, preference should be given to a vessel that is unused, easily detected by inspection and palpation, patent and healthy. These veins feel soft and bouncy and will refill when depressed (Weinstein 2007).

Influencing factors

- Injury, disease or treatment may prevent the use of a limb for venepuncture thereby reducing the venous access, e.g. amputation, fracture and cerebrovascular accident. Use of a limb may be contraindicated because of an operation on one side of the body, for example mastectomy and axillary node dissection, as this can lead to impairment of lymphatic drainage, which can influence venous flow regardless of whether there is obvious lymphoedema (Ernst 2005; Hoeltke 2006).

921

- The age and weight of the patient will also influence choice. Young children have short fine veins, and the elderly have prominent but fragile veins. Care must be taken with fragile veins and the largest vein should be chosen along with the smallest gauge device to reduce the amount of trauma to the vessel. Malnourished patients will often present with friable veins.

- If the patient is in shock or dehydrated there will be poor superficial peripheral access. It may be necessary to take blood after the patient is rehydrated as this will promote venous filling and blood will be obtained more easily.

- Medications can influence the choice of vein in that patients on anticoagulants or steroids or those who are thrombocytopenic tend to have more fragile veins and will be at greater risk of bruising both during venepuncture and on removal of the needle. Therefore choice may be limited by areas of bruising present or the inability to access the vessel without causing bruising.

- The temperature of the environment will influence venous dilatation. If the patient is cold, no veins may be evident on first inspection. Application of heat, e.g. in the form of a warm compress or soaking the arm in warm water, will increase the size and visibility of the veins, thus increasing the likelihood of a successful first attempt (Lenhardt *et al.* 2002; Weinstein 2007).

- Venepuncture itself may cause the vein to collapse or go into a spasm. This will produce discomfort and a reduction in blood flow. Careful preparation and choice of vein will reduce the likelihood of this and stroking the vein or applying heat will help resolve it.

- Patient anxiety about the procedure may result in vasoconstriction. The nurse's manner and approach will also have a direct bearing on the patient's experience (Garza & Becan McBride 2005). Approaching the patient with a confident manner and giving an adequate explanation of the procedure may reduce anxiety. Careful preparation and an unhurried approach will help to relax the patient and this in turn will increase vasodilatation (Weinstein 2007; Dougherty 2008). It is important to remember that patients may dread venepuncture (Ernst 2005; Lavery & Ingram 2005) and if a patient is particularly anxious, or for venepuncture in children, the use of a topical local anaesthetic cream may be appropriate (Ernst 2005; Weinstein 2007). Involving patients in the choice of vein, even if it is simply to choose the nondominant arm, can increase a feeling of control which in turn helps to relieve anxiety (Hudek 1986).

Improving venous access

There are a number of methods of improving venous access:

- Application of a tourniquet: this promotes venous distension. The tourniquet should be tight enough to impede venous return but not restrict arterial flow. The tourni-

quet should be placed about 7–8 cm above the venepuncture site. It may be more comfortable for the patient to position it over a sleeve or paper towel to prevent pinching the skin. The tourniquet should not be left on for longer than 1 minute as it may result in haemoconcentration or pooling of the blood, leading to inaccurate blood results (Hoeltke 2006).
There are several types of tourniquet available. A good-quality, buckle closure, single hand release type is most effective but the choice will depend on availability and operator. Consideration should be given to the type of material and the ability to decontaminate the tourniquet (Golder 2000; RCN 2005).

- The patient may be asked to clench the fist and encourage venous distension but should avoid 'pumping' as this action may affect certain blood results, e.g. potassium (Ernst 2005; Garza & Becan McBride 2005).

- Lowering the arm below heart level also increases blood supply to the veins.

- Light tapping of the vein may be useful but can be painful and may result in the formation of a haematoma in patients with fragile veins, e.g. thrombocytopenic patients (Dougherty 2008).

- The use of heat in the form of a warm pack or by immersing the arm in a bowl of warm water for 10 minutes helps to encourage venodilatation and venous filling (Lenhardt *et al.* 2002).

- Ointment or patches containing small amounts of glyceryl trinitrate have been used to improve local vasodilatation to aid venepuncture (Weinstein 2007).

Choice of device

The intravenous devices commonly used to perform a venepuncture for blood sampling are a straight steel needle and a steel winged infusion device. The optimum gauge to use is 21 swg (standard wire gauge), which measures internal diameter: the smaller the gauge size, the larger the diameter. Standard wire gauge measurement is determined by how many cannulae fit into a tube with an inner diameter of 1 inch (2.5 cm), and uses consecutive numbers from 13 to 24. This enables blood to be withdrawn at a reasonable speed without undue discomfort to the patient or possible damage to the blood cells.

Equipment available will depend on local policy (Table 46.1), but with increasing concern about the possibility of contamination to the practitioner, blood collection systems with integrated safety devices are now readily available and should be used wherever possible (Infection Control Nurses Association 2003). However, the nurse must always select the device after assessing the condition and accessibility of the vein.

Skin preparation

Asepsis is vital when performing a venepuncture as the skin is breached and a foreign device is introduced into a

Table 46.1   Choice of intravenous device.

Device	g	Advantages	Disadvantages	Use
Needle	21	Cheaper than winged infusion devices. Easy to use with large veins	Rigid. Difficult to manipulate with smaller veins in less conventional sites. May cause more discomfort Venous access only confirmed when sample tube attached	Large, accessible veins in the antecubital fossa. When small quantities of blood are to be drawn
Winged infusion device with or without safety shield	21	Flexible due to small needle shaft. Easy to manipulate and insert at any site. Increases the success rate of venepuncture and causes less discomfort (Hefler *et al.* 2004) Usually shows a 'flashback' of blood to indicate a successful venepuncture	More expensive than steel needles The 12–30 cm length of tubing on the device may be caught and dislodge the needle	Veins in sites other than the antecubital fossa When quantities of blood greater than 20 ml are required from any site
	23	Flexible due to small needle shaft. Easy to manipulate and insert at any site. Causes less discomfort. Smaller swg and therefore useful with fragile veins	More expensive than steel needles, plus there can be damage to cells which can cause inaccurate measurements in certain blood samples, e.g. potassium	Small veins in more painful sites, e.g. inner aspect of the wrist, especially if measurements are related to plasma and not cellular components

sterile circulatory system. The two major sources of microbial contamination are:

- Cross-infection from practitioner to patient.
- Skin flora of the patient.

Good hand washing and drying techniques are essential on the part of the nurse; gloves should be changed between patients (see Chapter 5).

To remove the risk presented by the patient's skin flora, firm and prolonged rubbing with an alcohol-based solution, such as chlorhexidine 0.5% in 70% alcohol, is advised (Walther *et al.* 2001). This cleaning should continue for about 30 seconds, although some authors state a minimum of 1 minute or longer (Weinstein 2007). The area that has been cleaned should then be allowed to dry to: (i) facilitate coagulation of the organisms, thus ensuring disinfection; and (ii) prevent a stinging pain on insertion of the needle due to the alcohol on the end of the needle. The skin must not be touched or the vein repalpated prior to venepuncture.

Skin cleaning is a controversial subject and it is acknowledged that a cursory wipe with an alcohol swab does more harm than no cleaning at all as it disturbs the skin flora.

Safety of the practitioner

It is recommended that well-fitting gloves are worn during any procedure that involves handling blood and body fluids, particularly venepuncture and cannulation (Infection Control Nurses Association 2003; NHS Employers 2007; RCN 2005). This is to prevent contamination of the practitioner from potential blood spills. Whilst it is recognized

that gloves will not prevent a needlestick injury, the wiping effect of a glove on a needle may reduce the volume of blood to which the hand is exposed, thereby reducing the volume inoculated and the risk of infection (Mitchell Higgs 2002; Infection Control Nurses Association 2003; National Audit Office 2003). However, there is no substitute for good technique and practitioners must always work carefully when performing venepuncture.

A range of safety devices are now available for venepuncture which can reduce the risk of occupational percutaneous injuries among health care workers, in particular vacuum blood collection systems (CDC 1997). A vacuum system consists of a plastic holder which contains or is attached to a double-ended needle or adaptor. It is important to use the correct Luer adaptor to ensure a good connection and avoid blood leakage (Garza & Becan McBride 2005). The blood tube is vacuumed in order that the exact amount of blood required is withdrawn, when the tube is pushed into the holder. Filling ceases once the tube is full which removes the need for decanting blood and also reduces blood wastage. The system can also be attached to winged infusion devices (Dougherty 2008).

Used needles should always be discarded directly into an approved sharps container, without being resheathed (Infection Control Nurses Association 2003; RCN 2005). Specimens from patients with known or suspected infections such as hepatitis or human immunodeficiency virus (HIV) should have a biohazard label attached. The accompanying request forms should be kept separately from the specimen to avoid contamination (Health Service Advisory Committee 2003). All other non-sharp disposables should be placed in a universal clinical waste bag.

Removal of the device

It is important to ensure that the needle is removed correctly on completion of blood sampling and that the risk of haematoma formation is minimized. Pressure should be applied as the needle is removed from the skin. If pressure is applied too early, it causes the tip of the needle to drag along the intima of the vein, resulting in sharp pain and damage to the lining of the vessel.

The practitioner should ensure that firm pressure is maintained until bleeding has stopped. The patient should also be instructed to keep his or her arm straight and not bend it as this also results in an increased risk of bruising (Ernst 2005). A longer period of pressure may be necessary where the patient's blood may take longer to clot, for example, if the patient is receiving anticoagulants or is thrombocytopenic. The practitioner may choose to apply the tourniquet over the venepuncture site to ensure even and constant pressure on the area (Perdue 2001). Alternatively they can elevate the arm slightly above the heart to decrease venous pressure (Garza & Becan McBride 2005).

The practitioner should inspect the site carefully for bleeding or bruising before applying a dressing to the site, and the patient leaving the department. If bruising has occurred the patient should be informed of why this has happened and given instructions for what to do to reduce the bruising and any associated pain. Initially the application of an ice pack may help to soothe and decrease bruising. The application of Hirudoid cream, which is used for the treatment of thrombophlebitis, may be helpful (BMA & RPS 2008).

Summary

In order to perform a safe and successful venepuncture, it is important that the practitioner:

- Considers carefully the choice of vein and device.
- Applies the principles of asepsis.
- Adheres to and understands safe technique and practices.

Recently there has been an increase in the number of cases of litigation involving injuries, which have occurred as a result of venepuncture (Garza & Becan McBride 2005). It is therefore vital that nurses receive accredited and appropriate training, supervision and assessment by an experienced member of staff (RCN 2005). The nurse is then accountable and responsible for ensuring that his or her skills and competence are maintained and his or her knowledge is kept up to date, in order to fulfil the criteria set out in the *The Code* (NMC 2008).

Procedure guidelines Venepuncture

Equipment

1 Clean tray or receiver.
2 Tourniquet or sphygmomanometer and cuff.
3 21 swg multiple sample needle or 21 swg winged infusion device and multiple sample Luer adaptor.
4 Plastic tube holder, standard or for blood cultures.
5 Appropriate vacuumed specimen tubes.
6 Swab saturated with chlorhexidine in 70% alcohol, or isopropyl alcohol 70%.
7 Low-linting swabs.
8 Sterile adhesive plaster or hypoallergenic tape.
9 Specimen request forms.
10 Non-sterile well-fitting gloves.
11 Plastic apron (optional).
12 Sharps bin.

A number of vacuum systems are available that can be used for taking blood samples. These are simple to use and cost effective. The manufacturer's instructions should be followed if one of these systems is used. Vacuum systems reduce the risk of health care workers being contaminated, because they offer a completely closed system during the process of blood withdrawal and there is no necessity to decant blood into bottles (Dougherty 2008). This makes them the safest method for collecting blood samples using venepuncture. If not available, the following items replace the vacuum system:
1 21 swg needle or 21 swg winged infusion device.
2 Syringe(s) of appropriate size.
3 Appropriate blood specimen bottle(s).

Procedure

Action	Rationale
1 Approach the patient in a confident manner and explain and discuss the procedure with the patient.	To ensure that the patient understands the procedure and gives his/her valid consent (DH 2001: C; NMC 2008: C).
2 Allow the patient to ask questions and discuss any problems which have arisen previously.	Anxiety results in vasoconstriction; therefore, a patient who is relaxed will have dilated veins, making access easier (E).

3 Consult the patient as to any preferences and problems that may have been experienced at previous venepunctures.	To involve the patient in the treatment. To acquaint the nurse fully with the patient's previous venous history and identify any changes in clinical status, e.g. mastectomy, as both may influence vein choice (Dougherty 2008: E).
4 Check the identity of the patient matches the details on the request form by asking for their full name and date of birth and checking their identification bracelet.	To ensure the sample is taken from the correct patient (E).
5 Assemble the equipment necessary for venepuncture.	To ensure that time is not wasted and that the procedure goes smoothly without unnecessary interruptions (E).
6 Carefully wash hands using bactericidal soap and water or bactericidal alcohol handrub, and dry before commencement.	To minimize risk of infection (DH 2005: C).
7 Check hands for any visibly broken skin, and cover with a waterproof dressing.	To minimize the risk of contamination to the practitioner (DH 2005a: C).
8 Check all packaging before opening and preparing the equipment on the chosen clean receptacle.	To maintain asepsis throughout and check that no equipment is damaged (E).
9 Take all the equipment to the patient, exhibiting a competent manner.	To help the patient feel more at ease with the procedure (E).
10 In both an inpatient and an outpatient situation, lighting, ventilation, privacy and positioning must be checked.	To ensure that both patient and operator are comfortable and that adequate light is available to illuminate this procedure (E).
11 Support the chosen limb on a pillow.	To ensure the patient's comfort and facilitate venous access (E).
12 (a) Apply a tourniquet to the upper arm on the chosen side, making sure it does not obstruct arterial flow. If the radial pulse cannot be palpated then the tourniquet is too tight (Weinstein 2007). The position of the tourniquet may be varied, e.g. if a vein in the hand is to be used it may be placed on the forearm. A sphygmomanometer cuff may be used as an alternative.	To dilate the veins by obstructing the venous return (Dougherty 2008: E).
(b) The arm may be placed in a dependent position. The patient may be asked to clench their fist.	To increase the prominence of the veins (E).
(c) The veins may be tapped gently or stroked.	
(d) If all these measures are unsuccessful, remove the tourniquet and apply moist heat, e.g. a warm compress, soak limb in warm water or, with medical prescription, apply glyceryl trinitrate ointment/patch.	To promote blood flow and therefore distend the veins (Lenhardt et al. 2002: R 3; E).
13 Select the vein using the aforementioned criteria (see Action figure 13).	To prevent haemocentration and pooling of the blood (Hoeltke 2006: E).
14 Release the tourniquet.	To ensure patient comfort (E).
15 Select the device, based on vein size, site, etc.	To reduce damage or trauma to the vein (RCN 2005: C; Dougherty 2008: E).

925

Procedure guidelines *(cont.)*

16 Wash hands with bactericidal soap and water or bactericidal alcohol handrub.	To maintain asepsis, and minimize the risk of infection (DH 2005a: C).
17 Reapply the tourniquet.	To dilate the veins by obstructing the venous return (Dougherty 2008: E).
18 Put on gloves.	To prevent possible contamination of the practitioner (NHS Employers 2007: C).
19 Clean the patient's skin carefully for 30 seconds using an appropriate preparation, e.g. chlorhexidine in 70% alcohol, and allow to dry. Do not repalpate or touch the skin (see Action figure 19).	To maintain asepsis and minimize the risk of infection (DH 2005a: C). To prevent pain on insertion (DH 2005a: C; RCN 2005: C; Dougherty 2008: E).
20 Remove the cover from the needle and inspect the device carefully.	To detect faulty equipment, e.g. bent or barbed needles. If these are present place them in a safe container, record batch details and return to manufacturer (MHRA 2005: C; RCN 2005: C).
21 Anchor the vein by applying manual traction on the skin a few centimetres below the proposed insertion site (see Action figure 21).	To immobilize the vein. To provide countertension to the vein which will facilitate a smoother needle entry (Dougherty 2008: E).
22 Insert the needle smoothly at an angle of approximately 30°. However, this will depend on size and depth of the vein (also see Action figure 21).	To facilitate a successful, pain-free venepuncture (E).
23 Reduce the angle of descent of the needle as soon as a flashback of blood is seen in the tubing of a winged infusion device or when puncture of the vein wall is felt. If you are using a needle and syringe, pull the plunger back slightly prior to venepuncture and a flashback of blood will be seen in the barrel on vein entry.	To prevent advancing too far through vein wall and causing damage to the vessel (E).
24 Slightly advance the needle into the vein, if possible.	To stabilize the device within the vein and prevent it becoming dislodged during withdrawal of blood (E).
25 Do not exert any pressure on the needle.	To prevent a puncture occurring through the vein wall (E).
26 Withdraw the required amount of blood using a vacuumed blood collection system or syringes (see Action figure 26). Collect blood samples in the following order: ■ Blood culture. ■ Coagulation. ■ Serum tube with or without clot activator or gel separator. (Glass, non-additive tubes can be filled before the coagulation tube.) ■ Additive tubes such as: (a) gel separator tubes (may contain clot activator or heparin); (b) heparin tubes; (c) EDTA. ■ All other tubes (National Committee for Clinical Laboratory Standards 2003 cited in Garza & Becan McBride 2005, pp. 277–8).	To minimize the risk of transferring additives from one tube to another and bacterial contamination of blood cultures (Manufacturer's guidelines: C).

27	Release the tourniquet. In some instances this may be necessary at the beginning of sampling as inaccurate measurements may be caused by haemostasis, e.g. when taking blood to assess calcium levels.	To decrease the pressure within the vein (E).
	Remove tube from plastic tube holder.	To prevent blood spillage caused by vacuum in the tube (Campbell *et al.* 1999: E).
28	If using a needle and syringe withdraw a small amount of blood into the syringe.	To reduce the amount of static blood in the vein and therefore the likelihood of leakage at the venepuncture site on removal of the needle (E).
29	Pick up a low-linting swab and place it over the puncture point.	To apply pressure (E).
30	Remove the needle, but do not apply pressure until the needle has been fully removed.	To prevent pain on removal and damage to the intima of the vein (E).
31	Activate safety device, if applicable, and then discard the needle immediately in sharps bin.	To reduce the risk of accidental needlestick injury (NHS Employers 2007: C).
32	Apply digital pressure directly over the puncture site. Pressure should be applied until bleeding has ceased; approximately 1 minute or longer may be required if current disease or treatment interferes with clotting mechanisms.	To stop leakage and haematoma formation. To preserve vein by preventing bruising or haematoma formation (E).
33	The patient may apply pressure with the finger but should be discouraged from bending the arm if a vein in the antecubital fossa is used.	To prevent leakage and haematoma formation (Ernst 2005: E).
34	Where a syringe has been used, transfer the blood to appropriate specimen bottles as soon as possible, making sure that the correct quantity is placed in each container.	To prevent clotting in the syringe. To ensure that an adequate amount is available for each test (E).
35	Gently invert tube at least six times.	To prevent damage to blood cells and to mix with additives (Manufacturer's guidelines: C).
36	Label the bottles with the relevant details.	To ensure that the specimens from the right patient are delivered to the laboratory, the requested tests are performed and the results returned to the correct patient's records (E).
37	Inspect the puncture point before applying a dressing.	To check that the puncture point has sealed (E).
38	Ascertain whether the patient is allergic to adhesive plaster.	To prevent an allergic skin reaction (E).
39	Apply an adhesive plaster or alternative dressing.	To cover the puncture and prevent leakage or contamination (E).
40	Ensure that the patient is comfortable.	To ascertain whether patient wishes to rest before leaving (if an outpatient) or whether any other measures need to be taken (E).

41 Remove gloves and discard waste, making sure it is placed in the correct containers, e.g. sharps into a designated receptacle.

To ensure safe disposal and avoid laceration or other injury of staff. (DH 2005b: C). To prevent reuse of equipment. (MDA 2000: C).

42 Follow hospital procedure for collection and transportation of specimens to the laboratory.

To make sure that specimens reach their intended destination (E).

Action 13   Palpating the vein.

Action 19   Cleaning the skin.

Action 21   Anchoring the skin.

Action 26   Attach sample bottle to holder.

Problem solving: Venepuncture

Problem	Cause	Prevention	Suggested action
Pain.	Puncturing an artery.	Knowledge of location of an artery. Palpate vessel for pulse.	Remove device immediately and apply pressure until bleeding stops. Explain to patient what has happened. Inform patient to contact doctor if pain continues or there is increasing swelling or bruising. Document in the patient's notes. Provide information leaflet.
	Touching a nerve (sharp, shooting pain along arm and fingers).	Knowledge of location of nerves. Avoid excessive or blind probing after needle has been inserted.	Remove the needle immediately and apply pressure. Explain to the patient what has happened and that the pain or numbness may last a few hours. Document in the patient's notes. Inform patient to contact doctor if pain continues or becomes worse. Provide information leaflet.

Problem	Cause Anxiety.	Prevention (See below.)	Suggested action (See below.)
	Use of vein in sensitive area (e.g. wrist).	Avoid using veins in sensitive areas wherever possible. Use local anaesthetic cream.	Complete procedure as quickly as possible.
Anxiety.	Previous trauma.	Minimize the risk of a traumatic venepuncture. Use all methods available to ensure successful venepuncture.	Approach patient in a calm and confident manner. Listen to the patient's fears and explain what the procedure involves. Offer patient opportunity to lie down. Suggest use of local anaesthetic cream (Lavery & Ingram 2005).
	Fear of needles.		All of the above and perhaps referral to a psychologist if fear is of phobic proportions.
Limited venous access.	Repeated use of same veins.	Use alternative sites if possible.	Do not attempt the procedure unless experienced.
	Peripheral shutdown.	Ensure the room is not cold.	Put patient's arm in warm water. Apply glycerol trinitrate patch.
	Dehydration.		May be necessary to rehydrate patient prior to venepuncture.
	Hardened veins (due to scarring and thrombosis).		Do not use these veins as venepuncture will be unsuccessful.
Bruising and/or haematoma.	Needle has punctured the posterior wall of the vein. Inadequate pressure on removal of needle.	Lower angle of insertion. The practitioner should apply pressure.	Remove the needle and apply pressure at the venepuncture site until bleeding stops. The following actions apply regardless of cause: (a) Elevate the limb. (b) Apply ice pack if necessary. (c) Apply Hirudoid cream or arnica cream (as per instructions) with pressure dressing.
	Forgetting to remove the tourniquet before removing the needle.		Explain to patient what has happened. Inform patient to contact doctor if area becomes more painful as haematoma may be pressing on a nerve. Do not reapply tourniquet to affected limb. Provide information leaflet. Document.
	Poor technique/choice of vein or device.	Ensure correct device and technique are used.	
Infection at the venepuncture site.	Poor aseptic technique.	Ensure good hand washing and adequate skin cleaning.	Report to doctor as patient may require systemic or local antibiotics.

Problem solving *(cont.)*

Problem	Cause	Prevention	Suggested action
Vasovagal reaction.	Fear of needles. Pain.	Spend time listening to patient's fears in a calm, confident manner.	Place patient's head between his/her legs if patient is feeling faint. Encourage patient to lie down. Call for assistance. It may be appropriate to secure the device (short term) in case it is required for the administration of medication.
	Warm environment.	Ensure environment is comfortable temperature.	Open a window or door.
Needle inoculation of or contamination to practitioner.	Unsafe practice. Incorrect disposal of sharps.	Maintain safe practice. Activate safety device if applicable. Ensure sharps are disposed of immediately and safely.	Follow accident procedure for sharps injury, e.g. make site bleed and apply a waterproof dressing. Report and document. An injection of hepatitis B immunoglobulin or triple therapy may be required.
Accidental blood spillage.	Damaged/faulty equipment.	Check equipment prior to use.	Report within hospital and/or MHRA.
	Reverse vacuum.	Use vacuumed plastic blood collection system. Remove blood tube from plastic tube holder before removing needle.	Ensure blood is handled and transported correctly.
Missed vein.	Inadequate anchoring. Poor vein selection. Wrong positioning. Lack of concentration. Poor lighting.	Ensure that only properly trained staff perform venepuncture or that those who are training are supervised. Ensure the environment is well lit.	Withdraw the needle slightly and realign it, providing the patient is not feeling any discomfort. Ensure all learners are supervised. If the patient is feeling pain, then the needle should be removed immediately.
	Difficult venous access.		Ask experienced colleague to perform the procedure.
Spurt of blood on entry.	Bevel tip of needle enters the vein before entire bevel is under the skin; usually occurs when the vein is very superficial.		Reassure the patient. Wipe blood away on removal of needle.
Blood stops flowing.	Through puncture: needle inserted too far.	Correct angle.	Draw back the needle, but if bruising is evident, then remove the needle immediately and apply pressure.
	Contact with valves.	Palpate to locate.	Withdraw needle slightly to move tip away from valve.
	Venous spasm.	Results from mechanical irritation and cannot be prevented.	Gently massage above the vein or apply heat.

Problem	Cause	Prevention	Suggested action
	Vein collapse.	Use veins with large lumen. Use a smaller device.	Release tourniquet, allow veins to refill and retighten tourniquet.
	Small vein.	Avoid use of small veins wherever possible.	May require another venepuncture.
	Poor blood flow.	Use veins with large lumens.	Apply heat above vein.

References and further reading

BMA & RPS (2008) *British National Formulary*. British Medical Association and Royal Pharmaceutical Society of Great Britain, London.

Campbell, H., Carrington, M. & Limber, C. (1999) A practice guide to venepuncture and management of complications. *Br J Nurs*, 8(7), 426–31.

Castledine, G. (1996) Nurses' role in peripheral venous cannulation. *Br J Nurs*, 5(20), 1274.

CDC (1997) Evaluation of safety devices for preventing percutaneous injuries among health care workers during phlebotomy procedures. *JAMA*, 277(6), 449–50.

DH (2001) *Good Practice in Consent Implementation Guide: Consent to Examination or Treatment*. www.dh.gov.uk. Accessed 24/9/07.

DH (2005a) *Saving Lives: A Delivery Programme to Reduce Healthcare Associated Infection including MRSA*. Department of Health, London.

DH (2005b) *Hazardous Waste (England) Regulations*. Department of Health, London.

Dougherty, L. (2008) Obtaining vascular access. In: *IV Therapy in Practice* (eds L. Dougherty & J. Lamb), 2nd edn. Blackwell Publishing, Oxford.

Ernst, D. & Ernst, C. (2001) *Phlebotomy for Nurses and Nursing Personnel*. Health Star Press, Indiana.

Ernst, D.J. (2005) *Applied Phlebotomy*. Lippincott, Williams & Wilkins, Baltimore.

Garza, D. & Becan McBride, K. (2005) *Phlebotomy Handbook: Blood Collection Essentials*. Prentice Hall, New Jersey.

Golder, M. (2000) Potential risk of cross infection during peripheral venous access by contamination of tourniquets. *Lancet*, 355, 44.

Health Service Advisory Committee (2003) *Safe Working and the Prevention of Infection in Clinical Laboratories and Similar Facilities*. HMSO, London.

Hefler, L. *et al.* (2004) To butterfly or to needle: the pilot phase. *Ann Intern Med*, 140(11), 935–6.

Hoeltke, L.B. (2006) *The Complete Textbook of Phlebotomy*, 3rd edn. Thomson Delmar Learning, New York.

Hudek, K. (1986) Compliance in IV therapy. *J Can Intraven Nurs Assoc*, 2(3), 3–8.

Hyde, L. (2008) Legal and professional aspects of IV therapy. In: *IV Therapy in Practice* (eds L. Dougherty & J. Lamb). Churchill Livingstone, Edinburgh.

Infection Control Nurses Association (2003) *Reducing Sharps Injury – Prevention and Risk Management*. Infection Control Nurses Association, London.

Intravenous Nursing Society (2006) *Standards for Infusion Therapy*. Intravenous Nursing Society & Becton Dickinson and Company, New York.

Lavery, I. & Ingram, P. (2005) Venepuncture: best practice. *Nurs Stand*, 19(49), 55–65.

Lenhardt, R. *et al.* (2002) Active hand warming eases peripheral intravenous catheter insertion. *BMJ*, 325, 409–12.

Masoorli, S. (2002) Catheter related nerve injury: inherent risk or avoidable outcome? *J Vasc Access Devices*, 7(4), 49.

McCall, R.E. & Tankersley, C.M. (2003) Blood collection variables and procedural errors. In: *Phlebotomy Essentials*, 3rd edn. Lippincott, Williams & Wilkins, Philadelphia.

Medical Devices Agency (MDA) (REFA) (2000) Single-use medical devices: implications and consequences of reuse. In: *Device Bulletin 2000, 04*. Department of Health, London.

MHRA (2005) *Alert MDA 2005/01 and Device Bulletin DB 2005 (01), Reporting Adverse Incidents and Disseminating Medical Device Alerts*. Medicines and Healthcare Products Agency, London.

Mitchell Higgs, N. (2002) Personal protective equipment – improving compliance. All Points Conference, Safer Needles Network, London, May.

National Audit Office (2003) *A Safer Place to Work – Management of Health and Safety Risks in Trusts*. National Audit Office, London.

NHS Employers (2007) Needlestick injury. In: *The Healthy Workplaces Handbook*. National Health Service, London, Chapter 19.

NMC (2008) *The Code: Standards of Conduct, Performance and Ethics for Nurses and Midwives*. Nursing and Midwifery Council, London.

Perdue, M.B. (2001) Intravenous complications. In: *Infusion Therapy in Clinical Practice* (eds J. Hankin *et al.*), 2nd edn. W.B. Saunders, Philadelphia, pp. 418–45.

RCN (1995) *Universal Precautions*. Royal College of Nursing, London.

RCN (2005) *Standards for Infusion Therapy*. Royal College of Nursing, London.

Smith, J. (1998) The practice of venepuncture in lymphoedema. *Eur J Cancer Care*, 7, 97–8.

Walther, K. *et al.* (2001) IV therapy in the older adult. In: *Infusion Therapy in Clinical Practice* (eds J. Hankin *et al.*), 2nd edn. W.B. Saunders, Philadelphia, pp. 592–603.

Waugh, A. & Grant, A. (2006) The cardiovascular system. In: *Anatomy and Physiology in Health and Illness*, 10th edn. Churchill Livingstone, Edinburgh, p. 101.

Weinstein, S.M. (2007) *Plumer's Principles and Practice of Intravenous Therapy*, 8th edn. Lippincott, Williams & Wilkins, Philadelphia.

Chapter 47

Violence: prevention and management

933 Reference material
938 *Procedure guidelines:* Violence: prevention and management
940 References and further reading

Definition

Violence is endemic in our health care system and is, for many staff working in certain areas, an almost daily occurrence (NMC 2002). Violence at work can be defined as:

> Any incident in which a health care employee is verbally abused, threatened or assaulted by a patient or member of the public in the circumstances of their employment.

(HSE 2000: 1)

The Royal College of Nursing (RCN) recommends the following definition of violence orientated towards staff members:

> Any incident in which a health professional experiences abuse, threat, fear or the application of force arising out of the course of their work, whether or not they are on duty.

(RCN 1998: 3)

However, as violence is also directed towards other individuals and objects, the local policy should encompass these aspects. The Nursing and Midwifery Council (NMC) advises nurses to be aware of their individual organizational policies on assessment and management of violence. This should extend to being aware of what support is available should an incident occur.

It can therefore be concluded from the above definitions that violence is an act or type of behaviour that may take the form of aggression, abuse, threat or assault (with or without injury).

Reference material

Prevalence

In 1999, the government developed the National Health Service (NHS) 'Zero Tolerance' Campaign in England with the aim of tackling the issue of violence and intimidation against NHS staff. The target was to reduce incidents of violence in all trusts by 30% by 2003. However, violent crime in the UK is steadily increasing and nearly 650 000 workers had experienced at least one violent incident during 1997 (Mahar 2002). In 1999 there were 65 000 reported violent incidents in British hospitals. By 2001 the number had increased by 30% to 85 000 (DH 2001). In April 2003 the NHS Security Management Service was set up to work with the Crown Prosecution Service taking legal action against those who assault health care workers. Donnelly (2006) described the figures released, showing 51 prosecutions in 2002/03 compared to 759 in 2004/05. With improved reporting systems there has been a 15-fold increase in the number of prosecutions (DH 2006). Official figures for 2005 showed 60 385 NHS staff physically assaulted, i.e. one assault for every 22 NHS staff (DH 2006). The RCN's Working Well Survey (RCN 2005) showed 79% of Accident and Emergency (A&E) nurses reported being victims of violent attack during 2005/06 compared to ward (52%) and care home (48%) nurses.

Moreover, there is evidence to suggest that acts of violence against NHS staff, for a variety of reasons, are still underreported (Arnetz & Arnetz 2000; Rippon 2000; Beech 2001; Paterson et al. 2001; Fern 2006). Nonetheless, assaults in the UK are now the third most common type of reported accident after slips, falls and needle accidents. Nurses, ambulance and A&E staff, and those caring for psychologically disturbed patients, are particularly vulnerable (Dobson 1999). Incidents range from threats and abuse to permanently disabling injuries and, rarely, loss of life. Wells and Bowers (2002) carried out a systematic literature search focusing on data of the prevalence of violence towards nurses in general hospitals in the UK; they concluded a majority of assaults occur outside the A&E, citing Whittington et al. (1996). They also identified differences in definition of violence and suggested a three category classification; namely, abuse, threats and assaults (with or without injury). The issue of underreporting was also highlighted.

This chapter aims to consider assessment and management of violence in non-psychiatric hospital settings. It is set out following the National Institute for Health and Clinical Excellence (NICE) guideline on violence (NICE 2005) considering: prediction, prevention, intervention and post-incident review. Firstly, a reference to legislation.

Legislation

The law on health and safety at work applies to risks from violence, just as it does to other risks at work. Key points are summarized as follows.

1 *Health and Safety at Work Act* (Department of Employment 1974):
   Employers must:
   (a) Protect the health and safety at work of their employees
   (b) Protect the health and safety of others who might be affected, such as visitors, contractors, students and patients.
2 *Management of Health and Safety at Work Regulations* (HSE 1999):
   Employers must:
   (a) Assess the risks to the health and safety of their employees
   (b) Identify the precautions needed to reduce the risks of violence
   (c) Make arrangements for the effective management of risks
   (d) Appoint competent people to advise them on health and safety
   (e) Provide information and training to employees.
3 *The Reporting of Injuries, Diseases and Dangerous Occurrences Regulations* (HSE 1995):

These Regulations state that employers must report cases in which employees have been off work for 3 days or more following an assault which has resulted in physical injury. This should be in conjunction with the local incident policy in which any psychological injury is also documented.

4 *The Safety Representatives and Safety Committees Regulations 1977 and The Health and Safety (Consultation with Employees) Regulations 1996 (HSE 1996):*
Employers must consult with safety representatives and employees on health and safety matters (Health Services Advisory Committee 1997).

5 *Employment Rights Act (1996)* (Department of Employment 1996):
Outlines staff member's right to withdraw from his/her care environment if he/she feels seriously under threat.

6 In 2003, the NHS Security Management Service instigated a new reporting system based on clear definitions of violence. Special investigators and NHS legal protection units work now with the Crown Prosecution Service.

Policy formation

NHS Trusts must establish targets for reducing violence against their staff. In addition, NHS Trusts will be expected to have systems in place to monitor and record violence against staff and have published strategies in place to achieve a reduction in such incidents (Dobson 1999).

In forming a policy for managing aggression or violence, the following aspects need to be considered:

- Anticipation and prevention of violence.
- Environmental and organizational factors.
- Action following an incident.

Prediction

The NICE guidance for the short-term management of violence (NICE 2005) refers to a list of risk factors to predict potential violent behaviour. The risks are divided into the following categories: demographic or personal history; clinical variables; situational variables; antecedents and warning signs:

Demographic/personal history

- History of violent behaviour.
- History of substance/alcohol misuse.
- Previous expression of violent intent.
- Known personal triggers.
- Verbal threats of violence.
- Recent severe stress.

Clinical variables

- Active symptoms, e.g. hallucinations, agitation.
- Substance misuse.

- Poor collaboration with treatment.
- Antisocial, impulsive personality traits.
- Organic dysfunction.

Situation variables

- Extent of social support.
- Availability of weapon.
- Relationship to potential victim especially if previous difficulties known.
- Access to potential victim.
- Limit settings.
- Staff attitudes.

Antecedents/warning signs

- Tense angry facial signs.
- Increased restlessness.
- General overarousal of body systems (increased heart rate, breathing, muscle twitching, dilating pupils).
- Increased volume of speech.
- Prolonged eye contact.
- Discontentment, refusal to communicate, fear.
- Unclear thought process.
- Delusions or hallucinations.
- Verbal threats.
- Similar behaviour to previous incidents of violence.
- Reporting angry feelings.
- Blocking escape routes.

Prediction of violence may also be understood in terms of factors that may combine to explain or produce a violent act. These are reviewed by Harrington (1972) and Gunn (1973). Generally, theories of violence may be classified as biological (Lorenz 1966; Gray 1971; Montague 1979), psychological (Freud 1955; Dollard & Miller 1961) or socio-cultural (Bandura & Walters 1963; Wertham 1968; Gelles 1972). Although the latter of these cannot be completely divorced from organic or biological predisposition, certain factors may increase the risk of violent or aggressive behaviour. Glasser (1998) also discusses the psychoanalytical perspective of violent acts which may be characterized as one of two types: self-preservation violence or sado-masochistic violence. Self-preservation violence is given as an instinctive, primitive response to danger or threat, whereas sado-masochistic violence is premeditated, usually sustained and pleasure is derived from the suffering of the object (Glasser 1998). In the hospital setting where reactions to stress, illness and treatment are prevalent, prediction, assessment and prevention will help to manage potentially violent situations.

It is important to realize that each visitor, contractor, outpatient or relative visiting the hospital will have individual needs, anxieties and expectations. Tension may be released in terms of anger, and on occasions violence, towards other members of their family or staff that they encounter.

Factors such as poor sign-posting, failure to find a parking space, long waiting times for an appointment, inadequate welfare facilities, perceived queue-jumping and inadequate information can all increase the risk of conflict and aggression (Royal Marsden Hospital 2002).

Under certain circumstances patients may have little or no ability to exercise control over their aggression. In these instances aggression may be related to pathological physiology. Internal stressors may include endocrine imbalance such as hyperthyroidism and hyperglycaemia. Krakowski and Czobor (1994) confirmed an association between persistent violence and neurological impairment, e.g. convulsive disorders, human immunodeficiency virus (HIV), encephalopathy, dementia and brain tumours. The effects of alcohol and substance abuse should also be considered. One study showed that rates for people with schizophrenia perpetrating violent acts were four times those of populations without mental disorders. For the so-called dual diagnosis populations (with co-existing mental illness and drug/alcohol misuse), rates were four times higher than for people with schizophrenia, i.e. 16 times higher than the general population (NMC 2002). Among the physiological causes given by Kerr and Taylor (1997) are pain, side-effects of medication (including neuroleptic-induced akathisia) and childhood disorders such as autism and mental retardation.

Common antecedents include patients' boredom, inadequate staffing levels, lack of opportunity for patients to participate in therapy and social groups, and staff attitudes, including physical abuse, racism, ridicule of service users and matters of confidentiality (NMC 2002).

Incidents of verbal or physical abuse are more likely to happen in long-term care and emergency areas and may be directed towards nurses and nursing assistants rather than doctors. In the UK, of all health care professions and grades, student nurses were at the greatest risk of being the victim of a work-related violent incident (Beech 1999). Furthermore, male staff were more involved in actual recorded incidents than expected in the given population (Vanderslott 1998). Violence may be viewed as behaviour influenced by various factors including personality, environment and social culture. Each perspective may add to the development of a body of knowledge about the problem of violence in the hospital setting.

Risk assessment

The purpose of risk assessment of violence is to identify how and why conflict can occur and consider what measures can be taken to reduce the risks of such events within the workplace. The risk assessment process for the identification and control of violence can be separated into the following steps: environmental; organizational; situational and attitudinal (NICE 2005).

It is helpful if there is an assessment form for the risks that are being assessed which can be completed in discussion with staff within the department. A review of past incidents will provide an opportunity to identify potential sources of conflict, potential aggressors and likely risk factors. For example, the assessment should consider whether any particular areas present a higher risk of violence such as:

- Front-line reception areas.
- Inpatient clinical areas.
- Outpatient clinical areas.
- Communal areas.
- Community.
- Lone working, e.g. interview rooms, isolated offices.

Regular and comprehensive risk assessments will ensure the clinical environment remains safe. Assessments can also highlight specific interventions which may be required in the management of an ongoing violent situation.

Structured and sensitive interviews ascertaining the patient's view and their level of awareness in relation to their trigger factors and early warning signs. Multidisciplinary involvement appropriate to the clinical setting should also be reflected in the assessment.

Cultural awareness is important specifically in relation to behaviours which may be misinterpreted as being aggressive.

Following assessment, if the risk of violent behaviour is identified intervention and management strategies should be recorded within a care plan and in the medical records. High risk assessments may necessitate searching the person identified as a risk. This must only happen according to local policy.

Prevention

Preventing situations of violent and aggressive behaviour include consideration of the following factors:

- Use of communication skills including de-escalation techniques.
- Training.
- Formulating a care plan.
- Deciding upon the appropriate level of observation.
- Environmental and organizational.

Signs of high arousal (boisterousness), irritability, confusion and anger (threats or attacks on inanimate objects) are reliable predictors of imminent assaults on staff (Whittington 1997). Responding to these cues to violence with an appropriate verbal interaction and non-verbal behaviour can prevent the escalation of an incident (NMC 2002).

Sheffield University has developed a model for de-escalation called 'CASE', the acronym standing for Calming, Accessing and Self Enabling, which takes into account the internal (thoughts and feelings) and external (behaviour) communication factors for both the nurse and the patient (Walker 2002). The nurse uses verbal and non-verbal skills to calm the situation down and access his or her own thoughts and feelings whilst encouraging the patient to do the same. For example, the nurse asks the angry patient if he would like to sit down and talk about what is upsetting him. This enables the nurse to assess not only the patient's level of emotion but also his cognitive ability to help resolve the conflict. When the patient sits down as offered and is ready to engage in conversation, the enabling phase comes into effect. There may be more negotiating language in the communication which gives an indication that the anger is subsiding to a level where he is more able to think and behave rationally (Walker 2002).

Knowledge of the propensities of individual patients will enable a nurse to recognize many of the signs of impending violence, thus allowing steps to be taken to help patients find alternative outlets for their aggressive feelings. These can be documented in the patient's care plan.

The way in which staff are deployed influences the likelihood and outcome of any violent incident. Teaching sessions on the management of violence should be held on a regular basis so that staff benefit from controlled practice of the required techniques for avoiding or containing violence. Topics may include assessment and prediction of risk factors, the do's and don'ts of verbal and non-verbal interaction and breakaway skills training (Beech 1999).

The NICE guidance for the short-term management of violence (2005) describes four different levels of observation: general; intermittent; within eyesight; and within arm's length. The least intrusive level should be adopted as appropriate.

Hospital environments can be stressful places and so certain design features can help to maximize a tranquil ambience. Calming features include creating a perception of space, ensuring there is natural daylight and fresh air and noise levels are controlled, providing smoking and non-smoking areas and ensuring privacy in toilet and bathroom areas. In creating a secure environment (in psychiatric settings) there must be a safe room for severely disturbed people. This list is not exhaustive and many other features are possible when considering environmental factors (Royal College of Psychiatrists 1998).

The response of staff to aggressive situations may be influenced by factors such as workload, stress, illness, confidence and experience. When long hours are worked, or a heavy workload is undertaken, staff may feel under increased stress. Misunderstandings, failure to clarify task requirements or requests can lead to verbal abuse or aggression. It should not be seen as a weakness of staff if they try to avoid violence. The level of training provided for staff (in terms of undertaking the work required, customer care skills, dealing with aggression, how to diffuse awkward situations, etc.) can also influence the degree of risk (Royal Marsden Hospital 2002).

Once the hazards and risks have been identified, the next step required is a review of the procedures already in place to reduce the risks. Any additional precautions, procedures or control measures required can then be implemented:

- Providing comfortable seating.
- Providing access to refreshment.
- Providing appropriate facilities for the disabled.
- Improving communication systems and multilingual notices and signposts.
- Reducing waiting times.
- Providing staff training.
- Increasing personal security systems, such as closed-circuit television.
- Providing staff support.
- Introducing an incident reporting system.

Intervention

Agreement within the policy should be considered concerning what criteria are used before calling the police to attend an incident. This will depend on the severity of the situation and persons or property at risk (RCN 1998). The involvement of the police and the criminal justice system is discussed at greater length in the NMC (2002) document. To summarize:

- Summoning police assistance generally means that the police will assume responsibility for the control of the violent incident, rather than seeing themselves as assisting nursing staff. The police will then deal with the situation as they see fit.
- The police are obliged to take action after any crime, which may take the form of a warning, a caution or a charge.
- The victim may be asked if they wish to take part in proceedings but does not have the responsibility, as is often thought, of 'pressing charges'.

Taking police action is often thought of as a last resort because of staff feeling that they have failed to manage the incident effectively or that the patient's medical or mental health needs will be overlooked, or fearing that a police presence will inflame the situation. However, there may be several benefits: it would increase the likelihood of the incident being recorded in the medical notes; it may lead to more appropriate future treatment; it may also communicate and enforce a firm message that violence will not be tolerated and that the patient is to be held responsible for his or her behaviour (NMC 2002).

Perhaps the most significant advance in the management of violence in recent years is the documentation on physical restraint. This has been comprehensively reviewed by Wright (1999) and is recognized as being a controversial and emotive topic. Since the mid-1980s, staff in health care and local authority settings have received training in methods for physically managing violence and aggression, termed 'control and restraint' (C&R). The use of this procedure has expanded to such an extent that in a survey of inpatient care in inner London (Gournay *et al.* 1998, cited in Wright 1999), only one of 11 inner London trusts surveyed did not routinely train acute nursing staff in C&R. However, there are safety, ethical and legal implications to be considered before embarking on these methods. There have been instances of accidental death of patients resulting from restraint procedures being inappropriately or incorrectly applied (Wright 1999). This is particularly relevant when working with patients who are elderly, infirm or sedated. It is also worth noting that while physical restraint may be seen as potentially damaging to a patient's physical or mental well-being, the consequences of not restraining a patient who is attempting to harm themselves or others may be even more damaging to the patient's self-esteem and may preserve life and/or minimize harm in the short term (Wright 1999). Whatever physical restraint method is employed, it is vital to apply it uniformly and it should only be conducted by appropriately trained and accredited staff. If there is an incident team in the hospital that is expected to respond to urgent situations where there is violence or the threat of violence, then each member of that team should have received training commensurate with their role and contact with patients (NMC 2002).

Once violence has occurred, the following may be regarded as important management decisions that need to be implemented:

- Medical personnel should be informed immediately because medication may be required as part of the management of the situation.
- Some nurses must be delegated to attend to the needs of the remaining patients, to telephone for help and to prepare any required medication.
- If immobilization is needed, the agreed local policy for seclusion of the patient, physical intervention of a patient or rapid tranquillization must be implemented.

Post-incident review

The law regarding assault and self-defence is complicated and often inconsistent. There is further complication in that, while certain responses to violence may be permissible under the law, the actions of health care staff are also regulated by codes of professional practice (Wright 1999). At all times *The NMC Code* must be adhered to (NMC 2008). This is discussed in further detail in *Dealing with Violence against Nursing Staff* (RCN 1998) but Point 5.3 on confidentiality and information disclosure and Point 8 on identifying and minimizing risk are particularly pertinent. If legal advice needs to be obtained in a particular case, such as financial compensation or prosecution following personal injury or damage to property, this should be obtained from a solicitor, barrister, health and safety representative and/or trade union representative.

Following the incident, staff should be given an opportunity to discuss their feelings about the aggressor(s), other members of staff involved and the way the incident was managed. This should happen as soon as possible after the

incident has resolved and with as many of the staff concerned as possible. There should be discussion on:

- What happened during the incident.
- Any trigger factors.
- Roles of the people involved in the incident.
- How they feel now and may feel in the near future.
- What can be done to address concerns.
- Any measures that can be taken to avoid a repeat of the situation (RCN 1998).

Emotional debriefing aims to recognize potential stress, acknowledge it as a normal response and provide a supportive and structured setting to allow people to cope more effectively. Discussion should not be focused on any person's performance but address the effects on them as individuals (Health Services Advisory Committee 1997). In addition to the debriefing procedure, the physical and psychological well-being of the staff involved and the team as a whole need to be addressed. Staff injured as a result of their involvement in the incident may be entitled to industrial injuries benefit or a payment under the criminal injuries compensation scheme and will need to be informed of their rights by the appropriate body (RCN 1998). Consideration must be given to the risk of infection in cases where injury has occurred; for example, bites or needlestick injuries. Staff must receive continued support when returning to work after a violent incident (RCN 1998). Debriefing can be supplemented by making confidential counselling available through in-house counsellors, occupational health departments or independent external bodies (Health Services Advisory Committee 1997).

Some staff view reporting of incidents as admission of failure, especially if violence is rare in the area in which they work, therefore debriefing becomes particularly relevant in order to promote reporting of incidents (Rippon 2000; Paterson *et al.* 2001; NMC 2002).

All documentation required by law (such as the reporting of staff off work for 3 days or more following an assault) or hospital policy (such as completing an incident form) should be completed and forwarded to the appropriate departments. Specific and accurate written records will aid recall if it is required, perhaps years later (RCN 1998).

Summary

Violent incidents often arise from a patient feeling vulnerable and attack may become the preferred means of defence. The manner in which a patient is approached may be crucial in determining whether the patient will feel secure enough to cease the behaviour or to continue to feel threatened, perhaps leading on to violent behaviour. The need for rapid tranquillization, seclusion or physical intervention should be seen as the application of the appropriate technique in a particular situation and not as a failure of other methods. Protection against any administrative or legal problems lies in following the appropriate guidelines and applying them in good faith and with due restraint.

Procedure guidelines   Violence: prevention and management

This guideline is based on the NICE guideline, *Violence. The Short-Term Management of Disturbed/Violent Behaviour in Psychiatric In-Patient Settings and Emergency Departments* (NICE 2005). This evidence is graded C, E.

Prediction of violence

Procedure

Action
Multidisciplinary team assessment for:
1 Demographic/personal history:
  ■ History of violent/disturbed behaviour.
  ■ Misuse of substances.
  ■ Evidence of social restlessness.
  ■ Known personal triggers.
  ■ Verbal threats of violence.
  ■ Recent severe stress especially loss.

Rationale
To reduce risk of a violent situation developing. If risk identified, steps should be taken to avoid violence arising.

2 Clinical variables:
  ■ Organic dysfunction, e.g. endocrine imbalance, convulsive disorders, dementia, neurological impairment, encephalopathy.
  ■ Drug toxicity.
  ■ Alcohol and substance misuse.
  ■ Psychiatric factors, e.g. personality disorder, symptoms of schizophrenia, antisocial impulsive behaviour.

3 Situational variables:
  ■ Staff attitudes.
  ■ Extent of social support.
  ■ Limit settings.

4 Antecedents/warning signs:
  ■ Tense angry facial signs.
  ■ Increased restlessness.
  ■ General overarousal of body systems (increased heart rate, breathing, muscle twitching, dilating pupils).
  ■ Increased volume of speech.
  ■ Prolonged eye contact.
  ■ Discontentment, refusal to communicate, fear.
  ■ Unclear thought process.
  ■ Delusions or hallucinations.
  ■ Verbal threats.
  ■ Similar behaviour to previous incidents of violence.
  ■ Reporting angry feelings.
  ■ Blocking escape routes.

5 Process of risk assessment considering:
  ■ Environmental.
  ■ Organizational.
  ■ Situational.
  ■ Attitudinal.

To identify why and how conflict can occur.

Prevention of violence

Procedure

Action	Rationale
Consideration of the following factors: 1 Environmental/organizational: ■ Perception of space. ■ Natural daylight. ■ Noise levels. ■ Provide smoking and non-smoking areas. ■ Privacy in toilet/bathroom and changing room areas.	To maintain a safe environment for all patients, staff and visitors present and to avoid aggravating the situation further.
2 Use of communication skills: ■ Respond to cues with measured and reasonable action. ■ Consider appropriate de-escalation technique. ■ Avoid provocation. ■ Develop staff and patient awareness of triggers and document in care plan.	
3 Observation: ■ Consider level of observation according to local policy.	

Intervention and management of violence

Procedure

Action	Rationale
1 A staff member should assume control and consider the need for further personnel to assist with the management of the situation.	To effectively manage the situation and inform staff and distressed individual who is taking responsibility for resolving the issues.
2 Remove other patients and relatives from area.	To minimize the risk of physical injury to patients and others.
3 Staff should ensure their non-verbal communication is non-threatening and non-provocative.	To de-escalate the risk of violence.
4 Use appropriate alarm to enlist help and contact patient's medical team.	To ensure the patient is given the appropriate treatment if required.
5 Consider contacting police if local policy indicates.	To maintain safe environment and contain violence if occurring.
6 If necessary apply physical intervention, seclusion, consider rapid tranquillization.	Physical and/or medical restraint may be required in the management of the patient.

Post-violent-incident review

Procedure

Action	Rationale
1 Attend to patients and staff injured during the incident.	To provide care and support to those involved.
2 A post-incident review should occur within 72 hours to address psychological concerns of patients and staff.	To comply with legal obligations and hospital policy.
3 Document Incident.	
4 Identify risk factors and/or triggers.	To prevent a repeat of the incident.

References and further reading

Arnetz, J.E. & Arnetz, B.B. (2000) Implementation and evaluation of a practical intervention programme for dealing with violence towards health care workers. *J Adv Nurs*, **31**(3), 668–80.

Bandura, A. & Walters, R. (1963) *Social Learning and Personality Development*. Holt, Rinehart & Winston, New York.

Beech, B. (1999) Sign of the times or the shape of things to come? A 3-day unit of instruction on 'aggression and violence in health settings for all students during pre-registration nurse training'. *Nurse Educ Today*, **19**(8), 610–16.

Beech, B. (2001) Zero tolerance of violence against health care staff. *Nurs Stand*, **15**(16), 39–41.

Briant, A. (2003) Developing a risk assessment policy. *Prim Health Care*, **13**(4), 39–41.

Brockmann, M. (2002) New perspectives on violence in social care. *J Soc Work*, **2**(1), 29–44.

Cembrowicz, S. (1989) Dealing with difficult patients: what goes wrong? *Practitioner*, **233**(5), 486–9.

Department of Employment (1974) *Health and Safety at Work Act*. www.hse.gov.uk/legislation/hswa.pdf. Accessed 30/11/07.

Department of Employment (1996) *Employment Rights Act*. www.opsi.gov.uk/acts/1996/1996018.htm.

DH (2001) *Withholding Treatment from Violent and Abusive Patients in NHS Trusts: NHS Zero Tolerance Zone*. HSC 2001/18. HMSO, London.

DH (2006) *Bullies Who Threaten NHS Staff are Shown Red Card as New Figures Reveal 1 in 22 NHS Workers Suffer Violence*. Press Release, ref. 2006/0214, HMSO, London.

Dobson, F. (1999) *Dobson Steps Up Major Drive to Protect NHS Staff from Assaults: Violence and Security*. Memorandum from NHS Executive. Press Release, 15 April. Stationery Office, London.

Dollard, J. & Miller, N.E. (1961) *Frustration and Aggression*. Yale University Press, New Haven.

Donnelly, C. (2006) Tackling violence head on. *Emerg Nurse*, **13**(10), 5.

Fern, T. (2006) Underreporting of violent incidents against nursing staff. *Nurs Stand*, **20**(40), 41–5.

Freud, S. (1955) *The Complete Psychological Works of Sigmund Freud*, Vol. 18. Hogarth Press, London.

Gelles, R.J. (1972) *The Violent Home*. Sage, Beverly Hills.

Glasser, M. (1998) On violence: a preliminary communication. *Int J Psycho-Analysis*, **79**(5), 887–902.

Gray, J.A. (1971) Sex differences in emotional behaviour in mammals including man: endocrine basis. *Acta Psychol*, **35**, 29–44.

Gunn, J. (1973) *Violence*. David & Charles, Newton Abbot.

Harrington, J.A. (1972) Violence: a clinical viewpoint. *Br Med J*, **1**, 228–31.

Health Services Advisory Committee (1997) *Violence and Aggression to Staff in Health Services: Guidance on Assessment and Management*, 2nd edn. Health and Saftey Executive Books, Suffolk.

HSE (1995) *A Guide to the Reporting of Injuries, Diseases and Dangerous Occurrences Regulations 1995 (RIDDOR)*. L73. HMSO, London.

HSE (1996) *A Guide to the Health and Safety (Consultation with Employees) Regulations 1996*. Guidance on Regulations L95. HMSO, London.

HSE (1999) *Management of Health and Safety at Work Regulations 1999*. Approved Code of Practice L21. HMSO, London.

HSE (2000) *Violence at Work*. LAC 88/1. HMSO, London.

Kerr, I.B. & Taylor, D. (1997) Acute disturbed or violent behaviour: principles of treatment. *J Psychopharmacol*, **11**(3), 271–7.

Krakowski, M. & Czobor, P. (1994) Clinical symptoms, neurological impairment, and prediction of violence in psychiatric inpatients. *Hosp Commun Psychiatry*, **45**(7), 711–13.

Leather, P. *et al.* (2005) Weighing up the benefits of training programmes. *Prof Nurse*, **20**(5), 6–7.

Lorenz, K. (1966) *On Aggression*. Harcourt, Brace & World, New York.

Montague, M.C. (1979) Physiology of aggressive behaviour. *J Neurosurg Nurs*, **11**, 10–15.

Morgan, S. (2001) The problems of aggression and violence for health-care staff. *Prof Nurse*, **17**(2), 107–8.

Mulholland, H. (2003) Analysis. Why are nurses still being attacked? *Nurs Times*, **99**(14), 10–11.

NICE (2005) *Violence. The Short-Term Management of Disturbed/Violent Behaviour in Psychiatric In-Patient Settings and Emergency Departments*. National Institute for Health and Clinical Excellence, London.

NMC (2002) *The recognition, prevention and therapeutic management of violence in mental health care*. Nursing and Midwifery Council. www.nmc-uk.org. Accessed 8/10/03.

NMC (2008) *The Code: Standards of Conduct, Performance and Ethics for Nurses and Midwives*. Nursing and Midwifery Council, London.

Paterson, B., Leadbetter, D. & Bowie, V. (2001) Zero in on violence. *Nurs Manage*, **8**(1), 16–22.

Paterson, B., Leadbetter, D. & Miller, G. (2005) Workplace health. Beyond zero tolerance: a varied approach to workplace violence. *Br J Nurs*, **14**(15), 810–15.

Pinker, S. (2002) The killer instinct. *The Times*, T2, 3 September; Suppl, pp. 2–3.

RCN (1998) *Dealing with Violence against Nursing Staff: an RCN Guide for Nurses and Managers*. Royal College of Nursing, London.

RCN (2005) *At Breaking Point? A Survey of the Well-Being and Working Lives of Nurses in 2005*. Royal College of Nursing, London.

Reilly, P. *et al.* (1994) Anger management and temper control: critical components of post traumatic stress disorder and substance abuse treatment. *J Psychoactive Drugs*, **26**(4), 401–7.

Rew, M. & Ferns, T. (2005) Conflict management. A balanced approach to dealing with violence and aggression at work. *Br J Nurs*, **14**(4), 227–32.

Rippon, T.J. (2000) Aggression and violence in health care professions. *J Adv Nurs*, **31**(2), 452–60.

Robinson, L. (1983) *Psychiatric Nursing as a Human Experience*. W.B. Saunders, Philadelphia.

Royal College of Psychiatrists (1998) *Management of Imminent Violence – Clinical Practice Guidelines: Quick Reference Guide*. Royal College of Psychiatrists, London.

Royal Marsden Hospital (2002) *The Violence at Work Policy*. Royal Marsden Hospital, London.

Strachan-Bennett, S. (2005) Managing violent patients. *Nurs Times*, **101**(13), 18–20.

Vanderslott, J. (1998) A study of incidents of violence towards staff by patients in an NHS trust hospital. *J Psychiatr Mental Health Nurs*, **5**, 291–8.

Walker, J. (2002) Safety first. *Nurs Times*, **98**(9), 20–1.

Wells, J. & Bowers, L. (2002) How prevalent is violence towards nurses working in general hospitals in the UK? *J Adv Nurs*, **39**(3), 230–40.

Wertham, D.J. (1968) *A Sign for Cain*. Hale, New York.

Whittington, R. (1997) Violence to nurses: prevalence and risk factors. *Nurs Stand*, **12**(5), 49–56.

Whittington, R., Shuttleworth, S. & Hill, L. (1996) Violence to staff in a general hospital setting. *J Adv Nurs*, **24**, 326–33.

Worthington, K. (2000) Violence in the health care workplace. *Am J Nurs*, **100**(11), 69–70.

Wright, S. (1999) Physical restraint in the management of violence and aggression in in-patient settings: a review of issues. *J Mental Health*, 8(5), 459–72.

Chapter 48

Wound management

943 **Wound healing and management**
943 Reference material
955 **Pressure ulcers or decubitus ulcers**
955 Reference material
960 **Fungating wounds**
960 Reference material
964 **Radiotherapy skin damage**
965 Reference material
965 **Plastic surgery wounds**
966 Reference material
968 **Scarring**
968 Reference material
969 **Methods of wound closure**
970 *Procedure guidelines:* Wound dressings change for acute and surgical wounds
971 *Procedure guidelines:* Suturing a simple wound
974 *Procedure guidelines:* Sutures, clips or staples removal
975 *Procedure guidelines:* Wound drain dressing (Redivac: closed drainage systems)
976 *Procedure guidelines:* Change of vacuum drainage system
977 *Procedure guidelines:* Wound drain removal (Yeates vacuum drainage system)
978 *Procedure guidelines:* Wound drain shortening (Penrose: open drainage systems)
978 *Procedure guidelines:* Topical negative pressure (TNP) therapy
980 References and further reading

Definition of a wound

A wound can be defined as an injury to the body that involves a break in the continuity of tissues or of body structures (Martin 2002). Wounds can be divided into six basic categories:

1 contusion (bruise);
2 abrasion (graze);
3 laceration (tear);
4 incision (cut);
5 puncture (stab);
6 burn.

Both external and internal factors can contribute to the formation of a wound. These may include:

- *External*: mechanical (friction, shear, surgery); chemical, electrical, temperature extremes (burns); radiation; micro-organisms.
- *Internal*: circulatory system failure (venous, arterial, lymphatic); endocrine (diabetes); neuropathy; haematological (porphyria cutanea tarda, mycosis fungoides); malignancy (fungating wound, Marjolin's ulcer) (Naylor *et al.* 2001).

Wound healing and management

Reference material

Classification of wounds

There are many different wound classification systems available and choice depends on the type of information required. A wound may be classified simply according to the method of healing, for example primary, secondary or tertiary intention (Miller & Dyson 1996), but this does not provide any information about the wound's characteristics. Further simple classification systems include whether the wound is acute (of short duration), chronic (of long duration) or according to the amount of tissue loss (Dealey 2005). A classification system that contains an appraisal of tissue loss is considered most useful (Flanagan 1996). Superficial, partial-thickness wounds are usually traumatic and painful, but retain the hair follicles or sweat glands and part of the dermis, and are usually considered **acute wounds**, whilst full-thickness wounds destroy the dermis and some deeper layers may also be involved (Dealey 2005). Full thickness wounds take longer to heal and can be life threatening if necrosis or infection complicate healing (Hampton & Collins 2004) and are therefore **chronic wounds**.

Wound healing

Wound healing is the process by which tissues damaged or destroyed by injury or disease are restored to normal function. Healing may occur by first, second or third intention. Healing by **first intention** involves the union of the edges of a wound under aseptic conditions without visible granulation, for example, a laceration or an incision that is closed with sutures, clips or skin adhesive (Miller & Dyson 1996; Dealey 2005).

Healing by **secondary intention** occurs when the wound's edges cannot be brought together. In this case the wound is left open and must fill with new tissue (granulate) until the level of intact epidermis is reached. When this is achieved epithelial cells will begin to migrate over the wound surface to restore integrity of the skin (Flanagan 1998). Wounds that heal by secondary intention include surgical or traumatic wounds where a large amount of tissue has been lost, heavily infected wounds, chronic wounds (leg or pressure ulcers) or, in some cases, where a better cosmetic or functional result will be achieved (Miller & Dyson 1996; Calvin 1998).

Healing by **tertiary intention** (sometimes referred to as delayed primary intention) may be employed when there is considerable infection or contamination of the wound. The wound is left open until it is clean or free of infection and then the edges are brought together, as with primary intention healing (Sussman 1998).

Phases of wound healing

Wound healing is a complex series of physiological events which occur in a predictable sequence (Flanagan 1999). These descriptive phases are dynamic, highly complex, dependent upon each other and overlap (Dealey 2005; Timmons 2006). It is important to support a wound healing environment that encourages progression from one phase to the next without bacterial contamination, which increases slough and necrosis (Hampton & Collins 2004).

The generally accepted stages of healing are:

1 Haemostasis.
2 Inflammatory phase.
3 Proliferation or reconstructive phase.
4 Maturation or remodelling phase.
   (Miller & Dyson 1996; Calvin 1998; Moore & Foster 1998; Ehrlich 1999; Flanagan 2000)

There are a number of internal and external factors that may have an influence on normal wound healing and cause a delay in progress through these stages (Table 48.1). Growth factors are involved throughout these phases and are listed in Table 48.2.

Haemostasis (minutes)

Vasoconstriction occurs within a few seconds of tissue injury and damaged blood vessels constrict to stem the blood flow. When platelets come into contact with exposed collagen from damaged blood vessels they release chemical messengers that stimulate a 'clotting cascade' (Flanagan 2000; Hampton & Collins 2004; Timmons 2006). Platelets adhere to vessel walls and edges and are stabilized by a network of fibrin to form a clot. Bleeding ceases when the blood vessels

Table 48.1 Factors that may delay wound healing. (From Hampton & Collins 2004; Convatec Wound Therapeutics 2005; Bale & Jones 2006.)

Extrinsic factor	Action	Intrinsic factor	Action
Cold	Any drop in temperature delays healing by up to 4 hours (Lock 1979)	Age	Elderly have a gradual thinning of the dermis and underlying structural support for the wound (i.e. less moisture and subcutaneous fat) and the metabolic process and circulation also slows with age
Excessive heat	Temperature over 30°C reduces tensile strength and causes vasoconstriction	Medical and general health conditions	Diabetes, cardiopulmonary disease, hypovolaemic shock, rheumatoid arthritis, anaemia, obesity
Chronic excessive exudate	Wounds should not be too wet or too dry (see moisture balance section in Table 48.3)	Malnutrition or protein–energy malnutrition	Poor healing, decreased tensile strength and higher risk of wound dehiscence and infection Low serum albumin causes oedema
Poor dressing application and techniques	If dressings are too tight or compression therapy is inadequate, adherence of dressings to wound bed, etc.	Psycho-social factors	Alcohol and smoking (carbon monoxide affects the blood vessels and circulation of oxygen), poor mobility, stress, isolation, anxiety and altered body image
Poor surgical technique	Prolonged operating time, inappropriate use of diathermy and drains can lead to 'dead space' haematomas and infection	Drugs	Steroids and non-steroidal anti-inflammatories, anti-inflammatories, immunosuppressives, cytotoxic chemotherapy

Table 48.2 Growth factors involved in wound healing. (From Timmons 2006; Hampton & Collins 2004.)

Growth factor	Actions
Epidermal growth factor (EGF)	Influences the rate of epithelialization
Fibroblast growth factor 2 (FGF-2)	Promotes angiogenesis, stimulates proliferation of epithelial cells and fibroblasts
Transforming growth factor (TGF-β)	Sustains fibrotic process that leads to scar formation
Insulin-like growth factor 1 (IGF-1)	Presence of these low molecular peptides predicts presence of underlying conditions and nutritional status.
Platelet derived growth factor (PDGF)	Triggers clotting cascade and promotes cell migration and repair at the injured site
Vascular endothelial growth factor (VGF)	Stimulates angiosentesis (formation of new cells)
Nerve growth factor (NGF)	Accelerates healing and is produced by fibroblasts and epithelial cells
Keratinoctye growth factor (KGF)	Stimulates keratinoctye proliferation and migration through the extra cellular matrix (during re-epithelialization)

thrombose, usually within 5–10 minutes of injury (Hampton & Collins 2004).

Inflammatory phase (1–5 days)

With the activation of clotting factors comes the release of histamine and vasodilatation begins (Flanagan 1996, Dowsett 2002). The liberation of histamine also increases the permeability of the capillary walls, and plasma proteins, leucocytes, antibodies and electrolytes exude into the surrounding tissues. The wound becomes red, swollen and hot. These signs are accompanied by pain and tenderness at the wound site, last for 1–3 days and can be mistaken for wound infection (Hampton & Collins 2004).

Polymorphonuclear leucocytes (neutrophils) and macrophages are chemotactically attracted to the wound to defend against infection and begin the process of repair (Hart 2002). The macrophage is also known as the 'director cell' of wound healing (Silver 1994). If the number and function of macrophages is reduced, as may occur in dis e.g. diabetes (Springett 2002), or due to treatment chemotherapy in cancer patients (Souhami & Tobias healing is seriously affected.

Neutrophils and macrophages combine to dest gest bacteria, debris and devitalized tissue. T great deal of cellular activity which requires up to the normal resting rate of oxygen of phagocytic cells (Timmons 2006). Patients with hypoxic wounds are, therefore, more susceptible to wound infection. The degradation of unwanted material causes an increased osmolarity within the area, resulting in further swelling.

This phase of wound healing requires energy and good nutrition and complications or infection will both delay the process and can be debilitating for the patient (Dealey 2005). A chronic wound can get stuck in this phase of wound healing (Collier 2002) with prolonged healing, tendency to infection and high levels of exudate (Timmons 2006).

Proliferative phase (3–24 days)

Acute wounds will start to granulate within 3 days, but the inflammatory and proliferative phases can overlap with both granulation and sloughy tissue present (Timmons 2006). The macrophage secretes a fibroblast-stimulating factor known as vascular endothelial growth factor (VEGF) which, in the presence of a platelet derived growth factor released by the dead platelets, causes the fibroplast to migrate into the wound soon after damage has occurred (Silver 1994; Calvin 1998).

The fibroblasts are activated to divide and produce collagen by processes initiated by the macrophages (Timmons 2006). This develops a network of poorly organized collagen which increases the strength and elasticity of the wound. Newly synthesized collagen creates a 'healing ridge' below an intact suture line, thus giving an indication of how wound healing is progressing. This mechanism is dependent on the presence of iron, vitamin C and oxygen. Vitamin C (ascorbic acid) and lactate are stimulants for fibroblast activity (Hampton & Collins 2004). Fibroblasts are also dependent on the local oxygen supply (Dealey 2005).The wound surface and the oxygen tension within encourages the macrophages to instigate the process of angiogenesis; forming new blood cell vessels (Hampton & Collins 2004; Dealey 2005). These vessels branch and join other vessels forming loops. The fragile capillary loops are held within a framework of collagen. This complex is known as granulation tissue. At this stage the wound will appear pink and moist with raised red bumps (Hampton & Collins 2004).

The process of wound contraction can significantly reduce the size of the wound and the area that new tissue must cover. It is extremely important, and only observable, in open wounds healing by secondary intention. There is debate about the exact method by which wound contraction occurs (Tejero-Trujeque 2001). The cell contraction theory proposes that an altered fibroblast, called a myofibroblast (which has similar properties to a smooth muscle cell), has the ability to contract and pull collagen fibrils towards itself, thereby reducing the size of the wound (Flanagan 1996; Calvin 1998).

Re-epithelialization of the wound usually begins within 24 hours of injury (Garrett 1997; Calvin 1998). Macrophages produce a number of growth factors including keratinocyte growth factor (KGF) which stimulates a proliferation of cells within the wound bed (Timmons 2006). Epithelial cells (keratinocytes) may migrate from hair follicles and sweat glands within the wound or from the perimeter of the wound (Moore & Foster 1998). The migration of epithelial cells across the wound surface may occur via single cell migration or 'leap-frogging' where a cell moves forward and stops while other cells move over the top of it (Calvin 1998). Epithelial cells will burrow under contaminated debris and unwanted material (Waldorf & Fewkes 1995) while also secreting an enzyme that separates the scab from underlying tissue. Dissolving dry eschar requires nearly 50% of the cell's metabolic energy (Messer 1989; Dealey 2005). Through a mechanism called contact inhibition epithelial cells will cease migrating when they come into contact with other epithelial cells (Garrett 1997).

The ability of the epithelium to cover the wound surface is limited to approximately 2 cm^2. This means that the process of contraction is of vital importance to healing wounds (Messer 1989). Epithelialization (migration, mitosis and differentiation) occurs at an increased rate in a moist wound environment, as do the synthesis of collagen and formation of new capillaries (Winter 1972; Eaglstein 1985; Dyson et al. 1988; Miller 1998a; Flanagan 1999). A hypoxic (low oxygen) environment has also been shown to increase the motility of epidermal cells (O'Toole et al. 1997). The rate of epithelialization is also influenced by growth factors (Timmons 2006). However, little is known about the reality of growth factor activity in chronic wounds (Hampton & Collins 2004).

Maturation phase (21 days onward)

This stage begins at around 21 days following the initial injury. Maturation or remodelling of the healed wound may last for more than a year. Collagen is reorganized, the fibres becoming enlarged and orientated along the lines of tension in the wound (at right angles to the wound margin) (Silver 1994). This occurs via a process of lysis and resynthesis. Intermolecular cross-linking aids the tensile strength of the wound. The reorganization of collagen may result in further contraction of the wound, which may potentiate contraction deformities (Silver 1994; Moore & Foster 1998). During this phase the number of blood vessels within the scar is reduced. Maximum strength is reached in approximately 3 months, although the scar will only achieve about 70–80% of normal skin strength (Calvin 1998; Ehrlich 1999). At the end of the maturation phase the delicate granulation tissue of the wound will have been replaced by stronger avascular scar tissue.

For acute wounds these phases flow relatively smoothly, however chronic wounds may get stuck in one phase or heal very slowly. It is necessary to bring a chronic wound back into the acute phase for it to heal. This process is termed 'wound bed preparation' (S. Hampton, pers. comm., October 2006).

Table 48.3 TIME principles for wound bed preparation. (Adapted from Schultz *et al.* 2003; permission granted by Smith & Nephew.)

TIME	Status	Problem	Solution
Tissue	Tissue not viable	Defective matrix Cell debris impairing healing	Debridement
Inflammation and infection	Colonized → infection continuum	Wound healing delayed	Topical anti-microbials dependent on bacterial load
Moisture balance	Dry → excessive moisture	Maceration potential	Restore moisture balance Prevent maceration to peri-wound margins May require compression/drug therapy
Edge of wound	Non-migrating keratinocytes	Wound not closing	Reassess cause Removal of callus

Wound bed preparation

Wound bed preparation (WBP) focuses on controlling and optimizing the wound environment for healing (Falanga 2000). It provides a means of bringing together a cohesive plan of both patient and wound care (Vowden & Vowden 2002).

Doctors have always applied the principles of wound bed preparation, even before it was given a name as, when they debrided a wound, they would cut through to healthy bleeding tissues. This would initiate the clotting cascade and the wound would become acute. Today, there are improved methods of achieving the same end through assessment and appropriate dressing selection (S. Hampton, pers. comm., October 2006).

In order to provide a method of assessment and a simplistic selection of appropriate dressings, an international group of wound care experts developed this concept using 'TIME' (tissue, infection, moisture and edge advancement) as an acronym to identify the key barriers to healing (Dowsett & Ayello 2004). See Table 48.3 for overview of TIME principles.

Tissue factors affecting wound healing

The rate of wound healing varies depending on the general health of the individual, the location of the wound, the degree of damage and the treatment applied.

Factors that may delay healing include systemic variables such as disease, poor nutritional state and infection. Other influences involve the local microenvironment of the wound, including temperature, pH, humidity, air gas composition, oxygen tension, blood supply and inflammation (Dyson *et al.* 1988; Cutting 1994; Benbow 1995; Collier 1996; Thomson 1998). Whether this influence is positive or negative may depend on the stage of wound healing that has been reached. Other important considerations are external variables such as continuing trauma, possibly caused by treatment or the presence of foreign bodies.

It is necessary when treating a wound to appraise all potential detrimental factors and minimize them, where possible, in order to provide the optimum systemic, local and external conditions for healing. Factors known to affect wound healing are listed in Table 48.1.

Nutrition and wound healing

Nutrition regulates wound healing as an extrinsic factor via two concepts: firstly that wound-related complications are more likely in the malnourished, and secondly, nutritional supplements can accelerate healing (Mandal 2006). A dietitian's assessment is advisable to set specific goals (Dealey 2005). Patients are considered 'at risk' for wound healing if they have lost 20% or more of their body weight within the previous 6 months or 10% in the previous 2 months (Messer 1989). These patients should be screened holistically and offered interventions to prevent wound failure postoperatively, as most wounds heal adequately despite preoperative fasting (Dealey 2005; Mandal 2006). Patient's age, debilitating disease, current medications, usual diet and methods of cooking and preparing food are all considerations (Dealey 2005).

Many concurrent conditions affect diet, and both protein and calorie malnutrition are possible in patients with chronic or acute malabsorption. This includes diabetes, Crohn's disease, alcohol abuse, gastrointestinal surgery, liver disease and long-term steroid therapy. Malignancy, major trauma, fever, inflammatory disease, smoking, drug use, stress and iatrogenic starvation are associated with deficient intake or high energy demands (Lewis 1996; Casey 1998).

Patients who are elderly, malnourished, have severe diabetes or rheumatoid arthritis or who have suffered significant injury (especially burns) or surgery may be deficient in vitamin A (Messer 1989; Hamilton 1995; Ferguson *et al.* 2000). Therefore vitamin A supplementation may be beneficial as a means of speeding wound healing in these patient groups. Vitamin A has also been shown to reduce the adverse effects of corticosteroids (slowed wound healing, increased rate of infection and weaker scars), when given orally or applied topically to the wound (Ehrlich & Hunt 1968; Smith *et al.* 1986; Hamilton 1995).

Vitamin C is necessary for collagen synthesis during the proliferative stage of the wound healing process. Deficiency

Table 48.4 Suitability of products used on wounds. (From Miller & Dyson 1996; Lawrence 1997; Hampton 1999; Morgan 2000; Royal Marsden Wound Management Guidelines 2000; Hess 2005; BNF 2006.)

Product type	Suitability	Caution
Normal saline solution (sodium chloride 0.9%)	All types of wounds and sterile for aseptic technique on acute wounds	Should be warmed to avoid cooling wound surface and for comfort
Tap water	Chronic wounds. A shower may be used to remove old dressings, or affected limb soaked in a bucket of water	Ensure water is correct temperature and patient is suitable
Antiseptic solutions (i.e. chlorhexidine, hydrogen peroxide, acetic acid, povidone iodine, proflavin)	Not ideal as can cause sensitization, irritation and delay healing. Proflavin cream may be used as second line treatment for moist desquamation in radiotherapy induced skin reactions	Hydrogen peroxide can cause an air embolism and is only used to clean very dirty wounds (i.e. road traffic accidents, or those contaminated by foreign matter). Iodine and proflavin stain clothing and are not for prolonged use
Topical antibiotics ■ Fusidic acid ■ Metronidazole ■ Mupirocin (Bactroban)	Penicillin-resistant staphylococci Antibacterial (anaerobes), odour For MRSA treatment, seek advice first after positive wound swab	Not recommended on open wounds Nausea when used systemically Can burn or itch (consult microbiologist before use)

of vitamin C is also associated with lowered resistance to infection (Lewis 1996; Casey 1998; Russell 2001). Patients with poor nutritional status may benefit from zinc supplements because of the role of zinc in DNA synthesis and the immune response (Wells 1994; Lewis 1996).

Promotion of wound healing

Wound care begins with the care of the patient. The psychological care of the patient is important to ensure acceptance of the wound and reduction in stress. It is also imperative to assess and treat pain. Apart from the obvious unpleasantness for the patient, this will also lead to stress which will then delay wound healing (Kiecolt-Glaser et al. 1995; Moore & Foster 1998). A holistic assessment is very important (Collier 2002; Hampton 2004).

Achieving a well-vascularized wound bed

Improving the blood flow to the wound bed will increase the availability of nutrients, oxygen, active cells and growth factors within the wound environment (Collier 2002). This may be achieved through the use of compression therapy, topical negative pressure therapy or wound management products that exert an osmotic pull on the wound bed, increasing capillary growth, e.g. Vacutex (Collier 2002).

Principles of wound cleaning

The aim of wound cleaning is to help create the optimum local conditions for wound healing by removal of excess debris, exudate, foreign and necrotic material, toxic components, bacteria and other micro-organisms.

If the wound is clean and little exudate is present, repeated cleaning is contraindicated since it may damage new tissue,

decrease the temperature of the wound unnecessarily and remove exudate (Morison 1989). A fall in the temperature of the wound of 12°C is possible if the procedure is prolonged or the lotions are cold. It can take 3 hours or longer for the wound to return to normal temperature, during which time the cellular activity is reduced and therefore the healing process slowed (Collier 1996).

Sodium chloride (0.9%) is a physiologically balanced solution that has a similar osmotic pressure to that already present in living cells and is therefore compatible with human tissue (Lawrence 1997). Used at body temperature, it is the safest and best cleaning solution for non-contaminated wounds (Miller & Dyson 1996; Fletcher 1997). Although sodium chloride has no antiseptic properties it dilutes bacteria and is non-toxic to tissue (Morgan 2000). Tap water is also advocated for cleaning chronic wounds (Riyat & Quinton 1997). A study demonstrated that, in comparison with sterile 0.9% sodium chloride, lower rates of infection were found in the group where tap water was used (Angeras et al. 1992).

A number of other solutions have been used traditionally to clean wounds, some of which need to be used with caution (Table 48.4).

Debridement of devitalized tissue

Surgical debridement is the most effective method of removing necrotic tissue (debridement) (Hampton 1999). It is performed by a surgeon and usually involves excision of extensive or deep areas of necrosis. This is usually performed to the point of bleeding viable tissue to 'kickstart' healing (Hampton & Collins 2004). While this option is very effective it carries the risks associated with general anaesthesia. An alternative method of rapid debridement is 'sharp' debridement, which may be utilized for the removal of loose, devitalized,

947

superficial tissue only (Vowden & Vowden 1999). Sharp debridement can be performed at the patient's bedside by an experienced health care professional with relevant training (Poston 1996). However, this can be a dangerous practice in inexperienced hands and is controversial (Fairbairn *et al.* 2002). Potentially ligaments may be severed as they can have the appearance of sloughy tissue or vascular damage could occur (Hampton & Collins 2004). Guidelines for sharp debridement have been drawn up and presented but have not been adopted yet (Davies 2004). It is also acknowledged that informed patient consent is required as this is an invasive procedure with potential risks and complications (Fairbairn *et al.* 2002).

Autolytic debridement is recommended as a less invasive technique which utilizes the body's natural debriding mechanism. This process involves the removal of necrotic tissue by neutrophils and macrophages. This effect is enhanced in a moist wound environment, which can be achieved through the use of hydrogel dressings or semi-occlusive dressings that maintain moisture at the wound surface (Bale 1991; Hofman 1996; Freedline 1999) (Table 48.5). A holistic wound assessment is needed to decide appropriate methods of debriding devitalized tissue (Davies 2004).

The National Institute for Health and Clinical Excellence (NICE) guidance (NICE 2001) suggests that less robust studies favour autolytic debridement or bio-surgical interventions (sterile maggots) which are more comfortable and acceptable methods for patients. The sterile larvae (maggots) are applied to and retained at the wound bed and are used generally in chronic wounds (Hinshaw 2000). The larvae move over the surface of the wound, secreting a powerful mixture of proteolytic enzymes which break down necrotic tissue. They remove devitalized tissue by this method (the enzymes are neutralized by live tissue) while at the same time ingesting and destroying bacteria.

This action may cause a significant increase in exudate production due to the rapid debridement of necrotic tissue. It has been proposed that the larval secretions may also change the wound pH and may stimulate healing (Hinshaw 2000). Maggots are also obtainable in 'tea bag' form where they are encased and unable to escape. This method is often more acceptable to nurses (S. Hampton, pers. comm., October 2006). Patient compliance is also an important consideration and a detailed explanation is required (Jones & Thomas 2000; Thomas *et al.* 2001).

Indications for sterile larvae use include:

- Gangrenous or necrotic tissue (the necrotic tissue needs to be softened before applying therapy [S. Hampton, pers. comm., October 2006]).
- Infected diabetic foot ulceration.
- Arterial leg ulceration.
- Traumatic infected ulcers.
- Chronic wounds with underlying co-morbidities (Steenvoorde *et al.* 2005).

In a study by Kitching (2004) participants were positive about the effects of using the larvae and had been previously disillusioned by the failure of other treatments. Pain

management was also an issue as the larvae grew and patients were controlled on durogesic plasters (Steenvoorde *et al.* 2005). Both studies reported good rates of debridement, reduction in malodour and exudate (Kitching 2004; Steenvoorde *et al.* 2005).

Inflammation and infection (or bacterial burden)

It is generally agreed that all chronic wounds harbour a variety of bacteria to some degree and this can range from contamination through colonization to infection. There is also a stage between colonization and infection called 'critical colonization' where the bacterial load has reached a level just below clinical infection (Collier 2002). When a wound becomes infected it will display the characteristic signs of heat, redness, swelling, pain, heavy exudate and malodour. The patient may also develop generalized pyrexia. However, immunosuppressed patients, diabetic patients or those on systemic steroid therapy may not present with the classic signs of infection. Instead they may experience delayed healing, breakdown of the wound, presence of friable granulation tissue that bleeds easily, formation of an epithelial tissue bridge over the wound, increased production of exudate and malodour, and increased pain (Miller & Dyson 1996; Cutting 1998; Miller 1998b; Gilchrist 1999). Careful wound assessment is essential to identify potential sites for infection, although routine swabbing of the area is not considered to be beneficial (Donovan 1998). Methods available for the management of wound infection or to decrease the bacterial burden in the wound include debridement, antimicrobial dressings, e.g. those containing iodine or silver, topical negative pressure therapy and antibiotic therapy. Honey and essential oils have also been used and there is a growing body of literature to this effect (see fungating wounds section). Appropriate antibiotic treatment of the infection should be determined from a positive wound swab(s).

Moisture balance

Wound exudate usually performs a useful function of cleaning the wound and providing nutrients to the healing wound bed. However, in the presence of excess exudate the process of wound healing can be adversely affected. This is especially so in chronic wounds where wound fluid may actually prevent the proliferation of cells vital to wound healing, such as fibroblasts, keratinocytes and endothelial cells (Phillips *et al.* 1998; White 2001; Vowden & Vowden 2002).

The control of oedema or lymphoedema and lessening the bacterial burden on the wound will undoubtedly help in the reduction of wound exudate. However, if the methods for achieving these goals are unsuccessful or contraindicated then exudate must be managed through the use of wound management products. These include such products as absorbent wound dressings (e.g. alginates, hydrofibre, foams), non-adherent wound contact layers with a secondary absorbent pad, wound manager bags and topical negative pressure therapy (White 2001). Immunosuppressive drugs or

Table 48.5 Dressing groups. Please refer to manufacturer's recommendations with regard to individual products (Dealey 2005; Hess 2005).

Dressings	Description	Advantages	Disadvantages
Activated charcoal	Contain a layer of activated charcoal that traps odour-causing molecules thereby reducing/removing wound odour	Easy to apply as either primary or secondary dressing; work immediately to reduce odour	Need to obtain a good seal to prevent leakage of odour; some dressings lose effectiveness when wet
Adhesive island	Consist of a low adherent absorbent pad located centrally on an adhesive backing	Quick and easy to apply; one-piece design negates need for multiple product use; protect the suture line from contamination and absorb exudate/blood	Only suitable for light exudate; some can cause skin damage (excoriation, blistering) if applied incorrectly
Alginates	A textile fibre dressing made from the calcium salt of an alginic acid polymer derived from brown seaweed; contain mannuronic and guluronic acids in varying amounts; available as a sheet, ribbon or packing	Provide a moist wound environment; suitable for moderate to heavy exudate; can be used on infected wounds; useful for sinus and fistula drainage; have haemostatic properties; can be irrigated out of wound with sodium chloride (0.9%)	Cannot be used on dry wounds or wound with hard necrotic tissue (eschar); sometimes a mild burning or 'drawing' sensation is reported on application; secondary dressing required
Antimicrobials	These topical dressings can be used as primary or secondary dressings and are available as alginates, hydrocolloids, alginates, charcoal impregnated and creams	Suitable for chronic wounds with heavy exudate that need protection from bacterial contamination by providing a broad range of antimicrobial activity; can reduce or prevent infection	Cannot be used during radiotherapy, sometimes sensitivity occurs with the use of silver and some skin staining can occur; instructions vary with products and dressings are expensive
Capillary wound dressings	Composed of 100% polyester filament outer layers and a 65% polyester and 35% cotton woven inner layer; outer layer draws exudate, interstitial fluid and necrotic tissue into the inner layer via a capillary action Example: 'Vacutex'	Suitable for light to heavy exudate; debride necrotic tissue; protect and insulate the wound; maintain a moist environment and prevent maceration; encourage development of granulation tissue; can be cut to any shape and are available in large rolls; can be used as a wick to drain sinus and cavity wounds	Can be hard to cut and are quite stiff to fit into wounds; cannot be used on malignant wounds or where there is the risk of bleeding due to the 'drawing' action and resultant increase in blood flow to the wound bed
Collagens	This protein is fibrous and insoluble and produced by fibroblasts. Collagen encourages collagen fibres into the granulation tissue. It is available in sheets/gels	Conforms well to wound surface, maintains a moist environment, suitable for most wounds to accelerate healing (example: Promogran). Supports ECM	Requires a secondary dressing and not recommended for necrotic wounds
Cadexomer bead dressings	Consist of hydophilic beads which contain iodine in powder or paste form, which swell and form a gel on contact with exudate	Useful in the treatment of infected, sloughy and necrotic wounds	Require retaining dressing; may be difficult to apply, caution in using products containing iodine. Should only be used for 3 months at a time. Not suitable for people with thyroid disorders
Foams	Produced in a variety of forms, most being constructed of polyurethane foam and may have one or more layers; foam cavity dressings are also available	Suitable for use with open, exuding wounds; highly absorbent, non-adherent and provide a moist, thermally insulated wound environment	May be difficult to use in wounds with deep tracts
Honey	Available as impregnated dressing pads or tubes of liquid honey; most widely used is Manuka honey	Suitable for acute and chronic infected, necrotic or sloughy wounds; provide a moist wound environment; non-adherent; antibacterial; assist with wound debridement; eliminate wound malodour; have an anti-inflammatory effect	Can be messy to use and cause leakage if excess exudate is present; caution in diabetes due to absorption of glucose and fructose

949

(continued on p. 950)

Table 48.5 (*continued*)

Dressings	Description	Advantages	Disadvantages
Hydrocolloids	Usually consist of a base material containing gelatin, pectin and carboxymethylcellulose combined with adhesives and polymers; base material may be bonded to either a semi-permeable film or a film plus polyurethane foam; some have an adhesive border	Suitable for acute and chronic wounds with low to no exudate; provide a moist wound environment; promote wound debridement; provide thermal insulation; waterproof and barrier to micro-organisms; easy to use	May release degradation products into the wound; strong odour produced as dressing interacts with exudate; some hydrocolloids cannot be used on infected wounds
Hydrogels	Contain 17.5–90% water depending on the product, plus various other components to form a gel or solid sheet	Suitable for light exudate wounds; absorb small amounts of exudate; donate fluid to dry necrotic tissue; reduce pain and are cooling; low trauma at dressing changes; can be used as carrier for drugs	Cool the wound surface; use with caution in infected wounds; can cause skin maceration due to leakage if too much gel is applied or the wound has moderate to heavy exudate
Hydrofibre	A soft, non-woven dressing composed of 100% hydrocolloid fibres (sodium carboxymethylcellulose); available as sheet or ribbon	Suitable for highly exuding wounds (able to absorb up to 30 times its weight in fluid); holds exudate within its structure and keeps it away from surrounding skin; very easy to remove, gels more easily than alginates	Requires a secondary dressing
Semi-permeable films	Polyurethane film with a hypoallergenic acrylic adhesive; have a variety of application methods often consisting of a plastic or cardboard carrier	Only suitable for shallow superficial wounds; prophylactic use against friction damage; useful as retention dressing; allow passage of water vapour; allow monitoring of the wound	Possibility of adhesive trauma if removed incorrectly; do not contain exudate and can macerate, slip or leak
Skin barrier films	Alcohol-free liquid polymer that forms a protective film on the skin	Non-cytotoxic; do not sting if applied to raw areas of skin; high wash-off resistance; protect the skin from body fluids (including urine, diarrhoea, saliva and wound exudate), friction and shear and the effects of adhesive products	Require good manual dexterity to apply; may cause skin warming on application

steroids may be indicated in the treatment of inflammatory exudate produced by wounds such as pyoderma gangrenosum or rheumatoid ulcers (Vowden & Vowden 2002). It is also vital to protect the skin surrounding the wound from maceration by excess exudate and excoriation from corrosive exudate. Useful products for skin protection include ointments/pastes (e.g. zinc oxide BP), alcohol-free skin barrier films and thin hydrocolloid sheets used to 'frame' the wound.

Principles of dressing a wound

With the exception of wounds where the main aim is to ameliorate symptoms such as malignant wounds, an ideal wound dressing must be capable of fulfilling the following functions:

- Removes excess exudate and toxic components.
- Maintains a high humidity at the wound–dressing interface.
- Allows gaseous exchange.
- Provides thermal insulation.
- Be impermeable to bacteria.
- Be free from particulate or toxic components.
- Allows change without trauma.
- Be acceptable to the patient.
- Be highly absorbent (for heavily exuding wounds).
- Be cost-effective.
- Provide mechanical protection.
- Be conformable and mouldable.
- Be able to be sterilized.
  (Field & Kerstein 1994; Hampton 1999; Morgan 2000)

In addition, the dressing should minimize pain, odour and bleeding and be comfortable when in place.

Occlusive dressings achieve many of these criteria. They affect the wound and healing in several ways. Occlusive dressings have the ability to maintain hydration and prevent the formation of an eschar.

A moist wound environment has been shown to affect a wound in the following ways. It:

- Increases rate of epithelial migration.
- Reduces the lag phase between epithelial cell proliferation and differentiation.
- Encourages synthesis of collagen and ground substance.
- Promotes formation of capillary loops.
- Decreases length of inflammatory phase.
- Reduces pain and trauma due to dressing adherence.
- Promotes breakdown of necrotic tissue.
- Speeds wound contraction.
   (Miller & Dyson 1996; Garrett 1997; Flanagan 1998; Williams & Young 1998)

Dry dressings (such as gauze) do not provide most of the criteria for an ideal dressing and should not be used as a primary contact layer (Dealey 2005).

This depends on the definition of 'dry' dressing as Aquacel, alginates, etc. can be considered dry. The wound itself has the ability to produce moisture and make the dressings into 'wet' dressings. Wet dressings, such as first generation amorphous hydrogels, can make a wound too wet if used inappropriately. Compare the 'wetness' of first generation hydrogel with second generation hydrogel (such as ActiFormCool). The amorphous gels do not absorb and donate fluid to already wet wounds. This means they could be responsible for maceration if used inappropriately. Second generation hydrogel (ActiFormCool) is in a sheet and absorbs large amounts. First generation hydrogel should be used on dry eschar to soften. Second generation hydrogel can be used on wet and dry wounds (S. Hampton, pers. comm., October 2006).

Care should be taken with wounds that are difficult shapes to treat. These include long, narrow cavities which require a dressing that can be comfortably inserted into the space but removed easily without leaving any fibres behind and without trauma (Bale 1991). (See Table 48.5 for details of groups of dressings.)

Edge non-advancement

The clearest sign that the wound is failing to heal is when the epidermal edge is not advancing over time (Dowsett & Ayello 2004). In this case a thorough assessment should recommence using the TIME principles and interventions.

Wound assessment

The wound should be evaluated each time a dressing is applied or if it gives rise for concern. The aim of evaluating the wound is to assess healing and to establish which treatment will best provide the ideal environment for healing. The surface area or volume of the wound should be measured. This can be carried out using a number of methods; for example, planimetry measurements using a ruler, tracing the wound onto grid paper or Vistrak, a box similar to a child's Etch a Sketch but one that converts the tracing into measurement of surface area or through the use of a computer mapping program (S. Hampton, pers. comm., October 2006). Photography also provides a useful record of wound progression (Vowden 1995). The amount and type of drainage are also important, in both traumatic and surgical wounds, but difficult to assess (S. Hampton, pers. comm., October 2006).

A simple method is to use dressing change. Change dressings daily exudates. Change alternate days to every 3rd day medium exudates. Change weekly low exudates (S. Hampton, pers. comm., October 2006).

A list of variables that require regular assessment is shown in Table 48.3. Figure 48.1 is an example of a wound assessment chart. Teare & Barrett (2002) recommend that the underlying cause of the wound should also be assessed, with the primary focus on details such as size and depth as well as the stage of healing. Links can then be made between the wound dressing and the optimal healing environment. The use of this type of documentation to assist in the assessment process is recommended to:

- Facilitate continuity of care by providing a central reference point for wound progression.
- Facilitate appropriate evaluation of all relevant parameters.
- Fulfil legal and professional requirements (Teare & Barrett 2002).

Other treatments

Other treatments for wounds include the use of hyperbaric oxygen therapy, topical negative pressure therapy (TNP), bio-engineered skin substitutes, topical wound treatments and complementary therapies.

Hyperbaric oxygen therapy

Wound hypoxia is common in patients with chronic wounds and may be exacerbated by diabetes, venous stasis, vascular insufficiency, cardiopulmonary disease or smoking (Messer 1989). Hyperbaric oxygen therapy has been used successfully in healing these wounds (Barr et al. 1990). Treatment involves the patient breathing 100% oxygen while in a chamber where the pressure is elevated above atmospheric pressure, thus increasing the amount of oxygen in solution and therefore the quantity of oxygen reaching the wound bed (Simmons 1999). Topical hyperbaric oxygen can also be used (S. Hampton, pers. comm., October 2006).

Topical negative pressure therapy

Topical negative pressure therapy (TNP) is the application of a uniform negative pressure across the wound bed. The benefits of TNP therapy are recognized as promotion of healing, improved exudates management, reduction of odour and bacteria.

THE ROYAL MARSDEN WOUND ASSESSMENT CHART
Complete one chart for each wound

Patient name:					
Hospital number:					
Date of assessment (weekly)					
Wound dimensions					
Max length (cm)					
Max width (cm)					
Max depth (cm)					
Wound bed – approximate % cover (enter %)					
Necrotic (BLACK)					
Slough (YELLOW)					
Granulating (RED)					
Epithelializing (PINK)					
Skin around wound					
Intact					
Healthy					
Fragile					
Dry					
Scaly					
Erythema					
Maceration					
Oedema					
Eczema					
Skin nodules					
Skin stripping					
Dressing allergy					
Tape allergy					
Other (please state)					
Exudate level					
None					
Low					
Moderate					
High					
Amount increasing					
Amount decreasing					
Odour (see over for rating scale)					
None					
Slight					
Moderate					
Strong					
Bleeding					
None					
Slight					
Moderate					
Heavy					
At dressing change					
Pain from wound (see over for rating scale)					
Level (0–10)					
Continuous					
At specific times (specify)					
Wound infection suspected					
Swab taken (Y/N)					
Swab result					
Treatment					
Assessment review date					
Initials of Assessor					

Figure 48.1   Wound assessment chart. (Courtesy of The Royal Marsden Hospital.)

Location (mark diagram):	Visual Analogue Scale (VAS) for Patient's Rating of Pain.

Right   Left   Left   Right

| 0 | 1 | 2 | 3 | 4 | 5 | 6 | 7 | 8 | 9 | 10 |

No pain   Worst pain imaginable

Rating Scale for Odour	
Score	Assessment
None	No odour evident, even when at the patient's bedside with the dressing removed.
Slight	Wound odour is evident at close proximity to the patient when the dressing is removed.
Moderate	Wound odour is evident upon entering the room (1.5 to 3 metres from patient) with the dressing removed.
Strong	Wound odour is evident upon entering the room (1.5 to 3 metres from patient) with the dressing intact.

Diagram of wound if appropriate (or attach tracing/photograph):

Date: _____	Date: _____
Date: _____	Date: _____
Date: _____	Date: _____

Notes on use
Use one chart per wound.
Complete a wound assessment at least once a week.
Measure the wound at its widest points using a clean ruler, use a sterile wound swab or blunt probe to measure wound depth.
For the 'skin around wound' assessment more than one box may be ticked.
Odour and pain should be assessed using the scales at the top of page 2.
Following the assessment a wound management care plan should be written and updated if necessary after each reassessment.

Figure 48.1   (*continued*)

This technique involves sealing a sterile foam or gauze dressing into the wound cavity and applying a controlled sub-atmospheric pressure. The negative pressure is achieved through a closed system, removing fluid from open wounds through sealed tubing which is connected to a container. Pressures are set at the level best suited to the wound type and can be set on continuous or intermittent according to the therapy required (Benbow 2006). Maintaining the vacuum seal is essential in providing this therapy (Kaufman & Pahl 2003). It has proven to be cost efficient, safe and effective as a treatment modality for wound care.

TNP therapy is indicated for:

- Chronic wounds.
- Diabetic foot ulcers.
- Pressure ulcers.
- Dehisced wounds and incisions.
- Partial thickness burns.
- Flaps and grafts.

(Kaufman & Pahl 2003; KCI International 2004)

This therapy is contraindicated in grossly contaminated wounds, malignant wounds, untreated osteomyelitis, non-enteric and unexplored fistula or necrotic tissue with eschar present (KCI International 2004).

Precautions should be exercised when there is active bleeding in the wound, difficult haemostasis or when the patient is taking anticoagulants (Benbow 2006). Careful assessment of the wound site must be made to ensure that TNP therapy is indeed the appropriate treatment modality (Kaufman & Pahl 2003).

Bio-engineered skin substitutes

Bio-engineered skin substitutes have arisen from a need to find an alternative to skin grafts (autograft, allograft or xenograft) and dressings in the management of extensive burns (Boyce *et al.* 2002; Harding *et al.* 2002; Pouliot *et al.* 2002). Original cultures of human epidermis have been replaced by new skin-equivalent products that contain living cells, predominantly keratinocytes and fibroblasts, within natural or synthetic scaffolding. Examples of these products are:

- Apligraf (Graftskin): a cultured human skin equivalent containing viable dermal and epidermal cells (Morgan 2000; Harding *et al.* 2002).
- Dermagraft: a bio-absorbable mesh containing living neonatal fibroblasts, which produce normal dermal proteins and cytokines (Gentzkow *et al.* 1996).

Topical wound treatment dressings

Currently there are several dressing products, Hyalofill and Promogran, Catrix, Cadesorb and Prisma, which are classified as 'topical treatments' although they are not classed as medicines (S. Hampton, pers. comm., October 2006). Hyalofill is a soft conformable fleece composed entirely of HYAFF, an ester of hyaluronic acid (Edmonds & Foster 2000; Baxter & Ballard 2001). It has been shown to increase angiogenesis and the phagocytic response of macrophages; when used as a wound dressing, it promotes granulation and contraction (Chen & Abatangelo 1999; Hollander *et al.* 2000).

Proteases have an important role in regulating the balance between tissue synthesis and degradation. However, in chronic wounds, this regulation may be defective and healing problems will result (Derbyshire 2003) and, if their activity becomes uncontrolled, proteases can mediate devastating tissue damage and consequently have been implicated in chronic wound pathophysiology (Cullen *et al.* 2002). Collagen can inactivate potentially harmful factors such as proteases, oxygen free radicals and excess metal ions present in chronic wound fluid (Cullen *et al.* 2002). Collagen dressings bind excess proteases and other inflammatory proteins to its structure and lower the wound pH to around pH5 which, in turn, helps to reduce the harmful protease activity (S. Hampton, pers. comm., October 2006).

Collagen is the most abundant protein in the human body and its synthesis plays a very important role in the early phases of the process of healing and formation of granulation tissues, which afterwards will form a healing tissue. Inside this process the collagen formation is due to the action of cytokines and the interaction between extra cellular mould and fibroblasts (Torra I Bou *et al.* 2001). The macrophages control the liberation of collagen by fibroblasts by means of so-called growth factors: platelet derived growth factor (PDGF), epidermal growth factor (EGF), fibroblast growth factor (FGF) and transforming growth factor (TGF-β) (Torra I Bou *et al.* 2001).

Catrix is designed to reduce protease levels in wound fluids by providing a competitive substrate (collagen) for the proteases. It thereby reduces proteolytic destruction of essential extracellular matrix ECM components and platelet-derived growth factors (S. Hampton, pers. comm., October 2006).

Cadesorb is a protease modulating ointment, which contains an absorbent starch based polymer, polythene Glycol and poloxamer. In the presence of exudate, Cadesorb transforms into a soft moist gel to promote an ideal wound-healing environment. The ointment has been designed specifically for non-healing wounds to rebalance the levels of protease activity in the wound and by removing excess exudate and slough from the wound bed.

Promogran is a matrix of freeze-dried collagen (55%) and oxidized regenerated cellulose (45%) (Morgan 2002; Thomas 2002). It forms a gel on contact with wound exudate and interacts with products found in wound exudate that impair healing, specifically binding to and inactivating metalloproteases that degrade growth factors. Promogran also binds to and protects growth factors, which are released back into the wound as the dressing is absorbed (Morgan 2002). Prisma has a similar makeup but has the addition of silver (S. Hampton, pers. comm., October 2006).

Complementary therapies

The use of complementary therapies in wound management is based very much on anecdotal evidence. However, there have been trials using essential oils in wound care, in particular for the relief of pain and wound odour (Price & Price 1995; Baker 1998). Complementary therapies such as relaxation, massage, visualization, imagery and distraction may be very useful in the reduction of wound pain, especially that associated with procedures such as dressing changes (Naylor 2001). Other complementary therapies that may be useful in the management of wound pain include acupuncture, acupressure, autogenic therapy, biofeedback and hypnosis (Rankin-Box 2001).

Complementary therapies should only be administered by health care professionals with the relevant training and qualifications (Stone 2001). When used alongside conventional management treatments, these therapies can be extremely beneficial in reducing pain or the response to pain.

Pressure ulcers or decubitus ulcers

Definition

Pressure ulcers (decubitus ulcers) are areas of localized tissue damage caused by excess pressure, shearing or friction forces (Benbow 2006). The extent of this damage can range from persistent erythema to necrotic ulceration involving muscle, tendon and bone (Reid & Morison 1994).

Pressure ulcers are a serious problem in health care systems, and are associated with pain, prolonged hospital stay, and if not prevented, can result in fatalilty (Schoonhoven *et al.* 2002). Clark (2002) discusses the significant reduction in quality of life for patients with pressure ulcers. He acknowledged that factors such as social isolation, pain and limitations on activity can have detrimental effects on patients and their families.

The Nursing and Midwifery Council's (NMC's) *The Code* states that nurses must act without delay if the patient is put at risk (NMC 2008). It was suggested that the focus of attention for pressure ulcers should be on prevention of initial tissue damage, prevention of progression of an ulcer to a more severe grade and prevention of infection (Bennett *et al.* 2004). There is a need to monitor and treat pressure ulcers effectively because they are generally avoidable, and this will prevent unnecessary pain and suffering for the patient (Grewal *et al.* 1999). It must be emphasized that the prevention of pressure ulceration is a multidisciplinary responsibility, and not solely for nursing staff (Beldon 2006).

Reference material

Prevalence

Pressure ulcers represent a significant financial burden on health care systems (Benbow 2006). Approximately 412 000 individuals will develop a new pressure ulcer annually in the UK: one in every 150 in the general population and one in 23 of the population over 65 years of age (Bennett *et al.* 2004). While the total cost of presssure ulcer care in the UK between 1999 and 2000 was £1.4–2.1 billion, 90% of this cost is nurse time (Bennett *et al.* 2004). The National Service Framework for Older People (DH 2001a) has identified the need to reduce the risk of pressure damage in older persons in both community and inpatient settings, and highlighted the importance of specialist care for this vulnerable group of people.

Aetiology

The three major extrinsic factors that were identified as being significant contributory factors in the development of pressure ulcers include pressure, shearing and friction. These factors should be removed or diminished to prevent injury (NICE 2003).

- *Pressure.* The blood pressure at the arterial end of the capillaries is approximately 35 mmHg, while at the venous end this drops to around 16 mmHg (the average mean capillary pressure equals about 17 mmHg) (Guyton & Hall 2000; Tortora & Grabowski 2008). Any external pressures exceeding this will cause capillary obstruction as the capillaries close when the pressure between the bed surface and the bony prominence exceeds the 16–32 mmHg (Landis 1930; S. Hampton, pers. comm., October 2006). Tissues that are dependent on these capillaries are deprived of their blood supply. Eventually, the ischaemic tissues will die (Bridel-Nixon 1999; Tong 1999). The pressure as it approaches the bony prominences can be up to five times greater and is known as the 'cone of pressure': it explains why a surface redness can hide extensive tissue damage nearer the bone. It also explains why a small ulcer can open into a large, undetermined ulcer with overhanging edges and sinus formation (S. Hampton, pers. comm., October 2006). Bliss (1993) identifies that the formation of undermined tissues and sinuses are not due to infection but are produced by lysis of necrotic tissue produced during the original ischaemic episode (S. Hampton, pers. comm., October 2006).
- *Shearing.* This may occur when the patient slips down the bed or is dragged up the bed. As the skeleton moves over the underlying tissue the microcirculation is destroyed and the tissue dies of anoxia. In more serious cases, lymphatic vessels and muscle fibres may also become torn, resulting in a deep pressure ulcer (Simpson *et al.* 1996; Collier 1999; Clay 2000).
- *Friction.* This is a component of shearing, which causes stripping of the stratum corneum, leading to superficial ulceration (Waterlow 1988; Johnson 1989). Poor lifting and moving techniques may be a major contributory factor (NICE 2001).

The most common sites for pressure ulcer development are areas where soft tissue is compressed between a prominence (such as the sacrum) and an external surface (such as a mattress or seat of a chair) (Hess 2005).

Identifying at-risk patients

Assessing a patient's risk of developing pressure ulcers should involve both informal and formal assessment procedures (NICE 2003). A patient's risk of developing a pressure ulcer should be assessed either on admission to hospital or in the community when the patient first comes into contact with health services. The NICE guidelines suggest that this should take place within 6 hours of the start of admission to the episode of care (NICE 2003). The European Pressure Ulcer Advisory Panel (EPUAP 2003) pointed out that assessment should be ongoing and frequency of reassessment

Table 48.6   The Norton scale (From Norton *et al.* 1985 and Braden & Bergstrom 1996).

Physical condition	Score	Mental condition	Score	Activity	Score	Mobility	Score	Incontinent	Score
Good	4	Alert	4	Ambulant	4	Full	4	Not	4
Fair	3	Apathetic	3	Walk/help	3	Slightly limited	3	Occasionally	3
Poor	2	Confused	2	Chairbound	2	Very limited	2	Usually/urine	2
Very bad	1	Stuporous	1	Bedfast	1	Immobile	1	Doubly	1

should be dependent on change in the patient's condition with the environment.

Many predisposing factors are involved in the development of pressure ulcers. An individual's potential to develop pressure ulcers may be influenced by the following intrinsic factors (NICE 2003):

- Reduced mobility or immobility.
- Acute illness.
- Level of consciousness.
- Extremes of age.
- Vascular disease.
- Severe, chronic or terminal illness.
- Previous history of pressure damage.
- Malnutrition and dehydration.

Skin inspection should occur regularly and frequency must be established according to the patient's medical condition (NICE 2003). Patients who are willing to be involved should be taught and encouraged to inspect their own skin. A mirror can be provided for patients to inspect areas that they cannot see easily.

Grades of pressure ulcers

If a pressure ulcer develops then classification of the wound may assist in determining the most appropriate treatment. These are valuable in describing the state of the ulcer and the most pertinent care required by the patient.

The EPUAP (2003) outlined four grades for risk of tissue damage:

- *Grade 1*: non-blanchable erythema of intact skin.
- *Grade 2*: presents clinically as an abrasion or blister.
- *Grade 3*: superficial lesions.
- *Grade 4*: deep lesions, extensive destruction, tissue necrosis, or damage to muscle, bone or supporting structures.

Assessment tools

There are several risk assessment tools in pressure ulcer development such as those developed by Norton, Braden and Waterlow (Norton *et al.* 1985; Braden & Bergstrom 1987; Waterlow 1991; Waterlow1998). Deeks (1996) suggested that no single tool is considered reliable and valid for universal use. It has become common for particular areas of care to construct their own hybrid assessment tool as a result of professional discussion and tailoring to specific patient needs (Birtwistle 1994; Chaplin 2000; Lindgren *et al.* 2002). NICE

(2001) cautions professionals to use risk assessment tools as an *aide mémoire* and recommends their use in conjunction with clinical judgment (Chaplin 2000; RCN 2001).

Some of the most commonly used tools include the following:

Norton scale

With the Norton scale (Table 48.6) patients with a score of 14 or below are considered to be at greatest risk of pressure ulcer development. A score of 14–18 is not considered at risk but will require reassessment and a score of 18–20 indicates minimal risk.

The 'cut off' point for 'at risk' patients was later raised to 15 or 16 by Norton (Norton *et al.* 1985; Papanikolaou *et al.* 2006). Norton acknowledged that the tool was not intended as a universal tool, otherwise age and nutrition would have formed part of the criteria (Waterlow 2005).

Waterlow scale

The Waterlow scale (Figure 48.2) defines a score of 11–15 as being 'at risk', 16–20 as 'high risk' and over 20 as 'very high risk' (Waterlow 2005). In a study of the Norton and Waterlow scales, 75.7% of patients identified as 'at risk' by the Waterlow scale developed a pressure ulcer, whereas 62% of those with a score of 16 or less on the Norton scale developed ulcers (Smith *et al.* 1986). This suggests that the Waterlow scale may give a more accurate prediction of patient risk.

Braden scale

The Braden scale (Table 48.7) consists of six subscores (sensory perception, activity, moisture, nutrition, mobility, and friction and shearing) which are scored from 1 to 4 depending on the severity of the condition (with the exception of friction and shearing which is scored 1–3). The total score is then added up with a range possible from 6 to 23. The lower the score, the higher the risk of developing a pressure ulcer. Hospital patients are considered to be at risk if their score is 16 or below. It has been tested in a variety of settings and validated by expert opinion (Bergstrom *et al.* 1987; Bergstrom & Braden 1992).

The Braden scale was originally designed as a pressure ulcer predictor, unlike the Norton and Waterlow scales which assess risk (Waterlow 2005). This distinction is important to note when tools are used, or compared. Targeted interventions are likely to differ; for instance, Braden, although used

Name: _____   Hospital No: _____

Instruction for use:
1. Score on admission and update weekly or if significant change in patient's condition
2. Add scores together and insert total score
3. Document actions taken in the evaluation section
4. If total score is 10+ initiate core care plan At Risk of Pressure Damage/Pressure Ulcer Formation

10+ AT RISK   15+ HIGH RISK   20+ VERY HIGH RISK

	Date (Day/Month/Year)									
	Time									
GENDER	Male	1								
	Female	2								
AGE	14–49	1								
	50–64	2								
	65–74	3								
	75–80	4								
	81+	5								
BUILD	Average	0								
	Above average	1								
	Obese	2								
	Below average	3								
APPETITE (select one option ONLY)	Average	0								
	Poor	1								
	NG Tube/fluids only	2								
	NBM/anorexic	3								
VISUAL ASSESSMENT OF AT RISK SKIN AREA (may select one or more options)	Healthy	0								
	Thin and fragile	1								
	Dry	1								
	Oedematous	1								
	Clammy (Temp↑)	1								
	Previous pressure sore or scarring	2								
	Discoloured	2								
	Broken	3								

Figure 48.2   Waterlow pressure ulcer risk assessment. (Adapted from the Waterlow Pressure Sore/Ulcer Risk Assessment Scoring System [available from www.judywaterlow.fsnet.co.uk] with permission and acknowledgement of the copyright holder, J. Waterlow 1991, revised 1995, 1998 & 2005.)

MOBILITY (select one option ONLY)	Fully	0							
	Restless/fidgety	1							
	Apathetic	2							
	Restricted	3							
	Inert (due to ↓ consciousness/traction)	4							
	Chairbound	5							
CONTINENCE (select one option ONLY)	Continent/catheterized	0							
	Occasional incontinence	1							
	Incontinent of urine	2							
	Incontinent of faeces	2							
	Doubly incontinent	3							
TISSUE MALNUTRITION (may select one or more options)	Smoking	2							
	Anaemia	2							
	Peripheral vascular disease	5							
	Cardiac failure	5							
	Cachexia	8							
NEUROLOGICAL DEFICIT (score depends on severity)	Diabetes, CVA, MS, motor/sensory paraplegia epidural	4–6							
MAJOR SURGERY TRAUMA (up to 48 hours post surgery)	Above waist	2							
	Orthopaedic, below waist, spinal > 2 hours on theatre table	5							
MEDICATION	Cytotoxics, high dose steroids, anti-inflammatory	4							
TOTAL SCORE									
NURSE SIGNATURE									

Figure 48.2 (*continued*)

Table 48.7 Braden scale for predicting pressure sore risk.

				Date of assessment
Sensory perception Ability to respond meaningfully to pressure related discomfort	**1. *Completely limited*:** Unresponsive (does not moan, flinch or grasp) to painful stimuli, due to diminished level of consciousness or sedation *or* limited ability to feel pain over most of body surface	**2. *Very limited*:** Responds only to painful stimuli. Cannot communicate discomfort except by moaning or restlessness *or* has a sensory impairment that limits the ability to feel pain or discomfort over half of the body	**3. *Slightly limited*:** Responds to verbal commands, but cannot always communicate discomfort or need to be turned *or* has some sensory impairment that limits ability to feel pain or discomfort in 1 or 2 extremities	**4. *No impairment*:** Responds to verbal commands. Has no sensory deficit that would limit ability to feel or voice pain or discomfort
Moisture Degree to which skin is exposed to moisture	**1. *Constantly moist*:** Skin is kept moist almost constantly by perspiration, urine etc. Dampness is detected every time patient is moved or turned	**2. *Very moist*:** Skin is often, but not always moist. Linen must be changed at least once a shift	**3. *Occasionally moist*:** Skin is occasionally moist, requiring an extra linen change approximately once a day	**4. *Rarely moist*:** Skin is usually dry, linen only requires changing at routine intervals
Activity Degree of physical activity	**1. *Bedfast*:** Confined to bed	**2. *Chairfast*:** Ability to walk severely limited or non-existent Cannot bear own weight and/or must be assisted into chair or wheelchair	**3. *Walks occasionally*:** Walks occasionally during day, but for very short distances, with or without assistance. Spends majority of each shift in bed or chair	**4. *Walks frequently*:** Walks outside the room at least twice a day and inside room at least once every 2 hours during waking hours
Mobility Ability to change and control body position	**1. *Completely immobile*:** Does not make even slight changes in body or extremity position without assistance	**2. *Very limited*:** Makes occasional slight changes in body or extremity position but unable to make frequent or significant changes independently	**3. *Slightly limited*:** Makes frequent though slight changes in body or extremity position independently	**4. *No limitations*:** Makes major and frequent changes in position without assistance
Nutrition Usual food intake pattern: 1 NBM: nothing by mouth 2 IV: intravenously 3 TPN: total parenteral nutrition	**1. *Very poor*:** Never eats a complete meal. Rarely eats more than 1/3 of any food offered. Eats 2 servings or less of protein (meat or dairy products) per day. Takes fluids poorly. Does not take a liquid dietary supplement *or* is NBM 1 and/or maintained on clear fluids or IV 2 for more than 5 days	**2. *Probably inadequate*:** Rarely eats a complete meal and generally eats only about 1/2 of any food offered. Protein intake includes only 3 servings of meat or dairy products per day. Occasionally willl take a dietary supplement *or* receives less than the optimum amount of liquid diet or tube feeding	**3. *Adequate*:** Eats over half of most meals. Eats a total of 4 servings of protein (meats, dairy products) each day Occasionally will refuse a meal, but will usually take a supplement if offered *or* is on a tube feeding or TPN 3 regimen that probably meets most of nutritional needs	**4. *Excellent*:** Eats most of every meal Never refuses a meal Usually eats a total of 4 or more servings of meat and dairy products. Occasionally eats between meals. Does not require supplementation
Friction and shear	**1. *Problem*:** Requires moderate to maximum assistance in moving. Complete lifting without sliding against sheets is impossible. Frequently slides down in bed or chair, requiring frequent repositioning with maximum assistance. Spasticity, contractures or agitation lead to almost constant friction	**2. *Potential problem*:** Moves feebly or requires minimum assistance. During a move skin probably slides to some extent against sheets, chair, restraints, or other devices. Maintains relatively good position in chair or bed most of the time but occasionally slides down	**3. *No apparent problem*:** Moves in bed and in chair independently and has sufficient muscle strength to lift up completely during move. Maintains good position in bed or chair at all times	

Total score Total score of 12 or less represents **high risk**

Assess	Date	Evaluator/signature/title		Assess	Date	Evaluator/signature/title
1	//			3	//	
2	//			4	//	

Name: last, first, middle | Attending physician | ID number

High risk: Total score <12 Moderate risk: Total score 13–14 Low risk: Total score 15–16 if under 75 years old or 15–18 if over 75 years old.

widely in the USA, has been criticized for being difficult to use in a working environment (RCN 2003; Waterlow 2005).

Treatment and prevention

Treatment of pressure ulcers is the same as for any other wound. The aetiology and underlying or related pathology, as well as the wound itself, must be assessed in order to provide the most appropriate treatment. Care should be aimed at relief of pressure, the minimization of symptoms from predisposing factors and the provision of the ideal microenvironment for wound healing.

When positioning patients, it must be ensured that prolonged pressure on bony prominences is minimized. An awareness of interface pressures, e.g. creased bed linen and night clothing, is also important to avoid increased friction and further skin breakdown. Repositioning is recommended by the NICE (2003) but with taking into consideration other factors such as patient's medical condition, comfort, overall plan of care and the support surface. NICE (2003) also suggested that a repositioning schedule must be available. This must be agreed with the patient and recorded. If patients are able, they should be taught the underlying principles of pressure relief and enabled to manage repositioning themselves (NICE 2001) (see Chapter 34). It has also been suggested that consideration must be given to whether sitting time should be restricted to less than 2 hours per session (NICE 2003). It is important to seek specialist advice for assessment for positioning, aids and equipment to use.

It was suggested that nurses should possess a basic level of knowledge relating to the underlying principles of pressure ulcer prevention, healing and treatment in order to reduce unnecessary occurrence and discomfort (Mockridge & Anthony 1999).

Devices used for relief of pressure

A wide variety of devices are available to help relieve pressure over susceptible areas, e.g. cushions, overlays, static/dynamic mattresses and replacement beds. These devices differ in function and complexity, and choice must be based on meeting the patient's individual need, sound criteria for decision-making and effective use of available resources (Table 48.8). NICE (2003) emphasized that the quality of data currently available to evaluate the clinical effectiveness of pressure-relieving devices is variable.

The following are recommendations from NICE (2001):

- Patients with pressure ulcers should have access to pressure-relieving support surfaces and strategies, for example mattresses and cushions, 24 hours a day and this applies to all support surfaces.
- All individuals assessed as having a grade 1–2 pressure ulcer should, as a minimum provision, be placed on a high-specification foam mattress or cushion with pressure-reducing properties. Observation of skin changes,

documentation of positioning and repositioning scheme must be combined in the patient's care.

- If there is any potential or actual deterioration of affected areas or further pressure ulcer development, an alternating pressure (AP) (replacement or overlay) or sophisticated continuous low pressure (CLP) system (e.g. low air loss, air fluidized, air flotation, viscous fluid) should be used.
- For patients who require bed rails, AP overlay mattresses should be placed on a reduced-depth foam mattress to maintain their safety.
- Depending on the location of ulcer, individuals assessed as having grade 3–4 pressure ulcers (including intact eschar where depth, and therefore grade, cannot be assessed) should be, as a minimum provision, placed on an AP mattress or sophisticated CLP system.
- If AP equipment is required, the first choice should be an overlay system. However, circumstances such as patient weight or patient safety indicate the need for a replacement system.
- Create the optimum wound healing environment by using modern dressings (e.g. hydrocolloids, hydrogels, hydrofibres, foams, films, alginates, soft silicones) in preference to basic dressing types such as gauze, paraffin gauze and simple dressing pads.

In 2005, NICE in collaboration with the Royal College of Nursing (RCN) created a clinical guideline in pressure ulcer management (NICE 2005; RCN 2005). This included data looking at evidence-based practice, cost-effectiveness and economic evaluations in the different devices, drugs, procedures, among others in the management of pressure ulcers (see Table 48.8).

Fungating wounds

Definition

A fungating wound is the result of a cancerous mass that infiltrates the epithelium and surrounding lymph and blood vessels (Grocott 2000a). It can present as an ulcerating crater with a distinct margin or a raised fungating nodule (Bennett & Moody 1995).

Reference material

Aetiology

Fungating wounds can occur almost anywhere on the body. They arise most commonly from cancer of the breast (62%) or head and neck (24%), melanoma, soft tissue sarcoma and some cancers of the genito-urinary system (Thomas 1992; Naylor 2001; Wilkes *et al.* 2001). The resulting lesion could be a local tumour or metastatic spread from a primary tumour (Hampton & Collins 2004). Each patient responds

Table 48.8 A selection of mechanical methods for relieving pressure. It is important to remember the risk of cross-infection with the use of special beds. Most companies provide adequate cleaning/sterilizing of their equipment. Sheepskin is not a pressure relieving device and can become hard and matted with washing although it has been commended for helping with shearing in the past. (Hampton & Collins 2004; NICE 2005 Guidelines: www.nice.org.uk/page.aspx?o=cg029fullguideline.)

Aid	Use	Advantages	Disadvantages
Silicone-filled mattress pad/cushion (e.g. Transoft)	Waterlow 10 or patients on prolonged bedrest, able to move spontaneously	Relieves pressure by distributing it over a greater area. Comfortable. Machine (industrial) washable. Acceptable in community settings as well as in hospital. Can be used for incontinent patients. Relatively cheap purchase price. Plastic protective covers available	If the patient is very incontinent of urine, even if the plastic side is uppermost, there is seepage into the core material. Stitching comes undone after several launderings. Not recommended for routine use in pressure ulcer prevention
Roho air-filled mattress/cushions	High–medium-risk patients, Waterlow 10–15	Interlinked air cells transfer air with movement. Patient can be nursed sitting or recumbent. Non-mechanical. Washable	Can be punctured and is expensive to repair. Often incorrectly inflated due to lack of understanding and education. Can be mechanically cleaned in sterile supply department
Alternating pressure beds	High–medium-risk patients, Waterlow 15 r	Mechanical alteration of pressure. Reduce the frequency of (but not need for) repositioning. Available on hire at short notice	Must be checked and maintained. May increase pressures in very thin patients. Punctures possible. Patients may complain of nausea due to movement of cells
Pressure redistributing foam mattress	Moderate-risk as above	Two-way multi-stretch foam and flexible covers, less expensive than beds	Should be audited 6 monthly for cross-infection risk. Should be placed on meshed mattress board, not solid, and turned monthly
Dynamic air mattress or low air loss bed	Moderate–high-risk patients, Waterlow 15–20	Equalizes pressure and weight and can be programmed to adjust air support to give optimal pressure redistribution. Warm	Expensive to buy, but can be hired. Makes some patients feel 'sea-sick'. Reduces self-motivated movement. Cells can become quite hard
Air fluidized bed	High-risk patients, Waterlow 20, or indicated because of medical condition	As near to levitation as possible. Warm, sterile air produces a beneficial environment for healing wounds. One nurse can manage even a very heavy or debilitated patient on his/her own. Can be used for incontinent patients or those with heavy wound exudate. May help to alleviate severe pain	Expensive to hire. Need to reinforce floors before it can be installed Minimizes self-motivation. Can be difficult for the patient to get in and out of bed even with help. Available on hire basis only

individually to having such a wound, the consequences of which impinge on physical, psychological, social, sexual as well as spiritual well-being. The highest level of nursing expertise is required.

It has been estimated that around 5–10% of people with metastatic cancer will develop such a wound (Haisfield-Wolfe & Rund 1997). Fungating wounds tend to occur in older patients (60–70 years old) with advanced cancer, and usually develop during the last 6 months of life (Ivetic & Lyne 1990; Haisfield-Wolfe & Rund 1997).

Assessment

Assessment and evaluation of a wound are discussed earlier in the chapter, but it is important to emphasize that an ac-

curate history of a malignant lesion should be taken, and that the management of the wound should be documented clearly from the beginning. The aim of management is to improve the patient's quality of life and based on the control of symptoms as opposed to the ability and progress of the wound to heal (Laverty et al. 1997). A wound assessment tool to record the amount and type of odour/exudate/pain, and the dressings used, is a helpful means of evaluating care strategies (see Figure 48.1). Dressings for managing fungating wounds are listed in Table 48.9.

Physical

The four most common symptoms associated with fungating wounds are:

961

Table 48.9 Dressings for management of fungating wounds. Normal wound principles in choosing dressings applies, only the management aim is towards palliating symptoms rather than healing. (From Mallett *et al.* 1999; Naylor *et al.* 2001; Naylor 2002; Dealey 2005; Hampton 2006.)

Wound type	Aim	Suggested intervention
Necrotic	Debridement of eschar	Hydrogel (Surgical intervention if appropriate)
Sloughy	Debride slough Prevent infection	Hydrogel (with absorbent secondary dressing, i.e. Allevyn) Alginate/hydrofibre (if high exudate is present)
Infected	Treat infection Prevent associated symptoms (odour, exudate)	Metronidazole gel (topical) (can be mixed with hydrogel or hydrocolloid gel to manage associated symptoms) Antibiotics for clinical infection as indicated by microbiology proven wound swab Manuka honey and ensure an absorbent secondary dressing as exudate will increase
Malodorous	Remove odour	Metronidazole gel (topical) Activated charcoal dressings with or without silver (if undergoing radiotherapy)
Highly exuding (cavity)	Contain exudate	Alginate (sheet/ribbon) Hydrofibre (sheet/ribbon) Foam sheet Foam cavity dressings (NB. Silver dressings combined with above are helpful, i.e. Acticoat, Aquacel Ag)
Lightly exuding	Contain exudate Prevent increase	Hydrocolloid Hydrogel/hydrocolloid gel With foam/foam with adhesive border
Bleeding	Control bleeding	Alginate Tranexamic acid Adrenalin 1% (as prescribed, topically with caution)
Itching	Control itching	Hydrogel sheets Aqueous cream with menthol

- Pain/discomfort.
- Heavy exudate.
- Malodour/infection.
- Bleeding (superficial or large vessel).
(Grocott 2000a; Lund-Nielsen *et al.* 2005)

Psychosocial

The nurse needs to be aware of these psychosocial issues and allow the patient to express his or her fears and concerns. Excellent communication skills coupled with empathy and sensitivity can be of great benefit to the patient when having

to cope, adapt and readjust to their changing situation (Naylor *et al.* 2001). It is impossible to completely understand the impact that a fungating wound has on patients and their family, but it is possible to offer a realistic and holistic approach to their care that affords them the opportunity to live as full a life as possible within the limitations of their wound and their disease.

Nurses must ensure that patients are aware that comfort, not cure, is the aim, and respond to patients' needs sensitively. The chronic nature of malignant wounds means that patients are involved in an ongoing process of adjustment. Wounds are also a constant reminder to patients of advanced disease and possible impending death (Laverty *et al.* 1997; Naylor *et al.* 2001). They may also feel embarrassment, especially with regard to their relationship with their partner (Bird 2000). Leakage of exudate and strong odour may lead them to live separate lives, and may make the continuation of a sexual relationship extremely difficult, if not impossible (Hallett 1995).

Management of symptoms

1 *Pain/discomfort.* Localized pain is sometimes experienced with wounds in addition to generalized pain which is addressed separately (see Chapter 27). Assessment provides a means to determine the underlying cause of the pain, e.g. infection, pressure on structures, heightened anxiety, invasion of nerves (Naylor 2001). A short-acting analgesic such as dextromoramide (e.g. Palfium) or nitrous oxide (e.g. Entonox) may be required to supplement the regular analgesic, for instance when dressings are changed (Hollinworth 1997). Similarly, a breakthrough dose of the patient's regular analgesia may be administered 20–30 minutes before the dressing change (Naylor *et al.* 2001). The use of morphine or diamorphine mixed with a hydrogel (to form a 0.08–0.10% mixture) and applied topically to the wound has been found to be an effective method of pain relief in ulcerating wounds, including fungating wounds (Back & Finlay 1995; Stein 1995; Krajnik & Zylicz 1997; Twillman *et al.* 1999; Grocott 2000b). This is based on the fact that peripheral opioid receptors are present. The results (although on a small group of patients) suggest that the use of topically based analgesia may have a clinically useful analgesic effect.

2 *Heavy exudate.* Exudate from a fungating lesion can act as a reservoir for infection (especially bacterial infection) (Collinson 1992; White 2000). Plastic surgical procedures are often not feasible because of local invasion by the tumour (Moss 1989). Less invasive measures (e.g. radiotherapy) may be beneficial in the short term (Thomas 1992; Fairbairn 1993). Wound dressings should be absorbent and non-adhesive (Fairbairn 1994), but can be bulky. The social and psychological effects of large, conspicuous dressings must be taken into account when selecting a suitable dressing (Thomas 1992;

White 2000). A high absorbency dressing (e.g. Aquacel) may provide adequate management for a heavily exuding wound (Williams 1999; Robinson 2000). Care needs to be taken to monitor the condition of the surrounding skin. Medium to high exudate levels can lead to excoriation and maceration of the periwound area. Avoiding maceration around the wound with a skin barrier (Cavilon) should help prevent pruritis and reduce discomfort at dressing changes (Hampton & Collins 2004).

3 *Malodour/infection.* Malodour in malignant wounds has been found to be significantly stressful for both the patient and the nurses managing them with maintaining emotional rapport very difficult. In a qualitative study nurses found building rapport with patients difficult as they hid their true feelings of revulsion. This can be detrimental to the nurse patient encounter and increase feelings of isolation (Wilkes *et al.* 2001).

Charcoal dressings are also effective at controlling odour. They attract and bind the molecules which cause odour and prevent their escape from the local area (Thomas 1992; Kelly 2002). If using a hydrogel or alginate for comfort and absorption at the wound bed, apply first and then cover with a charcoal sheet (Naylor 2002). Kaltocarb combines these with a secondary dressing; however there are limits regarding size and formability (Grocott 2000b). Silver dressings are also used in managing exudate and malodour, for example, Actisorb Silver 220, which combines a charcoal layer with silver (Wilson 2005) and should be used as a primary dressing. Using it as a secondary dressing is wasteful of the silver and not cost-effective (S. Hampton, pers. comm., October 2006). Aquacel Ag also combines silver and can absorb up to 30 times its weight (Wilson 2005).

Lund-Nielsen *et al.* (2005) evaluated a regimen for advanced breast cancer patients and found that use of a systematic and structured tool was beneficial in the care of the 12 women. A malodour assessment was used with a scale from none to strong (odour evident upon entering the room with intact dressing in place). Following the intervention, 50% felt there was an improvement and had a desire for social contact.

Malodour is often an indication that a wound is infected (Dealey 2005) or colonized (Hampton & Collins 2004). In the case of fungating wounds, these will often be colonized by anaerobic bacteria and that will be ongoing due to the poor vascular supply in the wound which leads to consistent necrosis (S. Hampton, pers. comm., October 2006). If infection is suspected, swabs can be taken to identify the causative organism before systemic measures are adopted. Malodour is commonly caused by anaerobic organisms that flourish in the necrotic tissue. They release volatile fatty acids as an end product, which are thought to be responsible for the characteristic smell. Metronidazole as a gel has proved an effective agent for deodorization of fungating lesions (Newman *et al.* 1989; Thomas & Hay 1991; Bower *et al.* 1992;

Finlay *et al.* 1996; Kelly 2002). Systemic metronidazole can also be beneficial if the odour is extreme. It inhibits anaerobic colonization and decreases associated odours. This should be used with caution in order to avoid any side-effects. Sparrow *et al.* (1980) conducted a small-scale study that showed systemic metronidazole could be given in the lower dose of 200 mg three times daily (as opposed to 400 mg) with equal effectiveness and fewer side-effects.

Small studies have been conducted on some other topical applications:

(a) *Sugar paste.* Useful for debridement of/and to aid regranulation of tissue. Twice daily application has been recommended for 'optimum antibacterial effect' (Middleton 1990; Topham 2000).

(b) *Honey.* This has antibacterial properties related to its sugar content and the presence of hydrogen peroxide and plant-derived antibacterial agents. These properties inhibit anaerobe activity, but the antibacterial effect can be destroyed by heat. Frequent dressing changes may be required if there is an increase in the amount of exudate produced, as this makes the honey too dilute and, therefore, affects its activity. The honey is applied directly to the wound and left on with a secondary dressing. It is important to use gamma-irradiated honey in wound care, as this is correctly sterilized. Care should be taken of the surrounding skin, which may be friable and break down easily (Dunford 2000). It can also be messy (Lund-Nielsen *et al.* 2005).

(c) *Tea tree and essential oils.* In a recent review (Carson *et al.* 2006) found a wealth of *in vitro* data supporting its use but pointed to the lack of evidence demonstrating clinical efficacy against bacterial, fungal, or viral infections and the need for randomized controlled trials. There is little evidence to support its long-term use in wound management or the potential systemic uptake when it is applied directly to a wound (Carson *et al.* 2006). Any treatments that are homeopathic in nature should be undertaken by a qualified homeopathic practitioner (S. Hampton, pers. comm., October 2006).

Some promising recent research (Warnke *et al.* 2004, 2005, 2006) has demonstrated the antibacterial and anti-inflammatory effect of essential oil mixtures, most recently eucalyptus-based, on malodorous necrotic ulcers in patients with malignant fungating wounds in head and neck. The product was applied twice daily with improvements noted in these areas and shrinkage of the wound due to minimizing of slough, and this greatly improved the patients' quality of life. This was a small study and further trials on a named-patient basis are planned. Again, until the research is complete, these treatments should be undertaken by a qualified homeopathic practitioner (S. Hampton, pers. comm., October 2006).

(d) *Deodorizers and environmental air fresheners.* These may help to reduce the odour around the patient but

963

are not particularly effective at masking the odour. Similarly, good ventilation, essential oils and scented candles may be of limited benefit.

4 *Bleeding/haemorrhage.* Because of their fragile vascular condition and capillary ooze, fungating wounds frequently bleed (Wilson 2005). Haemostasis can be achieved by simple compression (Wilson 2005) and using alginate dressings. If bleeding is profuse, measures with an immediate effect may be taken:

(a) *Adrenaline 1 : 1000.* Acts as a vasoconstrictor when applied topically, but must be applied with caution because it is absorbed systemically (Dealey 2005; BNF 2006).

(b) *Tranexamic acid.* Given orally as a tablet or applied topically to the wound, it stems bleeding and reduces re-bleeding by inhibiting fibrinolysis (breakdown of blood clots) (Dean & Tuffin 1997; Pudner 1998).

(c) *Haemostatic swabs.* Stimulate rapid capillary coagulation. They can be left in place and covered with a secondary dressing. They are most commonly applied in surgical procedures, but are also useful in controlling bleeding in chronic wounds and may be used in primary care as they are easy to apply to the wound and can be left in place under the usual dressing (Naylor 2002).

(d) Alginates are excellent as haemostats, as they exchange calcium in the wound with sodium, and this intitiates the clotting cascade. Sorbsan silver Plus would be useful for a wound that potentially can bleed as it has silver to fight colonization, high absorption capacity and is an alginate to act as a haemostat (S. Hampton, pers. comm., October 2006).

5 *Radiotherapy.* This can reduce the amount of exudate and control bleeding in malignant wounds. It is given either as a single fraction, to avoid frequent hospital visits, or in divided doses over 2–3 weeks. Occasionally, radiotherapy is used prophylactically to prevent fungation if the skin is intact. If fungation has already occurred, radiotherapy may still be of value in reducing tumour bulk and enabling a degree of healing (Souhami & Tobias 1998; Bale & Jones 2006).

6 *Hormone therapy.* Hormone therapy can reduce the rate at which a fungating wound progresses and deteriorates (Fairbairn 1993). Chemotherapy is occasionally used for this purpose, but hormone therapy has fewer side-effects and can enhance the patient's sense of well-being.

Securing dressings

Tapes should only be applied to healthy skin in order to avoid further tissue damage. Care should be taken to leave a large margin around the wound including any existing cutaneous nodules. Plain bandaging or the use of Netelast/Tubifast is helpful where a wound is positioned in a difficult area (Naylor *et al.* 2001).

Radiotherapy skin damage

Definition

Radiotherapy skin reaction may present as skin irritation, erythema and/or flaking or peeling of skin within a field of radiotherapy treatment. These reactions develop over a period of weeks as repeated ionizing radiation causes an inflammatory response (Simonen *et al.* 1998). Radiation impairs stem cell division within the basal layer of the epidermis, disrupting or sometimes halting the normal process of skin regeneration (Archambeau *et al.* 1995). Patients undergoing radiotherapy treatment will receive some degree of skin damage. Internationally there are many preventative and treatment options recommended, with evidence showing varying degrees of success (Maddocks-Jennings *et al.* 2005; S. Hampton, pers. comm., October 2006).

It has been estimated that the incidence of radiotherapy skin reactions experienced in patients at some level is around 85–95% (Porock & Kristjanson 1999; Fisher *et al.* 2000). There are four main types, which are classified according to the appearance of the skin (Table 48.10).

The degree of skin reaction depends on a number of factors:

- High total dose of radiation.
- Low-energy radiation or electrons.
- Treatment of areas with skin folds (i.e. the head and neck, breast or pelvic area) which are prone to increased moisture and friction.
- Large volume of normal tissue included in the area of treatment.
- Tangential treatment fields.
- Use of 'bolus' materials (e.g. a wax blanket to increase the dose of radiotherapy to the skin).
- Older age.
- Immunosuppression.
- Concurrent chemotherapy or steroid therapy.
- Poor nutritional status.
- Tobacco smoking.

Table 48.10   Categories of acute radiotherapy skin reactions

Category	Description
Erythema	Reddened skin, which may be oedematous and feel hot and irritable
Dry desquamation	Dry, flaky or peeling skin that may be itchy
Moist desquamation	Peeling skin with exposure of the dermis and exudate production, often painful and may become infected
Necrosis	Death of tissue; skin may darken and turn black

- Chronic sun exposure.

  (Rigter *et al.* 1994; Blackmar 1997; Porock *et al.* 1998; Maher 2005; Naylor *et al.* 2001; Wells & MacBride 2003).

Reference material

Assessment

Assessment of the treatment area is imperative and should be ongoing. A baseline assessment should note the current condition of the skin, the risk factors listed above and the educational needs of the patent and their family or carers (Maher 2005). Measures to minimize and delay skin breakdown and promote comfort should be initiated early on in the treatment plan. Special note should be made of concurrent illness (i.e. diabetes) or skin changes (i.e. scars, eczema) which may affect healing (Noble-Adams 1999).

Skin care during radiotherapy

Preventive measures to help maintain skin integrity during radiotherapy include:

- Gentle washing of the skin using warm water and non-perfumed mild soap.
- Avoiding friction on the skin (from, for example, wet shaving, tight clothing or scratching).
- Wearing comfortable cotton garments and silk scarves around the neck area (as long as skin remains intact).
- Protecting the skin from sunlight, wind or extremes of temperature.
- Avoiding perfumed or metallic products such as make up and deodorants.
- Using a simple moisturizer such as aqueous cream from the start of treatment.

  (Mallett *et al.* 1999; Westbury *et al.* 2000; Glean *et al.* 2001; Roy *et al.* 2001)

Symptom management

Surveys of skin care practice for radiotherapy reactions in the UK and abroad have concluded that there are a variety of approaches and products in use based largely on historical precedent and personal preference rather than clinical evidence (Lavery 1995; Glean *et al.* 2001; D'Haese *et al.* 2005; Nystedt *et al.* 2005). Similarly, reviews of published literature have found a lack of randomized controlled trials evaluating treatments for acute skin reactions (Glean *et al.* 2001; Naylor & Mallett 2001; Wickline 2004). Recent recommendations emphasize the importance of moist wound healing, for moist desquamation in particular (Table 48.11).

Plastic surgery wounds

Definition

Plastic surgery is the collective term that refers to surgical procedures that are performed to restore function and assist

Table 48.11 Recommended treatments for acute radiotherapy skin reactions. (From Shell *et al.* 1986; Margolin *et al.* 1990; Pickering & Warland 1992; Crane 1993; Strunk & Maher 1993; Boots-Vickers & Eaton 1999; Glean *et al.* 2001; Naylor & Mallett 2001; Heggie *et al.* 2002; Patwardhan *et al.* 2002; Wells & MacBride 2003; Wickline 2004.)

Category of skin reaction	Suggested treatment
Erythema and dry desquamation (may be managed in the same way)	■ Hydrophilic and moisturizing creams, e.g. aqueous cream: provide symptomatic relief ■ 1% hydrocortisone: for itchy, irritable or burning feelings of the skin within the treatment field; should be applied sparingly, 2–3 times a day, but *not to areas of broken or infected skin (use of moisturising creams should continue)*
Moist desquamation	■ Hydrogel sheets: reduce discomfort and promote healing (soothing and cooling) ■ Amorphous hydrogels: useful in skin-folds or the perineum ■ Semi-permeable film dressings: may be applied to areas of low or no exudate and left in place during treatment; reduce pain and are easy to remove ■ Modern absorbent dressings, e.g. alginate, hydrofibre, foam ■ Hydrocolloid sheets: may be applied to areas of moist desquamation *once radiotherapy treatment has finished*; provide an aesthetically acceptable dressing that promotes comfort and healing
Necrosis	Debride eschar/slough; use appropriate dressings to promote healing (see Table 48.4)

in the healing of exposed or nonunion fractures, soft tissue defects or to improve natural contours. Patients whose lives have changed following excision of a cancerous tumour or other misfortunes can be reconstructed and made whole again (Dinman 1999). This is achieved by using flaps and skin grafts for reconstruction purposes, in addition to using the natural elasticity and mobility of the skin. A surgical flap is a strip of tissue, usually consisting of skin, underlying fat, fascia, muscle and/or bone, which is transferred from one part of the body (known as the donor site) to another (known as the recipient site) (Edwards 1994; Brown *et al.* 1998).

A skin graft is living, but devascularized (separated from its blood supply), tissue consisting of all or some of the layers of the skin which is removed from one area of the body and applied to a wound on another area of the body. The three types of skin graft are full-thickness skin graft (FTSG), in which the entire epidermis and dermis is removed, split-thickness or split skin graft (SSG), which consists of the epidermis and the upper part of the dermis only (Francis 1998; Young & Fowler 1998), and pinch grafting, which

965

Name: .... Hospital No: .... Ward:.......................................

THE ROYAL MARSDEN

Flap Observation Chart

Instructions	Criteria for Assessment	Normal	Arterial Insufficiency	Venous Congestion
1. **Confirm with the surgeon the frequency of flap observations** (see medical notes / nursing care plan) Suggested immediate post-op assessment frequency: • every 15 minutes for first 4 hours, • every 30 minutes for the next 4 hours, • hourly for 24–36 hours, • then 2–4 hourly thereafter 2. **If signs of venous or arterial occlusion seek immediate help** 3. **At each handover, confirm flap status/observations at the bedside**	**Colour** • If it is an external flap then check with the donor site or original colour • If it is an internal flap then monitor for extremes of colour	Usual skin tone	Paler than usual skin tone	Blue / Purple / Mottled
	Temperature • An external or internal flap should always feel warm to touch • If the flap feels cool or has increased warmth, *seek medical assessment immediately* • A warmer flap may be due to an abnormal inflammatory response, e.g. infection	Warm	Cold	Increased warmth
	Turgidity (Texture) • The flap should usually feel soft (spongy), not hard or flaccid • Hard or swollen flap indicates possible oedema or haematoma	Soft	Flaccid	Turgid (hard)
	Capillary Refill (Blanching) • If possible this should be timed (in seconds) • If timing not possible and an alteration in perfusion is suspected, *seek medical assessment immediately*	2–3 seconds	Absent / Sluggish > 6 seconds	Brisk < 3 seconds
	Specific Monitoring Instructions (*e.g. Monitor the tension on the flap and check for kinking*)			

Type & Location of Flap: .... **Donor Area (if appropriate):** ....

....

Timing		Colour (*tick one*)			Temperature (*tick one*)			Turgidity (Texture) (*tick one*)			Capillary Refill (Blanching) (*tick one*)			Specific Instructions (specify):	Signature and Print Name
Date	Time	Usual skin tone	Paler than usual skin tone	Blue / purple / mottled	Warm	Cold	Increased warmth	Soft	Flaccid	Turgid (hard)	2–3 seconds	Absent / sluggish > 6 seconds	Brisk < 3 seconds		

Title: Flap Observation Chart	Version No: 2 Issue Date: March 2005 Unique Identification Number: NR027		Document Type: Clinical Record - Chart
Department: Nursing & Rehabilitation – Nursing	Page 1 of 2		© 2005 The Royal Marsden Hospital

Figure 48.3 Flap observation chart.

can be undertaken by a nurse educated in the procedure (S. Hampton, pers. comm., October 2006).

Reference material

Aetiology

Surgical reconstruction is often required following extensive surgery for cancers of the breast, head and neck, skin (melanoma), soft tissue (sarcomas) and genitourinary system. The aim is to perform the simplest procedure that will provide the best aesthetic and functional outcome (Clamon & Netscher 1994). Each patient will require individually planned, and therefore unique, surgery. Reconstructive surgery of this type often results in altered anatomy, in both appearance and function, which may impact upon the psychological and physical well-being of the patient.

Assessment

Preoperative patient assessment must be as detailed as possible; this should include information on past and present medical conditions that may delay wound healing (see Wound assessment and Tissue factors affecting wound healing sections, above). For certain patient groups, e.g. those with recurrence of head and neck cancer, anatomy may already have been altered, through previous surgery, thereby narrowing down the possible options for reconstruction.

Postoperative observation of the wound sites, dressings and drains is crucial as deterioration of a wound can occur suddenly, e.g. fluid-filled seromas, necessitating the need for prompt nursing action. The main aim following flap reconstruction is to allow easy access for observation and to ensure circulation and overall care is monitored efficiently during the crucial first 72 hours. Figure 48.3 shows a flap observation chart.

Associated problems

Split skin graft donor site

The two most common problems associated with a split skin graft donor site are slipping of dressing and infection.

Timing		Colour (tick one)			Temperature (tick one)			Turgidity (Texture) (tick one)			Capillary Refill (Blanching) (tick one)			Specific Instructions (specify):	Signature and Print Name
Date	Time	Usual skin tone	Paler than usual skin tone	Blue / purple / mottled	Warm	Cold	Increased warmth	Soft	Flaccid	Turgid (hard)	2–3 seconds	Absent / sluggish > 8 seconds	Brisk < 3 seconds		

Title: Flap Observation Chart — Version No: 2 Issue Date: March 2005 Unique Identification Number: NR027 — Document Type: Clinical Record - Chart
Department: Nursing & Rehabilitation – Nursing — Page 2 of 2 — © 2006 The Royal Marsden Hospital

Figure 48.3 (*continued*)

Slipping of dressing, resulting in pain and discomfort
The donor sites chosen for SSG harvesting are usually the upper thigh, upper arm or upper buttock. Less conspicuous areas of the body are chosen wherever possible. The excision of the thin layer of skin leaves nerve endings exposed, resulting in pain at the donor site (Wilkinson 1997). Traditionally paraffin gauze combined with an absorbent layer of gauze padding and a bandage have been applied to donor sites in theatre and left intact for 10 days. However, adherence to the wound bed, complicated by slipping of the secondary dressing once heavy with exudate, commonly occurs causing pain and delaying healing. Beldon (2003) observed four different dressings on donor sites in a sample of 40 patients and found healing and comfort were improved in the alginate combined with a semi-permeable film group. (The comparison groups used a film alone, paraffin gauze or alginate as a primary dressing and padding with a bandage as a secondary dressing [Beldon 2003].)

Infection
A high amount of exudate on the dressing, evident by new and excessive strikethrough, can indicate the presence of infection (Beldon 2003). The entire dressing should be soaked off in order to assess the wound site, and the site should be swabbed for microbial culture and sensitivity. While infected, the wound site should be dressed daily. *Pseudomonas aeruginosa* is a common infecting organism of donor sites and is often evidenced by a strong musty smell and bright blue–green exudate.

Flamazine (silver sulphadiazine) is usually an effective treatment for *Pseudomonas* when applied topically to the donor site and covered with a non-adherent dressing (Hamilton-Miller *et al.* 1993), but this is not commonly used today as there is a dearth of dressings containing silver which are used instead of creams. There are also products, such as Cadesorb, which modulate the pH of a wound and drop the pH from >8 to <6. *Pseudomonas aeruginosa* survives in a pH of 8.4 but not in an acidic pH (S. Hampton, pers. comm., October 2006).

If the patient experiences a raised temperature, increased pain or appears unwell, this may indicate the presence of a systemic infection and they will require a course of antibiotics (Wilkinson 1997).

Split skin recipient site (flap donor site)

When a flap is transferred from its original site or a tumour is widely excised, it leaves a deficit of tissue. Split skin is applied

967

to this site, as primary closure is not usually possible. The most common problem with SSG recipient sites is fluid-filled seromas.

Fluid-filled seromas

On removing the dressing after 5 days, the SSG should be smooth and pink or red in colour. Any seromas, characterized by blisters containing air and haemoserous fluid, must be expelled. Without performing this, the graft will not 'take'. A sterile needle is used to evacuate the fluid, enabling the graft to be carefully rolled from the centre outwards (Coull 1991). This can be performed by using a cotton bud and enables the graft to adhere to the underlying tissue. A tulle dressing, low-linting gauze and a bandage, or a tape-less dressing are then applied. The pressure from the dressing assists in expelling the blisters (Coull 1991).

Scarring

Definition

A scar is defined as the mark left after a wound has healed with the formation of connective tissue, giving rise to an altered appearance of the skin (Davis *et al.* 1993; Eisenbeiss *et al.* 1998). Initially the scar is red and raised; then over a period of 6–12 months this matures to produce a hypopigmented, flat scar (Davies 1985).

Hypertrophic and keloid scars

Occasionally the scar continues to become increasingly red, raised and itchy, defined as hypertrophic. If these symptoms continue, with the scar tissue invading surrounding unaffected tissue as well as increasing in height, a keloid scar is formed (Williams 1996; Eisenbeiss *et al.* 1998). The areas that are most susceptible are the upper back, shoulders, anterior chest, presternal area and the upper arms (Munro 1995a; Beldon 2000). Darker skinned people have a greater susceptibility to developing keloid scars than those who are lighter skinned (Eisenbeiss *et al.* 1998).

Reference material

Aetiology

There are a number of possible predisposing factors (Munro 1995a):

- Increased skin tension can contribute to the formation of keloid and hypertrophic scars; however, earlobes, which are free of tension, can also develop keloid scars.
- These scars appear to have a genetic basis. In addition to this, keloid formation is more common in females (3 : 1 female : male ratio).

- There is thought to be a relationship between endocrine changes and keloid formation, e.g. keloids have been known to occur after a thyroidectomy and with increased hypothalamic activity.
- The production of hypertrophic and keloid scars may have an immunological basis.
- Biochemical differences between healthy scars, keloid and hypertrophic scars have been found, indicating that collagen synthesis is altered.
- Growth factors may have a role in keloid formation. During the inflammatory stage several growth factors (collagenase, gelatinase and stromelysin) migrate into the wound and affect the collagen fibre formation of a matrix which enhances the strength of the wound. When they are overactive or these processes are interrupted, abnormal scarring can occur (Smith 2005).

Management

Patients may be offered a number of treatments to help prevent or improve an abnormal scar:

- *Finger massage* can improve the condition of the scar. A non-perfumed moisturizing cream should be used to prevent friction between the finger and scar. Finger massage can begin when the wound has completely healed and all bruising has subsided. Massage should be performed for 10 minutes, six times each day using firm pressure in a tight circular motion over the scar.
- *Pressure treatment* with individually tailored elastic garments may be used for both keloid and hypertrophic scars. This treatment is used to prevent secondary contractures and to restore flatness and smoothness to scars. Pressure must be applied continuously for at least 12 months and any break in pressure should not exceed 30 minutes per day (Munro 1995b; Puzey 2001). Enhancement of cosmetic appearance and an increased rate of scar maturation are promoted by compression (Smith 2005). Pressure must be applied continuously for at least 12 months and any break in pressure should not exceed 30 minutes per day (Munro 1995b; Puzey 2001).
- *Intralesional corticosteroid injections* may help reduce scar tissue deposition and to soften and flatten keloid scars (Munro 1995b). There is a risk of scar recurrence with this treatment and it is only suitable for small scars (Eisenbeiss *et al.* 1998).
- *Silicone gel sheeting* will soften, flatten and blanch keloid and hypertrophic scars (Carney *et al.* 1994; Williams 1996).
- *Glycerine-based hydrogel sheet* (Novogel) may be effective in the prevention and treatment of hypertrophic and keloid scars. It can soften, flatten and relieve itching, redness and burning of scars (Baum & Busuito 1998). CicaC is a recognized treatment for scar tissue (S. Hampton, pers. comm., October 2006).
- *Surgical excision* may be considered to release scar contractures; for example, a 'W' or 'Z' plasty to release a

Table 48.12   Advantages and disadvantages of methods of wound closure. (From Jay 1999; Elkin *et al.* 2004; Richardson 2007.)

Method:	Disadvantages
Sutures: Non-absorbable sutures are more widely used for skin closure where the material causes little reaction or rejection. A monofilament nylon is a strong single stranded nylon providing continued strength; silk is a braided strand and fairly easy to handle. Interrupted sutures are separate sutures each with its own knot and are used on the majority of wounds because they are the most versatile. They are not recommended for fragile skin. A continuous suture is one long thread that spirals along the entire suture line at evenly spaced intervals Absorbable sutures degrade rapidly and thus allow the deep tissues within a wound to be closed successfully. They are also useful for patients who may not remember they have had sutures or will not attend for follow up Sutures can be removed once healing has occurred normally 5–10 days after injury	Suturing must be performed by an experienced practitioner Requires local anaesthetic Suture material is a foreign body in the wound and thus increases the risk of infection Sutures tied too tightly can damage tissues Sutures too loose may delay healing If skin layers are not aligned then patients can be left with a scar Forceps used to lift skin may crush the tissue
Adhesive skin closure strips: Available in a variety of widths Useful for superficial wounds that are not subject to tension Strips are cheap and easy to use and remove No local anaesthetic required and tissue damage is minimal	Strips do not adhere to sweaty or hairy skin If there is tissue oedema it makes it difficult to achieve good apposition of the wound edges May be suitable over some joints but where skin is taut or subject to movement they do not provide optimum closure
Tissue adhesive: Surgical 'superglues' are now popular for emergency settings Good cosmetic results Less painful than suturing Wound complication rates are low	It is expensive Not suitable over joints and areas of high tension Need second person to assist in getting skin edges aligned
Metal clips and staples: Staples are made of stainless steel wire Provide greatest tensile strength Quick method and offers low level of tissue reactivity and better resistance to infection than sutures Can be performed without local anaesthetic	Staples are more expensive than sutures and may be confined to wounds where needlestick injury is a high risk Must be inserted by an experienced practitioner Failure to align tissue edges may cause scar deformity Only useful for superficial skin layers

scar contracture by cutting it in the line of relaxed skin tension (Allsworth 1985; Beldon 2000). In the case of larger scars, surgical excision with or without skin grafting may be performed but there is a high rate of scar recurrence especially with keloid scars. Postoperative radiotherapy may reduce the recurrence rate by up to 70% (Eisenbeiss *et al.* 1998).

■ *Cosmetic camouflage*, utilizing specialist cosmetic products, can be used to hide scarring; this is most successful in patients with atrophic (indented) and hypertrophic scars. This service is provided by appropriately trained professionals who also provide advice and education to enable patients to perform their own camouflage make-up.

Methods of wound closure

There are four main methods of wound closure:

(a) Sutures.
(b) Adhesive skin closure strips.
(c) Tissue adhesive.
(d) Metal clips and staples.

See Table 48.12 for advantages and disadvantages of each method.

Wounds may vary and therefore careful assessment is required before the method of closure is selected and attempted (Richardson 2007). Richardson (2007) lists the following guiding principles to assist with decision making:

1 What is the aim of the wound closure: e.g. eliminating dead space where a haematoma can develop, realigning tissue correctly, or holding aligned tissues until healing has occurred.
2 What is the history of the wound: this informs the practitioner about the depth of the wound and likelihood of infection.
3 What is the wound site pattern: this and biomechanical properties may rule out some methods of closure.

969

Suturing

This method is used to promote healing, realign tissue layers and hold the skin edges until they have healed by first intention and no longer require artificial support (Castille 1998). There are a number of common suturing errors as listed in Table 48.13.

Removal of sutures are usually performed between 7 and 10 days post-insertion, but this is dependent on where on the body the sutures were placed and if the practitioner has ascertained that the wound has healed. Routinely every other suture or staple is removed first, with the rest removed if the incision remains securely closed. If any sign of suture line separation is evident during the removal process, the remaining sutures are left in place and reported to the medical team (Elkin *et al.* 2004).

Table 48.13 Common suturing errors. (Adapted from Castille 1998.)

Error	Resulting problems
Sutures too loose	Fails to bring wound edges together leading to gaps Sutures may fall out
Sutures too tight	Does not allow for normal wound swelling May induce vascular compromise of the wound edges leading to necrosis, delayed healing, poor cosmetic results
Wound edge overlapping	Interferes with wound healing and may cause a ridge leading to a more obvious scar
Sutures too near the wound edge	These are likely to pull out

Procedure guidelines   Wound dressings change for acute and surgical wounds

Equipment

1 As for Procedure guidelines: Aseptic technique (see Chapter 5).

2 Cleaning fluid for irrigation (see Table 48.4).
3 Appropriate dressing (see Table 48.5).

Procedure

See Procedure guidelines: Aseptic technique (see Chapter 5) up to and including step 11, then loosen the dressing.

Action	Rationale
12 Where appropriate, loosen the old dressing.	The dressing can then be lifted off without causing trauma (E).
13 Clean hands with a bactericidal alcohol handrub.	Hands may become contaminated by handling outer packets, dressing, etc. (DH 2005: C).
14 Using the plastic bag in the pack, arrange the sterile field. Pour cleaning solution into gallipots or an indented plastic tray.	The time the wound is exposed should be kept to a minimum to reduce the risk of contamination. To prevent contamination of the environment. To minimize risk of contamination of cleaning solution (E).
15 Remove dressing by placing a hand in the plastic bag, lifting the dressing off and inverting the plastic bag so that the dressing is now inside the bag. Thereafter use this as the 'dirty' bag.	To reduce the risk of cross-infection. To prevent contamination of the environment (E).
16 Attach the bag with the dressing to the side of the trolley below the top shelf.	Contaminated material should be below the level of the sterile field (E).
17 Assess wound healing with reference to volume, amount of granulation tissue and epithelialization, signs of infection, underlying pathology, etc. (see Table 48.3/Figure 48.1). (Record assessment in relevant documentation at the end of the procedure.)	To evaluate wound care (Hampton & Collins 2004: E; Dealey 2005: E; Hess 2005: E).
18 Put on gloves.	To reduce the risk of infection to the wound and contamination of the nurse. Gloves provide greater sensitivity than forceps and are less likely to traumatize the wound or the patient's skin (E).

19 If necessary, gently clean the wound with a gloved hand using 0.9% sodium chloride, unless another solution is indicated (see Table 48.3). If appropriate, irrigate by flushing with water or 0.9% sodium chloride.

To reduce the possibility of physical and chemical trauma to granulation and epithelial tissue (Hess 2005: E).

20 Apply the dressing that is most suitable for the wound using the criteria for dressings (see Table 48.5).

To promote healing and/or reduce symptoms (E).

21 Remove gloves; fasten dressing as appropriate with hypoallergenic tape/Netelast/bandage/tapeless retention dressing.

To prevent irritation of skin and to avoid trauma to wound (E).

22 Make sure the patient is comfortable and the dressing is secure.

A dressing may slip or feel uncomfortable as the patient changes position (E)

Continue with steps 18–21 from the Procedure guidelines: Aseptic technique (see Chapter 5).

Procedure guidelines   Suturing a simple wound

Equipment

1 Plastic apron.
2 Sterile gloves.
3 Suture pack (containing needle holder, tissue forceps, dressing forceps, scissors, low linting swabs, gallipot).
4 Sutures in varying gauges and material.
5 Local anaesthetic, e.g. lidocaine 1%.
6 Sterile 0.9% sodium chloride solution.
7 10 ml syringe and needles (21 and 25 G).

Procedure

Action

1 Explain and discuss the procedure with the patient.

Rationale

To ensure that the patient understands the procedure and gives his/her valid consent (NMC 2006: C).

2 Follow the procedure for aseptic technique.

To reduce the risk of contamination (DH 2005: C).

3 Using a bright light, assess the wound and decide the type of material and gauge of needle to use.

To ensure that the wound is closed using most appropriate material to promote healing (E).

4 If appropriate, wound cleansing can be done by patient putting affected area under running water.

To remove any dirt and debris from wound (Castille 1998: E).

5 The wound must then be thoroughly cleansed using sterile solution of 0.9% sodium chloride.

To prevent possible wound infection (Castille 1998: E).

6 Contaminated wounds may need to be cleansed with a broad spectrum antibiotic, scrubbing or a solution to remove tar- or oil-based solutions.

To prevent possible wound infection (Castille 1998: E).

7 The area surrounding the wound may require shaving.

To prevent hairs from becoming trapped in the closed wound (Castille 1998: E).

8 Draw up and administer the local anaesthetic, checking that the areas are anaesthetized by testing with a small needle.

To prevent any pain during the procedure, but explain that a slight tugging sensation will still be felt (Castille 1998: E).

9 Inspect the site.

To ascertain how to match the wound edges (Castille 1998: E).

Procedure guidelines (*cont.*)

10 With linear wounds, suturing should begin at the centre.	To create good apposition of the edges (Castille 1998: E).
11 Select the tissue forceps, needle and needle holder.	To prepare the equipment for the procedure (E).
12 The needle should be grasped in the needle holder on its flattened area about a third of the way along from the suture material (see Action figure 12).	To prepare the suture material for use (Jay 1999: E)
13 The needle holder should be held in dominant hand and support the wound edge with the tissue forceps.	To allow adequate control by the practitioner of the equipment and to support the tissue during the procedure (Castille 1998: E).
14 The needle should be inserted at a 90^0 angle to the skin, taking a full wound thickness 'bite' about 5 mm from the edge of the wound (see Action figure 14).	To create good apposition of the edges without excessive tension (Castille 1998: E)
15 Bring the needle up in between the wound edges and pull the suture through the tissue until a short tail remains at the initial skin entry site (see Action figure 15).	To ensure there is enough suture to use for knotting (E).
16 Reinsert the needle at a 90^0 angle from the base of the wound on the other side and pull the suture through the tissue (see Action figure 16).	To bring wound edges together (Jay 1999: E).
17 Hold the needle parallel to the skin and grasping the needle end of the suture, make two clockwise loops around the needle holder (see Action figure 17).	To begin to create a knot (Castille 1998: E).
18 Grasp the tail of the suture with the needle holder and pull it through the loop with the needle holder pulled towards you (see Action figure 18).	To 'set a throw' (Castille 1998: E).
19 Follow this by a single anti-clockwise loop around the needle holder and move the needle to the opposite side of the wound (see Action figure 19a, b).	To square the knot (Castille 1998: E).
20 Then create a third throw of one loop.	To ensure that the knot is tied securely but not too tightly (Castille 1998: E).
21 The suture can then be cut free from the knot, leaving tails of about 5 mm (see Action figure 21).	To enable easy removal of the suture (Castille 1998: E).
22 Insert each suture in the same way until completed.	To close the wound effectively (E).
23 Once completed, discard needle in sharps bin.	To prevent potential sharps injury to practitioner (NHS Employers 2005: C).
24 Clean any blood from the surrounding area.	To prevent any possible wound infection (E).
25 Apply a suitable dressing.	To protect the wound from further trauma or contamination (Castille 1998: E)
26 Record the date, time and name of the practitioner, amount of local anaesthetic used and size and type of suture material and number of sutures on the appropriate charts.	To maintain accurate records, provide a point of reference in the event of any queries (NMC 2005: C).

27 Provide the patient with written and verbal advice regarding wound care and when the sutures should be removed.

To ensure optimum care for the wound and correct removal (Castille 1998: E).

Action 12 Grasp the needle.

Action 14 Insert the needle at 90° angle.

Action 15 Bring needle up between wound edges.

Action 16 Reinsert the needle on the other side.

Action 17 Make two clockwise loops.

Action 18 Grasp tail of suture with needle holder.

Action 19a   Loop suture around needle holder.

Action 19b   Move needle to opposite side of wound.

Action 21   Suture can be free from the knot.

Procedure guidelines   Sutures, clips or staples removal

Equipment

1 As for Procedure guidelines: Aseptic technique (see Chapter 5).

2 Sterile scissors, stitch cutter, staple remover (E).
3 Sterile adhesive sutures (E).

Procedure

Action	Rationale
1 Explain and discuss the procedure with the patient.	To ensure that the patient understands the procedure and gives his/her valid consent (E; DH 2001b: C).
2 Perform procedure using aseptic technique.	To prevent infection (for further information see Procedure guidelines: Aseptic technique, see Chapter 5) (DH 2005: C).

3 Clean the wound with an appropriate sterile solution such as 0.9% sodium chloride (see Table 48.4).

To prevent infection (E).

For removal of sutures

4 Lift knot of suture with metal forceps. Snip stitch close to the skin. Pull suture out gently.

Plastic forceps tend to slip against nylon sutures (E).
To prevent infection by drawing exposed suture through the tissue (E).

5 Use tips of scissors slightly open or the side of the stitch cutter to gently press the skin when the suture is being drawn out.

To minimize pain by counteracting the adhesion between the suture and surrounding tissue (E).

For removal of clips

6 Squeeze wings of clips together with forceps to release from skin.

To release clips atraumatically from the wound (E).

7 If the wound gapes use adhesive sutures to oppose the wound edges.

To improve the cosmetic effect (E).

8 When necessary, cover the wound with an appropriate dressing (see Table 48.5).

To provide the best possible environment for wound healing to take place. To reduce the risk of infection. To prevent the suture line from rubbing against clothing (E).

For removal of staples

9 Slide the lower bar of the staple remover with the V-shaped groove under the staple at an angle of 90°. Squeeze the handles of the staple removers together to open the staple.
If the suture line is under tension, use free hand to gently squeeze the skin either side of the suture line.

To release the staple atraumatically from the wound. If the angle of the staple remover is not correct, the staple will not come out freely (E).

To reduce tension of skin around suture line and lessen pain on removal of staple (E).

10 If the wound gapes use adhesive sutures to oppose the wound edges.

To improve the cosmetic effect (E).

For all suture lines

11 Record condition of suture line and surrounding skin (amount of exudate, pus, inflammation, pain, etc.; see Table 48.3).

To document care and enable evaluation of the wound (Dealey 2005: E; NMC 2005: C; Bale & Jones 2006: E).

Procedure guidelines   Wound drain dressing (Redivac: closed drainage systems)

Equipment

1 As for Procedure guidelines: Aseptic technique (see Chapter 5).

2 Non-adherent, absorbent dressing.

Procedure

Action

1 Explain and discuss the procedure with the patient.

Rationale

To ensure that the patient understands the procedure and gives his/her valid consent (DH 2001b. C).

2 Perform procedure using aseptic technique.

To prevent infection (for further information on asepsis, see Procedure guidelines: Aseptic technique, see Chapter 5) (DH 2005: C).

Procedure guidelines (*cont.*)

3 Clean the surrounding skin with an appropriate sterile solution such as 0.9% sodium chloride (see Table 48.4).	To prevent infection and remove excess debris (E).
4 Check condition of surrounding skin.	To assess for any excoriation of the skin (E).
5 Ensure that the skin suture holding the drain site in position is intact.	To prevent the drain from leaving the wound (E).
6 Cover the drain site with a non-adherent, absorbent dressing.	To protect the drain site, prevent infection entering the wound and absorb exudate (E).
7 Tape securely.	To prevent drain coming loose (E).
8 Ensure that the drain is primed or that the suction pump is in working order.	To ensure continuity of drainage (E). Ineffective drainage can result in oedema/haematoma (Hess 2005: E).

Procedure guidelines   Change of vacuum drainage system

(See also Chapter 20.)

Equipment

1 Sterile topical swab.

2 Dressing pack.

Procedure

Action	Rationale
1 Explain and discuss the procedure with the patient.	To ensure that the patient understands the procedure and gives his/her valid consent (DH 2001b: C).
2 Perform procedure using aseptic technique.	To prevent infection (see Procedure guidelines: Aseptic technique, see Chapter 5) (DH 2005: C).
3 Wash hands using bactericidal soap and water or bactericidal alcohol handrub.	To minimize the risk of infection (DH 2005: C).
4 Ensure sterile drainage system is readily available.	To ensure sterility during change of system (E).
5 Measure the contents of the bottle to be changed and record this in the appropriate documents.	To maintain an accurate record of drainage from the wound and enable evaluation of state of wound (E).
6 Clamp the tube with the tubing clamps on the drainage tube and bottle connector and remove the bottle.	To prevent air and contamination entering the wound via the drain (E).
7 Clean the end of the tube and attach it to the sterile bottle.	To maintain sterility (E).
8 Unclamp the tubing clamps.	To re-establish the drainage system (E).
9 Place used vacuum drainage system into the clinical waste bag.	To safely dispose of used system (E).

Procedure guidelines   Wound drain removal (Yeates vacuum drainage system)

Equipment

1 As for Procedure guidelines: Aseptic technique (see Chapter 5).

2 Sterile scissors or suture cutter.

Procedure

Action	Rationale
1 Check the patient's operation notes.	To establish the number and site(s) of internal and external sutures (E).
2 Explain and discuss the procedure with the patient.	To ensure that the patient understands the procedure and gives his/her valid consent (DH 2001b: C).
3 If appropriate (in closed drainage systems) release vacuum.	To prevent pulling at wound tissue, causing pain and tissue damage (E).
4 Perform the procedure using aseptic technique.	To minimize the risk of infection (DH 2005: C). (For further information on asepsis, see Chapter 5.)
5 Where the wound is covered with an occlusive dressing (e.g. following lumpectomy in the breast), lift and snip the dressing from around the drain. Do not remove it from the entire wound.	To prevent disturbing the incision or contaminating the wound (E).
6 Only clean the wound if necessary, using an appropriate sterile solution, such as 0.9% sodium chloride (see Table 48.4).	To reduce risk of infection (E).
7 Hold the knot of the suture with metal forceps and gently lift upwards.	Plastic forceps tend to slip against nylon sutures. To allow space for the scissors or stitch cutter to be placed underneath (E).
8 Cut the shortest end of the suture as close to the skin as possible.	To prevent infection by allowing the suture to be liberated from the drain without drawing the exposed part through tissue (E).
9 Remove drain gently. If there is resistance, place free gloved hand against the tissue to oppose the tugging of the drain being removed. If the resistance is felt to be excessive, nitrous oxide (e.g. Entonox) may be required.	To minimize pain and reduce trauma (E).
10 Cover the drain site with a sterile dressing and tape securely.	To prevent infection entering the drain site (E).
11 Measure and record the contents of the drainage bottle in the appropriate documents.	To maintain an accurate record of drainage from the wound and enable evaluation of state of wound (NMC 2005: C).
12 Dispose of used drainage system in clinical waste bag.	To ensure safe disposal (E).

Procedure guidelines   Wound drain shortening (Penrose: open drainage systems)

Procedure

Action	Rationale
1 Follow steps 1–8 above (removal of drain), i.e. to the stage where the suture has been cut.	
2 Using gloved hand, gently ease the drain out of wound to the length requested by surgeons (usually 3–5 cm).	To allow healing to take place from base of wound (E).
3 Using gloved hand, place a sterile safety pin through the drain as close to the skin as possible, taking great care not to stab either the nurse or patient.	To prevent retraction into the wound and minimize the risk of cross-infection and sharps injury (E).
4 Cut same amount of tubing from distal end of drain as withdrawn from wound.	So there is a convenient length of tubing to drain into the bag. To ensure patient comfort (E).
5 Place a sterile, suitably sized drainage bag over the drain site.	To allow effluent to drain into the bag. To prevent excoriation of the skin. To contain any odour (E).
6 Check bag is secure and comfortable for the patient.	For patient comfort (E).
7 Record by how much the drainage tube was shortened.	To ensure the length remaining in the wound is known (NMC 2005: C).

Procedure guidelines   Topical negative pressure (TNP) therapy

Equipment

1 1 TNP therapy unit.
2 1 TNP dressing pack.
3 1 TNP canister and tubing.
4 Sterile scissors.
5 Sterile gloves.

6 Apron.
7 Dressing procedure pack.
8 Sterile 0.9% sodium chloride for irrigation (warmed to approx. 37°C in a jug of warm water).
9 Clamp (Spencer Wells forceps).

Additional materials as required (follow manufacturer's instructions as there are several systems)

- Extra semi-permeable film dressings to seal any leaks.
- Non-adherent wound contact layer to prevent foam adhering to wound bed.
- Alcohol-free skin barrier film to protect any fragile or macerated skin around the wound *or* thin hydrocolloid sheet to 'frame' the wound.

Procedure

Action	Rationale
1 Explain and discuss the procedure with the patient. Agree a time limit for the procedure. The nurse should have completed supervised practice in advance of TNP commencement.	To ensure the patient understands the procedure and other options available and gives his/her valid consent (DH 2001b: C). Ensure competency and correct complementary dressings are used in the wound bed (Beldon 2006: C).
2 Provide routine analgesia prior to dressing procedure.	To prevent unnecessary procedural pain (E).
3 Ensure there is adequate lighting and the patient is comfortable and in a position where the wound can be accessed and viewed easily. Assemble all necessary equipment (Beldon 2006: C).	To allow access to area for dressing change. Dressing application can be complicated and take a long time so the patient should be in a comfortable position for the procedure (E).

4 Perform steps 2–15 of the Procedure guidelines: Aseptic technique (see Chapter 5).	To reduce the risk of cross-infection and reduce the amount of time the wound is exposed (DH 2005: C; E).

TNP dressing removal

5 Put on a pair of non-sterile gloves.	To reduce the risk of cross-infection (E).
6 Clamp the dressing tubing and disconnect it from the canister tubing. Allow any fluid in the canister tubing to be sucked into the canister. Switch off the pump and clamp the canister tubing.	To prevent spillage of body fluid waste from the tubing or canister (E).
7 Remove and discard the canister (if full or at least weekly).	To prevent pump alarming and for infection control (E).
8 Carefully remove the occlusive film drape by gently lifting one edge and then stretching the drape horizontally and slowly pulling up from the skin.	To prevent damage to the peri-wound skin (E).
9 Carefully remove the foam dressing from the wound bed.	To prevent damage to newly formed tissue within the wound bed and prevent pain (E).
10 Clean the wound with an appropriate sterile solution such as 0.9% sodium chloride (see Table 48.4).	To prevent infection and remove surface debris/necrotic tissue (Dealey 2005: E).
11 Debride the wound if applicable.	To remove loose necrotic tissue that may be a focus for infection (Vowden & Vowden 2002: C).

TNP dressing application

12 Apply semi-permeable film over the outer foam dressing and cut a small hole for the drainage tubing prior to applying the suction device and tubing (Beldon 2006).	To prevent skin damage and ensure a good seal (Beldon 2006: E).
13 Cut the TNP foam to fit the size and shape of the wound, including tunnelling and undermined areas.	The foam should fit the wound exactly to ensure full benefit of the negative pressure therapy (KCI International 2004: C; Beldon 2006: E).
14 Avoid cutting the foam over the wound bed.	To prevent loose particles of foam falling into the wound (E).
15 Place the foam into the wound cavity. (*Note*: if the wound is bigger than the largest foam dressing, more than one piece of foam may be used as long as the edges of the foam are in contact with each other.)	The whole wound bed must be covered with foam. If the foam is touching it will transfer the negative pressure to the next piece (E).
16 Cut the occlusive film drape to size and apply over the top of the foam, ensuring a 3–5 cm border onto intact skin, TNP gel strip or hydrocolloid. (*Note*: do not compress the foam into the wound.)	To obtain a good seal around the wound edges (E).
17 Choose a location on the sealed occlusive film drape to apply the tubing where the tubing will not rub or cause pressure. Cut a hole through the film, approximately 2 cm in diameter, leaving the foam intact.	To reduce the risk of pressure injury to skin (E).
18 Place the TRAC pad on the film with the hole in the centre of the elbow joint directly over the hole in the film drape. Gently press around the TRAC pad (KCI International 2004).	To ensure correct position and seal of the pad. (NB. TRAC is for the vacuum-assisted closure [VAC] system; follow manufacturer's individual instructions: C.)

Commencing TNP therapy

20	Insert the canister into the pump until it clicks into place.	Indicates the canister is positioned correctly and is secure (Beldon 2006: E).
21	Connect the dressing tubing to the canister tubing and open clamps.	The pump will alarm if the tubing is clamped or not connected (E).
22	Press POWER button and follow the on-screen instructions to set the level and type of pressure required according to instructions from the patient's medical/surgical team.	To ensure the therapy is set to the individual requirements of the patient (E).
23	Start the pump by pressing THERAPY ON/OFF: the foam should contract into the wound.	Any small air leak will prevent the foam dressing from contracting and reassessment is required (E).

References and further reading

Allsworth, J. (1985) *Skin Camouflage. A Guide to Remedial Techniques.* Arnould–Taylor, Cheltenham.

Angeras, M.H. *et al.* (1992) Comparison between sterile saline and tap water for the cleaning of acute traumatic soft tissue wounds. *Eur J Surg*, 58, 347–50.

Archambeau, J.O., Pezner, R. & Wasserman, T. (1995) Pathophysiology of irradiated skin and breast. *Int J Radiat Oncol Biol Phys*, 31(15), 1171–85.

Back, I.N. & Finlay, I. (1995) Analgesic effect of topical opioids on painful skin ulcers. *J Pain Symptom Manage*, 10(7), 493.

Baker, J. (1998) Essential oils: a complementary therapy in wound management. *J Wound Care*, 7(7), 355–7.

Bale, S. (1991) A holistic approach and the ideal dressing. *Prof Nurse*, 6(6), 316–23.

Bale, S. & Jones, V. (2006) *Wound Care Nursing: a Patient Centred Approach*, 2nd edn. Mosby Elsevier, Edinburgh.

Barr, P.O. *et al.* (1990) Hyperbaric oxygen and problem wounds. *Care Sci Pract*, 8(1), 3–6.

Baum, T.M. & Busuito, M.J. (1998) Use of a glycerin-based gel sheeting in scar management. *Adv Wound Care*, 11(1), 40–3.

Baxter, H. & Ballard, K. (2001) A novel wound dressing containing HYAFF an ester of hyaluronic acid for the treatment of recalcitrant wounds. Poster presentation: Tissue Viability Society. 31st UK Conference. September 16-17, 1998.

Beldon, P. (2000) Abnormal scar formation in wound healing. *Nurs Times*, 96(10), 44–5.

Beldon, P. (2003) Comparison of four different dressings on donor site wounds. *Br J Nurs*, 13(6)(Tissue Viability Suppl), S38–45.

Beldon, P. (2006) Topical negative pressure dressings and vacuum-assisted closure. *Wound Essentials*, 1, 110–14.

Benbow, M. (1995) Parameters of wound assessment. *Br J Nurs*, 4(11), 647–51.

Benbow, M. (2006) An update on VAC therapy. *J Community Nurs*, 20(4), 28–32.

Bennett, G. & Moody, M. (1995) *Wound Care for Health Professionals*. Chapman & Hall, London.

Bennett, G., Dealey, C. & Posnett, J. (2004) The cost of pressure ulcers in the UK. *Age Aging*, 33(3), 230–5.

Bergstrom, N. & Braden, B. (1992) A prospective study of pressure sore risk among institutionalized elderly. *J Am Geriatr Soc*, 40(8), 747–58.

Bergstrom, N. *et al.* (1987) The Braden Scale for Predicting Pressure Sore Risk. *Nurs Res*, 36(4), 205–10.

Bird, C. (2000) Supporting patients with fungating breast wounds. *Prof Nurse*, 15(10), 649–52.

Birtwistle, J. (1994) Pressure sore formation and risk assessment in intensive care. *Care Crit Ill*, 10(4), 154–5, 157–9.

Blackmar, A. (1997) Focus on wound care: radiation-induced skin alterations. *Medsurg Nurs*, 6(3), 172–5.

Bliss, M. (1993) Aetiology of pressure sores. *Rev Clin Gerontol*, 3, 379–97.

BNF (2006) *British National Formulary*. British Medical Association and Royal Pharmaceutical Association, London.

Boots-Vickers, M. & Eaton, K. (1999) Skin care for patients receiving radiotherapy. *Prof Nurse*, 14(10), 706–8.

Bower, M. *et al.* (1992) A double-blind study of the efficacy of metronidazole gel in the treatment of malodorous fungating tumours. *Eur J Cancer*, 28(4/5), 888–9.

Boyce, S.T. *et al.* (2002) Cultured skin substitutes reduce donor skin harvesting for closure of excised, full-thickness burns. *Ann Surg*, 235(2), 269–79.

Braden, B.J. & Bergstrom, N. (1987) A conceptual schema for the study of aetiology of pressure sores. *Rehabil Nurs*, 12(1), 8–12.

Braden, B.J. & Bergstrom, N. (1996) Risk assessment and risk based programs of prevention in various settings. *Ostomy Wound Manage*, 42, 65–125.

Bridel-Nixon, J. (1999) Pressure sores. In: *Nursing Management of Chronic Wounds*, 2nd edn (eds M. Morison, C. Moffatt, J. Bridel-Nixon & S. Bale). Mosby, London.

Brown, A.S. *et al.* (1998) *Essentials for Students – Plastic and Reconstructive Surgery*, 5th edn. Plastic Surgery Information Service: www.plasticsurgery.org/profinfo/essen/essentia.htm. Accessed 17/12/01.

Calvin, M. (1998) Cutaneous wound repair. *Wounds*, 10(1), 12–32.

Campbell, J. & Lane, C. (1996) Developing a skin-care protocol in radiotherapy. *Prof Nurse*, 12(2), 105–8.

Carney, S.A. *et al.* (1994) Cica-care gel sheeting in the management of hypertrophic scarring. *Burns*, 20(2), 163–7.

Carson, C.F., Hammer, K.A. & Riley, T.V. (2006) Melaleuca alternifolia (Tea Tree) oil: a review of antimicrobial and other medicinal properties. *Clin Microbiol Rev*, 19(1), 50–62.

Casey, G. (1998) The importance of nutrition in wound healing. *Nurs Stand*, 13(3), 51–6.

Castille, K. (1998) Suturing. *Nurs Stand*, 12(41), 41–8.

Chaplin, J. (2000) Pressure sore risk assessment in palliative care. *J Tissue Viability*, 10(1), 27–31.

Chen, W.Y. & Abatangelo, G. (1999) Functions of hyaluronan in wound repair. *Wound Repair Regen*, 7, 79–89.

Clamon, J. & Netscher, D.T. (1994) General principles of flap reconstruction: goals for aesthetic and functional outcome. *Plastic Surg Nurs*, **14**(1), 9–14.

Clark, M. (2002) Pressure ulcers and quality of life. *Nurs Stand*, **13**(16), 74–80.

Clay, M. (2000) Pressure sore prevention in nursing homes. *Nurs Stand*, **14**(44), 45–50.

Collier, M. (1996) The principles of optimum wound management. *Nurs Stand*, **10**(43), 47–52.

Collier, M. (1999) Pressure ulcer development and principles for prevention. In: *Wound Management: Theory and Practice* (eds M. Miller & D. Glover). Nursing Times Books, London.

Collier, M. (2002) Wound care. Wound-bed preparation. *Nurs Times*, **98**(2), 55–7.

Collinson, G. (1992) Improving quality of life in patients with malignant fungating wounds. *Proceedings of the Second European Conference on Wound Management*. Macmillan, London.

Cornwall, J.V., Dore, C.J. & Lewis, J.D. (1986) Leg ulcers: epidemiology and aetiology. *Br J Surg*, **73**(9), 693–6.

Coull, A. (1991) Making sense of split skin grafts. *Nurs Times*, **87**(27), 54–55.

Cullen, B. *et al.* (2002) The role of oxidised regenerated cellulose/collagen in chronic wound repair and its potential mechanism of action. *Int J Biochem Cell Biol*, **34**(12), 1544–56.

Cutting, K. (1994) Factors influencing wound healing. *Nurs Stand*, **8**(50), 33–7.

Cutting, K.F. (1998) *Wounds and Infection*. Wound Care Society, Huntingdon.

D'Haese, S. *et al.* (2005) Management of skin reactions during radiotherapy: a study of nursing practice. *Eur J Cancer Care*, **14**, 28–42.

Davies, D.M. (1985) Plastic and reconstructive surgery. *Br Med J*, **290**, 1056–8.

Davies, P. (2004) Current thinking on the management of necrotic and sloughy wounds. *Prof Nurse*, **19**(10), 34–6.

Davis, M.H. *et al.* (1993) *The Wound Handbook*. Centre for Medical Education, Dundee, and Perspective, London.

Dealey, C. (2005) *The Care of Wounds: a Guide for Nurses*, 3rd edn. Blackwell Science, Oxford.

Dean, A. & Tuffin, P. (1997) Fibrinolytic inhibitors for cancer-associated bleeding problems. *J Pain Symptom Manage*, **13**(1), 20–4.

Deeks, J.J. (1996) Pressure sore prevention: using and evaluating risk assessment tools. *Br J Nurs*, **5**(5), 313–20.

Derbyshire, A. (2003) A case study to demonstrate the role of proteases in wound healing. *Prof Nurse*, **19**(2), 108–11.

DH (2001a) *National Service Framework for Older People*. Department of Health, London.

DH (2001b) *Good Practice in Consent Implementation Guide: Consent to Examination and Treatment*. www.dh.gov.uk. Accessed 24/9/07.

DH (2005) *Saving Lives: a Delivery Programme to Reduce Healthcare Associated Infection Including MRSA*. Department of Health, London.

Dinman, S. (1999) Flaps and grafts revisited: cross-leg and thigh flaps for lower extremity wounds. *Plast Surg Nurs*, **19**(2), 62–5.

Donovan, S. (1998) Wound infection and wound swabbing. *Prof Nurse*, **13**(11), 757–9.

Dowsett, C. (2002) The role of the nurse in wound bed preparation. *Nurs Stand*, **16**(44), 69–76.

Dowsett, C. & Ayello, E. (2004) TIME principles of chronic wound bed preparation and management. *Br J Nurs*, **13**(15), S16–22.

Dunford, C. (2000) The use of honey in wound management. *Nurs Stand*, **15**(11), 63–8.

Dyson, M. *et al.* (1988) Comparison of the effects of moist and dry conditions on dermal repair. *J Invest Dermatol*, **91**(5), 434–9.

Eaglstein, W.H. (1985) The effect of occlusive dressings on collagen synthesis and re-epithelialisation in superficial wounds. In: *An Environment for Healing: The Role of Occlusion* (ed. T.J. Ryan). Royal Society of Medicine, London.

Edmonds, M. & Foster, A. (2000) Hyalofill: a new product for chronic wound management. *Diabetic Foot*, **3**(1), 29–30.

Edwards, M. (1994) The reliability and validity of the Waterlow pressure sore risk scale when used within district nursing to assess elders nursed in a domiciliary setting. MSc dissertation, University of London, London.

Ehrlich, H.P. (1999) The physiology of wound healing: a summary of normal and abnormal wound healing processes. *Adv Wound Care*, **11**(7), 326–8.

Ehrlich, H.P. & Hunt, T.K. (1968) Effects of cortisone and vitamin A on wound healing. *Ann Surg*, **167**(3), 324–8.

Eisenbeiss, W. *et al.* (1998) Hypertrophic scars and keloids. *J Wound Care*, **7**(5), 255–7.

Elkin, M.K., Perry, A.G. & Potter, P.A. (2004) Skill 22.3 removing staples and sutures. In: *Nursing Interventions and Clinical Skills*, 3rd edn. Mosby, St Louis. Missouri.

EPUAP (2003) Pressure ulcer prevention guidelines. www.epuap.org.uk. Accessed 11/05.

Fairbairn, K. (1993) Towards better care for women. *Prof Nurse*, **9**(3), 204–12.

Fairbairn, K. (1994) A challenge that requires further research: management of fungating breast lesions. *Prof Nurse*, **9**(4), 272–7.

Fairbairn, K. *et al.* (2002) A sharp debridement procedure devised by specialist nurses. *J Wound Care*, **11**(10), 371–5.

Falanga, V. (2000) Classifications for wound bed preparation and stimulation of chronic wounds. *Wound Repair Regen*, **8**(5), 347–52.

Ferguson, M. *et al.* (2000) Pressure ulcer management: the importance of nutrition. *Medsurg Nurs*, **9**(4), 163–75.

Field, C.K. & Kerstein, M.D. (1994) Overview of wound healing in a moist environment. *Am J Surg*, **167**(Suppl 1a), S2–6.

Finlay, I. *et al.* (1996) The effect of 0.75% metronidazole gel on malodorous cutaneous ulcers. *J Pain Symptom Manage*, **11**(3), 158–62.

Fisher, J. *et al.* (2000) Randomized phase III study comparing best supportive care to Biafine as a prophylactic agent for radiation-induced skin toxicity for women undergoing breast irradiation: Radiation Therapy Oncology Group (RTOG). *Int J Radiat Oncol Biol Phys*, **48**, 1307–10.

Flanagan, M. (1996) A practical framework for wound assessment 1: physiology. *Br J Nurs*, **5**(22), 1391–7.

Flanagan, M. (1998) The characteristics and formation of granulation tissue. *J Wound Care*, **7**(10), 508–10.

Flanagan, M. (1999) The physiology of wound healing. In: *Wound Management: Theory and Practice* (eds M. Miller & D. Glover). Nursing Times Books, London, pp. 14–22.

Flanagan, M. (2000) The physiology of wound healing. *J Wound Care*, **9**(6), 299–300.

Fletcher, J. (1997) Update: wound cleansing. *Prof Nurse*, **12**(11), 793–6.

Francis, A. (1998) Nursing management of skin graft sites. *Nurs Stand*, **12**(33), 41–4.

Freedline, A. (1999) Types of wound debridement. Wound Care Information Network. www.medicaledu.com/debridhp.htm. Accessed 8/10/99.

Garrett, B. (1997) The proliferation and movement of cells during re-epithelialisation. *J Wound Care*, 6(4), 174–7.

Gentzkow, G.D. *et al.* (1996) Use of Dermagraft, a cultured human dermis, to treat diabetic foot ulcers. *Diabetes Care*, 19(4), 350–4.

Gilchrist, B. (1999) Wound infection. In: *Wound Management: Theory and Practice* (eds M. Miller & D. Glover). Nursing Times Books, London, pp. 96–107.

Glean, E. *et al.* (2001) Intervention for acute radiotherapy induced skin reactions in cancer patients: the development of clinical practice guidelines recommended for use by the College of Radiographers. *J Radiother Pract*, 2(2), 75–84.

Grewal, P.S. *et al.* (1999) Pressure sore prevention in hospital patients: a clinical audit. *J Wound Care*, 8(3), 129–31.

Grocott, P. (2000a) Palliative management of fungating malignant wounds. *J Wound Care*, 9(1), 4–9.

Grocott, P. (2000b) Palliative management of fungating malignant wounds. *J Commun Nurs*, 14(3), 31–2, 35–6, 38.

Guyton, A.C. & Hall, J.E. (2000) *Textbook of Medical Physiology*, 10th edn. W.B. Saunders, Philadelphia.

Haisfield-Wolfe, M.E. & Rund, C. (1997) Malignant cutaneous wounds: a management protocol. *Ostomy Wound Manage*, 43(1), 56–66.

Hallett, A. (1995) Fungating wounds. *Nurs Times*, 91(47), 81–3.

Hamilton, K. (1995) Wound healing and nutrition – a review. *J Aust Coll Nutr Environ Med*, 14(2), 15.

Hamilton-Miller, J.M.T., Shah, S. & Smith, C. (1993) Silver sulphadiazine: a comprehensive *in vitro* reassessment. *Chemotherapy*, 39, 405–9.

Hampton, S. (2004) Holistic Wound Care. Journal of Community Nurs, 18(8), 12–7.

Hampton, S. (1999) Choosing the right dressing. In: *Wound Management: Theory and Practice* (eds M. Miller & D. Glover). Nursing Times Books, London pp. 14–22.

Hampton, S. & Collins, F. (2004) *Tissue Viability: The Prevention, Treatment and Management of Wounds*. Whurr Publishers, London.

Harding, K.G., Morris, H.L. & Patel, G.K. (2002) Healing chronic wounds. *BMJ*, 324(7330), 160–3.

Hart, J. (2002) Inflammation 1: its role in the healing of acute wounds. *J Wound Care*, 11(6), 205–9.

Heggie, S. *et al.* (2002) A phase III study on the efficacy of topical aloe vera gel on irradiated breast tissue. *Cancer Nurs*, 25(6), 442–51.

Hess, C.T. (2005) Pressure ulcers. In: *Wound Care Clinical Guide*, 5th edn. Lippincott, Williams & Wilkins, Philadelphia, pp. 79–93.

Hinshaw, J. (2000) Larval therapy: a review of clinical human and veterinary studies. *World Wide Wounds*: www.worldwidewounds.com/2000/oct/Janet-Hinshaw/Larval-Therapy-Human-and-Veterinary.html. Accessed 20/12/02.

Hofman, D. (1996) Know how: a guide to wound debridement. *Nurs Times*, 92(32), 22–3.

Hollander, D., Schmandra, T. & Windolf, J. (2000) Using an esterified hyaluronan fleece to promote healing in difficult-to-treat wounds. *J Wound Care*, 9(10), 463–6.

Hollinworth, H. (1997) Less pain, more gain. *Nurs Times*, 93(46), 89–91.

Ivetic, O. & Lyne, P.A. (1990) Fungating and ulcerating malignant lesions: a review of the literature. *J Adv Nurs*, 15, 83–8.

Jay, R. (1999) Suturing in A&E. *Prof Nurse*, 14(6), 412–15.

Johnson, A. (1989) Granuflex wafers as a prophylactic pressure sore dressing. *Care Sci Pract*, 7(2), 55–8.

Jones, M. & Thomas, S. (2000) Larval therapy. *Nurs Stand*, 14(20), 47–51.

Kaufman, M. & Pahl, D. (2003) Vacuum-assisted closure therapy: wound care and nursing implications. *Dermatol Nurs*, 15(4), 317–20, 323–25.

KCI International (2004) *VAC Recommended Guidelines for Use: Physician and Caregiver Reference Manual*. KCI International, Oxfordshire.

Kelly, N. (2002) Malodorous fungating wounds: a review of current literature. *Prof Nurse*, 17(5), 323–6.

Kiecolt-Glaser, J.K. *et al.* (1995) Slowing of wound healing by psychological stress. *Lancet*, 346(4), 1194–6.

Kitching, M. (2004) Patients' perceptions and experiences of larval therapy. *J Wound Care*, 13(1), 25–9.

Krajnik, M. & Zylicz, Z. (1997) Topical morphine for cutaneous cancer pain. *Palliat Med*, 11(4), 326–30.

Landis, E.M. (1930) Micro-injection studies of capillary blood pressure in human skin. *Heart*, 15, 209–28.

Laverty, D. (2003) Fungating wounds: informing practice through knowledge/theory. *Br J Nurs*, 12(15), S29–S40.

Laverty, D., Mallett, J. & Mulholland, J. (1997) Protocols and guidelines for managing wounds. *Prof Nurse*, 13(2), 79–81.

Laverty, D. *et al.* (2000) *Wound Management Guidelines*. Royal Marsden Foundation Trust, London.

Lavery, B.A. (1995) Skin care during radiotherapy: a survey of UK practice. *Clin Oncol*, 7(3), 184–7.

Lawrence, J.C. (1997) Wound irrigation. *J Wound Care*, 6(1), 23–6.

Lewis, B. (1996) Zinc and vitamin C in the aetiology of pressure sores. *J Wound Care*, 5(10), 483–4.

Lindgren, M. *et al.* (2002) A risk assessment scale for the prediction of pressure sore development: reliability and validity. *J Adv Nurs*, 38(2), 190–9.

Lund-Nielsen, B., Muller, K. & Adamsen, L. (2005) Malignant wounds in women with breast cancer: feminine and sexual perspectives. *J Clin Nurs*, 14(1), 56–64.

Maddocks-Jennings, W., Wilkinson, J.M. & Shillington, D. (2005) Novel approaches to radiotherapy-induced skin reactions: a literature review. *Complement Ther Clin Pract*, 11(4), 224–31.

Maher, K.E. (2005) Radiation therapy: toxicities and management. In: *Cancer Nursing: Principles and Practice* (eds C. Henke Yarbro *et al.*), 6th edn. Jones and Barlett, Boston, pp. 283–314.

Mallett, J. *et al.* (1999) An integrated approach to wound management. *Int J Palliat Nurs*, 5(3), 124–32.

Mandal, A. (2006) Do malnutrition and nutritional supplementation have an effect on the wound healing process? *J Wound Care*, 15(6), 254–7.

Margolin, S.G. *et al.* (1990) Management of radiation-induced moist skin desquamation using hydrocolloid dressing. *Cancer Nurs*, 13(2), 71–80.

Martin, E.A. (2002) *Concise Colour Medical Dictionary*. Oxford University Press, Oxford.

Messer, M.S. (1989) Wound care. *Crit Care Nurs Q*, 11(4), 17–27.

Middleton, K. (1990) Sugar pastes in wound management. *Dressings Times*, 3(2): www.smtl.co.uk/WMPRC/DressingsTimes/vol3.2.txt. Accessed 27/6/00.

Miller, M. (1998a) Moist wound healing: the evidence. *Nurs Times*, 94(45), 74–6.

Miller, M. (1998b) How do I diagnose and treat wound infection? *Br J Nurs*, 7(6), 335–8.

Miller, M. & Dyson, M. (1996) *Principles of Wound Care*. Macmillan, London.

Mockridge, J. & Anthony, D. (1999) Nurses' knowledge about pressure sore treatment and healing. *Nurs Stand*, 13(29), 66–72.

Moore, P. & Foster, L. (1998) Acute surgical wound care 2: the wound healing process. *Br J Nurs*, 7(19), 1183–7.

Morgan, D.A. (2000) *Formulary of Wound Management Products: a Guide for Healthcare Staff*, 8th edn. Euromed Communications, Haslemere.

Morgan, D.A. (2002) Formulary of wound management products: a guide for healthcare staff, 8th edn (Internet update). Euromed Communications. www.euromed.uk.com/formulary6update.htm. Accessed 20/12/02.

Morison, M.J. (1989) Wound cleansing – which solution? *Prof Nurse*, 4, 220–5.

Moss, A. (1989) Treatment of terminal breast cancer. *Br Med J*, 298(6670): 388.

Munro, K.J.G. (1995a) Hypertrophic and keloid scars. *J Wound Care*, 4(3), 143–8.

Munro, K.J.G. (1995b) Treatment of hypertrophic and keloid scars. *J Wound Care*, 4(5), 243–5.

Naylor, W. (2001) Assessment and management of pain in fungating wounds. *Br J Nurs*, 10(22 Suppl), S33–56.

Naylor, W. (2002) Malignant wounds: aetiology and principles of management. *Nurs Stand*, 16(52), 45–53.

Naylor, W., Laverty, D. & Mallett, J. (2001) *The Royal Marsden Hospital Handbook of Wound Management in Cancer Care*. Blackwell Science, Oxford.

Newman, V. *et al.* (1989) The use of metronidazole gel to control the smell of malodorous lesions. *Palliat Med*, 3, 303–5.

NHS Employers (2005) *The Management of Health, Safety and Welfare Issues for NHS Staff*. National Health Service Employers, London.

NICE (2001) Technology appraisal guidance 24. Wound care – debriding agents. Guidance on the use of debriding agents and specialist wound care clinics for difficult to heal surgical wounds. April 2001, updated March 2004. National Institute for Health and Clinical Excellence, London. www.nice.org.uk/page.aspx?o=TA024guidance. Accessed 09/2006.

NICE (2003) Pressure ulcer risk assessment and prevention. National Institute for Health and Clinical Excellence. www.nice.org.uk. Accessed 11/11/06.

NMC (2005) *Guidelines for Records and Record Keeping*. Nursing and Midwifery Council, London.

NMC (2006) *A–Z Advice Sheet Consent*. www.nmc.org.

NMC (2008) *The Code: Standards of Conduct, Performance and Ethics for Nurses and Midwives*. Nursing and Midwifery Council, London.

Noble-Adams, R. (1999) Radiation-induced skin reactions 2: development of a measurement tool. *Br J Nurs*, 8(18), 1208–11.

Norton, D. *et al.* (1985) *An Investigation of Geriatric Nursing Problems in Hospital*. Churchill Livingstone, Edinburgh.

Nystedt, K.E. *et al.* (2005) The standardization of radiation skin care in British Columbia: a collaborative approach. *Oncol Nurs Forum*, 32(6), 1199–1206.

O'Toole, E.A., Marinkovich, M.P., Peavey, C.L. *et al.* (1997) Hypoxia increases human keratinocyte motility on connective tissue. *J Clin Invest*, 100(11), 288–91.

Papanikolaou, P., Lyne, P. & Anthony, D. (2006) Risk assessment scales for pressure ulcers: A methodological review. *International Journal of Nursing Studies*, 44(2), 285–96.

Patawardhan, A., Sharma, V. & Dinshaw, K.A. (2002) Duoderm CGF vs Gentian violet 1% dressing in the treatment of radiation induced ulcers. *World Council of Enterostomal Therapists Journal*, 22(2), 32–8.

Phillips, T.J., Al-Amoudi, H.O., Leverkus, M. & Park, H.y. (1998) Effect of chronic wound fluid on fibroblasts. *J Wound Care*, 7(10), 527–32.

Pickering, D. & Warland, S. (1992) The management of desquamative radiation skin reactions. *Dressing Times*, 5(1): www.smtl.co.uk/WMPRC/DressingsTimes/vol5.1.txt. Accessed 11/10/06.

Pickworth, J.J. & De Sousa, N. (1988) Differential wound angiogenesis: quantitation by immunohistological staining for factor VIII-related antigen. In: *Beyond Occlusion: Wound Care Proceedings* (ed. T.J. Ryan). Royal Society of Medicine, London.

Porock, D. & Kristjanson, L. (1999) Skin reactions during radiotherapy for breast cancer: the use and impact of topical agents and dressings. *Eur J Cancer Care*, 8, 143–53.

Porock, D. *et al.* (1998) Predicting the severity of radiation skin reactions in women with breast cancer. *Oncol Nurs Forum*, 25(6), 1019–29.

Porock, D., Nikcoletti, S. & Cameron, F. (2004) The relationship between factors that impair wound healing and the severity of acute radiation skin and mucosal toxicities in head and neck cancer. *Cancer Nurs*, 27(1), 71–8.

Poston, J. (1996) Sharp debridement of devitalised tissue: the nurse's role. *Br J Nurs*, 5(11), 655–62.

Pouliot, R. *et al.* (2002) Reconstructed human skin produced *in vitro* and grafted on athymic mice. *Transplantation*, 73(11), 1751–7.

Price, S. & Price, L. (1995) *Aromatherapy for Health Professionals*. Churchill Livingstone, New York.

Pudner, R. (1998) The management of patients with a fungating or malignant wound. *J Commun Nurs*, 12(9), 30–4.

Pudner, R. (2001) Low/non-adherent dressings in wound management. *J Commun Nurs*, 15(8), 12, 15–17.

Puzey, G. (2001) The use of pressure garments on hypertrophic scars. *J Tissue Viability*, 12(1), 11–15.

Rankin-Box, D. (2001) *The Nurse's Handbook of Complementary Therapies*, 2nd edn. Bailliere Tindall, London.

Reid, J. & Morison, M. (1994) Towards a consensus classification of pressure sores. *J Wound Care*, 3(3), 157–9.

Reynolds, T.M. (2000) The future of nutrition and wound healing. *J Tissue Viability*, 11(1), 5–13.

Rice, A.M. (1997) An introduction to radiotherapy. *Nurs Stand*, 12(3), 49–54.

Richardson, M. (2007) Exploring various methods for closing traumatic wounds. *Nurs Times*, 103(5), 30–1.

Rigter, B., Clendon, H. & Kettle, S. (1994) Dermatology. Skin reactions due to radiotherapy. *New Zealand Pract Nurse*, September 17–19, 21–2.

Riyat, M.S. & Quinton, D.N. (1997) Tap water as a wound cleansing agent in accident and emergency. *J Accid Emerg*, 14, 165–6.

Robinson, B.J. (2000) The use of a hydrofibre dressing in wound management. *J Wound Care*, 9(1), 32–4.

Rollins, H. (1997) Special focus: tissue viability – nutrition and wound healing. *Nurs Stand*, 11(51), 49–52.

Roy, L., Fortin, A. & Larochelle, M. (2001) The impact of skin washing with water and soap during breast irradiation: a randomised study. *Radiother Oncol*, 58, 333–9.

RCN (2001) *Pressure Sore Prevention*. Royal College of Nursing, London. Accessed via National Institute for Health and Clinical Excellence: www.nice.org.uk. Accessed 17/03/07.

RCN (2003) *Pressure Ulcer Risk Assessment and Prevention*. Royal College of Nursing, London.

RCN (2005) The management of pressure ulcers in primary and secondary care: a clinical practice guideline. www.nice.org.uk/page.aspx?o=cg029fullguideline. Accessed 24/11/06.

Royal Marsden Hospital (1999) *Radiotherapy: Your Questions Answered*. Royal Marsden Hospital, London.

Russell, L. (2001) The importance of patients' nutritional status in wound healing. *Br J Nurs*, 10(6 Suppl), S44–9.

Scholl, D. & Langkamp-Henken, B. (2001) Nutrient recommendations for wound healing. *J Intraven Nurs*, 24(2), 124–32.

Schoonhoven, L., Defloor, T. & Grypdonck, M.H.F. (2002) Incidence of pressure ulcers due to surgery. *J Clin Nurs*, 11(4), 479–87.

Schultz, G.S. *et al.* (2003) Wound bed preparation: systematic approach to wound management. *Wound ep Reg,* **11**, 1–28. wound.smith-nephew.com/ca_en/Standard.asp?NodeId=3077. Accessed 17/10/06.

Silver, I.A. (1994) The physiology of wound healing. *J Wound Care,* **3**(2), 106–9.

Simmons, S. (1999) Hyperbaric therapy. In: *Wound Management: Theory and Practice* (eds M. Miller & D. Glover). Nursing Times Books, London.

Simonen, P. *et al.* (1998) Do inflammatory processes contribute to radiation-induced erythema observed in the skin of humans? *Radiother Oncol,* **46**(1), 73–82.

Simpson, A., Bowers, K. & Weir-Hughes, D. (1996) *Clinical Care: Pressure Sore Prevention.*Whurr, London.

Smith, F.R. (2005) Causes of and treatment options for abnormal scar tissue. *J Wound Care,* **14**(2), 49–52.

Smith, K.P., Zardiackas, L.D. & Didlake, R.H. (1986) Cortisone, vitamin A, and wound healing: the importance of measuring wound surface area. *J Surg Res,* **40**(2), 120–5.

Souhami, R. & Tobias, J. (1998) *Cancer and Its Management.* Blackwell Science, Oxford.

Sparrow, G. *et al.* (1980) Metronidazole in smelly tumours. *Lancet,* **1**(8179), 1185.

Springett, K. (2002) The impact of diabetes on wound management. *Nurs Stand,* **10**(1), 72–4.

Steenvoorde, P., Budding, T. & Oskam, J. (2005) Determining pain levels in patients treated with maggot debridement therapy. *J Wound Care,* **14**(10), 485–8.

Stein, C. (1995) The control of pain in peripheral tissue by opioids. *N Engl J Med,* **332**(25), 1685–90.

Stone, J. (2001) Ethical and legal issues. In: *The Nurse's Handbook of Complementary Therapies* (ed. D. Rankin-Box), 2nd edn. Bailliere Tindall, London, pp. 51–56.

Sussman, C. (1998) Wound healing biology and chronic wound healing. In: *Wound Care: A Collaborative Practice Manual for Physical Therapists and Nurses* (eds C. Sussman & B.M. Bate-Jensen). Aspen Publishers, MD, pp. 31–47.

Teare, J. & Barrett, C. (2002) Using quality of life assessment in wound care. *Nurs Stand,* **17**(6), 59–68.

Tejero-Trujeque, R. (2001) How do fibroblasts interact with the extracellular matrix in wound contraction? *J Wound Care,* **10**(6), 237–42.

Thomas, S. (1992) *Current Practices in the Management of Fungating Lesions and Radiation Damaged Skin.* Surgical Materials Testing Laboratory, Bridgend.

Thomas, S. (2002) SMTL Dressings Datacard: Promogran. Surgical Materials Testing Laboratory, Bridgend. www.dressings.org/Dressings/promogran.html. Accessed 25/7/02.

Thomas, S. & Hay, N. (1991) The antimicrobial properties of 2 metronidazole-mediated dressings used to treat malodorous wounds. *Pharm J,* **246**(6625), 264–66.

Thomas, T. *et al.* (2001) The current status of maggot therapy in wound healing. *Br J Nurs,* **10**(22 Suppl), S5–12.

Thomson, P. (1998) The microbiology of wounds. *J Wound Care,* **7**(9), 477–8.

Timmons, J. (2006) Skin function and wound healing physiology. *Wound Essentials,* **1**, 8–14.

Tong, A. (1999) Back to basics wound care. *Nurs Times Nurs Homes,* **1**(1), 20–3.

Topham, J. (2000) Sugar for wounds. *J Tissue Viability,* **10**(3), 86–9.

Torra I Bou, J.E. *et al.* (2001) Clinical evaluation of the effect of a collagen dressing in the treatment of pressure ulcers. In: *Final Abstracts from the Fifth EPUAP Open Meeting. Le Mans, France,* 2001. European Pressure Ulcer Advisory Panel Review, **4**(1).

Tortora, G.J. & Grabowski, S.R. (2008) *Principles of Anatomy and Physiology,* 12th edn. John Wiley & Sons, Chichester.

Twillman, R.K. *et al.* (1999) Treatment of painful skin ulcers with topical opioids. *J Pain Symptom Manage,* **17**(4), 288–92.

Vowden, K. (1995) Common problems in wound care: wound and ulcer measurement. *Br J Nurs,* **4**(13), 775–9.

Vowden, K. & Vowden, P. (1999) Wound debridement, part 2: sharp techniques. *J Wound Care,* **8**(6), 291–4.

Vowden, K. & Vowden, P. (2002) Wound bed preparation. *World Wide Wounds:* www.worldwidewounds.com/2002/april/Vowden/Wound-Bed-Preparation.html. Accessed 20/12/02.

Waldorf, H. & Fewkes, J. (1995) Advances in dermatology. *J Wound Heal,* **10**, 77–97.

Warnke, P.H. *et al.* (2004) Tumour smell reduction with antibacterial essential oils. *Cancer,* **100**(4), 879–80.

Warnke, P.H. *et al.* (2005) Antibacterial essential oils reduce tumor smell and inflammation in cancer patients. *J Clin Oncol,* **23**(7), 158–9.

Warnke, P.H. *et al.* (2006) Antibacterial essential oils in malodorous cancer patients: clinical observations in 30 patients. *Phytomedicine,* **13**(7), 463–7.

Waterlow, J. (1988) Prevention is cheaper than cure. *Nurs Times,* **84**(25), 69–70.

Waterlow, J. (1991) A policy that protects. *Prof Nurse,* **6**(5), 258–64.

Waterlow, J. (1998) The treatment and use of the Waterlow card. *Nurs Times,* **94**(7), 63–7.

Waterlow, J. (2005) From costly treatment to cost-effective prevention: using Waterlow. *Wound Care,* **10**(9 Suppl), S25–30.

Wells, L. (1994) At the front line of care, the importance of nutrition in wound management. *Prof Nurse,* **9**(8), 525–30.

Wells, M. & MacBride, S. (2003) Radiation skin reactions. In: *Supportive Care in Radiotherapy* (eds S. Faithfull & M. Wells). Churchill Livingstone, Edinburgh, pp. 135–39.

Westbury, C. *et al.* (2000) Advice on hair and scalp care during cranial radiotherapy: a prospective randomised trial. *Radiother Oncol,* **54**, 109–16.

White, R. (2001) Managing exudate. *Nurs Times,* **97**(14), 59–60.

White, R.J. (2000) *The Management of Exuding Wounds.* Wound Care Society, Huntingdon.

Wickline, M.M. (2004) Prevention and treatment of acute radiation dermatitis: A literature review. *Oncol Nurs Forum,* **31**, 237–47.

Wilkinson, B. (1997) Hard graft. *Nurs Times,* **93**(16), 63–4, 66, 68.

Wilkes, L. *et al.* (2001) Malignant wound management: what dressings do nurses use? *J Wound Care,* **10**(3), 65–70.

Williams, C. (1996) Product focus. Cica-care: adhesive gel sheet. *Br J Nurs,* **5**(14), 875–6.

Williams, C. (1999) Product focus: an investigation of the benefits of Aquacel Hydrofibre wound dressing. *Br J Nurs,* **8**(10), 676–80.

Williams, C. & Young, T. (1998) *Myth and Reality in Wound Care.* Mark Allen, Dinton.

Williams, L. (2002) Assessing patients' nutritional needs in the wound-healing process. *J Wound Care,* **11**(6), 225–8.

Wilson, V. (2005) Assessment and management of fungating wounds: a review. *Br J Cancer Nurs* (Wound Care Suppl), **10**(3), 528–34.

Winter, G.D. (1972) Epidermal regeneration studied in the domestic pig. In: *Epidermal Wound Healing* (eds H.I. Maibach & D.T. Rovee). Year Book Medical Publishers, Chicago, pp. 71–112.

Young, T. & Fowler, A. (1998) Nursing management of skin grafts and donor sites. *Br J Nurs,* **7**(6), 324, 326, 328, 330, 332–4.

The Code

The Code
Standards of conduct, performance and ethics for nurses and midwives

The people in your care must be able to trust you with their health and wellbeing.

To justify that trust, you must

- make the care of people your first concern, treating them as individuals and respecting their dignity
- work with others to protect and promote the health and wellbeing of those in your care, their families and carers, and the wider community
- provide a high standard of practice and care at all times
- be open and honest, act with integrity and uphold the reputation of your profession

As a professional, you are personally accountable for actions and omissions in your practice and must always be able to justify your decisions.

You must always act lawfully, whether those laws relate to your professional practice or personal life.

Failure to comply with this Code may bring your fitness to practise into question and endanger your registration.

This Code should be considered together with the Nursing and Midwifery Council's rules, standards, guidance and advice available from www.nmc-uk.org.

Make the care of people your first concern, treating them as individuals and respecting their dignity

Treat people as individuals

- You must treat people as individuals and respect their dignity
- You must not discriminate in any way against those in your care
- You must treat people kindly and considerately
- You must act as an advocate for those in your care, helping them to access relevant health and social care, information and support

Respect people's confidentiality

- You must respect people's right to confidentiality
- You must ensure people are informed about how and why information is shared by those who will be providing their care
- You must disclose information if you believe someone may be at risk of harm, in line with the law of the country in which you are practising

Collaborate with those in your care

- You must listen to the people in your care and respond to their concerns and preferences
- You must support people in caring for themselves to improve and maintain their health
- You must recognise and respect the contribution that people make to their own care and wellbeing
- You must make arrangements to meet people's language and communication needs
- You must share with people, in a way they can understand, the information they want or need to know about their health

Ensure you gain consent

- You must ensure that you gain consent before you begin any treatment or care
- You must respect and support people's rights to accept or decline treatment and care
- You must uphold people's rights to be fully involved in decisions about their care
- You must be aware of the legislation regarding mental capacity, ensuring that people who lack capacity remain at the centre of decision making and are fully safeguarded
- You must be able to demonstrate that you have acted in someone's best interests if you have provided care in an emergency

Maintain clear professional boundaries

- You must refuse any gifts, favours or hospitality that might be interpreted as an attempt to gain preferential treatment
- You must not ask for or accept loans from anyone in your care or anyone close to them
- You must establish and actively maintain clear sexual boundaries at all times with people in your care, their families and carers

Work with others to protect and promote the health and wellbeing of those in your care, their families and carers, and the wider community

Share information with your colleagues

- You must keep your colleagues informed when you are sharing the care of others
- You must work with colleagues to monitor the quality of your work and maintain the safety of those in your care
- You must facilitate students and others to develop their competence

Work effectively as part of a team

- You must work cooperatively within teams and respect the skills, expertise and contributions of your colleagues
- You must be willing to share your skills and experience for the benefit of your colleagues
- You must consult and take advice from colleagues when appropriate
- You must treat your colleagues fairly and without discrimination
- You must make a referral to another practitioner when it is in the best interests of someone in your care

Delegate effectively

- You must establish that anyone you delegate to is able to carry out your instructions
- You must confirm that the outcome of any delegated task meets required standards
- You must make sure that everyone you are responsible for is supervised and supported

Manage risk

- You must act without delay if you believe that you, a colleague or anyone else may be putting someone at risk
- You must inform someone in authority if you experience problems that prevent you working within this Code or other nationally agreed standards
- You must report your concerns in writing if problems in the environment of care are putting people at risk

Provide a high standard of practice and care at all times

Use the best available evidence

- You must deliver care based on the best available evidence or best practice.
- You must ensure any advice you give is evidence based if you are suggesting healthcare products or services
- You must ensure that the use of complementary or alternative therapies is safe and in the best interests of those in your care

Keep your skills and knowledge up to date

- You must have the knowledge and skills for safe and effective practice when working without direct supervision
- You must recognise and work within the limits of your competence
- You must keep your knowledge and skills up to date throughout your working life
- You must take part in appropriate learning and practice activities that maintain and develop your competence and performance

Keep clear and accurate records

- You must keep clear and accurate records of the discussions you have, the assessments you make, the treatment and medicines you give and how effective these have been
- You must complete records as soon as possible after an event has occurred
- You must not tamper with original records in any way
- You must ensure any entries you make in someone's paper records are clearly and legibly signed, dated and timed
- You must ensure any entries you make in someone's electronic records are clearly attributable to you
- You must ensure all records are kept confidentially and securely

Be open and honest, act with integrity and uphold the reputation of your profession

Act with integrity

- You must demonstrate a personal and professional commitment to equality and diversity
- You must adhere to the laws of the country in which you are practising
- You must inform the NMC if you have been cautioned, charged or found guilty of a criminal offence
- You must inform any employers you work for if your fitness to practise is impaired or is called into question

Deal with problems

- You must give a constructive and honest response to anyone who complains about the care they have received
- You must not allow someone's complaint to prejudice the care you provide for them
- You must act immediately to put matters right if someone in your care has suffered harm for any reason
- You must explain fully and promptly to the person affected what has happened and the likely effects
- You must cooperate with internal and external investigations

Be impartial

- You must not abuse your privileged position for your own ends
- You must ensure that your professional judgment is not influenced by any commercial considerations

Uphold the reputation of your profession

- You must not use your professional status to promote causes that are not related to health
- You must cooperate with the media only when you can confidently protect the confidential information and dignity of those in your care
- You must uphold the reputation of your profession at all times

Information about indemnity insurance

The NMC recommends that a registered nurse, midwife or specialist community public health nurse, in advising, treating and caring for patients/clients, has professional indemnity insurance. This is in the interests of clients, patients and registrants in the event of claims of professional negligence.

Whilst employers have vicarious liability for the negligent acts and/or omissions of their employees, such cover does not normally extend to activities undertaken outside the registrant's employment. Independent practice would not be covered by vicarious liability. It is the individual registrant's responsibility to establish their insurance status and take appropriate action.

In situations where an employer does not have vicarious liability, the NMC recommends that registrants obtain adequate professional indemnity insurance. If unable to secure professional indemnity insurance, a registrant will need to demonstrate that all their clients/patients are fully informed of this fact and the implications this might have in the event of a claim for professional negligence.

Contributors to previous editions

First edition edited by

A. Phylip Pritchard
Research Assistant, Department of Nursing Research
Valerie-Anne Walker
Research Assistant, Department of Nursing Research

Second edition edited by

A. Phylip Pritchard
Assistant to the Director of In-Patient Services/
  Chief Nursing Officer
Jill A. David
Director of Nursing Research

Third edition edited by

A. Phylip Pritchard
Formerly Co-ordinator of European Educational Initiatives
The Royal Marsden Hospital
and
Executive Secretary, European Oncology Nursing Society
Jane Mallett
Research and Practice Development Co-ordinator

Fourth edition edited by

Jane Mallett
Research and Practice Development Manager
Christopher Bailey
Macmillan Research Practitioner, Macmillan Practice
  Development Unit, Centre for Cancer and Palliative Care
  Studies, Institute of Cancer Research

Fifth edition edited by

Jane Mallett
Research and Practice Development Manager
  The Royal Marsden Hospital
Lisa Dougherty
Clinical Nurse Specialist Intravenous Services, The Royal
  Marsden Hospital

Sixth edition edited by

Lisa Dougherty
Nurse Consultant Intravenous Therapy, The Royal
  Marsden Hospital
Sara E. Lister
Assistant Chief Nurse/Head of School, The Royal Marsden
  Hospital School of Cancer Nursing & Rehabilitation

Contributors

Emma Allum, Senior Staff Nurse (Wiltshaw Ward)
Sarah Aylott, formerly Practice Development Facilitator
Caroline Badger, formerly Senior Nurse (Lymphoedema)

Christopher Bailey, Macmillan Research Practitioner
  Institute of Cancer Research
Sophie Baty, Sister (Recovery Theatre)
Rachel Bennett, formerly Ward Sister (Wilson Ward)
Chris Berry, formerly Back Care Advisor
Judith Bibbings, formerly Sister
  (Gastro-intestinal/Genito-urinary)
Peter Blake, Consultant Clinical Oncologist
Yannette Booth, formerly Lecturer in Cancer Nursing
Derryn Borley, formerly Assistant Director of Nursing
  Services
David Brighton, Professional Development Facilitator (IT)
Monica Burchall, formerly Sister (High Dependency)
Nancy Burnett, Senior Nurse Manager
Susannah Button, formerly Ward Sister (Ellis Ward)
Antoinette Byrne, formerly Dietitian
Jill Carter, formerly Clinical Nurse Specialist
  (Palliative Care)
Neve Carter, Senior Staff Nurse (Horder Ward) and
  Practice Development Facilitator
Patrick Casey, formerly Clinical Nurse Specialist/
  Unit Manager (Gastro-intestinal/Genito-urinary)
Anne Chandler, Clinical Nurse Specialist in Pain
  Management
Belinda Crawford, Matron (Neurointensive Care),
  Atkinson Morley Hospital
Gay Curling, Clinical Nurse Specialist (Breast Diagnostic
  Unit)
Lisa Curtis, formerly Macmillan Lecturer, Institute of
  Cancer Research
Tonia Dawson, Clinical Nurse Specialist (Pelvic Cancer)
Barbara Dicks, Director of Patient Services/Chief Nursing
  Officer
Emma Dilnutt, formerly Clinical Nurse Specialist
  (Palliative Care)
Anne Doherty, formerly Staff Nurse (Operating Theatres)
Nuala Durkin, formerly Clinical Nurse Specialist/
  Unit Manager (High Dependency)
Jean Edwards, Senior Nurse Manager/Private Patient
  Co-ordinator
Stephen Evans, Radiation Protection Adviser
  (Physics Department)
Sarah Faithfull, CRC Nursing Fellow, Institute of Cancer
  Research
Deborah Fenlon, formerly Group Clinical Nurse Specialist
  (Breast Care Services)
Emma Foulds, Lecturer Practitioner, The Royal Marsden
  Hospital School of Cancer Nursing & Rehabilitation
Tracey Gibson, Senior Staff Nurse (Critical Care Unit)
Aileen Grant, Staff Nurse (Children's Unit)
Jacqueline Green, Senior Dietitian

Douglas Guerrero, Clinical Nurse Specialist (Neuro-oncology)

Rachel Hair, formerly Senior Nurse (Neuro-oncology)

Shujina Haq, Specialist Registrar (Occupational Health)

Cathryn Havard, formerly Senior Nurse (Gastro-intestinal/Genito-urinary)

Pauline Hill, Clinical Nurse Specialist (Community Liaison)

Sian Horn, formerly Sister (High Dependency)

Elizabeth Houlton, formerly Senior Nurse (Community Liaison/Self-Care Unit)

Nest Howells, formerly Information Officer, CancerLink

Jennifer Hunt, Director, Nursing Research Initiative for Scotland

Maureen Hunter, Rehabilitation Services Manager

Elizabeth Janes, formerly Dietitian

Margareta Johnstone, formerly Clinical Nurse Specialist (High Dependency Unit)

Penelope A. Jones, formerly Clinical Nurse Specialist (Community Liaison/Palliative Care)

Danny Kelly, formerly Lecturer in Cancer Nursing, Institute of Cancer Research

Betti Kirkman, formerly Clinical Nurse Specialist (Breast Diagnostic Unit)

Glynis Knowles, Senior Staff, Breast Care (OPD Sutton)

Diane Laverty, Clinical Nurse Specialist (Palliative Care)

Susan J. Lee, formerly Occupational Health Manager

Annie Leggett, formerly Clinical Nurse Specialist (Intravenous Therapy)

Anne Lister, formerly Clinical Nurse Specialist/ Unit Manager (Palliative Care)

Philippa A. Lloyd, Senior Staff Nurse (Wiltshaw Ward)

Nicholas Lodge, Clinical Group Research Nurse (Gynaecology)

E. Lopez-Verdugo, Senior Technician/Theatre Manager

Jane Machin, Specialist Speech and Language Therapist

Hazel Mack, formerly Acting Ward Sister (Horder Ward)

Elizabeth MacKenzie, Sister (Critical Care Unit)

Jean Maguire, Ward Sister/Specialist Sister for Lung Cancer

Jane Mallett, Research and Practice Development Manager

Glynis Markham, formerly Director of Nursing Services

Lisa Mercer, Senior Dietitian

Catherine Miller, formerly Senior Nurse (Continuing Care)

Marion Morgan, formerly Research Sister (Gynaecology)

Wayne Naylor, Clinical Nurse Specialist, Wellington Cancer Centre, New Zealand, formerly Wound Management Research Nurse, The Royal Marsden Hospital

Katrina Neal, formerly Clinical Nurse Specialist/ Unit Manager (Palliative Care)

Liz O'Brien, Clinical Team Leader, District Nursing Croydon Primary Care Trust

Emma Osenton, Ward Sister (Wiltshaw Ward)

Evelyn Otunbade, Backcare Adviser

Buddy Joe Paris, Staff Nurse (Critical Care Unit)

Rachelle Pearce, formerly Sister (Medical Day Unit)

Emma Pennery, formerly Senior Clinical Nurse Specialist/Honorary Clinical Research Fellow

Helen Jayne Porter, formerly Clinical Nurse Specialist (High Dose Chemotherapy)

Joanne Preece, formerly Head of Risk Management

Judith Pretty, formerly Clinical Nurse Specialist (Head and Neck)

Ffion M. Read, Senior Staff Nurse (Medical Day Unit)

Elizabeth Rees, formerly Research Nurse Palliative Care

Francis Regan, formerly Senior Staff Nurse (Burdett Coutts Ward)

Frances Rhys-Evans, formerly Clinical Nurse Specialist/Ward Manager (Head & Neck and Thyroid Cancer)

Jean Maurice Robert, Staff Nurse (Critical Care Unit)

Helen Roberts, formerly Senior Nurse (Head and Neck)

Tim Root, Chief Pharmacist

Corinne Rowbotham, Senior Staff Nurse (IV Services)

Ray Rowden, formerly Director of Nursing Services

Miriam Rushton, formerly Senior Nurse (Gynaecology)

Patricia Ryan, Senior Sister (Haemato-oncology Unit)

Lena Salter, formerly Patient Services Manager

Kate Scott, Clinical Nurse Specialist (Psychological Care)

James Smith, formerly Chaplain

Val Speechley, Patient Information Officer

Moira Stephens, Clinical Nurse Specialist (Haemato-oncology)

Mavis Stork, formerly Theatre Services Manager

June Toovey, formerly Sister (Intravenous Therapy Team)

Anne Topping, formerly Senior Nurse (Gastro-intestinal/Genito-urinary)

Jennie Treleaven, Consultant Haematologist

Robert Tunmore, formerly Clinical Nurse Specialist (Psychological Support)

Beverley van der Molen, formerly Clinical Nurse Specialist/Unit Manager (General Oncology)

Rebecca Verity, formerly Senior Staff Nurse (Bud Flanagan Ward)

Chris Viner, Clinical Nurse Specialist (Ambulatory Chemotherapy)

Clare Webb, Specialist Sister in Psychological Care

Richard Wells, formerly Rehabilitation Services Manager

Isabel White, Head of Undergraduate Cancer Care Studies

Jane Wilson, formerly Group Theatre Manager

Karen Wright, formerly Research Assistant Nursing Research Unit

Karen Young, formerly Physiological Measurement Technician

Index

Page numbers in *italics* refer to figures and those in **bold** to tables and boxes.

ABC of resuscitation 156–9, *157*
abdominal distension
  during bladder lavage/irrigation 321
  enterally fed patients **476**
abdominal pain
  after intraperitoneal chemotherapy 285
  during peritoneal dialysis 743–4
abdominal paracentesis 44–9
  defined 44
  indications 44
  preparatory investigations 46
  problem solving 48–9
  procedure guidelines 46–8
  see also intraperitoneal chemotherapy
ABO blood groups 833, **833**
ABO incompatibility 833, 834, 838
abscess, epidural 590, 602
accidents *see* incidents; spillages
ACGM *see* Advisory Committee on Genetic
      Modification
aciclovir (acyclovir) 122, 123, 269
  eye preparations 635
  oral herpes 651
Acinetobacter, antibiotic resistant 100–1
acquired immune deficiency syndrome (AIDS)
      90–9
  clinical presentation 92
  community care 98–9
  confidentiality 92
  cryptosporidiosis 107
  death 99
  defined 90
  nursing care 93–6
  prevention of further infections 99
  procedure guidelines 93–9
  psychological support 92–3, 97
  transfusion-related 841
  treatment 92
  see also human immunodeficiency virus
actinomycin D 286
Actisorb Silver 220 963
activated charcoal dressings **949**, 962, 963
activities of daily living (ADLs), spinal cord
      compression **797**
acupuncture 567
acute lung injury, transfusion-related (TRALI)
      839–40
acute normovolaemic haemodilution (ANH)
      833
acute pain 558
  assessment tools 559–60, *561*
  management 564–8
  need for effective control 560–3
  see also postoperative pain
acute renal failure (ARF) 736, 739
acyclovir *see* aciclovir

Adapt ring Convex inserts 370
adefovir dipivoxil 113
adenosine 163
adenovirus vectors 401
adhesive, tissue **969**
adhesive island dressings **949**
adhesive skin closure strips **969**
adjuvant analgesics **563**, 571
  epidural/intrathecal 588
administration of drugs *see* drug administration
Administration of Radioactive Substances
      Advisory Committee (ARSAC) 718, 723
administration sets
  blood 217, 845–6
  enteral feeding 474
  gravity flow 296–8
  infusion flow rates 293
  parenteral nutrition 217, 477
  reducing risks of infection 217–18
  volumetric infusion pumps 298
adrenaline (epinephrine)
  blood glucose regulation 533
  cardiopulmonary resuscitation 160, 163
  topical, bleeding wounds 964
advance directives 851
advanced beginner nurse 7
advanced life support (ALS) 156, 158, *158*,
      159–61
advanced practice 8–9
Advisory Committee on Genetic Modification
      (ACGM) Compendium of Guidance 402,
      403, **403**
aerosol containers, storage 206
aerosol generators, humidification 758
aerosolization 208
affirming 33
aflatoxin 104
afterloading brachytherapy *see* brachytherapy,
      afterloading
ageing, skin 662
aggression *see* violence
AIDS *see* acquired immune deficiency syndrome
air, inspired 751, 757
air conditioning and ventilation systems
  negative pressure 73, 74, 404
  positive pressure 73, 74, 85–6
air dryers, electric 54
air embolism
  intra-arterial chemotherapy-associated 287
  intravenous procedure-related 249
  prevention, CVC insertion/removal 871
  transfusion-related 839
  VAD-related 857, 900
air fluidized beds **961**
air fresheners, environmental 963–4
air leaks, chest drainage systems 432–3, 441

airborne infection 57, 72–3
  aspergillosis 104
  Clostridium difficile 106
  extra precautions **75**
  genetically modified micro-organisms 404
  Legionnaires' disease 123–4
  MRSA 102
air-in-line detectors 296, 307
airway
  assessment, postanaesthetic recovery 620–1
  basic life support 156–7, *157*
  defence mechanisms 517
  evaluation of ability to protect 551–2
  functions 512
  maintenance, during respiratory therapy 762,
      763
  resistance 515
  secretions *see* respiratory secretions
airway management
  cardiopulmonary resuscitation 157–8, 163
  postanaesthetic recovery 621, 623
airway obstruction
  emergency tracheostomy 810
  postoperative 618, 623
Aitken report (1958) 204
albumin
  plasma 470, **478**
  solutions, human (HAS) **836**
alcohol consumption, and violence 935
alcohol solutions/swabs
  injection site preparation 216, 229, 230
  VAD site cleaning 856–7, 862
alcoholic handrubs 54, 72
  procedure guidelines 63
aldosterone 505, 530
alfentanil 570
alginate wound dressings **949**, 962, 963, 964
Allen test 902, *903*, 905
allergic reactions
  intravenous infusions 247, 249
  local flare reaction 266
allodynia 568
alopecia 663
  chemotherapy-induced 767–8, 769–70, 772
  radiotherapy induced 768
  scalp cooling to prevent 767–72
ALS *see* advanced life support
alteplase 859, 892
alternating pressure (AP) system 960, **961**
alveoli 516, **516**
  gaseous exchange *751*, 751–2
Ambu bag and mask ventilation 158, 164
ambulatory blood pressure monitoring 509
ambulatory infusion devices 299–301
amethocaine, topical (Ametop) 863
amino acids, parenteral nutrition solutions 476

aminoglycoside antibiotics 778–9
amiodarone 161, 163, 635
ammonia, catheter encrustation and 312
amoebic dysentery 785
amphotericin 269
amputees, positioning 688–9
amsacrine 268
anaemia 516–17
    after bone marrow harvest 417, 426
    aplastic 85
    in malnutrition 470
anaesthesia
    bone marrow harvest 416–17
    pain management interventions 571
    preoperative fasting 606
    pumps 299
    see also local anaesthesia; postanaesthetic
        recovery; topical anaesthesia
anaesthetic room, procedure guidelines 616
anaesthetist 618
anal cancer, HIV-related 90
anal sphincter control, porridge test 351
analgesia
    acute/postoperative pain 564–6
    around the clock (ATC) 563
    bone marrow aspiration/biopsy 416
    breakthrough *see* breakthrough analgesia
    inhalation *see* Entonox
    intrapleural drainage 433
    oral mucositis 652
    spinal cord compression 799, 802
    wound care 962
    see also pain management
analgesic ladder 563, *563*, 568–70
analgesics
    acute/postoperative pain 564–6
    adjuvant (co-analgesics) **563**, 571
    chronic pain 568–70
    epidural/intrathecal use 587–8
    non-opioid 565–6, 568
    opioid *see* opioid analgesics
anaphylactic reactions, blood transfusions 838
anesthesia *see* anaesthesia
angiogenesis 945
angiotensin 505
animals
    carrying/transmitting infections 73
    Cryptosporidium spread 107, 108
anorexia, dietary advice **473**
antecubital fossa
    cytotoxic drug administration 263, **263**, 266
    veins for venepuncture 920, 920–1
antenatal screening, HIV infection 92
anthracyclines
    extravasation 269, 270
    scalp cooling 768, 769
antibacterial eye preparations 635
antibacterial surfaces and materials 77
antibiotics
    bladder lavage solutions 312
    Clostridium difficile infection and 106, 107
    empirical, febrile neutropenia 87
    immunosuppressed patients 84
    Legionnaires' disease 124
    listeriosis 125
    local oral delivery 652
    oral infections 651–2
    pain management **563**
    Pneumocystis carinii pneumonia (PCP) 126
    resistance 100–4
    sensitivity testing 777
    specimen collection and 775–6, 778
    therapeutic monitoring 778–9
    topical, wound management **947**, **949**
antibody testing 777
anticoagulants

epidural catheter removal 599
    intrapleural drainage and 431
    lumbar puncture risks 460
    toxicity, after apheresis 419
    see also heparin
anticonvulsants, pain management **563**
antidepressants 635
antidiuretic hormone (ADH) 530
antiembolic stockings 606–7
    contraindications 609
    daily care 610
    fitting 607, 609
    Lloyd Davies position and 607, 614
    postoperative use 626
    procedure guidelines 608–10
antifungal agents
    aspergillosis 105
    eye preparations 635
    oral infections 651
antihistamines, eye toxicity 635
antihypertensive drug therapy 506
anti-inflammatory drugs, eye 635
antimetabolites 635
antimicrobial agents *see* antibiotics
antimicrobial resistance 100
antimicrobial-resistant organisms 100–4
antimotility drugs 331
antipyretic agents 526
antiretroviral therapy 90, 92
    post-exposure prophylaxis 92, 94
    in pregnancy 92
antiseptics
    bladder lavage 311, 312
    specimen collection and 775–6
    wound cleaning 947, **947**
    see also chlorhexidine
antispasmodics **563**
antiviral therapy
    cytomegalovirus infection 120
    eye preparations 635
    hepatitis B 113
    herpes simplex virus (HSV) infection 121–2
    varicella zoster virus (VZV) infection 123
anxiety 35–6
    breast aspiration 149
    during CPAP 764
    effects on pain 558
    infected patients in isolation 78
    during venepuncture 922, 929
aperients 334
aphasic patients, communicating with 38–9
apheresis 413, 417–19
    complications 419
    donor 417, **418–19**, 833
    therapeutic 417, **418**
aplastic anaemia 85
Apligraf 954
apnoeustic respiration 519, **551**
Appeal wipes and spray 369
appointments, HIV-positive patients 96
aprons, plastic 56
    barrier nursing 76, 80
    procedure guidelines 57–8, *58–9*
Aquacel Ag 963
aqueous humour 631, *632*
arachis oil enema 336
arachnoid mater 586, *587*
arachnoiditis 462
arginine 475
argyria 381
arm *see* upper limb
arousability 546
arrhythmias 499–500
    causing cardiac arrest 156
    ECG features *500*
    tracheal suctioning-induced 819

art therapy 566
arterial blood gases (ABG)
    in asthma 521
    blood sampling 902, 904–6, 909–10
arterial cannulae 902–13
    back-flow of blood into 912
    blood sampling from 909–10, *910–11*
    choice of site 902–3
    complications **903**, 903–4
    defined 902
    displacement 287
    indications 507, 902
    insertion 907–8, *908*
    intra-arterial chemotherapy 286–7
    nursing considerations 904
    problem solving 912–13
    procedure guidelines 904–12
    removal 911–12
arterial disease, compression therapy and 170,
        171, 175, 176
arterial pressure monitoring
    arterial cannulation 507, 902–4
    nursing considerations 904
    problem solving 912–13
    procedure guidelines 907–8, *908*
arterial puncture 904
    accidental 928
    procedure guidelines 904–6
arterial spasm 913
arteries 921
    cannulation-induced damage 903–4, 913
    complications of intra-arterial chemotherapy
        287
arterioles 505
ascites
    abdominal paracentesis 44–9
    fluid specimens for analysis 44, 45, 47
    intraperitoneal drug administration 45,
        283–5
    malignant 44–5
    nursing care 45–6
    physiology of formation 44
    treatment 45
ascorbic acid (vitamin C) **532**, 536, 946–7
asepsis 51
aseptic technique 51–65
    airborne contamination 57
    compliance with 52–3
    defined 51
    dressing trolley 55
    environmental cleanliness 56
    hand washing 53–4
    inanimate objects 55
    indications 51
    intravenous drug administration 217
    medical or clean 51
    microbiological specimen collection 775,
        778
    non touch technique 54–5
    operating theatre 615
    patient hygiene 56–7
    personal protective equipment 55–6
    principles 53–7
    procedure guidelines 59–61
    surgical or sterile 51
    urinary catheterization 384–7
    vascular access devices 856
L-asparaginase 275
aspergillosis 104–5
Aspergillus flavus 104
Aspergillus fumigatus 104
aspiration
    bone marrow 414–16
    breast *see* breast aspiration
    enteral feeds **476**
    extravasated drug 269

aspiration of gastric contents
  to check enteral tube position 473, 483, 486
  during CPAP 756, 764
aspirin 532, 568
  mouthwashes 652
assessment 16–20, 24
  comprehensive **18**
  discharge planning 196–7
  documentation **23**
  focused **18**
  interviews 18, **19**
  methods 18–20
  ongoing **18**
  principles 16
  self- 20, **20**
  single 193
  structure 17–18
  tools 18–20, **20**
  types **18**
Association for the Advancement of Medical
    Instrumentation (AAMI) 508
Association of Perioperative Registered Nurses
    (AORN) 608, 615
asthma
  peak flow measurements 521
  recognition and assessment 521–2, **522**
asymmetrical tonic neck reflex 685
asystole 156, 161
ataxic breathing **551**
atelectasis 514
athletes, heart rate 498
atmosphere 516, **516**
atrial fibrillation 499
atrioventricular (AV) block, Mobitz type 2 *500*
atrioventricular (AV) bundle (bundle of His)
    499, 502
atrioventricular (AV) node *499*, 502
atropine 161, 163, 635
audit, resuscitation 162
autoclaving 95–6
autologous blood donation 832–3
autolytic wound debridement 948
automated external defibrillators (AEDs) 162
autonomic dysfunction, spinal cord
    compression 797
autonomic dysreflexia 342, 806
awareness, conscious 546
axillary temperature 527
azotaemia, parenteral nutrition 478

Babinski response 551, 555
bacille Calmette-Guérin (BCG) 278, 280
back pain (backache)
  intraoperative positioning and 614
  peritoneal dialysis 743
  post-lumbar puncture 462, 464, 465
  spinal cord compression 797, **797**, 798
bacteraemia 528
  blood cultures 778
  Gram-negative 100–1
bacteria
  aerobic 775
  anaerobic 775
  facultative 775
  fastidious 775
  oral cavity 649
  specimen collection 777
  wound colonization 948, 963
bacterial filters
  Entonox face masks 579
  epidural/intrathecal analgesia 592
bacterial infections
  antibiotic-resistant 100–4
  oral 651–2
  transfusion-transmitted 840
  see also specific infections

bacteriuria 530, *531*
bad news, breaking 37
Bahai faith, last offices 452
balloon catheters *see* Foley catheters
barrier nursing 71–90
  cohort *see* cohort barrier nursing
  defined 71
  gene therapy 404, 406, 408
  indications 71
  principles 75–9
  reverse *see* protective isolation
  sources of infection 72–3
  standard and extra precautions 75, **75**
  tuberculosis patients 128
  types 73–4
  see also source isolation
basal cell carcinoma (BCC) 275
  eyelids 636
basic life support (BLS) 156–9, *157*
basilic vein 862, *865*, 867, *867*
  venepuncture 920, *920*, 921
basins, hand 61, 72
basophils *413*, **414**
bathing 56, 663
  barrier-nursed patients 77, 81
  preoperative 611
  see also bed bathing; showering
baths, cleaning 77
battery-operated infusion devices 300–1
BCG (bacille Calmette-Guérin) 278, 280
BCNU (carmustine) 268, 286
becquerel (Bq) 692
bed(s)
  linen *see* linen/laundry
  positioning in 670–3
    amputees 688
    neurological patients 685–7
    side lying 672–3, *673*
    sitting up 671, 672
    supine 670–1
  pressure-relieving devices 960, **961**
bed bathing 77, 663
  procedure guidelines 664–6
bed rest 670
bedpans 325–6, 333
  radioactive patients 728
belladonna-like substances 635
benchmarks
  food and nutrition 471, **472**
  personal and oral hygiene 77, 648, 661
Benner's model of skill acquisition 7–8
benzodiazepines **563**
beta-blockers 636
beta radiation 694
Better Hospital Food programme 471
biliary sclerosis, intra-arterial
    chemotherapy-induced 287
biochemical tests
  nutritional status 470
  parenteral nutrition **478**
bioelectrical impedance analysis (BIA) 469
bio-engineered skin substitutes 954
biofilms 103, 312, 857
biohazard labels 96, 776
biological safety cabinets, cytotoxic drug
    reconstitution 255–6
Biological Safety Officer (BSO) 403
biopsy
  bone marrow 414–16
  breast 148–51
  radioactive sentinel node 723
Biot's respiration 519
bisacodyl 335, 339
bisphosphonates **563**, 571
bladder
  empty, catheterized patients 393

neuropathic 349
  perforation 743
  rectal 350–1, *351*, 353
  symptoms, spinal cord compression 797
bladder cancer 280–3
  radioactive seed implants 711
bladder irrigation (continuous)
  catheters for 314, *314*
  defined 311
  indications 311
  patient assessment 313
  problem solving 321
  procedure guidelines 318–19
  recording chart 319–20, *320*
  solutions 311
bladder lavage 311–13
  defined 311
  indications 311
  patient assessment 313
  problem solving 321
  procedure guidelines 314–16
  solutions 311
  see also intravesical drug instillation
blanching, in extravasation 269
bleeding/haemorrhage
  after bone marrow collection 416, **417**,
      426
  after VAD removal 901
  arterial cannulation-related 903, 912
  cardiopulmonary arrest 159
  fungating wounds **962**, 964
  hepatitis B-infected patients 114–15, 116
  HIV-positive patients 94
  intra-arterial chemotherapy-associated 287
  lumbar puncture-associated 462
  peritoneal dialysis catheters 743
  postoperative care 626
  radioactive patients 704
bleomycin 275, 278, 280, 283, 286
blind patients, communication with 37–8
blink reflex 550–1, *555*
  absent, eye care 634
blocking behaviour 35
Blom–Singer voice prostheses 815, 820–1
  changing, procedure guidelines 828–9
  duckbill valve *820*, 820–1
  indwelling valve *820*, 821
  low-pressure valve *820*, 821
blood
  accidental spillage 930
  hepatitis B-infected 114, 115
  pH 516
  return, extravasation **268**, 269
  spurting, during venepuncture 930
  testing, donors 832–4
  traceability 832
  viscosity 504–5
  warming devices 839
blood administration sets
  changing 217
  transfusion procedure 845–6
blood borne infections 73
  blood donor selection and 832
  hepatitis B 111, 114–15
  hepatitis C 117
  hepatitis E 118
  HIV 91
  infection control 93
blood cells **414**
  in CSF 461–2
blood clots
  bladder irrigation 314, 319
  VAD occlusion 858–9, 892
blood components/products
  donation 833
  requesting 843

traceability 832
used for transfusion 835–6
blood cultures 778
  procedure guidelines 784
  specimen storage 776
blood donation 832–3
  autologous 832–3
  via apheresis 417, **418–19**, 833
blood flow 504
  problems during venepuncture 930–1
  resistance to 504–5, *505*
  wound bed, improving 947
blood gases, arterial *see* arterial blood gases
blood glucose *see* glucose, blood
blood groups 833–4
  haemopoietic stem cell transplantation 834
  incompatibility 833–4
blood pack labelling *842*
blood pressure (BP) 504–12
  ambulatory monitoring 509
  continuous arterial monitoring *see* arterial
    pressure monitoring
  continuous venovenous haemodiafiltration
    745
  defined 504
  diastolic 506
  factors affecting 505, *506*
  measurement
    auscultatory method *507*, 507–10, *509*
    clinical aspects 509–10
    epidural/intrathecal analgesia 595
    indications 504
    manual evacuation of rectum 342, 343, 344
    methods and equipment 507–9
    neurological patients 552, 554
    postanaesthetic recovery 621
    practical aspects 509
    procedure guidelines 510–12, *512*
    top tips **510**
    see also sphygmomanometers
  normal 505
  regulation 505, *505*
  systolic 505–6
  see also hypertension; hypotension
blood products *see* blood components/products
Blood Safety and Quality Regulations 2005
  832
blood sampling 777–9
  arterial puncture for 904–6
  blood cultures 778, 784
  blood glucose monitoring 535, 537
  order of collection 926
  pre-transfusion 844
  therapeutic drug monitoring 778–9, 784–5
  venepuncture for *see* venepuncture
  via arterial cannula 909–10, *910–11*
  via CVADs *see under* central venous access
    devices
  via intravenous devices 922, **923**
blood transfusion *see* transfusion
blood vessels, resistance to blood flow 505
blood warmers 839
bloodstream infections, health care acquired
  71
B-lymphocytes *413*, **414**
body, care after death *see* last offices
body bag 446, 447, 449, 450
  radioactive patients 704, 732
body composition, measurement 469
body fluids
  cytotoxic drug-treated patients 260
  hepatitis B transmission 111
  HIV transmission 91, 94
  radioactive 722, 724, 728, 730
    spillages 731–2
  specimen collection 784–9

body image, altered
  chemotherapy-induced hair loss 767
  indwelling CVADs 877–8
  urinary diversion 354–5
body mass index (BMI) 468–9
body surface area, calculation 262
body weight 468–9
  loss 468–9
    percentage 468, 469
  measuring, procedure guidelines 479–80, *480*
Bohr effect 752
bone marrow 413
  filtration of harvested 422
  procedures 413, 414–17
bone marrow aspiration/trephine biopsy
  414–16, **415**
  complications 416
  indications 415–16
  method 415
  post-procedure care 416
  problem solving 425–6
  procedure guidelines 419–22
  sites 414–15, *415*
bone marrow harvest 416–17
  complications 417
  post-procedural care 417, **417**
  problem solving 425–6
  procedure guidelines 422–5
bone marrow transplantation (BMT)
  blood cultures 778
  bone marrow harvest 416–17
  cryopreserved bone marrow/peripheral blood
    stem cells 834
  cryptosporidiosis 107
  cytomegalovirus infection 120
  diet 87
  infection risks 84–5
  nursing care 87–8
  protective isolation 85, 86
  see also neutropenia; stem cell transplantation
bone metastases
  Re186 HEDP therapy 718–21
  spinal cord compression 796
bone scan, radionuclide **719**
bovine spongiform encephalopathy (BSE) 129,
  841
bowel
  anatomy and physiology 328
  perforation 743
bowel care 325–45
  bedpans 325–6
  commodes 326–7
  digital rectal examination 340–2
  enemas 335–8
  manual evacuation 342–4
  rectal irrigation 344–5
  spinal cord injuries 342, 343–4
  suppositories 338–40
bowel function
  spinal cord compression 797
  unconscious patients 850–1
bowel habit
  factors affecting 331–3
  history taking 333
  normal 331
  see also constipation; diarrhoea
bowel preparation
  brachytherapy 705, 713
  continent urinary diversion 352
  rectal irrigation 344–5
BP *see* blood pressure
B/P. sphyg. *see* sphygmomanometers
bracelets, medical alert 353
brachial artery, blood pressure recording 507,
  509, 511
brachial plexus injury, after VAD insertion 900

brachytherapy (sealed source radiotherapy)
  692–714
  afterloading 696–7
    manual systems 697, 698
    procedure guidelines 705–6
    remote systems 697, 698–700, *699*
    see also microSelectron; Selectron
  application methods 696–8
  contamination monitors 692
  death during 451, 703–4
  defined 692
  incident procedure 692
  indications 692
  interstitial (implants) 694
    complications 695, 696
    insertion methods 696
    perineal template *695*, 695–6
    problem solving 708
    procedure guidelines 711–14
    radioactive sources *694*, 694–6, *695*
    removal of caesium and iridium wires
      706–7
  intracavitary 694
    applicators 696, 697, 697–8
    complications 700
    follow-up care 701
    patient discharge 701
    patient preparation 700–1
    procedure guidelines 705–6, 708–10
    radioactive sources 694
    vaginal care after 701
  patient assessment 692
  problem solving 710
  procedure guidelines 702–14
  radioactive isotopes 693–6
Braden scale 956–60, **959**
bradycardia 498
  postoperative 624
bradypnoea 518
brainstem
  damage 549, *550*
  herniation, after lumbar puncture 462, 465
breaking bad news 37
breakthrough analgesia 568, 569, 570
  via syringe driver 306
breakthrough pain 558, 570
breast
  anatomy and physiology 147, *147*
  benign conditions 147, 148
  core biopsy 148
breast aspiration (fine needle aspiration; FNA)
  147, 148–51
  accuracy 148
  application 148
  classification of results **149**
  patient's experience 149
  procedure guidelines 149–51, *151*
breast cancer 147–8
  diagnosis 148–9
  fungating wounds 963
  interstitial brachytherapy 695, *695*, 711,
    712
  lymphoedema 170, 171
  postoperative seromas 151–2
  radioactive sentinel node biopsy 723
  spinal cord compression 796
breast cysts 147
  aspiration 148, 150
breast feeding
  Entonox use 581
  HIV-positive women 92
  radiation exposure 730
breast lumps
  diagnostic methods 148
  fine needle aspiration *see* breast aspiration
  triple assessment 148

breast surgery
  blood pressure measurement and 510
  seroma drainage **152**, 152–3
  seroma formation after 151–2
breathing
  agonal 157
  cardiopulmonary resuscitation 157–8, *158*
  positioning to minimize work of 682, *682*
  see also respiration
breathlessness *see* dyspnoea
Brief Pain Inventory (BPI) 560
Bristol Stool Form Chart *330*, 333
British Committee for Standards in
    Haematology (BCSH) 85, 834, 844
British Humanist Association 453
British Hypertension Society 506, 508
British Medical Association (BMA), do not
    attempt resuscitation guidance 162–3
British Thoracic Society, intrapleural drainage
    guidelines 431
bronchitis, chronic 513, 758–60
Broviac catheters *see* skin-tunnelled catheters
bruising, after venepuncture 924, 929
BSE (bovine spongiform encephalopathy) 129,
    841
buccal tablets 206, 223
Buddhism, last offices 452
Buddhist Hospice Trust 452
buffy coat **835**
building work, *Aspergillus* spread 104, 105
bundle of His (AV bundle) *499*, 502
bupivacaine, epidural/intrathecal 588,
    591–2
buprenorphine 570
Burial Society of the United Synagogue 454
Burkitt's lymphoma 120
burn out 88
burns, diathermy 613
butterfly devices *see* winged infusion devices

Cadesorb 954, 967
Cadexomer bead dressings **949**
caesium-137 694
  gynaecological sources 694
    problem solving 710
    procedure guidelines 705–7
  remote afterloading systems 698, 699
  removal 706–7
  oral implants 694, *694*
calcium, plasma **478**
calcium chloride 161, 163, 269
calcium gluconate 269
calf compression boots, intermittent 607,
    614
Campylobacter food poisoning 73
cancer
  AIDS-related 90
  ascites 44–6
  aspergillosis 105
  communication 29, 35–7
  dietary modification 471, **473**
  fungating wounds *see* fungating wounds
  gene therapy 401–10
  health care acquired infections 71
  lymphoedema 170, 171
  mouth care 650–1
  nutritional assessment 469, 470
  oral assessment 649
  oral complications 648–9
  patient assessment 17, 19–20, **20**
  personal hygiene 77
  plastic surgery 966
  protective isolation 83–4
  radionuclide imaging **720**
  secondary *255*, 354
  skin complications 662

specimen collection for microbiological
    analysis 775
  spinal cord compression 796, *796*
  see also tumours; *specific types of cancer*
Cancer Action Team, assessment guidance 17
cancer nurses, stress and burn out 88
cancer pain 559
  assessment 559, **559**, *562*
  management 568–71
  pain chart 560, *562*, 573
  spinal analgesia 586, 591–9
  see also chronic pain
candidiasis (*Candida albicans* infections)
  oral 651
  specimen collection 777
  voice prostheses 821, 822
cannabis 570
cannulae
  arterial *see* arterial cannulae
  peripheral (venous) *see* peripheral cannulae
capillary wound dressings **949**
caps
  scalp cooling 768
  see also head coverings
capsules 206
  administration guidelines 221–3
  cytotoxic drugs 274–5
  opening 206, 275
  storage 206
carbohydrates
  parenteral nutrition solutions 477
  supplements 471
carbon dioxide
  control of respiration 513
  excretion 753
  narcosis 758–60
  pulmonary exchange 516, **516**, *751*, 751–2
  transport 516–17, *517*
carbon dioxide partial pressure (PCO_2) 751
  in blood ($PaCO_2$) 516, 758
carbon monoxide (CO) poisoning 519
carboplatin 283
cardiac arrest 156
  agonal breathing 157
  arrhythmias causing 156
  assessment 156
  management *see* cardiopulmonary
      resuscitation
  post-resuscitation care 165–7
  potentially reversible causes 159–60
  radioactive patients 703, 732
  team 161–2, 165
cardiac arrhythmias *see* arrhythmias
cardiac failure, compression therapy and 171,
    176
cardiac massage *see* chest compressions
cardiac nuclear medicine studies **719**
cardiac output (CO) 497
cardiac tamponade
  cardiopulmonary arrest 160
  complicating bone marrow aspiration/biopsy
    416
cardiopulmonary arrest *see* cardiac arrest
cardiopulmonary resuscitation (CPR) 156–67
  advanced life support (ALS) 156, 158, *158*,
      159–61
  assessment 156, *156*
  basic life support 156–9, *157*
  decision making 162–3
  defibrillation 161
  drugs 160–1, 163
  equipment 162, 163
  ethics 162
  indications 156
  in-hospital algorithm *157*
  post-procedure care 165–7

potentially reversible causes of arrest 159–60
  principles 156
  procedure guidelines 163–7
  radioactive patients 703, 732
  standards and training 161–2
  tracheostomy patients 819
cardiovascular disease
  positioning patients with 684
  pulse monitoring 500
cardiovascular function
  during CPAP 763
  epidural/intrathecal analgesia 595
  postanaesthetic assessment 618, *619*, 621
  unconscious patients 851
care 22–5
  communicating (handover) 25
  documentation **23**, 25
  evaluating 23–5
  implementing 22–3
  planning 22–3, **23**
care homes, discharge to 195
care of body after death *see* last offices
carers, informal
  discharge planning and 189, 198
  see also family
carmustine (BCNU) 268, 286
carotid pulse, checking 158, *159*
carpets 82
CASE method, prevention of violence 935–6
caspofungin 105
cathartics 334
catheter specimen of urine (CSU) 390–1, *391*
catheter tips
  embolism 901
  microbiological examination 874, 896, 899
catheter-associated infections, urinary *see*
      urinary catheter-associated infections
catheters
  continent urinary diversion 352–3, *353*
  defined 378
  intermittent self-catheterization of urinary
      stoma 355
  intrapleural drainage 431
  peritoneal *see* peritoneal catheters
  tracheal suctioning 819, *819*
  urinary *see* urinary catheters
Catrix 954
Cavilon barrier film 369, 963
CDs *see* controlled drugs
CE mark
  gloves 56, 64, 76
  medical devices 55
cefotaxime 269
cell salvage, intra-operative (ICS) 833
cellulitis
  compression therapy and 170, 175
  intravenous infusion-related 247
central lines *see* central venous catheters
central venous access devices (CVAD) 866
  blood sampling 778, 779
    blood cultures 784
    discard method 889
    procedure guidelines 889–91
    push–pull/mixing method 889
    reinfusion method 889
  complications 877
  cytotoxic drug administration 262–3
  defined 866
  discharge home with in situ 876–7, *877*
  extravasation 266
  hazards of insertion **866**
  indications 866
  infections related to 778
  maintaining a closed system 857
  maintaining patency 888
  occlusion 245

unblocking, procedure guidelines 891–3, 893
  see also under vascular access devices
problem solving 899–901
  procedure guidelines 887–91
quality of life issues 877–8
vesicant drug administration 267
see also central venous catheters; peripherally inserted central catheters
central venous catheters (CVCs)
  complications of indwelling 866
  damage and repair 859–60
  dressings 857
    changing 887–8
  maintaining patency 858
  microbiological examination of tip 874, 896, 899
  parenteral nutrition 476
  short-term percutaneous non-tunnelled **856**, 869–72
    care and management in situ 871–2
    choice of vein 870–1
    cleaning 857
    defined 869
    devices 869–70, *870*
    indications 869
    insertion 871, *871*
    procedure guidelines 887–8, 896
    removal 872, 896
  skin tunnelled see skin-tunnelled catheters
central venous pressure (CVP) 538–41
  defined 538
  monitoring 538–41, 869
    problem solving 540–1
    procedure guidelines 539–40
  normal 539
Centre for Evidence Based Nursing 10
Centre for Reviews and Dissemination, York 10
cephalic vein
  cannulation 861–2, 868
  venepuncture 920, *920*, 921
cerebral oedema *550*
cerebrospinal fluid (CSF) 460–1, 586
  abnormalities 461–2
  investigations 460, 462
  leakage from lumbar puncture site 464, 465
  pressure 461
  sampling 460, 461
Cervex-Brush® 780, 792
cervical cancer
  brachytherapy 697, 697–8, 701
  screening 780
  see also gynaecological cancer
cervical ('Pap') smear 779–80, **780**, *780*
  liquid-based cytology 780, 792
  procedure guidelines 789–92
cervical spine injuries, assessment 156
cervix, uterine *780*
chair
  positioning in *675*
  standing up from 675–6, *676*
chalazion 636
chapters, structure of 7
charcoal dressings **949**, *962*, 963
charrière (ch) 379
charting by exception (CBE) 23–5
chemical irritation, intravenous infusion-induced 247
Chemocap 768
chemotherapy 255
  cancer pain management 571
  induced alopecia see under alopecia
  for spinal cord compression 799, 803
  see also cytotoxic drugs

chest compressions
  cardiopulmonary resuscitation 158, *159*, 164
  intubated patients 165
chest drains see intrapleural drains
chest pain, after VAD insertion 900
chest X-rays
  enteral tube feeding 473, 483, 486
  post-CPR 166
Cheyne–Stokes respiration 519, **551**
chickenpox (varicella) 122, 123
Chief Nursing Officer's '10 key roles' for nurses 8
children see paediatric patients
Chiron barrier cream 369
chloramphenicol 635
chlorhexidine
  bladder lavage 311, 312
  chewing gum 653
  cleaning VAD insertion sites 856–7, 862
  mouthwash 650–1
  MRSA eradication 101
Christianity, last offices 453
chromosomal abnormalities, cytotoxic drug-induced 255
chronic obstructive pulmonary disease (COPD)
  Entonox and 578
  hypoxic drive 513, 758–60
  peak flow measurements 521
chronic pain 558
  assessment **559**, 559–60
  management 563, 568–71
  non-pharmacological techniques 566–8
  pain chart 560, *562*, 573
  procedure guidelines 573
  spinal analgesia 586, 590, 591–9
  see also cancer pain
chronic wasting disease 129, 841
Church of Jesus Christ of the Latter Day Saints, last offices 455
chylothorax 430
ciprofloxacin 635
circulation
  cardiopulmonary resuscitation 158, *159*
  postanaesthetic recovery 621
  postoperative monitoring 626
circulatory (fluid) overload
  apheresis 419
  bladder irrigation 311
  blood pressure monitoring 510
  blood transfusion 839
  during CPAP 764
  intravenous infusions 293–4, **295**, 901
    problem solving 248
    see also overinfusion
  parenteral nutrition 477
  peritoneal dialysis 744
cirrhosis of liver 44
cisplatin 283, 286
citrate toxicity, apheresis 419
citric acid 3.23% and magnesium oxide solution (Suby G) 311, 312–13
citric acid 6% solution (solution R) 311, 312–13
CJD see Creutzfeldt–Jakob disease
clamps, infusion devices 293, 859–60
clarifying 33–4
classified persons, radiation 717
clean technique, intermittent self-catheterization 388–90
cleaning
  baths 77
  environmental 56, 72, 77
    Clostridium difficile infections 107
    gene therapy 408–9
    hepatitis B 113
    HIV infection 96–7
    MRSA 102

protective isolation rooms 86, 88
source isolation rooms 78–9, 82, 83
  see also domestic staff
non-disposable equipment 95–6
radioactive treatment rooms 725
skin see skin preparation
stoma 369
vascular access devices 857
wounds 947, *947*, 971
cleanliness, environmental 56, 72
clients see patients
clinical experience/expertise 11, 12
clinical governance 9
clinical nurse specialists 8
clips, metal **969**
  removal 974–5
clonidine, epidural/intrathecal 588
Clostridium difficile 105–7
  diagnosis 106
  nursing care 107
  prevention of spread/management 106–7
  transmission 106
clothing
  cytotoxic drug spillages 259
  deceased patient 446, 448
  protective see protective clothing
cluster breathing **551**
coagulopathies
  lumbar puncture 460
  spinal analgesia 586
co-analgesics **563**, 571
cockroaches 73
co-codamol 568
Code, The (NMC) 4–5, 7, 937, 955, 986–92
codeine phosphate 331, 365, 568, 713
coffee 333
cohort barrier nursing 71, 75
  MRSA-infected patients 102
cold sores 121
cold therapy (cryotherapy)
  extravasation 270, 273
  oral 653
  pain management 568
  see also scalp cooling
colectomy, total 362
collaboration, with patients 988
collagen 945, 954
  dressings **949**, 954
Colledge silver laryngectomy tube 814, *815*
collusion 36–7
colon 328
colonic conduits 362–3
colonization, wound 948
colony stimulating factors 275, 652
colorectal cancer
  interstitial brachytherapy 695–6
  liver metastases 285, 286
colostomy 362
  defunctioning or loop 362, *362*
  end or terminal 362, *362*
  indications 363
  irrigation 365
  plugs 365, 368
  postoperative care 365–6
  postoperative function 365
  pouches 368, *368*
  problem solving 374–5
  see also stoma(s)
comatose patients see unconscious patients
Comfeel wafers 369
comfort measures, for pain management 566
Committee on Medical Aspects of Food Policy (COMA) report 470–1
commodes 326–7

communication 29–39
  aids 33
  aphasic patients 38–9
  during assessment 18
  barriers to effective 29–30
  blind and partially sighted 37–8
  breaking bad news 37
  deaf and hard of hearing 38
  de-escalation of violence 935–6
  defined 29
  discharge planning and 189–93, **193**
  guidelines 30–1
  intershift (handover) 25
  language and cultural issues 35
  laryngectomy patients 816
  non-verbal 32–3
  recognizing own agenda 31–2
  respiratory therapy and 763, 765
  skills 32–5
  specific problems 35–9
  specific therapeutic 4
  tracheostomy patients 816
  training 35
  verbal 32
community care
  AIDS/HIV-positive patients 98–9
  home enteral feeding 475
  MRSA-infected patients 103
Community Care (Delayed Discharges) Act 189,
  193
community nurses
  continent urinary diversion 353
  discharge planning **194–5**, 198
  see also district nurses
compartment syndrome 614
competence
  Benner's model of acquisition 7–8
  definition 7
  to give consent 5
  nursing staff 7–8
competent nurses 7–8
complaints, dealing with 991
complementary therapies, wound management
  954
Complex Discharge Coordinator **189**, 193,
  194–5
compliance
  aseptic technique 52–3
  hand washing 54, 72
  self-administration of medicines 209
  tuberculosis therapy 128
compression, intermittent pneumatic 607,
  614
compression bandaging 170, 175–7
  contraindications 176
  indications 176, *176*
  principles 177
  procedure guidelines 179–84, *181–2,*
  184
compression garments
  elastic 170, 174–5
    applying, procedure guidelines 178–9
    choosing correct 175
  inelastic 170
compression stockings, graduated elastic *see*
  antiembolic stockings
compression therapy 170–84
  contraindications 170
  definitions 170
  indications 170
  intensive phase 175–7
  limb volume measurement 171–4
  maintenance phase 174–5
  procedure guidelines 178–84
computed tomography (CT) 460, 799
conduction system, heart *499*

confidentiality
  HIV/AIDS patients 92
  respect for 988
conformable catheters 381
Conformité Europèene mark *see* CE mark
confusion
  evaluation 547
  radioactive patients 704
consciousness 546–9
  arousability 546
  assessment 547–9, *553*, 850
    cardiopulmonary arrest 156, *156*, 166
    postanaesthetic recovery 618, *619*, 622
    see also Glasgow coma scale
  awareness 546
  defined 850
  level 546
Conseal plugs 365
consent 5–7, 988
  components of valid 5
  cytotoxic drug administration 262
  documentation 5–7
  forms 6–7
  gene therapy 405
  HIV antibody testing 91
  implied 6
  unsealed radioactive source administration
    725
  verbal 6, **6**
  written 6, 6–7
constipation 331–5
  assessment 331–3
  causes 328, 331, *332*
  defined 325, 331
  enemas 335
  enterally fed patients **476**
  management 333–5, **334**
  opioid-induced 568
  unsealed radioactive source administration
    and 725
contact lenses 633
  care of 633, 639–40, *640*
  eye preparations and 633
  surgical patients 612
  unsealed radioactive source therapy 728
contact tracing, tuberculosis patients 127–8
contact transmission of infection 55, 72
  extra precautions 75
  hepatitis B 111
containers
  medicine 206
  specimen 775, 776
context
  as evidence source 11, 12
  nursing 4–12
continent urinary diversion 349–59
  bowel preparation 352
  with catheterizable stomas **349**, 349–51, *350*
  complications 354
  discharge advice 354
  flushing drainage tubes 352–3, 357–8
  indications 349
  intermittent self-catheterization 350, *350*
    problem solving 358–9
    teaching, procedure guidelines 355–7
    tubing types 355
  orthotopic neobladder *see* neobladder,
    orthotopic
  patient education before discharge 353
  patient selection 351
  postoperative care 352–3, *353*
  preoperative counselling 352
  principles 349
  procedure guidelines 355–8
  psychological effects 354–5
  second admission 350, 353–4

sexual dysfunction after 352
surgical procedures 349–51
continuous ambulatory peritoneal dialysis
  (CAPD) 736
continuous arteriovenous haemofiltration
  (CAVH) 739
continuous intravenous infusions *see under*
  intravenous infusions
continuous low pressure (CLP) system 960
continuous positive airway pressure (CPAP)
  756
  indications 756
  problem solving 763–5
  procedure guidelines 760–1
continuous renal replacement therapy (CRRT)
  739–40
continuous venovenous haemodiafiltration
  (CVVHDF) 736, 739, 739–40
  commencement 745–6
  procedure guidelines 744–6
contractures 687, 688–9
control and restraint (C&R) 936–7
Control of Substances Hazardous to Health
  (COSHH) regulations
  cytotoxic drugs 255, 257
  gene therapy 402, 403
  infectious agents 76, 93, 96, 128
controlled area, radiation 704, 717, 724
controlled drugs (CDs) 203–4
  legal requirements 204, **205**
  procedure guidelines 223–4
  register 204
  safe practice guidance 204
controlled-release tablets 206
conveens *see* penile sheaths
cooling
  in pyrexia 526
  scalp 767–73
coping mechanisms 36–7
coring, multidose vials 227, *228*
corneal (blink) reflex 550–1, *555*
corticosteroids (steroids)
  as analgesics **563**
  epidural/intrathecal 588
  for extravasation 270
  eye drops 635
  intra-articular injections 213
  intralesional, hypertrophic and keloid scars
    968
  spinal cord compression 799
  toxic effects on eye 635
  see also hydrocortisone
cortisol 533
COSHH regulations *see* Control of Substances
  Hazardous to Health (COSHH)
  regulations
cosmetic camouflage, scars 969
cost effectiveness 9–10
costs, health care-acquired infections 52, 71
co-trimoxazole 126
cough **518**
counselling
  after violent incidents 937
  AIDS/HIV infection 92–3
  continent urinary diversion 352
  before stoma surgery 363–4
  see also psychological support
covert drug administration 209–10
CPAP *see* continuous positive airway pressure
CPR *see* cardiopulmonary resuscitation
C-reactive protein (CRP) 470, **478**
creams 207
  cytotoxic drugs 275–6
  storage 206
creatinine 530
  plasma, parenteral nutrition 478

Creutzfeldt–Jakob disease (CJD) 129–30
  transmission in blood 129–30, 832, 841
  variant (vCJD) 129, 841
cricothyroidotomy 811
critical care
  arterial cannulation 902
  last offices 449–50
critical colonization, wounds 948
critical thinking 16
critically ill patients
  blood pressure measurement 510
  pulse monitoring 500
  renal replacement therapy 739–40
  respiratory monitoring 519
  sedation 850
  temperature monitoring 528
crockery/cutlery
  gene therapy 407
  hepatitis A-infected patients 110
  HIV-positive patients 98
  source barrier nursing 78, 80
  unsealed radioactive source therapy 728
cross-infection 72
  prevention see infection control
crutches, elbow 679–80
cryo-depleted plasma 836
cryogel caps 768
cryoprecipitate 836
cryopreservation, bone marrow/peripheral
    blood stem cells 834
cryotherapy see cold therapy
cryptosporidiosis 107–8
Cryptosporidium 88, 107
CSF see cerebrospinal fluid
CSU (catheter specimen of urine) 390–1, 391
cues, non-verbal 31, 32
cuff, sphygmomanometer 508, 511
cultural issues
  communication 35
  last offices 445, 452–6
  personal hygiene 661, 663
Cushing reflex 552
cushions, pressure-relieving 960, 961
cutaneous T-cell lymphoma 275
cutlery see crockery/cutlery
CVAD see central venous access devices
CVCs see central venous catheters
CVP see central venous pressure
CVVHDF see continuous venovenous
    haemodiafiltration
cyanosis 517
cyclizine 214
cyclophosphamide, scalp cooling 768,
    769
cycloplegics 634
cylinders
  Entonox 579, 579
  oxygen 753, 755
cytarabine (cytosine arabinoside) 275, 277
cytology
  cervical see cervical smear
  CSF 462
cytomegalovirus (CMV) 119–20
  congenital infection 119–20
  prevention 120
  transfusion-related infection 841
cytosine arabinoside (cytarabine) 275, 277
cytotoxic drugs 255–87
  administration 262–87
    body surface area calculation 262
    information provision 262
    patient consent 262
    patient fitness for 262
    routes 262–87
  classification 255
  defined 255

environmental protection 255–6, 261
  procedure guidelines 257–60
extravasation see extravasation
eye toxicity 635
hair loss 663
handling 255–7
  procedure guidelines 257–61
  protective clothing 256, 256–7
  risk assessment 257
  staff health surveillance 257, 257
intra-arterial administration 285–7
  methods 286
  problem solving 287
intramuscular injections 275
intraperitoneal administration 44, 283–5
  indications 45, 283
  problem solving 285
  procedure guidelines 284–5
  see also abdominal paracentesis
intrapleural administration 278–80
  problem solving 280
  procedure guidelines 279–80
intrathecal administration 276–8, 277, 462
intravenous administration 262–5
  choosing device 262–3, 263
  extravasation see extravasation
  indications 262
  methods 263–4
  prevention of extravasation 266–8
  procedure guidelines 264–5
intravesical instillation 280–3
  problem solving 282–3
  procedure guidelines 281–2
occupational hazards 255
oral administration 274–5, 276
oral damage 648, 649, 649, 654
routes of administration 262
scalp cooling to prevent alopecia see scalp
    cooling
skin complications 662
spillages 259–60, 261
subcutaneous injections 275
topical application 275–6
vesicant 268
  see also vesicant drugs
waste disposal 260
Cytotoxic Health Questionnaire 257, 260
Cytotoxic Health Surveillance Programme
  257

dacarbazine 268
dactinomycin 268
Dansac washers 369
danthron 335
daunorubicin 268
dead space, anatomical 516
deaf patients, communication with 38
death
  AIDS/HIV infection 99
  confirmation 446
  hepatitis B 112, 116
  last offices 445–56
  radioactive patients 451, 703–4, 732
debridement, wound 947–8
debriefing, after violent incidents 937
decannulation plug, tracheostomy 814, 814
decision making 20–2
decubitus ulcers see pressure ulcers
deep vein thrombosis (DVT)
  compression therapy and 170, 176
  postoperative care 626
  prophylaxis see thromboprophylaxis
  signs 610
  see also venous thromboembolism
defecation 328
  advice for patients 333

assisting, procedure guidelines 325–7
  digital stimulation 342
defibrillation 158, 161, 165
  placement of paddles/electrodes 161
  safe practice 161
defibrillators 162
dehydration
  blood glucose testing 536
  during CPAP 763
  in diarrhoea 329
  dysphagia and 492
  infusion-related 294, 295
  peritoneal dialysis 744
  venepuncture in 922
delegation, effective 989
delta (hepatitis D) virus 109, 118
deltoid muscle injections 215, 215
dendritic cell collection 418
denial 36–7
dental crowns/bridges 612
dentures 655, 656
  surgical patients 612
  unsealed radioactive source therapy 726, 728
deodorizers
  fungating wounds 963–4
  stoma 368, 370
depression 35–6
  infected patients in isolation 78
  urinary diversion and 354–5
Dermagraft 954
dermatomes 587, 587
dermis 662
detergent
  bactericidal 54, 63–4, 72
  see also soap
dexamethasone, subcutaneous infusions 214
Dexrazoxane 270
diabetes mellitus 533–4
  blood glucose monitoring 535–7
  consequences of hyperglycaemia 534–5, 535
  foot care 664
  odour of urine 531
diabetic ketoacidosis 519, 534–5, 535
diagnosis, nursing 20–2
  concept 21, 21
  example 21
  process 20
dialysis 736
  blood glucose testing 536
  see also peritoneal dialysis
diamorphine
  acute/postoperative pain 564, 565
  chronic pain 570
  epidural/intrathecal 587–8
  nasal spray 570
  safer practice guidance 204
diarrhoea 328–31
  assessment 329
  causes 328–9
  Clostridium difficile 106
  cryptosporidiosis 107
  defined 325
  enterally fed patients 476
  intracavitary brachytherapy and 705
  management 329–31
  specimen collection 777, 785
  stoma patients 329, 365
  unsealed radioactive source administration
    and 725
  vancomycin-resistant enterococci 104
diastolic blood pressure 506
  measurement 509, 511–12
diathermy 613–14
diazepam 269
diclofenac 565
dicrotic notch 904

diet
  constipation management 333
  in dysphagia 493
  history 468
  immunocompromised patients 87, 89
  modification 468, 471, **473**
  stoma patients 366–7
  see also food; nutrition
dietary reference values 470–1
dietary supplements 471
  indications 468
diffusion 737, *737*, 751
digital rectal examination (DRE) 333, 340–2
  precautions 340
  procedure guidelines 341–2
digital (rectal) stimulation, spinal cord injury
    342
digital veins, hand 862, *920*
dignity, respect for 4–5
digoxin 635
dihydrocodeine 568
dimethylsulfoxide (DMSO) 270, 273
2, 3-diphosphoglycerate (2,3-DPG) 752
dipstick (reagent) tests, urine 531–2, **532**, *533*
discharge
  to a care home 195
  complex 193, **194–5**
  delay monitoring form *190*
  delays 189, **193**, 196
  gene therapy 410
  hepatitis B 115–16
  HIV infection 97–8
  intermediate care 193–5
  against medical advice 189, **189**
  neutropenic patient 90
  NHS Continuing Healthcare 196
  nurse-led 193
  patients with particular care needs **188**
  postanaesthetic recovery 618, *619*
  protective isolation 88, 90
  radioactive patients 701, 725
  source isolation 83
  urgent, for palliative care at home 189, *191–2*
  with vascular access device in situ 876–7
Discharge Coordinators **189**, 189–93, **194–5**,
    197
discharge planning 188–200
  aims 188
  communication and 189–93, **193**
  complex cases 193, **194–5**
  defined 188
  epidural/intrathecal analgesia 592, 597–8
  principles 188
  procedure guidelines 196–200
  process 188–9
  role of informal carers 189
  single assessment process 193
  spinal cord compression **800**, 805
  stoma patients 366–7
dishwashing
  HIV-positive patients 98
  source barrier nursing 78, 80
  see also crockery/cutlery
disinfection
  non-disposable equipment 95–6
  spillages 98
disseminated intravascular coagulation (DIC)
    833, 838
district nurses
  care of indwelling VADs 876, 877
  discharge planning **194–5**, 198
  see also community nurses
diuretics 45
DNA (deoxyribonucleic acid) 401
do not attempt resuscitation (DNAR) 162–3
Dobbie applicators 697, 698

docetaxel, scalp cooling 767, 768, 769
doctors
  discharge against advice **189**
  white coats 76
documentation
  blood transfusion 846
  consent 5–7
  controlled drugs **205**
  CPR decisions 162–3
  extravasation incidents 272, 273–4
  NMC code 990
  nursing care **23**, 25
  refusals 31
  specimen collection 776
  subcutaneous infusions 306
  violent incidents 937
docusate sodium (dioctyl sodium
    sulphosuccinate)
  enema 335
  laxative 334
domestic staff
  barrier nursing 78–9, 82
  gene therapy 408–9
  HIV infection 96–7
  radiation protection 704
  see also cleaning
l-dopa **532**
dorsal venous network of hand 862
dorsalis pedis cannulation 903
dorsogluteal intramuscular injections *215*, 216
douching, after intracavitary brachytherapy 701
doxorubicin
  administration 278, 280, 286
  extravasation 267, 268, 270
  scalp cooling 767, 768, 769
2, 3-DPG (2,3-diphosphoglycerate) 752
drainage
  intraperitoneal 46–8
  intrapleural *see* intrapleural drainage
  seroma **152**, *152–3*
  vacuum, changing, procedure guidelines 976
  see also urine drainage bags
drains *see* wound drains
dressing trolley 55
dressings
  barrier-nursed patients 81
  changing
    acute and surgical wounds 970–1
    aseptic technique 55
    CVC insertion site 887–8
    epidural/intrathecal exit site 596
    total laryngectomy 818
    tracheostomy 817, 822
  chest drain insertion site 433
  peripheral cannulae 864
  short-term non-tunnelled CVCs 872
  skin-tunnelled CVCs 873–4, 899
  VADs 857, 876–7
  see also wound dressings
drinks
  assisting patients 481
  disguising medication in 209–10
driving, opioids and 571
droplet transmission 72–3
  extra precautions 75
  tuberculosis 126–7
drops per minute, calculation 297
drug administration 203–4, 208–50
  covert 209–10
  cytotoxic drugs 255–87
  defined 203
  errors 208–9
  indications 203
  legal and professional context 203–4
  in parenteral nutrition solutions 477
  procedure guidelines 220–50

  self- 209, 220–1
  single nurse 209
  verbal orders 208
  via enteral feeding tubes 489–90
  via infusion devices 291–308
drug intoxication, cardiopulmonary arrest 160
drug users, injecting *see* injecting drug users
drugs *see* medicines
dry lips 652, 657
dry mouth 648–9
  during respiratory therapy 762, 764
  treatment 652, 656
dry skin 662
drying
  hand 54, 63
  skin 662
dual diagnosis 935
dura mater 586, *587*
dural puncture, inadvertent 590, 601
Durogesic *see* fentanyl
Duthie Report (1988) 204
DVT *see* deep vein thrombosis
dying, care of *see* terminal care
dysphagia
  dietary advice **473**
  problem solving 491–3
  see also swallowing difficulties
dysphasia 547
dyspnoea 518
  complicating VAD insertion 900
  exertional 518
  paroxysmal nocturnal 518
dysuria, catheterized patients 395

ear care 664
ear drops, administration guidelines 234–5
ear swabs 781, *781*
eating
  assisted, procedure guidelines 481
  difficulties 491–3
ECG *see* electrocardiogram
eczema, nursing staff precautions 94
Einthoven's triangle *504*
elastic compression garments *see* compression
    garments, elastic
elastic compression stockings, graduated *see*
    antiembolic stockings
elastomeric balloons, infusion devices 300
elderly
  blood pressure measurement 509, 510
  discharge planning 193–5
  hypothermia 525
  pressure ulcers 955
  skin changes 662
  thermoregulation 524
  venepuncture 922
electric hand dryers 54
electrocardiogram (ECG) 499–500
  12-lead 502–3, *504*
  cardiopulmonary resuscitation 165, 166
  examples *500*
  procedure guidelines 502–3
  tracings 502, *502*
electro-larynx device 816
electrolytes
  monitoring, during parenteral nutrition **478**
  parenteral nutrition solutions 477
  postoperative management 626–7
  unconscious patients 851
electronic records 25
elemental feeds 475
elixirs 207
embolism
  arterial cannulation-associated 903–4, **904**,
    913
  intravenous procedure-related 249

see also air embolism; pulmonary embolism; venous thromboembolism
embolus *see* embolism
EMLA cream 863
emollients 662
empathy 34
emphysema 513, 515
peak flow measurements 521
Employment Rights Act 1996 934
empyema 430
endocervical brush 780, *780*, 791
end-of-life care *see* terminal care
endometrial cancer (cancer of body of uterus), brachytherapy 697, 697–8
endotracheal intubation, cardiopulmonary resuscitation 158, 165
endotracheal tube, drug administration via 160
end-stage renal failure (ESRF) 736
enemas 207, 335–8
contraindications 335
evacuant 335
indications 335
problem solving 338
procedure guidelines 336–7
retention 336
energy
requirements 470, **470**
supplements 471
enteral feeding tubes 472–4
blocked **476**
drug administration via 489–90
unblocking 490–1
see also gastrostomy tubes; nasogastric tubes
enteral tube feeding 472–5
complications 475, **476**
equipment 474, **474**
feeds 474–5
home 475
indications 468
monitoring 475
nasal care 664
procedure guidelines 482–91
termination 475
unconscious patients 850–1
enteric coated tablets 206, 223
enterococci 77, 103
see also vancomycin-resistant enterococci
Enterococcus faecalis 103
Enterococcus faecium 77, 103
Entonox (nitrous oxide and oxygen) 565, 578–83
cautions 579
complications 581
contraindications 578
duration and frequency of use 580
equipment 579, *579*, *580*
indications 578
mode of action 578
patient assessment for 579
in pregnancy and lactation 581
prescribing 580–1
principle of administration 579–80
problem solving 582–3
procedure guidelines 581–2
removal of brachytherapy applicators 707, 710
staff training 581
Envair Mino-Iso isolator 257–8, *261*
environment (health care)
cleaning *see* cleaning, environmental
cleanliness 56, 72
Clostridium difficile reservoirs 106
enterococcal survival 77, 104
MRSA contamination 102
prevention of violence 936

protection, cytotoxic drugs 255–6, 257–60, *261*
protective isolation 86
as reservoir of infection 72
eosinophils *413*, **414**
epidermal growth factor (EGF) **944**, 954
epidermis 662
epidural abscess 590, 602
epidural analgesia 586–603
acute pain 564
advantages 586
bolus injections 589, 597
checking height of block 590
complications 590, 601–2
continuous infusion 588
contraindications 586
defined 586
drug-related side-effects 589, 599–601
drugs used 587–8
indications 586
intractable chronic and cancer pain 571, 591–9
catheter insertion 593–4
catheter removal 599
discharge planning 592, 597–8
exit site dressing change 596
minimizing infection 592
post-insertion management 592, 595
preinsertion management 592
problem solving 599–603
procedure guidelines 592–9
setting up ambulatory pump 594
top up (bolus) 597
troubleshooting 602–3
monitoring 589, 595
pain assessment 589–90, 595
patient controlled (PCEA) 589
problem solving 601–3
pumps 299
safety checks 590, **591**
epidural catheter
disconnection 602–3
insertion, procedure guidelines 593–4
migration 590, 601, 602
occlusion 602
optimal position 588, **588**
removal, procedure guidelines 599
tunnelling 592
epidural haematoma 590, 602
epidural space 586–7
epileptic seizures 555
epinephrine *see* adrenaline
epirubicin
administration 267, 268, 280
scalp cooling 767, 768, 769
Epstein–Barr virus (EBV) 120–1
equipment
cleaning and disinfection 95–6
as reservoirs of infection 72
spread of infection via 55, 72
errors
blood pressure measurement 508, 509
infusion-related 291–2, 301
intrathecal chemotherapy 277
medication 208–9
transfusion 834, 837, 838, *838*
tympanic temperature measurement 528
see also incidents; spillages
erythema
extravasation **268**, 269
intravenous infusion site 246
staff handling cytotoxic drugs 261
erythrocytes *see* red blood cells
erythropoietin (EPO) 414, 426
Escherichia coli, antibiotic resistant 100–1
Essence of Care benchmarks 77, 471, 648, 661

essential oils 954, 963
ethambutol 635
ethical issues
cardiopulmonary resuscitation 162
HIV infection 92
unconscious patients 851
ethnic minorities, blind or partially sighted 38
ethylene oxide disinfection 96
Eton scale 331
etoposide 263, 264
eugenics 401
European Association of Palliative Care (EAPC) 563
European Medicines Evaluation Agency (EMEA) 203
European Pressure Ulcer Advisory Panel (EPUAP) 955–6
European Society of Hypertension 508
European Union (EU)
CE mark *see* CE mark
Directive 92/27/EEC 204
evaluating care 23–5
evidence
grading 11–12
levels 12, **12**
sources 10–11
evidence-based practice 10–12, 990
defined 10
implementation 12
Ewing's sarcoma 796
excreta
barrier-nursed patients 81
cytotoxic drug-treated patients 260
see also faeces; urine
exercise
constipation management 333
pain management 566–7
respiration during 513, 518
expert nurse 8
expert opinion 11
expiration 514, *514*
expiratory reserve volume (ERV) 515, *515*
exposure-prone procedures (EPP)
hepatitis B and 112
hepatitis C and 118
HIV and 91
see also invasive procedures
external jugular vein 870
extravasation 246, 266–74
defined 266
documentation and follow up 272
informing patient 271
intra-arterial chemotherapy 287
kits 271, 272
management 269–71, *271*
mixed vesicant 271
prevention 266–8
procedure guidelines 272–4
at risk patients 267, **267**
signs and symptoms 267, **268**, 269
wound management 271–2
exudate, wound 948–50
assessment 951
fungating wounds **962**, 962–3
eye(s)
anatomy and physiology 630, 630–2, *632*
artificial 634, 638–9, *639*, 664
cytotoxic drug exposure 255, 261
irrigation 633–4, 643–4, *645*
opening, Glasgow coma scale 547, **547**
oxygen toxicity 636, 760
swabbing 637–8, *781*
toxic effects of systemic drugs 635–6
tumours 636–7

eye care 630–45, 664
  comatose patient 637, 645, 664, 851
  during CPAP 764
  general principles 632
  indications 630
  insensitive eye 634
  procedure guidelines 637–45
eye drops
  contact lenses and 633
  instillation 632–3, 641, 642
  storage 206
eye medications 634–5
eye ointments
  contact lenses and 633
  instillation 633, 642–3, 643
  storage 206
eye patches 636
eye protection (goggles)
  barrier nursing 76, 80
  cytotoxic drug handling 256
  operating theatre 615
eyelids
  closure, comatose patients 645
  tumours 636

face masks *see* masks
faecal continence, porridge test 351
faecal incontinence 662
faecal–oral route of infection 108, 118
faecal (stool) softeners 334, **334**
faeces (stools) 328
  assessment 329, 330, 333
  leakage, stomas 374
  manual evacuation 342–4
  produced by stomas 365
  source barrier nursing 78, 81
  specimen collection 785
fainting, during venepuncture 930
famciclovir 121–2
family
  collusive behaviour 37
  communication 29
  deceased patients 446, 447, 451
  discharge planning and 189, 198
  long-term epidural/intrathecal analgesia and 591, 598
  spinal cord compression 802
  stoma patients 366
  viewing body after removal from ward 452
  see also visitors
fasting, preoperative 606
fat
  dietary supplements 471
  emulsion, parenteral nutrition solutions 477
fatal familial insomnia 129
fatigue
  after bone marrow harvest 417, 426
  personal hygiene and 86
  positioning and 670
feeding, procedure guidelines 481
feet, care of 664
feline spongiform encephalopathy 129, 841
female patients
  intermittent self-catheterization 388–9
  midstream specimen of urine 788–9
  urinary catheterization 378, 381, 386–8
  urinary catheters 379
femoral artery
  cannula, blood sampling from 909
  cannulation 903, **903**
femoral vein
  continuous renal replacement therapy 739
  short-term CVCs 870–1
  skin-tunnelled catheters 873
fentanyl (Durogesic) 564, 569
  epidural/intrathecal 587–8

oral transmucosal 569
  transdermal patches 569, **569**
ferritin, serum **478**
fever 526
  non-haemolytic transfusion reactions 839
  transfusion reactions 837, 847
  see also pyrexia
fibre, dietary 333
fibrillation, heart 499
fibrin sheath, VAD occlusion 245, 858–9
fibrinolytic agents, occluded VADs 859, 892–3
fibroblast growth factor 2 (FGF-2) **944**, 954
fibroblasts 945
fibrosing alveolitis 515
film badges, radiation 702, 724, 724, 730
filtration 737, 737
fine needle aspiration (FNA), breast *see* breast aspiration
finger massage, abnormal scars 968
finger pricking, blood glucose monitoring 535, 537
fires
  oxygen safety 753
  radiation safety 703, 733
fistulas, catheterized patients 394
Flamazine (silver sulphadiazine) 967
flaps, surgical 965
  donor site problems 967–8
  observation chart 966–7
flare reaction 266
  vs. extravasation **268**, 269
flashback
  midline catheter insertion 883
  venepuncture 926
  venous cannulation 859, 863, 881
flatus (wind), bowel stoma patients 365, 366
Fletcher applicators 697, 698
floors, protection from radioactive contamination 725
flossing, tooth 656
flowers, protective isolation facilities 85
flowmeters 753
floxuridine (5-FUDR) 286
fluconazole 651
fluid balance
  postanaesthetic recovery 618, 619
  postoperative management 626–7
  unconscious patients 851
fluid deficit *see* dehydration
fluid intake
  after intracavitary brachytherapy 706
  after intravesical drug therapy 281, 282
  after lumbar puncture 465
  catheterized patients 395
  constipation management 333
  continent urinary diversion 353, 354, 355
  daily requirements 470, **470**
  unsealed radioactive source therapy 728
  urostomy 367
fluid overload *see* circulatory overload
fluids
  dying patients 214
  in hypovolaemia 159
  intravenous, safe administration 217–18
  subcutaneous infusion 213–14
  see also infusion fluids
fluoride 651, 652
5-fluorouracil (5-FU)
  administration 264, 275, 283, 286
  prevention of oral complications 653
  skin complications 662
  toxic effects on eye 635
flushing
  after i.v. drug administration 219, 240, 243, 265
  CVADs 888, 890

enteral feeding tubes 489, 490, 491
  implantable ports 876, 894–5
  to maintain VAD patency 858
  midline catheters 865, 883
  negative pressure technique 892, 893
  occluded VADs 245, 892
  peripheral cannulae 880, 881
  PICCs 868
  positive pressure technique 858
  pulsatile (push pause) technique 858
  short-term non-tunnelled CVCs 872
  urinary diversion drainage catheters 352–3, 357–8
foam wound dressings **949**
foamsticks 650, 655, 657
folate, serum **478**
Foley (balloon) catheters 378, **378**, 380
  balloon deflation problems 395
  balloon size 378–9
  suprapubic catheterization 383
  see also urinary catheterization
food
  benchmarks 471, **472**
  charts 468
  disguising medication in 209–10
  oral drug administration and 222–3
  stoma patients 366
  see also diet; meals; nutrition
food-borne infections 73
  cryptosporidiosis 107
  hepatitis A 108–9
  hepatitis E 118
  listeriosis 124–5
  vancomycin-resistant enterococci 104
food hygiene 73, **73**
  immunocompromised patients 87, 89
  listeriosis prevention 125
food poisoning 73
foot care 664
footwear
  barrier nursing 76
  operating theatre staff 615
  protective 56
  radiation protection 727, 729
forceps 54, 55
forearm
  blood pressure measurement 509–10
  veins for venepuncture 920, 920–1
foscarnet 122
fractures
  complicating bone marrow aspiration/biopsy 416
  pathological, positioning and 670
fresh frozen plasma (FFP) **836**
FreshAire 370
friction 955
5-FU *see* 5-fluorouracil
full blood count **478**
fully weight bearing (FWB) 676–7
Functional Health Patterns, Gordon's 17, **17**, 19
functional mobility, spinal cord compression **797**
functional residual capacity (FRC) 515, 516, 756
funeral arrangements, AIDS patients 99
funeral directors 451
fungal infections
  aspergillosis 104–5
  feet 664
  oral 651
  pneumocystosis 125–6
  specimen collection 777, 778
  voice prostheses 821–2
fungating wounds 960–4
  aetiology 960–1
  assessment 961

defined 960
management **962**, 962–4
securing dressings 964
symptoms 961–2
fusidic acid, topical **947**

gag reflex 551, 555
gamma rays 694
ganciclovir 120, 122, 269
gargles 233, 652
gas and air *see* Entonox
gaseous exchange 516, *516*, *517*, *751*, 751–2
gastric contents
    aspiration *see* aspiration of gastric contents
    pH, enterally-fed patients 473, 483, 486
gastric distension, during CPAP 756, 764
gastrointestinal bleeding, radionuclide imaging **721**
gastrointestinal function, unconscious patients 850–1
gastrostomy 473–4
gastrostomy tubes 473–4
    percutaneous endoscopically placed (PEG) 473, 474
        procedure guidelines 486–7
    radiologically inserted (RIG) 473, 474
        procedure guidelines 488
GCS *see* Glasgow Coma Scale
Gelclair 652
Gel-X capsules 370
gene therapy 401–10
    administration 407–8
    consent 405
    defined 401
    ex vivo 401
    future options 405
    in vivo 401
    nursing care 404–5
    procedure guidelines 405–10
    regulatory controls 402–4, **403**
    risk assessment 403–4
    specimens 404, 406, 776
    standard operating procedures 404
Gene Therapy Advisory Committee (GTAC) 402, 405
general anaesthesia *see* anaesthesia
general sales list (GSL) medicines 203
genetic modification 401
Genetic Modification Safety Committee 403, 404
genetically modified micro-organisms (GMM) 402, 403
    classification 403, **403**
Genetically Modified Organisms (Contained Use) Regulations 402–4
Genetically Modified Organisms (Deliberate Release and Risk Assessment – Amendment) Regulations 402
genital herpes 121
genitourinary function, unconscious patients 851
genome 401
gentamicin 779
Gerstmann–Straussler–Scheinker syndrome 129
gingivitis 470
gingivostomatitis, herpetic 121
Glasgow Coma Scale (GCS) 166, 546–9, 850
    form *548*
    procedure guidelines 553
    scoring **547**
glaucoma 631
glomerular filtration 530, *530*
glomerular filtration rate (GFR) 531, **721**
gloves 56
    barrier nursing 76–7, 80
    clean non-sterile (examination)

indications for use 56, 58, 77
    procedure guidelines 64–5, 66
cytotoxic drug handling 256
    disposal of used 65
    materials 56
    operating theatre staff 615
    sterile
        aseptic technique 54–5, 61
        indications for use 56, 58, 77
        venepuncture 923
gloving, double 77, 256, 615
glucagon 533
glucose
    50% solution 269
    blood 533–7
        indications for measuring 533
        monitoring 535–7
        parenteral nutrition **478**
        procedure guidelines 536–7
        see also hyperglycaemia; hypoglycaemia
    parenteral nutrition solutions 477
    peritoneal dialysis solutions 737
    in urine 534
glucose polymers
    dietary supplements 471
    enteral feeds 475
glutamine 475
gluteus muscle injections *215*, 216
glycerine-based hydrogel sheet 968
glycerol (glycerin) suppositories 334, 339
glyceryl trinitrate, to improve venous access 922
glycopeptide-resistant enterococci (GRE) *see* vancomycin-resistant enterococci
goggles *see* eye protection
goitre 470
gold-198 696
Gordon's Functional Health Patterns 17, **17**, **19**
gowns
    aseptic technique 56, 58
    barrier nursing 76, 80, 81
    cytotoxic drug handling 256
    operating theatre staff 615
graduated elastic compression stockings *see* antiembolic stockings
Graftskin 954
graft-versus-host disease (GVHD) 85
    transfusion-associated (TA-GVHD) 840
Gram-negative bacteria, antibiotic resistant 100–1
Gram-positive bacteria, antibiotic resistant 101–4
granulation tissue 945
granulocyte colony-stimulating factor (G-CSF) 414, 652, 721
granulocyte macrophage colony-stimulating factor (GM-CSF) 270, 652
granulocytes 414
    apheresed **835**
    collection (apheresis) **418**
gravity drip rate controllers 298
gravity flow infusions 296–8
gray (Gy) 692
Gröningen type voice prosthesis 821
Groshong catheter 873, *873*
group protocols 210
    see also patient group directions
growth factors
    abnormal scarring 968
    haematopoietic 413–14
    oral mucositis 652
    wound healing **944**, 945, 954
gynaecological cancer
    brachytherapy 694, *695*, 695–8
        applicators 697, 697–8
        complications 700
        discharge from hospital 701

follow-up care 701
    patient preparation 700–1
    problem solving 708, 710
    procedure guidelines 705–10
    remote afterloading systems 698–700, *699*
    removal of caesium and iridium wires 706–7
    removal of Selectron applicators 709–10
    vaginal care after 701
    see also Selectron
lymphoedema 170

haematocrit, blood glucose testing and 536
haematological malignancies
    bone marrow harvest 416
    infection risks 84–5
    levels of care 85
    oral complications 654
    see also leukaemia; lymphoma
haematological procedures 413–26
haematoma
    after venepuncture 929
    epidural 590, 602
    spinal cord compression 796
haematopoiesis 413
haematopoietic stem cell transplantation *see* stem cell transplantation
haematuria
    after intravesical drug instillation 282
    bladder irrigation 319
haemodialysis 736
haemodilution, acute normovolaemic (ANH) 833
haemoglobin
    concentration 470
    oxygen transport 516, *517*, *752*, 752
haemolytic disease of the newborn (HDN) 834
haemolytic transfusion reactions
    acute 838
    delayed 840
haemopneumothorax 430
haemorrhage *see* bleeding/haemorrhage
haemostasis 943–4
haemostatic swabs, bleeding wounds 964
haemothorax 430
    complicating VAD insertion 900
    drainage 431, 432
haemovigilance 832
hair care 663–4, 770
hair loss *see* alopecia
hair removal
    preoperative 606
    prior to VAD insertion 862
hairdryers 663
halitosis 649
Hammersmith hedgehog *see* interstitial perineal template
hand(s)
    assessing arterial blood supply 902, *903*, 905
    Clostridium difficile spread 107
    cuts and abrasions 62
    drying 54, 63
    MRSA transmission 102
    radioactive contamination 732
    spread of infection 53, 72
    veins for venepuncture *920*, 920–1
hand washing 53–4, 72
    after glove removal 65, 77
    areas frequently missed 53, *53*–4
    barrier nursing 79, 87
    compliance with 54, 72
    cryptosporidiosis control 108
    equipment and facilities 61
    methods 54
    MRSA control 102
    operating theatre 64, 615

hand washing (*cont.*)
  by patients 77
  procedure guidelines 61–4
  surgical procedures 64
handling, manual *see* manual handling
handover 25
handrubs, alcoholic *see* alcoholic handrubs
Hazard Analysis Critical Control Points
    (HACCP) 73, 125
Hazardous Waste (England and Wales)
    Regulations 2005 78
HCAI *see* health care-acquired infections
head and neck tumours
  enteral tube feeding 473, 474
  interstitial brachytherapy 694–5, *695*
  swallowing difficulties 491
  see also oral cancer
head coverings
  barrier nursing 76
  operating theatre staff 615
head injury
  conscious level assessment 546
  neurological observations 552
head lice 663
head tilt/chin lift manoeuvre 156, *157*, 158
headache
  after inadvertent dural puncture 601
  post-lumbar puncture 462, 464, 465
  scalp cooling 772
healing, wound *see* wound healing
health and safety, occupational
  Creutzfeldt–Jakob disease 129
  cytomegalovirus infection 120
  cytotoxic drug handling 255–7
  cytotoxic drug spillages/accidents 260, 261
  diathermy smoke 614
  gene therapy 402, 403, 408
  hepatitis B 112
  hepatitis C 118
  HIV infection 91–2, 93
  intravenous drug administration 218
  MRSA 102
  radiation protection 692–3, 702–4
  tuberculosis 128
  venepuncture 923
  see also inoculation accidents; personal
    protective equipment; violence
Health and Safety at Work, etc. Act 1974 93,
    933
Health and Safety Executive (HSE)
  Advisory Committee on Genetic Modification
    (ACGM) Compendium of Guidance 402,
    403, **403**
  cytotoxic drug handling 257
  gene therapy 402, 403
  patient group directions 210, *211*
  radiation protection 717, 723
The Health and Safety (Consultation with
    Employees) Regulations 1996 934
health care assistants 9, 661
health care-acquired infections (HCAI) 51–3,
    71–3
  consequences to patients 52, 71
  costs 52, 71
  defined 51
  diagnosis 52
  prevention *see* barrier nursing; infection
    control
  reservoirs 72
  risk assessment 71, 84
  risk factors 52, 53, 71, 84–5
  routes of spread 72–3
  sites involved 71
  sources 72
Health Protection Agency (HPA) 91, 692, 723
hearing, testing 555

hearing aids 38, 612
hearing-impaired patients, communication with
    38
heart 497
  apical beat assessment 500
  conduction system *499*
  rhythm 499
heart rate 497–8
  factors affecting 498, *498*
  see also pulse
heat and moisture exchanger (HME) 758, *758*,
    759, 815–16
heat therapy
  extravasation 270, 273
  to improve venous access 922, 925
  pain management 567–8
heel supports, during surgery 607
hemiparesis/hemiplegia
  prevention of shoulder pain 685
  spinal cord compression 797
heparin 599
  continuous venovenous haemodiafiltration
    745
  'lock' 858
  maintaining VAD patency 858, 876
  occluded VADs 892
  peritoneal dialysis fluid 741
  spinal cord compression 801
hepatitis 108–19
  chemical, intra-arterial
    chemotherapy-induced 287
  non-A non-B (NANB) 116–17
  viruses **109**
hepatitis A 108–10, **109**
  procedure guidelines 110
  vaccine 109
hepatitis B **109**, 111–16
  death 112, 116
  prevention of spread 112–13
  procedure guidelines 113–16
  screening 111–12
  transfusion-related 841
  transmission 111, 112
  vaccine 112
hepatitis B e antigen (HBeAg) 111, 112
hepatitis B immunoglobulin (HBIg) 112
hepatitis B surface antigen (HBsAg)
    111–12
hepatitis B virus (HBV) 111, 118
  genotype F **109**, 119
hepatitis C **109**, 117–18
  transfusion-related 841
hepatitis D **109**, 118
hepatitis E **109**, 118–19
hepatitis G **109**, 119
herpes
  genital 121
  oral 121, 651
herpes simplex virus (HSV) 121–2
  type 1 (HSV 1) 121
  type 2 (HSV 2) 121
herpes zoster (shingles) 122, 123
herpesviruses 119–23
herpetic whitlow 121
Hickman lines *see* skin-tunnelled catheters
highly active antiretroviral therapy (HAART)
    90, 92
Hinduism
  last offices 453
  washing and personal hygiene 663
Hirudoid cream 924
histamine 944
HIV *see* human immunodeficiency virus
home
  enteral feeding 475
  indwelling VADs 876–7

oxygen therapy *see under* oxygen therapy
parenteral nutrition 479
homosexual men 112
honey **949**, 963
hormonal therapy
  fungating wounds 964
  spinal cord compression 799
Hospital Chaplaincies Council 453
hospital-acquired infections *see* health
  care-acquired infections
hot packs, for extravasation 270, 273
human immunodeficiency virus (HIV) 90
  antenatal screening 92
  antibody tests 91, 92
  confidentiality 92
  drug resistance 92
  infection 90–9
    atypical mycobacterial infections 126
    clinical presentation 92
    confidentiality 92
    cytomegalovirus infection 120
    diagnosis 91
    increased-risk patients 94
    low-risk patients 94
    nursing care 93–6
    nutritional assessment 469
    prevention of further infections 99
    procedure guidelines 93–9
    psychological support 92–3, 97
    treatment 92
    tuberculosis co-infection 127, 128
    women and children 92
    see also acquired immune deficiency
      syndrome
  infection control 93
  mother-to-child transmission 92
  occupational hazards 91–2
  p24 antigen test 91
  post-exposure prophylaxis 92, 94
  transmission 91–2, 841
  type 2 (HIV 2) 93
  vaccine 92
human leucocyte antigens (HLA) 834
human normal immunoglobulin (HNIg) 109
Human Rights Act 1998 162
human T-leukaemia/lymphoma virus type 1
    (HTLV-1) 841
Humanism, last offices 453
humidification 757–8
  devices 758, *758*, *759*
  procedure guidelines 761–2
  tracheostomy/laryngectomy patients 815–16,
    824–5
humidifiers
  cold water 758, *758*, *759*
  water bath 758, *758*, *759*
humidity 757
humour, using 566
Hyalofill 954
hyaluronidase
  extravasation injuries 270, 272
  subcutaneous fluid infusions 214
hydration
  in dysphagia 492
  terminally ill patients 214
  see also fluid intake
hydrocolloid wound dressings **950**, **962**
hydrocortisone 163
  cream, for extravasation 272, 273
hydrofibre wound dressings **950**, **962**
Hydroframe 370
hydrogel wound dressings **950**, **951**, **962**, 963
hydrogel-coated catheters 380–1
hydrogen peroxide **947**
hydromorphone 569
hydrothorax 900

hygiene
  bed bathing *see* bed bathing
  food *see* food hygiene
  hospital 56
  personal *see* personal hygiene
  see also cleaning
hyperbaric oxygen therapy 951
hyperbaric respiratory therapy 757
hypercalcaemia, spinal cord compression 801
hypercapnia 750, 758–60
hyperglycaemia 534–5, *535*
  parenteral nutrition 478
hyperkalaemia 160, 840
hyperlipidaemia, blood glucose testing and 536
hyperpyrexia **526**
  malignant 625
hypertension 506
  blood pressure measurement 510
  postoperative 623–4
hyperthermia 526, **526**
  postoperative 624–5
hyperthyroidism 528
  see also thyrotoxicosis
hypertonic fluid contraction 294, **295**
hypertonic solutions 269
hypertrophic scars 968–9
hyperventilation 519
  central neurogenic **551**
hypodermoclysis 213–14
hypoglycaemia 478, 534
hypokalaemia 160
hypophosphataemia 478
hypotension 506
  ascitic fluid drainage causing 45, 48
  blood pressure measurement 510
  complicating arterial cannulation 913
  epidural/intrathecal analgesia 589, 600
  orthostatic 506
  postoperative 623
hypothalamus, thermoregulation 524, *525*, 526
hypothermia 524–5
  cardiopulmonary arrest 160
  postoperative 622, 624
  scalp *see* scalp cooling
  transfusion-associated 839
hypothyroidism 528
hypotonic fluid contraction 294, **295**
hypoventilation, postoperative 623
hypovolaemia
  arterial pressure monitoring 904
  cardiopulmonary arrest 159
  complicating arterial cannulation 903, 912
hypoxaemia 750
hypoxia 517, 750, 752
  cardiopulmonary arrest 156
  tracheal suctioning-related 818–19
  wound healing and 945, 951
hypoxic drive 513, 760

ibuprofen 565
ice
  Cryptosporidium spread 107
  immunocompromised patients 87
  scalp cooling 768
  therapy *see* cold therapy
idarubicin 268
identification, patient 9
  blood transfusions 834, 843, 844, 845
  dead body 449
  radioactive procedures 731
  surgery 612, 616
ifosfamide 275
ileal–anal pouch 362
ileal conduits 362–3
  postoperative function 365
  psychological effects 354–5

urine specimen collection 372–3, 375
  see also urinary diversion; urostomy
ileal loops 362–3
ileostomy 362, *362*
  indications 363
  postoperative care 365–6
  postoperative function 365
  pouches 368, *368*
  problem solving 374–5
  see also stoma(s)
imaging, radionuclide 717, 718, **719–21**
immobility
  bed rest 670
  dependency oedema 170
  unconscious patients 850
  see also mobility
immunoadsorption **418**
immunocompromised patients 83–5
  aspergillosis 104–5
  blood cultures 778
  cryptosporidiosis 107, 108
  cytomegalovirus infection 119, 120
  diagnosis of infections 86–7
  diet 87, 89
  discharge home 88, 90
  Epstein–Barr virus reactivation 121
  herpes simplex virus (HSV) infections 121
  infection control 53, 108
  infection risks 52, 84
  intramuscular injections 216
  Legionnaires' disease 124
  listeriosis 125
  microbiological specimen collection 775
  oral complications 649
  Pneumocystis carinii pneumonia (PCP) 125–6
  procedure guidelines 88–90
  protective isolation 85–90
  sources of infection 72
  Staphylococcus epidermidis infections 103
  temperature monitoring 528
  tuberculosis 126
  varicella zoster virus (VZV) infection 122, 123
  water supplies 87, 89, 108
  wound infections 948
immunoglobulin
  human normal (HNIg) 109
  intravenous, *Clostridium difficile* infection 106
immunosuppression
  causes 53, 84
  infection risks 83–4
  to prevent chemotherapy-induced hair loss 767
impartiality 991
implantable peritoneal ports 284
implantable ports **856**, 874–6
  care and management in situ 876
  choice of vein 876
  device information 874, 875, *875*
  indications 874
  insertion 876
  insertion/removal of non-coring needles 894–5, *895*
  maintaining patency 858
  removal 876
implantable pumps, intra-arterial chemotherapy 286
incidents (accidents)
  inoculation *see* inoculation accidents
  radioactive contamination 693, 703–4, 731–2
  transfusion reactions and events 832
  violent *see* violence
  see also errors; spillages
incompatibilities, drug 218, 219
incongruence 32, 33

incontinence
  HIV-positive patients 94
  radioactive patients 730, 731–2
  skin care 662
  vancomycin-resistant enterococci 104
  see also urinary incontinence
Incorrect Blood Component Transfused (IBCT) 837, 838, 840
independent prescribing 210
individuals, treating people as 988
indomethacin 635
infection control
  AIDS/HIV infection 93
  aseptic technique 51–65
  education 53
  extra precautions 75, *75*
  microbiological specimens 776
  operating theatre 615
  principles 53–7
  rationale 51–3
  standard precautions 75, *75*
  vascular access devices 856–7
  see also barrier nursing
Infection Control Standards Working Party 52
infections
  antimicrobial-resistant organisms 100–4
  arterial cannula-associated 904
  blood borne *see* blood borne infections
  blood pressure monitoring 510
  central venous access device (CVAD)-related 778
  complicating abdominal paracentesis 49
  complicating bone marrow procedures 416, 417, 425
  complicating spinal analgesia 590, 592, 603
  compression therapy and 170, 175, 176
  diagnosis in immunocompromised patients 86–7
  endogenous (self-) 72
  exogenous (cross-infection) 72
  health and safety at work *see under* health and safety, occupational
  health care (hospital)-acquired *see* health care-acquired infections
  intra-arterial chemotherapy-associated 287
  intravenous infusion-related 247
  isolation of sources *see* source isolation
  lumbar puncture site 460
  notification 78
  peritoneal dialysis-associated 742–3
  prevention in HIV-positive patients 99
  pulse monitoring 500
  radionuclide imaging **720**
  reservoirs 72–3
  routes of spread 72–3
  sources 72
  specimen collection for microbiological analysis 775
  surgical risk categories **51**
  temperature monitoring 528
  tracheal suctioning-related 819
  transfusion-transmitted 111, 117, 129–30, 832, 840–1
  VAD-associated 901
  venepuncture site 929
  wound *see* wound infections
  see also sepsis
infectious diseases 90–130
  barrier nursing *see* barrier nursing
  isolation of patients with *see* source isolation
  last offices 447, 450
  purpose-built wards 74
  see also specific diseases
infectious mononucleosis 120–1
infertility, cytotoxic drug-induced 255

infiltration 246, 248
  defined 266
inflammation, wound 948
inflammatory phase, wound healing 944–5
inflammatory reactions, pulse monitoring 500
information provision 30–1
  breaking bad news 37
  colleagues 989
  continent urinary diversion 352
  cytotoxic drug administration 262
  at discharge 199–200
  extravasation incidents 271, 274
  procedure guidelines 30–1
  source barrier nursing 78
  vesicant drug administration 268
  see also communication; patient education
infusion(s) 212–19
  complications **291**, 293–4, **295**
    groups at risk **291**
  containers, height 293
  defined 212
  epidural/intrathecal analgesics 588, **588**
    procedure guidelines 594
  parenteral 207
  process of delivery 291
  routes of administration 213–19
  see also intravenous infusions; subcutaneous
    infusions
infusion devices 291–308
  ambulatory 299–301
  battery-operated 300–1
  decision tree for selecting 297
  defined 291
  factors affecting flow rates 293
  gravity 296–8
  indications 291
  mechanical 300
  MHRA classification 294–5, **296**
  paediatric patients 294
  problem solving 307–8
  requirements 295–6
  safe use **292**, 292–3, 301
  selection criteria 292
  user errors 292, 301
  winged *see* winged infusion devices
  see also infusion pumps
infusion flow rates
  calculations 218, 297
  factors affecting 293
  slowing/stopping 244–6
infusion fluids
  addition of drugs to 218, 219
  effects on flow rate 293
  visual inspection 218
infusion pumps 298–301
  accuracy of delivery 295
  alarm systems 296, 298, 307–8
  ambulatory 299–301
  battery-operated 300–1
  MHRA categories 294–5, **296**
  occlusion response and pressure 295–6
  parenteral nutrition 477
  problem solving 307–8
  specialist 299
  syringe *see* syringe pumps
  user errors 292
  volume calculations 218
  volumetric 298
inhalation analgesia 578–83
  see also Entonox
inhalations 208
  procedure guidelines 233
inhalers 208
injecting drug users
  hepatitis A 92
  hepatitis B 111

hepatitis C 117
HIV infection 91, 92
injections 207, 212–19
  defined 212
  direct intermittent intravenous *see*
    intravenous injections, direct intermittent
  equipment 224
  multidose preparations 207, 226–8, *228*
  procedure guidelines 224–31, *228*
  routes of administration 213–19
  single-dose preparations 207, 225–6
inoculation accidents 930
  gene therapy 408
  hepatitis B transmission 111, 112
  management guidelines 94, 114
  prevention 93, 113, 218
insect-borne infections 73
insertion, skin-tunnelled catheters 873
insomnia, fatal familial 129
inspiration 513–14, *514*
inspiratory capacity (IC) *515*, 516
inspiratory reserve volume (IRV) *515*, *515*
Institute of Jainology 454
instruments, sterile 55
insulin
  blood glucose regulation 533
  continuous subcutaneous infusion 214
  deficiency 534, *535*
  intravenous infusion 534
  subcutaneous injection 213
insulin-like growth factor 1 (IGF-1) **944**
insurance, indemnity 992
integrity, personal 991
interferon 275
interferon-α 113, 117, 118, 119
intermediate care 193–5
intermittent catheterization catheters **378**
intermittent pneumatic compression 607,
  614
intermittent self-catheterization (ISC) 383
  continent urinary diversion stoma *350*
    problem solving 358–9
    teaching, procedure guidelines 355–7
    tubing types 355
  procedure guidelines 388–90
internal jugular vein 739, 870
International Association for the Study of Pain
  (IASP) 558
International Council of Nursing, definition of
  nursing 4
International Normalized Ratio (INR),
  parenteral nutrition **478**
interpersonal aspects of care 4
interpreters 35, 38
interstitial brachytherapy *see* brachytherapy,
  interstitial
interstitial perineal template (Hammersmith
  hedgehog) *695*, 695–6, 712
  procedure guidelines 712–14, *714*
interviews, assessment 18, **19**
intra-arterial drug administration 213
  accidental 903, 913
  cytotoxic drugs 285–7
intra-articular drug administration 213
intracranial pressure (ICP), raised 460, 498
  tracheal suctioning-induced 819
  vital signs 552
intradermal drug administration 213
intramuscular injections 215–17
  cytotoxic drugs 275
  needles 216
  opioid analgesics 565
  pain 216–17
  procedure guidelines 230–1
  sites *215*, 215–16
  skin preparation 216

technique 216
  Z-track technique 216, 275
intraoperative care 613–17
  diathermy 613–14
  infection control and asepsis 615
  laparoscopic surgery 615
  patient positioning 614–15
  procedure guidelines 616–17
  see also operating theatre
intra-operative cell salvage (ICS) 833
intraperitoneal chemotherapy 44, 283–5
  indications 45, 283
  problem solving 285
  procedure guidelines 284–5
  see also abdominal paracentesis
intraperitoneal drain
  insertion 46–7
  removal 47–8
  see also abdominal paracentesis
intrapleural drainage 429–42
  changing bottle 438
  definitions 429
  indications 429, 430–1
  maintenance 432–3, 436–7
  pain control 433
  problem solving 441–2
  procedure guidelines 434–40
  suction 433, 436
  systems 431–2, *432*
intrapleural drains (chest drains) 429, *429*
  clamping 431
  dressings for insertion site 433
  insertion procedure 434–6
  insertion site 431
  removal 433–4, 439–40
  securing 431
  size 431
  stripping/milking 431, 437
intrapleural drug instillation 278–80
  indications 278
  problem solving 280
  procedure guidelines 279–80
intrapleural pressure 430
intrathecal analgesia 571, 586–603
  advantages 586
  bolus injections 589
  complications 590, 601–2
  continuous infusion 588, **588**
  contraindications 586
  defined 586
  drug-related side-effects 589, 599–601
  drugs used 587–8
  indications 586
  intractable chronic and cancer pain 591–8
    catheter insertion 593–4
    changing exit site dressing 596
    discharge planning 592, 597–8
    drugs and doses 591–2
    minimizing infection 592
    post-insertion monitoring 592, 595
    preinsertion management 592
    procedure guidelines 592–8
    setting up infusion 594
    troubleshooting 602–3
  monitoring 589, 595
  pain assessment 589–90, 595
  problem solving 599–603
intrathecal catheter
  disconnection 602–3
  insertion, procedure guidelines 593–4
  migration 590, 602
  occlusion 602
  optimal position 588, **588**
intrathecal drug administration 213
  cytotoxic drugs 276–8, **277**, 462
  lumbar puncture 460

intrathecal (subarachnoid) space 460, *461*, 586–7, *587*
intravenous access *see* venous access
intravenous administration sets 217–18
  changing 217–18
  intermittent infusions 219
intravenous bolus injections 219
  cytotoxic drugs 263–4
  procedure guidelines 241–4
  vesicant drugs 267
intravenous drug administration 212, 217–19
  acute/postoperative pain 564, 565
  asepsis/prevention of infection 217–18
  calculations 218
  in chronic pain 563
  comfort 218
  cytotoxic drugs *see under* cytotoxic drugs
  drug compatibilities 218, 219
  methods 218–19
  patient comfort 218
  principles 217–18
  pros and cons 217
  safety 218, 903
intravenous fluids, safe administration 217–18
intravenous infusions
  blood pressure monitoring 510
  continuous 218–19
    to keep vein open (KVO) 858
    parenteral nutrition 477
    procedure guidelines 235–7
  cytotoxic drug administration 264
  drug calculations 218
  drug injections into 219, 241–4
  flow rates
    calculations 218
    factors affecting 293
    slowing/stopping 244–6
  intermittent 219
    flushing to maintain patency 858
    procedure guidelines 238–41
  postanaesthetic recovery 622
  problem solving 244–9
  reducing risk of infection 217–18
intravenous injections, direct intermittent 219
  cytotoxic drugs 263–4
  problem solving 244–9
  procedure guidelines 241–4
intravenous push 219
  procedure guidelines 241–4
intravesical drug instillation 280–3
  problem solving 282–3
  procedure guidelines 281–2
  see also bladder irrigation; bladder lavage
invasive procedures
  aseptic technique 51
  hepatitis B 115
  HIV infection 94, 95, 96
  see also exposure-prone procedures
iodine, oral 722
iodine-123-labelled mIBG 722
iodine-125 seed brachytherapy 696
  procedure guidelines 711
iodine-131 (I-131) 718, 721–2
  administration 726
  emergency procedures 731–3
  labelled mIBG 722, 727
  patient preparation 726
  procedure guidelines 726–7
  radiation protection policies 722
  therapeutic uses 721–2
Ionising Radiation Regulations 1999 (IRR99) 692–3, 717, 723
Ionising Radiation (Medical Exposure) Regulations 2000 (IRMER) 692
  operator 717, 718

practitioner 717
  referrer 717
iontophoresis, local anaesthetics 863
IQRA Trust 455
iridium-198 692, 694–5
  gynaecological sources 695, *695*
    problem solving 710
    procedure guidelines 705–7
    removal 706–7
  implant types 694–5, *695*
  remote afterloading 700
IRMER *see* Ionising Radiation (Medical Exposure) Regulations 2000
iron
  overload 840
  serum **478**
iron lungs 757
irritants, defined 266
irritation, intravenous infusion-induced 247
ischaemia
  complicating arterial cannulation 904, 913
  pressure-induced 955
Islam
  last offices 455
  washing and personal hygiene 663
isolation *see* protective isolation; source isolation
isolators
  barrier nursing 74, 86
  cytotoxic drug preparation 255–6, 257–8, *261*
isotonic fluid expansion 293–4, *295*
  see also circulatory overload
ispaghula husk 334
itch, fungating wounds **962**
itraconazole 105

Jackson's silver tracheostomy tube 813, *813*
Jain Centre 454
Jainism, last offices 453–4
jaundice, blood glucose testing 536
Jehovah's Witnesses
  blood transfusion 837
  last offices 454
jejunostomy feeding tubes 474
  procedure guidelines 488–9
jewellery
  deceased patients 448
  nursing staff 54, 62
  surgical patients 612
joint protection, neurological patients 685
Judaism, last offices 445, 454

Kaltocarb 963
Kapitex Tracoetwist fenestrated tracheostomy tube 814, *814*
Kaposi's sarcoma 90, 91, 275
Kegel exercises *see* pelvic floor exercises
keloids 968–9
keratinocyte growth factor (KGF) **944**, 945
ketones 534
kidneys 530, *530*, 736
Klebsiella pneumoniae, antibiotic resistant 100–1
knee-jerk reflex 555
Kock nipple 349
Kold Kap 768
Korotkoff's sounds 507, 508–9, *509*
kuru 129
Kussmaul's respiration 519

labelling
  blood pack *842*
  medicines 206
  microbiological specimens 776
laboratory specimen collection *see* specimen collection
lacrimal apparatus 631, *632*

lactation *see* breast feeding
lactic acid 750
lactulose 334
lamivudine 113, 118
language
  nursing 21–2
  patients speaking different 35
laparoscopic surgery 615
large intestine 328
larval therapy 948
laryngectomy 810–30
  communication methods 816
  general nursing care 817–18
  humidification 815–16, 824–5
  stoma 810
    care 818
    suctioning via 818–19, 823–4
  stoma buttons (and vents) 815, *815*, 821
  swallowing difficulties 817
  total 810, *810*
  tubes 814–15, *815*, 821
  voice rehabilitation 819–22
  see also tracheostomy
laryngotomy 811
Lassa fever, isolation facilities 86
last offices 445–56
  critical care patients 449–50
  different religious faiths 452–6
  equipment 446
  problem solving 451–2
  procedure guidelines 446–9
  radioactive patients 451, 703–4, 732
  see also death
latex
  allergy 56, 379
    assessment 607, **607**
    management 607–8
  gloves 56
  urinary catheters 379
laundry *see* linen/laundry
laxatives 334, 334–5
  abuse 331
  bulking agents 334, **334**
  opioid-treated patients 568
  osmotic agents **334**, 334–5
  stimulant **334**, 335
  stool softeners 334, **334**
laying out *see* last offices
LBF barrier film 369
LDL apheresis **418**
lead shields 702, 724, 730
Leeds Assessment of Neuropathic Symptoms and Signs (LANSS) 560
leflunomide 120
left bundle branch *499*, 502
leg *see* lower limb
leg drainage bags 382
leg straps, catheterized patients 382
legal advice, after violent incidents 937
Legionella pneumophila 123–4
Legionnaire's disease 73, 123–4
legislation
  Creutzfeldt–Jakob disease 130
  gene therapy 402
  tuberculosis 128
  violence against staff 933–4
lethal response 294
leucoagglutination 839
leucocytes *see* white blood cells
leukaemia
  infection risks 84–5
  intrathecal drug administration 277, 462
  lumbar puncture 462
  oral complications 654
  protective isolation 85, 87
  scalp cooling 767

levomepromazine 214
liability, vicarious 992
lice, head 663
lidocaine (lignocaine)
 cardiopulmonary resuscitation 161, 163
 gel, urinary catheterization 381
 oral care 652
 peripheral cannulation 863
lifestyle changes, constipation 333
light source, eye care 632
lignocaine *see* lidocaine
limb
 elevation, extravasation 270
 misshapen, compression therapy 176, *176*
 movements, intraoperative 614
 selection for venepuncture 921–2
 size measurement 171–2
 volume measurement 171–4
  methods 172, **172**
  procedure guidelines 173–4
 see also lower limb; upper limb
Limone 370
linctuses 207
linen/laundry
 AIDS/HIV-positive patients 98
 cytotoxic drug spillages 259
 gene therapy 409
 hepatitis A infection 110
 hepatitis B infection 113
 radioactive patients 702, 728–9, 731
 source barrier nursing 78, 81
lip reading 38, 816
lipid emulsions, changing administration sets
  217
liposuction, extravasated drug 271
lips, dry 652, 657
liquid paraffin 334
liquid-based cytology (LBC) 780, 792
listening 32
Listeria monocytogenes 124–5
listeriosis 124–5
lithotomy position 614
litigation, extravasation injuries 266
liver function tests **478**
liver metastases 285, 286
Lloyd Davies position 614
 antiembolic stockings and 607, 614
local anaesthesia
 arterial puncture/cannulation 906, 908
 bone marrow aspiration/biopsy 420
 breast aspiration 149
 midline catheter insertion 882, 883
 peripheral venous cannulation 863, 878
 PICC insertion 868, 884
 postoperative blocks 565–6
 postoperative care 618
 removal of skin-tunnelled CVCs 898
 suturing wounds 971
 see also topical anaesthesia
local anaesthetic agents
 epidural/intrathecal 588, 591–2
 eye 633, 634
 iontophoresis 863
 side effects 589, 599–600
long lines *see* peripherally inserted central
  catheters
long-chain triglycerides (LCT)
 dietary supplements 471
 enteral feeds 474–5
loop of Henle 530
loperamide 331
lower limb
 amputees 688–9
 applying elastic compression garments
  178
 blood pressure measurement 509–10

compression bandaging 182–3, *184*
 lymphoedema 170
 size measurement 172
 veins for venepuncture 920
 volume measurement 173
lozenges 207
LP *see* lumbar puncture
lubricating gels, urinary catheterization 381
Luer-Lok connections 857
lumbar puncture 460–5
 anatomy 460, *461*
 complications 462
 contraindications 460
 defined 460
 indications 460
 intrathecal chemotherapy 277, 462
 leakage from site 464, 465
 nurse's role 462
 problem solving 465
 procedure guidelines 463–5, *465*
lung
 compliance and elasticity 515
 defence mechanisms 517
 gaseous exchange 516, **516**, *517*
 radioactive seed implants 711
 ventilation/perfusion scans **719**
lung cancer, spinal cord compression 796,
  799
lung infections
 health care acquired 71
 see also pneumonia
lung volumes 515–16
 measurement 514, *515*
lying position *see* side lying position; supine
  position
lymph nodes
 radioactive seed implants 711
 sentinel, radioactive biopsy 723
lymphatic drainage
 manual 176
 simple 174
lymphocytes 414
 collection (apheresis) **419**
 count, total 470
 in CSF 462
lymphoedema 170–1
 assessment of patient 171
 blood pressure measurement 510
 compression therapy *see* compression therapy
 intensive phase of treatment 174, 175–7
 maintenance phase of treatment 174–5
 measurement of limb volume 171–4
 phases of treatment 174–7
 severe 176
lymphoid progenitor cells *413*, 414
lymphoma
 AIDS-related 90
 intrathecal drug administration 277, 462
 oral complications 654
 scalp cooling 767
 spinal cord compression 799
lymphorrhoea *175*, 176

macrophages *413*, **414**, 944–5
maggots 948
magnesium
 deficiency 470
 plasma **478**
magnesium salts, laxative 334–5
magnesium sulphate 161, 163
magnetic resonance imaging (MRI) 797–9
Mainz Sigma II pouch 351, *351*, 354
malabsorption
 dietary supplements 471
 enteral feeds 475
malaria 841

male patients
 facial shaving 665
 intermittent self-catheterization 389–90
 midstream specimen of urine 788
 penile sheaths 395–7
 urinary catheterization 378, 381, 384–6
malignant hyperpyrexia 625
malnutrition
 assessment 468–70
 biochemical investigations 470
 poor wound healing 946
 postoperative prevention 626–7
 refeeding syndrome 478, **478**
 screening 468
malnutrition universal screening tool (MUST)
  468
malodour *see* odour
Management of Health and Safety at Work
  Regulations (MHSWR) 402, 403, 933
Manchester applicators 697, *697*, 698
mandelic acid solutions 311, 313
mandible, radionecrosis of 653
mannitol 269
manual evacuation of faeces 342–4
manual handling 669
 spinal cord compression 800–1
 surgical patients 614–15
 see also positioning; transfers
masks
 aseptic technique 56
 barrier nursing 76, 80
 complications of long-term use 763, 764
 cytotoxic drug handling 256
 Entonox 579
 grading 76
 MRSA control 102
 operating theatre 615
 oxygen *see* oxygen masks
 ventilation, CPR 158
massage, abnormal scars 968
mast cell activation syndrome 900
Matron Charter 77
mattresses, pressure-relieving 960, **961**
McGill Pain Questionnaire (MPQ) 560
meals
 barrier nursing 80
 oral drug administration and 222–3
 unsealed radioactive source therapy 728
 see also food
mean arterial pressure (MAP) 507
mean cell volume **478**
meatal cleaning, catheterized patients 382
mechanical irritation, intravenous
  infusion-induced 247
mechanical ventilation 757
mechlorethamine 268
median cubital vein
 cannulation 868
 venepuncture *920*, 920–1
medical alert bracelets 353
medical devices, CE mark 55
Medical Devices Agency (MDA) *see* Medicines
  and Health Care Products Regulatory
  Agency
medicinal products, defined 203
medicines
 addition to intravenous fluids/diluents 218,
  219
 administration *see* drug administration
 combinations, subcutaneous infusions 214
 compatibilities 218, 219
 containers 206
 defined 208
 disposal of unused 78, 204
 formulations 206–8
 general sales list (GSL) 203

labelling 206
legislation 203–4
mixtures 206, 207
off label 203
patient's own 206, 209
pharmacy (P) 203
prescription only (POM) 203
reconstitution *see* reconstitution
stability 206
stock control 206
storage 204–6
therapeutic monitoring 778–9, 784–5
unlicensed 203
Medicines Act 1968 203, 210
Medicines and Health Care Products Regulatory
 Agency (MHRA) (formerly Medical
 Devices Agency) 203
 blood transfusion practice 832
 classification of infusion devices 294–5, **296**
 mercury sphygmomanometers 507
 safe use of infusion devices **292**, 292–3
 thermometers 527
Medicines (Administration of Radioactive
 Substances) Regulations 1978 692
medium-chain triglycerides (MCT)
 dietary supplements 471
 enteral feeds 474–5
meibomian cysts 636
melanoma, eye 636
melphalan 286
meningitis, complicating spinal analgesia 590
menstruation, surgical patients 611, 615
mental illness, and violence 935
mercury
 sphygmomanometers 507–8
 thermometers 527
mesenteries 44
metabolic disorders
 cardiopulmonary arrest 160
 peritoneal dialysis 744
metacarpal veins
 cannulation 862
 venepuncture 920, 920, 921
meta-iodobenzylguanidine (mIBG) 718, **720**,
 722–3
 procedure guidelines 727
methadone 569
methicillin *see* meticillin
methotrexate 275, 286
 intrathecal 277, 462
 toxic effects on eye 635
meticillin-resistant *Staphylococcus aureus*
 (MRSA) 52, 100, 101–3
 colonization 101
 community care 103
 epidemic (EMRSA) 101
 eradication therapy 101
 isolation of infected patients 74
 psychological effects 78
 risk assessment 103
 risk factors 101, 103
 screening 101–2
 therapeutic drug monitoring 778–9
 transmission 102–3
metronidazole 963
 topical **947**, **962**, 963
MHRA *see* Medicines and Health Care
 Products Regulatory Agency
mIBG *see* meta-iodobenzylguanidine
microbiological examination
 catheter tips 874, 896, 899
 specimen collection for *see* specimen
 collection
microbore infusion sets 293
microSelectron (high dose rate; HDR) 698,
 699–700

follow-up care 701
 see also Selectron
midclavicular catheter 866
midline catheters **856**, 865–6
 care and management in situ 865
 choice of vein 865
 indications 865
 insertion 865
 problem solving 899
 procedure guidelines 882–3
 removal 866
midstream specimen of urine (MSU) 779, 788–9
millisieverts (mSv) 692, 693
minerals
 dietary requirements 470–1
 parenteral nutrition solutions 477
 serum levels 470
 supplements 471
mini assessment **18**
mini-tracheostomy 811
minoxidil 767
minute ventilation (MV) 514
miotics 634, *635*
Misuse of Drugs Act 1971 203–4
mithramycin 268
mitomycin C 268, 280, 283, 286
mitoxantrone 278, 280, 283
Mitrofanoff pouch 349, 350, *350*
mixtures of medicines 206, 207
mobility
 functional, spinal cord compression **797**
 nutritional status and 469
 see also immobility
mobilization 673–81
 amputees 688
 from lying to sitting 674, *674*
 patients on bed rest 670
 positioning in chair 675
 postoperative 626
 from sitting to standing 675–6, *676*
 spinal cord compression 800–1, 804
 walking 676–81
 see also transfers
modified-release tablets 206
moisturizers 662–3
monocytes 414, **414**
 in CSF 462
mood, in undernutrition 469
Morform sachet 370
Mormons, last offices 455
morphine
 acute/postoperative pain 564, 565
 breakthrough pain 568, 569, 570
 chronic pain 568–9
 conversion to fentanyl **569**
 epidural/intrathecal 591
 safer practice guidance 204
motor blockade, epidural/intrathecal analgesia
 589, 600
motor control 673
motor function
 assessment 550–1, 554
 spinal cord compression 797, **797**
motor response, Glasgow coma scale 547,
 547–9
mouth 648
 dry *see* dry mouth
 painful 652
mouth care 648–57
 advances 652–3
 agents 650–1
 defined 648
 equipment 650
 frequency 649–50
 intraoral brachytherapy 704–5
 oral problems 651–2

problem solving 656–7
 procedure guidelines 654–6
 unconscious patients 851, 852, 853
mouth-to-face mask ventilation 158
mouth-to-mouth ventilation 157–8, *158*
mouthwashes 650–1, 652
movements, abnormal 551
 positioning neurological patients with 686–7,
 687
MRSA *see* meticillin-resistant *Staphylococcus
 aureus*
MSU (midstream specimen of urine) 779, 788–9
mucositis, oral *see* oral mucositis
mucous membranes
 cytotoxic drug exposure 255, 261
 hepatitis B exposure 111, 112
 HIV exposure 95
 mouth 648
mucus, continent urinary diversion 352–3, 355
multidisciplinary approach
 discharge planning 189–93, **193**, **194–5**,
 197–8
 home enteral feeding 475
 nutritional support 479
 spinal cord compression 799–800, **800**, 804
mupirocin cream 101, **947**
muscle
 atrophy, unconscious patients 850
 co-ordination testing 550, 554
muscle strength 550
 testing 554
 unconscious patients 850
muscle tone
 defined 686
 positioning patients with abnormal 686–7,
 687
 testing 550, 554
muscle weakness
 assessment 554
 spinal cord compression 797, **797**
music, for pain management 566
Muslims
 last offices 455
 washing and personal hygiene 663
mustine 275, 278
mycobacteria, atypical 126
Mycobacterium bovis 126
Mycobacterium tuberculosis 126
mycosis 777
mydriatics 634, *634*
myelography 460
myeloid progenitor cells *413*, 414
myelopathy 796
myocardial perfusion imaging **719**
myofibroblasts 945

nail bed pressure, neurological assessment 549
nail brushes 62
nail varnish/polish 62
nails 62
 artificial 54, 62
 care 664, 666
nalidixic acid **532**
naloxone 163, 204, 623
name (wrist) bands 9
 see also identification, patient
nasal analgesia 570
nasal cannulae, oxygen via 754, *754*
 discomfort 763
 oxygen flow rates **754**
 problem solving 762–3
nasal care 664
nasal drops 233–4
nasal wash, syringe method 785–6, *786*
nasoduodenal feeding 472–3
nasogastric feeding 472–3

nasogastric tubes
    checking position 473, 483–4, 486
    enteral feeding 472–3
    insertion using an introducer 482–4, *484*
    insertion without an introducer 484–6
    see also enteral feeding tubes; Ryle's tube
nasojejunal feeding 472–3
nasopharyngeal specimen collection 785–7
    nasal wash: syringe method 785–6, *786*
    nose swab 782, *782*
    vacuum-assisted nasal aspirate method
        786–7, *787*, **787**
National Cancer Institute Common Toxicity
    Criteria (NCI-CTC) 649
National Collaborating Centre for Acute Care,
    parenteral nutrition 475–6, 477, **477**,
    478, 479
National Council of Hindu Temples 453
National Health Service (NHS)
    Continuing Healthcare 196
    health care-acquired infections 71
    isolation facilities 74
    management of violence 933, 934
    Security Management Service 934
National Institute for Health and Clinical
    Excellence (NICE) 10
    cervical cytology guidance 780
    on communication 29, 35
    pressure ulcer guidance 955–6, 960
    tuberculosis guidelines 127
    violence guideline 933, 936, 938–9
    wound management guidance 948
National Patient Safety Agency (NPSA) 9, 204,
    473
National Prescribing Centre (NPC) 212
National Service Framework for Older People
    discharge planning 188, 193–5
    self-administration of medicines 209
National Spiritual Assembly of the Bahais of the
    United Kingdom 452
natural killer lymphocytes **414**
Naturcare 370
nausea and vomiting
    during CPAP 764
    dietary advice **473**
    enterally fed patients **476**
    opioid-induced 589, 601
    postanaesthetic control 618, *619*, 624
    radioactive material 731–2
    source barrier nursing 78
nebulization 208
necrosis 266
    complicating arterial cannulation 913
    debridement methods 947–8
    drugs causing 268–9
        see also vesicant drugs
    fungating wounds **962**
    radiotherapy skin reactions **965**
needle sampling port, urinary catheter system
    391, *391*
needleless injection systems 239, 858
needleless sampling port, urinary catheter
    system 391
needles
    disposal of used 923
    injections 224
    intramuscular injections 216
    non-coring, implantable ports *874*, 875,
        894–5, *895*
    removal from vein 924
    venepuncture 922, *923*
needlestick injuries *see* inoculation accidents
needs, patient 21
negative pressure therapy *see* topical negative
    pressure therapy
Negus's silver tracheostomy tube 813, *813*

nelaton catheters 355, **378**, *380*, 383
neobladder, orthotopic 351, *351*
    postoperative patient education 353, 354
neonates
    haemolytic disease 834
    herpes simplex virus (HSV) infection 121
    infusions 294, **296**
    oxygen toxicity 636
    thermoregulation 524
    see also premature infants
nephron *530*
nerve blocks 571
nerve growth factor (NGF) **944**
nerve injuries
    after bone marrow harvest 426
    complicating venepuncture 928
neuroblastoma 722, 796
neuroendocrine tumours 722
neurogenic (spinal) shock 806
neurological disorders
    positioning 684–8
        abnormal tone and movement patterns
            686–7, *687*
        environment and 687
        joint protection 685
        soft tissue changes and contractures 687
    rehabilitation 687–8
    spinal analgesia 586
    swallowing difficulties 492, 493
neurological impairment
    spinal cord compression 797, **797**
    violence and 935
neurological observations (and assessment)
    546–55
    after lumbar puncture 464, *465*
    consciousness 546–9
    emergency *555*
    frequency 552, **552**
    general points 552
    indications 546
    motor function 550–1
    procedure guidelines 553–5
    pupillary activity 549
    sensory function 551
    unconscious patients 853
    visual acuity/visual fields 552, *552*
    vital signs 551–2
neuromuscular blockade, persistent 623
neuropathic bladder 349
neuropathic pain 560, 568
neurosurgery, for spinal cord compression 799,
    803
neutropenia
    aspergillosis 104–5
    blood pressure monitoring 510
    care guidelines 88–90
    diagnosis of infections 87
    diet 87, 89
    health care-acquired infections 52, 71
    infection risks 84, 85
    level of care required 85
    protective isolation 86
    sources of infection 72
    temperature monitoring 528
neutrophil count 84, **414**
neutrophils *413*, **414**, 944–5
NHS *see* National Health Service
The NHS Plan (2000), discharge planning
    193–5
NICE *see* National Institute for Health and
    Clinical Excellence
nil by mouth, preoperative 606
nitrogen
    dietary requirements 470, **470**
    parenteral nutrition solutions 476, 477
    partial pressure 751

nitrous oxide and oxygen *see* Entonox
NMC *see* Nursing and Midwifery Council
Nodor S drops 370
non-A non-B hepatitis (NANB) 116–17
non-invasive ventilation 756
non-steroidal anti-inflammatory drugs
    (NSAIDs) **563**, 568
    acute/postoperative pain 565
    COX 2-specific 565
non-touch technique 51, 54–5
    oral cytotoxic drug formulations 274–5
non-verbal communication 32–3
non-verbal cues 31, 32
noradrenaline 533
Norton scale 956, **956**
nose care 664
nose swab 782, *782*
Nosocomial Infection National Surveillance
    Service (NINSS) 52
nosocomial infections *see* health care-acquired
    infections
notification of infections 78
novice nurses 7
Novogel 968
NSAIDs *see* non-steroidal anti-inflammatory
    drugs
nuclear medicine 717–18
nurse consultants 8
nurse practitioners 8
nurse prescribing 210–12
    evaluation **212**
nurses
    blocking behaviour 35
    psychological support 35
    stress and burn out 88
nursing
    context 4–12
    defined 4
    language 21–2
    patients' perspective 4–8
    requirements of organizations 8–11
Nursing and Midwifery Council (NMC)
    Code, The 4–5, 7, 937, 955,
        986–92
    consent guidance 5
    consultation on advanced practice 8–9
    dealing with violence guidance 933
    drug administration guidance 208–10,
        212–13, 219–20
    nurse prescribing 210, 212
nursing assessment *see* assessment
nursing care *see* care
nursing diagnosis *see* diagnosis, nursing
nursing homes, discharge to 195
nursing models 17, 661
nutrients
    deficiencies 469
    intake, assessment 468
nutrition
    assessment of status 468–70
    benchmarks 471, **472**
    during CPAP 764
    laryngectomy patients 817
    oral complications and 653
    screening 468
    subjective global assessment (SGA) 468,
        470
    wound healing and 946–7
    see also diet; food
nutritional requirements **470**
    calculation 470–1
    causes of increased 468
nutritional support 468–93
    defined 468
    in dysphagia 493
    indications 468

multidisciplinary team 479
planning 471
problem solving 491–3
procedure guidelines 479–91
unconscious patients 850–1
see also dietary supplements; enteral tube feeding; parenteral nutrition
nystatin 651

obesity, nutritional assessment 469
observations 497–541
12-lead ECG 502–3
blood glucose 533–7
blood pressure 504–12
central venous pressure 538–41
neurological *see* neurological observations
peak flow 521–3
pulse 497–501
respiration 512–20
temperature 522–8
urinalysis 528–32
see also vital signs
occupational health and safety *see* health and safety, occupational
occupational therapy
discharge planning 197
spinal cord compression **800**, 805
octreotide 331
oculocephalic reflex 551
odour
fungating wounds **962**, 963–4
offensive oral (halitosis) 649
stomas 367–8, 375
urine 531, **531**
oedema
after VAD insertion 900
dependency or gravitational 170
intravenous infusion/injection-related 248
nutritional assessment 469
see also lymphoedema
oesophageal speech 816
oesophageal tumours
enteral tube feeding 473, 474
swallowing difficulties 492
oestrogen 147
ointments 207
cytotoxic drugs 275–6
eye *see* eye ointments
older people *see* elderly
oliguria, postoperative 625
Omaha nursing classification system 22
omega-3 fatty acids 475
Ommaya reservoir 277
Omnopon 565
one-handed technique, peripheral cannulation 863
one-step technique, peripheral cannulation 863
operating room (OR) *see* operating theatre
operating theatre 613–17
hand washing 64, 615
infection control and asepsis 615
patient transfers 613
procedure guidelines 616–17
see also intraoperative care; postanaesthetic recovery room
opioid analgesics
acute pain 564–5
chronic pain 568–70
driving and 571
epidural/intrathecal 564, 587–8, 591
intramuscular injections 565
intravenous 564
mild to moderate pain 568
moderate to severe pain 568–70
nasal 570

oral 565
oral mucositis pain 652
in renal failure 571
side effects 568, 589, 599–600
subcutaneous 564–5
transdermal patches 569, 570
optic nerve 631
OR *see* operating theatre
Orabase paste 369
Orahesive powder 369
oral assessment 649, **649**
Oral Assessment Guide (OAG) 649
oral cancer 653–4
brachytherapy
procedure guidelines 704–5
radioactive sources 694, 694–5, 695
see also head and neck tumours
oral cavity *see* mouth
oral complications 648–9
haematological malignancies 654
nutrition and 653
prophylaxis and treatment 651–3
oral contraceptives 635
oral drug administration
acute/postoperative pain 565
chronic pain 563
cytotoxic drugs 274–5, **276**
formulations 206–7
procedure guidelines 221–4
oral hygiene *see* mouth care
oral infections 649, 651–2
haematological malignancies 654
oral mucosa 648
oral mucositis 648
prevention 650–1
treatment 651, 652
Oral Mucositis Index (OMI) 649
oral temperature 527
Oramorph 565, 568
see also morphine
orbital tumours 636–7
orientation, evaluation of 547
orthopnoea 518
orthotopic neobladder *see* neobladder, orthotopic
osmosis 737, **737**
osteoporosis, spinal cord compression 796
osteoradionecrosis, of mandible 653
Ostobon deodorant powder 370
Ostoclear sachets or spray 369
Ostofix tape 370
OstoSorb gel 370
outcomes, patient 22, **22**
ovarian cancer 44, 45
overinfusion 292, 293–4
complications **291**
problem solving 248, 308
see also circulatory overload
overshoes, barrier nursing 76
oxycodone
acute/postoperative pain 565
chronic pain 568, 570
oxygen
consumption 752–3
liquid 755
pulmonary exchange 516, **516**, *751*, 751–2
supply 753
toxicity 636, 760
transportation 516–17, *517*, 750–1, 752
uptake 750, **751**, 751–2
utilization 751, 752
oxygen condensers (concentrators) 755
oxygen cylinders 753, 755
oxygen masks
discomfort 763

fixed performance/high-flow (Venturi-type) 755, *755*, **755**
non-rebreathing 755
partial rebreathing 754–5
problem solving 762–3
simple semi-rigid plastic 754, **754**, *754*
tracheostomy 755
oxygen partial pressure (PO$_2$) 751
in blood (PaO$_2$) 516, 752
oxygen saturation (SaO$_2$) 519, 752
factors affecting 752, *752*
measurement 752–3
monitoring 519, 520, *521*
oxygen therapy 753–5
delivery systems 754, 754–5, *755*
equipment 753–5
hazards 758–60
home (domiciliary) 755
discharge planning **194**
humidification 757–8, 825
hyperbaric 951
nasal cannulae catheters 754, **754**, *754*
nasal care 664
oral care 650
postanaesthetic recovery 620, 621, 623
problem solving 762–3
safety measures 753, 763
T-piece circuit 755
oxygenation
adequacy, during respiratory therapy 762
cellular 750
positioning to maximize 683, *683*
tissue 750–2
oxyhaemoglobin dissociation curve 752, *752*

paclitaxel
administration 268, 269, 283
scalp cooling 767, 768
paediatric patients
blood pressure measurement 509
enteral feeds 475
HIV infection 92
infusion devices 294
nasopharyngeal specimen collection 787
nutritional assessment 469
nutritional requirements 471
oral drug administration 223
pulse measurement 501
urinary catheters 378, 379
venepuncture 922
see also neonates; premature infants
pain
acute *see* acute pain
during bladder lavage/irrigation 321
bone marrow collection 416, 417, 426
breakthrough 558, 570
cancer *see* cancer pain
chronic *see* chronic pain
defined 558
evoked 560
extravasation **268**, 269
incident 570
intensity 558–9
intramuscular injections 216–17
intrapleural drainage 433
intravenous infusion site 248
location 558
lumbar puncture 465
neuropathic 560, 568
positioning and 670
postoperative *see* postoperative pain
skin graft donor sites 967
spinal cord compression 797, **797**
spontaneous 560, 570
total, concept of 559
during venepuncture 928–9

pain assessment 558–60
  chronic/cancer pain 559, **559**, *562*, 573
  epidural/intrathecal analgesia 589–90, 595
  procedure guidelines 572–3
  RMH patient held pain chart 560, *562*, 573
  spinal cord compression 802
  surgical patients 558–9, 572, 627
  tools 559–60, *561–2*
pain management 560–71
  acute pain 564–8
  anaesthetic interventions 571
  chronic pain 563, *563*, 568–71
  fungating wounds 962
  need for effective 560–3
  non-pharmacological measures 566–8
  peripheral cannulation 863
  postanaesthetic recovery 618, *619*
  postoperative pain 563–4, 627
  preoperative preparation 572
  principles 564
  see also analgesia
painful stimuli, response to, Glasgow Coma
    Scale 549
palifermin 653
Palladone *see* hydromorphone
palliative care
  compression therapy 176–7
  nutritional assessment 469
  spinal cord compression 799–800, 802
  urgent discharge home 189, *191–2*
  see also terminal care
palmar-plantar erythrodysesthesia syndrome
    662
palpation, veins 921
panic attacks 36
Pap smear *see* cervical smear
paper towels 54, 63
  dispensers 54, 61
  disposal of used 63
paracentesis, abdominal *see* abdominal
    paracentesis
paracetamol 565, 568
  combination preparations 565
  gargles 652
paralytic ileus 743
paraphimosis, catheterized patients 394
paraphrasing 33
paraplegia, spinal cord compression 797, 799
parasites 841
parasympathetic nervous system 498, *498*
parathyroid scan, radionuclide **720**
parenteral infusions 207
parenteral nutrition (PN) 475–9
  changing administration sets 217, 477
  choice of regimen 477
  delivery and management 477
  home 479
  indications 468, 475–6
  metabolic complications 477–9, **478**
  monitoring 477, **477**, **478**
  route of administration 476
  solutions 476–7
  termination 479
Parsees, last offices 456
partial pressure (P) 751
partial (persistent) withdrawal occlusion (PWO)
    858–9, *859*, 891
partially sighted patients, communication with
    37–8
partially weight bearing (PWB) 676–7
particle embolism, intravenous
    procedure-related 249
Passy Muir speaking valve 813
pastilles 207
patient education
  continent urinary diversion 353, 354, 355–7

epidural/intrathecal analgesia 592
  hepatitis A 110
  hepatitis B carriers 112–13
  indwelling VADs 876, 877, *877*
  oral anti-cancer chemotherapy 276
  as pain control measure 566
  preoperative 572, 606
  stomas 363–4, 365, 366
  see also information provision
patient group directions (PGD) 210–12
  defined 210
  flowchart *211*
  off label medicines 203
  unlicensed medicines 203
patient hygiene *see* personal hygiene
patient problems 21
patient-controlled analgesia (PCA) 564
  epidural (PCEA) 589
  postoperative pain 606
  pumps 299
  see also Entonox
Patient-Generated Subjective Global Assessment
    470
patients
  expectations 4
  identification *see* identification, patient
  involvement 11
  own drugs 206
  perspective of nursing 4–8
  positioning *see* positioning
  problems/needs 21
  providing information to *see* information
    provision
  safety 9–10
  self-administration of medicines 209, 220–1
  as sources of evidence 11, 12
  tampering with infusion devices 293
peak flow (peak expiratory flow rate, PEFR)
    521–3
  factors affecting 521–2
  normal values 522
  procedure guidelines 522–3, *523*
  timing of readings 521
PEG enteral feeding tubes *see* gastrostomy tubes,
    percutaneous endoscopically placed
pelvic floor exercises, continent urinary
    diversion 351, 353, 354
penciclovir 121–2
Penguin cap 768
penile pain on erection, catheterized patients
    394
penile sheaths 395–7
  procedure guidelines 396–7
penile swabs 782
Penrose drain, shortening 978
pentamidine 126
percutaneously endoscopically placed
    gastrostomy (PEG) tubes *see* gastrostomy
    tubes, percutaneous endoscopically
    placed
perianal area
  examination 340, 341
  hygiene/care 331, 663
perinatal transmission
  hepatitis A 109
  hepatitis B 111
  hepatitis E 118
  HIV 92
perineal care 663
perineal template, interstitial *see* interstitial
    perineal template
periodontitis 652
perioperative care 606–27
  see also intraoperative care; postoperative
    care; preoperative care
peripheral blood stem cells (PBSC) 417, **418**

peripheral cannulae **856**, 860–5
  care and management in situ 863–4, *864*
  choice of vein 861–2
  cytotoxic drug administration 262–3, **263**,
    266
  defined 860
  discharge home with indwelling 876
  extravasation of vesicants 266, 272–4
  flow rates 860, **860**
  indications 860
  insertion (cannulation) 862–3
    advancement techniques 863
    pain relief 863
    procedure guidelines 878–80, *880–1*
    repeat 863
    for subcutaneous infusions 304–6
    techniques 862–3
  over the needle 861
  ported 861, *861*
  removal and dwell times 864–5
  safety non-ported 861, *861*
  taping 864, *864*
  types and dimensions **860**, 860–1, *861*
  winged *see* winged infusion devices
peripheral resistance 505
peripheral vascular access devices
  occlusion 245
    see also under vascular access devices
  parenteral nutrition 476
  problem solving 899–901
  removal, after extravasation 270
  venepuncture 922, **923**
  vesicant drug administration 267
  see also midline catheters; peripheral cannulae
peripherally inserted central catheters (PICCs)
    856, 866–9
  care and management in situ 868, *869*
  choice of vein 867, 867–8
  cleaning 857
  defined 866
  design and types 867
  discharge home with in situ 876–7
  indications 866
  insertion 868
    length measurement 868, **868**, 884, *886*
    problem solving 899
    procedure guidelines 884–6
  malposition of tip 899
  parenteral nutrition 476
  pros and cons 866–7
  removal 868–9, 886
peristalsis 328
peritoneal catheters 739
  cytotoxic drug administration 283–4
  infectious complications 743
  insertion 740–1
  kinking 743
  leakage around 285, 743
peritoneal cavity 44, 737
  drug administration into *see* intraperitoneal
    chemotherapy
peritoneal dialysis (PD) 736–9
  anatomy and physiology 737, 737–8
  continuous ambulatory (CAPD) 736
  cycle 738, *738*
  fluids 737–8, 741–2
  indications 736
  problem solving 742–4
  procedure guidelines 740–2
  technique 739
peritoneal fluid 737
  withdrawal for analysis (peritoneal tap) 44,
    45, 47
peritoneovenous shunt 45
peritoneum 44, *44*, 737
peritonitis 742

persistent (partial) withdrawal occlusion (PWO)
        858–9, *859*, 891
personal hygiene 661–6
    aseptic technique 56–7
    barrier nursing 77, 86
    bed bathing *see* bed bathing
    defined 661
    eye care 630–45
    hepatitis A 110
    mouth care 648–57
    oxygen therapy and 763
    procedure guidelines 664–6
    skin care 661–3
    unconscious patients 851
    unsealed radioactive source therapy 728–9
personal protective equipment (PPE) 55–6
    barrier nursing 76–7, 80
    last offices 447
    operating theatre 615
    radiation protection 724, 727, 729
    see also aprons, plastic; eye protection;
        gloves; protective clothing
*Personal Protective Equipment at Work
        Regulations* 55
pessaries, vaginal 207
    procedure guidelines 231–2
pest control 73
pethidine *565*
pets, immunocompromised patients 88, 108
PGD *see* patient group directions
pH
    blood 516
    gastric contents, enterally-fed patients 473,
        483, 486
    urine *see under* urine
phaeochromocytoma 722
pharmacists, covert drug administration and
        210
pharmacy (P) medicines 203
phase angle 469
phenazopyridine (pyridium) **532**
phenytoin 269
phlebitis
    arterial cannulation-related 913
    intravenous infusion-related 246
    mechanical 900
    VIP scale *250*
phosphate
    enemas 335
    plasma **478**
photon radiation 694
photopheresis **418**
physical activity, constipation management 333
physical restraint 936–7
physiotherapist 677, 685
physiotherapy
    patients on bed rest 670
    spinal cord compression **800**, 805
pia mater 586, *587*
PICCs *see* peripherally inserted central catheters
pilocarpine 653
pinch-off syndrome 858, 891
pin-cushion technique, extravasation injury 270
pituitary gland tumours 631
planning
    care 22–3, **23**
    nutritional support 471
plantar reflexes 551
plants, protective isolation facilities 85
plasma 414
    cryo-depleted **836**
    fresh frozen (FFP) **836**
    oxygen transport 752
    proteins 470
plasma exchange **418**
plasma volume, radionuclide studies **721**

Plasmodium falciparum 841
plastic catheters 379
plastic surgery 965–8
    assessment 966
    associated problems 966–8
platelet derived growth factor (PDGF) **944**, 945,
        954
platelets *413*, 414, **414**
    apheresis **418**, **419**
    transfusion **835**
    wound healing 943–4
pleura 429, *429*
pleural effusion *278*, 278–80, 430
    drainage 430, 431
    intrapleural drug therapy 278–80
    malignant 278
pleural space 430
plugholes, hand basin 62, 63
plugs, colostomy 365, 368
pneumatic compression, intermittent 607, 614
pneumococcus (*Streptococcus pneumoniae*) 103
Pneumocystis carinii (jiroveci) (PC) 125–6
pneumocystosis 125–6
pneumonia
    health care acquired 71
    Legionnaires' disease 123, 124
    Pneumocystis carinii (PCP) 125, 126
    prevention, unconscious patients 852
    see also respiratory tract infections
pneumothorax 429, 430, 441, 514
    complicating VAD insertion 900
    intrapleural drainage 431, 432, 433
    spontaneous 430
    tension 160, 430, 441
point-of-care testing (POCT) 535–6
poisoning, cardiopulmonary arrest 160
police 936
polydipsia 534
polymorphonuclear leucocytes *see* neutrophils
polytetrafluoroethylene (PTFE)-coated catheters
        379
polyurethane tubes, enteral feeding 473
polyuria 534
polyvinylchloride (PVC)
    catheters 379
    tubes, enteral feeding 473
porridge test, anal sphincter control 351
Portacaths *see* implantable ports
Portex cuffed tracheostomy tube 811, *811*
positioning 669–88
    amputees 688–9
    assisting patients to move 673–81
    in bed 670–3, *672*, *673*
    in cardiorespiratory compromise 684
    CVC insertion 871, *871*
    CVP measurement 538, 539
    defined 669
    eye care 632
    infusion flow rate and 293
    interstitial perineal brachytherapy *714*
    intraoperative 614–15
    intrapleural drain insertion 435
    lumbar puncture 463, *465*
    medical considerations 669–70
    in neurological impairment 684–8
    postoperative period 625
    pressure ulcer prevention 960
    principles 669
    pulse rate and 497
    unconscious patients 852
    see also manual handling
positron emission tomography (PET) **720**
postanaesthetic recovery 617–25
    assessment for discharge 618, *619*
    defined 617
    local and regional anaesthesia 618

problem solving 623–5
    procedure guidelines 620–2
postanaesthetic recovery room 617
    equipment 618, 620
    handover to 617
posterior popliteal artery, blood pressure
        measurement 509–10
postherpetic neuralgia 122
post-mortem examination 451
postoperative care 617–27
    blood pressure measurement 510
    continent urinary diversion 352–3, *353*
    plastic surgery 966–7, 966–8
    procedure guidelines 625–7
    pulse monitoring 500
    respiratory monitoring 519
    stomas 365–6
    temperature monitoring 528
    total laryngectomy 818
    tracheostomy 817
    see also postanaesthetic recovery
postoperative complications
    prevention on ward 625–7
    recovery room 617–18, 623–5
Postoperative Observation and Pain Assessment
        Chart 560, *561*
postoperative pain
    assessment 558–9, 627
    epidural analgesia 586, 589–90
    management 563–8, 625, 627
    need for effective control 560–3
    patient education and 572, 606
    postanaesthetic recovery 624
    see also acute pain
postural alignment 673
potassium, peritoneal dialysis fluid 741
potassium chloride 163, 269
potassium iodate 722
powder, reconstitution for injection 226–7, *228*
preadmission clinics, discharge planning 188,
        196–7
prealbumin 470
precipitates, VAD occlusion 858, 892
precordial thump 156, 163
prednisolone enema 336
pregnancy
    breast changes 147
    cytotoxic drug exposure 255, 261
    Entonox use 581
    HIV testing 92
    listeriosis 125
    preoperative checks 611
    radiation exposure 730
    varicella 122, 123
    see also breast feeding; perinatal transmission
premature infants
    nasopharyngeal specimen collection **787**
    retrolental fibroplasia 760
premedication 613
preoperative autologous donation (PAD) 833
preoperative care 606–13
    bowel preparation 344–5
    continent urinary diversion 352
    fasting 606
    latex allergy 607–8
    patient education and pain control 572,
        606
    procedure guidelines 611–13
    skin preparation 606
    stoma creation 363–5
    thromboprophylaxis 606–7, 608–10
prescribing
    Entonox 580–1
    independent 210
    nurse 210–12, **212**
    supplementary 210–12

prescription only medicines (POM) 203
prescriptions
  controlled drugs 204, **205**
  drug administration without 208
pressure
  effects on tissues 955
  treatment, abnormal scars 968
pressure area care 960
  positioning and 669
  spinal cord compression 805
  unconscious patients 853
pressure ulcers (sores) 955–60
  aetiology 955
  assessment tools 956–60
  defined 955
  grades 956
  identifying at-risk patients 955–6
  prevalence 955
  treatment and prevention 960
  unconscious patients 851
  undernourished patients 469
pressure-activated safety valve (PASV) 873
pressure-relieving devices 960, **961**
  during surgery 614
primary health care team
  complex discharge planning **194–5**
  discharge planning 188–9
  epidural/intrathecal analgesia 591, 598
prion diseases 128–30, 841
Prisma 954
privacy 661
probenecid **532**
probiotics, *Clostridium difficile* infection 106
procedures
  consent to 5–7, **6**
  exposure-prone *see* exposure-prone
    procedures
  invasive *see* invasive procedures
  providing information on 30–1
professional boundaries, maintaining 988
professional reputation, upholding 991
proficient nurses 8
proflavin cream **947**
progesterone 147
prolactin 147
Promogran 954
proprioception, testing 555
proptosis 636
prostaglandins 526
prostate carcinoma
  interstitial brachytherapy 696, 711
  spinal cord compression 796
prostatic surgery, bladder irrigation after 311,
    314
proteases 954
protective clothing 55–6
  cytotoxic drug handling 256–7
  gene therapy 404, 406, 407
  HIV-positive patients 98
  intravenous drug administration 218
  source barrier nursing 76–7
  see also personal protective equipment
protective isolation 71, 74, 83–90
  defined 83
  environment 86
  facilities 85–6
  indications 83–5
  principles 86–8
  procedure guidelines 88–90
  rooms 86
    cleaning 86, 88
    entering 89
  visitors 89
protein, dietary
  requirements 470, **470**
  supplements 471

proteins
  CSF 462
  plasma 470
Proteus mirabilis
  antibiotic resistant 100–1
  catheter encrustation and 312
protozoa 777
Provox type indwelling voice prosthesis 821
pruritus, opioid-induced 589, 601
pseudomembranous colitis 106
Pseudomonas (aeruginosa) 967
  antibiotic resistant 100–1
  urine of catheterized patients 313
psychological disorders 35–6
psychological implications
  cancer nursing 88
  fungating wounds 962
  protective isolation 87
  scalp cooling 769, 772
  source isolation 71, 78
  stoma surgery 367
  unsealed radioactive source therapy 724–5
  urinary diversion 354–5
psychological interventions, pain management
    566
psychological support 32, 36
  after violent incidents 937
  AIDS/HIV infection 92–3, 97
  chemotherapy-induced alopecia 769–70
  communication issues 29, 30
  for nursing staff 35
  spinal cord compression 802
psychosocial factors
  acute pain 558
  chronic pain 559, **559**
pulmonary embolism (PE)
  cardiopulmonary arrest 160
  catheter tip as cause 901
  postoperative care 626
  prophylaxis *see* thromboprophylaxis
  signs 610
pulse 497–501
  amplitude 500
  assessing gross irregularity 500
  defined 497
  indications 497
  during manual evacuation of rectum 342, 344
  neurological patients 552, 554
  palpation sites 497, *497*
  paradoxical 500
  postanaesthetic recovery 621
  postoperative monitoring 625
  procedure guidelines 501, *501*
  rate **497**, 497–8, *498*
  rhythm 499–500
pulse oximetry 519, 753
  postanaesthetic recovery 620
  procedure guidelines 520, *521*
pulseless electrical activity (PEA) 156, 159, 161
pulsus paradoxus 904
pupils, examination 549, **549**, 553–4
purgatives 334
Purkinje fibres *499*, 502
pus, specimen collection 775
pyrexia 526, 528
  grades **526**
  during interstitial brachytherapy 708
  intravenous procedure-related 249
  time for recording 527
  of unknown origin, CVAD-related 901
  see also fever

quality assurance
  point-of-care testing (POCT) 535–6
  radiation protection 693, 724
quality improvement 9

quality of life, indwelling VADs 877–8
questioning 33
questions, open and closed 33

radial artery 902
  blood pressure measurement 903
  cannulation 902, **902**
    procedure guidelines 907–8, *908*
  pulse 497, *501*
  puncture, procedure guidelines 904–6
radiation
  dose 692
  dosimetry 724, *724*, 730
  ionizing 692
    regulations 692–3, 723
  measures 692
radiation controlled area 704, 717, 724
radiation employer 717
radiation film badges 702, 724, *724*, 730
radiation protection 723–4
  emergency procedures 693, 703–4, 731–3
  principles 723
  procedure guidelines 702–4, 727–9, 730–1
  regulations 692–3, 723–4
  terminology 717
radiation protection adviser 693, 717
radiation protection supervisor 693, 704, 717,
    723
radiation warning signs 702, 724
radiculopathy 796
radioactive contamination
  control 724
  deceased patients 451, 703–4, 732
  emergency procedures 693, 703–4, 731–3
  monitors 693
radioactive isotopes *see* radionuclides
radiologically inserted gastrostomy (RIG) tubes
    see gastrostomy tubes, radiologically
    inserted
radionecrosis, mandible 653
radionuclides (radioactive isotopes) 717–18
  defined 717
  definition of terms 717
  diagnostic investigations 717–18, **719–21**
    procedure guidelines 730–1
  sealed source therapy 694–6
  unsealed source therapy 717–33
    emergency procedures 731–3
    patient discharge 725
    patient preparation 725
    post-procedure care 727–9
    procedure guidelines 726–33
    radiation protection 723–4
    room preparation 724–5
  see also specific radionuclides
radiopharmaceuticals 717, 718, **719–21**
radiotherapy
  for cancer pain management 571
  fungating wounds 964
  induced hair loss 768
  lymphoedema complicating 170
  oral complications 648–9, 653
  sealed source *see* brachytherapy
  skin care during 965
  skin reactions 662, **964**, 964–5, **965**
  spinal cord compression 799, 803
  tracheostomy and 811
  unsealed radionuclides *see under*
    radionuclides
randomized controlled trials (RCTs) 11, 12,
    12
Rastafarians, last offices 455
RCN *see* Royal College of Nursing
Re186 HEDP *see* rhenium-186
    hydroxyethylidene diphosphonate
reagent sticks (dipsticks), urine 531–2, **532**, *533*

reconstitution
  cytotoxic drugs 255–6, 257–8
  powders for injection 226–7, *228*
reconstructive surgery *see* plastic surgery
records *see* documentation
recovery
  postanaesthetic *see* postanaesthetic recovery
  postoperative 625–7
recovery position 157, *157*
rectal bladder 350–1, *351*, 353
rectal cancer, interstitial brachytherapy 695–6
rectal drug administration 338–40
  procedure guidelines 339–40
  see also enemas; suppositories
rectal drug preparations 207
rectal examination, digital *see* digital rectal
    examination
rectal irrigation (lavage) 344–5
  contraindications 345
  fluid 345
rectal swabs 782
rectal temperature 527
rectum 328
  manual evacuation 342–4
  pain, peritoneal dialysis 743
rectus femoris injections *215*, 216
rectus sheath, stoma siting 364, *364*
red blood cells **414**
  in CSF 462
  exchange (apheresis) **418**
  formation *413*, 414
  frozen **835**
  in SAGM **835**
  for transfusion **835**
  washed **835**
red cell mass, radionuclide studies **721**
Redivac, drain dressing 975–6
5-α reductase inhibitors 767
refeeding syndrome 478, **478**
reference nutrient intake (RNI) 471
referrals, discharge planning 197–8
reflecting back 33
reflexes 550–1, *555*
  primitive developmental 685
Reform Synagogues of Great Britain 454
refrigeration, food **73**, 124–5
refusals
  respect for 31
  to take medication 209
regional anaesthesia, postoperative care 618,
    622
regional nerve blocks 571
rehabilitation
  laryngectomy voice 819–22
  mobilization *see* mobilization
  neurological patients 687–8
  spinal cord compression 799–800, **800**,
    804–5
relatives *see* family
relaxation techniques, pain control 566, **567**
religious practices
  last offices 445, 452–6
  personal hygiene 661, 663
renal clearance 531
renal failure
  acute (ARF) 736, 739
  end-stage (ESRF) 736
  opioid analgesia 571
renal function
  parenteral nutrition 478, **478**
  radionuclide imaging **721**
  tests 531
renal nuclear medicine scans **719**
renal replacement therapy 736–48
  continuous (CRRT) 739–40
  defined 736

procedure guidelines 740–6
types 736
  see also continuous venovenous
    haemodiafiltration; peritoneal dialysis
renal transplantation 736
renin 505
renogram **719**
The Reporting of Injuries, Diseases and
    Dangerous Occurrences Regulations
    1995 933–4
reproductive risks, cytotoxic drug exposure
    255
research evidence 10, 12
residential care homes
  discharge to 195
  MRSA control 103
residual volume *515*, 516
resistance
  airway 515
  to blood flow 504–5, *505*
respiration 512–20
  control 513, *513*
  defined 512
  depth 518
  external 750
  gas transport 516–17, *517*, 750
  history taking **518**
  internal (cellular) 513, 517, *517*, 750
  pattern 518–19, **551**, 551–2
  physiology 750
  see also breathing
respiratory assessment 753
respiratory capacities 516
respiratory centre 513
respiratory depression
  opioid-induced 589, 599–600
  postoperative 623
respiratory disease
  lung compliance 515
  non-invasive ventilation 756
  see also chronic obstructive pulmonary
    disease
respiratory effort, signs **518**
respiratory failure 750
  CPAP 756
  type 1 (hypoxaemic) 750
  type 2 (hypercapnic) 750
respiratory observations 517–20, **518**
  epidural/intrathecal analgesia 595
  indications 512
  neurological **551**, 551–2, 554
  postanaesthetic recovery 618, *619*, 621
  postoperative 625
  procedure guidelines 520, *521*
respiratory problems
  peritoneal dialysis 744
  positioning in 684
  spinal cord compression 806
  unconscious patients 851
respiratory pump failure 750
respiratory rate 518, **518**
  body temperature and 518, 526
  indications for assessing 512
  neurological patients 552
  normal 518, **518**
respiratory secretions
  eating difficulties 492
  humidification and 757
  during oxygen therapy 762
  positioning to maximize drainage 684
  suctioning via tracheostomy/laryngectomy
    818–19, 823–4
  tracheostomy/laryngectomy patients 817,
    818, 827
  see also sputum
respiratory system 512, 750

respiratory therapy 750–65
  CPAP 756
  defined 750
  equipment 753–4
  humidification 757–8
  hyperbaric 757
  indications 750
  mechanical ventilation 757
  non-invasive ventilation 756
  problem solving 762–5
  procedure guidelines 760–2
  see also oxygen therapy
respiratory tract infections
  tracheostomy patients 828
  viral 777
  see also pneumonia
rest, in pain management 567
restraint, physical 936–7
resuscitation
  cardiopulmonary *see* cardiopulmonary
    resuscitation
  do not attempt (DNAR) 162–3
  equipment 162, 163
  training 161
resuscitation committee 161
Resuscitation Council UK (RCUK) 161–2
Resuscitation Training Officer (RTO) 161
reticular activating system (RAS) 546, *546*
retinoblastoma 636
retinol binding protein 470
retrolental fibroplasia 760
rhenium-186 hydroxyethylidene diphosphonate
    (Re186 HEDP) 718–21
  therapy of bone metastases 718–21
rhesus (Rh) blood group system 833
rhesus (Rh) incompatibility 833–4
ribavirin 117, 118, 119
rifampicin **532**, 635
RIG enteral feeding tubes *see* gastrostomy tubes,
    radiologically inserted
right bundle branch 499, 502
rigors 280, 526
Riker scale 850
rings
  nursing staff 54, 62
  surgical patients 612
risk, defined 9
risk assessment
  cytotoxic drug handling 257
  gene therapy 403–4
  health care-acquired infections 71, 84
  MRSA infection 103
  pressure ulcers 956–60
  variant Creutzfeldt–Jakob disease 129
  violence 935
risk management 9–10, 989
rituals
  last offices 445–6
  nursing 10
Roberts catheters 379, *380*
role development 8–9
roller clamps 293
Royal College of Nursing (RCN)
  Advanced Practice Programme 8–9
  do not attempt resuscitation guidance
    162–3
  pressure ulcer guidance 960
  on violence 933
Royal National Institute of the Blind (RNIB) 38
Royal National Institute of the Deaf (RNID) 38
Rusch speaking valve 813, *813*
Ryle's tube, insertion 484–6

SABRE reporting system 832
Safe Handling of Hazardous Therapeutic
    Substances (SHOHTS) Committee 257

safety
  occupational *see* health and safety,
    occupational
  patient 9–10
The Safety Representatives and Safety
    Committees Regulations 1977 934
salicylates 519, **532**
saline, normal *see* sodium chloride, 0.9%
    solution
saline flush-out technique, extravasation injury
    271
saliva 648
  artificial 651, 656
  autologous 652
  reduced flow 648–9, 652
salivary gland dysfunction 648–9
Salmonella food poisoning 73
Saltair No-roma 370
Saltair solution 369
Salts cohesive seals 369
SARS (severe acute respiratory syndrome) 76
satiety, early **473**
scalp cooling 767–73
  defined 767
  factors influencing success 769
  indications 767
  limitations of studies 769
  machines 768–9
  patient selection 769
  problem solving 772
  procedure guidelines 770–1, *771*
  scientific rationale 767–8
  supportive care 769–70
  techniques 768–9
  types of drugs 768
scalp metastases 767
scalp tourniquets 767
scanning, radionuclide 717, 718
scars 945, 968–9
  hypertrophic and keloid 968
  management of abnormal 968–9
schizophrenia, and violence 935
sciatica, intraoperative positioning and 614
scintigraphy (radionuclide imaging) 717, 718,
    719–21
sclerosing agents, intrapleural instillation 278
The Scope of Professional Practice (UKCC
    1992) 8
scopolamine 635
Scotts catheters **378**
scrapie 129, 841
screw clamps 293
scrub nurse 617
SecuPlast 370
security, stored medicines 204–6
sedation
  bone marrow aspiration/biopsy 416, 420
  critically ill patients 850
  opioid-induced 589, 600
segmentation, intestinal 328
seizures 555
Selectron (low dose rate; LDR) 698–9, *699*
  operating 699
  patient preparation 700–1
  problem solving 710
  procedure guidelines 708–10
  removal of applicators 709–10
  see also microSelectron
self-catheterization, intermittent *see* intermittent
    self-catheterization
semen, specimen collection 787
semi-permeable films, wound management **950**
senna 335
sensory function
  assessment 551, *555*
  spinal cord compression 797, *797*

sepsis
  central venous catheter-related 778
  intravenous infusion-associated 246
  transfusion-associated 839
  see also infections
septic shock 100–1, 528
septicaemia 249
septicaemic shock 510
Serious Adverse Blood Reactions and Events
    (SABRE) reporting system 832
Serious Hazards of Transfusion (SHOT) scheme
    837
serological testing 777
seromas 151–3
  causes 151–2
  defined 151
  drainage **152**, 152–3
  flap donor site 968
severe acute respiratory syndrome (SARS) 76
Sevredol 565, 568
  see also morphine
sexual dysfunction
  after continent urinary diversion 352
  after intracavitary brachytherapy 701
  stoma patients 367
sexual transmission
  hepatitis A 109
  hepatitis B 111
  hepatitis C 117
  herpes simplex virus 121
  HIV 91, 92
shampoo 770
sharps disposal 78, *881*, 923
  radioactive 730
  see also inoculation accidents
shaving
  facial, male patients 665
  surgical site 606
  VAD insertion site 862
Shaw's silver laryngectomy tube 815, *815*
shearing 955
Shiley laryngectomy tube 814, *815*
Shiley tracheostomy tubes 811–13, *812*
  cuffed 811–12, *812*
  cuffed fenestrated *812*, 812–13
  cuffless 811, *812*
  fenestrated 812, *812*
shingles (zoster) 122, 123
shivering 524, 526
  postoperative 622, 624
shock
  blood glucose testing 536
  induced by abdominal paracentesis 48
  septic 100–1, 528
  septicaemic 510
  spinal 806
  venepuncture in 922
short bowel syndrome 479
SHOT (Serious Hazards of Transfusion) scheme
    837
shoulder, positioning in hemiplegia 685
showering 56–7, 77, 663
  preoperative 611
  unsealed radioactive source therapy 728
shroud 446, 448–9
side lying position 672–3, *673*
  neurological patients 687, *687*
  sitting up from 674, *674*
sigma-rectum (Mainz II) pouch 351, *351*, 354
Sikh Educational and Cultural Association 455
Sikh Missionary Society 455
Sikhism
  last offices 455
  personal hygiene 663
Silastic laryngectomy tube 815, *815*, 821
silicone catheters 379–80

silicone elastomer-coated catheters 379
silicone gel sheeting, hypertrophic and keloid
    scars 968
silicone tubes, enteral feeding 473
silver alloy-coated catheters 381
silver dressings **962**, 963, 967
silver sulphadiazine 967
silver toxicity 381
Sims (Graseby) Medical MS16A syringe driver
    300–1
Sims (Graseby) Medical MS26 syringe driver
    300–1, *301*
  calculating rate settings 302, *302*
  preparing syringe and priming infusion set
    303–4
Single Assessment Process 193
single rooms
  availability in NHS hospitals 74
  protective isolation 86, 88
  source isolation 74–5
sinoatrial (SA) node 499, *499*, 502
sinus rhythm 499
sip feeds 471
siphonage 294, 298–9
sitting position
  amputees 688
  in bed 671, *672*
  in chair 675
  moving from lying to 674, *674*
  standing from 675–6, *676*
skill acquisition, Benner's model of 7–8
skin 661–2
  ageing 662
  assessment 662
  bio-engineered substitutes 954
  cytotoxic drug exposure 255
    management 259, 260, 261
  dry 662
  fragile, compression therapy 175, 176
  non-intact
    aseptic technique 62
    hepatitis B exposure 111, 112, 113
    HIV exposure 94
    radioactive contamination 732
  radiation reactions 662, **964**, 964–5, *965*
  soreness, stoma site 374
  stabilization
    for venepuncture 926, *928*
    for venous cannulation 862
skin barrier products
  stoma 369
  wound management **950**, 963
skin cancer 275
skin care 661–3
  diarrhoea 331
  oxygen therapy 763
  during radiotherapy 965
  stoma patients 369
  subcutaneous infusion sites 214
  unconscious patients 851
skin cleaning *see* skin preparation
skin closure strips, adhesive **969**
skin grafts 965–6
  donor site problems 966–7
  recipient site problems 967–8
skin infections, lumbar puncture site 460
skin preparation (cleaning)
  intramuscular injections 216
  midline catheter insertion 882–3
  peripheral venous cannulation 862, 879, *880*
  PICC insertion 885
  preoperative 606
  VADs 856–7
  venepuncture 922–3, 926, *928*
skinfold thickness 469
Skinsafe non-sting protective film 369

skin-tunnelled catheters **856**, *872*, 872–4
  care and management in situ 873–4
  choice of vein 873
  defined 872
  device types and design 872, 873
  discharge home with indwelling 876–7
  indications 872
  parenteral nutrition 476
  removal 874
    procedure guidelines 897–9
slough, fungating wounds **962**
small intestine 328
smell *see* odour
soap
  bactericidal 54, 63–4, 72
  dispensers 61, 63
  hand washing 54, 62–3, 72
  patient skin care 662
  perineal/perianal area 663
social interaction, during procedures 4
social services
  discharge planning 188–9, **193**, 197
  spinal cord compression **800**, 805
sodium bicarbonate
  cardiopulmonary resuscitation 161, 163
  extravasation hazard 269
  mouthrinse 653
sodium chloride, 0.9% solution (normal saline)
  bladder washout 311, 312
  as drug diluent 214
  eye irrigation 633
  flushing
    after i.v. drug administration 219, 240, 243, 265
    midline catheters 865
    urinary diversion drainage catheters 352–3
    VADs 245, 858, 892
  mouth care 650
  nasopharyngeal specimen collection 785–6
  wound cleaning 947, **947**
sodium citrate enema 335
sodium fluoride mouthwash 652
Soft Seal products 370
soft tissue changes, neurological patients 687
SOLER acronym 32–3
solution R *see* citric acid 6% solution
Sorbsan silver Plus 964
sore mouth, dietary advice **473**
source isolation 71, 73, 74–83
  Clostridium difficile infection 107
  cohort *see* cohort barrier nursing
  cryptosporidiosis 108
  defined 74
  discharge from 83
  facilities required 74–5
  gene therapy 406–7, 408
  general principles 75–9
  guidelines 79–83
  hepatitis A 109
  indications 74
  MRSA-infected patients 102
  procedure guidelines 79–83
  psychological effects 71, 78
  rooms 74–5
    cleaning 78–9, 82, 83
    entering 80
    leaving 81
    preparation 79–80, 88
    transporting patients in/out 83
  standard and extra precautions 75, **75**
  strict 71
  tuberculosis patients 128
spacer devices 208
spasticity
  defined 686
  patient positioning 686–7, *687*

speaking valves *813*, 813–14
  leaking/fallen out 817
  see also voice prostheses
specimen collection 775–94
  blood *see* blood sampling
  body fluids 784–9
  cytology 779–80
  defined 775
  documentation 776
  indications 775
  procedure guidelines 781–92
  swabs 781–3
  types of investigation 777
  urine *see* urine specimen collection
specimens
  gene therapy 404, 406, 776
  hepatitis B-infected 115
  HIV-positive patients 96
  radioactive patients 729, 731
  storage 776
  transport containers 775, 776
  transportation 776
spectacles 612
speculum, vaginal 790
speech and language therapists (SLT) 491, 492, 493
speech deficits 33, 547
speed shock 249, 294
sphygmomanometers 507–8
  aneroid 508
  components 508
  mercury 507–8
  non-invasive automated 508
  postanaesthetic recovery 620
  servicing 509
  using *507*, 509, 511–12
SPIKES model 37
spillages
  blood 930
  cytotoxic drugs 259–60, 261
  gene therapy 408
  hepatitis B-positive material 114
  HIV-positive material 98
  microbiological specimens 776
  radioactive fluids 731–2
  source barrier nursing 81
spinal anaesthesia/analgesia 460
  postoperative care 622
  see also epidural analgesia; intrathecal analgesia
spinal cord 460, 586–7, *587*
  tumours 796, *796*
spinal cord compression (SCC) 796–808
  assessment 801–2
  classification 796–7
  clinical presentation 797, **797**
  defined 796
  incidence and aetiology 796
  investigations 797–9
  management protocol 798
  moving and handling patient 800–1
  problem solving 806
  procedure guidelines 800–5
  prognosis and predictors 799
  rehabilitation 799–800, **800**, 804–5
  treatment 799, 803
spinal cord injuries 797
  bowel management 342, 343–4
spinal nerves 587
spinal shock 806
spinal stability, positioning and 669
spirometry 514, *515*
spondylosis 796
spring coil piston syringes 300
sputum
  assessment **518**

collection 788
infected, tracheostomy patients 828
positioning to maximize drainage 684
see also respiratory secretions
squamous cell carcinoma (SCC)
  cutaneous 275, 636
  oral cavity 653
staff
  allocation to infected patients 79
  health and safety *see* health and safety, occupational
  training *see* training
  violence against *see* violence
standard operating procedures, gene therapy 404
standard precautions 75, **75**
  see also universal precautions
standing, assistance with 675–6, 676
Staphylococcus aureus 101
  coagulase-negative 103
  coagulase-positive 101–3
  glycopeptide intermediate (GISA) 101
  meticillin-resistant *see* meticillin-resistant *Staphylococcus aureus*
  meticillin-sensitive (MSSA) 101
  on nurses' uniforms 76
  vancomycin intermediate (VISA) 101
  vancomycin resistant (VRSA) 101
Staphylococcus epidermidis, antibiotic resistance 100, 103
staples **969**
  removal 974–5
stem cell transplantation (SCT)
  blood groups in 834
  bone marrow harvest 416–17
  cryopreserved bone marrow/peripheral blood stem cells 834
  infection risks **84**, 84–5
  levels of care required 85
  nursing care 87–8
  oral complications 654
  Re186 HEDP therapy 721
  see also bone marrow transplantation
stem cells, haematopoietic *413*, 413–14
  harvest from bone marrow 416–17
  peripheral blood (PBSC) 417, **418**
Stenotrophomonas maltophila, antibiotic resistant 100–1
sterculia 334
sterile supplies, aseptic technique 55
sterilization, non-disposable equipment 95–6
sternal rub, neurological assessment 549
steroid 5-α reductase inhibitors 767
steroids *see* corticosteroids
stethoscope
  apical heart beat assessment 500
  blood pressure measurement 508–9, 510–12, *512*
  postanaesthetic recovery 620
stock control, medicines 206
Stockholm applicators *697*, 697–8
  modified 697, 698
stockings, graduated elastic compression *see* antiembolic stockings
stoma(s) 362–75
  accessories 368–70
  bridges or rods 362, *362*
    removal 373–4, *374*
  cleaning solutions 369
  defined 362
  deodorants 370
  diarrhoea management 329, 365
  diet 366–7
  discharge plans 366
  fear about malodour 367–8
  indications 362, 363

stoma(s) (*cont.*)
management systems 367–70
postoperative care 365–6
preoperative care 363–5
problem solving 374–5
procedure guidelines 370–4
sexual function and 367
siting 364, *364–5*
types 362–3
see also colostomy; gastrostomy; ileal
conduits; ileostomy; laryngectomy;
urostomy
stoma appliances 367–8
changing, procedure guidelines 370–1
obtaining supplies 366
plug systems 368
postoperative period 365–6
pouches 367–8, *368*
skin barriers 369–70
stoma nurse/therapist 355
postoperative care 365
preoperative counselling 352
Stomahesive products 369
stomatitis 648, 657
prevention 653
see also oral mucositis
stool softeners 334, **334**
stools *see* faeces
storage
controlled drugs **205**
medicines 204–6
microbiological specimens 776
patient's own medicines 206, 209
Streptococcus pneumoniae 103
streptozocin 268
stress
cancer nursing 88
hormones 533
response to surgery 560–3
see also psychological implications
stroke
joint protection 685
positioning 685, 687
stroke volume 497
subarachnoid (intrathecal) space 460, *461*,
586–7, *587*
subclavian vein 870, 873
subcutaneous infusions 213–14, 302–8
calculating rate settings 302, *302*
choice of sites 214
connecting syringe to 304–7, *307*
drugs 214
equipment 302
fluids (hypodermoclysis) 213–14
infusion devices 300–1
preparing syringe and priming infusion set
303–4
problem solving 307–8
procedure guidelines *302*, 302–7, *307*
site care 214
subcutaneous injections 213
cytotoxic drugs 275
procedure guidelines 229–30
sites 213
subcutaneous layer 662
subcutaneous route of administration 213–14
acute/postoperative pain management 564–5
chronic pain management 563
subjective global assessment (SGA) 468, 470
sublingual tablets 206, 223
substance abuse, and violence 935
Suby G *see* citric acid 3.23% and magnesium
oxide solution
sucralfate 651, 652
suction
intrapleural drainage 433, 436

postanaesthetic recovery 620, 621
tracheal *see* tracheal suctioning
sudden cardiac death 156
sugar paste 963
summarizing 34
supervised area, radiation 717
supervision, drug administration 209
supine position
in bed 670–1
neurological patients 685, 686, *687*
sitting up from 674, *674*
supplementary prescribing 210–12
supportive care *see* psychological support
suppositories 207, 338–40
administration 338–9
contraindications 338
defined 338
indications 338
types available 339
supraorbital pressure, neurological assessment
549
suprapubic catheterization 383
SurePath®792
surfaces
antibacterial 77
cytotoxic drug spillages 259
surgery 606–27
for cancer pain management 571
for extravasation injury 270–1
hypothermia risk 525
infection risk categories **51**
pain after *see* postoperative pain
for spinal cord compression 799, 803
stress response to 560–3
see also intraoperative care; plastic surgery;
postoperative care; preoperative care
surgical instruments, sterile 55
surgical wounds
changing dressings 970–1
exposure to water 55, 56
infection risk categories **51**
infections 52
plastic surgery 965–8
postanaesthetic recovery 622
postoperative care 626
see also wound drains
suspensions, drug 207
sustained-release tablets 206
sutures
chest drains 431
removal 970, 974–5
VADs 868, 876
wound closure **969**
suturing 970
common errors **970**
procedure guidelines 971–3, *973–4*
swabs 775, 781–3
ear 781, *781*
eye 637–8, 781
haemostatic 964
nose 782, *782*
penile 782
rectal 782
throat 782–3, *783*
vaginal 783
wound 783
swallow reflex 551
swallowing, normal *493*
swallowing difficulties 491–3
laryngectomy patients 817
problem solving 491–3
tracheostomy patients 491, *492*, 816–17
see also dysphagia
Swedish nose *see* heat and moisture exchanger
swelling, extravasation 268, *269*
symmetrical tonic neck reflex 685

sympathetic nervous system 498, *498*
syphilis, CSF testing 462
syringe drivers 300–1
calculating rate settings 302, *302*
connecting syringe to 304–7, *307*
preparation for 24-h drug administration
303–4
problem solving 307–8
procedure guidelines 302–7, *307*
syringe pumps 298–9
alarm systems 296, 298
ambulatory 300
anaesthesia 299
patient-controlled analgesia 299
pros and cons 298–9
siphonage 294, 298–9
user errors 292
syringes
blood sampling via CVADs 890
oral drug administration 223
syrups 207
systemic inflammatory response syndrome
(SIRS) 839
systolic blood pressure 505–6
measurement 509, 511–12

tablets 206
administration guidelines 221–3
crushing or breaking 206, 223, 274, 275, 490
cytotoxic drugs 274–5
storage 206
via enteral feeding tube 490
tachycardia 498
junctional *500*
postoperative 624
transfusion reactions 837
tachypnoea 518
tamoxifen, toxic effects on eye 635
tamponade *see* cardiac tamponade
tampons, during surgery 611, 615
tapeworms 785
taps, for hand washing 54, 61, 72
taste changes 652
taxanes
scalp cooling 767, 768
see also paclitaxel
tea tree oil 963
team working 989
tears 631–2, *632*
artificial 635
technetium-99m colloid 718
radioactive sentinel node biopsy 723
TED stockings *see* antiembolic stockings
TEDS *see* antiembolic stockings
teeth, loose 612
Teflon
coated catheters 379
peripheral cannulae 860–1
temperature
body 522–8
conditions requiring monitoring 528
core 524, *524*
defined 522–4
indications for measuring 524
neurological patients 552, 554
postanaesthetic recovery 622
postoperative monitoring 625
procedure guidelines 529
recording sites 526–7
regulation 524, *525*
respiratory rate and 518, 526
time for recording 527
transfusion reactions 837
chemotherapy-induced hair loss and 768
food safety and 73, 124–5
inspired gases 757, 758

Legionella survival 123
  skin *524*
  venepuncture and 922
  wound 944, 947
Tenckhoff catheter 283–4
tendon reflexes 555
terminal care
  communication problems 30
  hydration 214
  unconscious patients 850
  urgent discharge home 189, *191–2*
  see also death
theatre, operating *see* operating theatre
therapeutic drug monitoring 778–9, 784–5
therapeutic relationships, trusting 566
thermometers 527–8, *528*
thermoregulation 524, *525*
thiamine deficiency 469
thinking, critical 16
Thinprep® 792
thiotepa 277, 278, 280
thoracic duct injury, after VAD insertion 900
thoracotomy tube, drainage 280
threadworms 782
three-way taps
  arterial blood sampling 909–10, *910–11*
  infection risk 217
  unblocking occluded VADs 892, *893*
throat swabs 782–3, *783*
thrombocytes *see* platelets
thromboembolic deterrent stockings *see*
    antiembolic stockings
thrombolytic agents, occluded VADs 859, 892–3
thrombopoietin 414
thromboprophylaxis
  patients on bed rest 670
  spinal cord compression 801
  surgical patients 606–7, 608–10
  see also antiembolic stockings
thrombosis
  arterial cannula-associated 287, 903–4, 913
  indwelling VADs 877, 900
  intravenous infusion-related 248
  see also deep vein thrombosis; venous
      thromboembolism
thyroid cancer
  iodine-131 therapy 721, 722, 726
  treatment programme 722
thyroid eye disease 636
thyroid scan, radionuclide **720**
thyroidectomy 722
thyrotoxic crisis 528
thyrotoxicosis
  iodine-131 therapy 721, 726
  see also hyperthyroidism
tidal volume (TV) 514, *515*
Tieman-tipped catheters 379, *380*
Tilley's forceps 818
TIME principles, wound bed preparation **946**
tissue adhesive **969**
tissue integrity, impaired
  aetiology 955
  respiratory therapy 756, 763, 764
  unconscious patients 851
  see also pressure ulcers
tissue necrosis *see* necrosis
tissue oxygenation 750–2
T-lymphocytes *413*, **414**
TNP *see* topical negative pressure therapy
Todd's paralysis 555
toilets, barrier-nursed patients 81
tone *see* muscle tone
tongue
  interstitial brachytherapy 694
  tumours 653
tonic labyrinthine reflex 685

tonic neck reflex
  asymmetrical 685
  symmetrical 685
toothbrushes 650
toothbrushing 650, 655, 657
topical anaesthesia
  eye drops 633
  peripheral cannulation 863
  urinary catheterization 381
topical applications of drugs
  cytotoxic drugs 275–6
  procedure guidelines 232
topical negative pressure therapy (TNP) 951–4
  procedure guidelines 978–80
topical preparations 207
topical wound treatment dressings 954
topitriol, topical 767
total lung capacity (TLC) *515*, 516
touch, without consent 5
tourniquets
  after venepuncture needle removal 924
  to improve venous access 878–9, 922, 925–7
towels, paper *see* paper towels
toxic shock syndrome 615
toxicity, cardiopulmonary arrest 160
T-piece circuit *755*
trace elements, parenteral nutrition solutions
    477
tracheal dilators 817
tracheal suctioning (via tracheostomy) 818–19
  catheters 819, *819*
  indications 818–19
  procedure guidelines 823–4
tracheo-oesophageal puncture 817, 818, 820
  see also voice prostheses
tracheostomy 810–30
  communication methods 816
  defined 810
  dressing changes 817, 822
  emergency 810
  general nursing care 817
  humidification 758, 815–16, 824–5
  indications 810
  mini 811
  oxygen masks 755
  percutaneous 810
  permanent 810, *810*
  problem solving 827–8
  procedure guidelines 822–7
  resuscitation 819
  suctioning via 818–19, 823–4
  surgical 810–11
  swallowing problems 491, 492, 816–17
  temporary 810, *810*
  see also laryngectomy
tracheostomy tubes 811–14, 817
  changing 817, 825–7
    problem solving 827–8
  decannulation plug 814, *814*
  dislodgement 827
  insertion difficulties 827
  Jackson's silver 813, *813*
  Kapitex Tracoetwist fenestrated 814, *814*
  laryngectomy tubes 814–15, *815*
  Negus's silver 813, *813*
  occlusion 827
  Portex cuffed 811, *811*
  Shiley 811–13, *812*
  speaking valve *813*, 813–14
  stoma button 815, *815*
  total laryngectomy 818
  see also voice prostheses
trachphone 816, *816*
traction method, skin-tunnelled catheter
    removal 874
training

blood glucose monitoring 536
cardiopulmonary resuscitation 161–2
communication 35
Entonox use 581
infusion device use 292
prevention of violence 936
radiation safety 693
tramadol 565, 568
tranexamic acid 964
transcutaneous electrical nerve stimulation
    (TENS) 567
transdermal patches 207
transfers
  brachytherapy patients 702, 703
  interhospital, MRSA-infected patients 103
  spinal cord compression 805
  to/from operating table 614–15, 616
  to/from operating theatre 613
  see also manual handling; mobilization
transforming growth factor-β (TGF-β) 652,
    944, 954
transfusion 832–48
  appropriate use 834
  blood and blood products used **835–6**
  blood pack labelling *842*
  blood sampling prior to 844
  care during 834–7
  defined 832
  incompatible 833–4
  indications 834, **835–6**
  Jehovah's Witnesses 837
  observations during 500, 528, 834–7, 846
  pre-administration checks 838, *838*, 845
  problem solving 847
  procedure 841, 845–6
  procedure guidelines 843–7
  process 834
  requesting blood 843
  safety and quality of practice 832
transfusion reactions 837–41
  apheresis 419
  Blood Safety and Quality Regulations 832
  bone marrow transplantation 426
  delayed 840
  immediate 838–40
  infectious complications 111, 117, 129–30,
    832, 840–1
  major 837–8, **838**
  management 837–8, **838**, *838*, 847
  minor 837
  monitoring for 846
transfusion-associated circulatory overload
    (TACO) 839
transfusion-associated graft-versus-host disease
    (TA-GVHD) 840
transfusion-related acute lung injury (TRALI)
    839–40
transmissible mink encephalopathy 129
transmissible spongiform encephalopathies
    (TSEs) 128–30, 841
transmission based precautions *see* source
    isolation
transplant co-ordinators 451
transplant donors 451
transplant recipients
  cytomegalovirus infection 120
  infection risks 84, **84**
  protective isolation 83–4, 85
  see also bone marrow transplantation
transportation
  discharge planning 199
  hepatitis B-infected patients 115
  infected patients 83
  MRSA-infected patients 103
  specimens 776
trapezium squeeze, neurological assessment 549

trauma
   bone marrow procedure-related 426
   cardiopulmonary arrest 156, 160
   Entonox analgesia 578
   epidural analgesia 586
   spinal cord compression 797
   tracheal suctioning 819
   urethral mucosal, catheterized patients 394
Trendelenburg position
   CVC insertion 871, *871*
   CVC removal 896
   during surgery 614
tricyclic antidepressants 563
triglycerides
   dietary supplements 471
   in enteral feeds 474–5
trusting therapeutic relationships, creating 566
tuberculosis (TB) 126–8
   last offices 450
   multi-drug resistant (MDR-TB) 127, 128
   nursing care 128
tubing
   infusion administration sets 293
   intermittent self-catheterization of urinary
      stoma 355
tubular reabsorption 530, *530*
tubular secretion 530, *530*
tumour suppressor genes 401–2
tumours
   radionuclide imaging **720**
   spinal cord compression 796, *796*
   susceptibility genes 402
   see also cancer
tunica adventitia 921
tunica intima 921
tunica media 921
two-handed technique, peripheral cannulation
   863
tympanic membrane thermometers 526–7, 528,
      528
   procedure guidelines 529

ulceration, extravasation injuries **268**, 271–2
ulcerative colitis 362
ultrasound guidance
   CVC insertion 871
   PICC insertion 867
umbilical cord, haematopoietic stem cells 417
unconscious patients 850–4
   defined 850
   ethical issues 851
   eye care 637, 645, 664, 851
   physiological changes 850–1
   procedure guidelines 852–3
   see also consciousness
underinfusion 294, **295**
   complications **291**
   problem solving 308
undertakers 451
uniforms, nurses 55–6
   barrier nursing 76
Union of Liberal and Progressive Synagogues
   454
universal precautions 93
   operating theatre 615
   see also standard precautions
upper limb
   amputees 688, 689
   applying elastic compression garments 178–9
   compression bandaging 179–81, *181–2*
   lymphoedema 170, 171
   oedema, after VAD insertion 900
   size measurement 172
   veins for cannulation 861–2
   veins for venepuncture *920*, 920–1
   volume measurement 173–4

urea, plasma 478, **478**
urease-secreting micro-organisms 312
ureteric stents, continent urinary diversion 352,
   353, *353*
ureterosigmoidostomy 350–1, *351*
ureterostomy 363
urethral catheterization *see* urinary
   catheterization
urethral meatus
   cleaning, catheterized patients 382
   crusting around, catheterized patients 394
urethral mucosal trauma/irritation, catheterized
   patients 394
urinals, radioactive patients 728
urinalysis 528–32
   dipstick (reagent) tests 531–2, *533*
   drugs affecting results **532**
   indications 529
   procedure guidelines 532, *533*
urinary catheter-associated infections 311–12,
      381–2, 395
   bladder lavage 312
   management 393
   sites of entry 381, *382*
   specimen collection 779
urinary catheterization 378–97
   anaesthetic lubricating gel 381
   defined 378
   drainage bags *see* urine drainage bags
   indications 378
   intermittent self- *see* intermittent
      self-catheterization
   intracavitary brachytherapy 697, 700–1
   intravesical drug instillation 282
   leg straps 382
   meatal cleaning 382
   postanaesthetic recovery 618
   problem solving 393–5
   procedure guidelines 384–8
   spinal cord compression 801
   suprapubic 383
   unconscious patients 851, 853
   unsealed radioactive source therapy 718–21,
      728
   urine specimen collection 390–1, *391*
urinary catheters 378–81
   bags *see* urine drainage bags
   balloon size 378–9
   biofilm formation 312
   bladder irrigation 314, *314*
   continent urinary diversion 352–3, *353*
   encrustations and blockages 312–13
   leakage around 283, 321
   length 379
   maintenance solutions 311
      clinically-based studies 313
      defined 311
      indications 311
      patient assessment 313
      problem solving 321
      procedure guidelines 316–18
   materials 379–81
   removal 392–3
   size 379
   suprapubic 383
   three-way 313, *313*, **378**, *380*
   tip design 379, *380*
   types **378**, *380*
   valves 382–3
urinary diversion 362–3
   continent *see* continent urinary diversion
   defined 349
   psychological effects 354–5
   see also ileal conduits; urostomy
urinary incontinence 662
   penile sheaths 395–7

see also incontinence
urinary retention
   catheterized patients 395
   epidural/intrathecal analgesia 589, 601
urinary stones, continent urinary diversion 354
urinary tract infections (UTIs) 530
   catheter-associated *see* urinary
      catheter-associated infections
   continent urinary diversion 355
   dipstick tests 531–2
   health care-associated 71
   observations 530, **531**
   predisposing factors *531*
urine 530–1
   colour 530, **531**
   formation 530, *530*
   HIV-positive patients 95
   leakage
      around catheters 394
      urinary stomas 374
   observations 530–1, **531**
   pH 530
      catheter encrustation and 312, 313
   radioactive 722, 728, 730
   smell 531, **531**
   source barrier nursing 78, 81
urine drainage bags 382
   body-worn 382
   changing 381
   emptying 392
   leg 382
   positioning 381–2
urine output/production
   impaired
      after intravesical drug instillation 282, 283
      catheterized patients 393, 394
      postoperative 625
   urostomy 365
urine specimen collection 779
   catheter (CSU) 390–1, *391*
   ileal conduit or urostomy 372–3, 375
   midstream (MSU) 779, 788–9
   procedure guidelines 788–9
   twenty-four hour 789
urokinase 859, 892
urostomy 362–3, *363*
   fluid intake 367
   indications 363
   postoperative care 365–6
   postoperative function 365
   pouches 368, *368*
   problem solving 374–5
   urine specimen collection 372–3, 375
   see also stoma(s); urinary diversion
urticaria, transfusion-induced 840
uterine corpus cancer, brachytherapy 697,
   697–8

vaccines, storage 206
vacs system *see* topical negative pressure therapy
vacuum blood collection systems 923
   procedure guidelines 924, 926
   sampling via CVADs 890
vacuum drainage system
   changing 976
   removal 977
VADs *see* vascular access devices
vaginal care, after brachytherapy 701, 713–14
vaginal drug preparations 207
   procedure guidelines 231–2
vaginal speculum 790
vaginal swabs 783
valacyclovir 121
Valsalva manoeuvre
   chest drain removal 433, 439
   CVC insertion 871

neobladder emptying 351
valves, venous 921
vancomycin 778–9
vancomycin-resistant enterococci (VRE) 100, 103–4
  barrier nursing 76, 77
  environmental survival 104
varicella (chickenpox) 122, 123
varicella zoster immunoglobulin (VZIg) 123
varicella zoster virus (VZV) 122–3
vascular access devices (VADs) 856–918
  blood pressure measurement and 509–10
  central *see* central venous access devices
  clamping 859–60
  damage and repair 859–60
  defined 856
  direct intermittent injections 219, 241–4
  discharge home with 876–7
  dressings 857
  flushing techniques 858
  infusion flow rate and 293
  inspection of insertion site 857
  kinking 858
  maintaining a closed intravenous system 857
  maintaining patency 857–9
  occlusion 245, 858–9
    partial withdrawal (PWO) 858–9, *859*, 891
    total 859
    unblocking, procedure guidelines 891–3, *893*
  peripheral *see* peripheral vascular access devices
  prevention of infection 856–7
  principles of care 856–60
  procedure guidelines 878–99
  quality of life issues 877–8
  securing 857
  types **856**
  see also specific types of devices
vascular endothelial growth factor (VEGF) **944**, 945
vasovagal reaction, venepuncture 930
vastus lateralis injections *215*, 216
vector-borne infections 73
vectors, gene 401
veins
  anatomy and physiology 920–1
  cannulation methods 862–3, 926
  injuries, during intravenous infusions 245
  irritation, *vs.* extravasation **268**, 269
  missed 930
  palpation 921, *928*
  selection
    cytotoxic drug administration 263, **263**
    implantable ports 876
    midline catheters 865
    peripheral cannulation 861–2
    PICCs 867, 867–8
    short-term non-tunnelled percutaneous CVCs 870–1
    skin-tunnelled catheters 873
    venepuncture 921–2
    vesicant drug administration 266
  stabilization methods 862, 926, *928*
  tapping 922
  for venepuncture *920*, 920–1
  visual inspection 921
venepuncture 920–31
  choice of device 922, **923**
  choice of vein 921–2
  defined 920
  improving venous access 922
  indications 920
  problem solving 928–31
  procedure guidelines 924–8, *928*
  removal of device 924

safety of practitioner 923
  skin preparation 922–3
Venflons *see* peripheral cannulae
venipuncture *see* venepuncture
venous access
  apheresis 419
  cardiopulmonary resuscitation 160, 165
  continuous renal replacement therapy 739, 744
  limited, problem solving 929
  methods for improving 922
  parenteral nutrition 476
  see also central venous access devices; peripheral cannulae; vascular access devices
venous disease, chronic 170
venous pressure, infusion flow and 296
venous spasm
  effect on flow rate 293
  during intravenous infusions 245
  PICC removal 869
  during venepuncture 922, 930
venous thromboembolism (VTE)
  cardiopulmonary arrest 160
  postoperative care 626
  prophylaxis *see* thromboprophylaxis
  risk factors 606–7, 608
  unconscious patients 851
  see also deep vein thrombosis; pulmonary embolism
venous valves 921
ventilated patients
  enteral feeds 475
  humidification of inspired gases 758
  positioning 683, *683*
  tracheal suctioning 819
ventilation 513–15, *514*
  Ambu bag and mask 158, 164
  mechanical 757
  minute (MV) 514
  mouth-to-face mask 158
  mouth-to-mouth 157–8, *158*
  non-invasive 756
  pulmonary 750
  see also continuous positive airway pressure; respiratory therapy
ventilation systems *see* air conditioning and ventilation systems
ventilation/perfusion *(V/Q)* ratio
  effect of CPAP 756
  positioning and 683, *683*
ventilation/perfusion *(V/Q)* scanning **719**
ventilators
  negative pressure 757
  positive pressure 757
ventricular fibrillation (VF) 499, *500*
  cardiopulmonary resuscitation 156, 161
ventricular rupture, after VAD insertion 900
ventricular tachycardia (VT), pulseless 156, 161
ventrogluteal intramuscular injections *215*, 216
Venturi-type oxygen masks 755, *755*
verbal communication 32
verbal orders, drug administration 208
verbal response, Glasgow coma scale 547, **547**
vertebral fractures, spinal cord compression 797
vesicant drugs 268–9
  antidotes 270
  defined 266
  extravasation 266–74
    see also extravasation
  method of administration 263, 267
  prevention of extravasation 266–8
  sequencing **266**, 267
Vialon peripheral cannulae 860–1

vicarious liability 992
vigilance 9
vinblastine 268
vinca alkaloids 268, 269
vincristine 268, 286
  scalp cooling 767, 769
vindesine 268, 767
vinorelbine 263, 268
violence 933–41
  defined 933
  intervention and management 936–7, 939
  legislation 933–4
  policy formation 934
  post-incident review 937, 939
  prediction 934–5, 938
  prevalence 933
  prevention 935–6, 939
  procedure guidelines 939–40
  risk assessment 935
viral infections
  oral 651
  specimen collection 777
  transfusion-transmitted 840–1
  see also specific infections
virus vectors 401
viscosity, blood 504–5
visitors
  HIV-positive patients 97, 99
  protective isolation facilities 89
  radioactive patients 693, 703, 723, 729
  source isolation facilities 76, 78
  tuberculosis patients 128
  see also family
visual acuity testing 552, 555
visual field defects 552, *552*, 631
visual fields *631*
visual pathways 631, *631*
visually impaired patients, communication with 37–8
vital capacity (VC) *515*, 516
vital signs
  epidural/intrathecal analgesia in chronic setting 595
  neurological assessment 551–2, 554
  postanaesthetic recovery 621–2
  see also blood pressure; observations; pulse; respiratory observations; temperature
vitamin A 946
vitamin B_{12}, serum **478**
vitamin C (ascorbic acid) **532**, 536, 946–7
vitamin D deficiency 469
vitamins
  dietary requirements 470–1
  parenteral nutrition solutions 477
  serum levels 470
  supplements 471
vitreous humour 631
voice prostheses 819–22
  changing, procedure guidelines 828–9
  defined 819–20
  drink and/or food leaks around 822
  inability to make sound with 822
  indications for replacing 821–2
  leaking 817, 821–2
  'lost' or dislodged 817, 822
  Silastic laryngectomy tube for use with 821
  types *820*, 820–1
  wear and tear 821
  see also speaking valves
voice rehabilitation, laryngectomy 819–22
volumetric infusion pumps 298
  ambulatory 300
vomiting *see* nausea and vomiting
voriconazole 105
VRE *see* vancomycin-resistant enterococci

walking 676–81
  assistance, procedure guidelines 681
  using elbow crutches **679–80**
  using sticks 677–8
  using walking frame **680–1**
walking aids 677, 677–81
walking frame **680–1**
walking sticks **677–8**
wards
  cleaning see cleaning, environmental
  protective isolation facilities 86
  purpose built infectious disease 74
  see also single rooms
waste
  cytotoxic drug-contaminated 260
  domestic 78
  gene therapy 407
  hepatitis B-infected patients 113
  HIV-positive patients 95, 98
  radioactive 702, 724, 730
  source barrier nursing 77–8, 79, 81
  venepuncture 923, 928
The Watch Tower Bible and Tract Society 454
watches, removal 54, 62
water
  balloon catheters 379
  drinking
    Cryptosporidium removal 107, 108
    immunocompromised patients 87, 89, 108
  exposure of wounds to 55, 56–7
  eye irrigation 633
  filtration 108, 124
  flushing enteral feeding tubes 489, 490, 491
  hand washing 54, 62, 63–4, 72
  rectal irrigation 345
  wound cleaning 947, **947**
water baths, blood warming 839
water systems, *Legionella* survival 123–4
water vapour 751, 757
water-borne infection
  cryptosporidiosis 107
  hepatitis A 108–9
  see also droplet transmission
Waterlow scale 956, 957–8
weighing, procedure guidelines 479–80, 480
weight, body see body weight
weight bearing
  fully (FWB) 676–7
  partially (PWB) 676–7
wheezing **518**
whistle-tipped catheters 379, 380
white blood cells **414**
  in CSF 462
  depletion (apheresis) **418**

formation 413, 414
for transfusion 835
white coats, doctors' 76
WHO see World Health Organization
wigs 770
winged infusion devices 861, 922, **923**
  cytotoxic drug administration 262–3
  insertion for subcutaneous infusions 304–6
WISECARE project 19
women
  HIV infection 92
  see also female patients
World Health Organization (WHO)
  analgesic ladder 563, 563, 568–70
  Mucositis Scale 649
wound(s)
  acute 943, 945
    changing dressings 970–1
  assessment 951, 952–3
  bacterial colonization 948, 963
  chronic 943, 945
  classification 943
  cleaning 947, 947, 971
  contraction 945
  debridement 947–8
  defined 943
  exudate see exudate, wound
  fungating see fungating wounds
  improving blood flow to 947
  inflammation and infection 948
  moisture balance 948–50, 951
  re-epithelialization 945
  surgical see surgical wounds
  swabs 783
wound bed preparation (WBP) 946, **946**
wound closure **969**, 969–70
  procedure guidelines 971–3, 973–4
  see also sutures
wound drains
  after continent urinary diversion 352–3, 353
  dressing, procedure guidelines 975–6
  removal, procedure guidelines 977
  shortening, procedure guidelines 978
wound dressings **949–50**
  changing, procedure guidelines 970–1
  closed drainage systems (Redivac) 975–6
  dry and wet 951
  fungating wounds **962**, 962–3, 964
  moisture balance control 948–50, 951
  occlusive 950
  principles of use 950–1
  promoting autolytic debridement 948
  radiotherapy skin reactions **965**

slipping, skin graft donor sites 967
topical treatments 954
  see also dressings
wound healing 943–7
  assessment 951
  edge non-advancement 951
  factors affecting **944**, 946
  by first intention 943
  growth factors **944**, 945, 954
  haemostasis 943–4
  inflammatory phase 944–5
  maturation phase 945
  nutrition and 946–7
  phases 943–5
  poor 469
  proliferative phase 945
  promotion of good 947–50
  by secondary intention 943
  by tertiary intention 943
wound infections 948
  fungating wounds **962**, 963–4
  health care acquired 71
  skin graft donor sites 967
wound management 943–84
  bio-engineered skin substitutes 954
  bone marrow aspiration/biopsy 416
  complementary therapies 954
  extravasation injuries 271–2
  fungating wounds **962**, 962–4
  hepatitis B infection 115
  hyperbaric oxygen therapy 951
  moisture balance 948–50, 951
  pressure ulcers 960
  procedure guidelines 970–80
  radiotherapy skin reactions 965, **965**
  topical negative pressure therapy (TNP) 951–4, 978–80
  topical treatment dressings 954
wrist bands 9
  see also identification, patient

xerostomia (dry mouth) 648–9, 652, 656
X-rays 694

Yeates vacuum drainage system, removal 977

zinc 947
Zoroastrian Trust Funds of Europe 456
Zoroastrianism, last offices 456
zoster (shingles) 122, 123
Z-track technique, intramuscular injections 216, 275